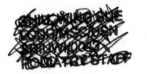

Comprehensive Textbook of

Foot Surgery

Volume Two

SECOND EDITION

Comprehensive Textbook of
Foot Surgery

Volume Two

SECOND EDITION

Editors

E. Dalton McGlamry, D.P.M.

Alan S. Banks, D.P.M.

Michael S. Downey, D.P.M.

Authors' Editors

Rebekah McGlamry, B.A.

Nancy Sinnott Vickers, B.M.

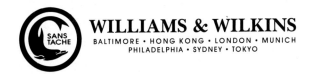

WILLIAMS & WILKINS

BALTIMORE • HONG KONG • LONDON • MUNICH
PHILADELPHIA • SYDNEY • TOKYO

Editor: John P. Butler
Associate Editor: Linda Napora
Designer: Karen S. Klinedinst
Production Coordinator: Charles E. Zeller

Copyright © 1992
Williams & Wilkins
428 East Preston Street
Baltimore, Maryland   21202,   USA

Accurate indications, adverse reactions, and dosage schedules for drugs are provided
in this book, but it is possible that they may change. The reader is urged to review
the package information data of the manufacturers of the medications mentioned.

Chapter reprints are available from the publisher.

Printed in the United States of America

First Edition 1987

Library of Congress Cataloging-in-Publication Data

Comprehensive textbook of foot surgery/editors, Alan S. Banks, Michael S. Downey,
   E. Dalton McGlamry; authors' editors, Rebekah McGlamry, Nancy Sinnott
   Vickers.—2nd ed.
      p.   cm.
   Includes bibliographical references and indexes.
   ISBN 0-683-05857-6
   1. Foot—Surgery.   I. McGlamry, E. Dalton   II. Banks, Alan S.
III. Downey, Michael S.
   [DNLM: 1. Foot—surgery.   WE 880 C7375]
RD563.C657   1992
617.5′85059—dc20
DNLM/DLC
for Library of Congress   91-30507
                                                             CIP

                                    92   93   94   95   96
                          1   2   3   4   5   6   7   8   9   10

Foreword

Webster defines *contribution* as "to furnish something for a common benefit." The second edition of *Comprehensive Textbook of Foot Surgery* is a contribution of unequaled proportion and uncommon benefit.

It has been said that a profession is judged by what it writes. If true, the central beacon for podiatric medicine will no doubt shine on the legacy that has been provided by Dr. McGlamry and his associates by this monumental effort. This text represents more than just a compilation of ideas by the authors. It is a synopsis of an unparalleled experience in podiatric medical writing, teaching, research, lecturing, investigation, and inter-professional and intra-professional communication. From the lecture platform, in resident training, study sessions, articles, CME programs, monographs, treatises, and texts, this edition of *Comprehensive Textbook of Foot Surgery* has been fashioned as an artist develops a statue, building layer upon layer. Each layer defining more finitely the image that the artist chooses to portray. The printed word, likewise, gives rise to the opportunity for modification, refinement, and depth. This process has clearly evolved in the production of this text.

The dynamics of technology in health care, and in podiatric medical care particularly, is proceeding with such speed that words can hardly be set to print before modification is indicated. Dr. McGlamry leaves no doubt of his awareness of this fact. The development of this edition is the embodiment of the creativity of Dr. McGlamry. It covers the subjects in detail and with an appreciation of the opportunity presented to challenge the health care community's understanding of this area of interest.

The work has grown beyond its scope, as has the influence of its author. Any collection of information on this portion of human anatomy is incomplete without including this keystone. It should be required of every student for study and is the definitive research tool for private practioners and resident training programs.

The previous edition has proven to be the most often utilized reference in podiatric journals. It so broadly covers the subject that review of the literature on related subjects often contains quotes from within the covers of this "standard." Undoubtedly, the response to this work will continue to prove its merit. *Comprehensive Textbook of Foot Surgery* will be viewed as the *Campbell's* of podiatry.

An interesting vignette regarding the text is that in addition to being a tribute to Dr. McGlamry's individual capability and accomplishment, it is also a family accomplishment produced by loving parents to, and for, and with, appreciative children—an unmatched family dedication.

As Webster said, "It is for a common benefit." That benefit being education and the highest perception and understanding of quality in health care that will stand for many years to come.

IRVIN O. KANAT, D.P.M.

Preface

Like the first edition, this edition of *Comprehensive Textbook of Foot Surgery* is intended as a resource for students, residents, and practitioners of foot, ankle, and leg surgery. The two volumes that make up the second edition replace both *Comprehensive Text Book of Foot Surgery* volumes one and two and *Fundamentals of Foot Surgery*. The reader will note that sections have been reorganized, chapters revised, rewritten, and updated, and new chapters added to provide complete coverage of the subject of foot surgery.

Section 1, Technical Principles, incorporates a new chapter, Power Instrument Skills. The skills demonstrated in this chapter may prove of value to the most experienced surgeons. Section 3, Fundamental Conditions and Procedures, covers those procedures generally performed by most foot surgeons. Section 4, First Ray, Hallux Abducto Valgus, and Related Deformities, is significantly revised and updated. New chapters include Osteotomy of the First Metatarsal Shaft in Hallux Abducto Valgus Surgery, First Metatarsophalangeal Joint Arthrodesis, Geriatric Hallux Valgus Deformity, and Hallux Varus. This section provides a much more complete review of procedures that are currently in vogue for repair of first ray deformities. Section 5, Compound Deformities, contains twelve chapters that discuss more advanced conditions and procedures. All of these chapters are substantially rewritten, and a new chapter on Charcot-Marie-Tooth disease has been added. A new section, Section 6, deals with major arthrodesis procedures. Rather than discuss various components of arthrodesis in separate areas of the text, the technical aspects of each procedure are presented in detail for any particular condition that might require a major fusion. Certain conditions that may require more refined techniques are detailed in Special Surgery, Section 7. New chapters in this section include Reflex Sympathetic Dystrophy Syndrome, Elective Diabetic Foot Surgery, Limb Salvage, and Amputations in the Foot. Management of Acute Tendon Trauma, Midfoot Fractures, and Pilon Fractures are topics that have been added to complete Section 8, Trauma of the Foot and Leg. Many of the complications that may be encountered after foot surgery are discussed in Section 9, Postoperative Complications and Considerations.

To complete such a text demands a dedicated cadre of individuals. Our thanks is extended to each of the authors for their work. A special thank you is in order for the members of The Podiatry Institute. These individuals have either directly contributed to the text as authors or indirectly assisted through their contributions to the authors. The collaborative talents and energies of Institute members cannot be overemphasized.

Finally, the residents of Northlake Regional Medical Center contributed untold thousands of hours. They did much of the literature search and medical photography. They sat with the illustrators to advise on details of surgical techniques. And they generally assisted in any and everything necessary in the production of a textbook. We especially express our thanks to these residents for helping to make the book possible.

E. Dalton McGlamry, D.P.M.
Alan S. Banks, D.P.M.
Michael S. Downey, D.P.M.

Contributors

Alan S. Banks, D.P.M.
Private Practice, Peachtree Podiatry Group, P.C.
Tucker, Georgia
Director of Podiatric Medical Education and Residency
Training, Northlake Regional Medical Center
Tucker, Georgia
Diplomate, American Board of Podiatric Surgery
Faculty, The Podiatry Institute, Tucker, Georgia

Gary R. Bauer, D.P.M.
Assistant Professor of Surgery, Pennsylvania College of
Podiatric Medicine
Philadelphia, Pennsylvania
Diplomate, American Board of Podiatric Surgery

Robert E. Bergman, D.O.
Anesthesiologist, Northlake Regional Medical Center
Tucker, Georgia
Director, Anesthesia Training, Podiatry Residents,
Northlake Regional Medical Center
Tucker, Georgia
Chairman, Department of Anesthesia, Northlake Regional
Medical Center
Tucker, Georgia
Member, Advisory Board and Instructor for Emergency
Medical Technicians
Dekalb County, Georgia
Member, American College of Osteopathic
Anesthesiologists
Member, American Society of Anesthesiologists

Maria Bidny, D.P.M.
Private Practice, Chicago, Illinois

Jeffrey Boberg, D.P.M.
Private Practice, Cahokia, Illinois
Diplomate, American Board of Podiatric Surgery
Fellow, American College of Foot Surgeons
Faculty, The Podiatry Institute, Tucker, Georgia
Director, Residency Training, St. Mary's Hospital
East St. Louis, Illinois
Visiting Clinical Instructor, Ohio College of Podiatric
Medicine
Cleveland, Ohio

William A. Boegel, D.P.M.
Staff Podiatrist, Virginia Mason Medical Center
Seattle, Washington
Diplomate, American Board of Podiatric Surgery
Fellow, American College of Foot Surgeons
Education Director, Waldo Surgical Residency, Fifth Ave.
Hospital
Seattle, Washington
Podiatric Advisor, Northwest Podiatric Foundation for
Research and Education

James L. Bouchard, D.P.M.
Private Practice, Roswell, Georgia
Diplomate, American Board of Podiatric Surgery
Fellow, American College of Foot Surgeons
Chairman, Board of Directors, The Podiatry Institute
Tucker, Georgia
Faculty, The Podiatry Institute, Tucker, Georgia

Thomas D. Cain, D.P.M.
Private Practice, Tucker, Georgia
Chairman, Department of Podiatric Surgery, Northlake
Regional Medical Center
Chairman, Board of Trustees, Northlake Regional
Medical Center
Tucker, Georgia
Diplomate, American Board of Podiatric Surgery
Fellow, American College of Foot Surgeons
Faculty, The Podiatry Institute, Tucker, Georgia

Bradley D. Castellano, D.P.M.
Private Practice, Fort Myers, Florida
Faculty, The Podiatry Institute, Tucker, Georgia

Raymond G. Cavaliere, D.P.M.
Private Practice, New York, New York
Assistant Professor, Division of Surgical Sciences, New
York College of Podiatric Medicine
New York, New York
Faculty, The Podiatry Institute, Tucker, Georgia
Fellow, American College of Foot Surgeons

Stephen V. Corey, D.P.M.
Private Practice, Decatur, Georgia
Consultant, National Naval Medical Hospital
Bethesda, Maryland
Director, Post Graduate Program, The Podiatry Institute
Tucker, Georgia
Faculty, The Podiatry Institute, Tucker, Georgia

D. Richard DiNapoli, D.P.M.
Private Practice, Bedford, New Hampshire
Faculty, The Podiatry Institute, Tucker, Georgia

Bruce Dobbs, M.S., D.P.M.
Private Practice, Daly City, California
Professor, Department of Surgery, California College of
Podiatric Medicine
San Francisco, California
Diplomate, American Board of Podiatric Surgery
Fellow, American College of Foot Surgeons
Editor, *Journal of the American Podiatric Medical Association*

Gary L. Dockery, D.P.M.
Private Practice, Seattle Foot and Ankle Clinic
Seattle, Washington
Diplomate, American Board of Podiatric Surgery
Fellow, American College of Foot Surgeons
Diplomate, American Board of Podiatric Orthopedics
Director, Northwest Podiatric Foundation for Education
and Research

Michael S. Downey, D.P.M.
Associate Professor and Chairman, Department of
Surgery, Pennsylvania College of Podiatric Medicine
Philadelphia, Pennsylvania
Faculty, The Podiatry Institute, Tucker, Georgia
Diplomate, American Board of Podiatric Surgery
Fellow, American College of Foot Surgeons

Charles F. Fenton, III, D.P.M.
Private Practice, Atlanta, Georgia
Diplomate, American Board of Podiatric Surgery
Fellow, American College of Foot Surgeons
Staff, Northlake Regional Medical Center
Tucker, Georgia

Brian D. Gale, D.P.M.
Attending Staff and Externship Director, The
Permanente Medical Group, Inc.
Hayward, California

James V. Ganley, D.P.M.
Founder and Past President, American College of
Podopediatrics
Editor, Author, *Clinics in Podiatry—Podopediatrics,* Dec.
1984
W.B. Saunders, Philadelphia, Pennsylvania

Theodore J. Ganley, M.D.
Surgical Resident, Orlando Regional Medical Center
Orlando, Florida

Joshua Gerbert, M.S., D.P.M.
Professor and Former Chairman, Department of Podiatric
Surgery, California College of Podiatric Medicine
San Francisco, California
Diplomate, American Board of Podiatric Surgery
Fellow, American College of Foot Surgeons
Surgical Editor, *Journal of the American Podiatric Medical
Association*

Flair D. Goldman, D.P.M.
Chief, Department of Podiatric Surgery, Kaiser
Foundation Hospital
Santa Clara, California
Clinical Association Professor, Department of Basic
Medical Science, California College of Podiatric Medicine
San Francisco, California

Donald R. Green, D.P.M.
Private Practice, San Diego, California
Clinical Instructor, Department of Orthopedics,
University of California
San Diego, California
Diplomate, American Board of Podiatric Surgery
Fellow, American College of Foot Surgeons
Podiatric Residency Director, Mercy Hospital and Medical
Center
San Diego, California

Jim L. Gregory, D.P.M.
Private Practice, San Antonio, Texas
Clinical Instructor, Orthopedic Department, University of
Texas Health Science Center
San Antonio, Texas

George Gumann, D.P.M.
Chief, Podiatric Service, Martin Army Hospital
Ft. Benning, Georgia
Diplomate, American Board of Podiatric Surgery
Fellow, American College of Foot Surgeons

Lawrence B. Harkless, D.P.M.
Clinical Professor, Department of Orthopaedics/Podiatry
Service, University of Texas Health Science Center at San
Antonio
Director, Podiatry Residency Training Program

Vincent J. Hetherington, M.S., D.P.M.

Associate Dean for Academic Affairs, Ohio College of
Podiatric Medicine
Cleveland, Ohio
Past Chairman Department of Surgery, Ohio College of
Podiatric Medicine
Cleveland, Ohio
Past Associate Dean, Clinical Affairs, College of Podiatric
Medicine and Surgery
Des Moines, Iowa
Diplomate, American Board of Podiatric Surgery
Fellow, American College of Foot Surgeons

Allen M. Jacobs, D.P.M.

Fellow, American College of Foot Surgeons
Chairperson, Department of Podiatry, Deaconess Hospital
St. Louis, Missouri
Director of Podiatric Residency Training, Deaconess
Hospital
St. Louis, Missouri
Director of Residency Training, Central Medical Center,
St. Louis, Missouri

A. Louis Jimenez, D.P.M.

Private Practice, Snellville and Tucker, Georgia
Faculty, The Podiatry Institute, Tucker, Georgia
Chairman, Continuing Education Committee, The
Podiatry Institute
Tucker, Georgia

Stanley R. Kalish, D.P.M.

Senior Attending Podiatric Surgeon, Northlake Regional
Medical Center
Tucker, Georgia
Professor, Department of Surgery (Traumatology), New
York College of Podiatric Medicine
New York, New York
Faculty, The Podiatry Institute, Tucker, Georgia

Patrick Landers, D.P.M.

Private Practice, Cuyahoga Falls, Ohio
Diplomate, American Board of Podiatric Surgery
Former Assistant Professor of Surgery, Ohio College of
Podiatric Medicine
Cleveland, Ohio
Consultant, Kaiser Medical, Akron, Ohio

Francis R. Lynch, D.P.M.

Diplomate, American Board of Podiatric Surgery
Fellow, American College of Foot Surgeons

Kieran T. Mahan, M.S., D.P.M.

Vice President for Academic Affairs and Dean,
Pennsylvania College of Podiatric Medicine
Philadelphia, Pennsylvania
Diplomate, American Board of Podiatric Surgery
Faculty, The Podiatry Institute, Tucker, Georgia
Consultant, National Naval Medical Center
Bethesda, Maryland
Fellow, American College of Foot Surgeons

D. Scot Malay, D.P.M.

Assistant Professor, Department of Surgery, Pennsylvania
College of Podiatric Medicine
Philadelphia, Pennsylvania
Co-Director of Podiatric Education, North Philadelphia
Health System
Staff Surgeon, North Philadelphia Health System and
The Graduate Hospital
Philadelphia, Pennsylvania

David Edward Marcinko, D.P.M.

Private Practice, Peachtree Podiatry Group, P.C.
Atlanta, Georgia
Editor, *A.P.M.A. Textbook of Podiatric Medicine and Surgical
Practice*
Editor, *Comprehensive Textbook of Hallux Abducto Valgus
Reconstruction*
Special Editor, *Journal of Foot Surgery*
Diplomate, American Board of Podiatric Surgery
Fellow, American College of Foot Surgeons

Jeffrey A. Marks, D.P.M.

Former Chief Resident, St. Joseph's Hospital
Philadelphia, Pennsylvania
Private Practice,
Mechanicsburg, Pennsylvania

Dennis E. Martin, D.P.M.

Private Practice, North Charleston, South Carolina
Faculty, The Podiatry Institute, Tucker, Georgia
Staff, Trident Regional Medical Center
Charleston, South Carolina

Michael W. McDonough, D.P.M.

Private Practice, Ormond Beach, Florida
Diplomate, American Board of Podiatric Surgery
Fellow, American College of Foot Surgeons

E. Dalton McGlamry, D.P.M., D.Sc. (Hon.), D.H.L.

Peachtree Podiatry Group, P.C.
Atlanta, Georgia
Diplomate, American Board of Podiatric Surgery
C.E.O., The Podiatry Institute, Tucker, Georgia
Faculty, The Podiatry Institute, Tucker, Georgia
Attending Staff, Northlake Regional Medical Center
Tucker, Georgia
Former Editor, *Journal of the American Podiatric Medical Association*
Past President, American Podiatric Medical Association

Thomas J. Merrill, D.P.M.

Associate Professor of Surgery, Barry University School of Podiatric Medicine
Miami Shores, Florida
Diplomate, American Board of Podiatric Surgery
Faculty, The Podiatry Institute, Tucker, Georgia

Stephen J. Miller, D.P.M.

Private Practice, Anacortes, Washington
Diplomate, American Board of Podiatric Surgery
Diplomate, American Board of Podiatric Orthopaedics
Fellow, American College of Foot Surgeons
Faculty, The Podiatry Institute, Tucker, Georgia
Active Staff, Island Hospital, Anacortes, Washington
Trustee, Northwest Podiatric Foundation,
Seattle, Washington

Jerome S. Noll, D.P.M.

Assistant Professor of Surgery, Barry University School of Podiatric Medicine
Miami Shores, Florida
Diplomate, American Board of Podiatric Surgery

Robert G. O'Keefe, D.P.M.

Private Practice, Chicago, Illinois

Michael Perlman, D.P.M.

Diplomate, American Board of Podiatric Surgery
Fellow, American College of Foot Surgeons
Director of Medical Education and Residency Training
Committee, Meadowlands Hospital, Medical Center
Surgical Residency Program

Verdon Peters, D.P.M.

Diplomate, American Board of Podiatric Surgery
Diplomate, American Board of Podiatric Orthopedics
U.S. Army-Health Services Command—Podiatry
Consultant
Clinical Professor and Consultant, Department of
Orthopaedics, University of Texas Health Science Center
San Antonio, Texas

Alfred J. Phillips, D.P.M.

Private Practice, Scituate, Massachusetts
Faculty, The Podiatry Institute, Tucker, Georgia
Active Staff, Carney Hospital, Dorchester, Massachusetts
Active Staff, Southshore Hospital
Weymouth, Massachusetts

Irving Pikscher, D.P.M.

Private Practice, Evergreen Park, Illinois

Timothy Pitts, D.P.M.

Northlake Regional Medical Center, Tucker, Georgia
Third Year Resident, Northlake Regional Medical Center
Tucker, Georgia

Mitchell A. Pokrassa, D.P.M.

Co-Director, Baja Project for Crippled Children
Diplomate, American Board of Podiatric Surgery
Diplomate, American Board of Podiatric Orthopedics
Attending Staff, Los Angeles County/University of
Southern California Medical Center
Los Angeles, California
Associate Clinical Professor, California College of
Podiatric Medicine
San Francisco, California
Attending Staff, Podiatry, St. Vincent's Medical Center
Los Angeles, California

Gene K. Potter, D.P.M., Ph.D.

Medical Affiliate Member, American Society of Clinical
Pathologists
Associate Member, American Society of
Dermatopathology
Member, International Society for Experimental
Hematology
Former Research Associate, Memorial Sloan-Kettering
Cancer Center
New York, New York
Fellow, American Society of Podiatric Medicine
Fellow, American Society of Podiatric Dermatology

Catherine A. Purdy, D.P.M.

Private Practice, Salem, Oregon
Director of Podiatric Services, Valley Community Hospital
Dallas, Oregon
Diplomate, American Board of Podiatric Surgery
Fellow, American College of Foot Surgeons
Adjunct Clinical Assistant Professor, College of Podiatric
Medicine and Surgery
Des Moines, Iowa

Richard P. Reinherz, D.P.M.

Assistant Clinical Professor of Family Medicine, Medical College of Wisconsin
Diplomate, American Board of Podiatric Surgery
Editor-in-Chief, *The Journal of Foot Surgery*
Fellow, American College of Foot Surgeons
Former Residency Director, American International Hospital
Zion, Illinois

John A. Ruch, D.P.M.

Private Practice, Tucker, Georgia
Faculty, The Podiatry Institute, Tucker, Georgia
Diplomate, American Board of Podiatric Surgery
Fellow, American College of Foot Surgeons
Director 1967-1988, Podiatric Residency Program, Doctors Hospital
Tucker, Georgia

Barbara S. Schlefman, D.P.M.

Private Practice, Tucker, Georgia
Faculty, The Podiatry Institute, Tucker, Georgia
Diplomate, American Board of Podiatric Surgery
Fellow, American College of Foot Surgeons
Past President, American Association for Women Podiatrists

Barry L. Scurran, D.P.M.

Chief, Podiatric Surgery and Chief Medical Staff Education, The Permanente Medical Group, Inc.
Hayward, California
Diplomate and Director, American Board of Podiatric Surgery
Clinical Associate Professor, Department of Surgery, California College of Podiatric Medicine
San Francisco, California
Clinical Instructor, Stanford University School of Medicine
Palo Alto, California

Ann M. Seifert, D.P.M.

Assistant Director, Deaconess Hospital, Department of Podiatric Medicine and Surgery
St. Louis, Missouri

Stephen Silvani, D.P.M.

Chief, Podiatric Surgery Department, Permanente Medical Group
Walnut Creek, California
Residency Director, Second Year Surgical Program, Kaiser Foundation Hospital
Walnut Creek, California
Clinical Assistant Professor, Surgery Department, California College of Podiatric Medicine
Diplomate, American Board of Podiatric Surgery
Fellow, American College of Foot Surgeons

Michael E. Smith, D.P.M.

Private Practice, Orlando, Florida
Podiatric Surgery Residency Training Committee, Orlando General Hospital
Orlando, Florida

Thomas F. Smith, D.P.M.

Diplomate, American Board of Podiatric Surgery
Fellow, American College of Foot Surgeons
Acting Chief, VA Medical Center
Augusta, Georgia
Past President, Region X, American Podiatric Medical Association
Faculty, The Podiatry Institute, Tucker, Georgia

G. Clay Taylor, D.P.M.

Northlake Regional Medical Center, Tucker, Georgia
Third Year Resident, Northlake Regional Medical Center
Tucker, Georgia

Michael Trepal, D.P.M.

Professor and Chairman, Department of Surgery, New York College of Podiatric Medicine
New York, New York
Diplomate, American Board of Podiatric Surgery

John A. Vanore, D.P.M.

Private Practice, Chicago, Illinois
Diplomate, American Board of Podiatric Surgery
Residency Director, Podiatric Surgical Program, Hyde Park Hospital
Chicago, Illinois
Auxiliary Clinical Professor, William M. Scholl College of Podiatric Medicine
Chicago, Illinois

George R. Vito, D.P.M.
Private Practice, Macon, Georgia
Podiatric Staff, Northlake Regional Medical Center
Tucker, Georgia
Faculty, The Podiatry Institute, Tucker, Georgia

Harold W. Vogler, D.P.M.
Visiting Professor of Orthopaedic Surgery, Malmo
General Hospital, Lund University
Malmo, Sweden
Professor, Department of Surgery, Pennsylvania College
of Podiatric Medicine
Philadelphia, Pennsylvania
Fellow, American College of Foot Surgeons
Diplomate, American Board of Podiatric Surgery
Immediate Past Chairman, Department of Foot and
Ankle Surgery, St. Joseph's Hospital
Philadelphia, Pennsylvania

Katherine A. Ward, D.P.M.
First Year Resident, St. Joseph's Hospital,
Flushing, New York

Gerard V. Yu, D.P.M.
Associate Professor and Former Chairman, Department
of Surgery, Ohio College of Podiatric Medicine and The
Cleveland Foot Clinic
Cleveland, Ohio
Diplomate, American Board of Podiatric Surgery
Fellow, American College of Foot Surgeons
Director of Residency Training, The Mt. Sinai Medical
Center
Chief, Division of Podiatry, Department of Surgery,
Meridia Huron Hospital
Faculty, The Podiatry Institute, Tucker, Georgia

Richard J. Zirm, D.P.M.
Private Practice, Coeur D'Alene, Idaho
Faculty, The Podiatry Institute, Tucker, Georgia

Contents

Volume One

SECTION **1**

Technical Principles

SECTION **4**

First Ray, Hallux Abducto Valgus, and Related Deformities

SECTION **5**

Compound Deformities

Volume Two

SECTION **6**

Major Arthrodesis Procedures

SECTION **7**

Special Surgery

SECTION **8**

Trauma of the Foot and Leg

SECTION **9**

Postoperative Complications and Considerations

Major Arthrodesis Procedures

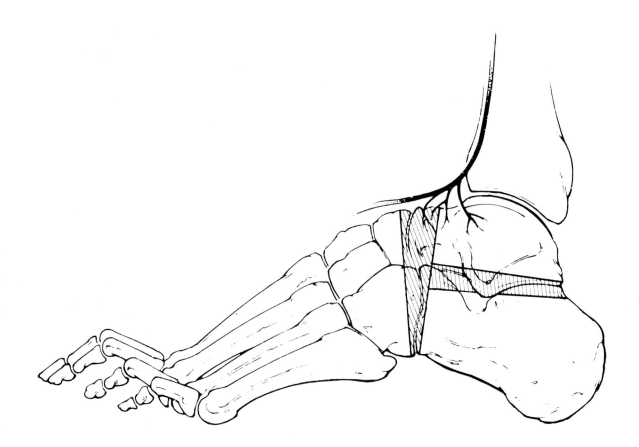

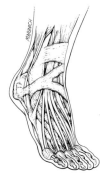

CHAPTER 41

Lisfranc's Joint Arthrodesis

Bradley D. Castellano, D.P.M.

Fusions of the tarsometatarsal joints (Lisfranc joint) have been used to alleviate pain, correct deformity, and stabilize the forefoot (1-3). Often, however, the Lisfranc level is either overlooked or circumvented by use of less direct methods for treatment of midfoot symptoms (Fig. 41.1). The relative difficulty in dissecting the midfoot, with its maze of tendon and neurovascular structures, may explain the reluctance of some surgeons. Once dissection is achieved, fixation at the tarsometatarsal junction may also prove to be demanding. All things considered, misdiagnosis is probably the most common reason the area is neglected.

INDICATIONS FOR SURGERY

Posttraumatic arthritis is probably the single most common reason for arthrodesis of Lisfranc's joint (4). Unfortunately, many of these advanced cases might have been avoided if proper initial therapy had been instituted at the time of the injury. Because spontaneous reduction of fracture-dislocations at this level often occur, a high index of suspicion is required for diagnosis. In most cases, the metatarsals are laterally deviated. However, medial subluxation of the first metatarsal base is not uncommon. Whenever injury to this joint is suspected, radiographic evaluation, including dorsoplantar, medial oblique, and lateral views, is essential. If the radiographs are inconclusive, stress evaluation should be considered to completely rule out the injury inasmuch as delayed diagnosis and early weight bearing is often disastrous (Fig. 41.2). Closed or open reduction with realignment of the involved joints has been shown to significantly lower the likelihood of posttraumatic degenerative arthritis. However, in some cases of severe injury, primary arthrodesis may be indicated (Fig. 41.3).

Chronic stress may also cause structural breakdown of the tarsometatarsal joint. The forces of weight bearing and propulsion may easily destroy the foot that is structurally unsound. The level at which this destruction occurs will be at the weakest link as the forces progress from heel strike to toe-off. In a foot with mechanically stable subtalar and midtarsal joints, pathological pronatory force is transferred distally to the smaller tarsal joints and to the tarsometatarsal level. When peripheral neuropathy is added to this situation, the result is marked destruction as seen in the Charcot joint (Fig. 41.4). Banks and McGlamry (2) have supported the use of arthrodesis for correction of the neuropathic joint.

There are some congenital and acquired foot deformities that may be treated with arthrodesis at the tarsometatarsal level. These include pes cavus and severe cases of metatarsus adductus in the adult. However, in most cases, joint-sparing procedures, such as osteotomies at the metatarsal bases, are preferable.

PREOPERATIVE EVALUATION

Misdiagnosis is common in dealing with Lisfranc's joint. Trauma and chronic injury are both subject to misinterpretation because the joint is not easily visualized on standard radiographs. Localization of pain to the midfoot region is usually a presenting symptom. However, in some cases, the patient will have difficulty localizing the area of discomfort. Symptoms may be referred to other areas such as the metatarsophalangeal joints. In most cases, a planovalgus deformity is seen. The metatarsal may be elevated distally when significant degenerative disease is present at its proximal articulation. This results in lesser metatarsophalangeal joint limitus, complicating the presenting condition (Fig. 41.5).

Special studies such as tomography may be used if Lisfranc's joint arthritis is suspected despite equivocal radiographs (Fig. 41.6). Bone scans have also been used to delineate the involved articulations. Stress radiographic evaluation of the joint(s) may be performed to determine the degree of instability in the acute and chronic situation.

Accurately determining the articulations involved is important in deciding which joints are suitable for arthrodesis. Single or multiple joint involvement may be present. However, fusion of uninvolved joints may also be necessary to allow angular correction or to provide additional stability. In a significant number of cases, the medial joints are involved and the more lateral articulations (metatarsocuboid joints) are spared.

TECHNIQUES

Two basic techniques have been described for arthrodesis of Lisfranc's joint. Arthrodesis with the insertion of graft material is the first method. The technique described in 1986 by Johnson and Johnson (5) involves the use of dowel grafts from the iliac crest. The second method is primary end-to-end arthrodesis following joint resection. The goals of the procedure include (*a*) achieving fusion of the bones involved in a reasonable period of time, (*b*) providing correction of significant deformities, and (*c*) alleviating symptoms. Other considerations include the degree of difficulty

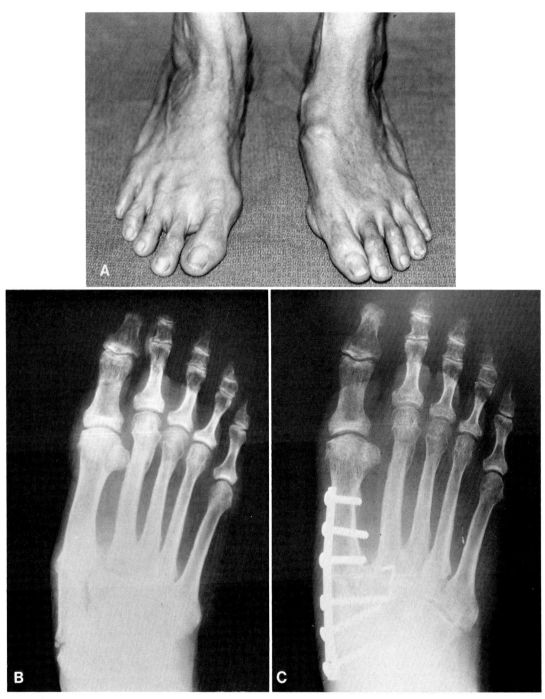

Figure 41.1. Patient suffered a fracture-dislocation injury of the Lisfranc's joint during a motorcycle crash. Initial therapy included compression bandage and non–weight bearing for a few days. Several years later, surgery was performed to relieve painful callouses beneath the second and third metatarsal heads. **A.** Prominence of the entire medial cuneiform is seen. **B.** Radiograph revealing that second and third metatarsal oste-otomies were performed despite the presence of obvious deformity at medial tarsometatarsal and intertarsal joints. **C.** Arthrodesis was later nec-essary to alleviate continued pain at the midfoot level.

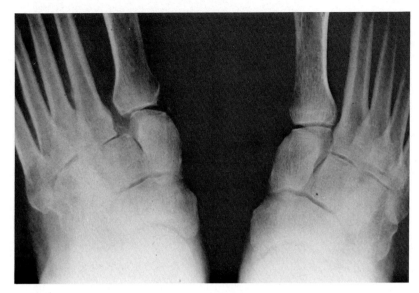

Figure 41.2. Patient, who had fallen while jumping from a moving truck, was seen in emergency room for chief complaint of pain and swelling of left foot. After an initial diagnosis of "foot sprain," patient was discharged with a compression wrap and crutches. Later examination by the author and review of radiographs revealed significant lateral fracture-dislocation requiring reduction. Proper therapy included open reduction and cast immobilization to prevent the posttraumatic degenerative arthritis.

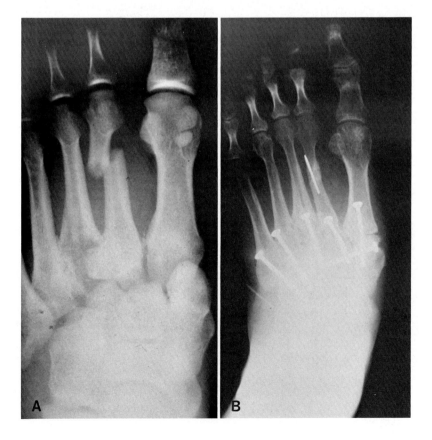

Figure 41.3. Severe crush injury resulting in multiple fracture-dislocations. **A.** Comminution of the metatarsal bases with lateral dislocation required open reduction. **B.** Arthrodesis of Lisfranc's joint and internal fixation of the second metatarsal fracture were performed. However, noncompliance during postoperative period resulted in failure of screws at first three joints, requiring revision to achieve fusion of arthrodesis sites.

Figure 41.4. Severe dislocation and joint destruction at Lisfranc's joint in diabetic Charcot's foot. Reduction and fixation in these severe cases are demanding and often require autogenous bone graft to supplement areas of bone loss.

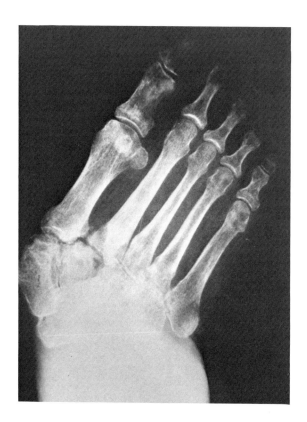

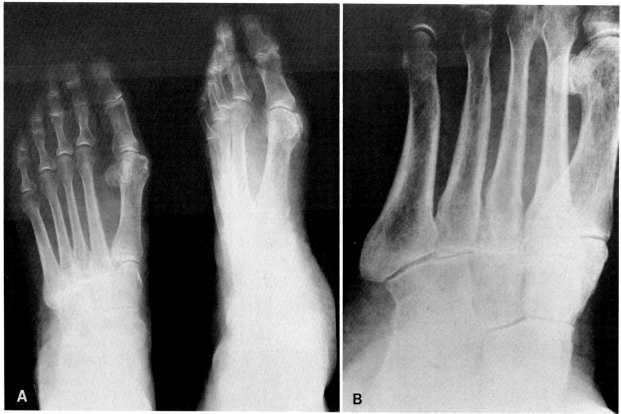

Figure 41.5. A 77-year-old female with 3-year history of left foot pain following jamming of third and fourth toes against chair leg. Pain while ambulating was poorly localized to ball of foot, occasionally radiating to plantar arch. Range of motion examination revealed pain and limitation of dorsiflexion at third and fourth metatarsophalangeal joints. Further ex- amination elicited pronounced pain with passive motion at third and fourth tarsometatarsal joints. **A.** Dorsoplantar view appeared essentially normal findings. **B.** Oblique films revealed degenerative arthritis at third and fourth tarsometatarsal joints, with resulting elevatus of third and fourth ray segments.

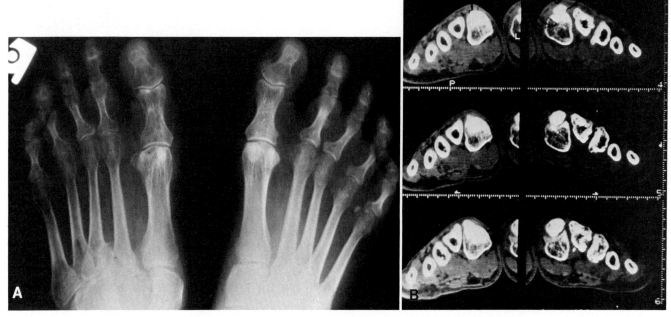

Figure 41.6.   Several months after subtle fracture-dislocation of left foot. **A.** Lisfranc's joint posttraumatic arthritis. **B.** CT findings reveal severe destruction of metatarsocuneiform joints, requiring arthrodesis.

involved in performing the procedure, the availability of graft material, and the method of fixation to be used.

Soft Tissue Dissection

Dissection of the midfoot may be performed without significant soft tissue disturbance. Thigh tourniquet hemostasis, although not essential, is very helpful in expediting the process. Proper placement of the incision lines will allow access to the targeted joints without the need for tenotomy, neurectomy, or major vessel ligation. Care is taken not to place longitudinally aligned incisions in close proximity in order to avoid vascular demise of intervening dorsal skin (Fig. 41.7)

Medial dissection is performed through an incision that parallels the medial aspect of the extensor hallucis longus tendon. The medial marginal vein is generally ligated distally as it joins the dorsal venous arch. This allows medial retraction of the vessel and avoids ligation of multiple tributaries extending from the plantar aspect. Blunt dissection through the superficial fascia with a Metzenbaum scissors may reveal branches of the medial dorsal cutaneous nerve. It may be necessary to sacrifice small branches of this nerve to achieve adequate exposure (Fig. 41.8). The deep fascia is incised medial to the extensor hallucis longus, and the tendon is retracted laterally. Dissection of the first ray segment is then performed subperiosteally. Joint capsule of the first metatarsocuneiform joint should be preserved with the longitudinal line of dissection. Lateral subcapsular dissection onto the dorsal surface of the intermediate cuneiform and second metatarsal base may be possible through this

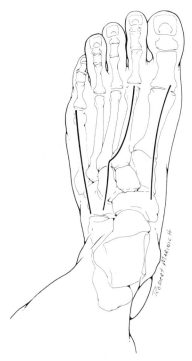

Figure 41.7.   Incision placement for arthrodesis of Lisfranc's joint. Care must be taken to avoid superficial undermining of narrow skin islands created by closely approximated parallel incisions. First metatarsocuneiform joint is approached through medial incision. The second, third, and, occasionally, fourth tarsometatarsal joints are exposed through midline incision. The fifth and, occasionally, fourth metatarsocuboid joints are accessed through dorsolateral incision.

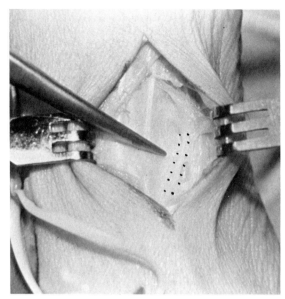

Figure 41.8. Dorsomedial incision over first metatarsocuneiform joint often reveals small branches of medial dorsal cutaneous nerve. These nerve branches may have to be excised to allow access to underlying tissues.

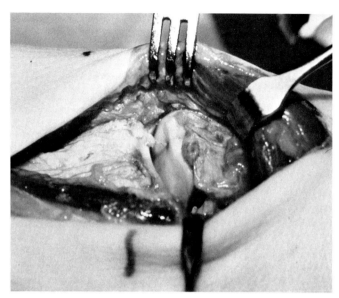

Figure 41.9. Deep fascia over first metatarsocuneiform joint is incised just medial to extensor hallucis longus tendon. Tendon is then retracted laterally. Subperiosteal and subcapsular dissection reveals joint surfaces to be arthrodesed.

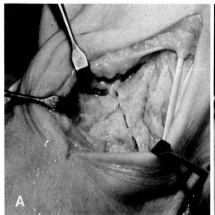 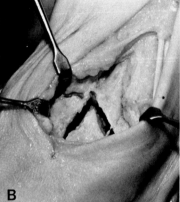 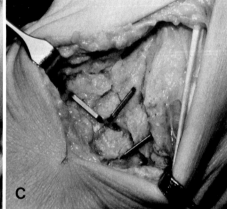

Figure 41.10. Central incision is made between second and third metatarsal bases. **A.** Markedly arthritic joints of lesser tarsus are seen. **B.** Joint resection has been performed at metatarsocuneiform and intertarsal joints between second and third cuneiforms. **C.** Power-driven staples are used for fixation between adjacent cuneiforms and at metatarsocuneiform joints.

incision. In extending the dissection laterally in this manner, caution must be observed to avoid the dorsalis pedis artery and deep peroneal nerve located in the more superficial tissues (Fig. 41.9).

Very often a second incision will be required to expose the second and third metatarsocuneiform joints. This incision may be made in a slight lazy-S fashion over the articulation between the second and third metatarsal bases. Dissection over the midfoot region necessitates caution to protect the medial and intermediate dorsal cutaneous nerves. Extensor tendons are retracted medially or laterally as necessary to allow access to the underlying joints (Fig. 41.10).

Subcapsular and subperiosteal dissection is performed as already described. A lateral incision aligned over the bases of the fourth and fifth metatarsal joints is used if the entire Lisfranc's joint is to be exposed (Fig. 41.11).

Joint Resection

The first step in appropriate joint resection is identification of the joints themselves. In cases with exuberant exostosis formation, joint identification may be difficult. Osteotomes or rongeurs are helpful in removing dorsal exostoses. Manual rather than power instrumentation is recommended for this task in order to preserve the boundaries of each articulation. The joints to be identified should include all articulations about the base of the metatarsal to be arthrodesed: the intermetatarsal, the metatarsocuneiform, and the metatarsocuboid joints.

If in situ arthrodesis is to be performed, it is done without excision of the ligaments about the articulation. No attempt is made to reposition the metatarsals. The dowel graft procedure advocated by Johnson and Johnson (5) involves the trephining of bicortical bone plugs centered over the joint to undergo arthrodesis (Fig. 41.12). These joints must first be carefully identified to allow proper placement of the trephine. Power or manual trephines measuring approximately 7.5 mm in diameter are best suited for this procedure. The cylinder of bone trephined from the tarsometatarsal joint is then replaced with the same-sized dowel of autogenous bone graft. These bicortical graft cylinders are harvested from the patient's anterior iliac crest with the same instrumentation.

The in situ dowel method provides good potential for rapid healing in an area that otherwise may be slow to consolidate. The need for internal fixation is diminished because of the partially intact ligamentous structures. Johnson and Johnson (5) recommend two smooth Kirschner wires (K-wires) inserted in a crossing fashion across Lisfranc's joint. Cast immobilization is used to supplement the fixation. This method should be restricted for use in those patients who do not require correction of severe deformities. Patients

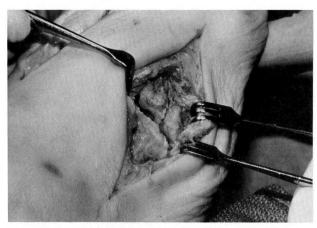

Figure 41.11. Dissection of metatarsocuboid joints. Sural nerve is carefully protected in full-thickness tissue retracted on lateral side of incision.

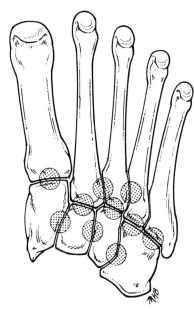

Figure 41.12. Placement of dowel grafts for in situ arthrodesis of lesser tarsus and Lisfranc's joints. (Modified with permission from Johnson JE, Johnson KA: Dowel arthrodesis for degenerative arthritis of the tarsometatarsal [Lisfranc] joints. *Foot Ankle* 6:243-253, 1986 © by American Orthopaedic Foot Society.)

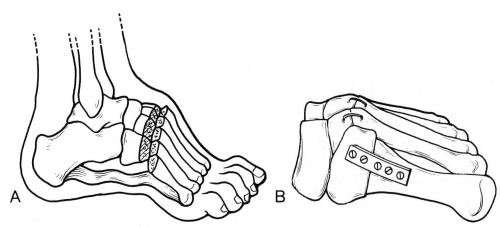

Figure 41.13. **A** and **B.** Dorsiflexory truncated arthrodesis of Lisfranc's joint for correction of cavus foot deformity. (From Green DR, Lepow GM, Smith TF: Pes cavus. In McGlamry ED [ed]: *Comprehensive Textbook of Foot Surgery,* vol 1. Baltimore, Williams & Wilkins, 1987, p 314.)

with a less than optimal potential for healing may also benefit from this procedure.

In cases that require correction of deformity along with arthrodesis, joint mobilization is necessary. Ligamentous attachments of the Lisfranc articulations are excised to allow free mobility during joint resection and fixation. The involved joints may be resected with power instrumentation. A precise instrument with a thin, sharp blade is required for accurate joint resection. Careful preoperative planning will help determine the degree of correction necessary. In any case, minimal joint resection to normal cancellous bone is first performed (Fig. 41.10B). More bone may be resected as needed to allow appropriate forefoot to rearfoot realignment. Although bone graft material may be used to augment the arthrodesis, it should be kept to a minimum because the risk for nonunion increases with graft size.

Correction of cavus deformities with Lisfranc's joint arthrodesis requires that a truncated wedge be resected (Fig. 41.13). This procedure is used when the apex of the cavus deformity is at the tarsometatarsal joint level. Jahss (1) warns that triangular, rather than truncated, wedge resection will not allow relaxation of the plantar fascia, causing difficulty in the approximation of arthrodesis surfaces. In this procedure, it is easy to resect an excessive amount of bone, resulting in an undesirable rocker-bottom deformity.

In posttraumatic degenerative arthritis and in Charcot's joint destruction, significant abduction deformity of the forefoot usually exists. If adduction is needed for realignment, the metatarsocuneiform joints will usually require a greater amount of bone resection relative to the metatarsocuboid joints. When severe deformities are present, a compromise should be made between bone resection medially and bone grafting laterally. This is done to prevent excessive shortening of the medial metatarsals (Fig. 41.14).

The use of bone graft to augment the arthrodesis has been extremely helpful in allowing reconstruction of defects at the midfoot level. In some cases of Charcot's joint destruction, entire lesser tarsus bones may be lost. In these cases autogenous, tricortical iliac crest grafts have been used to replace the destroyed bone (2). In cases in which autogenous graft is not available, allogeneic graft may be substituted. However, significant increases in the healing time should be expected when large defects must be substituted with nonviable bone graft.

Temporary Fixation

In some cases it will be tempting to place temporary fixation prior to completing all the joint resections. However, in most instances this fixation will need to be removed for final positioning. In the relatively small cancellous bones of the midfoot, inserting and removing fixation cause a significant compromise of the bone integrity. This may result in difficulty in achieving adequate bone purchase with the permanent fixation devices. Therefore, all joint resections and most forefoot to rearfoot correction should be obtained prior to inserting any form of fixation.

When the entire Lisfranc's joint is to undergo arthrodesis, it is helpful to temporarily fixate the first metatarsocuneiform and fifth metatarsocuboid arthrodesis sites prior to intraoperative x-ray examination. Temporary fixation then allows evaluation of metatarsal length pattern, declination, and degree of angular correction. Smooth 0.062-inch K-wires are used as temporary fixation. Careful planning and placement of these K-wires permit later substitution with screws if desired. In any event, the temporary fixation should not interfere with the placement of permanent fixation devices.

Optimal positioning of the first and fifth metatarsals results in a relatively straight medial and lateral border of the foot (Fig. 41.15). Intraoperative dorsoplantar x-ray views

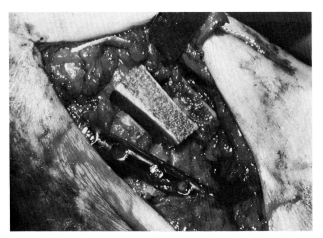

Figure 41.14. Large autogenous iliac crest graft used to fill lateral defect. Grafts of this size may be used with fixation in patients who have lost entire segments of lesser tarsus such as occurs in Charcot's joint destruction.

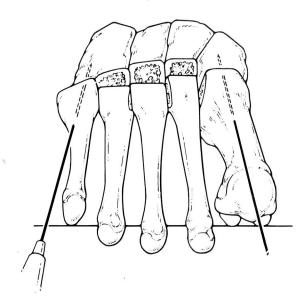

Figure 41.15. Temporary fixation of first metatarsocuneiform and fifth metatarsocuboid arthrodesis sites allows evaluation of forefoot declination, metatarsal parabola, and forefoot alignment.

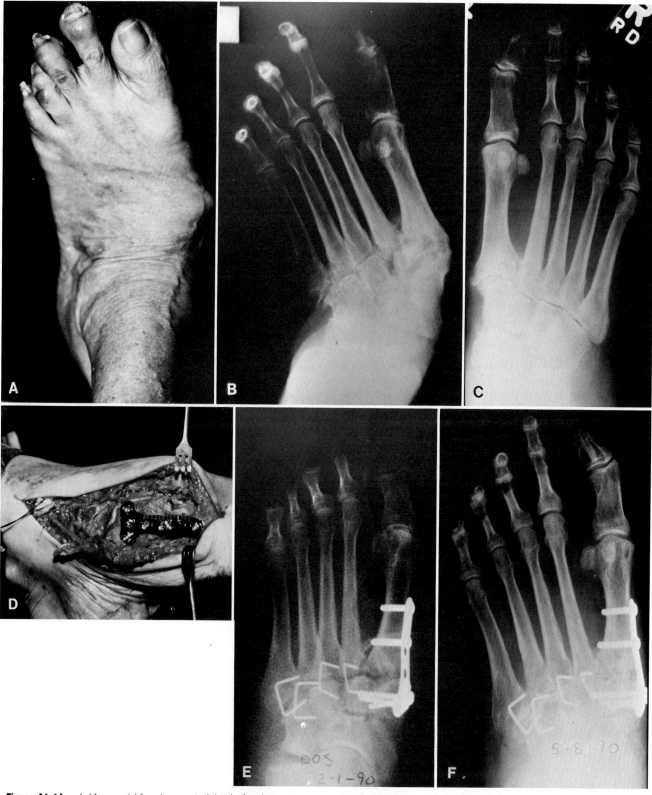

Figure 41.16. A 61-year-old female reported that before knee surgery (performed 2 years before this presentation) her feet appeared similar. Examination revealed bilateral gastrocsoleus equinus with mild weakness of pretibial muscles of left leg. **A.** Marked forefoot abduction and medial prominence resulted in aching pain and difficulty in wearing shoes. **B.** Radiograph of left foot shows serious deterioration and subluxation of Lisfranc's joint. **C.** Contralateral limb showed early degenerative changes at first metatarsocuneiform joint. However, knee surgery was not performed in this extremity. It is speculated that injury to the common peroneal nerve, which had evidently resulted from knee surgery, accentuated muscle imbalance of left-sided equinus. This illustrates the significant influence equinus imparts on structurally weak foot. **D.** Plate fixation of first metatarsocuneiform joint provides significant stability across Lisfranc's joint. **E.** Power-driven staples were used to fixate remainder of Lisfranc's joint. Note compression screw fixation is used between medial and intermediate cuneiforms. Autogenous cancellous bone graft taken from patient's iliac crest was used to augment fixation. Closed suction drain tube is also visible in this radiograph. **F.** Approximately 12 weeks after surgery, consolidation across arthrodesis sites is achieved. Gradual return to full weight bearing was allowed at this point.

should reveal the longitudinal bisection of the talus to be parallel or slightly medial to the first ray bisection. However, in some instances, this degree of correction will not be obtainable. Lateral views should reveal mild plantarflexion of the first metatarsal relative to the midfoot. The first and fifth metatarsal heads should appear on the same transverse plane. Excessive plantarflexion of the first ray segment relative to the remaining metatarsals results frequently in a painful forefoot valgus deformity.

As previously stated, any additional bone resection necessary to achieve proper alignment should be performed toward the more cancellous of the bone surfaces. In many cases this will be the cuneiform or the cuboid, because significant bone resection at the metatarsal base results in entering the more cortical diaphyseal region. Permanent fixation is placed after (a) satisfactory degree of correction is obtained and (b) the first and fifth metatarsals are plantarflexed to approximately the same weight-bearing plane.

Permanent Fixation

Many types of internal fixation have been described for Lisfranc's joint arthrodesis. Most authors agree that some period of cast immobilization and non–weight bearing to augment the internal fixation is necessary (2, 3, 5). Stable fixation with pins, staples, screws, or plates in some combination is necessary to provide the patient the best chance for healing in a reasonable period of time. In both posttraumatic and Charcot's joint cases the bone quantity and quality may be significantly compromised. This complicates the fixation process but should not preclude the use of internal fixation.

The order of fixation will vary from patient to patient depending on the situation. However, in most cases, initially stabilizing the first metatarsocuneiform joint will allow manipulation of the remainder of the metatarsals without disruption of the fixation already applied. The greater size of the first metatarsocuneiform arthrodesis segment allows a greater latitude for use of various forms of fixation. The

most stable of the fixation devices for this application is the combination of compression plate and interfragmental screw fixation. However, this is also one of the more difficult methods.

Generally, plate fixation of the first metatarsocuneiform joint requires a straight or T-plate (Fig. 41.16). Some contouring of the medial surface of the first metatarsal base and medial cuneiform may be necessary to allow the plate to rest evenly against the bone surfaces. A smooth 0.062-inch K-wire temporarily fixates the arthrodesis site. This wire is inserted from distal-superior to proximal-inferior or from distal-inferior to dorsal-superior depending on contours of the bones. This K-wire may later be replaced by a partially threaded 4.0-mm cancellous screw, providing additional stability. The plate is applied using standard AO technique to achieve axial compression across the arthrodesis site. Note that the temporary fixation should be removed prior to completing the final tightening of the compression plate.

Other less technically demanding methods of fixating the first metatarsocuneiform joint include crossed K-wires, multiple small bone staples, or intraosseous wire loop fixation. External splintage and strict non–weight bearing become more important when less stable forms of internal fixation are employed.

The bases of the lesser metatarsals and the corresponding tarsal surfaces are relatively narrow, requiring the use of small fixation devices. Crossed pin fixation is one of the simpler methods used by many surgeons for these sites of arthrodesis. However, significant compression at the arthrodesis site is not obtained. Single compression screw fixation affords good compression but requires sufficient bone quality for adequate purchase of the screw threads (Fig. 41.17). In less optimal conditions staple fixation is better suited to these areas.

The development of power-driven staples has significantly improved the ability to achieve rapid and effective fixation at the Lisfranc's joint level (Fig. 41.10C). Caution must be taken to avoid trying to use staples when cortical

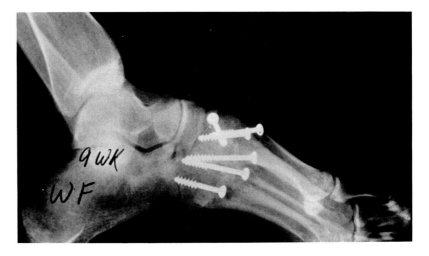

Figure 41.17. Use of multiple lag screws for fixation is effective means of stabilization. However, this method is best reserved for those patients with minimal or no evidence of osteopenia.

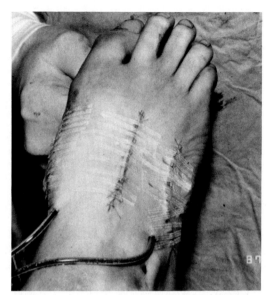

Figure 41.18. Closed suction drains are employed to prevent excessive postoperative edema and hematoma. Drains are usually discontinued by third postoperative day.

bone must be penetrated. Predrilling of the more dense bone surface may be helpful if staples are to be used in this situation.

Wound Closure and Bandaging

The incisions are closed in layers. The periosteal and capsular tissue is reapproximated with an absorbable suture such as 3-0 Dexon or Vicryl. Prior to deep fascial closure, a closed suction drain is inserted and exited through a separate puncture site. Deep fascia and superficial fascia are approximated over the drain. Skin is finally reapproximated with suture of the surgeon's preference (Fig. 41.18).

A modified Jones compression dressing is applied for 2

to 3 days. Closed suction drains are generally removed at 48 hours, but longer periods are necessary in some cases. Once postoperative edema has begun to resolve, a cast is applied. A below-knee cast is used in cases of arthrodesis alone. If the procedure was combined with a tendoachillis lengthening or if there is questionable stability or patient compliance, then an above-knee cast may be used.

POSTOPERATIVE MANAGEMENT

Generally, 12 weeks is considered a normal period of time for healing to occur. However, in some cases, significantly longer periods of time may be necessary to achieve solid bony union. Some authors have suggested an early return to weight bearing to prevent healing of an uneven plantar surface (1). However, most agree that strict non–weight bearing in all cases is necessary to prevent delayed or nonunion at the arthrodesis sites (2, 3, 5). Weight bearing is allowed after there is sufficient radiographic evidence of healing.

Arthrodesis of the Lisfranc's joint level is considered by most to be a salvage procedure. The late results of arthrodesis are based on subjective and objective interpretation. The success of the procedure is usually judged by patients being relatively free from pain, by absence of nonunion, and by good functional results.

References

1. Jahss MH: Tarsometatarsal truncated wedge arthrodesis for pes cavus and equinovarus deformity of the fore part of the foot. *J Bone Joint Surg* 62:712-722, 1980.
2. Banks AS, McGlamry ED: Charcot foot. *J Am Podiatr Med Assoc* 79:213-235, 1989.
3. Sangeorzan BJ, Veigh RG, Hansen ST: Salvage of Lisfranc's tarsometatarsal joint by arthrodesis. *Foot Ankle* 10: 193-200, 1990.
4. Granberry WM, Lipscomb PR: Dislocation of the tarsometatarsal joints. *Surg Gynecol Obstet* 114:467-469, 1962.
5. Johnson JE, Johnson KA: Dowell arthrodesis for degenerative arthritis of the tarsometatarsal (Lisfranc) joints. *Foot Ankle* 6:243-253, 1986.

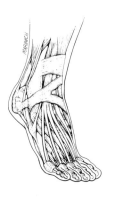

CHAPTER **42**

Triple Arthrodesis and Subtalar Joint Fusions

D. Richard DiNapoli, D.P.M.
John A. Ruch, D.P.M.

Seventy years ago Edwin W. Ryerson (1) said of triple arthrodesis, "The essential aim of this kind of reconstructive surgery is the improvement of the function of the foot."

Triple arthrodesis is an extremely effective procedure that offers gratifying and predictable results when performed for a vast assortment of foot deformities and disorders. The procedure is just one tool that is available for stabilizing the foot and ankle.

HISTORICAL OVERVIEW

The procedure known today as triple arthrodesis was first described by Ryerson in 1923 (Fig. 42.1). At that time he was seeking an alternative procedure that would produce satisfying long-term results in those patients affected by infantile paralysis or similar disabilities. Ryerson was not content with the tendon transpositions that were being used at that time because of their inability to maintain long-term control of varus and valgus deformities. His procedure was based on the success and insight of Gwilyn Davis' efforts in stabilizing the foot through resection of the joint surfaces of the talocalcaneal and talonavicular joints. Ryerson's greatest concern was avoiding a postoperative lateral deformity of the foot. This resulted in his decision to fuse the calcaneocuboid joint in addition to the subtalar and talonavicular joints. The term *triple arthrodesis* was thus appropriate (1).

A number of other triple arthrodesis procedures had been developed during that period, including those of Hoke (Fig. 42.2), Lambrinudi (Fig. 42.3), the Brewster countersinking procedure (Fig. 42.4), the Dunn modification (Fig. 42.5)(2), and the Seiffert, or beak, modification (Fig. 42.6)(3). Each procedure offered certain advantages in achieving a desired result, although the common goal was to achieve a plantigrade foot. Ryerson indicated that the solution was evident in individuals with artificial limbs because the device was capable of only flexion and extension, the only motion that he believed was essential in ordinary walking (4-6).

A sharp divergence of opinion exists regarding many aspects of triple arthrodesis. The indications for the procedure have all but remained the same since Ryerson's time: improved foot function. This is a rather broad term, but any disorder that causes pain, deformity, or instability of the rearfoot on the leg may lend itself to correction by triple arthrodesis.

Since its introduction as a stabilizing procedure for the foot, triple arthrodesis has attracted considerable attention in the literature, not only for its attributes but also for its complications (7-32). The pitfalls and disadvantages of the procedure have led many surgeons to avoid using triple arthrodesis except as a last resort. The technical performance of the procedure may appear at the outset to be relatively straightforward. However, that view is far from accurate, and before identifying all the significant variables likely to provide a satisfactory result, the hazards and detriments of the procedure need to be discussed.

Classically, the problems associated with triple arthrodesis can include pseudoarthrosis and nonunion, recurrence of the deformity, development of degenerative joint disease in joints either proximal or distal to the arthrodesis site, avascular necrosis, ankle instability, alteration on overall growth when performed in children, and callous formation. Additional complications have been noted including scarring, chronic edema, postincisional entrapment neuropathy, muscle atrophy, and weakness.

The two most consistent complications noted are pseudoarthrosis and recurrence of deformity. A significant factor cited for dissatisfaction and failure of the procedure is the rather high rate of pseudoarthrosis. Williams and Menelaus (22) reported the rate of nonunion to be as low as 3.5% with their modification of the procedure. They noted that the midtarsal joint was the culprit in each case; however, they failed to identify specifically which component. Others cite an incidence of pseudoarthrosis ranging from 7% to 23% (2, 9, 15).

One of the most comprehensive reviews, published by Patterson and associates 1950 (2), noted an overall pseudoarthrosis rate of 18% for all forms of triple arthrodesis. A total of 36 nonunions were encountered in 200 cases. In addition they further delineated the nonunions by procedure: Hoke, 7%; Ryerson, 16%; Brewster, 20%; and Lambrinudi, 33%. In reviewing their work, the authors identified the culprit as poor apposition of the osseous surfaces of the resected joints at the time of surgery. Otherwise pseudoarthrosis most often was due to technical error rather than to a failure of the procedure itself.

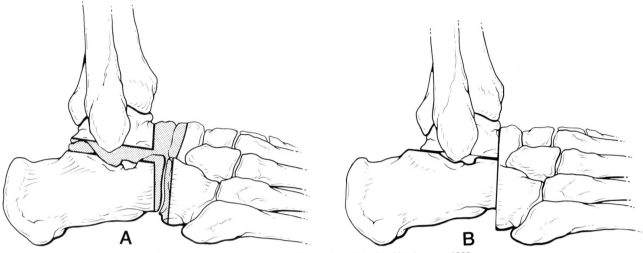

Figure 42.1. **A** and **B.** Triple arthrodesis as described by Ryerson, 1923.

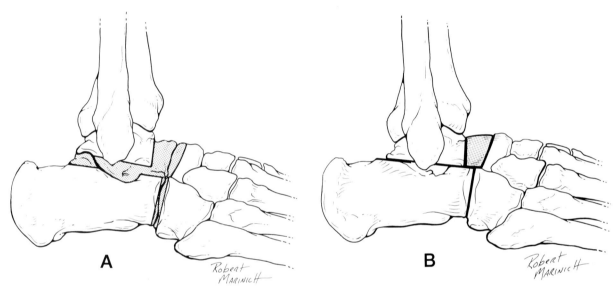

Figure 42.2. **A** and **B.** In the Hoke triple arthrodesis the head and neck of the talus are used as a bone graft.

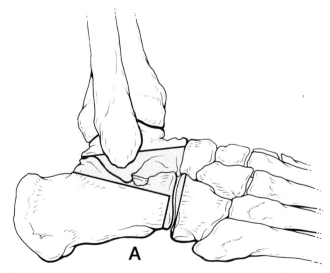
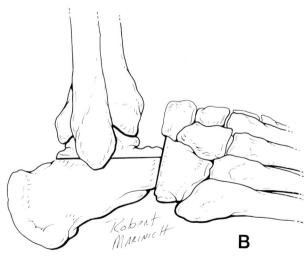

Figure 42.3. **A** and **B.** The Lambrinudi stabilization is most effective in dealing with a drop foot provided adequate muscles are available for concurrent transfer. When the foot attempts to plantarflex, the posterior process of the talus serves as a stop against the posterior malleolus of the tibia.

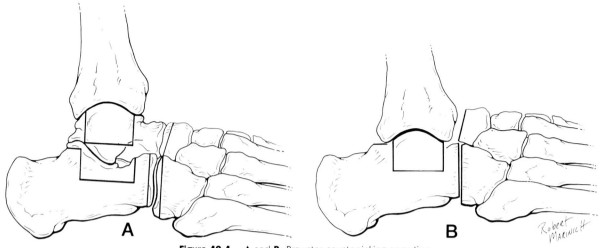

Figure 42.4.   **A** and **B.** Brewster countersinking operation.

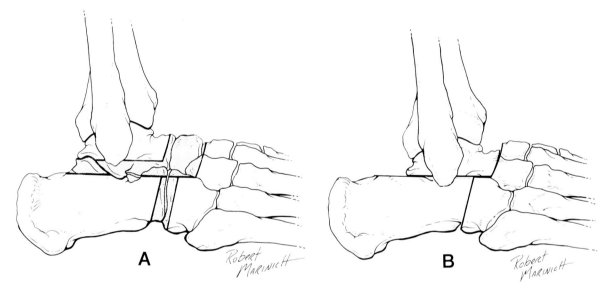

Figure 42.5.   **A** and **B.** Dunn modification.

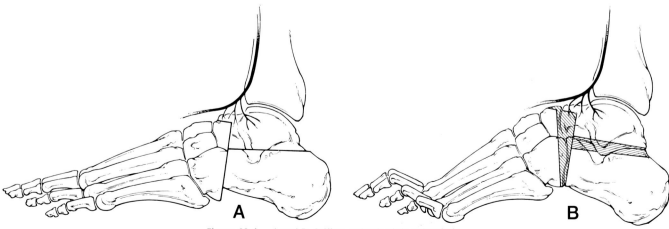

Figure 42.6.   **A** and **B.** Seiffert, or beak, triple arthrodesis.

At the time of Patterson and associates (2) the various methods of internal fixation as practiced today were not used. Wilson et al. in 1965 (11) identified the factors that influenced the development of pseudoarthrosis to include lack of internal fixation, poor apposition of the surgical sites, and early weight bearing. As a retort, Angus and Cowell (9) reviewed 80 triple arthrodeses and noted that 18 were affected by pseudoarthrosis. Their rate of 23% was well within that described by other authors. In their series, 12 cases were performed by means of internal fixation, three of which resulted in nonunions. This was almost the same rate as the rest of their series. They did not identify the type of fixation or further delineate the cause of the nonunions.

Further studies identify age as a contributing factor to the development of pseudoarthrosis, particularly at the talonavicular joint. Patterson and co-workers (2) indicated that stabilization procedures performed prior to the age of 9 years were associated with a failure rate of 47%. Procedures performed after that age demonstrated only a 9% failure rate. The authors did not identify the number of pseudoarthroses for those procedures performed prior to age 9 years, but the overall pseudoarthrosis rate for the group of children aged 12 years and younger was 12%. This contrasts with the report by Galindo and associates (15) of a nonunion rate of only 7%.

Residual deformity has been reported by numerous authors (2, 9, 12, 17, 19). Patterson and associates (2), in 1950, reported 38 recurrences in a series of 305 rearfoot stabilizations (12%). For triple arthrodesis the overall recurrence rate was also 12%, or 25 cases of 210. The authors identified the most common causes for residual deformity as undercorrection, an inadequate period of immobilization, failure to align the foot with the ankle joint, loss of position during cast changes, failure of fusion, muscle imbalance, and surgery at too early an age. Even though residual deformities appear multifactorial the primary component was undercorrection. The investigators did not delineate the foot types associated with undercorrection, but it appears to have been in cavovarus and equinus foot deformities.

Hill and associates (12), in 1970, reported a 12% recurrence rate following triple arthrodesis in children. In all cases the need for revision was the result of residual heel varus. Through further analysis they were able to conclude that inadequate correction at the time of the original surgery was responsible for the recurrence rather than a return of the deformity by growth through a solid fusion. Severe clubfoot deformity was associated with four out of five of their revisions.

Angus and Cowell (9), in 1986, reported a recurrence rate of 62% in 80 feet undergoing triple arthrodesis. The greatest percentage of these individuals had a planovalgus deformity. This was similarly reported by Seitz and Carpenter in 1974 (10). The remaining patients with recurrent deformity had either a rigid equinovarus or a cavo adductovarus foot before surgery. Other authors recounted similar findings following triple arthrodesis in cavovarus feet associated with Charcot-Marie-Tooth disease (17, 19).

The occurrence of degenerative disease in adjacent joints is a favorite target of those who caution against triple arthrodesis in either a primary role or as a salvage procedure. MacKenzie (30) was one of the first to report degenerative changes in the foot and ankle in a long-term follow-up of triple arthrodesis. He reviewed 100 Lambrinudi-type procedures and noted that 15 had developed painful osteoarthritis. Bernau (20) in 1977 reviewed 50 triple arthrodeses and found that painful osteoarthritis occurred in only three of 50 feet. He concluded that this was a rare and exceptional occurrence.

Since that time much more attention has been directed to the incidence of osteoarthritic changes, yet without significant regard to the preoperative deformity. A number of conditions, such as the painful collapsing pes planovalgus deformity, are often associated with significant osteoarthritic changes at more proximal joints (ankle, knee, hip) because of the faulty biomechanical function of the foot. The same may be said of uncompensated rigid cavovarus deformities. Without surgery, arthritic changes can occur in these patients.

Duncan and Lovell (31) in 1978 reported on 109 cases in which there was no evidence of ankle joint malfunction, instability, or degeneration secondary to the procedure. They did note in 14 patients with myelomeningocele that there was an acceleration of degenerative change in the ankle, but no incidence of Charcot's joint. They postulated that three factors could contribute to the development of degenerative changes in the ankle. The first two are the loss of motion from fusion of the subtalar and midtarsal joints. The third was the presence of excess compressive forces at the end of ankle dorsiflexion, or residual equinus.

Hill and associates (12) failed to find degenerative changes in the ankle after an average of 9½ years following 43 triple arthrodesis procedures performed in children. There was no mention of degenerative changes in other proximal joints.

Southwell and Sherman (18), in 1981, reported a 58% incidence of degenerative changes in the foot or ankle after triple arthrodesis. However, they noted that most cases were asymptomatic at an average of 8 years after surgery. They also performed force plate gait analysis in the 24 patients and compared this with results in 12 normal control subjects. One of their conclusions was that triple arthrodesis results in a statistically significant increase in midfoot load-bearing regardless of the extent of heel valgus that may be present. In reviewing their paper one finds no mention of preoperative force plate gait studies. Furthermore, their conclusion was based on comparisons made with normal individuals. One should also note that most patients in their study had some neurological disease; 71% had neuromuscular disorders and 21% had congenital deformities. Therefore it seems that the conclusions of increased weight-bearing stress within the midfoot is poorly documented. In addition, for many patients with cavus and cavovarus deformities, increased midfoot weight bearing is desirable.

The idea that increased compressive forces with ankle dorsiflexion could lead to osteoarthrosis was further emphasized by Angus and Cowell (9). They reported that degenerative changes occurred in the ankle at a rate of 39% and that there was an overall incidence of degenerative change of 54%. They believed that this high rate was also due to the lack of midtarsal and subtalar joint motion. This high rate of degenerative joint changes was not specifically correlated to the preoperative condition, that is, rigid cavovarus, rigid pes valgus, or collapsing pes valgus, or the presence or absence of ankle equinus.

In 1989 two separate studies detailed the incidence of arthritic changes in patients with Charcot-Marie-Tooth disease. Wetmore and Drennan (19) reported radiographic evidence of osteoarthritic changes in 23 of 30 feet (76%). However, there was clinical evidence of this condition in only 19 of 30 feet (63%). Although this rate appears high, Wukich and Bowen (17) reported overall degenerative changes of the midfoot to be 62%. In addition, they reported 24% cases of osteoarthrosis in the ankle. They did not specify whether the degenerative changes were present preoperatively or what percentage of feet had both foot and ankle osteoarthrosis.

Another criticism of triple arthrodesis cited by a number of authors is the effect on immature subjects. Crego and McCarroll (13), in 1938, stated that the procedure should not be used in children younger than 8 years of age for fear that a secondary deformity would result as well as overall difficulties with fusion. This was further supported by Patterson and associates (2) who reported a failure rate of 47% when the procedure was performed in children 8 years and younger. They attributed their failures to the small size of the structures, the difficulty in maintaining correction in plaster, poor evaluation of muscle power with subsequent muscle imbalance, and the influence of the osseous structures. Their overall failure rate was only 9% in patients aged 9 to 20 years. In examining the long-term effect on foot length and growth, they determined that the difference was insignificant and that growth was not deterred. Duncan and Lovell (31) indicated that if the procedure were performed in children younger than 12 years of age for girls and 14 years for boys, the foot size would be significantly smaller compared with older patients. However, they did not provide specific data to support their findings.

In contrast, Hill and associates (12) advocated that triple arthrodesis be performed at as early an age as possible when that surgery is the only alternative. In their opinion, postponing a procedure for several years until a child reaches skeletal maturity was not necessary, especially in cases in which the patient would continue to use braces and casts that were ineffective. They did emphasize that the ossification center of the talar head needed to be present to ensure adequate fusion. Overall their results seem satisfactory. In reporting on 43 triple arthrodeses performed in children between the ages of 5 and 8 years, they noted a 12% revision rate for persistent deformity, rather than recurrence through growth, and a pseudoarthrosis rate of 12%. The average shortening was 0.75 inches. However, the authors commented that overall foot length was difficult to evaluate because many of the feet that required arthrodesis and stabilization were short initially. This view is further supported by Galindo and associates (15) who performed 19 triple arthrodeses in children 10 years and younger. In each case the surgery was undertaken as a salvage procedure and an alternative to talectomy. Overall the shortening that they recorded was 0.81 inches, which was not statistically significant when compared with a control group of patients with clubfoot. In addition, they did not record an increase in the rate of nonunion or a recurrence of deformity.

One of the remaining reported hazards of triple arthrodesis is avascular necrosis (AVN) of the talus, navicular, or cuneiforms. The predominant tarsal bone affected is the talus. It was noted by Duncan and Lovell (31) that AVN occurred about 6.5% of the time when the Hoke triple arthrodesis was used and in those cases performed prior to 1948. After that time the resection of the head and neck of the talus was modified to preserve the artery of the tarsal canal.

CRITICAL REVIEW

Upon initial review, the complications that have been reported to occur with triple arthrodesis would seem substantial. However, most authors have apparently condemned the procedure without objectively reviewing their own work to determine how the surgery could be improved. With such a cursory examination almost any procedure would probably appear to fare poorly. Over the years the members of The Podiatry Institute have consistently searched for ways to improve the techniques and results of triple arthrodesis. As a result, they have concluded that triple arthrodesis is a suitable, reliable means of stabilizing the foot and improving function.

One of the primary reasons for failure of the triple arthrodesis may be the surgeon's underestimation of the complexity of the procedure. Many factors must be constantly assessed and reassessed intraoperatively inasmuch as triple arthrodesis requires full attention to detail.

Many complications may be related to the single lateral incision often employed for the exposure of joint surfaces. It is difficult to resect or to position the talonavicular joint adequately from the lateral side of the foot, because this approach does not provide consistent visualization or mobility of the tissues. Thus incomplete resection of the joint surface may result in poor positioning or in pseudarthrosis due to incomplete resection of the joint surface. Two previous reports have attributed the failure to achieve adequate correction of pes valgus deformity with triple arthrodesis to the use of the traditional Ollier approach (9, 10).

Bone resection is a critical part of triple arthrodesis. Historical procedures such as the Lambrinudi result in the resection of much of the talus, which may encourage impingement of the anterior tibia, the fibula, or pseudarthrosis as a result of the reduced viability of the remaining bone. Enough substance should be removed to provide the relaxation of the soft tissues required to achieve good positioning and healing. Additional bone resection may also cause unnecessary shortening.

Previous authors have cited residual or recurrent deformity as a fairly common complication (2, 9, 12, 17, 19). Provided the structures have completely healed, it is difficult to understand how the deformity recurs unless the fusion sites were not fixated. In this instance shifting may occur with changes in swelling or during cast changes. Residual deformity should not be interpreted as a consequence of the procedure but rather as incomplete realignment of the foot.

Proper positioning of the foot is vital to ensure good postoperative function. In many patients this is not an easy task, especially in the rigid cavus foot deformity. The mechanics of positioning the foot will be discussed later in this chapter, but the importance of the incisional approach and the dissection process must be appreciated because they relate to achieving good alignment.

Good bone apposition is necessary to ensure the optimum environment for healing. Although numerous authors indicate a fairly high rate of pseudarthrosis (2, 9, 15), this complication is a rare problem in the authors' experience. Improved power instrumentation and skills, in particular the use of reciprocal planing, have enabled surgeons to obtain flush-fitting bone interfaces. Furthermore, more rigid forms of internal fixation furnish good stability that is not easily disrupted, provided the patient abstains from weight bearing. Another key to successful healing is eliminating weight-bearing stress until adequate consolidation has been achieved. Otherwise, even with internal fixation, alignment may not be maintained and there is a high risk for complications.

Ankle arthrosis has been seen in rare instances following triple arthrodesis. Success with the procedure involves more than simply achieving fusion. Once again, good positioning and alignment are necessary to ensure function without introducing inordinate stress to the adjacent joints. In fact, realignment of the foot deformity may actually preclude future degeneration of the ankle. The position demonstrated in many reports of triple arthrodesis would be considered unacceptable by the authors of this chapter; it probably accounts for a variety of complications, including ankle arthrosis.

Avascular necrosis of the talus is another complication seen in only two or three cases following triple arthrodesis by Institute members over the past 20 years, involving well over 600 surgeries. This low incidence may be due to the judicious resection of bone and techniques of anatomical dissection.

INDICATIONS

Triple arthrodesis is performed for a wide variety of foot deformities and malformations. In the broadest sense the procedure is used to achieve four major goals: correction of deformity, relief of pain, stabilization, and improved function. These indications are essentially unchanged from the original goals proposed by Ryerson (1). The dominant deformity in the early twentieth century was flaccid paralysis, with instability of the foot secondary to poliomyelitis. Today a variety of conditions are implicated in producing a painful, deformed, and unstable foot that may require triple arthrodesis. Table 42.1 reflects the wide range of diagnoses in which this surgery is performed.

Many of the disease processes in Table 42.1 reflect a number of similar deformities. For simplicity, each of the major deformities will be addressed and categorized as in Table 42.2. This approach will enable the authors to identify particular situations that may warrant triple arthrodesis.

Valgus Foot Deformity

Valgus foot deformities are associated with a wide variety of conditions. In those circumstances in which the deformity is severe, there will be collapse of the entire rearfoot complex, both at the subtalar and midtarsal joints. Patients with this condition have often been relegated to a sedentary life-

Table 42.1.
Conditions Requiring Triple Arthrodesis

Idiopathic collapsing pes planovalgus deformity
Peroneal spastic flatfoot
Tarsal coalition
Congenital vertical talus
Rheumatoid arthritis
Degenerative arthritis
Posttraumatic degenerative arthritis
Ruptured tibialis posterior tendon
Idiopathic cavus and cavovarus deformities
Congenital clubfoot (uncorrected)
Poliomyelitis
Spina bifida
Friedreich's ataxia
Charcot-Marie-Tooth disease
Muscular dystrophy
Cerebral palsy
Myelodysplasia
Arthrogryposis

Table 42.2.
Indications for Triple Arthrodesis

Valgus Foot Deformity

1. Collapsing pes planovalgus
2. Ruptured tibialis posterior tendon
3. Tarsal coalition and arthritic deformities
   a. Congenital
   b. Rheumatoid
   c. Degenerative
   d. Posttraumatic

Varus Foot Deformities

1. Cavus
2. Cavovarus
3. Talipes equinovarus

Miscellaneous

1. Lateral ankle instability and ankle equinus
2. Neuromuscular disease
   a. Hereditary familial sensorimotor neuropathies
   b. Paralytic deformities
   c. Charcot joint deformities
   d. Other diseases affecting the spinal cord and brain

style because of the painful nature of the foot. Most often such patients fail to respond to conservative care. The poor biomechanical characteristics associated with this foot often produce symptoms and deterioration of the more proximal joint structures: ankle, knee, hip, and lumbar spine.

COLLAPSING PES VALGUS DEFORMITY

The collapsing pes valgus deformity typically represents an advanced stage of the flexible pes valgus foot (Fig. 42.7). This condition has been termed the end-stage flatfoot or recalcitrant equinovalgus deformity (16). The foot has surpassed any meaningful degree of biomechanical compensation. Most often the condition has been present since birth as a calcaneovalgus that goes untreated and has progressed. Through growth and development the rearfoot complex and the joint surfaces grow into a malaligned position, manifesting as a collapsed subtalar joint that remains in fixed pronation and a midtarsal joint in fixed abduction and dor-

siflexion. In addition, through normal activity the joint complex may produce significant degenerative changes, further exacerbating the deformity and symptoms.

Another important consideration is the function of the first ray and first metatarsophalangeal joint. Very often the first ray will be unstable. Other extensive pathomechanical changes may be noted in the forefoot as well.

This type of foot deformity is quite responsive to stabilization through triple arthrodesis. An important consideration in correcting the valgus foot is full knowledge of the amount of available ankle joint motion and its relative stability. A further consideration is the absolute necessity to address ankle equinus if it is present.

RUPTURED TIBIALIS POSTERIOR TENDON

Tibialis posterior tendon rupture and the end-stage dysfunctional tibialis posterior tendon generally occur with a severely pronated foot. The peroneus brevis gains mechan-

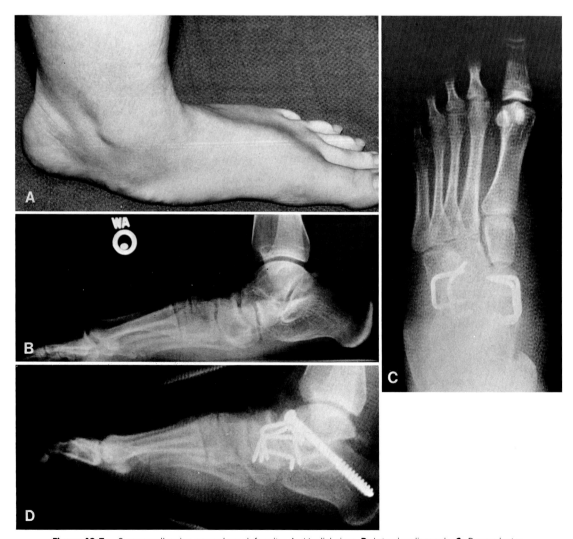

Figure 42.7. Severe collapsing pes valgus deformity. **A.** Medial view. **B.** Lateral radiograph. **C.** Dorsoplantar radiograph following triple arthrodesis. **D.** Lateral postoperative view.

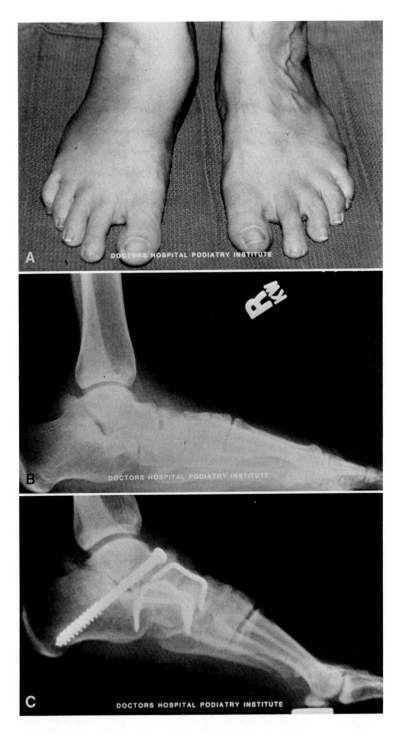

Figure 42.8. Collapsing pes valgus deformity as a result of a ruptured tibialis posterior tendon. This patient had markedly pronated feet of long-standing duration. **A.** Pre-operative clinical appearance. **B.** Preoperative radiograph; note the extensive degenerative changes in the midtarsal and subtalar joints. **C.** Postoperative radiograph following triple arthrodesis.

ical advantage, resulting in further collapse and medial column instability manifested as increased forefoot abduction and dorsiflexion at the midtarsal joint (Fig. 42.8). The condition has received some notoriety in the literature as a spontaneous pes valgus deformity. The truth is quite the contrary. The rupture of the tibialis posterior tendon most often is the result of chronic tenosynovitis in a pathological pes valgus foot type (32). The excessive loading of the mid-tarsal joint during active propulsion leads to further breakdown. The presence of chronic tenosynovitis sets the stage for weakening and eventual rupture of the tendon.

TARSAL COALITION

Tarsal coalitions may produce either a fixed valgus or a varus foot condition. Most often the patient has a painful tarsal coalition and secondary peroneal spastic pes valgus deformity (Fig. 42.9). Usually the foot is significantly more pronated than the contralateral extremity. The subtalar joint is fixed in eversion, and the midtarsal joint is often everted and abducted as well. The head of the talus is prominent medially and plantarly. There is reduced motion or a total absence of motion in the rearfoot complex. This may exist even if the peroneal spasm is alleviated. If there has been substantial osseous adaptation in the rearfoot complex as a result of the coalition, triple arthrodesis offers a suitable surgical correction.

TARSAL ARTHROSIS

Arthritic conditions that affect the ankle and rearfoot complex may be secondary to underlying systemic disorders such as rheumatoid arthritis or degenerative changes associated with pathological foot mechanics (Fig. 42.10). This is most often seen in the severe collapsing pes valgus foot deformity, especially one with significant ankle equinus. The tarsal area is subjected to a variety of deforming forces, resulting in significant arthrosis in the subtalar, midtarsal, or ankle joint region.

Any trauma to the rearfoot complex that results in intra-articular fractures of any of the four major tarsal bones can produce a high incidence of arthrosis. This is most often seen with fractures of the calcaneus, especially when the fracture involves the posterior and middle facets of the sub-talar joint. If the articular surfaces are not anatomically reduced, then the patient is highly susceptible to subsequent arthrosis. The progressive nature of this process produces sufficient pain and disability to warrant surgical repair. Calcaneal fractures that also produce intra-articular injury of the calcaneocuboid joint exhibit more rapid arthritic changes.

Triple arthrodesis offers permanent relief of pain while affording realignment and stability of the foot (Fig. 42.11). In the surgical repair of this deformity the presence of posterior equinus cannot be ignored. Old compression fractures of the calcaneus will often require bone grafting at the talocalcaneal joint level to restore the osseous segment to its proper height. This will effectively restore the soft tissue to preinjury length and improve the overall mechanical function.

DIABETIC CHARCOT FOOT

The collapsed diabetic Charcot's foot offers the surgeon perhaps the greatest challenge in surgical reconstruction. Usually a major component is the destruction of the midtarsal joint, possibly with dislocation. The principles used in reconstruction are covered in great depth in the chapter on diabetic foot surgery. Triple arthrodesis is but one step that may be employed in the repair and reconstruction of the diabetic Charcot foot.

Figure 42.9. **A.** Middle facet talocalcaneal coalition with extensive remodeling of the midtarsal joint. **B.** The patient required triple arthrodesis because of the secondary adaptive changes and disabling pain.

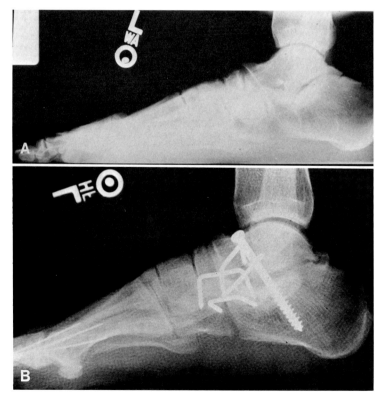

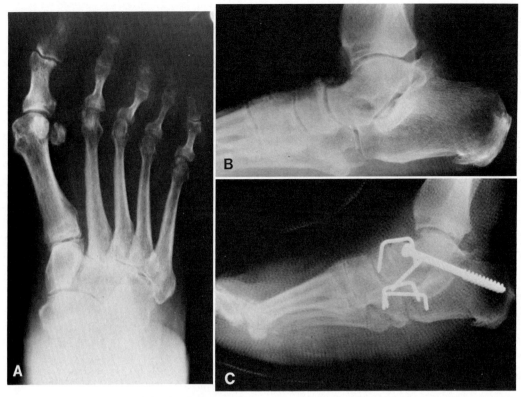

Figure 42.10. Severe collapsing pes valgus deformity. **A.** Dorsoplantar radiograph shows extensive degenerative changes present in the entire midfoot. **B.** Preoperative lateral radiograph shows extensive degenerative changes in the rearfoot. **C.** The foot was stabilized and the painful symptoms resolved through triple arthrodesis.

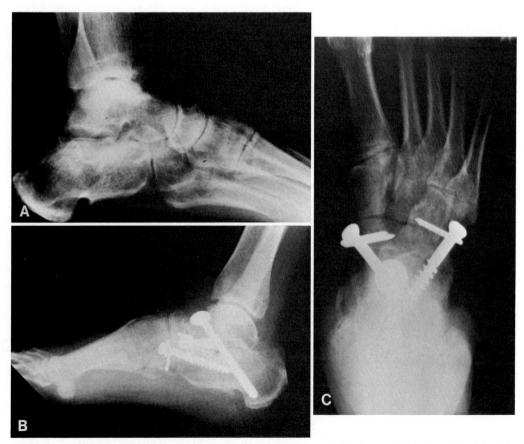

Figure 42.11. Posttraumatic arthrosis of the subtalar joint resulting from a joint depression fracture of the calcaneus. **A.** Close examination of lateral radiograph reveals extension of the fracture into the calcaneocuboid joint, as well as arthritic changes in the talonavicular joint. Lateral **(B)** and dorsoplantar **(C)** views following triple arthrodesis.

Varus Foot Deformity

The varus foot deformity is most commonly associated with a high arch and a rigid foot. There are many conditions responsible for this type of foot.

CAVUS FOOT

The cavus foot, which has various presentations and causative factors, may be the result of neuromuscular disease or an idiopathic process. The faulty biomechanics of this foot type are quite apparent. The rearfoot functions in fixed varus position and is not capable of adequate compensation. Associated postural symptoms include knee and lower-back strain as well as lateral ankle and foot pain. Not uncommonly, recurrent ankle sprains and instability are reported. As the foot continues to function in fixed varus, other deformities may develop, including claw toes, fixed plantar-flexion of the first ray, and painful hyperkeratoses beneath the metatarsal heads.

Triple arthrodesis offers a mechanism to reduce arch height, reposition the rearfoot at the subtalar joint, and abduct the forefoot at the midtarsal joint (Fig. 42.12). In fixed forefoot deformity (forefoot varus or valgus) derota-

tion may usually be accomplished as a part of the triple arthrodesis.

CAVOADDUCTO VARUS

The cavoadducto varus foot deformity is usually idiopathic but may be associated with neurological disease in which dynamic muscular imbalance is present. As in the cavus foot deformity, triple arthrodesis presents an opportunity to correct the osseous deformity and stabilize the foot. The procedure offers increased function and mobility to the patient and may be used in conjunction with muscle-tendon balancing procedures as necessary. This is addressed in the chapter on Charcot-Marie-Tooth disease.

TALIPES EQUINO VARUS

The recalcitrant talipes equinovarus is best treated by triple arthrodesis in conjunction with appropriate soft tissue releases (Fig. 42.13). The resection of the articular surfaces of the subtalar and midtarsal joints does not necessarily effect a complete release of the deformity. Soft tissue procedures and tendon transfers will at times be necessary as

Figure 42.12. A. Cavus foot. **B.** Note the relative arch-lowering effect and increased trochlear surface available at the anterior ankle following triple arthrodesis.

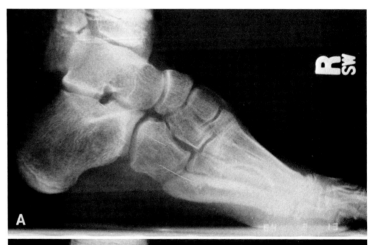

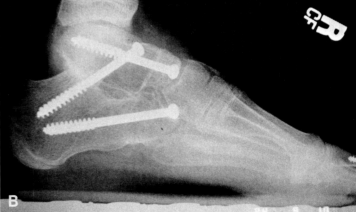

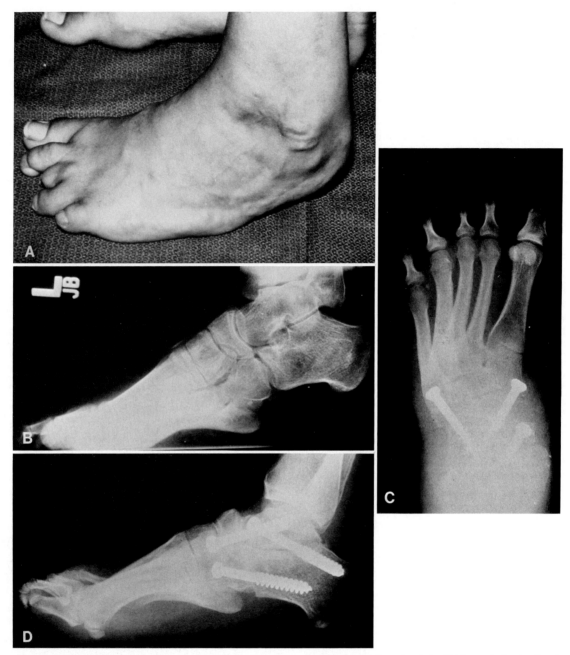

Figure 42.13. **A** and **B.** Neglected clubfoot deformity that had undergone previous selected soft tissue surgeries. **C** and **D.** Correction was obtained via triple arthrodesis, tibialis posterior tendon transfer, and Achilles tendon lengthening.

Lateral Ankle Instability

The fixed varus foot type is commonly associated with lateral and anterior ankle instability. The problem is amenable to stabilization by triple arthrodesis. It is essential that there not be a proximal osseous deformity such as tibial varum, which is a major influence. Restoration of stability is dependent on slight valgus alignment of the rearfoot and proper positioning of the forefoot in mild abduction. The lateral ankle ligaments may be repaired in conjunction with triple arthrodesis.

Ankle Equinus

Osseous equinus of the ankle may be addressed with triple arthrodesis. The surgical correction in this deformity depends on the resection of more bone from the anterior aspect of the underside of the talus than from the posterior surface (posterior facet). This maneuver results in plantarflexion of the head and neck of the talus and creates a reserve of the trochlear surface at the anterior ankle. This effectively increases the articulation of the tibia and the posterior dome of the talus, thereby increasing available dorsiflexion at the ankle joint.

Neuromuscular Disease

There are a wide variety of neuromuscular diseases and disorders that may produce any and all of the deformities discussed (Table 42.1). The resultant rearfoot and ankle deformity is often best treated with triple arthrodesis. Cerebral palsy may produce a spastic pes valgus deformity whereas spina bifida often produces a cavoadducto varus deformity. Charcot-Marie-Tooth disease usually results in

cavoadducto varus deformities as well. Poliomyelitis is responsible for a variety of complex foot conditions depending upon which muscles are affected.

Triple arthrodesis allows sufficient flexibility of design to correct the deformity of the rearfoot while restoring stability in most cases (Fig. 42.14). In many of the neuromuscular deformities tendon transfers are combined with rearfoot fusion to increase stability and function.

Pediatric Patient

Many of the deformities that have been discussed also occur in children. The decision to perform surgery for any podiatric or orthopedic problem in children involves many considerations. Perhaps the foremost is the degree of deformity present. Consideration must be given to surgical procedures that avoid, where reasonable, arthrodesis of the

Figure 42.14. A and **B.** Patient with severe Charcot-Marie-Tooth disease and associated cavoadducto varus deformity, claw toes, and plantarflexed first metatarsal. **C.** Major reconstructive surgery was performed, including triple arthrodesis, dorsiflexory osteotomy of first metatarsal, and digital stabilizations.

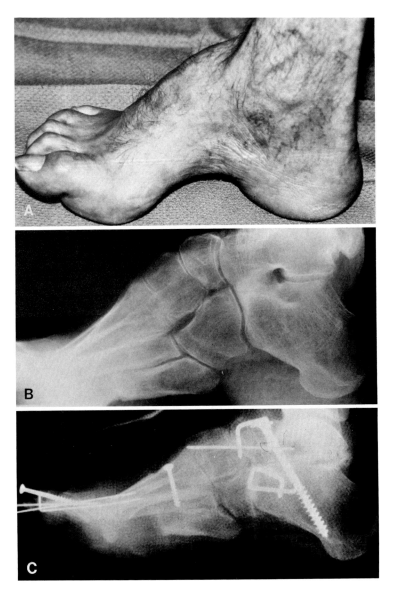

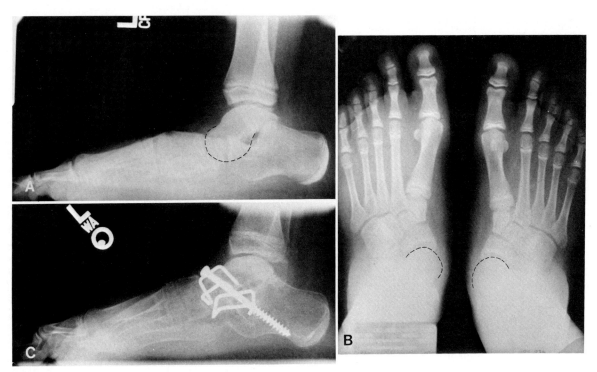

Figure 42.15. **A** and **B.** Preoperative radiographs of a pediatric patient with severe pes planovalgus deformity and marked forefoot supinatus. Note also the degree of metatarsus adductus. **C.** Postoperative radiograph showing excellent correction of deformity.

major tarsal joints. The age of the child is also a consideration. As the child grows, will the correction obtained at surgery be adversely affected? One should also consider the future effects on function at the more proximal joints as a result of the alteration of foot biomechanics. The effect on overall shape, length, and appearance of the operative foot compared with the contralateral foot is important. In addition, one must consider the normal surgical complications that may occur. Previous authors have noted that performing the procedure in children may affect the success rate.

The indications for triple arthrodesis in the child invariably overlap with those for the adult. Usually triple arthrodesis in children is reserved as a salvage procedure for previous, failed surgical attempts such as soft tissue releases in clubfoot, arthrogryposis, and myelodysplasia. It is occasionally used in the recurrent pes valgo planus, rigid pes valgo planus deformity, and spastic valgus deformity associated with tarsal coalition. Faculty members of The Podiatry Institute usually reserve the procedure for the adolescent patient (Fig. 42.15). Because the procedure affords correction in all three cardinal planes, as well as increasing the functional stability of the foot, it may produce very gratifying long-term results even in the child.

SURGICAL CONSIDERATIONS AND PREOPERATIVE EVALUATION

There still exist a number of other considerations that must be reviewed prior to performing triple arthrodesis. Included are patient expectations and selection, the desired goal of fusion and its functional effect, timing of the surgical intervention, biomechanical considerations of the subtalar and midtarsal joints, neurovascular status of foot and leg, bone quality, soft tissue quality, lower extremity evaluation and function, and gait evaluation.

Candidates selected for triple arthrodesis must be those patients who have proven resistance to conservative therapy or who cannot reasonably be expected to respond to it, and in whom the surgeon can expect an adequate result. The patient needs to be informed that the pronatory-supinatory motion in the rearfoot will be eliminated. The only motion that will remain after surgery is flexion and extension at the ankle joint and to some extent the tarsometatarsal joint. The elimination of subtalar and midtarsal joint motion will restrict the ability of the patient to adapt to uneven surfaces and terrain.

The biomechanics of the lower extremity need to be understood in relation to the effect of triple arthrodesis (33). The hip joint is normally positioned in neutral in both the transverse and sagittal planes and is tilted slightly anterior. There should be an equal amount of internal and external rotation available from the neutral position. The hip should be able to flex to approximately 130° and extend (hyperextend) to 10°. The femur is 10° degrees retroverted relative to the frontal plane. Deformities at the hip such as coxa vara and coxa valga, as well as degenerative arthrosis, will be significantly influenced by an alteration of rearfoot mechanics.

The knee joint is generally aligned in the sagittal plane and at full extension does not normally exhibit transverse plane rotation or motion. The knee does not hyperextend but should flex to 130°. When the knee is flexed, transverse plane motion is available.

The ankle is normally positioned 90° relative to the leg. It should be able to dorsiflex to approximately 10° with the knee extended and to plantarflex to between 30° and 50°. The axis of the ankle joint is slightly deviated from both the sagittal and transverse planes by approximately 10°. This effectively creates a triplanar axis, with supination and pronation occurring at the joint. However, because of the location of the axis, most of the motion occurs in the sagittal plane. Often the amount of motion available in a patient with a severe collapsing pes valgus deformity will appear adequate at first inspection because of the collapse of the midtarsal and subtalar joints. In contrast the ankle joint dorsiflexion in a cavus-type foot may first appear inadequate because of the increase in the osseous height from the maximally supinated position of the midtarsal and subtalar joints.

Proper evaluation of the quality and quantity of motion in the rearfoot and ankle complex is essential and is accomplished in the standard fashion by means of the Silfverskiold test. An errant impression will be obtained if the ankle joint is evaluated without regard to the positioning of the midtarsal and subtalar joints. In the severely collapsed pes valgus foot with ankle equinus, the calcaneus is everted from its neutral position and may be subluxed from beneath the talus. The foot will appear to have adequate dorsiflexion as a result of the increased motion at the midtarsal and subtalar joints.

In those individuals who have inadequate ankle joint motion, dorsiflexion may be enhanced through appropriately designed triple arthrodesis. However, there are instances in which the posterior equinus will need to be addressed in addition to the rearfoot fusion. Osseous ankle equinus, which may pose a challenge to the surgeon, can occur in a variety of foot types. During the surgical resection of the subtalar joint, more bone may be resected from the undersurface of the talus in the region of the middle and anterior facets. By plantarflexing the distal talus, one increases the available trochlear surface at the anterior ankle.

Subtalar joint evaluation and positioning are critical to the success of the procedure. The important point in evaluating the subtalar component of the arthrodesis is that the fusion should be performed with the joint in its neutral position or slightly pronated (calcaneus slightly everted) (34).

The midtarsal joint is composed of the talonavicular and calcaneocuboid joints. An important consideration during triple arthrodesis is the positioning of the midtarsal joint inasmuch as the alignment of the forefoot to the rearfoot is affected at this level. In the normal foot the midtarsal joint is usually in its neutral position. This is apparent with the frontal plane alignment of the metatarsal heads, which are perpendicular to the bisection of the rearfoot when the subtalar joint is in its neutral position. The greatest success

in triple arthrodesis has been achieved with the midtarsal joint positioned in slight valgus when fused, that is, with the medial column slightly plantarflexed relative to the lateral. This position increases the stability of the medial column and first ray, permitting enhanced first metatarsophalangeal joint motion. The valgus positioning may also be more easily accommodated with an orthotic device after surgery. If the medial column is dorsiflexed relative to the lateral column, the patient is left with a fixed forefoot varus deformity for which there is no suitable compensation. This provides a very painful complication in a foot with a rigid subtalar joint.

The first ray and the first metatarsophalangeal joint are important components of mechanical function. First metatarsophalangeal joint motion is essential to the normal transfer of weight through the forefoot once heel-off has been effected. After triple arthrodesis, any limitation of motion in the joint is more difficult to accommodate (35, 36).

There should be a full understanding between the surgeon and the patient as to the goal of the procedure. In those cases in which triple arthrodesis or subtalar joint fusion is performed for the relief of pain, the goal is simple. Regarding the improvement of function, if a patient can return to a prior activity level or exceed previous activity and function, then the surgery would be graded a success.

In the broadest terms the creation of a stable platform suitable for ambulation is a basic goal. The patients who are candidates for triple arthrodesis most often have poor mechanical function of the foot and lower extremity. After surgery they may require orthotic devices for optimum function.

After triple arthrodesis the patient usually is totally disabled for 3 months and partially disabled for another 3 to 6 months. The disability associated with the procedure reflects the normal healing time as well as the physical rehabilitation.

SURGICAL APPROACHES AND TECHNIQUES IN FUSIONS

Triple Arthrodesis

The incisional technique traditionally employed in triple arthrodesis has consisted of a single lateral approach. A number of variations have been described, but the incision typically begins proximal to the ankle joint along the course of the peroneal tendons, extending distally along the lateral aspect of the foot over the sinus tarsi, ending about the dorsal midfoot. This provides exposure to the undersurface of the talus and access to the lateral midtarsal joint. Unfortunately, it is almost directly perpendicular to most of the underlying vital structures.

This type of incision was more useful in cavus-type deformities in which most of the bone resection consisted of laterally based wedges from the subtalar and midtarsal joints. However, in pes valgus feet, especially the rigid type, access to the talonavicular joint was extremely poor. There was often a disregard for the soft tissue structures that would be encountered, especially the sural and the intermediate and lateral dorsal cutaneous nerves. Postincisional entrapments of these nerves were not uncommon. Other neuromuscular structures occasionally were disrupted as well.

The modification of the Ollier incision was more of a lateral approach that began over the posterior subtalar joint slightly beneath the lateral malleolus, crossed the sinus tarsi, and extended distally and medially to the base of the second metatarsal.

There are several disadvantages to the single lateral incisional approach. The first and most obvious is the poor exposure and access to the medial aspect of the talonavicular joint. In those cases that require medially based wedge resections, it is difficult, if not impossible, to perform such work accurately from a lateral approach. Also, proper fixation is limited by the single lateral incision.

Ryerson (1) described a two-incisional approach in his original publication. The medial incision permitted access to the anterior and middle facets of the subtalar joint, as well as easy access to the talonavicular joint. The lateral incision provided exposure to the posterior subtalar joint and the calcaneocuboid joint. It is the collective opinion of the faculty of The Podiatry Institute that the two incisional approach is more "physiological."

The techniques of fusion are all variations of the procedure as described by Ryerson. The modifications evolved from a need to meet new challenges as triple arthrodesis was applied to a greater variety of disorders.

The Podiatry Institute Technique

The faculty members of The Podiatry Institute primarily use a modification of the Ryerson technique. The following section will examine the technique employed, the basic principles of joint resection, bone sliding and wedging, and the application of internal fixation.

ANATOMICAL DISSECTION

The techniques of anatomical dissection have significantly enhanced the execution of triple arthrodesis. Anatomical dissection is a fundamental surgical skill that employs the use of natural tissue plane separation and the relationship of individual anatomical structures. The technique has been thoroughly illustrated in its application to the first metatarsophalangeal joint in the section on hallux abducto valgus deformity.

The fundamental components of anatomical dissection are as follows:

1. Skin incision
2. Dissection through the superficial fascia (subcutaneous layer)
3. Identification of the deep fascia
4. Separation of the superficial fascia from the deep fascia
5. Execution of the deep fascial incision and manipulation of deeper structures based upon specific procedure requirements
6. Closure by layer

Purpose

The general goals of anatomical dissection in triple arthrodesis include (*a*) exposure, (*b*) hemostasis, and (*c*) atraumatic technique. Although these goals may appear to be rather simple, they are both complex and comprehensive when expanded to their fullest potential.

Exposure

The primary purpose of surgical exposure in any procedure is to provide for unrestricted visualization and manipulation of critical structures and tissues. Although full exposure continues to be a primary goal, the authors have found the two-incision approach to satisfy the general needs of anatomical dissection.

Lateral and medial incisions are used to expose the rearfoot. The lateral incision extends from the tip of the fibular malleolus distally to the region of the base of the fourth and fifth metatarsals. This provides direct access to the subtalar and calcaneocuboid joints, with minimal disruption or transection of vital structures. The medial incision extends from the region of the medial malleolus distally to the level of the naviculocuneiform joint and provides exposure of the talonavicular joint, as well as access for fixation of the subtalar joint.

There are several significant advantages of the two-incision technique.

1. Direct access to the subtalar and calcaneocuboid joints is available laterally and the talonavicular joint medially for joint resection and fixation.
2. Direct visualization through medial and lateral approaches minimizes excessive tissue retraction and related wound complications.
3. The longitudinal orientation of the incisions runs parallel to most vital structures and tissues. The combination of the incision placement and the techniques of anatomical dissection significantly minimizes violation of the major blood and nerve supply to the tissues of the foot. The relationship and viability of the dorsal soft tissues are preserved as subperiosteal dissection extends between the two incisions.

An anatomical plan for exposure and manipulation of both soft tissues and osseous structures is very important to the success of the procedure. Accurate and delicate execution of these techniques will greatly facilitate the procedure and minimize damage to the vital supportive soft tissues. All of these techniques will limit pain and swelling and minimize wound complications such as hematoma, dehiscence, tissue slough, and infection.

Hemostasis

Hemostasis for triple arthrodesis was traditionally accomplished with a midthigh pneumatic tourniquet. Although this technique adequately controlled bleeding during the surgical procedure, it was common to see a blood-soaked cast within the first few postoperative hours. The techniques of anatomical dissection not only provide hemostasis during surgery but also reduce bleeding when the tourniquet is released as well as after surgery.

Anatomical dissection may be so effective that a tourniquet is not even necessary during some procedures. However, the tourniquet is a surgical tool and may be put to good use if properly employed in the execution of a triple arthrodesis.

The primary use of the tourniquet in triple arthrodesis is to speed the surgical procedure, especially during the initial phases of dissection and exposure of the osseous structures. Even with the tourniquet elevated, superficial and penetrating vessels are identified and secured. However, one of the primary areas of bleeding comes with the reflection of soft tissues from bone or the subperiosteal dissection. Bleeding from the bone surface cannot be ligated, and the use of the tourniquet greatly facilitates this phase of the surgical dissection.

Another phase of the procedure that elicits active bleeding is the resection of the primary joint surfaces. Exposure of the cancellous bone of the greater tarsals can create significant bleeding. Execution of this phase of the procedure without the use of the tourniquet is exceptionally difficult because of constant bleeding that obscures vision and requires continuous suctioning. Therefore it is highly recommended that the tourniquet be inflated for the primary resection of articular surfaces during the procedure.

In most cases the tourniquet may be safely inflated for 2 hours. This length of time is usually sufficient for completion of the initial dissection, joint exposure, bone resection, joint apposition, and temporary fixation. In a rapidly moving and uncomplicated case, even the permanent fixation may be accomplished within that time period. If permanent fixation can be accomplished within the initial tourniquet application, it is strongly recommended that it be released before wound closure. The medial and lateral wounds may be packed with moist saline sponges and temporary compression applied. The tourniquet is released, and 5 to 10 minutes are allotted to permit the return of normal blood flow, to allow reflex hyperemia to subside, and to encourage normal coagulation of bleeding surfaces. This time may be used to obtain intraoperative radiographs to evaluate fixation. The wounds are then carefully inspected to identify and coagulate any actively bleeding vessels. The wounds may then be closed in layers over standard suction tubing.

If final fixation has not been accomplished within the initial tourniquet application, the tourniquet may be released with the wound packed and dressed as described. A 15-minute period of breathing is allowed and the tourniquet may then be reinflated for completion of the procedure, or one may continue without the tourniquet if bone bleeding is not a major obstacle.

The use of closed suction drainage systems is standard in triple arthrodesis. It is not uncommon to collect 200 to 300 ml of hemorrhage after surgery even in a completely secured wound. Cancellous bone bleeding is responsible for this portion of the hemorrhage and may continue in some form for as long as 2 to 3 days.

A uniform and firm compression dressing, elevation of the extremity, and application of ice are also helpful and important in reducing the immediate postoperative bleeding, hematoma, and edema.

ATRAUMATIC TECHNIQUE. The topic of atraumatic technique introduces principles of gentle tissue handling, proper instrumentation, and a generally delicate touch to avoid bruising and additional insult to the soft tissues. Obviously, one of the requirements for primary bone healing is viable vascularized bone. The techniques of anatomical dissection detailed here involve skills that will ensure viability of both the bone and adjacent soft tissues.

The technique consists of the identification and separation of tissue layers rather than laceration, shredding, and tearing. This approach literally allows the surgeon to elevate the structures overlying the dorsum of the foot and ankle as a complete and intact layer, including the primary neural and vascular supply. With the vital soft tissues cleanly separated and retracted, the individual joints of the rearfoot may be freely manipulated, resected, and fixated. Essentially, all osseous work is performed within the protective envelope of the periosteum of the tarsal bones. Upon completion of the osseous work, the periosteum and other soft tissues are reapplied to the bony surfaces to allow additional revascularization of the underlying bone.

Technique

The patient is initially placed in a slight lateral position to facilitate the approach to the lateral aspect of the foot. A pneumatic-suction pack is helpful for positioning of the patient. A midthigh pneumatic tourniquet is inflated and routine cautery and suction is available as needed.

LATERAL INCISION. The lateral incision is used for exposure of the subtalar and calcaneocuboid joints (Fig. 42.16). The

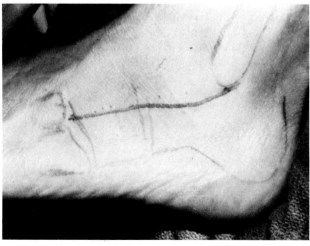

Figure 42.16. Podiatry Institute lateral approach to the subtalar and calcaneocuboid joints.

key landmarks for placement of the incision include tip of the fibular malleolus, the sinus tarsi, and the calcaneocuboid joint. Other key landmarks that may be appreciated by palpation include the peroneal tendons, the lateral process of the talus, the lateral margin of the floor of the sinus tarsi, the lateral wall of the calcaneus, and the bases of the fourth and fifth metatarsals.

The incision runs from just inferior to the distal tip of the fibular malleolus along the lateral margin of the floor of the sinus tarsi, across the calcaneocuboid joint to the junction of the fourth and fifth metatarsal bases. This incision placement will provide direct access to the subtalar and calcaneocuboid joints and will run longitudinally between the course of the intermediate dorsal cutaneous and sural nerves.

A controlled-depth incision technique is used to separate the skin and avoid laceration of underlying veins that may cross the surgical incision.

DISSECTION THROUGH THE SUPERFICIAL FASCIA. Once the skin edges have been freely separated, dissection is carried through the subcutaneous layers to the level of the deep fascia. The technique is performed in either a sharp or blunt manner during ligation of any superficial vessels.

The sural and the intermediate dorsal cutaneous nerves should be safely protected within the subcutaneous tissues below and above the primary incision, respectively. Occasionally, a communicating branch between the sural and the intermediate dorsal cutaneous nerves will be identified crossing the line of dissection. If the nerve can be safely retracted, it is preserved; if not, it is sacrificed.

SEPARATION OF THE SUPERFICIAL FASCIA FROM THE DEEP FASCIA. The deep fascia is exposed through the full length of the incision. A moderate degree of separation of the two tissue layers is then created before the deep fascia is incised. The primary purpose of this separation between the layers is to facilitate wound closure by making tissue-layer identification more readily visible at the completion of the procedure.

The superficial fascia or subcutaneous layer is easily separated from the deep fascia, especially over the extensor digitorum brevis muscle belly. This maneuver is readily performed by peeling the tissues away from the deep fascia with the use of a moist surgical sponge. This separation becomes more difficult over the sinus tarsi and may require a spreading technique with the use of a Metzenbaum scissors. Clean separation should be carried proximally to identify deep fascia over the tip of the fibular malleolus and inferiorly over the peroneal retinaculum at the proximal extent of the wound.

The inferior margin of the superficial fascia is rather firmly affixed to the underlying deep fascia. Minimal separation is required at this level, and care should be taken to avoid laceration of the peroneal retinaculum and sheath specifically over the peroneus brevis tendon as it crosses from the tip of the fibular malleolus to the base of the fifth metatarsal. The course of the peroneus brevis tendon along the lateral aspect of the calcaneus will be a key dissection landmark.

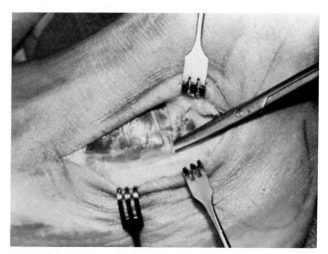

Figure 42.17. Demonstration of the deep fascia overlying the junction of the extensor digitorum brevis muscle belly and peroneal tendons.

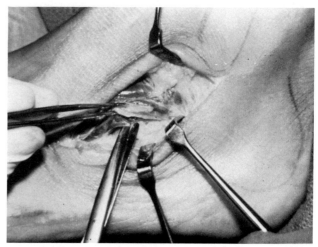

Figure 42.18. Elevation of the extensor digitorum brevis muscle belly from the dorsal surface of the calcaneocuboid joint.

DEEP FASCIAL INCISION. The primary relationship that determines the location of the deep fascial incision is the junction of the inferior edge of the extensor digitorum brevis muscle belly and the peroneus brevis tendon (Fig. 42.17). The deep fascia is initially penetrated at the distal extent of the wound over the extensor digitorum brevis muscle belly just superior to the peroneal retinaculum and sheath.

The incision is carried proximally along the inferior border of the muscle belly to the level of the fibrous plug at the sinus tarsi. Minimal dissection across the sinus tarsi is necessary at this time as the primary tissues within this area will be evacuated with the subperiosteal dissection.

A Metzenbaum scissors is used to gently tease and lift the inferior edge of the extensor digitorum brevis muscle belly from capsular tissues over the calcaneocuboid joint and neck of the calcaneus (Fig. 42.18). This clearly reveals the capsular and ligamentous covering on the calcaneocuboid joint and periosteum over the dorsolateral aspect of the neck of the calcaneus. The peroneus brevis tendon should still be totally ensheathed.

LATERAL PERIOSTEAL AND CAPSULAR INCISION. The lateral periosteal and capsular incision will expose the subtalar and calcaneocuboid joints. The tip of the fibular malleolus is easily palpated proximally. Just anterior to the tip of the fibular malleolus, the prominence of the anterior lateral corner of the lateral process of the talus is palpable.

The lateral process of the talus is a key structure for orientation within the subtalar joint. This forms a part of the body of the talus that articulates with the large posterior facet on the calcaneus. The anterior surface of the lateral process of the talus forms the posterior wall of the sinus tarsi. The anterior and inferior edge defines the anterior margin of the posterior facet of the subtalar joint. Intimate familiarity with the contours of the lateral process of the talus will greatly facilitate exploration and exposure of the subtalar joint.

The lateral capsular and periosteal incision employs an inverted L technique (Fig. 42.19). The incision courses inferiorly along the lateral process to the lateral margin of the calcaneus and then extends distally along the dorsolateral edge of the calcaneus. The incision is lengthened past the calcaneocuboid joint to the level of the metatarsocuboid articulation.

The subperiosteal dissection will then follow two different directions to fully expose the osseous structures on the lateral aspect of the foot. The dorsal route will lift all soft tissues from the dorsal surface of the cuboid, as well as the calcaneocuboid joint, and clean all tissues from the floor of the sinus tarsi. This will include the periosteum and capsule, the origin and main mass of the extensor digitorum brevis muscle belly, and the contents of the sinus tarsi.

The incision over the lateral process of the talus is actually a lateral capsulotomy to the posterior facet of the subtalar joint (Fig. 42.20). The anterior edge of the capsule may be reflected with a pickup, and the margin of the posterior facet is clearly visualized.

The subperiosteal dissection can begin with a clean intracapsular approach. The knife blade can be inserted across the anterior surface of the lateral process of the talus and directed inferiorly and then anteriorly to dissect the origin of the extensor digitorum brevis muscle belly and other soft tissues from the floor of the sinus tarsi (Fig. 42.21).

A similar technique may be used to initiate the reflection of soft tissues from the region of the calcaneocuboid joint. A proximal extension of this dissection will communicate with the sinus tarsi and begin the elevation of the dorsal tissues over the calcaneocuboid joint and sinus tarsi as an intact and viable tissue flap (Fig. 42.22).

Dissection across the dorsal surface of the cuboid extends

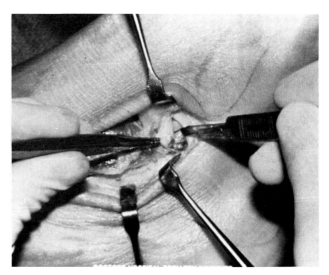

Figure 42.20. Proximal portion of the lateral capsular incision demonstrating the posterior subtalar joint.

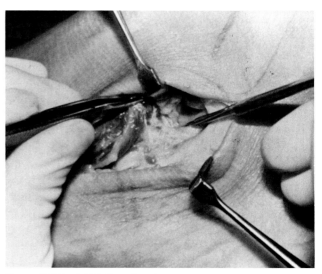

Figure 42.21. Initial dissection elevating capsule, periosteum, and the extensor digitorum brevis muscle belly from the superior surface of the sinus tarsi and calcaneocuboid joint.

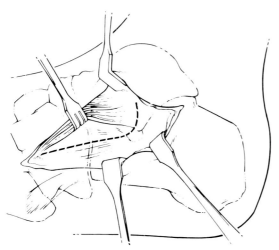

Figure 42.19. Capsular incision into the subtalar joint.

medially to the lateral surface of the navicular (Fig. 42.23). A proximal and medial extension across the neck of the calcaneus and into the sinus tarsi will expose the intertarsal ligament and elevate the proximal attachment of the bifurcate ligament from the dorsal surface of the calcaneus.

Care must be taken to follow the contour of the calcaneus to cleanly evacuate the sinus tarsi. The inferior attachment of the intertarsal ligament must be freed to allow separation of the subtalar joint and, more important, to provide access to the middle facet of the subtalar joint (Fig. 42.24). Excess fibroligamentous tissue may be excised from the sinus tarsi to aid in visualization. Resection of muscle tissue should be avoided.

Once the middle facet has been visualized, the subperiosteal dissection is extended to the lateral side of the head and neck of the talus where dissection aids in exposure of the talonavicular joint by communication with the dissection from the medial incision (Figs. 42.25 and 42.26). At this

point the subtalar joint is easily visualized. The lateral tissues of the calcaneocuboid region must then be reflected to fully expose this joint.

The soft tissues over the lateral aspect of the calcaneocuboid joint and the subtalar region are essentially intact from the skin to the level of the periosteum. There has been minimal separation of the subcutaneous tissues from the deep fascia and retinaculum over the peroneal tendons. The sural nerve and the lesser saphenous vein should be safely protected within this tissue layer.

The peroneus brevis tendon now becomes the primary structure used for orientation and preservation of the anatomical relationships as the capsule and periosteum are reflected from the lateral aspect of the calcaneocuboid joint. The internal surface of the peroneal sheath is actually tissue that includes the periosteum of the lateral wall of the calcaneus.

The subperiosteal dissection is extended inferiorly from the primary capsular and periosteal incision to cleanly expose the lateral surface of the calcaneocuboid joint. The peroneal tendons are totally maintained within their soft tissue covering (Fig. 42.27). Inferior release of the calcaneocuboid joint may be performed with sharp dissection or a curved Crego elevator (Fig. 42.28).

Proximal reflection of periosteum from the lateral wall of the calcaneus will begin to expose the calcaneal margin of the posterior facet. Full exposure of the posterior facet requires reflection of the peroneal tendons. The peroneal sheath is entered just inferior to the distal tip of the fibular malleolus, and an incision is extended proximally around the tip of the malleolus, sectioning the anterior portion of the peroneal retinaculum (Fig. 42.29). The peroneus brevis and longus tendons are then retracted posteriorly with the blade of a Senn retractor (Fig. 42.30).

Retraction of the peroneal tendons reveals the lateral capsular tissues covering the posterior facet of the subtalar joint. Two primary structures included in these lateral tissues are the calcaneofibular ligament and the lateral talocalcaneal ligament (Figs. 42.31 and 42.32).

Full exposure and visualization of the subtalar joint are

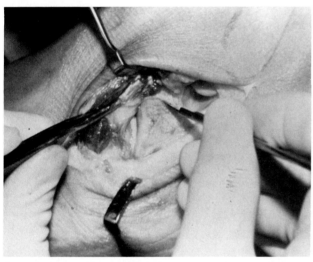

Figure 42.22. Additional dorsal dissection exposing the calcaneocuboid joint.

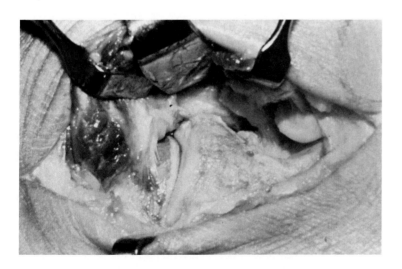

Figure 42.23. Close-up view of the calcaneocuboid joint, the sinus tarsi, and posterior facet on the calcaneus. Note the talocalcaneal ligament deep in the sinus tarsi.

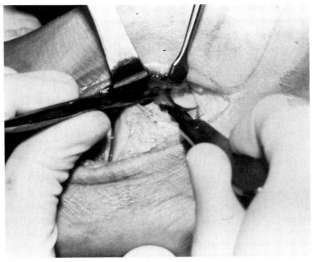

Figure 42.24. Sectioning of the talocalcaneal ligament.

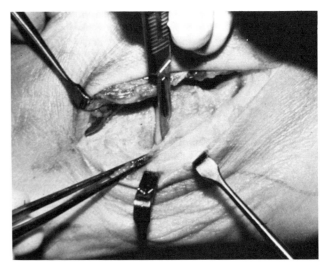

Figure 42.27. Reflection of the periosteum and capsular tissues from the lateral aspect of the calcaneocuboid joint.

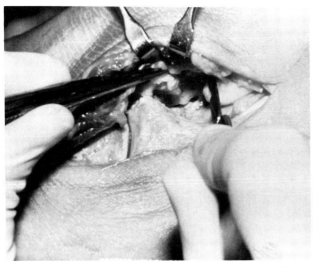

Figure 42.25. Initiation of the dissection across the anterior surface of the lateral process of the talus and along the lateral surface of the head and neck of the talus.

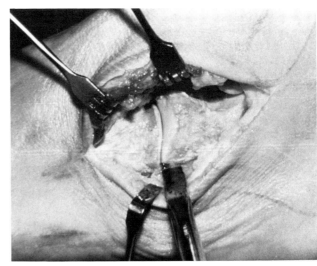

Figure 42.28. Full exposure of the calcaneocuboid joint.

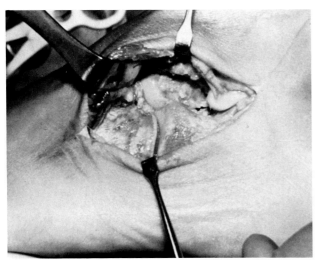

Figure 42.26. Lateral exposure demonstrating calcaneocuboid joint, posterior facet of subtalar joint, middle facet of subtalar joint, head and neck of talus, and talonavicular joint.

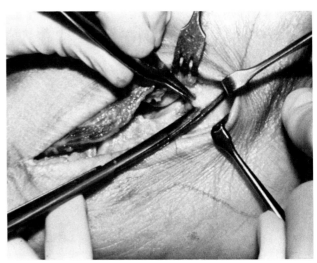

Figure 42.29. Incision through the peroneal retinaculum at the distal tip of the fibular malleolus.

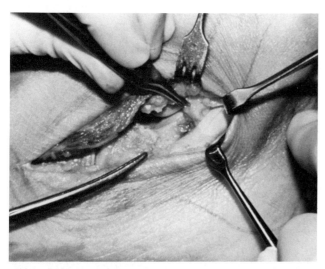

Figure 42.30. Exposure of the peroneal tendons before retraction.

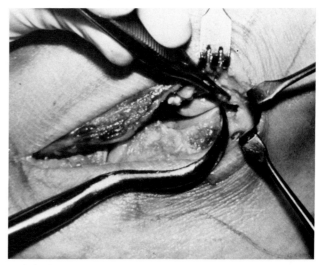

Figure 42.33. Insertion of a Crego elevator intracapsularly around the posterior contour of the subtalar joint.

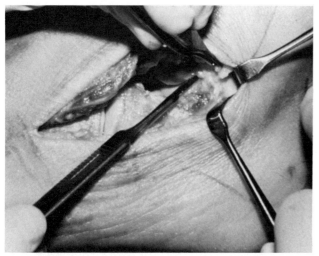

Figure 42.31. Incision of the lateral capsule of the posterior facet of the subtalar joint including the calcaneofibular ligament.

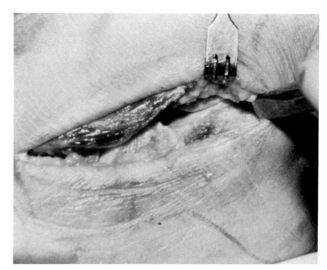

Figure 42.34. Full exposure of the posterior subtalar joint.

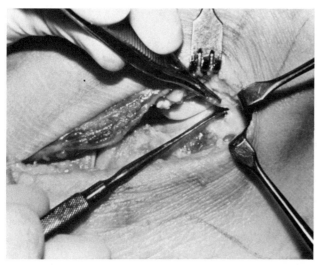

Figure 42.32. Demonstration of the sectioned calcaneofibular ligament.

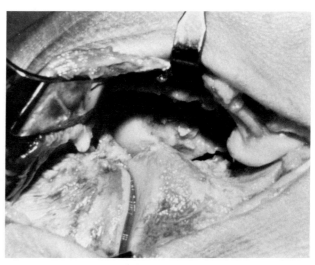

Figure 42.35. Completed lateral exposure, demonstrating calcaneocuboid joint, posterior facets of subtalar joint, middle facets of subtalar joint, head and neck of talus, and talonavicular joint.

aided by the ability to open the joint with inversion of the foot. Opening of the subtalar joint would be significantly hindered by the intact lateral ligamentous structures. The calcaneofibular ligament may be primarily repaired at the time of closure.

A Crego elevator may be passed intracapsularly around the posterior rim of the posterior facet to visualize the contour and extent of the joint (Figs. 42.33 and 42.34).

The subtalar and calcaneocuboid joints are now fully exposed (Fig. 42.35). The surgeon should evaluate the integrity of the joints and any related pathological finding. Attention is now directed medially as the procedure continues.

MEDIAL INCISION. The medial incision provides direct access to the talonavicular joint and exposure of the dorsal surface of the neck of the talus for fixation of the subtalar joint. The subperiosteal dissection from the medial incision is also extended laterally around the head and neck of the talus and the lateral surface of the navicular. The soft tissues over the dorsal aspect of the midtarsal region may then be cleanly retracted and protected as an intact and viable tissue layer.

The landmarks for the incision include the medial malleolus, the prominence of the navicular, and the naviculocuneiform joint (Fig. 42.36). The incision begins at the notch formed by the anterior medial junction of the medial malleolus and the medial aspect of the dome of the talus. The scalpel is directed inferiorly across the prominence of the navicular to the lower margin of the naviculocuneiform joint. The angulation of this incision allows for three specific technical executions:

1. Direct access to the talonavicular joint
2. A superior approach to the dorsal surface of the neck of the talus for instrumentation and fixation of the subtalar joint
3. An inferior approach to the distal surface of the navicular for instrumentation and fixation of the talonavicular joint

SUBCUTANEOUS DISSECTION. The dissection is extended through the subcutaneous tissues over the anterior aspect of the ankle, across the dorsal region of the talonavicular joint, and across the medial and inferior aspect of the naviculocuneiform joint. At the proximal extent of the incision, the surgeon will encounter the medial marginal vein. As the incision courses inferiorly, it is usually possible to retract this vessel without transection. Large communicating veins from the medial marginal vein should be isolated and ligated (Fig. 42.37). Dissection is carried again to the level of the deep fascia. The superficial tissues are gently separated from the surface of the deep fascia over the anterior aspect of the ankle and the medial and inferior aspects of the talonavicular region.

DEEP FASCIAL INCISION. The incision through the deep fascia is made along the medial border of the tibialis anterior tendon. The tendon is then retracted laterally. From the level of the talonavicular joint distally there is minimal areolar tissue between the deep fascia and the underlying joint capsule and periosteum. However, from the talonavicular

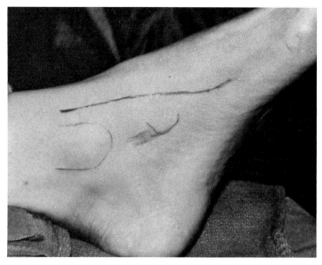

Figure 42.36. Medial skin incision for exposure of the talonavicular joint.

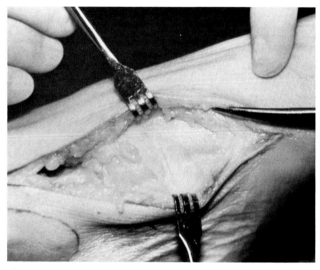

Figure 42.37. Retraction of the medial marginal vein and exposure of the deep fascia over the talonavicular and ankle joints.

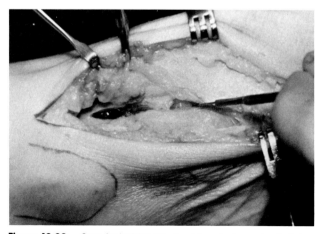

Figure 42.38. Capsular incision into the talonavicular and ankle joints.

joint proximally across the ankle, there is a significant layer of soft tissue and often a rather extensive network of vessels, including branches of the anterior medial malleolar artery and the deep venous complex or anteromedial malleolar veins. These rather large vessels must be individually isolated and secured to avoid significant bleeding upon release of the tourniquet.

MEDIAL PERIOSTEAL AND CAPSULAR INCISION. The deep incision through capsule and periosteum actually traverses both the ankle and the talonavicular joints (Fig. 42.38). The approach essentially follows the skin incision. It begins proximally at the medial notch of the ankle mortise, then courses distally over the dorsomedial aspect of the head and neck of the talus and talonavicular joint to the inferior aspect of the naviculocuneiform joint.

An intra-articular dissection technique then readily peels the capsular tissues from the dorsal surface of the neck of the talus. This subperiosteal plane reveals the talonavicular joint and is carried distally to expose the dorsal surface of the navicular. The intracapsular dissection across the anterior aspect of the ankle and the subperiosteal dissection across the dorsal surface of the midtarsal region elevate the soft tissues and protect the deep vessels, including the dorsalis pedis artery.

The contour of the head and neck of the talus and the navicular is followed laterally and inferiorly with the use of a Crego elevator as the periosteum and capsule are stripped from the lateral aspect of the midtarsal area (Figs. 42.39 and 42.40). The dissection extends laterally and communicates with the subperiosteal dissection from the lateral incision.

The communication of the dissection planes across the midtarsal region is of primary significance in providing full exposure of the midtarsal joint. It also preserves the viability of the dorsal soft tissue island that has been created between the medial and lateral incisions. If needed, a malleable retractor may be passed across the dorsal foot to protect the soft tissues during joint resection and fixation.

Inferiorly, the capsular tissues, including the primary insertion of the tibialis posterior tendon, are reflected from the navicular to the level of the naviculocuneiform joint. This provides the exposure for resection of the talonavicular joint and its fixation. When using a large cancellous bone screw in the fixation of the talonavicular joint, the surgeon will need to penetrate the navicular cortex at its distal and inferior surface as the course of the screw passes proximally and dorsally along the neck of the talus. Less exposure is needed if the midtarsal joint is to be fixated with staples.

JOINT RESECTION AND FIXATION. Once complete exposure of all joint areas has been accomplished, joint resection and fixation are performed. The details of this procedure are discussed later in this chapter.

WOUND CLOSURE. Once fixation has been completed, the medial and lateral incisions are closed in anatomical layers. Usually the tourniquet is released and any active bleeding is secured. The wounds are generously irrigated, as has been done repeatedly during the entire procedure. A closed suction-type drain is placed in both the medial and lateral in-

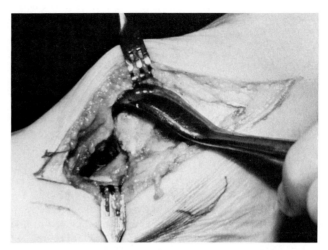

Figure 42.39. Insertion of a Crego periosteal elevator to elevate the periosteum and capsular tissues from dorsum and lateral surfaces of the talonavicular joint.

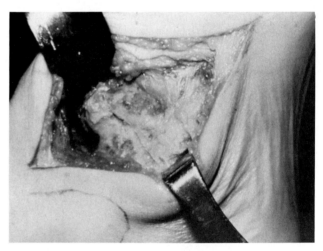

Figure 42.40. Full exposure of the talonavicular joint.

cisions to provide effective evacuation of internal bleeding from the resected joint surfaces. The capsular and periosteal layers are closed over the drain tubes.

The remaining tissue layers—deep fascia, superficial fascia, and skin—are then closed individually. The incisions are cleansed and covered with moist saline soaked sponges, and a surgical dressing is applied. The foot and lower extremity are then placed in a Jones compression cast and postoperative management is initiated.

JOINT RESECTION, POSITION, AND INTERNAL FIXATION

Traditionally, the procedure of triple arthrodesis involved resecting predetermined wedges of bone from the tarsal area, fitting the pieces together to obtain the desired correction, and maintaining the position with a plaster cast (1). Later surgeons added pins and staples to assist in maintaining correction. The early approaches often led to numerous postoperative complications, such as nonunion, poor alignment, loss of correction, pseudoarthrosis, and others already discussed.

It is important to plan the alignment of the forefoot to the rearfoot and the rearfoot to the leg. This is especially critical in determining the final position of fusion. The foot normally exhibits approximately 10° to 15° of abduction from the line of progression in gait. In arthrodesis of the rearfoot it is imperative to know the position of the knee during gait, as well as during surgery. Some authors have recommended that the foot be fused strictly in relationship to the ankle, disregarding the knee position. This approach could have dire consequences. The best function appears to result from a foot that is abducted approximately 10° to 15° laterally to the leg. If the knee functions medially rotated 15°, then it would be desirable to abduct the foot on the leg 30° thus resulting in a 15° abduction from the line of progression. The position of the foot is also important. It is not advisable to abduct a foot if the individual already possesses 15° to 30° lateral position of the knee in gait. In the latter instance the foot may be aligned directly with the knee (Fig. 42.41).

The technique preferred by faculty members of the Institute involves the principles of anatomical dissection, as well as several other simple concepts: minimal bone resection, joint manipulation and sliding, and rigid internal fix-

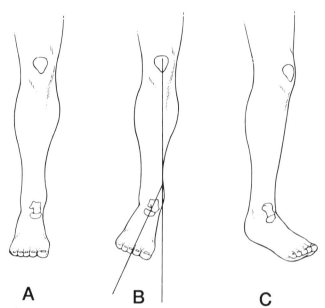

Figure 42.41. Relationship of the knee position to the foot. **A.** Rectus knee and foot. **B.** Rectus knee with foot abducted 30°. **C.** Internal knee position with adducted foot 25°.

Figure 42.42. A and **B.** Excessive bony resection may result in a short, fat foot.

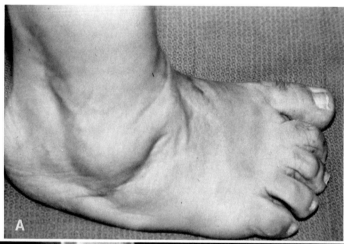

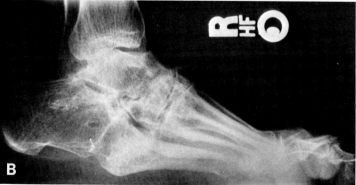

ation (7). In addition, the concept of accelerated aftercare may be applied to postoperative management.

The resection of the joint surfaces, repositioning, and realignment of the rearfoot complex initially may appear quite simple to the untrained surgeon. The process begins with a well-conceived tactical approach to bone resection and realignment. One of the more critical steps in the entire process is in determining the reducibility of the deformity. Much has been written that predetermined amounts of bone would need to be resected to achieve the desired position of the rearfoot in a triple arthrodesis. It has been the experience of the members of the Institute that correction of a flexible deformity will require a different approach than will a rigid fixed deformity. The entire procedure uses a number of relatively simple concepts that will be described and illustrated.

One of the primary characteristics of the technique employed by The Podiatry Institute faculty is minimal bone resection. It is wise to resect as little bone as possible in achieving the desired alignment. Excessive bone resection may produce undesirable results, as well as poor cosmetic appearance and function (Fig. 42.42). In the flexible deformity, the soft tissue dissection usually affords increased mobility to the entire rearfoot complex. The talus may be manipulated into full articulation with the navicular, and the same often holds true for the remaining joints. In these cases denuding of the articular surfaces to the level of good bleeding subchondral bone is often all the resection that is required. However, this method would not be applicable to

the rigid pes valgus deformity, the foot with a fixed tarsal coalition, or the rigid cavovarus foot. In rigid deformities bone resection further increases the mobility of the tarsal complex to permit reduction of the deformity. The same holds true for the posttraumatic foot with severe arthritic changes.

Triple arthrodesis permits correction of foot deformities in all three planes. Sagittal plane deformity (which may manifest as either a high arch or a low arch) may be corrected at all three joint surfaces. Correction at the midtarsal level (talonavicular and calcaneocuboid joints) is considered as one structure for simplicity. To effectively lower the arch, an increased amount of bone is resected from the opposing surfaces at the dorsal aspect of the midtarsal joint. When the joint surfaces are approximated, the distal foot will be located in a more dorsal position (Fig. 42.43). In a similar fashion, to recreate an arch, as in a severe flatfoot deformity, more bone will be resected from the plantar aspect of the midtarsal joint than from the dorsal side (Fig. 42.44). This may be visualized as plantarflexion of the forefoot on the rearfoot.

Sagittal plane correction may also be affected by resecting a greater amount of bone from the posterior facet region of the talus and calcaneus. This will effectively decrease arch height, although correction in this plane is usually most effectively performed at the midtarsal level.

Deformities in the sagittal plane may also be addressed through sliding and repositioning of the tarsal bones. This is often an overlooked technique. Repositioning of the talus

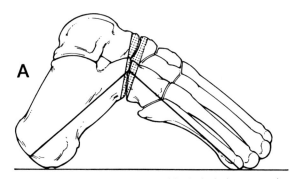
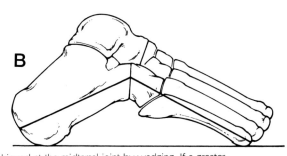

Figure 42.43. **A** and **B.** Sagittal plane correction may be achieved at the midtarsal joint by wedging. If a greater amount of bone is resected from the dorsal aspect of the joint surfaces, arch-lowering will be effected.

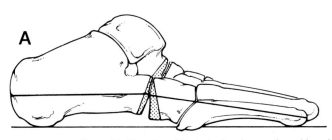
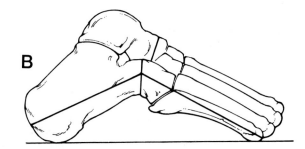

Figure 42.44. **A** and **B.** Arch elevation can be achieved if more bone is resected from the plantar aspect of the joint surface, resulting in plantarflexion of the forefoot upon the rearfoot, thus raising the arch.

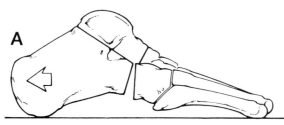 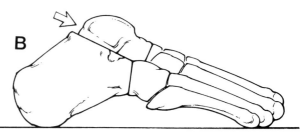

Figure 42.45. Sliding of the tarsal bones is difficult to achieve in the rigid deformity but is a useful tool. If the calcaneus is slid posteriorly on the talus, the forefoot will need to be plantarflexed to achieve good bone-to-bone contact, which will raise the arch. This is more commonly used in pes valgus.

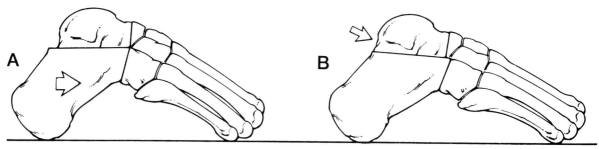

Figure 42.46. Sliding the calcaneus anteriorly will force the foot into dorsiflexion. This will decrease the arch height and is useful in the cavus-type foot correction.

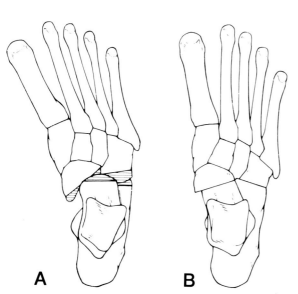

Figure 42.47. **A** and **B.** Laterally based wedge of the calcaneocuboid and talonavicular joints results in abduction of forefoot on the rearfoot.

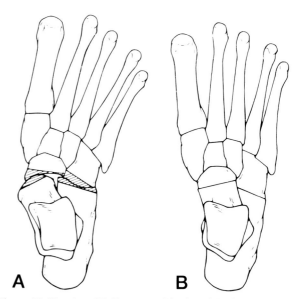

Figure 42.48. **A** and **B.** To create adduction of the forefoot a medially based wedge is resected from the midtarsal joint. Caution is required to prevent removing too much navicular.

can effectively raise and lower arch height. Sliding of the calcaneus posteriorly on the talus (Fig. 42.45) will result in plantarflexion of the forefoot in relationship to the rearfoot, thereby elevating the arch. In a similar fashion, sliding the calcaneus anteriorly on the talus (Fig. 42.46) will result in dorsiflexion of the forefoot on the rearfoot, or arch depression. The technique of sliding will also affect the fit of the midtarsal joint and usually requires more bone resection at this level.

Correction of transverse plane deformity, abduction or adduction of the forefoot, is attained in a similar fashion, but almost exclusively at the midtarsal joint. In the adducted forefoot (Fig. 42.47) the surgeon must visualize a laterally based wedge both in the talonavicular and the calcaneocuboid joints. This will effectively abduct the forefoot on the rearfoot. Similarly, the abducted forefoot may be repositioned and aligned in a more adducted position through resection of medially based wedges from these two joints. This is a more difficult maneuver to accomplish and is cited as one of the hazards of the procedure. More bone must be resected from the medial aspect of the articular surfaces (Fig. 42.48) so that upon completion, the forefoot may be rotated into a more adducted position. It is during this resection that the surgeon should proceed with great caution, especially in the pes valgus deformity because the talus is usually markedly adducted. The final position of the talus will also be determined by the subtalar joint resection.

Frontal plane deformity in the rearfoot may coincidently exist at both the subtalar and midtarsal joints. The subtalar joint should be positioned in slight valgus. It will be necessary to wedge the subtalar joint through joint resection in those cases in which severe or nonreducible deformity exists. It is prudent to minimize the amount of bone resection at this level inasmuch as excessive resection may significantly shorten the heel and result in constant irritation of the malleoli against the shoe counter when the patient returns to normal function. If a varus deformity exists in the subtalar joint, resection of a laterally based wedge is accomplished by resecting slightly more bone from the lateral aspect of the joint than from the medial. In addition, the calcaneus may be shifted slightly laterally beneath the talus to facilitate correction (Fig. 42.49). Another means to derotate the heel into a valgus position is to resect only the posterior facet of the subtalar joint and leave the more medial anterior and middle facets intact. Closure of the posterior facet will automatically reduce part if not all of the heel varus.

In a reverse fashion a severe valgus deformity may be addressed at the subtalar joint. The concept of a medially based wedge resection of the subtalar joint is illustrated in Figure 42.50. This process is often technically difficult to perform from the lateral incision. As in the varus deformity, the calcaneus may also be simultaneously shifted beneath the talus to improve the weight-bearing platform.

Caution must be exercised in positioning the subtalar joint inasmuch as a permanent varus deformity will result in a significant shift of weight bearing to the lateral side of the foot. Compensation for this deformity is very difficult.

Additional frontal plane abnormalities may exist at the midtarsal joint. Often a fixed forefoot varus or valgus will be encountered. Correction of the frontal plane deformity is accomplished through derotation of the forefoot as a unit. In each instance the forefoot must be derotated into a neutral or slight valgus position before fixation (Fig. 42.51).

Resection of the midtarsal joint is performed first. This will provide increased relaxation of the tissues and will further facilitate access to the subtalar joint. In flexible feet the process will be simplified if the foot is held in corrected alignment while the talonavicular and calcaneocuboid joints are resected. This simple procedure will permit resection of bone parallel to the articular surfaces, minimizing the amount of bone removed.

Once the midtarsal joint is resected, the subtalar joint may be addressed. This procedure may be performed with an osteotome and mallet or with a power saw. Special care should be exercised in resecting the subtalar joint because of its irregular contour. Very often the lateral process of talus (recall its intimate association with the posterior facet) must be removed to provide instrument access to the posterior subtalar joint. Additional separation of the talocalcaneal joint may be achieved with a baby lamina spreader to elevate the talus from the calcaneus. Care should be employed when using the lamina spreader as overzealous force has been known to fracture the neck of the talus. Once resection of the subtalar joint has been accomplished, then the fixation process may begin.

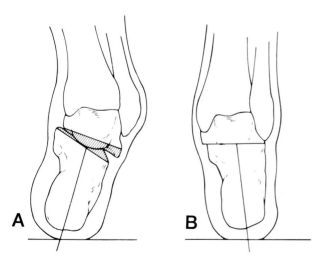

Figure 42.49. **A** and **B.** Frontal plane eversion is achieved by resection of a laterally based wedge of bone from the subtalar joint.

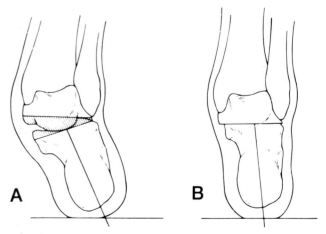

Figure 42.50. **A** and **B.** Correction in a varus direction in the frontal plane is sometimes necessary, but a truly varus rearfoot will not be tolerated. Change in a varus direction is accomplished by resecting a medially based wedge from the subtalar joint.

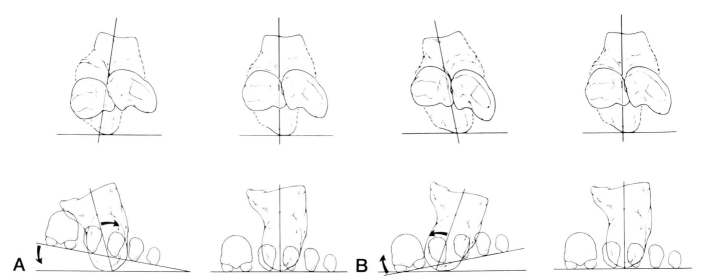

Figure 42.51.   Derotation of the forefoot. **A.** Supinatus or varus forefoot deformity of pes valgus derotated to rectus or slightly valgus position. **B.** Valgus forefoot deformity associated with pes cavus derotated to rectus or slight valgus position.

RIGID INTERNAL FIXATION IN TRIPLE ARTHRODESIS

The addition of rigid compression fixation to tarsal arthrodesis has led to more consistent joint fusion and to a decrease in nonunion. The cornerstone of rigid internal fixation in triple arthrodesis is the 6.5-mm cancellous bone screw. Other forms of fixation are often used for the midtarsal joint in conjunction with screw fixation of the subtalar joint. They include Blount staples and the pneumatic stapler designed by 3M Company. The primary stability of the rearfoot fusion is dependent on the large talocalcaneal compression screw. New changes in available fixation devices, such as the cannulated screw, also enhance the procedure by reducing the necessary steps in the fixation process. Our discussion here will focus on the standard 6.5-mm cancellous screw. The technique begins with accurate joint resection and alignment of the rearfoot.

SUBTALAR JOINT REDUCTION. The subtalar joint is fixated first. The surgeon or assistant manually reduces the calcaneus beneath the talus in the proper position. Because one is accustomed to treating excessive rearfoot pronation, there is a tendency to avoid pronation in almost all situations. This must *not* be the case in triple arthrodesis. When the subtalar and midtarsal joints have been fused, the foot has *no* mechanism to compensate for a varus alignment. Therefore it is imperative to avoid arthrodesis of the foot in a varus position. A mild valgus position is acceptable, even desirable, but a varus position results in a painful foot deformity that cannot be accommodated by shoe or orthosis.

Once the subtalar joint is suitably aligned, it is critical to maintain the reduction. Temporary fixation is achieved with large K-wires or small Steinmann pins. The pin is driven from the neck of the talus across the subtalar joint and into the body of the calcaneus. Placement of the Steinmann pin or K-wire is an important step in the fixation process. The surgeon must consider the placement of the fixation screw

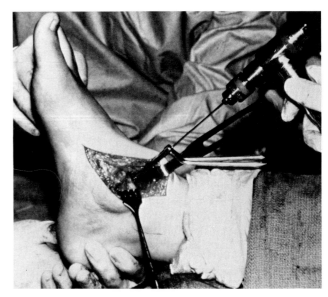

Figure 42.52.   Placement of the temporary talocalcaneal pin. The pin is driven from neck of the talus, across the joint, and through the calcaneus to exit plantarly and posteriorly.

prior to inserting the temporary wire. The permanent fixation device will generally be placed medial and parallel to the pin throughout its entire course across the subtalar joint. It is critical that the surgeon envision the path and exit site of the pin (Fig. 42.52). Usually the pin is placed in the lateral two thirds of the neck of the talus and angled slightly from dorsal, distal, and medial to plantar, proximal, and lateral. The goal is to have the pin traverse the lateral one half of the body of the calcaneus and exit the posterior aspect of the calcaneal tuberosity. The surgeon or the assistant should feel for the pin as it exits at the inferior aspect of the bone, but it need not exit the skin.

The pin may often be visualized through the lateral incision. Proper positioning of the pin is essential to the use of rigid internal fixation, because it serves as a template for the permanent fixation. It would be preferable if the pin crossed the subtalar joint directly perpendicular to the two surfaces. This will ensure that there will be no shift of the bones as the cancellous screw is tightened. Standard lateral and axial projection radiographs may be obtained at this time. As the surgeon becomes more familiar with the technique, radiographs may be obtained after all three joints have been temporarily stabilized.

After the subtalar joint is stabilized, the midtarsal joint is then inspected for alignment as well as for fit of the apposed surfaces. This is the point in the procedure when derotation of the forefoot is accomplished if needed. If derotation of the forefoot results in midtarsal joint surfaces that fail to fit perfectly, then reciprocal planing is performed to complete fitting. A large oscillating power saw blade is introduced into the joint to remove the irregularities from the adjacent bone surfaces. The power saw blade is passed completely through the center of the joint several times in order to collapse the high spots until a smooth flush interface is created.

Once there is adequate alignment and apposition at the talonavicular and calcaneocuboid joints, the midtarsal joint is stabilized (Fig. 42.53). A Steinmann pin or Kirschner wire is introduced from the distal medial surface of the navicular, crossing the talonavicular joint into the neck of the talus. The surgeon should exercise caution while inserting the talonavicular pin to avoid driving it through the talus and into the ankle joint.

By a similar approach another pin is driven across the calcaneocuboid joint. The pin is introduced into the dorsal-distal cuboid and driven proximally well into the calcaneus. The reader is referred to the chapter on power instrument skills for specific techniques on directing pins.

Once the temporary fixation process is completed, intraoperative radiographs are obtained. Radiographs are taken in the lateral, axial calcaneal, and dorsoplantar projections. The lateral projection confirms the proper position of the pin in the neck of the talus and the angle across the subtalar joint. An estimate of the length of screw needed for fixation and its position within the body of the calcaneus can also be acquired from the lateral projection. In addition, the lateral view serves to evaluate the sagittal plane alignment of the midtarsal joint, confirming joint congruity.

The axial projection is needed to ensure that the talocalcaneal pin is properly positioned within the calcaneus. If poor alignment exists, the pin may be withdrawn and reinserted and its position reconfirmed.

The dorsoplantar projection of the foot allows one to evaluate the positioning of the forefoot to the rearfoot, especially in the transverse plane. The actual placement of the pins in the midtarsal joint is not as critical as that through the talocalcaneal joint. The pin placement should be so positioned as to leave room for the permanent fixation.

SUBTALAR JOINT FIXATION. Fixation of the subtalar joint is facilitated by proper placement and alignment of the initial Steinmann pin. The screw position should parallel the placement of this wire provided the direction is suitable. The technique for insertion of the 6.5-mm screw is described in detail in the chapter on internal fixation (Fig. 42.54).

TALONAVICULAR JOINT FIXATION. Fixation of the talonavicular joint with a 6.5-mm screw is usually a difficult procedure. In order for a large compression screw to be employed, an extreme distal approach must be used. Surgical

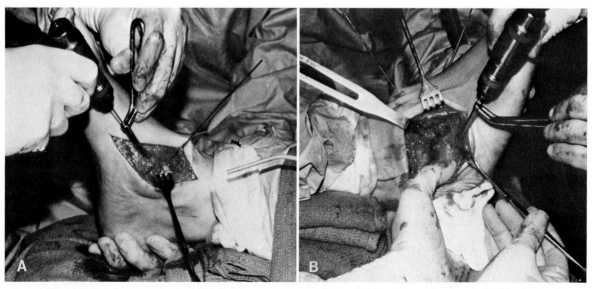

Figure 42.53.   A. Temporary fixation of midtarsal joint is achieved in a fashion similar to that for subtalar joint. **B.** The calcaneocuboid joint is then pinned.

dissection must be extended past the level of the medial cuneiform. When countersinking is performed in the distal margin of the navicular, a portion of the medial cuneiform is grooved as well. This allows the head of the screw to glide past the cuneiform and compress against the distal surface of the navicular (Fig. 42.55). The point of approach should be at the distal inferior surface of the navicular to allow proper angulation across the talonavicular joint and into the neck of the talus.

CALCANEOCUBOID FIXATION. A similar technique is then employed to fixate the calcaneocuboid joint. A distal approach on the cuboid is necessary. Penetration of the screw is usually just proximal to the base of the fifth metatarsal somewhat dorsally on the cuboid (Fig. 42.56).

ALTERNATIVE METHODS OF MIDTARSAL JOINT FIXATION. Alternative methods of fixation of the midtarsal joint include the use of Blount staples or the 3M power staplizer system. Often the placement of screws across the talonavicular and calcaneocuboid joints may be more traumatic or require more surgical dissection than is otherwise necessary. There are also times when the screws are inserted and one or both joints are not stable. In addition, when cancellous bone is not adequate to support a screw, staples provide rigid fixation.

Many members of the Institute faculty prefer staples for the midtarsal joint because of ease and speed of application.

When staples are used, it is preferable to place two in each joint, oriented 90° to one another. Care must be taken to ensure that the staples do not impinge on the adjacent joints. Their placement and positioning should be well planned and selected to achieve the most stable fixation possible.

Previous methods of fixation have included K-wires and Steinmann pins. These techniques are reserved as alternatives when more rigid fixation is not possible.

In recent years the use of cannulated screws has facilitated the fixation process. With cannulated screws the temporary fixation then serves as a true template for the permanent device, provided accurate alignment is achieved initially.

After stable fixation has been achieved, intraoperative radiographs are again obtained (Fig. 42.57), and the wound is closed in anatomical layers.

The use of rigid compression fixation has greatly enhanced the rate of successful fusion in triple arthrodesis. Rehabilitation may be initiated at a much earlier date because of the overall stability.

POSTOPERATIVE MANAGEMENT AND ACCELERATED AFTERCARE

Postoperative management of triple arthrodesis may be viewed as a sequence of phases beginning with the day of surgery and extending for up to 1 year. For simplicity the aftercare will be divided into five general phases (7).

Phase I: Initial Management (Days 0 to 5)

The initial management of the triple arthrodesis begins before closure of the incision with the placement of some type of closed suction drainage system, such as a TLS (Glasrock Corp., Atlanta, GA) drain. The use of a closed suction drainage system provides for the evacuation of hematoma that normally follows the resection of multiple bone surfaces. Extensive soft tissue reflection and exposure of well-vascularized cancellous bone are responsible for the large amount of hemorrhagic drainage that develops postoperatively. Placing a closed suction drain medially and laterally

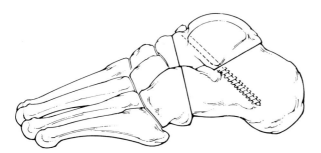

Figure 42.54. Fixation of talocalcaneal joint with 6.5-mm cancellous screw.

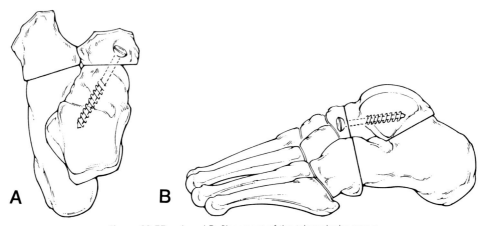

Figure 42.55. **A** and **B.** Placement of the talonavicular screw.

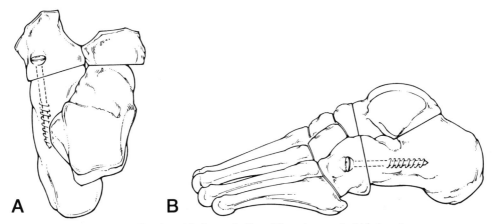

Figure 42.56. **A** and **B.** Screw fixation of the calcaneocuboid fusion site.

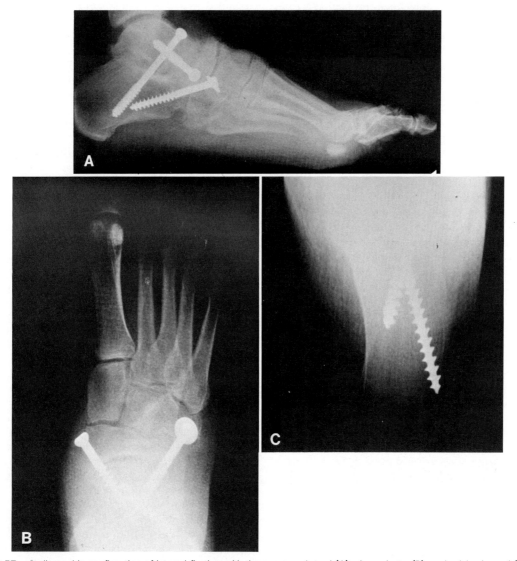

Figure 42.57. Radiographic confirmation of internal fixation with three screws. Lateral **(A),** dorsoplantar **(B),** and axial calcaneal **(C)** views.

will provide for evacuation of hemorrhagic and serous fluids during the immediate postoperative period and will considerably reduce edema. It is not uncommon for a triple arthrodesis to drain 200 to 300 ml of fluid over the first 3 postoperative days, with the lateral drain providing two thirds to three fourths of the fluids. The drains are placed against the periosteum to facilitate maximum effectiveness.

After wound closure, adhesive Steri-Strips, one-eighth or one-quarter inch, will provide extra support for the incision lines by decreasing the tension along the wound.

The patient will usually undergo a cast change on or about the third postoperative day. This is important for evaluating wound healing and possible wound infection, as well as allowing a preliminary evaluation of the extent of edema. If the foot proves to be too edematous for casting at that time, a second Jones-type compression cast is employed for an additional 2 to 3 days. Occasionally the initial cast will provide primary compression at the surgical site, forcing edema proximally and distally. This may prove detrimental in cases in which digital or forefoot work was performed in conjunction with the triple arthrodesis.

Once edema is adequately controlled, the foot is redressed and an appropriate cast applied prior to discharge. At that time phase II begins.

Phase II: Consolidation (Day 5 to 4 Weeks, Non-weight Bearing)

The second phase in the management of the triple arthrodesis may be considered as a period of wound healing and resolution of the inflammatory response. Casting may be of several forms: above-knee, below-knee, bivalved, synthetic, or plaster. Mitigating factors include the type of fixation employed, its stability, and patient compliance. The management of this phase is often as important as the surgical procedure. Inappropriate measures may actually compromise the surgical result. If there is any question about the stability of the fixation (bone quality, poor fixation) or patient compliance, then above-the-knee casting is an appropriate choice. The above knee cast with the knee flexed provides increased protection against the disruptive forces of torque that may affect the midtarsal joint. The cast tends to absorb this disruptive force at the level of the thigh.

A bivalved cast will be used for patients demonstrating high compliance. The cast may be split the day it is applied or at 3 weeks after surgery. This may be performed initially to facilitate wound care if additional dressing changes are required. Occasionally the patient may progress so that after the fourth week dressings are not needed. In these cases some type of elastic bandage is used to enclose the foot from the metatarsophalangeal joints to above the ankle. Experience has shown that it is better to wait until the third week to bivalve the cast if significant edema is present. The edema is more evenly controlled in a cast before bivalving.

Phase III: Preliminary Physical Therapy (Weeks 4 to 8, Non-weight Bearing)

After 1 month radiographs are obtained to assess the progress of osseous healing. This will be repeated at 2 and 3 months. During this phase the patient becomes involved with the rehabilitation. The previously bivalved cast is removed for a total of 1 to 2 hours once or twice per day. Active, unresisted range of motion exercises of the toes, foot, and ankle are performed. The patient begins soaking (provided wound healing is complete) in a tub or whirlpool. The goal of this phase is the reduction of edema through range of motion exercises and continuous compression. If an above-knee cast is used initially, it may be converted to below-the-knee.

Phase IV: Progressive Physical Therapy (Weeks 10 to 12)

This period is significant for more aggressive physical therapy. Radiographs are obtained at the eighth week (2 months) to assess healing. Orthotic molds or impressions are also prepared at this time provided swelling is not too great. The goal of the device is to minimize midtarsal stress once weight bearing is resumed. This is best accomplished using a rigid neutral shell with a three-sixteenths to five-sixteenths-inch heel lift on the rearfoot portion. One should still maintain compression for the reduction of edema.

The patient may begin partial weight bearing with crutches or walker at 10 to 12 weeks provided x-ray results indicate joint fusion. Weight bearing begins with 10% of body weight on the foot and is gradually increased. The patient performs isometric exercises to enhance range of motion of the ankle. As weight bearing is begun, new aches and pains will be experienced. These may be secondary to periods of disuse and renewed function in the realigned foot.

Phase V: Graduation (to Full Weight Bearing, Months 3 to 6)

At 3 months the patient is usually ready for full weight bearing, which usually begins in some type of padded high-top basketball shoe or padded work boot. The foot and ankle are continually compressed with a closed-heel elastic ankle support, Tubigrip, or elastic stocking. Elastic support with an open heel is avoided because the area becomes a site of edema and irritation. This routine is continued for 6 months at which time the patient and physician must evaluate a return to normal activities.

Footwear is important. If a low-cut oxford-type shoe is worn before 12 to 16 weeks, moderate to severe edema may develop at the shoe counter. This may be minimized with use of the elastic ankle support as described.

If the physician is not confident in the form of fixation used or fears that the patient is poorly compliant, then 12 weeks in an above-knee cast is an acceptable method of management. The postoperative physical therapy will need to be more aggressive because stiffness and disuse osteoporosis will be more pronounced.

SUBTALAR JOINT FUSION

Subtalar joint fusions with and without bone grafts are performed for a variety of disorders and dysfunction of talocalcaneal joint. The indications for subtalar joint fusion range from acute displaced intra-articular fractures of the calcaneus, late complications of displaced intra-articular calcaneal fractures, acquired adult flatfoot, isolated talocalcaneal arthrosis, tarsal coalition, and valgus rearfoot deformity.

Subtalar joint fusion has been reported for many years as a salvage procedure in those individuals with pain and dysfunction in the talocalcaneal joint. It is especially applicable in those individuals in whom there is distinct incongruity of the subtalar joint surfaces, often diminished rearfoot height (loss of calcaneal body height), tibiotalar impingement, peroneal muscle spasm and tendonitis, posterior muscle group weakness, widening of the heel, and occasionally calcaneofibular abutment. These patients are

good candidates for subtalar joint fusion provided that they do not have symptoms involving the midtarsal joint. It is also essential that such patients have a normal forefoot to rearfoot relationship.

Other patients who are good candidates for subtalar joint fusion are those individuals who have isolated talocalcaneal joint coalition without concomitant arthrosis of the midtarsal joint. A simple test in determining the extent of symptoms is to infiltrate a small amount of lidocaine into the subtalar joint. This will usually eliminate peroneal spasm or splinting.

Techniques for fusion of the subtalar joint are twofold, the in situ fusion and fusion involving bone grafts. Most of the techniques described in the literature have included bone grafting, especially in those cases of severe intra-articular calcaneal fracture. Gallie (37) described subtalar fusion using a bone graft obtained from the tibia and placed posteriorly into the talocalcaneal joint. Since that time there have been numerous reports in the literature regarding subtalar joint fusion as a salvage procedure for posterior talocalcaneal joint arthrosis (38-42).

Recently, Carr and associates (42) described a modifica-

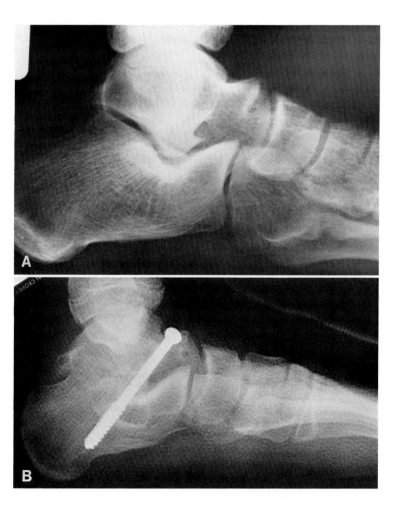

Figure 42.58. **A.** Preoperative lateral radiograph of an adolescent patient with a painful tarsal coalition of the subtalar joint. **B.** Postoperative lateral view following subtalar joint fusion using a 6.5-mm cancellous screw as fixation.

tion of the usual fusion technique. Its primary application is for the painful deformed calcaneus that results after severe comminuted joint depression fracture of the calcaneus. The technique uses subperiosteal resection of the lateral wall blow-out fracture. A femoral distractor is applied medially to the calcaneus and tibia. The subtalar joint is distracted to facilitate the resection of joint surfaces and to assist in correction of subtalar varus or valgus. The resultant gap is packed with a tricortical bone graft and internally fixated with 6.5-mm AO cancellous screws. Carr and colleagues report satisfactory results in 13 of 16 feet.

The advantage of this procedure is that it restores the normal talocalcaneal relationship and narrows the heel. This leads to an improvement in shoe fit, a decrease or resolution of tibiotalar impingement symptoms, relief of lateral rearfoot impingement between the calcaneus and fibula, and relief of chronic peroneal tendonitis.

In cases of chronic pain and dysfunction related to the subtalar joint as well as in other selected talocalcaneal coalitions, the in situ method of subtalar joint fusion is very applicable (Fig. 42.58).

The prerequisite for use of subtalar arthrodesis is the absence of tarsal arthrosis at the midtarsal joint. Even then there is considerable debate over the use of selected subtalar joint fusion. Isolation of symptoms to the subtalar joint by clinical means or through the use of selective anesthetic blocks or by careful radiographic examination is essential prior to making the decision to fuse an isolated joint.

The approach for arthrodesis of the subtalar joint varies from that described for triple arthrodesis in that the soft tissue dissection is not as extensive. The procedure does require two incisions. The medial incision allows access to the dorsal surface of the neck of the talus and facilitates insertion of screw fixation. Dissection on the lateral aspect of the foot is much as described in the previous section on triple arthrodesis, with the notable distinction that it does not extend into the calcaneocuboid joint area. Joint resection and fixation are quite similar. The use of the cannulated screw system will simplify this fixation.

The postoperative course and aftercare are similar to those for the triple arthrodesis except that primary fusion may be complete in 8 weeks. A longer period is needed for those in whom bone grafts are used. Most patients require an orthotic device, as well as a heel lift, to ensure adequate heel height.

SUMMARY

Triple arthrodesis and subtalar arthrodesis are time-tested and effective procedures in the treatment of a wide variety of foot deformities and malformations. Relief of pain, improvement of function, correction of deformity, and stabilization of the rearfoot are indications for these procedures. The hazards and complications may be minimized with effective planning, technical execution, and sensible postoperative management.

References

1. Ryerson EW: Arthrodesing operations on the feet. *J Bone Joint Surg* 5:453-471, 1923.
2. Patterson RL, Parrish FP, Hathaway EN: Stabilizing operations on the foot. *J Bone Joint Surg* 32A:1-26, 1950.
3. Seiffert RS, Forster RI, Nachamie B: "Beak" triple arthrodesis for correction of severe cavus deformity. *Clin Orthop* 45:101-104, 1966.
4. Hart VL: Arthrodesis of the foot in infantile paralysis. *Surg Gynecol Obstet* 64:794-797, 1937.
5. Hallgrinnsson S: Studies on reconstructive and stabilizing operations on the skeleton of the foot with special reference to subastragalar arthrodesis in treatment of foot deformities following infantile paralysis. *Acta Chir Scand* (Supp) 78:1-215, 1943.
6. Schwartz RP: Arthrodesis of the subtalus and midtarsal joints of the foot. Historical review, preoperative determinations and operative procedures. *Surgery* 20:619-635, 1946.
7. McGlamry ED, Ruch JA, Mahan KT, DiNapoli DR: Triple arthrodesis. In McGlamry ED, McGlamry RC (eds): *Reconstructive Surgery of the Foot and Leg—Update '87.* Tucker, GA, Podiatry Institute Publishing Co, 1987, pp 126-152.
8. Johnson MK, Kanat IO: Complications of triple arthrodesis with comparison to select rearfoot fusions. *J Foot Surg* 26:371-379, 1987.
9. Angus PD, Cowell HR: Triple arthrodesis, a critical long-term review. *J Bone Joint Surg* 68B:260-265, 1986.
10. Seitz DC, Carpenter EB: Triple arthrodesis in children: a ten year review. *South Med J* 67:1429-1424, 1974.
11. Wilson FC, Fay GF, Lamotte P, Wilson JC: Triple arthrodesis: a study of the factors affecting fusion after three hundred and one procedures. *J Bone Joint Surg* 47A:340-348, 1965.
12. Hill NA, Wilson HJ, Chevres F, Sweterlitsch PR: Triple arthrodesis in the young child. *Clin Orthop* 70:187-190, 1970.
13. Crego CH, McCarroll HR: A report of 1100 consecutive stabilizations in poliomyelitis. *J Bone Joint Surg* 20:609-620, 1938.
14. Marek FM, Schein AJ: Avascular necrosis of the talus in children. *J Bone Joint Surg* 27A:587-594, 1945.
15. Galindo MJ, Siff SJ, Butler JE, Cain TD: Triple arthrodesis in young children: a salvage procedure after failed releases in severely affected feet. *Foot Ankle* 7:319-325, 1987.
16. Vogler HW: Triple arthrodesis as a salvage for end-stage flatfoot. *Clin Podiatr Med Surg* 6:591-604, 1989.
17. Wukich DK, Bowen JR: A long-term study of triple arthrodesis for correction of pes cavovarus in Charcot-Marie-Tooth disease. *J Pediatr Orthop* 9:433-437, 1989.
18. Southwell RB, Sherman FC: Triple arthrodesis: a long-term study with force plate analysis. *Foot Ankle* 2:15-24, 1981.
19. Wetmore RS, Drennan JC: Long-term results of triple arthrodesis in Charcot-Marie-Tooth disease. *J Bone Joint Surg* 71A:417-422, 1989.
20. Brenau A: Long-term results following Lambrinudi arthrodesis. *J Bone Joint Surg* 59A:473-479, 1977.
21. Patterson RL: Various factors involved in triple arthrodesis. *Clin Orthop* 85:59-61, 1972.
22. Williams PF, Menelaus MB: Triple arthrodesis by inlay grafting—a method suitable for the underformed or valgus foot. *J Bone Joint Surg* 59B:333-336, 1977.
23. Sennara H: Triple arthrodesis: a modified new technique. *Clin Orthop* 83:237-240, 1972.
24. Sgarlato TE, Sharpe DA: Triple arthrodesis: a new approach. *J Am Podiatry Assoc* 65:41-49, 1975.
25. Jayakumar S, Cowell HR: Rigid flatfoot. *Clin Orthop* 122:77-84, 1977.
26. Morris HD: Arthrodesis of the foot. *Clin Orthop* 16:164-175, 1960.
27. Howorth MB: Triple subtalar arthrodesis. *Clin Orthop* 99:175-180, 1974.
28. Tang SC, Leong JCY, Hsu LCS: Lambrinudi triple arthrodesis for correction of severe rigid drop-foot. *J Bone Joint Surg* 66B:66-70, 1984.
29. Medhart MA, Krantz H: Neuropathic ankle joint in Charcot-Marie-Tooth disease after triple arthrodesis of the foot. *Orthop Rev* 17:873-880, 1988.
30. MacKenzie IG: Lambrinudi's triple arthrodesis. *J Bone Joint Surg* 41B:738-748, 1959.
31. Duncan JW, Lovell WW: Hoke triple arthrodesis. *J Bone Joint Surg* 60A:795-798, 1978.

32. Banks AS, McGlamry ED: Tibialis posterior tendon rupture. *J Am Podiatr Med Assoc* 77:170-176, 1987.

33. Burns MJ: Biomechanics. In McGlamry ED (ed): *Fundamentals of Foot Surgery*. Baltimore, Williams & Wilkins, 1987, pp 111-135.

34. Motion of the joints of the foot. In Root ML, Orien WP, Weed JH (eds): *Normal and Abnormal Function of the Foot*. Los Angeles, Clinical Biomechanics Corp, 1977, pp 1-61.

35. Dananberg HJ: Functional hallux limitus and its relationship to gait efficiency. *J Am Podiatry Assoc* 76:648-652, 1986.

36. Dananberg HJ, Lawton M, DiNapoli DR: Hallux limitus and non-specific gait related bodily trauma. In DiNapoli DR (ed): *Reconstructive Surgery of the Foot and Leg: Update '90*. Tucker, GA, Podiatry Institute Publishing Co, 1990, pp 52-59.

37. Gallie WE: Subastragular arthrodesis in fractures of the os calcis. *J Bone Joint Surg* 25:731, 1943.

38. Kalamchi A, Evans JG: Posterior subtalar fusion: a preliminary report on a modified Gallie's procedure. *J Bone Joint Surg* 59B:287-289, 1977.

39. Dennyson WG, Fulford GE: Subtalar arthrodesis by cancellous grafts and metallic internal fixation. *J Bone Joint Surg* 58B:507, 1976.

40. Johansson JE, Harrison J, Greenwood FAH: Subtalar arthrodesis for adult arthritis. *Foot Ankle* 2:294-298, 1982.

41. Mann RA, Baumgarten M: Subtalar fusions for isolated subtalar disorders. Preliminary report. *Clin Orthop* 226:260-265, 1988.

42. Carr JB, Hansen ST, Benirschke SK: Subtalar distraction bone block fusion for late complications of os calcis fractures. *Foot Ankle* 9:81-86, 1988.

43. Russotti GM, Cass JR, Johnson KA: Isolated talocalcaneal arthrodesis: a technique using moldable bone graft. *J Bone Joint Surg* 70A:1472-1478, 1988.

Additional References

Banks HH: The management of spastic deformities of the foot and ankle. *Clin Orthop* 122:70-76, 1977.

Chambers RB, Cook TM, Cowell HR: Surgical reconstruction for calcaneonavicular coalition: evaluation of function and gait. *J Bone Joint Surg* 69A:829-836, 1982.

Chieppa WA, Sydnor KH, Walter JH: Use of the cannulated bone screw in rearfoot surgery. *J Foot Surg* 28:333-334, 1989.

Cowell HR, Elener V: Rigid painful flatfoot secondary to tarsal coalition. *Clin Orthop* 177:54-60, 1983.

Fogel GR, Katho Y, Rand JA, Chao EYS: Talonavicular arthrodesis for isolated arthrosis, 9.5 year results and gait analysis. *Foot Ankle* 3:105-113, 1982.

Gellman H, Lenihan M, Halikis N, Botte MJ, Giordani M, Perry J: Selective tarsal arthrodesis: an in vitro analysis of the effect on foot motion. *Foot Ankle* 8:127-133, 1987.

Hall JE, Calvert PT: Lambrinudi triple arthrodesis: a review with particular reference to the technique of operation. *J Pediatr Orthop* 7:19-24, 1987.

Kuwada GT: Modification of fixation technique for a subtalar joint and triple arthrodesis. *J Am Podiatr Med Assoc* 78:482-485, 1988.

Olney BW, Menelaus MB: Triple arthrodesis of the foot in spina bifida patients. *J Bone Joint Surg* 70B:234-235, 1988.

Samilson RL, Dillin W: Cavus, cavovarus, and calcanealcavous: an update. *Clin Orthop* 177:125-132, 1983.

Scranton PE: Treatment of symptomatic talocalcaneal coalition. *J Bone Joint Surg* 69A:533-539, 1987.

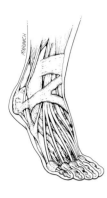

CHAPTER **43**

Ankle and Pantalar Fusion

Kieran T. Mahan, M.S., D.P.M., F.A.C.F.S.

Ankle fusion has been a useful treatment for more than 100 years. More than 40 techniques and modifications have been described. In appropriate circumstances the procedure can be quite successful in alleviating pain and deformity.

INDICATIONS

Fusion of the ankle joint is indicated primarily in patients with severe pain and/or deformity (Fig. 43.1). The specific indications include degenerative joint disease, rheumatoid arthritis, talar collapse, failed ankle joint prostheses, infection of the ankle joint, drop foot, tumors with joint invasion, and congenital deformities.

The most common indication for ankle fusion is now posttraumatic degenerative joint disease subsequent to inadequate or poorly executed management of ankle fractures. Degeneration of the ankle joint is correlated with lateral shift or shortening of the fibula. Ramsey and Hamilton (1) demonstrated that the initial 1 mm of lateral displacement of the fibula after fracture results in a 42% decrease in tibiotalar contact. Because a decrease in contact area means that greater force is transmitted per unit area, one may understand how fractures with small amounts of displacement can result in degenerative joint disease of the ankle. Proper management of ankle fractures requires accurate anatomical reduction to preserve joint function.

Patients with paralytic deformities may also benefit from ankle arthrodesis. At one time the most common paralytic condition associated with the procedure was poliomyelitis. The deformity and instability caused by this condition often respond well to pantalar arthrodesis to stabilize not only the ankle but the rearfoot as well. Fortunately, this surgery is needed much less frequently today because of mass immunization programs. Other paralytic deformities may respond well to ankle fusion, particularly in instances in which muscle tendon rebalancing is not possible. Examples include extremity trauma with nerve injury, deformity and paralysis following compartment syndrome, myelodysplasia, or spinal cord trauma. In paralytic deformities, pantalar arthrodesis is required more commonly than simple ankle fusion. However, the insensitive foot is more difficult to treat because of a much higher incidence of delayed and nonunion.

Ankle fusion is also performed when either side of the joint has been eroded or crushed. Examples include avascular necrosis of the talus, tumors, and crushing injuries.

Primary ankle arthrodesis is not commonly performed immediately after trauma but may be indicated when there is extensive comminution or bone loss (2). An unsuccessful total ankle implant can be salvaged only with fusion of the joint and bone grafting (Fig. 43.2).

Rheumatoid arthritis is not a frequent indication for ankle fusion. However, severe ankle pain and deformity associated with the disease can best be treated with arthrodesis. In a survey of 300 patients with an average duration of 10 years of rheumatoid arthritis, Gschwend and Stieger found that the ankle and subtalar joints were involved 52% of the time (3). Several caveats must be considered in patients with rheumatoid arthritis. After fusion of one joint, load and stress are shifted to adjacent joints. In rheumatoid arthritis these joints are often already painful and arthritic, reducing the ability of the joints to compensate for the ankle fusion. Some patients with rheumatoid arthritis may be poor candidates for ankle fusion because of osteoporosis, vasculitis, mononeuritis multiplex, and skin atrophy (4, 5).

Infection with joint destruction can be caused by osteomyelitis or septic arthritis. After infectious destruction of the ankle joint, fusion is the only alternative once the infection has been eradicated.

PREOPERATIVE EVALUATION

Patients selected for ankle fusion should be those for whom it will be reasonable to expect a significant reduction in pain, decrease in deformity, and increase in activity. Subjective indications for fusion include daily pain, significant limitation of activity, the desire to function free of braces, and the desire to reduce severe deformity for a more comfortable gait. The author has found that patients in severe pain preoperatively and those given an exhaustive trial of conservative therapy have the highest sense of satisfaction with their ankle fusion postoperatively (K. Mahan and G. Yu, unpublished observations). It is recommended that the surgeon offer the patient the option of nonoperative therapeutic measures before committing to destruction of the joint.

Before any fusion is performed, it is essential to evaluate the integrity of the adjacent joints. It is particularly important to evaluate the subtalar and forefoot joints before performing ankle fusion. The subtalar joint can frequently be involved in degenerative joint processes. If a degenerated

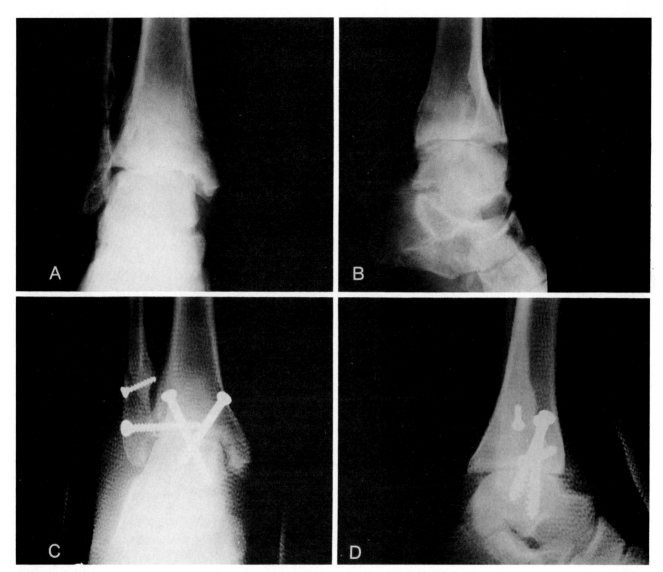

Figure 43.1. **A** and **B.** Preoperative views of an ankle 3 years after a fracture sustained during hang gliding accident. Note the obliteration of the joint. **C.** Anteroposterior view of ankle fusion with internal fixation. **D.** Lateral view of the fusion demonstrating good alignment and fixation.

subtalar joint is not fused, the resultant increase in stress to the area after the ankle arthrodesis will usually accelerate the degenerative process at the subtalar level (Fig. 43.3). Selective local anesthetic blocks of the subtalar and ankle joints can isolate the area of pain and aid in determining the necessity for ankle or pantalar fusion. Ahlberg and Henricson (6) reported that two thirds of the patients in their study reported pain in the region of the subtalar joint at long-term follow-up. A secondary subtalar fusion or, more commonly, triple arthrodesis may be required in the event of accelerated rearfoot symptoms or deformity.

The ankle joint is usually fused at a right angle to the leg. Compensation for heel height must then come from plantarflexion at the midtarsal and tarsometatarsal joints (7).

Available plantarflexion and forefoot deformity should be assessed preoperatively.

Gait analysis and biomechanical evaluation should be performed preoperatively. Before the position for fusion is determined, superstructural deformities should be noted. Deformities both proximal and distal to the level of the ankle joint may need to be compensated for by the position of the fusion. Stability at the knee joint is important for those patients who have a pantalar fusion.

Other important preoperative considerations include adequate vascular status, good bone stock, and good general health. Obese patients, those with sensory loss, and patients who are psychologically unprepared for loss of motion will have a higher incidence of complications during the peri-

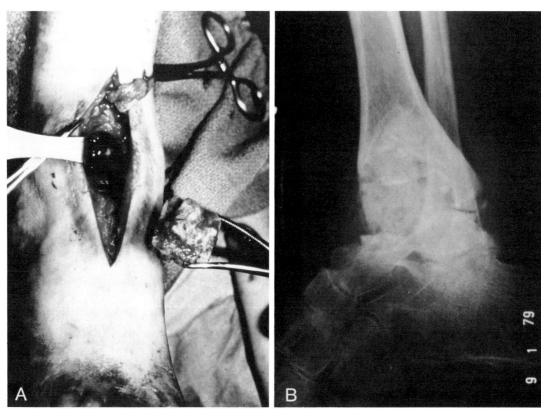

Figure 43.2.   A. Intraoperative photograph demonstrating the removal of an ankle implant (held in clamp). Note the large defect remaining after removal of the implant. **B.** Postoperative view showing the defect packed with large fenestrated bone graft. This went on to uneventful consolidation.

operative period. Patients with motion available at the midtarsal and tarsometatarsal joints of the affected limb and normal range of motion in the contralateral ankle have a better prognosis for functioning well in daily activities (8).

SURGICAL APPROACHES AND TECHNIQUES FOR FUSION

Numerous techniques and modifications for achieving ankle fusion have been described. Naturally, surgical approaches have been designed with specific arthrodesis techniques in mind. Nonetheless, it is worthwhile to examine the different approaches individually, because each may have some merit in a given situation.

Approaches

Charnley described a transverse anterior approach for access to the talus and lower surface of the tibia (9). The dissection results in transection of the extensor tendons and the anterior neurovascular bundle. Although this approach offers excellent anterior exposure, it is fraught with obvious potential complications. As described by Charnley, this method would involve extensive soft tissue dissection and meticulous repair of tendons, risk vascular embarrassment, and cause permanent sensory loss to the dorsum of the foot. Nonetheless, Charnley claimed good results and stated that the exposure was superior to that achieved with other approaches, such as the longitudinal anterior approach, the lateral approach, and the combined medial and lateral approach.

The midline longitudinal anterior approach provides good exposure to the anterior aspect of the joint, particularly at the lower end of the tibia. Exposure of the malleoli is adequate. This approach requires extensive soft tissue dissection, and there is inadequate visualization of the posterior ankle joint. However, the neurovascular complications of the transverse incision can be avoided with this longitudinal approach.

The lateral approach consists of an incision in the shape of a hockey stick, beginning over the lateral aspect of the fibula and coursing distally over the lateral aspect of the neck of the talus to end at the base of the fourth metatarsal. This gives excellent exposure of the lateral aspect of the ankle joint and, when combined with a fibular osteotomy, provides good exposure of the posterior, lateral, and anterior aspects of the ankle joint. Much of the dissection is subperiosteal and, with the exception of the perforating peroneal artery, neurovascular structures are not threatened.

A medial approach gives good exposure of the medial malleolus. In combination with a medial malleolar osteotomy, one achieves good exposure of the anteromedial, medial, and posteromedial aspects of the ankle joint.

Anteromedial and anterolateral approaches have been de-

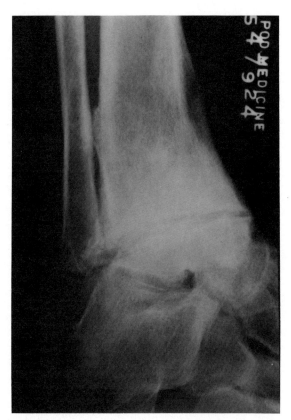

Figure 43.3. Incomplete union of an ankle fusion 12 years postoperatively. Note the narrowing of subtalar joint that has occurred because of increased load to the area. The patient complained of pain in the subtalar area.

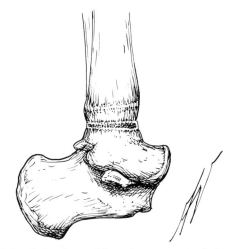

Figure 43.4. Chuinard type of distraction-compression fusion with bone graft. Note the preservation of the distal tibial growth plate.

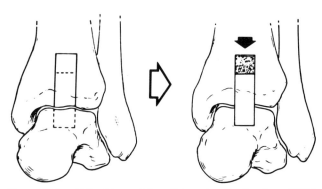

Figure 43.5. Sliding inlay graft from tibia as described by Soren (1968) for ankle fusion.

scribed, and these provide good exposure of the anterior ankle and the respective malleoli.

A posterior approach to the ankle joint is possible through a longitudinal incision parallel to the Achilles tendon. This is a poor method for total resection of ankle joint cartilage and should be reserved for those situations in which skin coverage is inadequate over other areas of the ankle and a subtotal fusion (dowel or other graft) is to be performed. The subtalar joint is intimately associated with the ankle joint posteriorly and must be carefully protected.

The surgical approach selected is based on the exposure needed to perform the desired technique and on the condition of the soft tissues. The lateral hockey-stick approach combined with the accessory medial incision is the method usually employed by the author.

Techniques

The extensive number of techniques and modifications for ankle arthrodesis can be simplified into several categories: articular wedging with or without grafting, anterior arthrodesis with inlay grafting, articular wedging combined with malleolar osteotomy, dowel fusions or other subtotal fusions, compression arthrodesis, and other miscellaneous techniques.

The simplest technique consists of the removal of articular cartilage from the talus and tibia. Bone graft may be used to pack any defect. Goldthwait (10), in 1908, performed this technique through a U-shaped incision and Hallock (11), in 1945, supplemented the technique with a tibial bone graft. Chuinard and Peterson (12) applied the technique to ankle fusion in children. After removing the articular cartilage, they impacted an autogenous iliac crest graft as an interpositional graft to achieve compression without damage to the epiphysis (Fig. 43.4).

Numerous authors have used anterior bone grafts across the ankle to facilitate fusion. Wescott (13) used a graft from the upper tibia and believed that it would provide sufficient stability to obviate the need for a cast. Campbell and associates (14) used autogenous iliac crest grafts across the talotibial space after excision of the joint. More commonly a sliding graft from the distal tibia is employed, as described by Hatt (15), Brittain (16), and Soren (17) (Fig. 43.5). Kennedy's modification of the Gallie ankle fusion uses anteromedial and anterolateral allogenic grafts with staple fixation and joint excision (18) (Fig. 43.6).

A third type of ankle fusion technique is joint resection

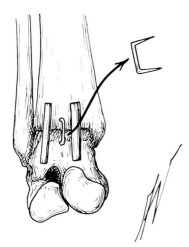

Figure 43.6. Modified Gallie fusion with joint resection, inlay grafts, and staple fixation, as described by Kennedy.

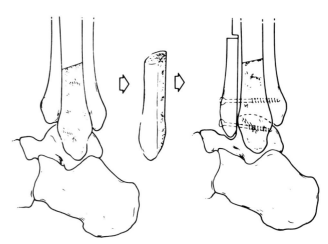

Figure 43.8. Bi-hemi-malleolar onlay grafts as described by Wilson (1969) for ankle fusion.

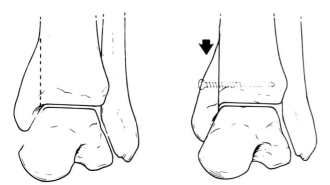

Figure 43.7. Glissan's technique (1949) for fusion included medial malleolar osteotomy for exposure of joint and for use as an onlay graft.

with malleolar osteotomy. Osteotomy of either malleolus increases exposure of the joint, facilitating resection of cartilage. In addition, the malleolus can be used as an onlay graft for stability and to promote fusion. It also allows for a better fit between the talus and the tibia without the need for interpositional grafting. Goldthwait (10) may have been the first to describe osteotomy of a malleolus for ankle fusion. Horwitz (19) described a lateral approach with osteotomy of the fibular malleolus. After resection of the joint cartilage, he divided the fibula in half longitudinally and applied one half anteriorly and the other half to the lateral side of the talus and the tibia as grafts. Adams (20) also discussed the transfibular approach, recommending the fibula as an onlay graft and advocating packing of cancellous chips into open spaces. Glissan (21) used a medial malleolar osteotomy. He removed a small section of bone from the medial malleolus to narrow the mortise and then secured the malleolus to the tibia (Fig. 43.7).

Wilson (22) describes a bimalleolar approach with a tibial graft medially and the lateral longitudinal half of the fibula as an onlay graft anterolaterally (Fig. 43.8). Verhelst and associates (23) advocate complete removal of the distal part

of the fibula rather than its use as a graft to "eliminate the risk of drainage . . . due to the presence of a large bone graft immediately underneath the skin." Anderson (24) also used a bimalleolar approach with resection of both malleoli, remodeling of their stumps, and crushing of the malleoli for use as cancellous grafts. Staples (25) used a posterior malleolar graft slid behind the ankle and subtalar joints for fusion of both sites. Mead (26), Marcus and associates (27), Stewart and associates (28), and Bingold (29) all describe modifications involving malleolar osteotomies.

The fourth category of ankle fusion modalities includes the subtotal techniques. These techniques accomplish fusion without total resection of the articular cartilage. This is clearly less than desirable in most situations but may be indicated in patients who might not be able to withstand more extensive dissection and lengthy surgery. The nature of these procedures dictates that extensive wedging not be required for subtotal fusion to be successful. A good example of this is the dowel fusion described by Pridie (30). This is performed from a medial approach with removal of the medial malleolus. A 1.5 inch auger bit is used to ream the central portion of the joint, and the cavity is filled with bone chips. Hone (31) modified this technique by cutting a dowel from anterior to posterior and rotating the dowel 90° to place bone across the joint and effect fusion.

Baciu and Filibiu (32) described a similar procedure. Graham (33) used cylindrical fibular grafts across the ankle joint from lateral to medial with reattachment of the remainder of the fibula to the tibia as an onlay graft. The procedure described by Ottolenghi and associates (34) is similar to both Graham's and Pridie's procedures in that a canal is reamed transversely across the ankle joint and the fibula is then used as a graft to fill the defect and create fusion.

Gallie (35) and Van Gorder and Chen (36) describe subtotal fusion with bone grafts. Gallie's procedure for ankle fusion involves anteromedial and anterolateral bone grafts across the joint without joint resection or fixation. Van Gorder and Chen also did not perform joint resection. They state that either an anterior or a posterior approach can be used, with a tibial bone graft being driven through the central portion of the talotibial articulation. This procedure was described for tuberculous arthritis, and Van Gorder and Chen state that, because joint degeneration and wasting are so extensive in this disease, total joint resection becomes unnecessary.

The fifth category of ankle fusion techniques is compression arthrodesis. This technique consists of total joint resection and compression fixation. Most commonly this has been achieved by external fixation devices. Anderson (24), in 1945, described ankle fusion with external fixation that may or may not have achieved compression. Numerous authors have described compression techniques (23, 37-41); however, Charnley (9, 42) is acknowledged as the father of compression arthrodesis. He believed that two clear advantages of compression arthrodesis were the prevention of a gap at the fusion site and resistance to shearing forces.

The last category of techniques consists of those miscellaneous procedures that do not fall into other categories. An example is the White posterior ankle fusion (43). Other examples include those procedures that are not truly ankle fusions, such as tibiocalcaneal fusions (44) and the Blair fusion for avascular necrosis of the talar body (45, 46) (Fig. 43.9).

PODIATRY INSTITUTE ANKLE ARTHRODESIS WITH INTERNAL FIXATION

Although numerous techniques are available for ankle fusion, as previously described, many can be readily discarded because of their failure to meet Glissan's four requirements for a successful fusion (21):

1. Complete removal of all cartilage, fibrous tissue, and any other material that may prevent contact of raw bone surfaces
2. Accurate and close fitting of the fusion surfaces
3. Optimal position of the ankle joint
4. Maintenance of the bone apposition in an undisturbed fashion until fusion is completed.

The Podiatry Institute technique of internal fixation for ankle fusions has evolved over many years with contributions from several surgeons. Retrospective studies have assisted in the evolution of this procedure (47). There are several advantages to internal fixation, including patient acceptance, resistance to rotary stresses, the avoidance of pin tract infections, and the one-stage nature of the procedure (removal of hardware is optional rather than mandatory).

The preferred approach for the technique is the lateral transfibular approach. The dissection, osteotomy, and fixation are usually performed with thigh tourniquet hemostasis. The incision begins over the lateral aspect of the fibula at the junction between the middle and distal thirds of the leg. The incision courses distally over the fibula and over the lateral surface of the talus. Dissection is carried down to the periosteum overlying the fibula. Subperiosteal dissection is then carried out over the anterior aspect of the ankle.

Osteotomy of the fibula is performed by one of several

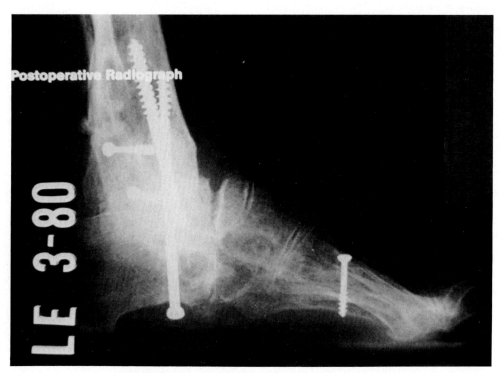

Figure 43.9. Tibiocalcaneal fusion with internal fixation.

possible techniques (e.g., oblique, transverse), depending on whether the fibula will be repaired. The fibula is then reflected distally, leaving the distal attachments of the fibula intact (Fig. 43.10). When the lateral exposure is completed, there is excellent visualization of the lateral and anterior aspects of the talotibial articulation. The articular cartilage on the talus is then removed with power instrumentation after visualization of the ankle in the desired position of fusion (Fig. 43.11). Cartilage on the tibial plafond is removed next, followed by any additional wedging that may be necessary and removal of cartilage off the medial side of the fibula.

An ancillary medial incision may be made next for removal of cartilage from the medial malleolus and placement of the medial screw.

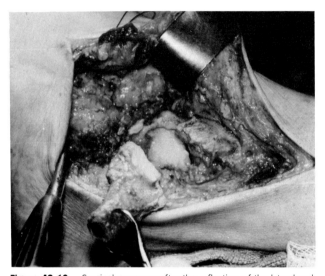

Figure 43.10. Surgical exposure after the reflection of the lateral malleolus. The fibula is held by a bone clamp.

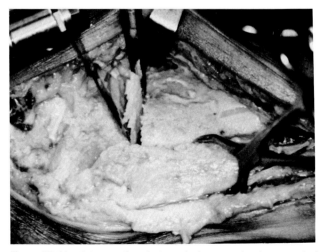

Figure 43.11. Intraoperative photograph demonstrating the removal of a wedge of cartilage from the ankle joint.

When the ankle appears to be in the desired position with flush bone surfaces, it is temporarily fixed and intraoperative radiographs are taken. As Scranton and associates (48) have noted, the value of the intraoperative radiograph "to confirm satisfactory ankle alignment cannot be overemphasized." Before the radiographs, the drill holes for the crossing lag screws can be made. The drill bit is left in one hole and the depth gauge in the other. With this technique the intraoperative radiographs assess not only the position of the ankle joint but also the position of the drill holes (Fig. 43.12). This is particularly helpful for checking the depth of the holes to ensure that the subtalar joint has not been violated. Alternatively, a cannulated screw system may be used with the guide pins inserted prior to intraoperative radiographs.

Numerous studies have demonstrated that the desired position of fusion is with the foot at a right angle (0° plantarflexion) to the leg (8, 37, 49), although up to 5° of plantarflexion can usually be tolerated well. Compensatory plantarflexion at the midtarsal and tarsometatarsal joints allows the patient to wear a heel (7, 8). Fusing the ankle in equinus can create a functional genu recurvatum in the stance phase of gait and results in a significantly less desirable gait pattern, particularly when the patient is barefoot (8). Fusion in calcaneus also produces an unsatisfactory gait. The transverse plane position of the fusion should be in line with the

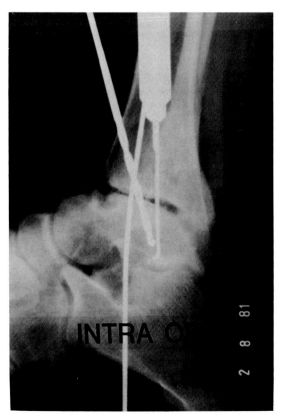

Figure 43.12. Intraoperative radiograph during ankle fusion. The drill bit and depth gauge demonstrate the position for screws.

normal transmalleolar axis of 15° of external rotation. The position of the knee should be visualized when the final transverse plane alignment is planned. The frontal plane position of the fusion should be such that the rearfoot is in slight valgus. The existing subtalar neutral position and frontal plane angulation from the tibia and femur will determine the ideal position for the ankle.

After satisfactory position of the ankle has been confirmed by the intraoperative radiographs, the final fixation can be performed. The fixation consists of two crossing 6.5 mm (or similar size) cancellous screws at the talotibial articulation, and fixation of the fibular onlay graft to the tibia with a 4.0 mm cancellous screw or 4.5 mm screw (malleolar or cortical). The two heavy screws are positioned to be crossing each other to cancel out any theoretical shift caused by the oblique angle of the screw. The medial screw begins above the medial malleolus and is positioned into the anteromedial aspect of the body of the talus. The lateral screw begins on the anterolateral aspect of the tibia and is directed posteriorly and distally into the posterolateral aspect of the body of the talus (Fig. 43.13). There are other acceptable variations for screw placement (Fig. 43.14). The 16 mm thread pattern is usually employed with the 6.5 mm screws. A considerable compressive force is generated by these screws. The fibula is then stabilized by interfragmentary compression against the tibia. The junction between the tibia and the fibula can

be decorticated in spots to facilitate bridging. Cannulated screw systems exist which permit application of the permanent fixation directly over the temporary fixation pin. This modification is particularly useful in a small talus.

Finally, the fibular osteotomy can be repaired, although this is not necessary. The author's own retrospective study (Mahan KT, Yu GV, unpublished observations) revealed that the fibular osteotomy site can be troublesome if inadequately fixated (Fig. 43.15). Small amounts of motion can cause the interfragmentary screw to back out, leaving a distracted osteotomy site that goes on to a delayed union or nonunion. A transverse osteotomy with no fixation is perfectly acceptable and creates less difficulty at the fibula.

Intraoperative radiographs are performed again and layer closure is accomplished over closed suction drainage. A compression cast is applied for 3 to 4 days followed by casting for 3 to 4 months with progressive weight bearing after stability of the ankle has been achieved. Although it is not absolutely necessary, removal of the screws is possible after 6 to 12 months, provided that fusion has been accomplished.

EXTERNAL FIXATION TECHNIQUE

The advantages of external fixation include substantial interfragmentary compression and relative ease of applica-

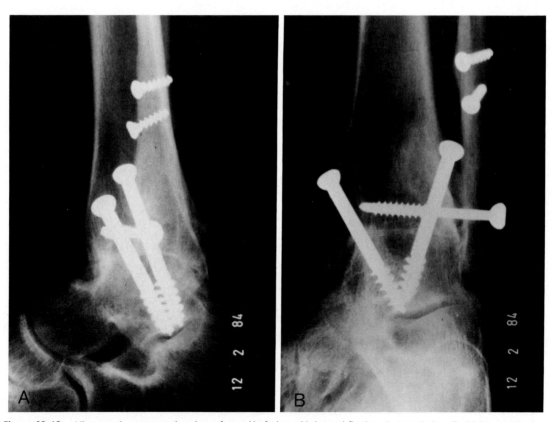

Figure 43.13. Nine-month postoperative view of an ankle fusion with internal fixation. **A.** Lateral view. **B.** Oblique ankle view.

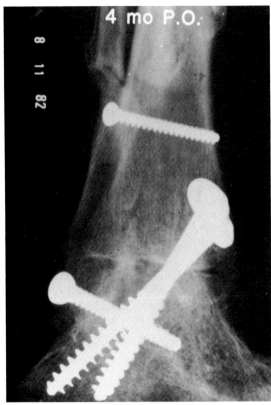

Figure 43.14. Four-month postoperative view of an ankle fusion in a postpoliomyelitis patient with a previous triple arthrodesis. Oblique ankle view demonstrates the use of crossing long-thread 6.5 mm cancellous screws. With previous subtalar fusion, longer screws can be used without fear of joint violation.

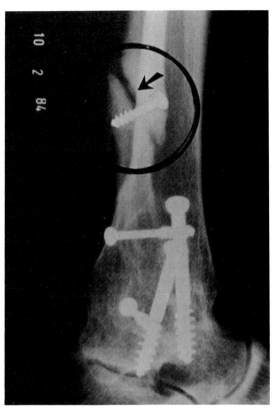

Figure 43.15. Nonunion at the fibular osteotomy site (circled).

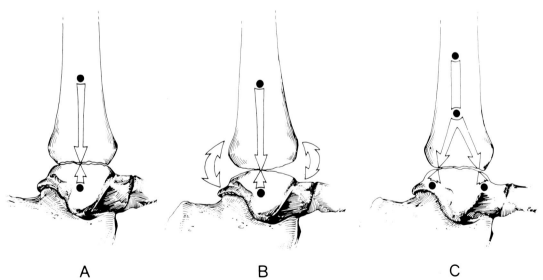

Figure 43.16. **A** and **B.** Two-pin fixation with uneven bone surfaces can create instability. **C.** Triangular compression or the four-pin Muller device creates increased osseous stability, although pin placement in the talus may be difficult in a small foot. (From Williams J, Marcinko D, Lazerson A, Elleby D: The Calandruccio triangular compression device. *J Am Podiatry Assoc* 73:536-539, 1983.)

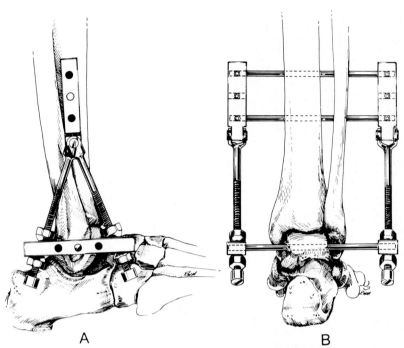

A   B

Figure 43.17. Lateral and posterior view of Calandruccio triangular compression device. (From Williams J, Marcinko D, Lazerson A, Elleby D:

The Calandruccio triangular compression device. *J Am Podiatry Assoc* 73:536-539, 1983.)

tion. Several devices are available for achieving external compression fixation. It is particularly critical in the one-plane fixation generated by most external fixators of the ankle that the bone surfaces be completely flush. Uneven bone surfaces may allow motion or creation of a hinge effect, particularly in two-pin fixation devices (Fig. 43.16).

The Charnley, Hoffman, Muller four-pin, Muller two-pin, and Calandruccio devices are examples of external fixators (Fig. 43.17). Scranton and associates (48) have noted poor results with use of the Charnley apparatus. The Hoffman device is rather large and is better suited to more proximal uses, although it has been used for ankle fusion (50-52). The four-pin Muller and the Calandruccio devices require placement of two pins in the talus. Therefore these devices must be used with caution in a foot with a small talus because of the danger of penetrating the medial neurovascular bundle. In the small talus this can be difficult. It may also be necessary to resect the posteroinferior aspect of the fibula to prevent pin impingement when the talus and the tibia are compressed (41) (Fig. 43.18).

The small two-pin Muller device does not provide as much rigidity as the larger devices, although patient acceptance is higher (Fig. 43.19). The talar pin should be placed slightly anterior to the ankle joint axis to prevent anterior gravity distraction (53). An aiming device can be used to assist with pin placement. This ensures that the pins are parallel and that they are placed at an angle of 15° of external rotation (Fig. 43.20). The pins must not transfix an intact malleolus because that will prevent the motion between the talus and the tibia necessary to generate compression. Pins should not

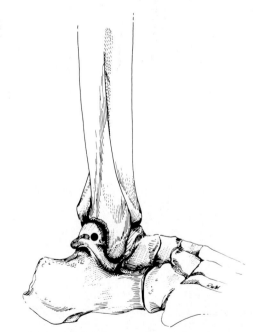

Figure 43.18. Resection of the lateral malleolus may be necessary to retard pin impingement with devices that use two pins in the talus. (From Williams J, Marcinko D, Lazerson A, Elleby D: The Calandruccio triangular compression device. *J Am Podiatry Assoc* 73:536-539, 1983.)

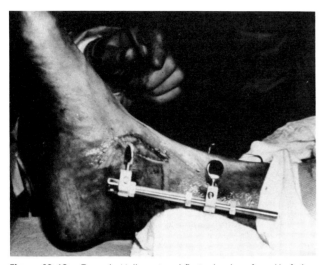

Figure 43.19.   Two-pin Muller external fixator in place for ankle fusion.

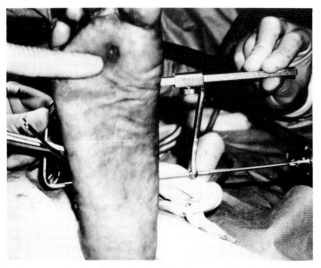

Figure 43.20.   An aiming device facilitates correct positioning of the external fixator pins. Note the transverse plane external rotation of the pin.

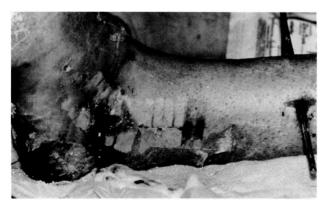

Figure 43.21.   Pin tract infection and drainage in the distal pin of a Charnley external fixator.

be placed through the calcaneus unless the subtalar joint is also being fused.

External fixators are usually maintained in position for 6 to 10 weeks, followed by another month of casting. The fixators are removed while the patient is under heavy sedation or general anesthesia. Meticulous care of the pin sites is critical, particularly when one considers the high incidence of pin tract infections (40) (Fig. 43.21). Cleansing with hydrogen peroxide and application of povidone-iodine ointment are essential for good pin care. To prevent the development of a forefoot equinus, the forefoot should be supported with a posterior splint, cast, or metatarsal transfixion pins attached to the conventional frame.

INTERNAL FIXATION TECHNIQUES

Various techniques that use internal fixation to produce compression arthrodesis of the ankle have been described. The recent literature has provided a variety of new techniques that use internal fixation. Scranton and associates (48) performed extensive research on the mechanical stability of the Charnley device, the Royal Air Force procedure, and a T-plate compression device. The external fixator generated massive interfragmental compression but provided almost no rotatory stability. Malposition of the talar pin was common in the clinical series, and this significantly reduced the effectiveness of the fixation. This led their group to develop plate fixation of the fusion. The T-plate can be applied medially or laterally, although medial placement was more common in their series. Two cortical screws are used to attach the plate to the talus, and three screws are used proximally on the tibia. It would appear that prebending of the plate along with additional stabilization with pins or wires would be necessary to prevent gaping opposite the plate. Scranton's clinical series with the plate fixation was small; however, the mechanical testing of the device is impressive.

In 1985 Scranton (54) reported the results of the above technique in 25 patients. All patients went on to achieve fusion, and Scranton reported that he now routinely uses this technique.

Internal fixation with the use of screws to create static interfragmentary compression has also been employed. Wanger and Pock (55) described the use of two to three 6.5 mm cancellous screws. Morgan and associates (56) (1985) reported a series of 101 ankle fusions in which they used two crossing cortical screws into the talus, one each from the tibia and the fibula. No malleolar osteotomy was performed, and the authors report that they now use cancellous screws in the technique. The nonunion rate was only 5%.

Gschwend and Steiger (3) modified the technique of Wagner and Pock by performing an osteotomy of the fibula for exposure and fixing it to the tibia and the talus as an onlay graft. Dennis and associates (57) (1990) used a similar technique and reported a 94% fusion rate in 16 patients.

Sowa and Krackow (58) (1989) described a different form of internal fixation ankle arthrodesis. From a lateral and anteromedial approach, they use a modified pediatric blade plate and an onlay fibular strut to achieve compression arthrodesis. They reported a union rate of 94% in 17 patients.

COMPARISON OF TECHNIQUES: INTERNAL VERSUS EXTERNAL FIXATION

There is no question that there is no single best approach or technique for all patients who require ankle fusion. One patient may need only joint resection, whereas another patient may require extensive wedging or grafting. Fixation is only one element of a procedure, but it is clearly an extremely important component. Therefore it is useful to review the characteristics of both internal and external fixation of ankle fusions to facilitate the selection of the appropriate technique.

External fixation has been the most common fixation technique for ankle fusion. It is well suited for the ankle because of the anatomy of the region. The fixator can generate substantial static interfragmentary compression because of the perpendicular relationship to the joint. The technique is relatively straightforward for those with experience in ankle surgery, although apposition of the fusion surfaces is quite critical. With external fixation, the compression can be adjusted during the postoperative period. This is not usually important for ankle fusion because of the relatively short period of time that the fixator is in place. It becomes more important for tibial fractures and other injuries where the device will be in place for a substantial period of time. With internal fixation, the result achieved on the table cannot be modified without reoperation, making intraoperative radiographs even more important.

Frequent pin tract infections, occasionally requiring reoperation, have been reported with external fixators (40). This requires vigilance on the part of the surgeon to ensure that a deep infection does not occur. Proper surgical technique (i.e., to avoid burning the skin with power equipment) and aggressive pin care can go a long way toward preventing pin tract infections. This problem is clearly not encountered with internal fixation, although one must be cautious about burying metal beneath atrophic skin.

Patient acceptance can be a problem with external fixators, particularly the larger devices. To most patients the devices can appear unwieldy, painful, and unsightly. Ankle fusion is most commonly an elective procedure, and good patient education is required so that the patient understands the nature and function of the device. The acceptance of internal fixation is much greater because the devices are not visible. However, patients must still be properly prepared so that they understand the nature of the implanted devices.

Although external fixators are capable of producing a great deal of interfragmentary compression, they do lack rotatory stability, as demonstrated by Scranton and associates (48). Therefore, these fixators are not superior to internal techniques on the basis of fixation properties. Crossed lag screws (e.g., 6.5 mm) generate substantial interfragmentary compression, resist anteroposterior forces better than the T-plate fixation of Scranton, and resist rotatory motion. Hagen (1986) notes that two-pin external fixators

"afford stability in only one plane and do not give rigid immobilization" (59).

The Podiatry Institute technique for internal fixation of ankle fusions has proved useful for almost a decade in the experience of many surgeons. It is the first choice in most situations. External fixation continues to be useful in patients with skin loss or atrophy, extensive osteoporosis, or in certain situations in which extensive bone grafting is required.

FOLLOW-UP CARE

Unsupported weight bearing should be delayed until fusion has occurred. The incompletely fused ankle is under tremendous strain and is incapable of resisting the forces of weight bearing. Supported weight bearing may begin earlier. When the patient is ready for ambulation, shoe modifications may be necessary, including a rocker-bottom sole and a heel lift (60).

PANTALAR FUSION

Pantalar fusion consists of fusion of the ankle, subtalar, and midtarsal joints. Lorthioir (61) originally described the procedure in 1911 as fusion of the ankle, subtalar, and talonavicular joints. The calcaneocuboid joint is now usually included in the procedure. Pantalar fusion is most often indicated when the subtalar joint is already degenerated and/or painful or when the rearfoot as well as the ankle is grossly unstable, such as can occur in poliomyelitis. Congenital equinovarus deformity is also a frequent indication. Pain, instability, and deformity are the three general indications for pantalar arthrodesis.

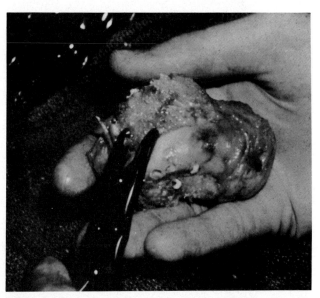

Figure 43.22. Intraoperative photograph demonstrating denuding of the talus before reinsertion as free bone graft in a Hunt-Thompson pantalar arthrodesis.

The procedure can be performed as either one-stage or two-stage (triple arthrodesis, ankle fusion) surgery. Liebolt (62) recommended that the procedure be performed in two stages because of the length of the surgery and the difficulty in correcting the deformity at all of the joints at one time. Although the procedure is undoubtedly more lengthy and complicated than ankle fusion alone, a surgeon experienced in the area will not have difficulty completing the procedure in one stage. It has been thoroughly demonstrated that there is no difference in fusion rates between the one-stage and two-stage procedures (63-67).

Lorthioir (61) and Hunt and Thompson (67) performed pantalar fusion by temporarily extirpating the talus, denuding it of cartilage and soft tissues, and replacing it in position as a free bone graft (Fig. 43.22). This technique creates less shortening, as less bone is removed to create flush surfaces. The stripping of blood supply to the talus does not appear to create problems in the sensitive foot, according to Barrett and associates (63). However, these authors reported a 50% increase in avascular necrosis and nonunion when extirpation of the talus was performed on the insensitive foot.

Steindler (68), in 1923, and Waugh and associates (69), in 1965, described one-stage pantalar fusion without removal of the talus. The procedure can be performed quite well with this technique. An extended lateral hockey-stick incision can be used for exposure of the ankle, subtalar, and calcaneocuboid joints. A medial incision is used for exposure of medial malleolar cartilage and the talonavicular joint. Internal fixation can be employed, with heavy cancellous screws traversing the ankle and subtalar joints, or the subtalar joint can be fixed separately with a 6.5 mm screw through the neck of the talus (Fig. 43.23). External fixation is performed with transverse pins in the tibia and calcaneus and the talus compressed between the two. With fusion of so many joints at one time, position must be perfect. Any time spent ensuring precise optimum position is well invested. Intraoperative radiographs are mandatory. Consolidation will take 3 to 4 months, although some authors report consolidation time approaching 7 to 9 months (67).

Pantalar fusion is quite successful in the flail or deformed sensitive foot with a stable knee (63, 66, 70, 71). However, the neurotrophic foot presents a myriad of problems including a high rate of initial nonunion and breakdown of surrounding joints after fusion of the ankle (63). Stuart and Morrey (64) report only 38% satisfactory results in ankle fusions performed on diabetic patients with radiographic evidence of neuropathic arthropathy.

BLAIR FUSION

Fusion in patients with avascular necrosis of the talus is difficult and unpredictable. The Blair fusion is a sliding graft

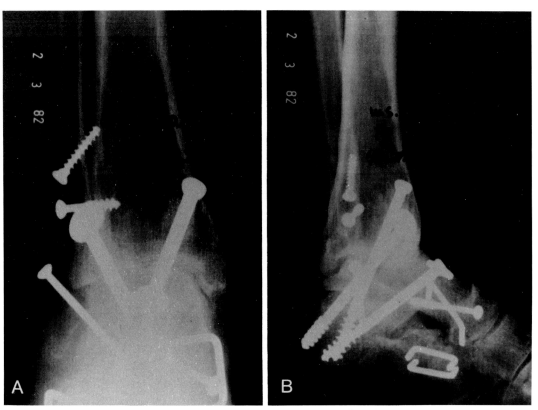

Figure 43.23. Pantalar fusion with internal fixation. **A.** Anteroposterior ankle view. **B.** Lateral view of foot and ankle. The midtarsal joint may also be fixed by means of large 6.5 mm cancellous screws.

from the tibia into the neck of the talus (45). Lionberger and associates (46) have described a modification that involves compression fixation of the tibia to the talar neck.

FUSION IN CHILDREN

When indicated, fusion in a child should be delayed until the child has reached the age of 8 (62) to 12 years (67). The distal tibial epiphyseal plate should be preserved. This can be done with the interpositional graft technique of Chuinard and Peterson (12) (Fig. 43.4). Compression should not be generated across the epiphyseal plate. Because of the continued growth of the foot and leg in the child, any error in execution of the fusion can be exaggerated with time (72). Wang and associates (73) reviewed 20 ankle fusions in children and observed the following: *(a)* growth status is not affected if the procedure is performed properly, *(b)* there is a high rate of nonunions when a bone graft is not used, and *(c)* procedures performed on patients under the age of 10 resulted in more complications and were more unpredictable.

ALTERNATIVE PROCEDURES

There are three alternatives to ankle fusion: implant arthroplasty, bone block procedures, and tendon anchoring. A number of devices have been used clinically for ankle joint replacement with some limited success (74-81). Newton (82) states that indications for ankle replacement with his design include *(a)* osteoarthritis in an ankle with good ligamentous stability, reasonably normal anatomy, and no significant frontal plane deformity, and *(b)* pain in rheumatoid arthritis patients who are not on long-term steroids and who have no significant bone erosions. McGuire and associates (83) (1988) reported poor results with total ankle arthroplasty in young patients with posttraumatic arthrosis.

Contraindications include significant talar tilt, failed ankle fusion, significant deformity, and avascular necrosis of the talus. The present indications for ankle replacement are quite limited.

Bone block procedures are somewhat intermediate in character and can be useful for the treatment of anterior group paralysis. These procedures are not useful in painful degenerative joint disease of the ankle. Some ankle motion is preserved (in contrast to fusion), but excess plantarflexion is blocked, preventing tripping. Campbell (84) described a procedure to raise shelves of bone from the calcaneus to the posterior aspect of the ankle and subtalar joints (85). This effectively limits plantarflexion, although subtalar motion is also compromised. Gill (86) described a bone block consisting of transfer of a wedge of bone from the calcaneus posteriorly to the posterior aspect of the talus, where it functions to block plantarflexion.

Tendon checkrein procedures have limited indications for the treatment of dropfoot. A nonfunctional anterior group tendon can be attached to the tibia under some tension to limit excess plantarflexion. Elongation of the soft tissues limits the time period that this can be functional.

COMPLICATIONS AND FAILURE

The literature regarding ankle fusions can be quite confusing. Some studies claim very few complications (28), whereas others report extensive problems (87-90). Fusion rates reported in the literature vary from 92.8% (28) to 50% in insensitive feet with pantalar fusion by talar extirpation (63). Most reports give a fusion rate of 80% to 85% (89), although in the author's experience it has been somewhat higher. This varies with the surgeon, the type of fusion, and many other factors (91-95). Appropriate treatment is based on the cause of the nonunion and may include bone grafting, electrical stimulation, and additional compression fixation (Fig. 43.24).

Infection has been reported to be present more than 20%

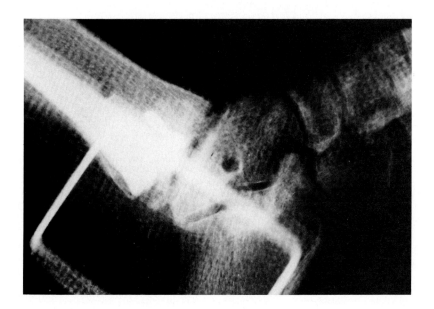

Figure 43.24. Nonunion of an ankle fusion successfully treated with an electrical stimulation device. (Note the outline of the locator block incorporated into the cast.)

of the time (87, 90). This is an unacceptable rate of infection. The author has not seen deep infection occur after ankle or pantalar fusion. It may be desirable to use short-term antibiotic prophylaxis because of the operating time required and the serious consequences that could occur with deep infection.

Other complications have also been reported. Davis and Millis (87) reported that 12% of the patients in their series went on to below-the-knee amputation and 56% of the patients had significant limitation of subtalar motion. Johnson and Boseker (88) reported an overall complication rate of 60%, although most of these complications were minor. Ahlberg and Henricson (6) reported that 68% of the patients in their series had long-term postoperative pain of some type.

Even though these reports do not reflect the author's experience with complications after ankle or pantalar fusion, they do serve to emphasize the major nature of this surgery. Patients should be well prepared for the surgery and should have a good understanding of the objectives and limitations of the procedure.

SUMMARY

Ankle and pantalar fusion has proved to be effective, time-tested procedures. Relief of pain and improvement in the ability to function in daily activities are reasonable expectations for patients undergoing these procedures. Limitation of activity when barefoot and subtalar symptoms may be seen.

References

1. Ramsey PL, Hamilton W: Changes in tibiotalar area of contact caused by lateral talar shift. *J Bone Joint Surg* 58A:356-357, 1976.
2. Stiehl J, Dollinger B: Primary ankle arthrodesis in trauma: report of three cases. *J Orthop Trauma* 2:277-283, 1989.
3. Gschwend N, Steiger U: Stable fixation in hindfoot arthrodesis, a valuable procedure in the complex RA foot. *Rheumatology* 11:114-125, 1987.
4. Iwata H, Yasuhara N, Kawashima K, Kaneko M, Sugiura Y, Nakagawa M: Arthrodesis of the ankle joint with rheumatoid arthritis. *Clin Orthop* 153:189-193, 1980.
5. Mahan K: Wound healing in the rheumatoid patient. In McGlamry ED, McGlamry R (eds): *Categoric Foot Rehabilitation, Fourteenth Annual Surgical Seminar*. Atlanta, Doctors Hospital Podiatric Education and Research Institute, 1985, pp 71-73.
6. Ahlberg A, Henricson A: Late results of ankle fusion. *Acta Orthop Scand* 52:103-105, 1981.
7. Jackson A: Tarsal hypermobility after ankle fusion—fact or fiction. *J Bone Joint Surg* 61B:470-473, 1979.
8. Mazur J, Schwartz E, Simon S: Ankle arthrodesis: long-term follow-up with gait analysis. *J Bone Joint Surg* 61A:964-975, 1979.
9. Charnley J: Compression arthrodesis of the ankle. In Charnley J (ed): *Compression Arthrodesis*. London, E & S Livingstone Ltd, 1953, p 133.
10. Goldthwait J: An operation for the stiffening of the ankle joint in infantile paralysis. *Am J Orthop Surg* 5:271-279, 1908.
11. Hallock H: Arthrodesis of the ankle joint for old painful fractures. *J Bone Joint Surg* 27:49-58, 1945.
12. Chuinard E, Peterson R: Distraction-compression bone-graft arthrodesis of the ankle. *J Bone Joint Surg* 45A:481-490, 1983.
13. Wescott HH: An operation for the fusion of the tibio-astragaloid joint. *Va Med Monthly* 61:38-39, 1934.
14. Campbell CJ, Rinehart WT, Kalenak A: Arthrodesis of the ankle: deep autogenous inlay grafts with maximum cancellous-bone apposition. *J Bone Joint Surg* 56A:63-70, 1974.
15. Hatt RN: The central bone graft in joint arthrodesis. *J Bone Joint Surg* 22:393-402, 1940.
16. Brittain HA: Arthrodesis of the ankle. In Brittain HA: *Architectural Principles in Arthrodesis*. Baltimore, Williams & Wilkins, 1942, pp 58-68.
17. Soren A: Safe inlay of bone graft in arthrodesis. *Clin Orthop* 58:147-152, 1968.
18. Kennedy JC: Arthrodesis of the ankle with particular reference to the Gallie procedure. *J Bone Joint Surg* 42A:1308-1316, 1960.
19. Horwitz T: The use of the transfibular approach in arthrodesis of the ankle joint. *Am J Surg* 60:550-552, 1942.
20. Adams JC: Arthrodesis of the ankle joint: experiences with the transfibular approach. *J Bone Joint Surg* 30B:506-511, 1948.
21. Glissan DJ: The indications for inducing fusion at the ankle joint by operation with description of two successful techniques. *Aust N Z J Surg* 19:64-71, 1949.
22. Wilson HJ: Arthrodesis of the ankle: a technique using bilateral hemimalleolar onlay grafts with screw fixation. *J Bone Joint Surg* 51A:775-777, 1969.
23. Verhelst MP, Mulier J, Hoogmartens M, Spaas F: Arthrodesis of the ankle joint with complete removal of the distal part of the fibula. *Clin Orthop* 118:93, 1976.
24. Anderson R: Concentric arthrodesis of the ankle joint. *J Bone Joint Surg* 27:37-48, 1945.
25. Staples OS: Posterior arthrodesis of the ankle and subtalar joints. *J Bone Joint Surg* 38A:50-58, 1956.
26. Mead NC: Arthrodesis of the ankle joint: a simple, efficient method. *Q Bull Northwest Univ Med School* 25:248-250, 1951.
27. Marcus R, Balourdas G, Heiple K: Ankle arthrodesis by chevron fusion with internal fixation and bone grafting. *J Bone Joint Surg* 65A:833-838, 1983.
28. Stewart M, Beeler TC, McConnell JC: Compression arthrodesis of the ankle: evaluation of a cosmetic modification. *J Bone Joint Surg* 65A:219-225, 1983.
29. Bingold AC: Ankle and subtalar fusion by a transarticular graft. *J Bone Joint Surg* 38B:862-870, 1956.
30. Pridie KH: Arthrodesis of the ankle. In Proceedings and Reports of Councils and Associations. *J Bone Joint Surg* 35B:152, 1953.
31. Hone MR: Dowel fusion of the ankle joint. *J Bone Joint Surg* 50B:678, 1978.
32. Baciu C, Filibiu E: Rapid arthrodesis of the ankle joint via verticalisation of the joint space. *Arch Orthop Trauma Surg* 93:261-264, 1979.
33. Graham CE: A new method for arthrodesis of an ankle joint. *Clin Orthop* 68:75-77, 1970.
34. Ottolenghi C, Animoso J, Burgo P: Percutaneous arthrodesis of the ankle joint. *Clin Orthop* 68:72-74, 1970.
35. Gallie WE: Arthrodesis of the ankle joint. *J Bone Joint Surg* 30B:618-621, 1948.
36. Van Gorder GW, Chen C-M: The central-graft operation for fusion of tuberculous knees, ankles, and elbows. *J Bone Joint Surg* 41A:1029-1046, 1959.
37. Ratliff A: Compression arthrodesis of the ankle. *J Bone Joint Surg* 41B:524-534, 1959.
38. Thomas FB: Arthrodesis of the ankle. *J Bone Joint Surg* 51B:53-59, 1969.
39. Reinherz RP, Sharon SM, Schwartz R, Pitzer S, Knudsen HA: Modification of the Charnley approach to ankle arthrodesis. *J Am Podiatry Assoc* 69:265-268, 1979.
40. Rothacker GW, Cabanela ME: External fixation for arthrodesis of the knee and ankle. *Clin Orthop* 180:101-108, 1983.
41. Williams JE Jr, Marcinko D, Lazerson A, Elleby D: The Calandruccio triangular compression device: a schematic introduction. *J Am Podiatry Assoc* 73:536-539, 1983.
42. Charnley J: Compression arthrodesis of the ankle and shoulder. *J Bone Joint Surg* 33B:180-191, 1951.
43. White A: A precision posterior ankle fusion. *Clin Orthop* 98:239-250, 1974.
44. Carmack JC, Hallock HH: Tibiotarsal arthrodesis after astragalectomy. *J Bone Joint Surg* 29:476-482, 1947.

45. Dennis MD, Tullos HS: Blair tibiotalar arthrodesis for injuries to the talus. *J Bone Joint Surg* 62A:103-107, 1980.

46. Lionberger DR, Bishop JO, Tullos HS: The modified Blair fusion. *Foot Ankle* 3:60-62, 1982.

47. Mahan KT, Yu GV: Ankle and pantalar fusion. In McGlamry ED, McGlamry R (eds): *Comprehensive Conference in Foot Surgery, Thirteenth Annual Surgical Seminar.* Atlanta, GA, Doctors Hospital Podiatric Education and Research Institute, 1984, pp 49-51.

48. Scranton PE, Fu FH, Brown T: Ankle arthrodesis: a comparative clinical and biomechanical evaluation. *Clin Orthop* 151:234-243, 1980.

49. King H, Watkins T, Samuelson K: Analysis of foot position in ankle arthrodesis and its influence on gait. *Foot Ankle* 1:44-49, 1980.

50. Newman A: Ankle fusion with the Hoffmann external fixation device. *Foot Ankle* 1:102-109, 1980.

51. Mears DC, Behrens F: Application and use of external fixation. In Mears DC (ed): *External Skeletal Fixation.* Baltimore, Williams & Wilkins, 1983, p 161.

52. Mears DC: Nonunions, infected nonunions and arthrodeses. In Mears DC (ed): *External Skeletal Fixation.* Baltimore, Williams & Wilkins, 1983, p 93.

53. Vogler H: Ankle arthrodesis: clinical and conceptual applications. *Clin Podiatry* 2:59-80, 1985.

54. Scranton P: Use of internal compression in arthrodesis of the ankle. *J Bone Joint Surg* 67A:550-555, 1985.

55. Wagner H, Pock, HG: Die verschraubungsarthrodese der Sprunggelenke, *Unfallheilkunde* 85:280-300, 1982.

56. Morgan C, Henke J, Bailey R, Kaufer H: Long-term results of tibiotalar arthrodesis. *J Bone Joint Surg* 67A:546-550, 1985.

57. Dennis D, Clayton M, Wong D, Mack R, Susman M: Internal fixation compression arthrodesis of the ankle. *Clin Orthop* 253: 212-220, 1990.

58. Sowa D, Krackow K: Ankle fusion: a new technique of internal fixation using a compression blade plate. *Foot Ankle* 9:232-240, 1989.

59. Hagen R: Ankle arthrodesis: problems and pitfalls. *Clin Orthop* 202:152-162, 1986.

60. Baker P: Brief note: SACH heel improves results of ankle fusion. *J Bone Joint Surg* 52A:1485-1486, 1970.

61. Lorthioir J: Huit ras d'arthrodese du pied avec extirpation temporaire de l'astragala. *Ann Soc Belge Chir* 11:184-187, 1911.

62. Liebolt FL: Pantalar arthrodesis in poliomyelitis. *Surgery* 6:31-34, 1939.

63. Barrett G, Meyer L, Bray E, Taylor R, Kolb F: Pantalar arthrodesis: a long-term follow-up. *Foot Ankle* 279-283, 1980.

64. Stuart M, Morrey B: Arthrodesis of the diabetic neuropathic ankle joint. *Clin Orthop* 253:209-211, 1990.

65. Hamsa WR: Panastragaloid arthrodesis. *J Bone Joint Surg* 18:732-736, 1936.

66. Browne M: Arthrodesis of the ankle. *Bull Hosp Special Surg* 3:25-40, 1960.

67. Hunt WS, Thompson HA: Pantalar arthrodesis: a one-stage operation. *J Bone Joint Surg* 36A:349-360, 1954.

68. Steindler A: The treatment of the flail ankle: panastragaloid arthrodesis. *J Bone Joint Surg* 5:284-294, 1923.

69. Waugh T, Wayner J, Stinchfield F: An evaluation of pantalar arthrodesis. *J Bone Joint Surg* 47A:1315-1322, 1965.

70. Ansart MB: Pan-arthrodesis for paralytic flail foot. *J Bone Joint Surg* 33B:503-507, 1951.

71. Natarajan M: Pan-talar arthrodesis for post polio flail foot. *Singapore Med J* 8:214-221, 1967.

72. Turner H: Deformities of the foot associated with arthrodesis of the ankle joint performed in early childhood. *J Bone Joint Surg* 16:423-431, 1934.

73. Wang C-J, Tambakis A, Fielding J: An evaluation of ankle fusion in children. *Clin Orthop* 98:233-238, 1974.

74. DeBastiani G, Vecchini L: Arthroprosthesis of the ankle joint. *Ital J Orthop Traumatol* 7:31-39, 1981.

75. Dini AA, Bassett FH III: Evaluation of the early result of Smith total ankle replacement. *Clin Orthop* 146:228-230, 1980.

76. Evanski PM, Waugh TR: Management of arthritis of the ankle: an alternative to arthrodesis. *Clin Orthop* 122:110-115, 1977.

77. Smith CL: Physical therapy management of patients with total ankle replacement. *Phys Ther* 60:303-306, 1980.

78. Spector EE: Ankle implants. *Clin Podiatry* 1:225-235, 1984.

79. Stauffer RN, Segal NM: Total ankle arthroplasty: four years' experience. *Clin Orthop* 160:217-221, 1981.

80. Stauffer RN: Total ankle joint replacement as an alternative to arthrodesis. *Geriatrics* March:79-85, 1976.

81. Newton SE: An artificial ankle joint. *Clin Orthop* 142:141-145, 1979.

82. Newton SE: Total ankle arthroplasty: clinical study of fifty cases. *J Bone Joint Surg* 64A:104-111, 1982.

83. McGuire M, Kyle R, Gustilo R, Premer R: Comparative analysis of ankle arthroplasty versus ankle arthrodesis. *Clin Orthop* 226: 174-181, 1988.

84. Campbell WC: End results of operation for correction of drop-foot. *JAMA* 85:1927, 1925.

85. Stewart M: Arthrodesis. In Edmonson A, Crenshaw A (eds): *Campbell's Operative Orthopaedics,* vol 1. St Louis, CV Mosby, 1980, p 1100.

86. Gill AB: An operation to make a posterior bone block at the ankle to limit foot-drop. *J Bone Joint Surg* 15:166, 1933.

87. Davis R, Millis M: Ankle arthrodesis in the management of traumatic ankle arthrosis: a long-term retrospective study. *J Trauma* 20:674-678, 1980.

88. Johnson E, Boseker E: Arthrodesis of the ankle. *Arch Surg* 97:766-773, 1968.

89. Lance E, Paral A, Fries I, Larsen I, Patterson R: Arthrodesis of the ankle joint: a follow up study. *Clin Orthop* 142:146-158, 1979.

90. Morrey B, Wiedeman G: Complications and long-term results of ankle arthrodeses following trauma. *J Bone Joint Surg* 62A:777-784, 1980.

91. Kivilaakso R, Langenskiold A, Salenius P: Arthrodesis of the ankle as a treatment for post-fracture conditions. *Acta Orthop Scand* 37:409-414, 1966.

92. Poss K, Kaplan EG, Kaplan G: Talectomy leading to an ankle fusion: a case history. *J Foot Surg* 18:76-80, 1979.

93. Said E, Hunka L, Sillger T: Where ankle fusion stands today. *J Bone Joint Surg* 60B:211-214, 1978.

94. Wagner FW: Ankle fusion for degenerative arthritis secondary to the collagen diseases. *Foot Ankle* 3:24-31, 1982.

95. Stauffer RN: Salvage of painful total ankle arthroplasty. *Clin Orthop* 170:184-188, 1982.

Additional References

Lynch A, Bourne R, Rorabeck C: The long-term results of ankle arthrodesis. *J Bone Joint Surg* 70B:113-116, 1988.

Helm R: The results of ankle arthrodesis. *J Bone Joint Surg* 72B:141-143, 1990.

Buck P, Morrey B, Chao E: The optimum position of arthrodesis of the ankle. *J Bone Joint Surg* 69A:1052-1062, 1987.

Russotti G, Johnson K, Cass J: Tibiocalcaneal arthrodesis for arthritis and deformity of the hind part of the foot. *J Bone Joint Surg* 70A:1304-1307, 1988.

Campbell P: Arthrodesis of the ankle with modified distraction-compression and bone grafting. *J Bone Joint Surg* 72A:552-556, 1990.

Special Surgery

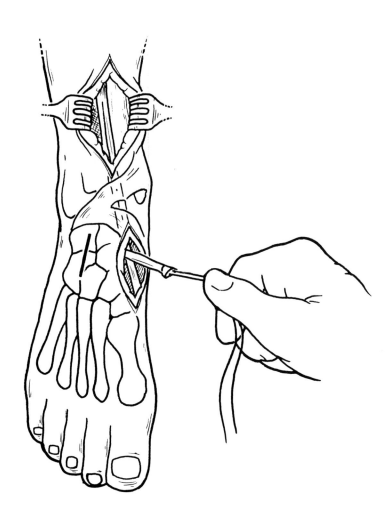

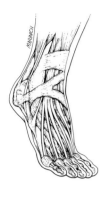

CHAPTER **44**

Acquired Neuropathies of the Lower Extremities

D. Scot Malay, D.P.M.
E. Dalton McGlamry, D.P.M.
Chester A. Nava, Jr., D.P.M.*

Acquired neuropathies in the lower extremities are common, and there are no nerves in the foot or leg that are immune to injury by entrapment, compression, traction, laceration, or incarceration in scar. Although the term *nerve entrapment* is frequently used to describe any type of localized acquired peripheral nerve trunk lesion, Kopell and Thompson (1) classically describe entrapment neuropathy as "a region of localized injury and inflammation in a peripheral nerve that is caused by mechanical irritation from some impinging anatomic neighbor." In practice, there are many local causes of acquired peripheral neuropathy, and clinical signs and symptoms vary according to the extent of neural damage and the specific nerve trunk involved. Although the literature is replete with reviews of the classic nerve entrapment syndromes (2, 3), there is still much to be learned about the diagnosis and treatment of the wide variety of painful and disabling acquired neuropathies that affect the lower extremities.

Anatomically speaking, all peripheral nerve trunks are mixed nerves containing sensory, motor, and autonomic fibers. Approximately 50% of the peripheral nerve trunk is made up of connective tissue (4) (Fig. 44.1). It is this intraneural connective tissue element that, when appropriately stimulated, may proliferate and disrupt the internal continuity of the nerve trunk. Resultant intraneural fibrosis, combined with extraneural scarring, may cause symptomatic neuritis. Diagnosis of such a nerve lesion requires a thorough knowledge of the segmental (dermatomal), as well as the specific cutaneous, nerve supply to the lower extremity (Fig. 44.2). Furthermore, an understanding of the motor innervation to the lower extremity aids in diagnosis when muscle weakness is present (Table 44.1).

ETIOLOGY OF LOCALIZED ACQUIRED PERIPHERAL NEUROPATHY

Localized acquired peripheral neuropathy may develop after acute gross trauma or recurrent microtrauma induced

by either endogenous or exogenous sources. The trauma induces an inflammatory response that infiltrates the nerve trunk and surrounding tissues. The gross continuity of the nerve trunk is generally maintained, and the nerve may swell proximal to the point of injury or constriction (5). In cases of nerve entrapment, a fusiform or eccentric neuroma incontinuity usually develops at the point of impingement. Intraneural fibrosis subsequently proceeds to disrupt axonal organization and impulse conduction, thereby inhibiting axonal remyelination (6). Distal Wallerian degeneration may ensue, and actual myxoid degeneration of intraneural connective tissue with multifocal ganglion formation may occur (7-10). Extraneural scarring and adhesion (perineural fibrosis) aggravate the neuritis, and as extraneural fibrosis and resultant compression progress, occlusion of the vasa nervorum ensues. Nerve ischemia adds to further degeneration, decreased conduction, and increased symptoms. The natural history of the untreated localized acquired peripheral neuropathy is unpredictable. Symptoms may spontaneously worsen, resolve, or resolve only to recur on an intermittent basis.

A variety of mechanisms cause localized acquired peripheral neuropathy (Table 44.2). Endogenous or spontaneous entrapments are very common. These develop after neighboring anatomical structures have repeatedly microtraumatized the adjacent nerve trunk by means of direct pressure and inhibition of normal peripheral nerve mobility. Neighboring anatomical structures include muscle bellies and fibrous bands, osseous surfaces, and combinations of soft tissue and bone. Congenital anatomical relationships become a source of nerve compression because of developmental anomalies or abnormal circumstances, such as conditions of overuse that surpass the nerve's ability to adapt to changes in the local environment. This concept has been referred to as the stress anatomy of a particular nerve trunk and pertains to conditions of excessive tension or compression on a nerve associated with motion of the extremity (1).

Other endogenous mechanisms of localized acquired peripheral neuropathy include neoplastic disorders, such as metastatic infiltration (11), neurilemoma (schwannoma) (12-18), ganglion cyst (8-10, 19), varix, and lipoma, to name a few. Moreover, microvascular dysfunction and subcuta-

*Appreciation is expressed to Chester A. Nava, Jr., D.P.M., who, along with D. Scot Malay, D.P.M., and E. Dalton McGlamry, D.P.M., wrote this chapter in the first edition.

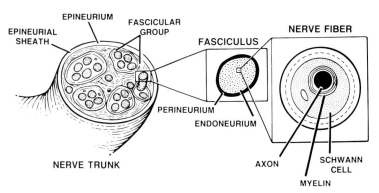

Figure 44.1. Peripheral nerve trunk functional and structural anatomy.

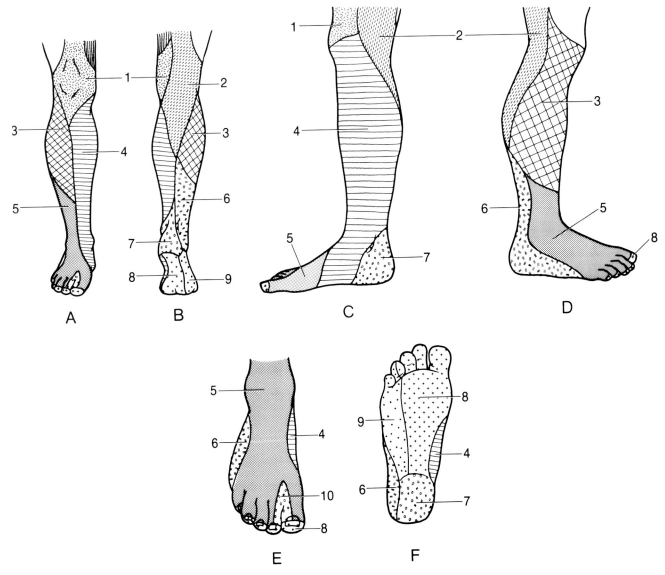

Figure 44.2. Peripheral nerve distribution. **A.** Anterior. **B.** Posterior. **C.** Medial. **D.** Lateral. **E.** Dorsal. **F.** Plantar. *1,* Medial and intermediate femoral cutaneous nerves (L2, 3). *2,* Posterior femoral cutaneous nerve (S1, 2, 3). *3,* Lateral sural cutaneous nerve (L5, S1, 2). *4,* Saphenous nerve (L3, 4). *5,* Superficial peroneal nerve (L4, 5, S1). *6,* Sural nerve (L5, S1, 2). *7,* Medial calcaneal branch of tibial nerve (S1, 2). *8,* Medial plantar nerve (L4, 5). *9,* Lateral plantar nerve (S1, 2). *10,* Deep peroneal nerve (L4, 5).

Table 44.1.
Motor Innervation to the Leg and Foot

Muscle	Peripheral Nerve	Spinal Level	Muscle	Peripheral Nerve	Spinal Level
Tibialis anterior	Deep peroneal	$L_{4,5}$	Abductor hallucis	Medial plantar	$S_{2,3}$
Extensor digitorum longus	Deep peroneal	$L_{4,5}$	Flexor digitorum brevis	Medial plantar	$S_{2,3}$
Extensor hallucis longus	Deep peroneal	$L_{4,5}$	First lumbricalis	Medial plantar	$S_{2,3}$
Peroneus tertius	Deep peroneal	$L_{4,5}$	Flexor hallucis brevis	Medial plantar	$S_{2,3}$
Gastrocnemius	Tibial	$S_{1,2}$	Abductor digiti quinti brevis	Lateral plantar	$S_{2,3}$
Soleus	Tibial	$S_{1,2}$	Quadratus plantae	Lateral plantar	$S_{2,3}$
Plantaris	Tibial	$S_{1,2}$	Second, third, fourth lumbricales	Lateral plantar	$S_{2,3}$
Popliteus	Tibial	$L_{4,5}S_1$	Adductor hallucis	Lateral plantar	$S_{2,3}$
Flexor hallucis longus	Tibial	$S_{2,3}$	Flexor digiti quinti brevis	Lateral plantar	$S_{2,3}$
Flexor digitorum longus	Tibial	$S_{2,3}$	Plantar interossei	Lateral plantar	$S_{2,3}$
Tibialis posterior	Tibial	$L_{4,5}$	Dorsal interossei		
Peroneus longus	Superficial peroneal	$L_5S_{1,2}$	First, second	Deep peroneal, lateral plantar	$S_{1,2,3}$
Peroneus brevis	Superficial peroneal	$L_5, S_{1,2}$	Third, fourth	Lateral plantar	$S_{2,3}$
Extensor digitorum brevis	Deep peroneal	$S_{1,2}$			

Table 44.2.
Etiology of Localized Acquired Peripheral Neuropathy

Endogenous	Exogenous

I. Congenital
  A. Anomalous development
  B. Overuse
	I. Traumatic
	  A. Laceration
	  B. Blunt trauma
	  C. Fracture/dislocation
	  D. Traction
	  E. Injection
	    1. Puncture
	    2. Chemical

II. Neoplastic
  A. Varix
  B. Ganglion cyst
  C. Lipoma
  D. Neurilemoma (schwannoma)
  E. Metastatic infiltration
	II. Iatrogenic
	  A. Tourniquet compression
	  B. Surgical positioning
	  C. Cast or bandage constriction
	  D. Surgical technique
	    1. Incision planning
	    2. Dissection
	    3. Hemostasis
	    4. Nerve handling
	    5. Suturing

III. Metabolic
  A. Diabetes mellitus
  B. Rheumatoid arthritis and other connective tissue diseases
  C. Peripheral vascular disease
  D. Thyroid dysfunction
  E. Hyperlipidemia
  F. Drug toxicity
	III. Infectious
	  A. Local abscess
	  B. Postinflammatory fibrosis

neous atrophy complicating such metabolic disorders as rheumatoid arthritis and other connective tissue disorders, diabetes mellitus, peripheral vascular disease (19), hyperlipidemia (20), and hypothyroidism may act as endogenous causes of peripheral nerve entrapment.

Exogenous causes of localized acquired peripheral neuropathy are also variable (Table 44.2). Gross traumatic episodes, including nerve trunk laceration (21-23), blunt trauma and compartment syndrome (24, 25), fracture or dislocation, injection injury (4, 26-30), and excessive traction with resultant intraneural hematoma, have been implicated (31-33). There are also many iatrogenic causes of nerve entrapment including tourniquet compression (34, 35), improper positioning of the anesthetized patient during surgery, bandage or cast pressure (36), and surgical technique (34, 37, 38). Postoperative scarring secondary to normal wound healing may also create an acquired neuropathy, even after proper incision planning, layer dissection, hemostasis, nerve manipulation, and wound closure. Finally, local infection causing postinflammatory fibrosis may effect peripheral entrapment neuropathy.

DIFFERENTIAL DIAGNOSIS

In general, the distribution of pain proximal to the point of nerve damage may make the accurate diagnosis of localized acquired peripheral neuropathy very difficult. In all cases one must distinguish lower extremity nerve entrapment from lumbosacral radiculopathy. In fact, a major diagnostic dilemma exists in the case of suspected nerve entrapment associated with unrelated lumbosacral arthritis (39). Furthermore, autonomic overtones with vasoconstriction, decreased skin temperature, distal cyanosis, and development of causalgia-like pain and reflex sympathetic dystrophy can easily cloud the clinical picture (40, 41). Similarly chronic tenosynovitis or a smoldering infection (abscess or osteomyelitis) may mimic the pain of nerve entrapment. Patients who may stand to secondarily gain from their symptomatic condition also pose a diagnostic problem. Finally, peripheral polyneuropathy associated with metabolic, toxic, or infectious processes must also be included in the differential diagnosis.

SIGNS, SYMPTOMS, AND DIAGNOSIS

The key diagnostic criterion associated with localized acquired peripheral neuropathy is pain created by irritation of a specific nerve. The pathologic condition may affect the entire nerve trunk or asymmetrically involve only a portion of its diameter. Sensory abnormalities tend to predominate over motor dysfunction. Pain is usually well localized over the sensory distribution of the involved nerve and typically has the nature of a sharp or burning sensation. Dysesthesia, hypesthesia, and hyperesthesia may also be present.

Pain associated with an entrapped motor component of the nerve is typically less well defined in terms of its distribution. Motor nerve pain takes the form of a dull, aching sensation associated with the muscle and joint innervated by the involved nerve. In the advanced case severe muscle tenderness may result in disuse atrophy and weakness. Pain caused by peripheral nerve entrapment is usually aggravated by limb motion and patient activity. Rest pain is also a frequent finding in chronic cases and may be severely debilitating.

The actual diagnosis of localized acquired peripheral neuropathy is made after a thorough history and physical examination. The patient may not recall a specific traumatic event to which the onset of signs and symptoms may be attributable. Objective evaluation centers around the sensorimotor examination (42). Decreased two-point tactile distinction over the sensory distribution of the involved nerve is an early finding. Usually, if the nerve trunk is not too deeply situated, palpation or percussion of the nerve at the suspected point of irritation can elicit pain and paresthesia. Distal radiation of pain and paresthesia along the sensory distribution of the nerve, Tinel's sign, is usually present from the early stages of localized acquired neuropathy. The Valleix sign, or proximal radiation of pain and paresthesia along the neuraxis on percussion at the point of nerve injury, may also be present. Moreover, active or passive manipulation of the extremity may exacerbate symptoms. Manual muscle testing is usually not very helpful unless the neuropathy is seriously advanced and muscle pain and atrophy are present. In the difficult case, nerve conduction velocity and electromyographic measurements may be helpful. Conduction velocity is decreased in most cases of nerve entrapment, whereas electromyography is of little use unless nearly complete conduction blockade is present (41). Electrodiagnostic findings should not override one's clinical assessment, because both nerve conduction velocity and electromyography vary with the patient's age, skin temperature, and other conditions that may effect false-negative values. Finally, diagnostic local steroid injection, combined with a local anesthetic agent, may be used as part of the evaluation. The local anesthetic rapidly inhibits impulse conduction, while the glucosteroid alleviates both perineural and intraneural inflammation and fibrosis when infiltrated around the nerve trunk. Immediate and dramatic resolution of symptoms indicates accurate localization of the nerve trunk lesion. Dramatic relief of symptoms is usually associated with a decrease in the local inflammatory process. Dramatic relief followed by recurrence of symptoms after a period of time points toward deep diffuse scarring or a permanent anatomical structure as the cause of nerve dysfunction.

PROGNOSIS, TREATMENT, COMPLICATIONS

Because a significant proportion of the anatomical continuity of the involved nerve trunk is usually preserved, the prognosis after nonsurgical treatment of localized acquired peripheral neuropathy is relatively good (21). Prognosis varies with the patient's age, cause and extent of the nerve defect, and location and duration of the lesion. The younger the patient, the more distal the site of injury; the shorter the duration of symptoms, the better the prognosis. In general, after 6 weeks the risk of peripheral nerve changes secondary to continued degeneration outweighs the risks associated with corrective surgical intervention (4).

Conservative measures should initially include removal of any direct extrinsic compression or tension placed on the nerve trunk and the use of nonsteroidal anti-inflammatory drugs (NSAIDs). Abnormal mechanical stress should be alleviated with the use of orthoses, careful casting or splinting, or application of a desensitizing shield as indicated (Fig. 44.3). Immobilization for 7 to 10 days to prevent any motion that may be perpetuating local inflammation, and hence nerve irritation, is often beneficial. Local infiltration of steroid (triamcinolone acetonide or some other highly soluble steroid) combined with a local anesthetic at the site of entrapment is very useful and is a mainstay of conservative therapy (38, 43). Perineural infiltration of glucosteroid decreases both intraneural and extraneural inflammation and fibrosis, allowing axonal reorganization and remyelination within the nerve trunk. The addition of hyaluronidase to the injected solution has also been reported to enhance

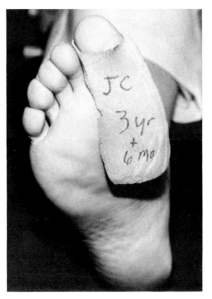

Figure 44.3. Polyurethane desensitization shield worn by 59-year-old woman with painful entrapment of the medial plantar nerve at the first metatarsophalangeal joint after hallux valgus repair. Complete symptomatic relief had been experienced for 3 years and 6 months following application of the shield as a therapeutic trial. The shield protected the hyperesthetic area from external stimuli and aided in softening scar tissue.

breakdown of perineural fibrosis, especially in cases involving hypertrophic scars (44). Electroacupuncture has also been reported to be of use in the treatment of recalcitrant stump neuromas (45).

In cases in which denervation is severe, range-of-motion exercises and electrical nerve stimulation may be used to maintain joint function and muscle tone. Generally, after neuroma formation caused by acute or chronic injury by means of entrapment, crush or contusion, partial laceration, or previous nerve suture, axon regeneration distalward through the area of injury takes about 7 to 14 days. Thereafter the nerve regenerates at the rate of approximately 1 mm per day or 1 inch per month, calculated by measuring the distance from the point of injury to the muscle belly or end organ being tested (46). Conservative therapy is continued if pain is alleviated, sensorium returns, and conduction velocity improves.

If the pain of entrapment is disabling and fails to respond to conservative treatment, if the clinical picture worsens with advancing sensory loss that threatens position sense or weight-bearing sensation, or if motor weakness and atrophy develop, then surgical intervention is indicated. At this point, the risk of permanent nerve damage far exceeds the risk of surgical intervention (4). It is important to inform the patient that symptoms may recur, or worsen, or that disturbing anesthesia may result after surgery. The primary surgical goal is pain relief.

Surgical management of localized acquired peripheral neuropathy evolves primarily around external neurolysis. It is most important to localize normal nerve trunk, either proximal or distal to a region of scar entrapment, in order to expedite and make adequate external neurolysis possible. After exposure of the involved nerve trunk, and before complete external neurolysis is performed, intraoperative electrical nerve stimulation both proximal and distal to the nerve trunk lesion or point of entrapment may be used to produce distal motor activity and thereby aid in evaluation of the degree of conduction blockade. External neurolysis entails freeing the entrapped nerve from any impinging local structures, incising any adjacent fibrous bands and, when present, dissecting and mobilizing the nerve trunk from surrounding scar tissue. Thorough inspection consists of visual and palpatory examination. Typically, some form of indurated neuroma incontinuity exists. Terminal bulb neuromas (amputation or stump neuromas) may also be present, especially when small branching sensory fibers are entangled in diffuse scar following previous surgery or trauma. This condition is often associated with recurrent intermetatarsal neuroma. Less commonly the nerve trunk appears completely normal; however, palpation reveals pathologic intraneural fibrosis.

Once an incontinuity nerve lesion is isolated, intraoperative direct nerve stimulation or evoked nerve action potentials (NAPs) may be recorded on major nerve trunk lesions. These tests are useful when one is performing external neurolysis on the tibial nerve in the leg or tarsal tunnel, the common peroneal nerve at the fibular neck, and the superficial and deep peroneal nerves in the leg and anterior tarsal tunnel. Direct nerve stimulation may be performed with a battery-powered stimulator grounded in adjacent soft tissues. Attention must be paid to tourniquet-induced nerve trunk ischemia as this may inhibit impulse conduction, usually within 20 minutes following exsanguination, and thereby cause a false-negative test response. Visualization of distal skeletal motor contraction upon direct nerve stimulation proximal to the lesion (e.g., pedal intrinsic musculature contraction on stimulation of the posterior tibial nerve or its branches in the tarsal tunnel) indicates axonal regeneration and the need for only external neurolysis.

In the absence of stimulated distal motor function, or when one is testing nerves that do not innervate skeletal muscle, evoked NAPs conducted through the lesion may be recorded (47). Measurement of evoked NAPs requires highly sensitive electrodiagnostic equipment that is readily available in most hospital operating rooms. Identification of evoked NAPs traversing the lesion indicates that axonal regeneration is in progress and that only external neurolysis is needed. Absence of both stimulated muscle function and evoked NAPs indicates the absence of axonal regeneration and strongly suggests the need for more than simple external neurolysis. When operative electrodiagnostic equipment is not available, the decision as to the adequacy of external neurolysis is based on intraoperative visualization and palpation. When external neurolysis is deemed adequate, it may be beneficial to transpose the freed nerve trunk to a nearby protected, well-vascularized, soft tissue bed, preferably between intact broad muscle bellies or into fatty tissue (48, 49) in those cases in which the nerve is predisposed to re-entrapment in scar tissue secondary to wound healing. Entubulation with a 0.02 or 0.01 inch thick silicone elastomer sheet may also be beneficial in preventing re-entrapment of a major nerve trunk, such as the posterior tibial nerve in the tarsal tunnel (50). In theory, entubulation or damming is designed to protect the nerve trunk from noxious extrinsic compressive forces and scar incarceration. Although silicone sheath entubulation is generally beneficial, our experience with it has yielded poor results in two patients who suffered recalcitrant tarsal tunnel syndrome after several previous surgical interventions (Fig. 44.4). In these two patients, intraneural edema and dysvascularity led to nerve trunk hypertrophy (Fig. 44.5), and recurrent symptoms resulted in the need for revisional neurectomy.

When external neurolysis reveals a palpable neuroma incontinuity of a major peripheral nerve trunk, internal neurolysis should be considered (4, 51, 52). This technique creates the potential for iatrogenic intraneural damage; however, it may be helpful in cases in which skeletal muscle function or plantar or contact-area sensation is at risk or in extremely debilitated or recalcitrant cases. Internal neurolysis entails release of interfascicular fibrosis and scarring (Fig. 44.6). After external neurolysis, the nerve trunk is gingerly manipulated with 0.25-inch Penrose drains and the intraneural lesion is isolated. It is helpful to inject a small amount of normal saline solution just under the epineurium

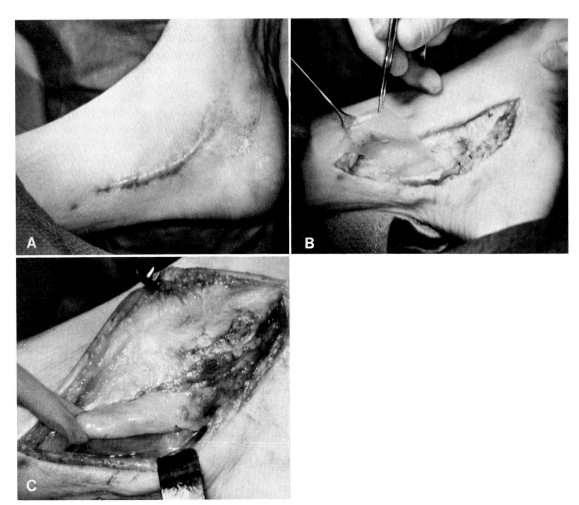

Figure 44.4. Silicone entubulation was used for treatment of recalcitrant left tarsal tunnel syndrome in a 53-year old woman with a diagnosis of reflex sympathetic dystrophy and yielded only 2 symptom-free months prior to recurrence of pain. The silicone sheath was removed 8 months after implantation. Prior to entubulation, treatment had included five previous tarsal tunnel decompressions, steroid injections, TENS, epidural blocks, Tegretol, and narcotic analgesics, as well as numerous hospital-izations for treatment of chronic pain. Approximately 1 year after removal of the silicone sheath, the patient continued to suffer and was considering posterior tibial neurectomy. **A.** Hypertrophic scar and dermatitis 8 months after silicone entubulation of the posterior tibial nerve. **B.** Hypertrophic scar excised and silicone sheath removed. **C.** Gross hypertrophy of the nerve trunk after 8 months of entubulation.

in an effort to inflate the epineurial sheath and allow easier identification of intraneural adherence between the perineurium and epineurium. The saline solution is used as an adjunct to internal neurolysis and does not itself effect neurolysis (4). Under loupe magnification, the epineurial sheath is then incised at the point of adherence and the individual fascicles are gently teased apart with microsurgical instrumentation. Intraoperative stimulated distal motor function and/or evoked NAPs may then be tested. If stimulated function or evoked NAPs are registered, then internal neurolysis effectively releases axonal entrapment and further functional improvement can be anticipated. If axonal conduction is not apparent at the time of surgery, it may still be beneficial to allow additional time for axonal regeneration and rehabilitation of the extremity after the operation, especially

if permanent loss of the nerve trunk would create a serious functional deficit. After internal neurolysis, the epineurial sheath is not closed with sutures.

In the case of severe incontinuity nerve trunk damage involving the smaller, distal sensory branches, perhaps with a history of recurrent symptoms after previous neurolysis, resection of the involved portion of the nerve is often the preferable method of treatment. Neurectomy is also the preferred method of treating a symptomatic stump neuroma. Neurectomy of an incontinuity lesion involves retracting the nerve trunk from surrounding tissues, then sharply sectioning it proximally and distally, and allowing the cleanly sectioned stumps to retract back into the protective surrounding soft tissues. When a stump neuroma is being resected, the lesion is dissected until normal proximal

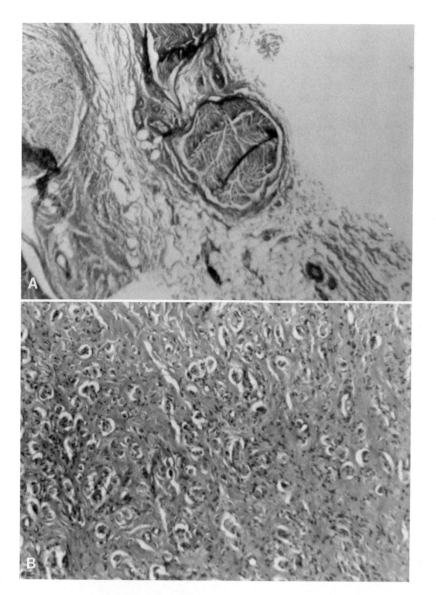

Figure 44.5. Histologic appearance of hypertrophic posterior tibial nerve after 1 year of silicone sheath entubulation for the treatment of recalcitrant tarsal tunnel syndrome (not the same patient as in Figure 44.4). **A.** Hyperplastic epineurial sheath fibrosis and perineural fibrofatty tissue (× 60). **B.** Intraneural fibrosis and vessel hypoplasia (× 160).

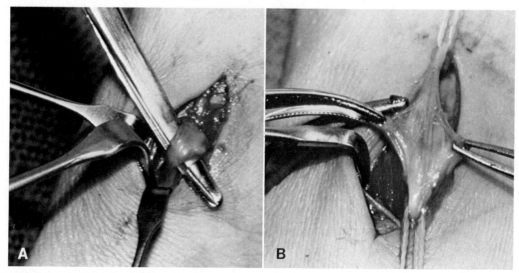

Figure 44.6. Internal neurolysis of deep peroneal neuroma-in-continuity in a 14-year-old boy who had suffered contusion of anterior tarsal tunnel 11 months earlier. Following endoneurolysis the patient experienced 95% symptomatic relief for only 12 weeks. Deep peroneal neurectomy was performed 5 months later, as symptoms worsened in spite of aggressive conservative management. **A.** Identification of deep peroneal neuroma-in-continuity. **B.** Epineurial sheath retracted and fascicular separation completed.

nerve trunk is identified, followed by sharp transection and visualization of the fresh proximal stump retracting into protective soft tissues. The experimental use of various tissue glues, such as cyanoacrylate or fibrin, has also been reported useful in preventing the development of painful stump neuromas secondary to excess neurite budding (Fig. 44.7) (53-55). Another useful technique in the prevention of formation of a symptomatic amputation neuroma is transposition of the free nerve stump into bone (Fig. 44.8). This technique satisfies the requirements for a well-vascularized and protected location necessary for unremarkable healing of a freshly sectioned nerve trunk. Neurectomy may serve as a last resort in patients who are severely debilitated by recalcitrant neuritis, even in cases of recurrent tarsal tunnel syndrome.

Occasionally, sharp resection of a neuroma-in-continuity followed by primary neurorrhaphy or cable grafting is indicated for recalcitrant lesions that affect the posterior tibial or common peroneal nerves or their skeletal muscular branches. This requires the use of microsurgical instrumentation and may be considered in cases involving extreme axonal damage with significant motor paralysis or plantar sensory deficit. Release of nerve trunk tension and appropriate splinting of the extremity are crucial to the successful completion of neurorrhaphy.

Following neurolysis, either external only or external and internal combined and perhaps including transposition or resection, a small amount of soluble steroid should be infiltrated about the remaining nerve trunk or stump. The placement of a percutaneous perineural indwelling neurocannula is also useful in the immediate postoperative phase and can be maintained for several days or weeks if the clinical situation warrants continued local pharmacological therapy. Periodic administration of local anesthetic and/or soluble steroid agent about the epineurium is sometimes necessary to effect sustained pain relief, especially in patients with a previous diagnosis of causalgia or chronic pain. Wound closure is performed in anatomical layers, typically leaving the fascia open or only partially closed if it is likely to impinge on the healing nerve. It is preferable to relocate the involved nerve trunk away from the vicinity of primarily closed deep fascia. Meticulous hemostasis is mandatory.

As long as the anatomical continuity of the nerve is maintained the postoperative prognosis is generally good. Usually the patient is allowed to freely move the extremity to tolerance. The patient may experience profound improvement in sensorimotor function almost immediately after neurolysis. Axonal conduction may further improve over the next few weeks to months as regeneration progresses. After transposition with epineurial anchoring in a new location, postoperative splinting for 2 weeks is recommended. After neurorrhaphy at or distal to the ankle, splinting for

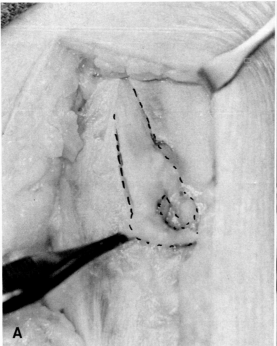
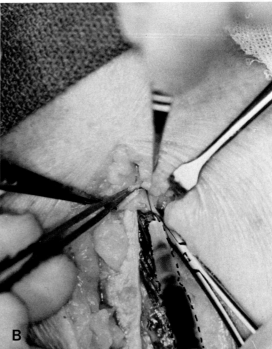
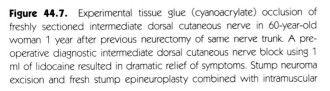

Figure 44.7. Experimental tissue glue (cyanoacrylate) occlusion of freshly sectioned intermediate dorsal cutaneous nerve in 60-year-old woman 1 year after previous neurectomy of same nerve trunk. A preoperative diagnostic intermediate dorsal cutaneous nerve block using 1 ml of lidocaine resulted in dramatic relief of symptoms. Stump neuroma excision and fresh stump epineuroplasty combined with intramuscular relocation resulted in immediate and total cessation of this patient's debilitating burning pain. **A.** Exposure of the intermediate dorsal cutaneous stump neuroma incarcerated in scar and adherent to deep crural fascia proximal to the ankle. External neurolysis reveals normal proximal nerve trunk. **B.** Application of tissue glue to seal epineurium over the tips of sectioned fascicles.

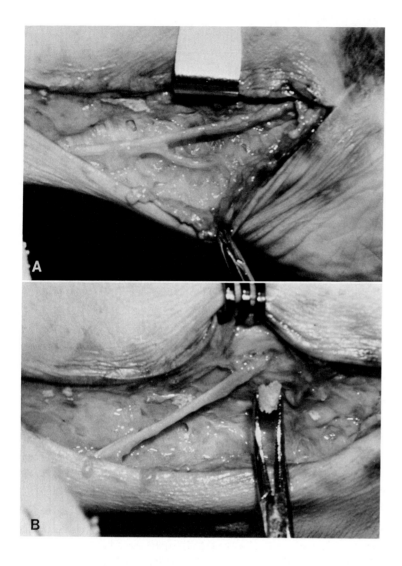

Figure 44.8. Sural nerve stump repositioned into fibula after revisional neurectomy. **A.** Right sural neuroma-in-continuity exposed. **B.** Sural nerve trunk sectioned and transplanted into the posterior aspect of the fibula proximal to the lateral malleolus. The epineurium is anchored to periosteum, and cancellous bone is delicately packed into any residual cortical cleft.

at least 3 weeks is recommended. Appropriate joint positioning may be very helpful in reducing tension on the nerve trunk after relocation or neurorrhaphy. Follow-up physical therapy may be used as indicated, and repeat conduction velocity measurements may be necessary to monitor regeneration if clinical improvement is less well marked.

LOCALIZED ACQUIRED NEUROPATHIES OF THE LOWER EXTREMITY

Saphenous Nerve

Acquired neuropathy of the saphenous nerve (L3, L4) caused by direct trauma is rather uncommon, except in certain contact sports such as football (1, 56). The nerve is mechanically vulnerable to injury where it emerges through the fascia interior to the sartorius muscle (Fig. 44.9). Spontaneous entrapment may develop secondary to chronic compression associated with genu valgum and medial tibial positioning. Postoperative scarification with subsequent en-

trapment after arthroscopy and arthrotomy of the knee may also occur. The authors have encountered entrapment of the nerve at the medial aspect of the first metatarsal base more frequently than elsewhere, although on occasion they have treated patients for neuropathy involving the nerve at the anterior aspect of the medial malleolus.

Saphenous nerve entrapment frequently affects obese, middle-aged individuals. Complaints of pain and altered sensorium inferior to the patella and along the medial aspect of the leg and foot are indicative of saphenous nerve compression. Focal nerve trunk tenderness at the point of emergence through the subsartorial fascia may be present, and palpation here may elicit both Tinel's and Valleix's signs. Local steroid infiltration at this location may prove both diagnostic and therapeutic. Differential diagnoses include compensatory knee changes secondary to faulty foot biomechanics, as well as actual internal derangements of the knee itself. At the level of the medial malleolus the differential diagnosis is facilitated by the superficial position of the nerve and by its immediate identification with the sa-

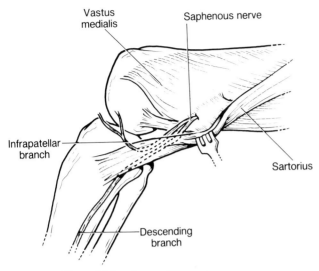

Figure 44.9. Course of the saphenous nerve.

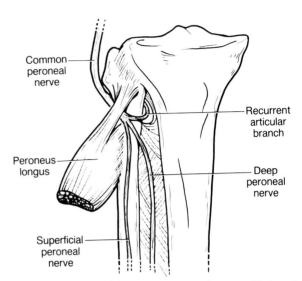

Figure 44.10. Course of the common peroneal nerve and its branches.

phenous vein. When the entrapment is present at the malleolar level, palpation readily produces pain and/or paresthesia. Entrapment medial to the base of the first metatarsal bone produces more of a diagnostic challenge. One must rule out synovitis, ligamentous strain, and degenerative joint disease of the first metatarsocuneiform joint, as well as acute tendonitis of the tibialis anterior tendon. The key diagnostic finding is pain on palpation, with the pain following a linear pattern along the course of the saphenous nerve. The nerve is usually acutely tender to palpation.

Conservative treatment consists of rest, as well as oral administration of NSAIDs. Local steroid infiltration is also recommended. When entrapment occurs at the base of the first metatarsal bone, a steroid injection should be combined with soft padding of the tongue and throat of the shoe.

Surgical repair entails external neurolysis at the point of entrapment. Exposure is achieved by means of a longitudinal medial curvilinear incision centered over the point of entrapment. Surgery should usually be done with the use of a tourniquet, and dissection should be as atraumatic as possible along anatomical planes. If the nerve shows substantial thickening, the authors have had better success with local neurectomy.

Neurectomy has proved to be a highly reliable procedure for the relief of chronic saphenous neuritis; however, re-entrapment may occur. There is usually little difficulty with loss of sensation related to neurectomy of the saphenous nerve distal to the ankle. The majority of the saphenous neurectomies that the authors have performed have been at the level of the first metatarsal base in association with chronic neuritis secondary to recurrent metatarsocuneiform exostosis.

Common Peroneal Nerve

Localized traumatic common peroneal (L4, L5, S1) neuropathy is common because the nerve trunk is vulnerable to injury, since it lies against fibular periosteum while it courses through a narrow fibrous hiatus in the origin of the peroneus longus (Fig. 44.10)(23, 57). Compression secondary to cast pressure (36), sitting for long periods with one's legs crossed, improper positioning on the operating room table (58), or decubitus pressure affecting the bedridden patient (59) are possible etiological factors. Moreover, popliteal cysts, osseous tumors of the fibula, traumatic ganglia at the fibular head (9, 10), an enlarged fabella (60), lepromatous infection, or changes associated with diabetes mellitus and rheumatoid arthritis have been associated with common peroneal nerve entrapment.

Traction secondary to sudden ankle supination or adduction of the leg commonly injures the common peroneal nerve at the fibular neck. In such cases, the entrapment has been attributed to intraneural hemorrhage caused by rupture of the vasa nervorum with resultant hematoma-induced nerve compression (32, 33). High fibular fractures (Maisonneuve) associated with pronation-eversion ankle injuries can directly traumatize the common peroneal nerve and its branches. However, such fractures are typically not treated with open reduction because of the risk of damage to the peroneal nerve during surgery.

Pain and altered sensation over the lateral aspect of the leg and dorsum of the foot are major complaints associated with common peroneal nerve entrapment. Weakness of ankle dorsiflexion and foot eversion may develop after longstanding nerve compression or after acute trauma about the neck of the fibula. Almost immediate footdrop may ensue. Percussion or rolling of the nerve trunk along the posterior aspect of the fibular neck may elicit Tinel's sign, or proximal radiation of pain and paresthesia may propagate along the sciatic neuraxis. The authors have seen several patients in whom profound dropfoot developed simply as a result of habitual sitting with one leg crossed over the other while at work, which caused compression of the common peroneal nerve against the neck of the fibula.

In the presence of weak or absent ankle dorsiflexion, one must distinguish between common peroneal nerve entrapment and lumbosacral radiculopathy. This is done by extending the knee to test the quadriceps femoris (L2, L3, L4), abducting and adducting the hip to test the gluteals (L5, S1) and thigh adductors (L2, L3, L4), inverting the foot to test the tibialis posterior (L4, L5), and plantarflexing the toes to test the flexor digitorum longus (S2, S3). A serious common peroneal nerve entrapment will cause weak ankle dorsiflexion and foot eversion while sparing the quadriceps femoris, hip abductors and adductors, foot inversion, and digital plantarflexion (58). Other considerations in the differential diagnosis include peroneal tenosynovitis, anterior crural compartment syndrome with resultant footdrop, and ruptured plantaris or partial tear of the lateral head of the gastrocnemius. One should also consider common peroneal nerve entrapment when dealing with chronic lateral ankle instability, a situation in which ankle stress radiographs may be helpful in ruling out entrapment neuropathy. A partial sciatic neuritis or sciatic nerve entrapment at the sciatic notch may also create signs and symptoms similar to those caused by common peroneal nerve entrapment, and electrodiagnostic testing is often helpful in isolating the locus of injury.

Conservative therapy focuses on decreasing local inflammation and reducing traction or pressure on the nerve trunk as it rounds the fibular neck and courses through the fibroosseous hiatus in the origin of peroneus longus. NSAIDs combined with orthoses to alleviate heel varus stress are often useful in chronic cases. In the acute case, careful casting or splinting with the ankle neutral or in slight dorsiflexion and the knee gently flexed can be used to alleviate tension on the nerve while it recovers. A spring brace to prevent footdrop and physical therapy to augment muscle rehabilitation are useful therapeutic adjuncts.

Operative neurolysis of the common peroneal nerve involves a posterolateral curvilinear approach about the fibular neck, allowing adequate visualization of the nerve proximally in the popliteal fossa, as well as distally beyond its trifurcation. It is usually necessary to incise the fascia at the inferior margin of the peroneus longus origin to obtain adequate freedom of the nerve trunk as it branches and changes direction to run distally in the leg.

Superficial Peroneal Nerve

Localized acquired neuropathy of the superficial peroneal nerve (L4, L5, S1) has been described as relatively uncommon (61-63), although its branches—the medial and intermediate (Lemont's nerve) (64) dorsal cutaneous nerves—are quite vulnerable to a variety of injuries because of their subcutaneous location. The superficial peroneal nerve may be subjected to traction injury caused by severe ankle supination. Specific sites of entrapment are superior at the fibular neck or distal where the nerve or its branches emerge through the deep crural fascia (Fig. 44.11). Entrapment at this location is typically related to athletic activity, particularly running and jumping. Biomechanically speaking,

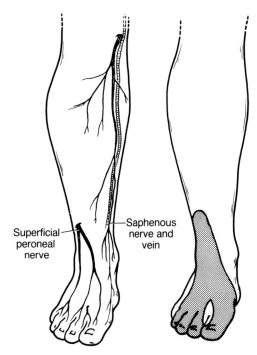

Figure 44.11. Emergence of the superficial peroneal nerve and its distribution. Note the course of the saphenous nerve and vein.

compression neuropathy of the superficial peroneal nerve or its terminal branches has been associated with a rigid forefoot valgus with a plantarflexed first ray (65). We have noted entrapment of the medial dorsal cutaneous nerve at the anterior ankle and, more frequently, at the base of the first metatarsal related to bony prominence and direct shoe irritation of the subcutaneous nerve.

Contusions to the front of the leg or dorsum of the foot (commonly seen in soccer players) or simply pressure from tight shoes, especially in elderly patients with subcutaneous atrophy complicating peripheral vascular disease, diabetes mellitus, or rheumatoid arthritis frequently result in localized acquired neuropathy of the superficial peroneal nerve or its terminal branches (Fig. 44.12). Furthermore, postoperative nerve entrapment after elective skin incision planning and surgical dissection and suturing techniques all too frequently affects Lemont's nerve just anterior to the lateral malleolus or on the dorsum of the foot, as well as the medial dorsal cutaneous nerve on the dorsum of the foot and at the medial aspect of the first metatarsophalangeal joint (37, 38).

Symptoms of entrapment of the superficial peroneal nerve, or its branches usually consist of sharp, burning pain and decreased sensory perception over the nerve's distribution. Tinel's sign may be elicited on percussion of the nerve trunk as it pierces the deep fascia about 7 to 10 cm superior to the ankle. Retrograde pain along the peroneal neuraxis is common, and lumbar radiculopathy as well as compartment syndrome must be considered in the differential diagnosis.

Conservative treatment focuses on alleviation of abnormal

Figure 44.12. Posttraumatic asymmetrical neuroma-in-continuity involving the common digital branch of the intermediate dorsal cutaneous nerve, left foot.

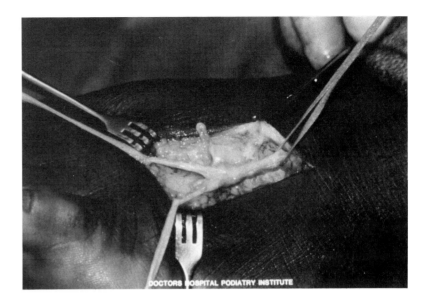

traction or pressure on the nerve trunk. Orthoses to balance rigid forefoot valgus or heel varus deformities can be used to decrease inversion stress and the resultant nerve traction. In the acute case, splinting or immobilization with the foot slightly everted is appropriate. Local infiltration of a highly soluble steroid is usually beneficial and may be of diagnostic and therapeutic value. Symptoms are typically alleviated or considerably reduced after two or three injections. In recalcitrant cases, external neurolysis at the point where the nerve or its branches emerge through the deep crural fascia is indicated (Fig. 44.13). A longitudinal anterolateral approach is used, and a 4 to 6 cm longitudinal fasciotomy is usually adequate. The superficial fascia and skin are closed, and the deep fascia is only partially reapproximated in an effort to avoid re-entrapment. Nerve trunk translocation and deep fascial closure may be necessary if muscle herniation poses a potential problem. Gentle range-of-motion exercise is started immediately in an effort to avoid any reincarceration. All efforts should be made to prevent the need to resect the entrapped nerve trunk or its branches proximal to the ankle, as this produces extensive anesthesia over the dorsum of the foot. When debilitating neuritis is localized to either of the terminal branches of the superficial peroneal nerve, surgical neurolysis or neurectomy may be necessary to alleviate pain (Figs. 44.14 to 44.16).

Deep Peroneal Nerve

Entrapment neuropathy of the deep peroneal nerve (L4, L5, S1), also known as the anterior tibial nerve, typically occurs at or just distal to the ankle. The nerve is situated in intimate proximity to the long extensor tendons and their binding retinacula, as well as the extensor digitorum brevis and its muscular slips, at the anterior aspect of the ankle and tarsus (Fig. 44.17). The resultant symptom complex has been termed the anterior tarsal tunnel or anterior tarsal syndrome (65-67). Acute injuries in the form of direct trauma, as well as chronic biomechanically induced microtrauma related to cavus foot deformity aggravated by tight shoes, are also frequent etiological factors. Severe ankle supination can place excessive traction on the deep peroneal nerve, either at its origin near the fibular neck or, more commonly, deep to the cruciate crural ligament (anterior tarsal tunnel). Distally, the branches of the deep peroneal nerve may become entrapped in resultant scar after surgery about the first metatarsophalangeal joint and hallucal sesamoid apparatus.

Deep peroneal nerve entrapment produces first interspace pain, sensory deficit, and paresthesia. Prolonged entrapment at or distal to the ankle may cause extensor digitorum brevis and interosseous atrophy with resultant weakness. Entrapment near the origin of the deep peroneal nerve can weaken the anterior compartment musculature and effect footdrop. The authors have treated four such cases in which complete function of the anterior muscles returned at various times 2 years and more after the original entrapment. Electromyography may be useful in localizing the level of entrapment. Differential diagnosis includes anterior compartment syndrome as well as sinus tarsitis.

Conservative treatment entails removal of any external aggravating factors, the use of NSAIDs, and local infiltration of steroid at the point of entrapment. Immobilization of the ankle is frequently necessary in the acute case of acute injury of the deep peroneal nerve. Often conservative management of anterior tarsal tendonitis will alleviate the symptoms of deep peroneal neuritis when the neuropathy is caused by impingement due to edematous anterior tendon sheaths. If conservative efforts fail, external neurolysis should be performed (Fig. 44.18). Visualization of the nerve proximal to the cruciate crural ligament is recommended, and care should be taken to identify the intermediate (Lemont's) and medial dorsal cutaneous nerves superficially. If the decision is made to section the deep peroneal nerve, it should be incised proximal to the cruciate crural ligament to avoid

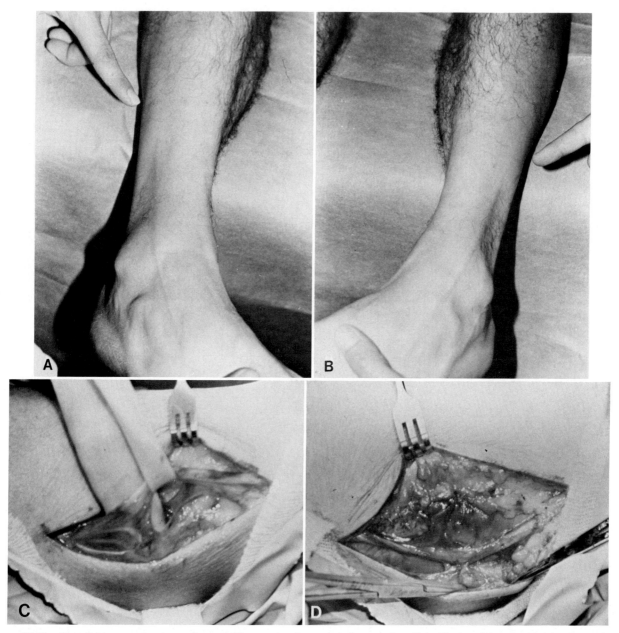

Figure 44.13. Superficial peroneal entrapment neuropathy associated with muscle herniation in a 58-year-old man. This patient had bilateral chronic burning pain and paresthesia, as well as a "lump" on the front of each leg, which began after he became a paratrooper more than 35 years earlier. Symptoms were immediately alleviated bilaterally after external neurolysis, nerve relocation, and herniorrhaphy, and there had been no recurrence of symptoms 18 months postoperatively. **A.** Clinical appearance of right leg. **B.** Clinical appearance of left leg. **C.** Superficial peroneal external neurolysis and identification of deep fascial defect. Peroneal musculature is being manually repositioned deep to the crural fascia. **D.** Deep crural fascia has been reapproximated, thereby containing the underlying muscles. The superficial peroneal nerve has been relocated posteriorly away from deep fascial wound and anchored with absorbable epineurial suture to the deep surface of the subcutaneous fat layer prior to wound closure.

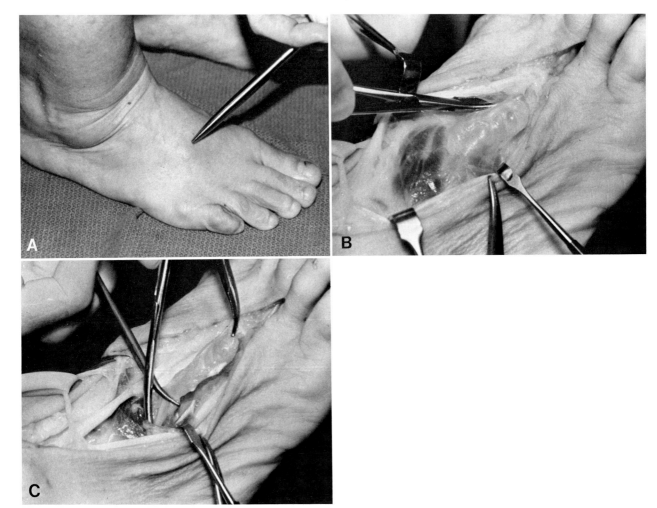

Figure 44.14. Chronic pain affecting the dorsum of right foot in a 55-year-old woman. Burning and paresthesia, as well as a "binding" sensation and the development of a "lump" in her foot began 2 years earlier after a severe inversion sprain of the right ankle. She subsequently could not work and suffered pain in her entire forefoot. Chronic lateral ligamentous instability persisted, and stress radiography indicated a ruptured anterior talofibular ligament. External neurolysis of the intermediate dorsal cutaneous nerve and ganglion cyst excision, as well as delayed primary repair of the anterior talofibular ligament produced immediate and complete relief. The freed intermediate dorsal cutaneous nerve was relocated with an epineurial anchor suture into robust subcutaneous fat, and an indwelling neurocannula was used to maintain neural blockade for the first 3 postoperative days. At 2 years postoperatively, a new ganglion developed and symptoms partially recurred. Subsequent ganglion excision yielded total alleviation of symptoms. **A.** Exquisitely tender, indurated, linear subcutaneous bulge situated over the dorsolateral aspect of the lesser tarsus. Palpation induced pain extending from the anterolateral aspect of the ankle to the forefoot. **B.** Ganglion cyst identified and noted to engulf the intermediate dorsal cutaneous nerve distally. **C.** Prior to excision, the stalk of the ganglion cyst is traced to the lateral margin of the talonavicular joint. The cyst probably resulted from rupture of joint capsule at the time of the severe sprain.

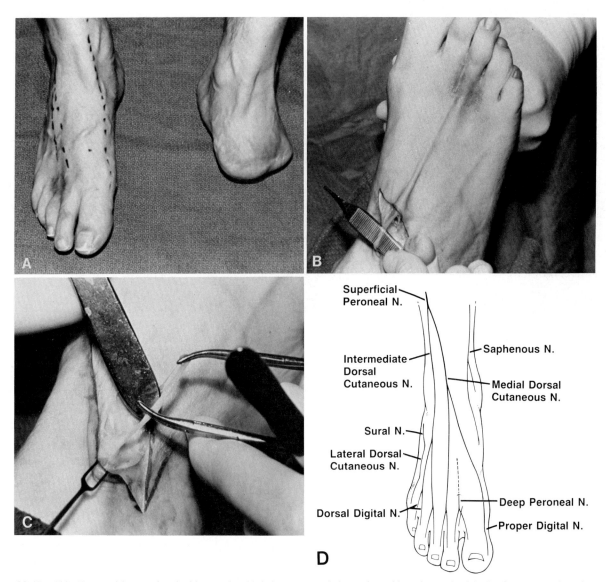

Figure 44.15. This 42-year-old man related a history of multiple inter-metatarsal neuroma operations on the left foot followed by chronic pain and eventual amputation for relief. The right foot subsequently developed neuromas of the second and third intermetatarsal spaces which were treated with excision, and painful stump neuromas followed. The painful stump neuromas were treated by revisional neurectomy. However chronic pain developed and the patient could not tolerate anything touching the dorsum of his right foot. En bloc resection of the incarcerated cutaneous nerve resulted in complete but temporary (3 months) relief of symptoms, and the patient ultimately sought right forefoot amputation. **A.** Dotted lines indicate areas at which the patient experienced severe pain, and the pigmented area at the base of the third toe was most sensitive. **B.** Proximal identification of cutaneous nerve confirms its course into the indurated area. **C.** Section of cutaneous nerve is excised proximally but fails to provide permanent relief. **D.** Chart depicting sensory distribution to dorsum of foot. Such charts fail to identify anomalous anastomoses between nerves, which may doom en bloc resections to failure unless the full nerve distribution is examined at the time of surgery.

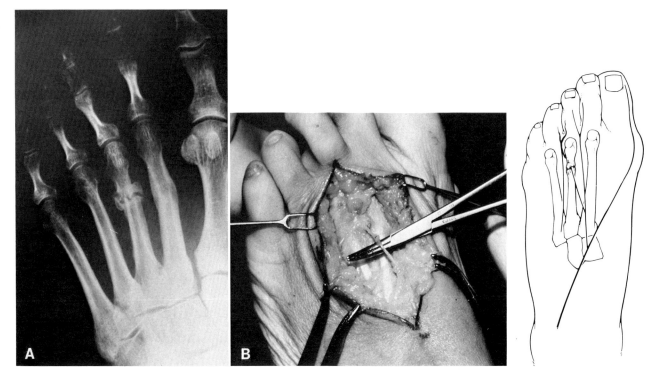

Figure 44.16. Postsurgical incarceration of the second metatarsal branch of the medial dorsal cutaneous nerve effecting RSD in a 52-year-old female 1 year after minimal-incision surgical second and third metatarsal osteotomies. The patient had failed to respond to chronic pain therapy in two pain clinics, TENS, and numerous epidural blocks. Although she complained of constant burning pain affecting the entire foot, examination revealed focal tenderness at the third metatarsal, and a field block infiltrated at the base of the metatarsal provided dramatic relief within minutes. Surgery revealed incarceration of the sensory nerve in bone callus and metatarsal nonunion. Proximal neurectomy and resection of the nonunion with plate fixation yielded significant partial relief of symptoms. Complete relief of symptoms coincided with settlement of a pending lawsuit. **A.** Radiograph showing healed osteotomy of second and hypertrophic nonunion of third metatarsal. **B.** Surgical exploration reveals sensory nerve incarcerated in bone callus. **C.** Schematic representation of nerve incarcerated in bone callus.

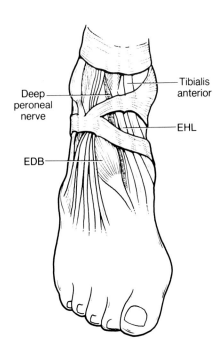

Figure 44.17. Course of the deep peroneal nerve. *EHL,* extensor hallucis longus; *EDB,* extensor digitorum brevis.

predisposing the patient to symptomatic stump neuroma irritation from the neighboring tendons in the anterior tarsal tunnel.

Sural Nerve

The sural nerve (L5, S1, S2) and its distal extension, the lateral dorsal cutaneous nerve, as well as the communicating branch between the sural nerve and Lemont's nerve, traverse the subcutaneous tissues in close proximity to the Achilles tendon, the lateral malleolus and fibular collateral ligaments, and the lateral aspect of the hindfoot and metatarsus (Fig. 44.19). Entrapment of the sural nerve or its branches usually follows direct trauma and, unfortunately, is commonly related to surgical intervention and postsurgical scarring about the Achilles tendon, the lateral malleolus, and the lateral aspect of the hindfoot (Fig. 44.20). Displaced fifth metatarsal base fractures can tent the sural nerve, causing posttraumatic entrapment, and the nerve is vulnerable to scar incarceration after surgical manipulation of fifth metatarsal fractures. Peroneal tendon sheath, and calcaneocuboid joint capsular degeneration with ganglion formation have also been implicated as causes of sural nerve compression neuropathy (68). Sural compression neuropathy may

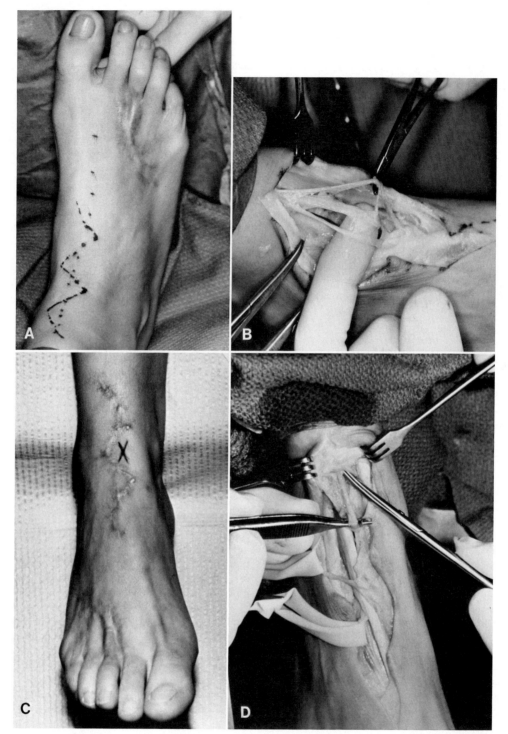

Figure 44.18. Chronic pain related to anterior tarsal tunnel syndrome in a 31-year old woman who suffered a severe contusion to the dorsum of the foot and anterior ankle 13 months earlier. RSD had been previously diagnosed and more than 20 local anesthetic/steroid injections, TENS, narcotic analgesics, and a 2-month course of weekly epidural blocks failed to alleviate her constant burning pain. Examination indicated deep peroneal neuritis, and a local anesthetic block of this nerve yielded major although incomplete relief. External neurolysis yielded complete relief that lasted only 2 months before symptoms gradually recurred and once again failed to respond to aggressive physical therapy and neurolytic injections. Nine months after external neurolysis, the patient returned to surgery, and a deep peroneal neurectomy was performed. Relief was prompt and complete, and the patient returned to full activities with no recurrence of symptoms at 1-year follow-up. **A.** First surgery: course of deep peroneal nerve and proposed Z incision line are marked. **B.** External neurolysis of deep peroneal nerve. **C.** Nine months after external neurolysis, X marks nidus of maximum pain that extends throughout the entire foot and ankle. **D.** Second surgery: neurectomy of the deep peroneal nerve from above ankle to the metatarsus.

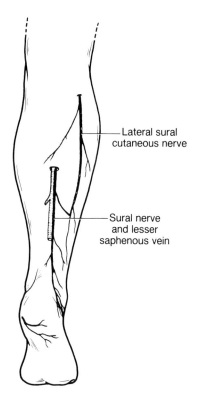

Figure 44.19. Emergence of the sural nerve and lesser saphenous vein.

also be acquired secondary to long-term chronic tendonitis of the Achilles or peroneal tendons and related induration of the peritendinous connective tissue. The authors have seen several cases in which enlargement of the peroneal tubercle on the lateral aspect of the calcaneus caused severe compression neuropathy.

Signs and symptoms include sensory alteration along the distribution of the sural nerve. Tinel's sign may be elicited on percussion at the point of entrapment. Conservative care entails the use of systemic anti-inflammatory medications and local steroid infiltration combined with gentle range-of-motion physical therapy. Because of the subcutaneous location of the nerve, phonophoresis of dexamethasone-lidocaine ointment has also proved to be a useful treatment modality, especially when injection therapy is not desirable.

Surgical intervention is frequently necessary when dense subcutaneous scarring incarcerates the sural nerve or its branches or when a bony prominence is responsible for direct compression. External neurolysis through a curvilinear skin incision over the point of entrapment may yield a good result; however, sharp nerve resection is commonly necessary to alleviate pain caused by sural nerve entrapment. When external neurolysis is performed, the incidence of re-entrapment appears to be directly related to the quality of the soft tissues in which the freed nerve can be relocated. If the soft tissue bed is of poor quality, there appears to be little value in neurolysis as the sole operative manipulation. In such cases, neurectomy usually provides relief of pain but should be performed far enough proximally to place

the stump of the remaining nerve trunk in a good-quality bed. Placement of the sural nerve stump into the protective and well-vascularized confines of the medullary canal of the fibula is a useful option, especially when one is dealing with recurrent sural entrapment or extensive subcutaneous scarring (Fig. 44.8). Whenever sural neurolysis is performed, care must be taken to ligate any damaged branches of the lesser saphenous vein because even a small hematoma may provide the mechanism for re-entrapment of the nerve.

Tibial Nerve

Proximal entrapment along the tibial neuraxis may occur anywhere from the posterior aspect of the lower thigh distally into the leg and is often the result of direct penetrating trauma. Most frequently tibial nerve (L4, L5, S1, S2, S3) entrapment occurs in the fibro-osseous tarsal tunnel, where the nerve runs deep to the laciniate ligament (Fig. 44.21). Compression neuropathy in this region produces a symptom complex commonly known as the tarsal tunnel, or medial tarsal tunnel, syndrome (69-72). The laciniate ligament forms the roof of the tarsal tunnel and, by means of individual fibrous septa, four canals are created deep to the ligament (Fig. 44.22). The tendons of the tibialis posterior, the flexor digitorum longus, and the flexor hallucis longus run in the first, second, and fourth canals, respectively. The tibial nerve and its branches, along with the posterior tibial artery and its venae comitans, occupy the third canal of the tunnel. Division of the posterior tibial nerve into the medial and lateral plantar nerves occurred deep to the laciniate ligament in 93% of dissected specimens and proximal to the ligament in the remaining 7% of specimens in a recent anatomical study (73, 74). The tarsal tunnel is typically most constricting at its distal margin (75), where the medial and lateral plantar nerves change direction and pass into the plantar vault. This region, at the distal margin of the laciniate ligament, is a key location for plantar nerve entrapment and is intimately related to tarsal tunnel syndrome.

The tarsal tunnel syndrome most commonly occurs in adults. However, when children are affected it is more prevalent in girls (76). Etiological factors that induce local tibial nerve compression with resultant ischemia and demyelination include excessive subtalar joint pronation, accessory or hypertrophic abductor hallucis muscle belly (75), tenosynovitis, or ganglion formation affecting the long flexor tendons or intraneural connective tissue (Fig. 44.23), as well as ankle synovitis or synovial cyst formation (19). Varix of the posterior tibial artery or its venae comitans, or simply prolonged venous stasis, can produce a tarsal tunnel syndrome. If posterior tibial arterial aneurysm or arteriovenous fistula is suspected, vascular consultation and arteriography are recommended. Other causes of tarsal tunnel syndrome include retromalleolar lipoma and hyperlipidemia (20) and complications associated with systemic diseases such as rheumatoid arthritis and ankylosing spondylitis, diabetes mellitus, and myxedema. The condition has even been associated with regional migratory osteoporosis (77). There are many reports of neurilemoma (schwannoma) of the tibial nerve

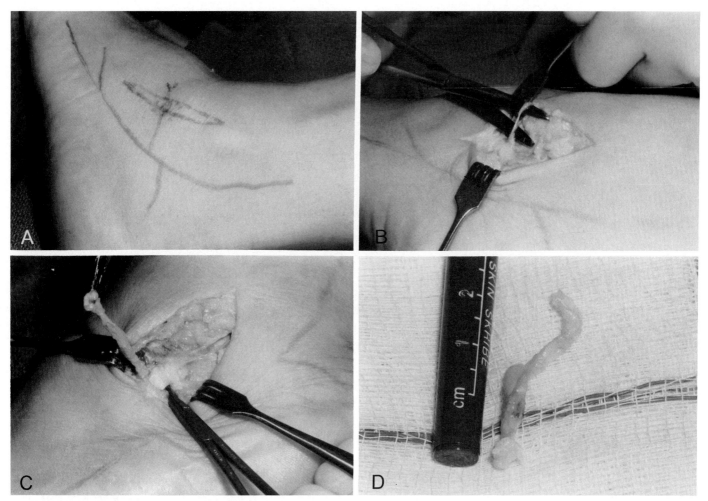

Figure 44.20. Posttraumatic neuroma-in-continuity of a communicating branch of the sural nerve. **A.** Dorsolateral aspect of the left foot and ankle marking the course of the sural nerve and area of paresthesia, and the point of a positive Tinel's sign, along the course of communicating branch.

B. Communicating branch isolated, with neuroma-in-continuity coming into view. **C.** Sharp resection of large neuroma-in-continuity. **D.** Posttraumatic neuroma after resection.

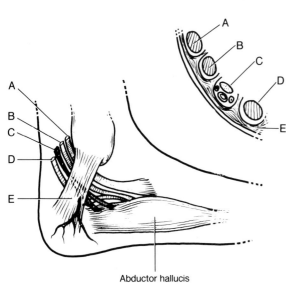

Abductor hallucis

Figure 44.21. Course of tibial nerve beneath the laciniate ligament and bifurcation into medial and lateral plantar nerves. Note medial calcaneal branch piercing the laciniate ligament. *A.* Tibialis posterior. *B.* Flexor digitorum longus. *C.* Tibial nerve, posterior tibial artery, and venae comitans. *D.* Flexor hallucis longus. *E.* Laciniate ligament.

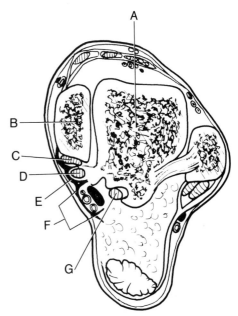

Figure 44.22. Transverse section through the talocrural joint and tarsal tunnel. *A.* Talus. *B.* Medial malleolus. *C.* Tibialis posterior. *D.* Flexor digitorum longus. *E.* Laciniate ligament. *F.* Tibial nerve and posterior tibial artery and venae comitans. *G.* Flexor hallucis longus.

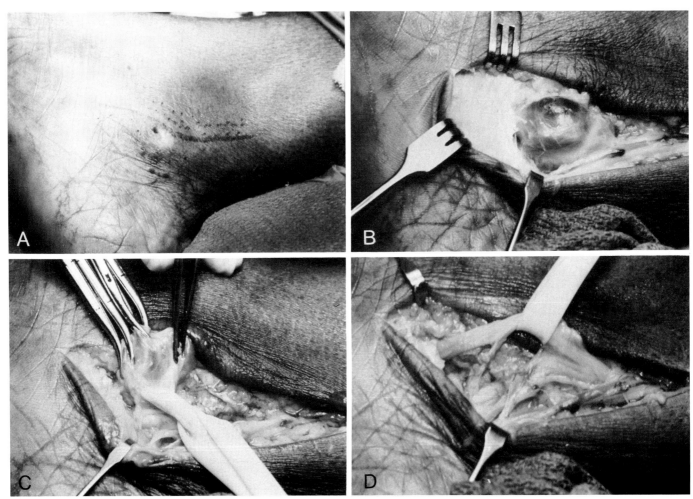

Figure 44.23. Tarsal tunnel syndrome caused by a ganglion cyst formation secondary to myxoid degeneration of epineurial connective tissue. **A.** Medial aspect of right tarsal tunnel showing nonpulsatile nodular mass posterior-plantar to the medial malleolus and the planned incision. **B.** Tarsal tunnel opened and cyst observed. **C.** Cystic structure carefully dissected from the medial plantar nerve trunk. **D.** Medial plantar nerve trunk after external neurolysis.

sheath creating nerve compression within the tarsal tunnel (15-18). Moreover, posttraumatic fibrosis and scarring after calcaneal, talar, and ankle fractures commonly cause incarceration of the tibial nerve and its branches. The medial calcaneal branches of the tibial nerve are very susceptible to direct trauma, often resulting in neurilemoma formation (12-14), and are commonly irritated in long-distance runners (78).

Symptoms usually center on a pins-and-needles sensation, burning pain, or numbness affecting the plantar aspect of the entire foot. Symptoms may be severe about the level of the metatarsal heads and medial arch. However, exquisite local tenderness in the tarsal tunnel is the most common symptom. Pain and paresthesia are aggravated by a variety of activities, such as prolonged standing or ambulation, long-distance running, wearing of tight shoes, or climbing the rungs of a ladder. Patients may also relate a feeling of arch fullness or tightness, and others complain of a feeling

of impending arch cramping (59). Symptoms are often worse at night. If the medial calcaneal branches are involved, symptoms will be most marked over the plantar and medial aspects of the heel. Proximal radiation of pain can ascend the leg and affect the thigh or buttock. Patients often state that relief is obtained with massage, ankle and foot motion, and elevation. Intrinsic muscular atrophy and associated hammertoes are late findings.

The diagnosis of tarsal tunnel syndrome is based on historical interview and physical findings. The distribution of sensorimotor alteration is the key to accurate diagnosis. Tinel's sign, as well as the Valleix sign, can almost always be elicited on percussion of the laciniate ligament. Nerve-conduction velocity and electromyographic measurements may be helpful in making the difficult diagnosis as well as in monitoring the therapeutic regimen (79, 80); however, one should not discount the clinical diagnosis of tarsal tunnel syndrome in the light of negative electrodiagnostic findings

(71). The differential diagnosis includes plantar fasciitis and heel spur syndrome, heel neuroma, acute or chronic myofascial foot strain, intermetatarsal neuroma or distal plantar nerve entrapment, lumbosacral radiculopathy, and pain associated with peripheral vascular disease, peripheral neuritis, or drug toxicity (thiazide diuretics and nitrofurantoin) (75).

Conservative therapy has traditionally revolved around the use of NSAIDs combined with the control of abnormal pronatory forces and possibly shoe modifications. These measures alone have typically met with limited success. Local infiltration of steroid into the third canal of the tarsal tunnel has proved to be beneficial, especially when combined with mechanical support. Surgical decompression of the tarsal tunnel with external neurolysis of the tibial nerve and its branches is often necessary in the recalcitrant case (81) and yields a good prognosis, provided excessive intrabundle fibrosis is not present.

Tarsal tunnel decompression is performed with or with-

out the use of a pneumatic thigh tourniquet. If a tourniquet is used, it should be deflated before wound closure so that absolute hemostasis is assured. The approach is by means of a retromalleolar curvilinear incision extending from approximately 2 cm superior to the laciniate ligament and gently curving distally to the proximal margin of the abductor hallucis. During subcutaneous dissection, attention should be directed toward avoidance of iatrogenic damage to the medial calcaneal branch or branches of the posterior tibial nerve as they emerge through the laciniate ligament and provide cutaneous sensation to the medial and plantar aspects of the heel. The incision is deepened by layer dissection to the laciniate ligament, where the pulse of the posterior tibial artery is palpated, if there is no tourniquet in use, or the tendons of tibialis posterior and flexor digitorum longus are palpated.

Care should be taken to accurately identify the third canal in an effort to prevent damage or postoperative instability affecting the adjacent tendons. The flexor hallucis longus

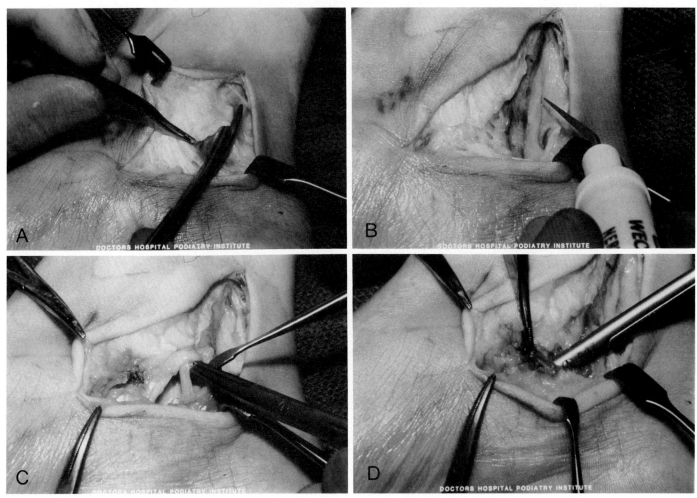

Figure 44.24. Tarsal tunnel decompression, right foot. **A.** Third canal of laciniate ligament being incised from distal to proximal. **B.** Intraoperative nerve stimulation of the lateral plantar nerve. **C.** Isolation of the medial and lateral plantar nerves. **D.** Incising the proximal margin of abductor hallucis muscle fascia to complete external neurolysis of the tarsal tunnel.

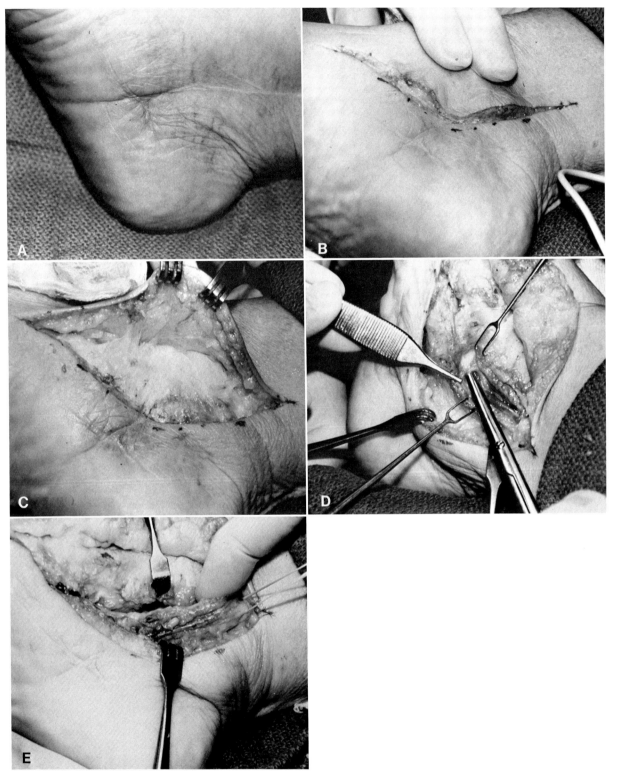

Figure 44.25. Recalcitrant tarsal tunnel syndrome in a 60-year-old woman in whom original tarsal tunnel symptoms developed following heel spur surgery. Patient subsequently underwent two surgical decompressions without relief. Examination revealed an indurated and tethered postsurgical scar, and led to a diagnosis of recurrent tarsal tunnel syndrome with medial calcaneal branch entrapment. Revisional exploration revealed incarceration of all branches of the posterior tibial nerve, and neurolysis of the medial and lateral plantar nerves and neurectomy of the medial calcaneal branch were followed by 3 days of continuous nerve block via epineurial cannula. This treatment effected almost total alleviation of symptoms and allowed full return to normal shoes and activities. One year later a significant portion of the patient's symptoms had returned. **A.** Immobile and indurated scar at medial aspect right heel. **B.** Retromedial malleolar incision extends along proximal border of abductor hallucis. **C.** Exposure of normal deep fascia allows controlled exploration of the fibrotic laciniate ligament and isolation of the medial calcaneal branch prior to incarceration in cicatrix. **D.** Lysis of the tarsal tunnel meets with little restriction until exploration of the porta pedis reveals a fibrocartilaginous consistency to the tendon of origin of abductor hallucis, which effectively strangulated the plantar nerves at the distal margin of the tunnel. **E.** Posterior tibial nerve and its branches free after external neurolysis.

tendon may also be deeply palpated while the hallux is passively manipulated at the first metatarsophalangeal joint. Once the third canal of the flexor retinaculum has been identified, the roof is incised in its entirety from proximal to distal, or vice versa, allowing access to its contents (Fig. 44.24). The tibial nerve and its branches are isolated and freed of any constricting connective tissue or scarring. Any benign local neoplasms are identified and excised. Great care should be taken during excision of a ganglion cyst because the lesion may stem from connective tissue degeneration within the nerve itself. Ligation and sectioning of varicose segments of the venae comitans may readily be performed; however, repair of aneurysmal dilatation of the posterior tibial artery should be performed with loupe magnification and an appropriate microsurgical technique.

Dissection of the tarsal tunnel is carried distal to the point where the medial plantar nerve passes between the abductor hallucis and the spring ligament and where the lateral plantar nerve passes between the abductor hallucis and the quadratus plantae en route to the plantar vault (Fig. 44.25). External neurolysis is performed at this level by sectioning muscle fascia and ligament and dilating each fibrous hiatus. This is a critical component of tarsal tunnel decompression. In treatment of severe cases of recurrent tarsal tunnel syndrome, silicone elastomer entubulation or damming of the posterior tibial nerve may be beneficial in an effort to avoid neurectomy and salvage plantar sensation and intrinsic muscle function (Fig. 44.26). We prefer the use of 0.01-inch silicone elastomer sheathing and recommend rolling the sheet about the nerve trunk in a concentric fashion while care is taken to avoid excessive constriction, overlapping, or telescoping of the elastomer. The material is anchored to itself with interrupted absorbable or nonabsorbable sutures. We now believe that the silicone sheeting should be left in place only 3 or 4 months and then removed. Posterior tibial neurectomy may be beneficial as a last resort when less drastic surgical manipulations have failed to alleviate the patient's disabling symptoms. Surgical excision of the medial

calcaneal branch of the posterior tibial nerve is often useful in the treatment of recalcitrant neuritis secondary to scarring of the medial or plantar aspects of the heel (Fig. 44.27).

After complete neurolysis the laciniate ligament is only partially reapproximated and the subcutaneous layer and skin are closed. A below-knee Jones compression dressing is applied and the patient is kept in a cast and allowed no weight bearing or only partial weight bearing for two weeks before active range-of-motion and weight bearing are resumed. It is wise to begin active dorsiflexion-plantarflexion exercises by 2 weeks to encourage free movement between the nerve and the related tissues in which it is embedded. Prolonged immobilization may risk a greater chance of reincarceration of the nerve.

Plantar Nerves

Plantar nerve entrapment most frequently occurs at the fibrous openings between the dorsal margin of the abductor hallucis or quadratus plantae and overlying structures where each nerve traverses the porta pedis and enters the plantar vault. An abnormally pronated subtalar joint or chronic pes valgus deformity effectively increases pressure and stretch on the nerve trunks secondary to impingement of the plantar-medial margin of the spring ligament and quadratus plantae against the abductor hallucis for the medial and lateral plantar nerves, respectively. Moreover, the inferior calcaneal branch of the lateral plantar nerve can readily become irritated by inflammatory changes localized at the attachment of the plantar fascia to the calcaneus or by direct pressure from the calcaneal tuberosity on the nerve itself (82–84).

Direct trauma affecting the plantar-medial arch, fractures or dislocations involving the calcaneus, or surgery performed on the hindfoot may damage nerve trunks and surrounding connective tissues, thus producing plantar nerve entrapment. Similarly, space-occupying lesions in the plantar vault may obliterate normal anatomy and create plantar

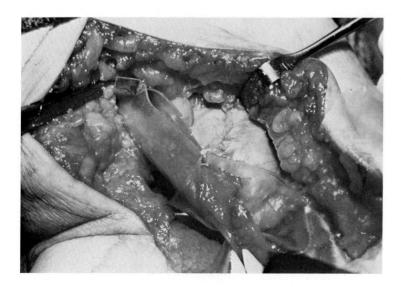

Figure 44.26. Silicone elastomer entubulation of posterior tibial nerve for treatment of recalcitrant tarsal tunnel syndrome. This technique may be useful when severe scar tissue composes the nerve's surrounding soft tissue bed.

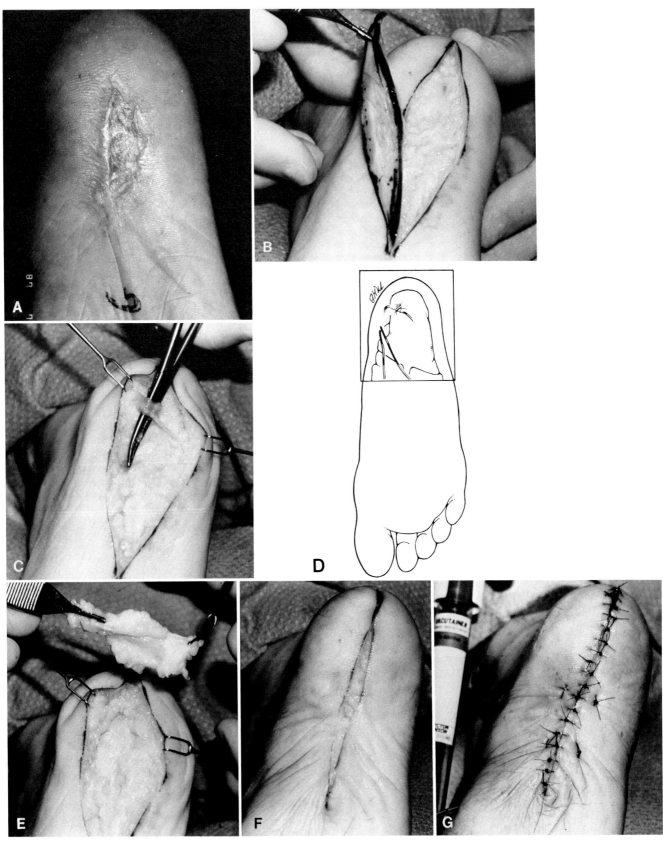

Figure 44.27. Chronic pain and inability to bear weight secondary to hypertrophic plantar scar incarceration of medial calcaneal branch of posterior tibial nerve in a 27-year-old woman who underwent laser treatment for plantar verruca several years earlier. Examination revealed exquisite local tenderness, paresthesia, and a thick, indurated, and immobile scar. Diagnostic local block of the medial calcaneal nerve at medial aspect of heel produced relief. Surgical treatment entailed scar revision and medial calcaneal neurectomy followed by 6 weeks of non-weight-bearing ambulation. Immediate and dramatic relief was experienced postoperatively and the patient returned to full activity, including daily jogging. At 32 months after surgery no recurrence of symptoms was reported. **A.** Severely painful full-thickness adherent plantar scar. **B.** Elliptical excision of scar. **C.** Entrapped medial calcaneal nerve isolated proximally in normal subcutaneous tissue, then traced distally into deep scar tissue. **D.** Schematic representation of nerve distribution. **E.** Dense fibrous central mass, including incarcerated nerve, excised and medial and lateral wound margins undermined at periosteal level. **F.** Careful undermining allows reapproximation of wound margins without the need for transpositional skin plasty. **G.** Despite being an antitension line incision, the wound closed under minimal tension and subsequently healed unremarkably. Weight bearing was avoided for the first 6 postoperative weeks.

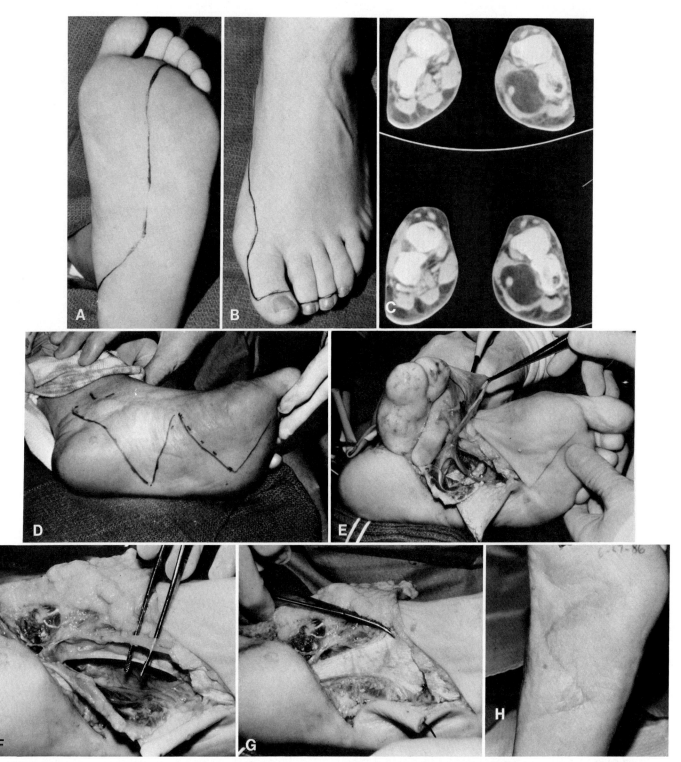

Figure 44.28. Rapidly progressing tarsal tunnel syndrome and suspected plantar mass in a 32-year-old woman with pain, paresthesia, and
numbness of the plantar-medial aspect of the left foot. She related that
her arch had enlarged over the previous 18 months. Examination revealed
moderate enlargement of the left foot relative to the right. The entire medial
arch and the tips of the first, second, and third toes were essentially
anesthetic. Ankle dorsiflexion induced radiation of pain into the medial
arch and first three toes, and Tinel's sign was evident at the left tarsal
tunnel. A CAT scan displayed a fibrous mass extending from the tarsal
tunnel to the first intermetatarsal space, and lesion calcification raised
suspicion of malignancy. A diagnosis of tarsal tunnel syndrome with tumor
of the plantar vault, was made and, after oncology consultation, excisional
biopsy via a plantar Z incision was performed. A fibrolipoma was excised,
and obliteration of the plantar intrinsic musculature and compression of
the medial plantar nerve were observed. The wound was primarily closed
and healed unremarkably after 6 weeks of no weight bearing. The patient
related 80% restoration of plantar sensation, with relief of pain 24 hours
postoperatively, and nearly complete recovery 4½ months postoperatively. She related no recurrence of symptomatology at 4 years postoperatively. **A.** Plantar area of primarily anesthesia with paresthesia, as outlined
by the patient. **B.** Dorsal view of symptomatic area as outlined by the
patient. Area is consistent with medial plantar nerve distribution. **C.** CAT
scan displays large mass in plantar vault with fibrous tissue density and
an area of calcification. **D.** Zigzag incision approximates relaxed skin tension lines to minimize scarring and maximize exposure. **E.** Large mass (13
× 5 cm) histologically designated as fibrolipoma. **F.** Apparently viable
medial plantar nerve identified along the margin of the lesion along with
atrophied muscle. **G.** Plantar fascia reapproximated and large void required the use of two closed-suction drains. **H.** Four and one half months
postoperatively, a fine-line scar is nontender, nearly full restoration of
plantar sensorium has returned, and paresthesias are absent.

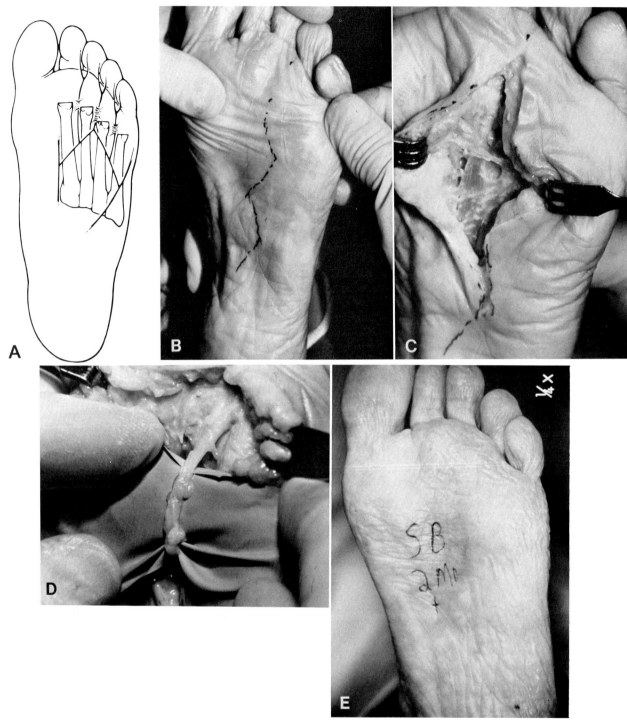

Figure 44.29. Chronic pain related to recurrent intermetatarsal stump neuroma in a 63-year-old woman after two previous operations for treatment of left third intermetatarsal neuroma. Aggressive conservative care failed to alleviate symptoms. Examination revealed maximum tenderness just proximal to the metatarsal heads in the third intermetatarsal space, and dorsiflexion of the toes induced pain in the second and third intermetatarsal spaces. A diagnosis of second and third plantar intermetatarsal nerve entrapment was made, and surgical exploration was undertaken via a plantar zigzag incision. The third intermetatarsal nerve was observed to be adherent to the fourth metatarsophalangeal joint and, therefore, aggravated by digital dorsiflexion. The second intermetatarsal nerve was found to be under traction because of its communicating branch with the third intermetatarsal nerve. Prompt and dramatic relief ensued, but a recurrent stump neuroma developed in the third intermetatarsal space several months later. Revisional neurectomy and cyanoacrylate epineuroplasty performed under loupe magnification yielded only partial relief. **A.** Schematic representation of plantar nerve supply to the second, third, and fourth intermetatarsal spaces. It is understandable that tethering of the nerve in the third interspace may affect the nerves in the second and fourth interspaces. **B.** Plantar zigzag incision allows proximal exposure of normal neural anatomy and distal exposure of nerve entrapment and scarring while accommodating relaxed skin tension lines. **C.** Dissection is carried deep to the plantar fascia before undermining to permit wide access to three interspaces. **D.** Nerve to the third interspace is seen to thicken as it proceeds distally, and a distal stump neuroma is adherent to a lumbricale tendon and joint capsule. **E.** Two months and one week postoperatively a fine-line scar is noted.

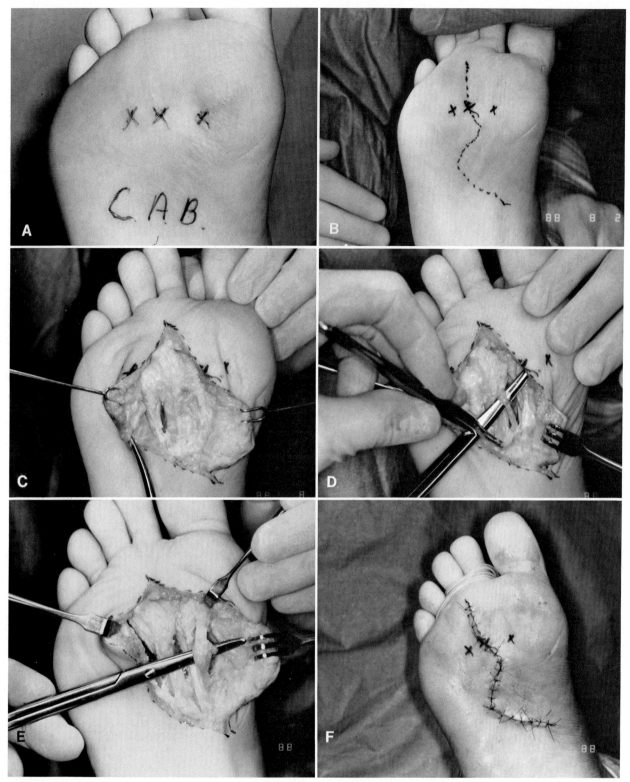

Figure 44.30. Recurrent intermetatarsal stump neuromas in a 25-year-old woman after two previous neuroma operations in the second and third interspaces. The patient also related a history of hallux valgus repair followed by neuroma pain in the first interspace. Neuritis redeveloped within 8 weeks after each previous surgical procedure and was more severe each time. All previous operations were performed through dorsal approaches. Examination revealed pain on digital and ankle dorsiflexion and was most severe in the first, second, and third intermetatarsal spaces. Pain radiated plantarly to the retromedial malleolar area. Surgical neurolysis was performed via a modified plantar zigzag incision, and incarcerated stump neuromas were resected from the first, second, and third intermetatarsal spaces. Intraoperative digital dorsiflexion displayed nerve trunk tethering. The residual freshly sectioned nerve trunk was allowed to retract proximally into the plantar vault. Pain relief was prompt and complete, and weight bearing was resumed at 6 weeks postoperatively. Twenty-

two months postoperatively there was no reported recurrence of symptoms. **A.** *X*s identify points of maximum tenderness. **B.** Incision designed to access three interspaces and allow identification of normal anatomy proximal to the region of scar tissue prior to the exploration of distal cicatrix. Moreover, the incision accounts for relaxed skin tension in an effort to minimize scar formation. **C.** Deep fascial layer obtained before medial, lateral, and distal undermining are performed. **D.** Intermetatarsal nerves are identified by separation of the digitations of the plantar fascia just proximal to the normal bifurcation. **E.** After identification of the normal nerve proximally, the nerve trunk is traced distally into scar. Here, the nerve is scarred to the flexor plate and tendon on the lateral plantar aspect of the joint. **F.** A thin plantar scar may be expected following primary closure, compression bandaging, closed-suction drainage, and 5 to 6 weeks of no weight bearing.

nerve compression (Fig. 44.28). Distally, branches of the medial plantar nerve can be iatrogenically entrapped after plantar fasciectomy or hallucal sesamoidectomy and, all too often, after dissection about the first metatarsophalangeal joint. Primary entrapment of the common and proper digital branches of the plantar nerves at the level of the deep transverse intermetatarsal ligament, causing Morton's neuroma is discussed in great detail elsewhere in this text. Symptomatic stump neuroma occurring at the level of, and proximal to, the deep transverse intermetatarsal ligament may develop secondary to nerve stump incarceration and/or tethering after surgical excision of the plantar nerve in the treatment of Morton's neuroma (85-87).

Symptoms associated with plantar nerve entrapment may be similar to those encountered with tarsal tunnel syndrome, Morton's neuroma, or radiculopathy. The cutaneous distribution over the sole of the foot, however, does not include the plantar-medial aspect of the heel. Complaints of sharp or burning pain, numbness, and paresthesia, along with plantar sensory deficit, are common. Diffuse, aching pain about the distal aspect of the calcaneal tuberosity may result from inferior calcaneal nerve entrapment, and the heel spur syndrome should be ruled out. Focal tenderness and Tinel's sign, even proximal radiation of pain, may be elicited on percussion along the dorsal margin of the abductor hallucis proximally. Intrinsic muscle weakness and digital contracture may develop after long-standing or severe entrapment.

Conservative treatment can be very gratifying, especially when abnormal subtalar joint pronation is the causative factor. The use of a soft insole pad, a flexible sole, and a low-heeled shoe may also be helpful. Orthoses combined with NSAIDs and local infiltration of steroid at the point of entrapment often effect a cure. Recalcitrant cases require surgical neurolysis. If the entrapment site is located proximally, the surgical approach is similar to that used for tarsal tunnel decompression. When the entrapment is located distally, deep in the plantar vault, or in the forefoot (usually of posttraumatic or iatrogenic nature), a plantar or dorsal approach is used, depending on the exact location of nerve incarceration. A plantar Z incision can be used to expose the entire plantar vault and readily allows exposure distally to the plantar digital sulcus (Figs. 44.29 and 44.30). It should be pointed out that external neurolysis is not always a satisfactory solution. In those instances in which significant fibrous invasion of the nerve has occurred or in which severe neural degeneration is present, patients may continue to have severe symptoms, even after the most thorough external neurolysis. In recalcitrant cases, neurectomy may offer the most benefit.

References

1. Kopell HP, Thompson WAL: *Peripheral Entrapment Neuropathies*, ed 2. Huntington, NY, Robert E Krieger Publishing Co, 1976, pp 1-88.
2. Kopell HP, Thompson WAL: Peripheral entrapment neuropathies of the lower extremity. *N Engl J Med* 262:56-60, 1960.
3. Carrel JM, Davidson DM: Nerve compression syndromes of the foot and ankle: a comprehensive review of symptoms, etiology, and diagnosis using nerve conduction testing. *J Am Podiatry Assoc* 65:322-341, 1975.
4. Brown BA: Internal neurolysis in traumatic peripheral nerve lesions in continuity. *Surg Clin North Am* 52:1167-1175, 1972.
5. Duncan D: Alterations in the structure of nerves caused by restricting their growth with ligatures. *J Neuropathol Exp Neurol* 7:261-273, 1948.
6. Birch R, St. Clair Strange FG: A new type of peripheral nerve lesion. *J Bone Joint Surg* 72B:312-313, 1990.
7. Brooks DM: Nerve compression by simple ganglia. *J Bone Joint Surg* 34B:391-400, 1952.
8. Ellis VH: Two cases of ganglia in the sheath of the peroneal nerve. *Br J Surg* 24:141-142, 1937.
9. Wadstein T: Two cases of ganglia in the sheath of the peroneal nerve. *Acta Orthop Scand* 2:221-231, 1932.
10. Jacobs RR, Maxwell JA, Kepes J: Ganglia of the nerve: presentation of two unusual cases, a review of the literature, and a discussion of pathogenesis. *Clin Orthop* 113:135-144, 1975.
11. Wilson RL: Management of pain following peripheral nerve injuries. *Orthop Clin North Am* 12:343-359, 1972.
12. Davidson MR: Heel neuroma: identification and removal. *J Am Podiatry Assoc* 67:431-435, 1977.
13. Davidson MR, Liston H, Jacoby RP, Cohen SJ, Beldon LM, Seidner AR, Bock RF: Heel neuroma. *J Am Podiatry Assoc* 67:589-594, 1977.
14. Altman MI, Hinkes MP: Heel neuroma: a case history. *J Am Podiatry Assoc* 72:517-519, 1982.
15. Brietstein RJ: Compression neuropathy secondary to neurilemoma. *J Am Podiatry Assoc* 75:160-161, 1985.
16. Dowling GL, Skaggs RE: Neurilemoma (schwannoma) as a cause of tarsal tunnel syndrome. *J Am Podiatry Assoc* 72:45-48, 1982.
17. Menon A, Dorfman HD, Renbaum J, Friedler S: Tarsal tunnel syndrome secondary to neurilemoma of the medial plantar nerve. *J Bone Joint Surg* 62A:301-303, 1980.
18. Levin AS, Titchnal WO, Clark J: Tarsal tunnel syndrome secondary to neurilemoma. *J Am Podiatry Assoc* 67:429-431, 1977.
19. Kenzora JE, Lenet MD, Sherman M: Synovial cyst of the ankle joint as a cause of tarsal tunnel syndrome. *Foot Ankle* 63:181-183, 1982.
20. Ruderman MI, Palmer RH, Olarte MR, Lovelace RE, Haas R, Rowland LP: Tarsal tunnel syndrome caused by hyperlipidemia. *Arch Neurol* 40:124-125, 1983.
21. Simeone FA: Acute and delayed traumatic peripheral entrapment neuropathies. *Surg Clin North Am* 52:1329-1337, 1972.
22. Seddon HJ: Three types of nerve injury. *Brain* 66:238-288, 1943.
23. Mathews GJ, Osterholm JL: Painful traumatic neuromas. *Surg Clin North Am* 51:1313-1324, 1972.
24. Subotnick SI: Compartment syndromes in the lower extremities. *J Am Podiatry Assoc* 65:342-348, 1975.
25. Matsen FA, Clawson DK: Compartment syndromes (symposium). *Clin Orthop* 113:2-110, 1975.
26. Schut L: Nerve injuries in children. *Surg Clin North Am* 52:1307-1312, 1972.
27. Bigos SJ, Coleman S: Foot deformities secondary to gluteal injection in infancy. *J Pediatr Orthop* 4:560-563, 1984.
28. Matsen DD: Early neurolysis in treatment of injury of peripheral nerves due to faulty injection of antibiotics. *N Engl J Med* 242:973-975, 1950.
29. Clark WK: Surgery for injection injury of peripheral nerves. *Surg Clin North Am* 52:1325-1328, 1972.
30. Preston D, Logigian E: Iatrogenic needle-induced peroneal neuropathy in the foot. *Ann Intern Med* 108:921-922, 1988.
31. Highet WB, Holmes W: Traction injuries to the lateral popliteal nerve and traction injuries to peripheral nerves after suture. *Br J Surg* 30:212-233, 1942.
32. Nobel W: Peroneal palsy due to hematoma in the common peroneal nerve sheath after distal torsional fractures and inversion ankle sprains: report of two cases. *J Bone Joint Surg* 48A:1484-1495, 1966.
33. Mansoor IA: Delayed incomplete traction palsy of the lateral popliteal nerve. *Clin Orthop* 66:183-187, 1969.
34. Seddon HJ: A classification of nerve injuries. *Br Med J* 2:237-239, 1942.
35. Denny-Brown D, Brenner C: Paralysis of nerve induced by direct pressure and by tourniquet. *Arch Neurol Psychiatry* 51:1-26, 1944.
36. Gordon SL, Dunn EJ: Peroneal nerve palsy as a complication of clubfoot treatment. *Clin Orthop* 101:229-231, 1977.
37. Joplin RJ: The proper digital nerve, Vitallium stem arthroplasty, and some thoughts about foot surgery in general. *Clin Orthop* 76:199-212, 1971.

38. Kenzora JE: Symptomatic incisional neuromas on the dorsum of the foot. *Foot Ankle* 5:2-15, 1984.

39. Banerjee T, Koons DD: Superficial peroneal nerve entrapment: report of two cases. *J Neurosurg* 55:991-992, 1981.

40. Edwards WG, Lincoln CR, Bassett FH, Goldner JL: The tarsal tunnel syndrome: diagnosis and treatment. *JAMA* 207:716-720, 1969.

41. Kopell HP, Goodgold J: Clinical and electrodiagnostic features of carpal tunnel syndrome. *Arch Phys Med Rehabil* 49:371-375, 1968.

42. Omer GE: Physical diagnosis of peripheral nerve injuries. *Orthop Clin North Am* 12:207-228, 1981.

43. Smith JR, Nery HG: Local injection therapy of neuromata of the hand with triamcinolone acetonide. *J Bone Joint Surg* 52A:71-83, 1970.

44. Grumbine NA, Radovic PA: Volume injection adhesiotomy. *J Am Podiatr Med Assoc* 79:121-123, 1989.

45. Sidlow CJ, Frankel SL, Chioros PG, Hamilton V: Electroacupuncture therapy for stump neuroma pain. *J Am Podiatr Med Assoc* 79:31-33, 1989.

46. Kline DG: Early evaluation of peripheral nerve lesions in continuity with a note on nerve recording. *Am Surg* 34:77-81, 1968.

47. Kline DG, Nulsen FE: The neuroma in continuity: its preoperative and operative assessment. *Surg Clin North Am* 52:1189-1209, 1972.

48. Madden JW, Peacock EE: Some thoughts on repair of peripheral nerves. *South Med J* 64:17-21, 1971.

49. Mackinnon SE, Dellon AL, Hudson AR, Hunter DA: Nerve regeneration through a pseudosynovial sheath in a primate model. *Plast Reconstr Surg* 75:833-837, 1985.

50. Malay DS: Update: peripheral entrapment neuropathy. In: McGlamry ED (ed): *Reconstructive Surgery of the Foot and Leg: Update '88*. Tucker, GA, The Podiatry Institute Publishing Co, 1988, pp 153-154.

51. Grabb WC: Management of nerve injuries in the forearm and hand. *Orthop Clin North Am* 1:419-431, 1970.

52. Gould N, Trevino S: Sural nerve entrapment by avulsion of the base of the 5th metatarsal bone. *Foot Ankle* 2:153-155, 1981.

53. Martini A, Fromm B: A new operation for the prevention and treatment of amputation neuromas. *J Bone Joint Surg* 71B:379-382, 1989.

54. Moss ALH: Ideas and innovations: the preparation of divided nerve ends. *Br J Plast Surg* 43:247-249, 1990.

55. Narakas A: The use of fibrin glue in the repair of peripheral nerves. *Orthop Clin North Am* 19:187-199, 1988.

56. Kopell HP, Thompson WAL: Knee pain due to saphenous nerve entrapment. *N Engl J Med* 263:351-353, 1960.

57. Fisher MA, Gorelick PB: Entrapment neuropathies: differential diagnosis and management. *Postgrad Med* 77:160-174, 1985.

58. Pickett JB: Localizing peroneal nerve lesions. *Am Fam Physician* 31:189-196, 1985.

59. Cozen L: Management of footdrop in adults after permanent peroneal nerve loss. *Clin Orthop* 167:151-158, 1969.

60. Mangierri JV: Peroneal nerve injury from an enlarged fabella: a case report. *J Bone Joint Surg* 55A:395-397, 1973.

61. Lowdon IMR: Superficial peroneal nerve entrapment: a case report. *J Bone Joint Surg* 67B:58-59, 1985.

62. Kernohan J, Levack B, Wilson JN: Entrapment of superficial peroneal nerve: three case reports. *J Bone Joint Surg* 67B:60-61, 1985.

63. McAuliffe TB, Fiddian NJ, Browett JP: Entrapment neuropathy of the superficial peroneal nerve: a bilateral case. *J Bone Joint Surg* 67B:62-63, 1985.

64. Lemont H: The branches of the superficial peroneal nerve and their clinical significance. *J Am Podiatry Assoc* 65:310-314, 1975.

65. Cangialosi CP, Schnall SJ: The biomechanical aspects of anterior tarsal tunnel syndrome. *J Am Podiatry Assoc* 70:291-292, 1980.

66. Adelman KA, Wilson G, Wolf JA: Anterior tarsal tunnel syndrome. *J Foot Surg* 27:299-302, 1988.

67. Gessini L, Jandolo B, Pietrangeli A: The anterior tarsal syndrome. *J Bone Joint Surg* 66A:786-787, 1984.

68. Pringle RM, Protheroe K, Mukherjee SK: Entrapment neuropathy of the sural nerve. *J Bone Joint Surg* 56B:465-468, 1974.

69. Keck C: The tarsal-tunnel syndrome. *J Bone Joint Surg* 44A:180-182, 1962.

70. Radin EL: Tarsal tunnel syndrome. *Clin Orthop* 181:167-170, 1983.

71. Gathier JC, Bruyn GW, Van Der Meer WK: The medial tarsal tunnel syndrome. *J Neurol Neurosurg Psychiatry* 73:87-96, 1970.

72. Johnson MK: The anatomy and electrodiagnosis of tarsal tunnel syndrome. *Cur Podiatr Med* January: 8-15, 1989.

73. Havel PE, Ebraheim NA, Clark SE: Tibial nerve branching in the tarsal tunnel. *Foot Ankle* 9:117-119, 1988.

74. Heimkes B, Posel P, Stotz S, Wolf K: The proximal and distal tarsal tunnel syndromes: an anatomical study. *Int Orthop* 11:193-196, 1987.

75. Edwards WG, Lincoln CR, Bassett FH, Goldner JL: The tarsal tunnel syndrome: diagnosis and treatment. *JAMA* 207:716-720, 1969.

76. Albrektsson B, Rydholm A, Rydholm U: The tarsal tunnel syndrome in children. *J Bone Joint Surg* 64B:215-217, 1982.

77. Byrd JW, Ricciardi JM, Jung BI: Regional migratory osteoporosis and tarsal tunnel syndrome. *Clin Orthop* 157:164-169, 1981.

78. Henricson AS, Westlin NE: Chronic calcaneal pain in athletes: entrapment of the calcaneal nerve. *Am J Sports Med* 12:52-54, 1984.

79. Goodgold J, Kopell HP, Spielholz NI: Tarsal tunnel syndrome: objective diagnostic criteria. *N Engl J Med* 273:742-745, 1965.

80. DiGiacomo MA, Bernstein AL, Scurran BL, Karlin JM: Electrodiagnosis of the tarsal tunnel syndrome. *J Am Podiatry Assoc* 70:94-96, 1980.

81. Stern DS, Joyce MT: Tarsal tunnel syndrome: a review of 15 surgical procedures. *J Foot Surg* 28:290-294, 1989.

82. Tanz SS: Heel pain. *Clin Orthop* 28:169-178, 1963.

83. Przylucki H, Jones CL: Entrapment neuropathy of muscle branch of lateral plantar nerve: a cause of heel pain. *J Am Podiatry Assoc* 71:119-124, 1981.

84. Arenson DJ, Cosentino GL, Suran SM: The inferior calcaneal nerve: an anatomical study. *J Am Podiatry Assoc* 70:552-560, 1980.

85. Malay DS: Recurrent intermetatarsal neuroma. In McGlamry ED (ed): *Reconstructive Surgery of the Foot and Leg: Update '89*. Tucker, GA, The Podiatry Institute Publishing Co., 1989, pp 321-324.

86. Beskin JL, Baxter DE: Recurrent pain following interdigital neurectomy—a plantar approach. *Foot Ankle* 9:34-39, 1988.

87. Johnson JE, Johnson KA, Unni KK: Persistent pain after excision of an interdigital neuroma. *J Bone Joint Surg* 70A:651-657, 1988.

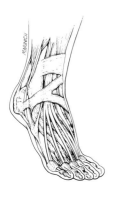

CHAPTER **45**

Reflex Sympathetic Dystrophy Syndrome

Catherine A. Purdy, D.P.M.
Stephen J. Miller, D.P.M.

Normally, the body will heal in an orderly fashion after trauma or disease. Occasionally, this does not occur and the patient will have an unexpected degree of pain, swelling, stiffness, and dysfunction, even though appropriate treatment was given. This symptom complex is known as reflex sympathetic dystrophy syndrome (RSDS). It is caused by an abnormal response in the sympathetic nervous system. There is not only an increase in the sympathetic nervous system activity but also an abnormal reflex that allows this increase in stimulation to perpetuate itself (1). The characteristic abnormality is vasomotor instability. The common denominator is pain in the extremity (2).

RSDS has been reported in adults, adolescents, and children (3). It represents a spectrum of disease (4). Sixty-five percent of the patients have an initial cause, while approximately 35% have no initial cause (5). The sciatic nerve and its distal branches are affected in approximately 40% of the cases. It has been suggested that the median and sciatic nerves (6, 7) are most frequently involved because they carry the vast majority of sensory and postganglionic sympathetic fibers to the extremities (8). An estimated 1% to 15% of peripheral nerve injuries eventually lead to RSDS (9). These patients are difficult to treat. Spontaneous remission is unusual in adults, occurring in fewer than 5% of the cases.

When an extremity is traumatized, a normal sympathetic reflex arc occurs. The painful stimulus travels through the afferent sensory fibers within the peripheral nerve. It then proceeds through the posterior root ganglion and synapses in the posterior horn. The impulse then moves to the lateral horn, where the sympathetic nerve body becomes excited and an impulse is sent via sympathetic efferent nerves out of the anterior root. Here the impulse synapses again in the sympathetic ganglia, traveling out the gray rami and into the somatic nerve to the periphery, causing vasoconstriction. However, as healing progresses, the vasoconstriction is not needed and the normal sympathetic reflex shuts down, promoting further healing by increasing vasodilatation.

With RSDS, this reflex is continued abnormally and is accelerated, causing an intense hypersympathetic condition in the peripheral tissues and resulting in ischemia and pain in the affected limb. This can be devastating to the patient's injured extremity and can result in severe pain and permanent disability.

Interestingly enough, the interval from the precipitating event to the onset of symptoms is highly variable. The average time interval in which symptoms occur is several weeks. However, the interval may be as short as 1 day or as long as several years. The causal association is less clear when several years have elapsed (3). Some authors report that the average incidence of RSDS in the population is 1% to 15% (9). All clinical forms of RSDS show a statistically higher incidence in the female, usually a 3:2 female/male ratio, and are more frequently seen in the middle-aged patient (age 30 to 60 years) (1, 9).

RSDS is a variable symptom complex characterized by chronic pain, hypersensitivity, abnormal vasomotor activity, and a muscle-splinting response that may progress to muscle and bone atrophy, chronic edema, and fibrosis, with tendon adhesions and joint contractures. Diagnosis must be prompt, and initiation of treatment must be immediate. Most authors agree that the sooner the treatment is started, the greater the likelihood that the condition will be halted or reversed. Treatment is directed at breaking up the abnormal sympathetic reflex. There is not one single treatment that has proved completely satisfactory for this (10).

RSDS: DEFINITIONS AND NOMENCLATURE

The term *causalgia* (from the Greek *kausos* = heat and *algos* = pain) was introduced in 1872 by Mitchell (11), although the burning pain syndrome he described had been identified by the end of the sixteenth century (12) (Table 45.1) (11-28). Several years earlier, Mitchell and his colleagues wrote the original brilliant clinical description of causalgia, which even today remains unsurpassed (19).

As knowledge and recognition of this syndrome have broadened and the basic sympathetic nervous dysfunction has been identified more clearly, many descriptive terms have evolved (Table 45.2) (11, 23, 24, 28-47). Often these terms describe only one or two aspects or types of the disorder, which is now known as reflex sympathetic dystrophy syndrome (28), an all-encompassing name that reflects a spectrum of painful sympathetic dysfunctions. The British literature uses a similarly inclusive term *algodystrophy* (30), sometimes referred to as *algoneurodystrophy* (31).

Causalgia is actually a subcategory of RSDS. It refers to

Table 45.1.
History of RSDS

1598	Pare (12)	First recorded awareness of the condition
Late 18th C	Pott (13, 14)	Surgeon at St. Bartholomew's Hospital; described RSDS as response to trauma
1813	Denmark (15)	Described terrible burning pain in the arm of one of Wellington's troopers after an injury at the Battle of Badajoz
1812	Bell (16)	
1832	Scarpa (16)	Reported on patients with painful extremities following injuries to nerves
1838	Hamilton (17)	
1864	Paget (18)	Wrote about the distressingly painful glossy fingers seen after injury to the radial nerve
1864	Mitchell, Moorehouse, Keene (19)	Gave classic description of a pain syndrome produced by gunshot nerve wounds in U.S. Civil War soldiers
1867	Dunglison (20)	Colleague of Mitchell credited with suggesting the term *causalgia* to describe the (burning) pain syndrome
1872	Mitchell (11)	Published a book on nerve injuries in which the word *causalgia* appears for the first time
1882	Volkmann (21)	First to describe posttraumatic rarefaction of bone
1898	Destot (22)	Noted osteoporosis following a long-standing, painful ankle sprain
1900	Sudeck (23)	Described acute atrophy of bone in the extremity and attributed it to inflammation
1901	Kienboch (24)	Related acute atrophy of bone to antecedent trauma
1938	Sudeck (25)	Accepted both inflammation and trauma as precursors of the osteoporosis that now bears his name
1930	Spurling (26)	Performed sympathectomy to treat circulatory disturbance of causalgia, confirming the role of the sympathetic nervous system in controlling vasomotor tone
1935	Kwan (27)	Duplicated sympathectomy treatment, documenting the presence of an incomplete peripheral nerve lesion as the primary source of injury
1947	Evans (28)	Reported on 57 cases and coined the term *reflex sympathetic dystrophy*

Table 45.2.
Terminology Used to Describe Reflex Sympathetic Dystrophy Syndrome

Term	Source
Acute atrophy of bone	Sudeck, 1900 (23)
Acute posttraumatic bone atrophy	Gurd, 1934 (29)
Algodystrophy	*British Medical Journal*, 1978 (30)
Algoneurodystrophy	Glick, 1973 (31)
Atypical posttraumatic pain syndrome	Turf and Bacardi, 1986 (32)
Causalgia	Mitchell, 1872 (11)
Causalgic state	DeTakats, 1945 (33)
Major causalgia	Echlin et al., 1949 (34)
Minor causalgia	Homan, 1940 (35)
Mimocausalgia	Thompson et al., 1975 (36); Black, 1980 (37)
Posttraumatic painful osteoporosis	Fontaine and Hermanne, 1933 (38)
Posttraumatic vasomotor disorder	Schumaker and Abramson, 1949 (39)
Reflex dystrophy of the extremities	DeTakats, 1937 (40)
Reflex hyperemic deossification	DeLorimer et al., 1946 (41)
Reflex neurovascular dystrophy	Steinbrocker and Argyros, 1947 (42)
Reflex sympathetic dystrophy	Evans, 1947 (28)
Reflex trophoneurosis	Kienböck, 1901 (14)
Shoulder-hand syndrome	Steinbrocker, 1947 (43)
Sudeck's osteodystrophy	Lenggenhager, 1971 (44)
Sympathetic-maintained pain syndrome	Roberts, 1986 (45)
Traumatic vasospasm	Lehman, 1933 (46)
Variable pain syndrome	Kleinert et al., 1973 (47)

Adapted from Malament IB, Glick JB: Sudeck's atrophy: A clinical syndrome. *J Am Podiatry Assoc* 73:362,1983.

a syndrome of sustained burning pain after a traumatic nerve lesion combined with vasomotor and sudomotor dysfunction and later trophic changes (48). Terms such as *minor causalgia* and *causalgic state* have been used to describe causalgia without major nerve injury but are now redundant within the RSDS spectrum. *Reflex sympathetic dystrophy* as coined by Evans (28) has been used to describe latent pain syndromes that are not related to nerve damage (8, 49).

Sudeck's atrophy of bone (23, 25) is actually a radiological finding that usually is seen later in the disease process. It is a type of osteoporosis caused by the sympathetically induced hyperemia.

All of these conditions (Table 45.3)(9) have the common features of sympathetic hyperactivity associated with persistent pain, and they usually respond to sympathetic interruption. Thus reflex sympathetic dystrophy is a syndrome of pain, hyperesthesia, vasomotor disturbances, and dystrophic changes, which usually improves with sympathetic denervation (50).

PATHOPHYSIOLOGY

No single hypothesis proposed to date explains all the features of RSDS (9), and the pathophysiology of RSDS is not well understood even today. Even more perplexing is how to explain a minor injury in which pain is greater than the pain produced by the initial injury and can persist long after the injury has healed (51).

One of the more plausible theories is a centrally mediated autonomic regulation theory proposed in 1943 by Livingston (52), who postulated that three factors were involved in the production of a vicious cycle of reflexes (Fig. 45.1). The first factor is chronic irritation of a peripheral sensory

Table 45.3.
Clinical Variants of Reflex Sympathetic Dystrophy

Condition	Description
Causalgia	RSD symptom complex that occurs after peripheral nerve injury
Minor causalgia	RSD symptoms with prominent hyperesthesia that occur after insult which does not cause demonstrable nerve injury
Major causalgia	RSD symptom complex that occurs after peripheral nerve injury
Minocausalgia	RSD symptom complex that occurs after insult to central nervous system
Sudeck's atrophy of bone	RSD symptom complex that occurs after soft-tissue trauma with *bony atrophy* as predominant finding
Algoneurodystrophy	RSD symptom complex that occurs after minor trauma
Shoulder-hand syndrome	RSD symptom complex with "frozen shoulder" that occurs after myocardial infarction, cardiovascular accident, or cervical radiculopathy
Reflex dystrophy	RSD symptom complex
Reflex neurovascular dystrophy	RSD symptom complex

From Schwartzman RJ, McLellan TL: Reflex sympathetic dystrophy: a review. *Arch Neurol* 44:555-561, 1987.

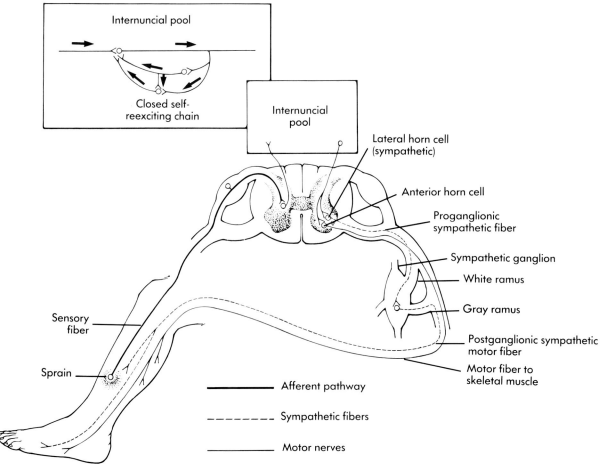

Figure 45.1. Theory of reverberating circuits. Livingston adopted the theory of Lorento de No relative to the "internuncial pool" to explain the vicious cycle of impulses within the spinal cord instigated by the afferent pain stimuli. (Adapted from Lorento de No R: Analysis of the activity of the chains of internuncial neurons. *J Neurophysiol* I:237, 1938, and Evans JA: Reflex sympathetic dystrophy; report on 57 cases. *Ann Intern Med* 26:417, 1947.)

nerve by trauma and soft tissue damage. This produces an increased afferent input and results in the second factor, which is an abnormal state of activity in the internuncial neuronal pool. This then creates a large intracord burst of activity and subsequently produces the third factor, a continuous stimulation of sympathetic and motor efferent fibers (51, 52). This is the so-called theory of reverberating circuits in the spinal cord to explain the phenomenon of RSDS (9). Headley advocated sympathectomy as one way to interrupt the negative feedback loop (20).

In 1965 the gate-control theory was developed by Melzak and Wall (53). They theorized that specialized cells in the dorsal horn called substantiae gelatinosa (SG) form a functional unit that is under constant cortical feedback. The substantiae gelatinosa modulate afferent transmissions carried by small (C) and large (A) fibers (Fig. 45.2). Activation of the small fibers suppresses the SG and the gate opens. Alternately, if the large-fiber activity is greatest in stimulating the SG, this further suppresses it, afferent impulses are blocked, and the gate closes. This means that dominant small-fiber input could result in unchecked transmission of pain through an open gate (53, 54). Since both of these systems operate at all times, the information that is relayed is a summation of all activity (9). This describes in technical terms what Mitchell's patients knew instinctively 100 years ago: counterirritation provides relief from pain (19, 20). Also, this is how transcutaneous nerve stimulation is thought to decrease pain in RSDS.

In contrast, Doupe and associates (55), in 1944, proposed a peripheral mechanism for this type of pain. Using laboratory studies, they postulated that in patients with traumatized peripheral nerves an artificial synapse (ephapse) developed between sensory afferents and sympathetic ef-

ferents, allowing direct cross-stimulation and cycle formation (54). This direct cross-stimulation of sensory fibers by efferent sympathetic impulses at the point where the nerve is injured furnishes an explanation for the increase in pain plus temperature changes. It also helps explain why emotional excitement increases pain, whereas sleep and a calm emotional state greatly diminish this pain (51, 55).

In 1983 Devor (56) reported experimental evidence that damage to Schwann cells or to the axons themselves results in local demyelination or sprout outgrowth. These localized areas can acquire an ectopic pacemaker capability, which may discharge spontaneously or in response to any depolarizing stimulus. Circulating catecholamines and those from sympathetic efferents start the pacemaker and increase its discharge (9, 56).

Most recently, advances in the nociceptive pain system have solved some of the problems with the earlier theories. The classic reflex arc or nociceptive loop is now well known. Afferent pain impulses move toward the spinal cord via the dorsal root ganglion. Substance P is a neurotransmitter of noxious stimuli at this level. Sympathetic efferents carry impulses that cause release of substances that excite (histamine and bradykinin) or stimulate (prostaglandins) skin nociceptors. This loop can be modified by local or encephalon-inhibitory systems within the dorsal horn of the medulla. Ephapses between sympathetic and nociceptive afferent nerves have been demonstrated in experimental animal models (57, 58).

The pathophysiology of the osteoporosis that may accompany RSDS is not well understood. One theory maintains that the alteration of hemodynamics associated with abnormal sympathetic activity causes hyperemia and that the resultant increased blood flow to the bone causes the char-

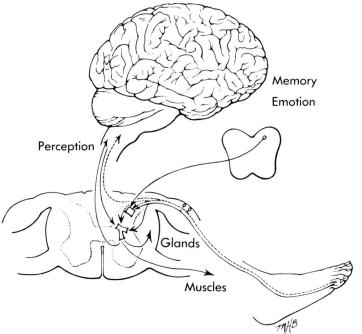

Figure 45.2. Gate control theory. Melzack and Wall postulated that spinal cord activity is modulated by a balance between the myelinated A fibers and the small unmyelinated C fibers. Thus, higher cortical centers, psychological factors, and other levels of the spinal cord influence this balance. (Redrawn from Wilson, RL: Management of pain following peripheral nerve injuries. *Orthop Clin North Am* 12:343, 1981.)

Memory
Emotion

Perception

Glands

Muscles

acteristic osteoporosis (51). Swezey (59) attributes continued osteoporosis in the latter stages of RSDS to lack of muscle action on bone. Huaus and associates (60) found that radiographic findings suggestive of RSDS are found frequently in patients with osteomalacia secondary to renal tubular disorders. They suggest that some patients with musculoskeletal complications of renal tubular acidosis may have a quick resolution of RSDS symptoms with the appropriate treatment. Furthermore, excitation of the nociceptive loop causes an increase in prostaglandins, which also affect bone metabolism (58).

Biopsies of synovium show proliferation of synovial lining cells accompanied by synovial edema, fibrosis, capillary proliferation and perivascular inflammatory infiltration. The histopathology of the involved bone shows increased vascularity and prominent osteoclastic activity (49, 61).

DIATHESIS

Lankford (62, 63) proposed three factors that must be present at the same time before RSDS can develop: (a) a persistent painful lesion (traumatic or acquired), (b) a diathesis, and (c) an abnormal sympathetic reflex. The diathesis, or predisposition, is a susceptibility to a certain disease status. With respect to diathesis, Lankford believes there are two types of patients.

The first type consists of the hypersympathetic reactors, the patients with evidence of increased sympathetic activity such as feet that are chronically cold or sweaty, summer or winter. They may exhibit pallor, slight cyanosis, or coolness of the toes in spite of palpable pulses. There may be a history of fainting, blushing easily, or migraine headaches.

The second type consists of patients who are described psychologically as having inadequate personality. These patients are fearful, suspicious, and emotionally labile and tend to be chronic complainers. Patients of this type can be difficult to treat, since they try to control their own treatment and habitually blame others for their problems.

In general, it has been suggested that patients with such a hypersympathetic diathesis have some common characteristics. Julsrud (64) described a background of vasomotor instability and a hyperemotional temperament as prerequisites to the development of RSDS. Owens (65), in reviewing the histories of such patients, believed them to have a different anatomic and physiologic makeup from the other 95% of the population, one that allows their sympathetic nervous systems to become hyperactive. He described these persons as sympathetic reactors.

Steinberg (66) recognized a sympathetic-sensitive patient type that he termed Raynaudian. This is a patient with a centrally induced hypertonicity of the sympathetic nervous system, similar to the hypersympathetic reactor described by Lankford. This condition is not the same as Raynaud's disease, which is a pathologically exaggerated response to cold exposure that results in prolonged vasoconstriction in the skin of distal parts. Another disorder with the common

trait of vasomotor instability is acrocyanosis frigida (pernio), the mildest form of cold injury. Patients with those conditions have a susceptibility to RSDS, especially after trauma or surgery.

CLINICAL PRESENTATION AND COURSE

Precipitating Factors

Even though RSDS is associated with a remarkable variety of triggering events (9) (Table 45.4), studies have shown that in as many as 35% of the cases no precipitating factor can be identified (5).

Exactly how all of these events cause the same clinical syndrome remains unknown. Trauma, even the most trivial, is a frequent instigator. The symptoms may appear gradually or within days or weeks and sometimes within hours after the incident.

Table 45.4.

Precipitating Factors and Diseases Associated With Reflex Sympathetic Dystrophy

Peripheral

Soft-tissue injury
Arthritides
Infection
Fasciitis, tendonitis, bursitis
Venous or arterial thrombosis
Fractures, sprains, dislocations
Operative procedures
Malignancy
Aortic injury
Myelography, spinal anesthesia
Paravertebral alcohol injection
Postherpetic
Brachial plexus pathosis, scalenus anticus syndrome
Radiculopathy
Immobilization with cast or splint
Vasculitis
Myocardial infarction
Weber-Christian disease
Polymyalgia rheumatica
Pulmonary fibrosis

Central

Brain tumor
Severe head injury
Cerebral infarction
Subarachnoid hemorrhage
Cervical cord injury
Subacute combined degeneration
Syringomyelia
Poliomyelitis
Amyotrophic lateral sclerosis

Other

Idiopathic
Prolonged bedrest
Familial

Modified from Schwartzman RJ, McLellan TL: Reflex sympathetic dystrophy: a review. *Arch Neurol* 44:555-561, 1987.

Pain

Pain in the extremity is the one denominator common to all stages and all patients affected with RSDS (16). All other symptoms, changes, or manifestations may or may not occur. They include vasomotor, sudomotor, and trophic changes and response to sympathetic blockade (48).

The pain is characteristically of a burning or aching nature. It is often accompanied by allodynia, pain due to a noxious stimulation of normal skin or painful sensation to touch (touch-pain), and hyperpathia, the delayed over reaction to a stimulus, especially a repetitive stimulus (45, 48, 67-69). The pain is usually out of proportion to the injury or precipitating event and progresses outside the dermatome of any involved nerves. As a result, the patient suffers greatly and tends to protect the affected extremity (11, 70, 71).

Stages

Many authors have classified RSDS into several stages based on objective, radiographic, and clinical signs rather than on subjective pain (16). Although there is disagreement as to the exact divisions, it is apparent that RSDS is a dynamic disease process that can have simultaneous involvement of skin, connective tissues, muscle, blood vessels, and bone.

Each stage was originally described as being from 3 to 6 months in duration (72). In the clinical setting, however, the actual length of each stage may vary remarkably, lasting from weeks to years. In addition, there may be considerable overlap of the stages.

STAGE I (ACUTE)

The constant pain, which may start immediately or not until several weeks after the incident, is of an intense burning or aching nature and is closely limited to the site of the injury. There may be edema of the foot and ankle, accompanied by hyperthermia or hypothermia, hyperhidrosis or anhidrosis, and muscle wasting as the patient protects the part against motion. The pain is aggravated by light touch, bed sheets, movement, and emotion as well as by auditory and visual stimuli. It is usually lessened in a quiet environment and by sleep or narcosis. Trophic changes are not yet apparent, although signs sufficient to be seen on radiographs may appear within 4 to 6 weeks. Symptoms may cease at this stage, or the dystrophy may advance into the second stage.

STAGE II (DYSTROPHIC)

The edema becomes more indurated over a somewhat larger area as the skin takes on a cool, pale, discolored, and frequently mottled or cyanotic appearance. It may even be hyperhydrotic. Hair loss may occur as the nails become cracked, brittle, and ridged. The pain is constant and is aggravated by any stimulus. Radiographs reveal a diffuse osteoporosis. This stage is still capable of improvement.

STAGE III (ATROPHIC)

Now the intractable pain spreads proximally to involve the entire limb, and trophic changes lead to irreversible tissue damage. Dermal blood flow is decreased, the skin is thin and shiny, and the toe-tips become wasted as the fat pads atrophy. The fascia becomes thickened, and joints stiffen, even to the point of ankylosis. Radiographs show a marked demineralization.

Clinical Course

Confusion in staging and determining the extent of the dystrophy revolves around the exaggerated sympathetic response. There are two principal variations related to sympathetic function (16, 64, 73). In one type, vasoconstriction predominates and the extremity skin is cold, thin, and shiny and perspires profusely. In the other type, vasodilatation predominates and the skin is warm, dry, and scaly.

There are various forms of this disorder, distinguished by the severity of the sympathetic response (74). In many cases the reaction borders so closely on the normal response of an extremity to trauma that the diagnosis is not made and the patient suffers through a natural course without treatment.

It is difficult, if not impossible, to predict the course of RSDS, once it has been identified. The disorder may be self-limiting, but not without much agony. There is agreement that early recognition and treatment will lead to a much better response to treatment, thus limiting the duration of the syndrome (9).

Patients afflicted with RSDS may seem emotionally unstable, anxious, and socially withdrawn (75). Unrelenting pain, distress, and discouragement can lead to chronic invalidism, drug addiction, psychiatric problems, and even suicide. Emotional sequelae and the disparity between the degree of pain and the physical examination findings may mislead clinicians to believe the pain is psychogenic. This erroneous belief, added to misguided therapeutic efforts at relieving the intractable pain, serves only to further aggravate the psychological symptoms. The increased anxiety then increases sympathetic discharge, which exacerbates the pain, and the vicious cycle continues (9) (Fig. 45.3).

Determining secondary gain motives can be all but impossible in the case of RSDS with emotional and psychological factors. It is also difficult when litigation or compensation is involved. When the possibility of malingering, somatization, or conversion disorder (hysterical neurosis) is suspected, a paravertebral sham block of the sympathetic chain can be performed (76, 77). If the patient reports relief, then the presence of RSDS is questionable. On the other hand, if a patient gets no relief from a paravertebral sympathetic nerve block with a local anesthetic, then the diagnosis of RSDS is doubtful and further investigation should be performed (4).

Figure 45.3. The vicious cycle of reflex sympathetic dystrophy. Pain causes reflex immobility leading to stasis and edema. Reactive fibrous tissue develops scar and muscle contracture. Persistent vasospasm produces ischemia, which magnifies the pain. All factors lead to a painful stiff dystrophic extremity. (Adapted from Wilson, RL: Management of pain following peripheral nerve injuries. *Orthop Clin North Am* 12:343, 1981.)

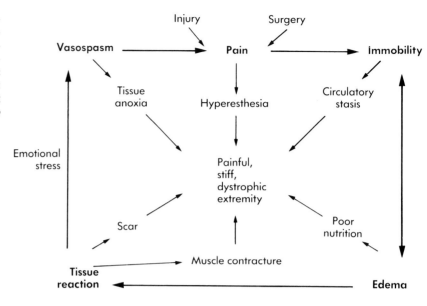

DIAGNOSIS

The diagnosis of RSDS must be distinguished from that of causalgia. The diagnostic criteria must be strict, as the two entities may exist together. Symptoms of causalgia are directly related to an injury to a specific peripheral nerve. This injury can be documented, and distribution of the burning pain is contained only along that specific peripheral damaged nerve. In RSDS, the symptoms of hyperalgesia are outside the distribution of any single peripheral nerve. Also, the pain must be grossly out of proportion to the injury. In no case can the patient's pain be completely accounted for by an injury to a specific injured peripheral nerve (1).

Diagnostic criteria for RSDS have been proposed by Kozin and associates (Table 45.5) (78). The signs and symptoms of RSDS include pain, hyperesthesia to light touch, swelling, discoloration and stiffness, and limitation of motion, which allows fibrosis secondary to formation of adhesions. There is a decrease in the gliding of the structures in the extremity and an increase in the thickness of the fascia, with resulting contractures (5, 54). RSDS is usually unilateral, but in 10% to 20% of the cases it may be bilateral (6). The differential diagnosis for RSDS is listed in Table 45.6.

In the lower extremity, the foot may become red with capillary vasodilatation, blue with vasoconstriction of the venous system, or white with pallor or vasoconstriction of the arterial system. There may be a generalized reddish purple mottling of the affected lower extremity called livedo reticularis as a further sign of vasomotor instability.

By far the most prominent clinical feature is pain out of proportion to the injury or trauma involved (62). The common denominator in all patients at all stages is pain in the extremity (51). In addition, the pain may appear within hours of an injury or sometime thereafter. Kirklin and co-workers (79) in their case descriptions, considered the pain to have begun immediately in 80% of the cases, with 20% beginning anywhere from 3 days to 4 weeks after injury.

Diagnosis of RSDS can be made when the four cardinal

Table 45.5.
Diagnostic Clinical Features and Supportive Criteria for RSDS

Definite RSDS

Pain and tenderness in an extremity
Signs and/or symptoms of vasomotor instability
Swelling in the extremity—often with periarticular prominence
Dystrophic skin changes usually present (late stages)

Probable RSDS

Pain and tenderness in an extremity and either
   vasomotor instability or swelling
Dystrophic skin changes often present (late stages)

Possible RSDS

Vasomotor instability and either
   swelling or tenderness
Dystrophic skin changes occasionally present

Doubtful RSDS

Unexplained pain and tenderness in an extremity
No evidence of vasomotor instability
No dystrophic skin changes

Supportive Criteria

Abnormal delayed-image bone scan showing increased periarticular activity in several joints
Radiographs of the affected distal extremity show localized patchy osteoporosis
Relief by sympathetic blockade

Data from Smith and Campbell (3) and Kozin et al. (78).

signs and symptoms (pain, swelling, stiffness, and discoloration) and most of the secondary signs and symptoms (osseous demineralization, pseudomotor changes, temperature changes, trophic changes, vasomotor instability, and plantar fasciitis) are present (1, 57, 80). The diagnosis is confirmed when there is diminution of the patient's signs and symptoms with interruption of the abnormal sympathetic reflex (1, 4, 9, 62, 81).

Testing for vasomotor instability may be performed in

Table 45.6.
Differential Diagnosis for RSDS

Tarsal tunnel syndrome
Raynaud's phenomenon
Long-standing diabetes—polyneuropathy
"Flare reaction" following injury/surgery
Lupus erythematosus
Polymyalgia rheumatica
Giant cell arteritis
Multiple sclerosis
Peripheral neuritis
Osteomyelitis
Thromboangiitis obliterans
Thrombophlebitis/deep vein thrombosis
Hypertrophic/inflammatory arthritis
Neurovascular entrapment
Early scleroderma
Mixed connective tissue disease
Acute arterial occlusion
Metastatic carcinoma
Multiple myeloma
Hyperparathyroidism
Cushing's syndrome
Paget's disease
Disuse atrophy
Migratory osteolysis of the lower extremity

the office by means of the cold water immersion test (82). An extremity placed in a container with water cooled to 8 to 10° C for about 20 minutes will produce pallor in the extremity, and the limb will also have increased pain. Subcapillary venous plexus filling time may be prolonged on the affected side (1). There can be sudomotor changes in the extremity, usually in the first few months. This can cause maceration of the skin and fungus or yeast infections in the web spaces, as well as hyperhidrosis.

Corresponding temperature changes may occur (83). Thermography is the best diagnostic instrument beyond the physical examination in the evaluation of RSDS and its treatment (84). One may see a decrease in temperature in either the early or late stages of the disease. Alternatively, there may be an increase in temperature, which may be localized to the joints, with a concomitant increase in redness (1). Trophic changes may be seen in the skin. In the late stages, the skin has a glossy, shiny appearance with absence of skin creases. The patient may have plantar fasciitis or acute nodules and thickening of the plantar fascia. In such circumstances surgery would be contraindicated.

Measurements of segmental blood pressures and Doppler waveform analysis aid in diagnosing the vasomotor changes in RSDS. Segmental pressures may vary, being up to 10 to 20 mm Hg lower on the affected side over the dorsalis pedis and posterior tibial arteries. Doppler waveform changes may be only trivial compared with the marked changes seen on physical examination (85). Sympathetic blockade is diagnostic if the pain in the affected limb improves, prompt peripheral warming occurs, and there is a loss of sweating. An accurate examination of the extremity can be made, and active mobilization and physical therapy may be performed during this pain-free interval.

In patients with RSDS blood tests will demonstrate a normal white blood cell count, erythrocyte sedimentation rate, and serum biochemistry estimations. Occasionally, an increased urinary excretion of calcium and hydroxyproline has been demonstrated. The hypercalciuria seems to be a less common, variable feature, but increased hydroxyprolinuria appears fairly often and may parallel the course of the disease (86). Local or regional nerve blocks similar to Bier blocks may also be used for this purpose. Prolongation of the pain-free interval is claimed when the Bier block technique is augmented with corticosteroids, guanethidine, reserpine, or bretylium (2, 9, 82, 86-93).

Radiographically, osteoporosis can be seen as early as the third week, but it usually appears after the sixth week. It can progress for about a year and may move proximally up the limb (1). It is also known as acute bone atrophy after trauma demonstrating punched-out areas followed by bone atrophy in the affected limb. This osteoporosis is not like senile osteoporosis, and it may decrease with use of the involved limb. The osteoporosis tends to be patchy and primarily in the juxta-articular regions initially, in the short bones of the feet, and becomes more diffuse as the disease progresses (3, 9). There are many cases of sympathetic dystrophy, however, in which there is no bone change (51). About 70% of patients with RSDS demonstrate osteopenia (3). Other bone diseases that demonstrate subperiosteal bone resorption, striation, and tunneling in the cortices, as well as large excavations and tunneling of the endosteal surface, include hyperparathyroidism, thyrotoxicosis, and other conditions associated with increased bone turnover (9).

Bone scans using methylene diphosphonate labeled with technetium (Tc 99m) in patients with RSDS often show increased blood flow and regional pooling, even if an x-ray film is normal (3). Comparatively speaking, Kozin and associates (78) found that the specificity of roentgenography was 71% whereas that of scintigraphy was 86%. The sensitivity of roentgenography was 69% and that of scintigraphy was 60% for RSDS patients. Delayed scintigraphic images almost invariably show increased justa-articular uptake in multiple joints in the affected extremity (3)(Fig. 45.4).

The diagnostic findings of RSDS in bone scans have yet to be clearly outlined. MacKinnon and Holder (57) do not consider a flow study positive if there are only focal increases in perfusion. They require a diffuse increase in perfusion in the extremity to determine the scan positive for RSDS. They also require that all joints be involved on the delayed image before they deem the result positive. It must be noted that abnormal perfusion scans may occur, resulting in diminished flow to the involved extremity. This is thought to be due to the vasomotor instability noted clinically (5). Helms and associates (94) described two cases of segmental RSDS that displayed positive bone scan findings in only two digits in an extremity.

When severe pain occurs, a person's ability to handle the situation may be complicated by any personality deficiencies, and a psychiatric consultation can be helpful to both the physician and the patient (95). Other important consulta-

Figure 45.4. Delayed image from a Tc-99 bone scan showing the characteristic periarticular uptake of the isotope, diagnostic of RSDS.

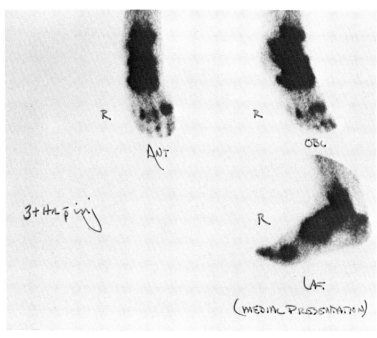

Table 45.7.
Treatments for RSDS

Pharmaceutical	Chemical Sympathectomy
Prednisone (3, 49, 58, 78)	Paravertebral block (1, 28, 45)
Elavil (95)	Bier block (9)
Prolixin (95)	Reserpine (82, 92)
Procardia (4, 85)	Guanethidine (82, 88, 90, 91, 93, 95)
NSAIDs (4)	Solu-Medrol (2, 54, 58)
Dibenzyline (8)	Lidocaine (3, 4, 8, 51, 98)
	Peripheral block
Physical Therapy	Bretylium (87, 88, 99)
Massage (4)	Raj technique epidural block (100)
Ultrasound (4, 96)	
Desensitization (8, 58)	*Surgery*
ROM exercises (1, 8, 9, 51)	Sympathectomy (58, 81, 98, 99)
Jobst extremity pump (20, 95)	
Splint (20, 95)	*Adjunct Therapy*
Hydrotherapy (20)	Psychotherapy
Contrast baths	Biofeedback (4, 20)
	In hospital physiatry (20, 58)
Interference With Neural Transmission	
TENS (8, 20, 95)	
Trigger point electrical stimulation (4, 81, 97)	
Acupuncture (97)	

tions include those with the radiologist, the vascular specialist, the rheumatologist, and the internist. These specialists will help rule out other diagnoses. An anesthesiologist can be consulted to perform the paraspinal sympathetic nerve blocks. It may also be helpful to enroll the patient in a pain clinic to learn such techniques as biofeedback or to wean the patient from narcotic analgesics (20).

TREATMENT

There are nearly as many treatments for RSDS as there are causes of the disease (Table 45.7)(1-5, 8, 9, 20, 49, 51, 54, 58, 78-81, 82, 85, 87-93, 95-100). Most important, it is essential to make the diagnosis as soon as possible so that treatment can be started immediately. The earlier the treatment, the better the chances of reversing or halting the disease process.

Rodriquez-Moreno and associates (101) state that RSDS can continue for years and that none of the therapeutic trials have shown true efficacy. Davis and associates (102), using dog studies, gave the first experimental proof that sympathectomy exerts a transient effect on blood flow in bone, with the largest increases seen in the metatarsals and proximal phalanges. Chemical or surgical sympathectomies have had relatively high rates of success (Fig. 45.5). However, even surgical sympathectomies may fail when an inappropriate level is selected or a contralateral procedure has to be performed, possibly because of reinnervation (103, 104). Inadequate or unsuccessful sympathectomy may also be caused by variations in the lumbar trunk (104). With end-stage RSDS, amputation may be the only means of relief (9).

RSDS in Children

Until 1985 only about 57 cases of childhood RSDS had been reported in the English language literature. Rush and co-workers (105) described three more children with the disease. They reported results unlike those previously published. Three patients had permanent roentgenographic changes similar to adult disease as well as permanent limb changes, including failure of growth, fixed flexion contractures, and muscle wasting.

Stilz and associates (106) described a 6-year-old girl with the disease, who was treated successfully with transcutaneous electrical nerve stimulator (TENS). They stated that this treatment modality was reintroduced on the basis of Melzak and Wall's gate control theory. The youngest child with RSDS was reported by Richlin and co-workers (107). They

described successful treatment of a 3½-year-old boy with TENS therapy and proposed it as the preferred treatment for RSDS in children.

Bernstein and associates (108) reported 24 more cases of RSDS in 23 children. All were given physical therapy in hospital rehabilitation centers on an inpatient or outpatient basis. Rigorous physical therapy modalities were used and seven of the children received psychotherapy as well. After treating more than 300 children under the age of 16 years, they concluded that certain aspects of RSDS are different in childhood. These differences include a lesser frequency of knee involvement, a rarity of chronic trophic changes, a paucity of radiographic findings, and excellent responses to treatment. Again, delayed or incorrect diagnosis may lead to chronic or permanent disability and prolonged suffering in affected children. RSDS may not be such a rare disease in children, which substantiates the need for an increased diagnostic awareness.

SUMMARY

RSDS is a very real and painful disorder that involves an exaggerated reaction of the sympathetic nervous system. It is widely agreed that early diagnosis is essential to prevent long-term morbidity. A heightened awareness of RSDS as

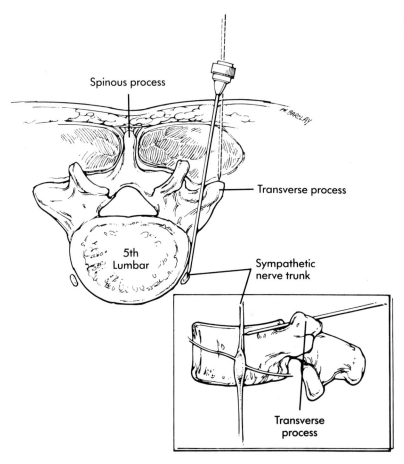

Figure 45.5. Technique for paravertebral nerve block (PNB). (Redrawn from Evans, JA: Reflex sympathetic dystrophy; report on 57 cases. *Ann Intern Med* 26:417, 1947.)

Spinous process

Transverse process

5th Lumbar

Sympathetic nerve trunk

Transverse process

a clinical spectrum, a knowledge of the wide array of precipitating events, and the prompt institution of therapy are needed to prevent protracted cases and to eliminate prolonged suffering and limitation of function.

The ideal situation when one is planning to inflict the iatrogenic trauma of surgery is to predict the susceptible patient, the one with the diathesis for RSDS. Ideally, in the future prophylactic measures might be designed for such patients in order to guard against triggering RSDS.

References

1. Lankford LL: Reflex sympathetic dystrophy. In Evarts CM (ed): *Surgery of the Musculoskeletal System.* London, Churchill Livingstone, 1983, vol I, pp 1, 145-174.

2. Poplawski K, Wiley A, Murray J: Post-traumatic dystrophy of the extremities. *J Bone Joint Surg* 65A:642-655, 1983.

3. Smith DL, Campbell SM: Reflex sympathetic dystrophy syndrome: diagnosis and management. *West J Med* 147:342-345, 1987.

4. Amadio TC: Current concepts review: pain dysfunction syndromes. *J Bone Joint Surg* 70A:944-949, 1988.

5. Kozin F, Soin J, Ryan L, Carrera G, Wortmann R: Bone scintigraphy in the reflex sympathetic dystrophy syndrome. *Radiology* 138:437-443, 1981.

6. Richards RL: Causalgia: a centennial review. *Arch Neurol* 16:339-350, 1976.

7. Jebara VA, Saade B: Causalgia: a wartime experience - report of twenty treated cases. *J Trauma* 27:519-524, 1987.

8. Hodges DL, McGuire TJ: Burning and pain after injury. *Postgrad Med* 83:185-192, 1988.

9. Schwartzman RJ, McLellan TL: Reflex sympathetic dystrophy: a review. *Arch Neurol* 44:555-561, 1987.

10. Malament IB, Glick JB: Sudeck's atrophy: the clinical syndrome. *J Am Podiatry Assoc* 73:362-368, 1983.

11. Mitchell SW: *Injuries of Nerves and Their Consequences.* Philadelphia, JB Lippincott, 1872, p 56.

12. Pare A: *Les Ouvres D'Ambroise Pare.* Paris, Gabriel Buon, 1598 (Histoire de defunct) Rl: Charles IX, 10th book, chap 41, p 401.

13. Pote P (cited by EM Webb and EW Davis). Causalgia: a review. *California Med* 69:412, 1948.

14. Ross JP: Causalgia. *St Barth Hosp Rep* 65:103-188, 1932.

15. Denmark A: An example of symptoms resembling tic douloureux produced by a wound in the radial nerve. *Med Chir Trans* 4:48, 1813.

16. Drucker WR, Hubay CA, Holden WD, Bukovnic JA: Pathogenesis of post-traumatic sympathetic dystrophy. *Am J Surg* 97:454-465, 1959.

17. Hamilton J: On some effects resulting from wounds of nerves. *Dublin J Med Sci* 13:38, 1838.

18. Paget J: Effects from a wound to the radial nerve. *Med Times* 612:1, 1864.

19. Mitchell SW, Morehouse GR, Keene WW: *Gunshot Wounds and Other Injuries of Nerves.* Philadelphia, JB Lippincott, 1864, p 164.

20. Headley B: Historical perspective of causalgia: management of sympathetically maintained pain. *Phys Ther* 67:1370-1374, 1987.

21. Volkmann R: Cited in Landoff GA: Experimentelle untersuchungen uber die "Knochenatrophie" infolge einer immobilization und einer akuten arthritis. *Acta Chir Scand Suppl* 71, 1942.

22. Destot: Nouvelle application de la radiographie et de la radioscopie diagnostic chirugical. *Echo Med Lyon* 3:12-15, 1898.

23. Sudeck P: Uber die akute entzundliche Knockentrophe. *Arch Klin Chir* 62:147, 1900.

24. Kienboch R: Über akute knochen und die eutzundungsprozesse an den extremitaten (falschlich sogenannte Inactivitastrophie der Knochen) und ihre diagnose nach dem rontgenbily. *Wien Med Wochenschr* 51:1345, 1901.

25. Sudeck P: Die kollaterallen entzundungsreaktionen an den gliedmassen (Sog akute knochen-atrophie). *Arch Klin Chir* 191:710, 1938.

26. Spurling RG: Causalgia of the upper extremity: treatment by dorsal sympathetic ganglionectomy. *Arch Neurol Neurosurg Psychiatry* 23:784, 1930.

27. Kwan ST: The treatment of causalgia by thoracic sympathetic ganglionectomy. *Ann Surg* 101:222-227, 1935.

28. Evans JA: Reflex sympathetic dystrophy; report on 57 cases. *Ann Intern Med* 26:417, 1947.

29. Gurd FB: Post-traumatic acute bone atrophy (Sudeck's atrophy). *Ann Surg* 99:449, 1934.

30. Algodystrophy (Editorial). *Br Med J* 1:461-462, 1978.

31. Glick EN: Reflex dystrophy (algoneurodystrophy): results of treatment by corticosteroids. *Rheumatol Rehabil* 12:84-88, 1973.

32. Turf RM, Bacardi BE: Causalgia: clarifications in terminology and a case presentation. *J Foot Surg* 25:284-295, 1986.

33. DeTakats G: Causalgia states in peace and war. *JAMA* 128:699, 1945.

34. Echlin F, Owens FM Jr, Wells WL: Observations on major and minor causalgia. *Arch Neurol Psychiatry* 62:183, 1949.

35. Homans J: Minor causalgia: a hyperesthetic neurovascular syndrome. *N Engl J Med* 222:870-874, 1940.

36. Thompson JE, Patman RD, Persson AV: Management of post-traumatic pain syndromes (causalgia). *Ann Surg* 41:599, 1975.

37. Black JR: Minocausalgia. *J Am Podiatry Assoc* 70:430, 1980.

38. Fontaine R, Herrmann LG: Post-traumatic painful osteoporosis. *Ann Surg* 97:26, 1933.

39. Schumaker HB, Abramson DI: Post-traumatic vasomotor disorders. *Surg Gynecol Obstet* 88:417, 1949.

40. DeTakats G: Reflex dystrophy of the extremities. *Arch Surg* 34:939, 1937.

41. DeLorimer AA, Minear WL, Boyd HB: Reflex hyperemic deossification regional to joints of the extremities. *Radiology* 46:227, 1946.

42. Steinbrocker O, Argyros TG: The shoulder-hand syndrome in reflex dystrophy of the upper extremity. *Ann Intern Med* 92:22, 1947.

43. Steinbrocker O: The shoulder-hand syndrome. *Am J Med* 3:402-407, 1947.

44. Lenggenhager K: Sudeck's osteodystrophy: its pathogenesis, prophylaxis and therapy. *Minn Med* 54:967-972, 1981.

45. Roberts WJ: A hypothesis on the physiological basis for causalgia and related pains. *Pain* 24:297-311, 1986.

46. Lehman EP: Traumatic vasospasm: a study of four cases of vasospasm in the upper extremity. *Arch Surg* 29:92-107, 1934.

47. Kleinert HE, Cole NM, Wayne L, Harvey R, Kutz JE, Atasoy E: Post-traumatic sympathetic dystrophy. *Orthop Clin North Am* 4:917-927, 1973.

48. Schott GD: Mechanisms of causalgia and related clinical conditions: the role of the central and of the sympathetic nervous systems. *Brain* 109:717-738, 1986.

49. Kozin F, McCarty DJ, Sims J, Genant HK: The reflex sympathetic dystrophy syndrome (RSDS). I. Clinical and histologic response to corticosteroids, and articular involvement. *Am J Med* 60:321-331, 1976.

50. Patman RD, Thompson JE, Persson AV: Management of post-traumatic pain syndrome: report of 113 cases. *Ann Surg* 177:780-787, 1973.

51. Drucker WR, Hubay CA, Holden WD, Bukovnic JA: Pathogenesis of post-traumatic sympathetic dystrophy. *Am J Surg* 97:454-465, 1959.

52. Livingston WK: *Pain Mechanisms. A Physiologic Interpretation of Causalgia and Its Related States.* New York, Macmillan, 1943, p 212.

53. Melzak R, Wall PD: Pain mechanisms: a new theory. *Science* 150:971-979, 1965.

54. Schutzer SF, Gossling HR: Current concepts review: the treatment of reflex sympathetic dystrophy syndrome. *J Bone Joint Surg* 66A:625-629, 1984.

55. Doupe J, Cullen CH, Chance GZ: Post-traumatic pain and the causalgic syndrome. *J Neurol Neurosurg Psychiatry* 7:33, 1944.

56. Devor M: Nerve pathophysiology and mechanisms of pain in causalgia. *J Auton Nerv Syst* 7:371-384, 1983.

57. McKinnon SE, Holder LE: The use of three-phase radionuclide bone scanning in the diagnosis of reflex sympathetic dystrophy. *J Hand Surg* 9A:556-563, 1984.

58. McKinnon SE, Dellon AL: *Surgery of the Peripheral Nerve.* New York, Theime Medical Publishers, 1988, pp 492-504.

59. Swezey RL: Transient osteoporosis of the hip, foot and knee. *Arthritis Rheum* 13:858-868, 1970.

60. Huaus JP, Malghem J, Maldague B, Devogelaer JP, Esselinckx W, Withofs H, Nagant de Deuxchaisnes C: Reflex sympathetic dystrophy syndrome: an unusual mode of presentation of osteomalacia. *Arthritis Rheum* 29:918-925, 1986.

61. Fahr LM, Sauser DD: Imaging of peripheral nerve lesions. *Orthop Clin North Am* 19:27-41, 1988.
62. Lankford L, Thompson J: Reflex sympathetic dystrophy, upper and lower extremity: diagnosis and management. *The American Academy of Orthopaedic Surgeons Instructional Lectures*, St. Louis, CV Mosby, 1977, vol 26, pp 163-178.
63. Lankford L: Reflex sympathetic dystrophy. In *Management of Peripheral Nerves*. Philadelphia, WB Saunders, 1980, pp 216-244.
64. Julsrud ME: A review of reflex sympathetic dystrophy. *J Am Podiatry Assoc* 70:512, 1980.
65. Owens JC: Causalgia. *Ann Surg* 23:636, 1957.
66. Steinberg M: Gout and Sudeck's atrophy. *J Am Podiatry Assoc* 65:379-383, 1975.
67. Kozin F: Reflex sympathetic dystrophy syndrome. *Bull Rheum Dis* 36:1-8, 1986.
68. Tahmoush AJ: Causalgia: a redefinition as a clinical pain syndrome. *Pain* 10:187-197, 1981.
69. Merskey H: Pain terms: a supplementary note. *Pain* 14:205-206, 1982.
70. Steinbrocker O, Argyros TG: The shoulder-hand syndrome: present status as a diagnostic and therapeutic entity. *Med Clin North Am* 42:1533-1553, 1958.
71. Wirth FP, Rutherford RB: A civilian experience with causalgia. *Arch Surg* 100:633-638, 1970.
72. Leriche R, Policard A: *Physiologic Pathologique, Chirugicale Inflammations, Effets des Tranmatismes, Reparation des Plaies, Greffes, Maladies, des Os, des Articulations, des Vaisseaux et des Nerfs.* Paris, Mason & Cie, 1930, p 178.
73. Casten DF, Betcher AM: Reflex sympathetic dystrophy. *Surg Gynecol Obstet* 100:97, 1955.
74. Casten DF, Betcher AM: Reflex sympathetic dystrophy: criteria for diagnosis and treatment. *Anesthesiology* 16:994-1003, 1955.
75. DeTakats G: Nature of painful vasodilation in causalgic states. *Arch Neurosurg Psychiatr* 50:318, 1943.
76. Omer GD: Management of the painful extremity. *Curr Pract Orthop Surg* 8:86, 1979.
77. Ghia J, Duncan G, Scott D, Gregg J: Therapeutic nerve blocks for chronic pain. *Am Fam Pract* 20:74, 1979.
78. Kozin F, Ryan LM, Carerra GF, Soin JS, Wortmann RL: The reflex sympathetic dystrophy syndrome (RSDS). III. Scintigraphic studies, further evidence for the therapeutic efficacy of systemic corticosteroids, and proposed diagnostic criteria. *Am J Med* 70:23-30, 1981.
79. Kirklin J, Chenoweth A, Murphey F: Causalgia: a review of its characteristics, diagnosis and treatment. *Surgery* 21:321, 1947.
80. Genant H, Kozin F, Beckerman C, McCarty D, Sims J: The reflex sympathetic dystrophy syndrome. *Radiology* 117:21-32, 1975.
81. Omer GE, Thomas SR: The management of chronic pain syndromes in the upper extremity. *Clin Orthop* 104:37-45, 1974.
82. McKain CW, Urban BJ, Goldner JL: The effects of intravenous regional guanethidine and reserpine. *J Bone Joint Surg* 65A:808-811, 1983.
83. Tahmoush AJ, Malley J, Jennings JR: Skin conductance temperature and blood flow in causalgia. *Neurology* 33:1483-1482, 1983.
84. Levine AM: Reflex sympathetic dystrophy (Letter to Editor). *Arch Neurol* 45:243, 1988.
85. Paulson RR: Reflex sympathetic dystrophy in a teenaged girl. *Postgrad Med* 81:66-67, 1987.
86. Glick EN: Algodystrophy. In Helal B, Wilson D (ed): *The Foot*. London, Churchill-Livingstone, 1988, vol II, chap 54, pp 1078-1087.
87. Ford SR, Forrest WH, Eltherington L: The treatment of reflex sympathetic dystrophy with intravenous regional bretylium. *Anesthesiology* 69:147-148, 1988.
88. Ford SR, Forrests WH, Eltherington, L: The treatment of reflex sympathetic dystrophy with intravenous regional bretylium. *Anesthesiology* 68:137-140, 1988.
89. Glynn CJ, Basedow RW, Walsh JA: Pain relief following post-ganglionic sympathetic blockade with IV guanethidine. *Br J Anesthesia* 53:1297-1301, 1981.
90. Hannington-Kiff J: Intravenous regional sympathetic block with guanethidine. *Lancet* 1:1132-1133, 1974.
91. Bonnelli S, Conoschente F, Movilia PG, Restelli L, Francucci B, Grossi E: Regional intravenous guanethidine vs. stellate ganglion blocks in reflex sympathetic cystrophies: a randomized trial. *Pain* 16:297-307, 1983.
92. Benzon HT, Chomka CM, Brunner EA: Treatment of reflex sympathetic dystrophy with regional intravenous reserpine. *Anesth Analg* 59:500-502, 1980.
93. Driessen JJ, Van der Werken C, Nicolai JPA, Crul JF: Clinical effects of regional intravenous guanethidine (Ismel) in reflex sympathetic dystrophy. *Acta Anesthesiol Scand* 27:505-509, 1983.
94. Helms C, O'Brien E, Katzberg R: Segmental reflex sympathetic dystrophy syndrome. *Radiology* 135:67-68, 1980.
95. Wilson RL: Management of pain following peripheral nerve injuries. *Orthop Clin North AM* 12:343-359, 1981.
96. Portwood MM, Lieberman JS, Taylor RG: Ultrasound treatment of reflex sympathetic dystrophy. *Arch Phys Med Rehabil* 68:116-118, 1987.
97. Melzak R: Prolonged relief of pain by brief, intense transcutaneous somatic stimulation. *Pain* 1:357-373, 1975.
98. Carlson T, Jacobs AM: Reflex sympathetic dystrophy syndrome. *J Foot Surg* 25:149-153, 1986.
99. Ford SR, Forrest WH, Elgherington L: The treatment of reflex sympathetic dystrophy with intravenous regional bretylium. *Anesthesiology* 67:218, 1987.
100. Kleinman D, Rosen RC, Cohen JM: Combined anesthetic and surgical treatment of RSD following a healed crush injury of the foot. *J Foot Surg* 29:55-58, 1990.
101. Rodriguez-Moreno J, Nolla JM, Ruiz LM, Juanola X, Roig D: Transient regional osteoporosis or reflex sympathetic dystrophy (Letter to the Editor). *Ann Intern Med* 107:262, 1987.
102. Davis RF, Jones LC, Hungerford DS: The effect of sympathectomy on blood flow in bone. *J Bone Joint Surg* 68A:1384-1390, 1987.
103. Erdemir H, Gelman S, Galbraith JG: Prediction of the needed level of sympathectomy for post-traumatic sympathetic dystrophy. *Surg Neurol* 17:353-354, 1982.
104. Munn JS, Baker WH: Recurrent sympathetic dystrophy: successful treatment by contralateral sympathetic dystrophy. *Surgery* 102:102-105, 1987.
105. Rush PJ, Wilmot D, Saunders N, Gladman D, Shore A: Severe reflex neurovascular dystrophy in childhood. *Arthritis Rheum* 28:952-945, 1985.
106. Stilz RJ, Carron H, Sanders DO: Case history number 96: Reflex sympathetic dystrophy in 6-year old: successful treatment by transcutaneous nerve stimulation. *Anesth Analg* 56:438-441, 1977.
107. Richlin DM, Carron H, Rowlinson JC, Sussman MD, Baugher WH, Goldner RD: Reflex sympathetic dystrophy: successful treatment by transcutaneous nerve stimulation. *J Am Podiatr Assoc* 84-86, 1978.
108. Bernstein BH, Singsen BH, Kent JT, Kornvich H, King K, Hicks R, Hanson V: Reflex neurovascular dystrophy in childhood. *J Pediatr* 93:211-215, 1978.

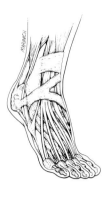

CHAPTER **46**

Tumors

Gene K. Potter, D.P.M., Ph.D.
Katherine A. Ward, D.P.M.

Steven J. Berlin, D.P.M.*

The word "tumor" engenders great fear. Education has raised awareness of the variety of foot tumors (1). Although uncommon, malignant primary or metastatic pedal tumors can be life threatening. Procedures for the investigation of tumors are initiated because of concerns of patients. It is to the patient's advantage to seek help early, inasmuch as early diagnosis and treatment of tumors increase chances for successful management and may preserve limb and life. A relevant, complete, and confirmed history is necessary, with the understanding that there often is a significant lag between lesion development and symptoms requiring diagnosis and treatment.

Modern diagnostic procedures have greatly increased the ability to locate tumors, to define visible borders and involvement of adjacent and/or distant structures, and to explain some physiological responses. Such procedures extend cooperation between the attending physician and the patient to include consultants and other specialists in a team effort. Other chapters of this book provide sources for radiological diagnosis and surgical approaches to extirpation of pedal tumors.

Two appropriate thoughts were enunciated over 120 years ago by Charles Moore, F.R.C.S., who was a consultant surgeon of the Middlesex Hospital of London: "In the performance of the operation, it is desireable to avoid not only cutting the tumour, but also seeing it . . . Recurrence is neither constitutional nor organic, nor regional, but that of an incompletely extirpated tumour."†

This chapter deals with pedal tumors and information relevant to their diagnosis and treatment. Related basic definitions concerning surgical oncology can be found in current pathology texts.

TUMOR GRADING

Malignant neoplasms are *graded* on the basis of microscopically determined cytological characteristics with higher numbers representing greater degrees of malignancy and anaplasia. Various grading systems exist, but a given system may not be applicable for all neoplasms. The factors of the

grading system, with clinical tumor characteristics (size, lymph node involvement, metastases), combine to suggest tumor *stage* (i.e., effects on the patient) and thus approaches to care and prognosis.

There are a number of systems used for staging of malignant tumors, but no particular one satisfies everyone. Union Internationale Contre Cancer (UICC) uses the TNM system, in which T represents presence, size, and extent of primary tumor, N indicates extent of regional lymph node involvement, and M describes extent of metastasis. Tumor stage is expressed as a combination of TNM factors, with descriptive numbers after each letter. Because the system varies for tumor types, oncology texts should be consulted for specific details. Generally, higher stage suggests larger tumor, more nodes involved, and more metastases.

The American Joint Committee on Cancer Staging and End Result Reporting (AJCCS) uses combinations of the same factors arranged in five stages (0 through 4). For soft tissue sarcomas one system depicts five stages (0 through 4) whose criteria are tumor size (smaller or larger than 5 cm), depth (superficial or deep), and histological grade (low or high). The best prognosis is therefore associated with small, superficial, low-grade neoplasms. No single system is used by all facilities for a given malignancy; thus clinicians must determine the system in use in their locale.

Names of neoplasms usually are based on the tissue of origin and the histological architecture. Details can be found in any current and standard pathology text. Because reclassification of tumor types occurs with new findings, one must keep up with results achieved by current cytological diagnostic techniques. Pathologists examine tissue and cell-containing fluids in laboratories established for specimen processing and evaluation. In most instances a definitive diagnosis can be derived. If required, tissue sections can be stained to demonstrate special features to aid in diagnosis. When neoplastic cells cannot be clearly identified with light microscopy examination, transmission electron microscopy (TEM) is used to seek cell-specific organelles, and even this may not be helpful.

Analysis of submitted tissue is neither a guessing game nor a test of the pathologist's skill. The pathologist must have information that includes biographical details (name, address, age, sex, occupation), nature of the patient's complaint (type, duration, association with other factors, prior treatment, related conditions), familial history (genetic pre-

*Appreciation is expressed to Steven J. Berlin, D.P.M., author of this chapter in the first edition.
†Med Chir Trans 50:245-252, 1867.

dispositions), description of the lesion area (color, size, consistency, number of areas involved, presence or absence of pain and tenderness, definition of borders), site of the sample's origin, and date of the sampling procedure. If more than one sample is taken, each must be described separately, specifically labeled, and placed in its own container. A specimen must be of reasonable size, undamaged by instruments, representative of the disease process, and well fixed to preserve cellular structure as closely as possible to the living state. The most frequently used fixative is 10% buffered formalin, usually supplied by the pathology laboratory. Certain reactions (determined by the pathologist) require special fixatives.

Tissue sample excision and the sample itself are colloquially called "biopsy" (*bios*, life; *opsis*, vision), a highly feared word to a patient because of its association with cancer. Biopsies are sources of such diagnoses, but in most cases biopsy determines the nature of an abnormality, of which cancer is only one. The procedure suggests a clinician's respectable index of suspicion as to the condition's nature and a desire to be as certain in diagnosis and subsequent procedures as is possible.

The biopsy site is a vital consideration in obtaining representative tissue without interfering with subsequent surgical intervention, if needed. A specimen is taken from the most active, untreated part of a *lesion* (a circumscribed area of pathological change, representing disease or injury to which the body is reacting). For most skin lesions, this usually represents the edge, whereas for blistering lesions, an intact, fresh vesicle with surrounding tissue is best. Tissue altered by chemicals, burning, or freezing provides a poor biopsy specimen. Skin biopsies must include complete dermal depth into subcutis, because some conditions show changes at deep levels. For malignant tumors, depth determination is required to judge metastatic potential, to determine treatment, and to define local metastases from elsewhere. The site of the incision for partial biopsy of deeper lesions should be one that will be included in the final surgical incision. Most states require by law or as part of a health code that all tissues, fluids, or foreign bodies be examined by a licensed pathologist and that a formal report be issued.

TYPES OF BIOPSIES

Detailed techniques on the many types of biopsies are found in the surgical sections of this or other texts. Techniques used and the manner of administration of local anesthetics should be considered carefully to avoid needle tracks, other artifacts, or implantation of tumor cells sublesionally. Regional anesthesia is a viable approach. Biopsy types include *excisional*, in which an entire lesion, usually not exceeding 2 cm in diameter, is removed with a clinically normal border of about 2 to 3 mm. A major exception to this is melanoma, to be discussed later. Biopsy may also be curative and allows for the apposition of wound edges. For each excisional biopsy, different instruments and gloves should be used. Punch biopsy is adequate for small (up to 0.5 cm), superficial skin lesions if the specimen bears the entire lesion, full depth, and a clinically normal border.

INCISIONAL. A piece of a large and/or a deep lesion is excised for study. This includes "pie wedge" and punch biopsies of large skin lesions. Multiple sites from a lesion should be labeled as if on a clock, for example 12-, 3-, 6-, or 9-o'clock position and center. For pie wedge or elliptical samples, different blades are used for each incision. Incisions proceed from clinically normal tissue into the lesion, preventing passage of abnormal cells to normal tissue. For deep or large lesions, sampling error is a risk (i.e., the specimen not representing the lesion). Some suggest a risk of spreading malignant cells through the tissue planes traversed. Unnecessary tumor manipulation during biopsy and hematoma formation present risks for dissemination of tumor cells.

CURETTAGE. This method (shave biopsy) has been used for superficial skin lesions but is not recommended. Samples are scant and may not represent the lesion. If underlying tumor has been cut, iatrogenic dissemination may be a risk.

ASPIRATION. This is a type of needle biopsy, in which fluid is withdraw antiseptically from a lesion or joint for analysis. Study of the cell content (*cytology*) may reveal malignant cells, other unusual cells, microorganisms, or crystals as in gout or chondrocalcinosis. Some claim ability to diagnose tumor types from cytological preparations; others believe that finding suspicious or malignant cells on properly prepared smears is sufficient and a prelude to definitive tissue examination. If content is scanty, cells may be concentrated (by centrifugation) and either a smear or a cell block made. Smears are fixed before drying, using any of a variety of products. The technique can be used to obtain a tissue core for examination, but it bears the risk of sampling error, and the needle does traverse tissue planes.

FROZEN SECTION. A prearranged intraoperative consultation with the pathologist is undertaken if there is strong suspicion that a lesion is malignant and anticipation of prompt and more extensive surgery. At operation, labeled, fresh, unfixed tissue is sent from the operating room to the laboratory for immediate examination after rapid processing (5 to 10 minutes). The report to the waiting surgeon helps determine the procedure. If the specimen does not represent the lesion, another may be requested. If diagnosis is not established, the surgeon may perform local excision, pending tissue examination. More surgery can be done within a few days. For some specimens, frozen section may be a choice procedure (e.g., lipomatous and liposarcomatous tumors that show intracellular lipids only in frozen sections after special procedures). However, cell and tissue warping resulting from rapid freezing/thawing may cause nevus cells to look malignant. Thus, many clinicians suggest that lesions clinically suggesting melanoma should not be diagnosed by frozen section.

For all tumors, the pathologist should indicate whether the clinically normal surrounding tissue is indeed tumor-free. Subsequent treatment depends on such issues. The patient should be promptly notified of findings for reassurance or to begin prompt and definitive therapy. Questions of diagnosis in context with a patient's overall presentation should be discussed with the pathologist and all information noted and passed to specialists.

TUMORS OF EPIDERMAL CELL ORIGIN

Skin tumors include benign and malignant tumors occurring (but not necessarily arising) in epidermis and dermis. Epidermal tumors arise from keratinocytes, Merkel's cells, and melanocytes. Most occur in the most superficial layers, above the dermoepidermal basement zone, or from the epidermal adnexa (sudoriferous or sebaceous glands and hair follicles). Most manifest some hyperkeratosis. Clinical appearance alone may not be a reliable criterion for diagnosis, even if other factors (such as age and location) seem right. Some lesions occur in specific areas even though epidermal (e.g., in a normal postnatal foot, pilosebaceous tumors do not originate from indigenous plantar tissues).

Verruca

A survey of pedal lesions (1) reveals that verrucae (viral papillomata, warts) are the most frequent, occurring in various forms (e.g., plantar myrmeciae, planar, filiform, mosaic). A given form of verruca is associated with the same human papillomavirus (HPV) serotype in all populations and locations (2). Although some HPV serotypes are associated with transformation of verrucous lesions to squamous carcinomas (3), those affecting the foot are not as firmly implicated. However, a plantar form of verrucous carcinoma is recognized (4), and there have been examples of plantar verruca merging into squamous cell carcinoma. Persons with various wart types have immunological defects (5, 6), as shown by studies in children immunosuppressed after renal transplantation, whose rate of development of verrucous lesions exceeded that of the general population of children by about three times (7). Similar lesions have systemic implications. For example, acrodermatitis verruciformis (a genetic defect, sometimes familial), angiokeratoma Fabry-type condition affecting the feet, which is associated with a metabolic defect and occurs as other types, and epidermodysplasia verruciformis (associated with two HPV serotypes, one frequently associated with in situ or invasive squamous carcinoma (8, 9). Therefore, surgical excision may be considered for single lesions and representative lesions from mosaic or multiple types, as well as for recurrent verrucae (Fig. 46.1).

Other lesions may also resemble verrucae, and appropriate texts (10) should be reviewed. Surgical excision of otherwise untreated verrucae is a definitive treatment (9) and is the only source for a clear histopathological diagnosis. Antiviral (11-13) and anticancer chemotherapeutic agents (11, 14) seem draconian for single lesions or small numbers of uncomplicated, true verrucae inasmuch as they may enhance immunosuppression. Local immunotherapy has helped in some cases of verruca and other lesions in which clinical (but not histopathological) diagnosis has been rendered (15, 16).

Seborrheic Keratosis

Seborrheic keratoses are benign lesions that appear in middle age in crops on body areas, including the feet (except

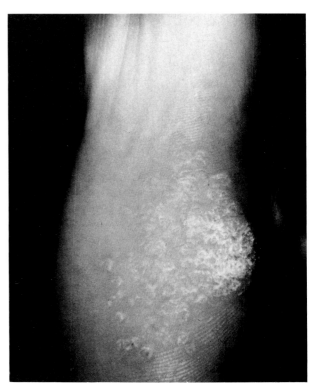

Figure 46.1. Mosaic verruca, posterior aspect of heel. These are difficult to manage conservatively.

the soles), usually as small, scaly, slightly hyperpigmented lesions that seem tacked onto the skin surface (an image based on growth pattern that is distinct peripherally and slightly elevated, with a slightly verrucous surface). The most common type in the ankle region is the off-white stucco keratosis. A darker form results in clinical and histological suspicion of melanoma (17) but is a benign melanoacanthoma (18). Similar lesions occasionally seen on the lower extremities of black patients fall into the dermatosis papulosa nigra variant, which occurs more frequently on the face. Unless unsightly to the patient or irritated by foot gear, no surgery is needed for any of these except as a diagnostic aid, which may be necessary for differentiation from the more dangerous and clinically similar solar keratoses. Irritated seborrheic keratoses may appear as small inflamed ulcerations ("sores that don't heal"), necessitating biopsy. Irritated forms may resemble squamous carcinoma histologically, but they are benign.

The Leser-Trélat sign consists of the sudden appearance of pruritic seborrheic keratosis crops (19), in association with a visceral malignant tumor. Such a history should prompt biopsy (which demonstrates keratoses histologically resembling early acanthosis nigricans that later develops into true acanthosis nigricans [19]) and appropriate consultation to seek visceral malignancy. Although colon adenocarcinomas are most frequently associated with these growths (20), there are reports of mycosis fungoides (21), melanoma (22), and a treated leukemia (23).

Acanthoma and Epidermolytic Acanthoma

Acanthomas show a predilection for the lower extremities but rarely the feet. These benign lesions, described in 1962 (24), may clinically resemble seborrheic keratoses; they are slow growing, reddish, elevated, demarcated lesions, each surrounded by a collarette. The reddish color is due to vascularity (25). Excision is curative, and there may be underlying hyperplastic and proliferative eccrine changes (26, 27). Epidermolytic acanthoma primarily occurs on more proximal body areas and may resemble a seborrheic keratosis or verruca.

Epidermal Adnexal Tumors

Tumors of epidermal adnexa in the feet have sometimes been reported. Symptoms are nonspecific, and patients report a slowly growing mass, discomfort in foot gear, or paresthesia such as "walking on a pebble." Clinically, a palpable mass is present, moving with the skin. Many may be present for years, and some may be large. In rare cases, such tumors appear as erosions, as an ulcer over an induration, or as fungating lesions. Some are benign but aggressive; some are slow growing yet malignant.

Pedal adnexal tumors are *papillary eccrine adenoma* (28) in the heel (29), *chondroid syringoma* (toes) (30) (Fig. 46.2), *eccrine poroma* (31, 32) (Fig. 46.3), *hidroacanthoma simplex* (eccrine poroma variant) with in situ *porocarcinoma* (33), and the rare plantar *mucinous syringometaplasia*, which can clinically resemble verruca (34). The eccrine origin of these lesions can be confirmed (35, 36). A very unusual case of plantar *sebaceous epithelioma* was reported (37). In most cases, these lesions can be removed as excisional biopsies. However, with suspicion of malignancy in large or chronic lesions, frozen section may be indicated, with results suggesting further treatment. Tumors arising in dorsal pedal

and digital hair follicles have been seen (*trichoepithelioma* and *pilomatrixoma*), as well as have *eccrine hidradenomas*. The authors are not aware of any pedal tumors with apocrine differentiation.

Cystic Tumor-Like Lesions

Cystic pedal lesions occasionally occur and may suggest a neoplasm. Epidermal cyst usually results from traumatic introduction of viable epidermal tissue subepidermally (38) (Fig. 46.4). Trauma involves penetrating wounds from mis-

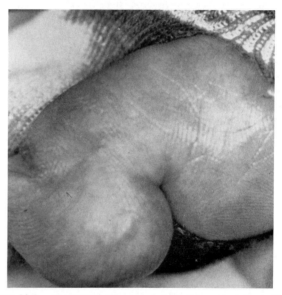

Figure 46.2. Chondroid syringoma causing painless enlargement of fifth toe distally. (From Potter GK, Baldinger HG, Boxer MC: Chondroid syringoma in a toe. *Cutis* 30:339-341, 1982).

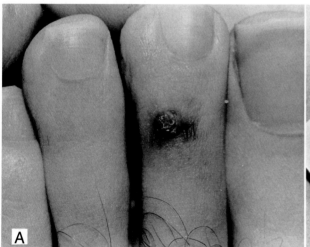
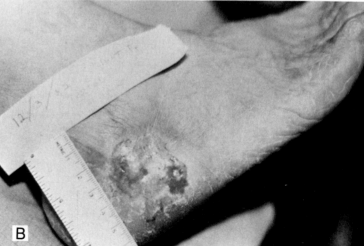
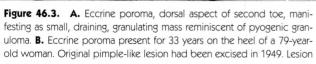

Figure 46.3. A. Eccrine poroma, dorsal aspect of second toe, manifesting as small, draining, granulating mass reminiscent of pyogenic granuloma. **B.** Eccrine poroma present for 33 years on the heel of a 79-year-old woman. Original pimple-like lesion had been excised in 1949. Lesion appeared as an erosion, and multiple-site biopsies were benign. Lesion was excised without recurrence. (**A** courtesy of E.D. McGlamry. **B** courtesy of A. Hernandez.)

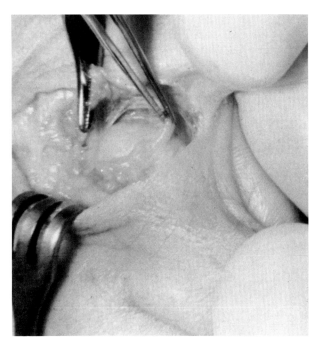

Figure 46.4. Epidermal inclusion cyst between fourth and fifth metatarsals. Clinical presentation was that of local callosity overlying the mass.

siles (e.g., bullets), industrial accidents, or even surgery or injections. The tissue acts like normal epidermis but produces keratin within and may grow as large as 5 cm, even affecting local bone. The slow-growing, palpable mass may be reported as a discomfort or lump that appeared suddenly, with no recalled associated trauma. The lesion may be fluctuant. If keratin escapes traumatically, it is an intradermal foreign body that causes inflammation. A sinus tract may develop, exuding cheesy material consisting of keratin and cell debris. This is especially true of those beginning as corns in the first metatarsophalangeal region over the extensor hallucis longus at the area of the break of the shoe, a result of improper fit (formerly known as vamp disease because of involvement of the vamp portion of the shoe).

Excision of the cysts and sinus tracts is usually curative. However, with vamp lesions, repair of the surgical defect should include interposition of fatty tissue between the extensor tendon and overlying skin to avoid fibrosis of tendon to dermis. Multiple epidermal inclusion cysts, especially on the face and scalp, may suggest *Gardner's syndrome,* which requires consultation for confirmation and for follow-up of other sequelae. Rarely, malignant epidermal tumors have occurred with these cysts (39-41).

Sebaceous (pilar, trichilemmal) cysts are extremely rare in the foot, only one having been reported by Podiatric Pathology Laboratories, Baltimore, MD, in 11 years. They occur in pilosebaceous structures on the dorsal aspect of the foot and toes and usually are small, round, whitish, firm, discrete lesions that are asymptomatic unless traumatized. They can be enucleated and not recur. Concurrent lesions, especially in the scalp, may suggest an autosomal dominant

problem requiring additional evaluation. Pilar cysts have been associated with *trichilemmomas* (42, 43), but as yet this association has not been made for either lesion in the foot. The significance of finding trichilemmomas in a young woman is that with multiple verrucous lesions on the face, *Cowden's disease* may be present, suggesting predilection for breast carcinoma. Acral keratoses and multiple fibrous hamartomas may also be present (44), as well as other visceral malignant tumors (45). Reports of Cowden's disease have not yet included foot lesions.

Hyperkeratoses with Local or Systemic Malignant Tumors

Epidermodysplasia verruciformis is uncommon, affecting the lower extremities with lesions resembling verruca plana. The causative factor is one (or both) of two HPV serotypes. Those with HPV-3 tend to be familial, occur in childhood, and do not transform to malignancy (46). Those with HPV-5 have been known to undergo malignant transformation in sun-exposed skin, manifesting as an in situ (Bowen's disease) or invasive squamous cell carcinoma (8, 9). Histological diagnosis of this lesion should lead to HPV serotyping to determine care and prognosis. Some lesions show both types of HPV.

Keratosis palmaris et plantaris (palmoplantar keratoderma) has been associated with various pulmonary carcinomas (47). Thus, if diffuse palmoplantar hyperkeratosis histologically reveals otherwise normal underlying epidermal structure (vs. epidermal changes of weight-bearing hyperkeratosis [48]), the patient should be referred for a complete medical workup.

Keratosis punctata (keratosis papulosa) on palms and soles may also suggest local or systemic malignancies. Ham-colored palmoplantar pits occur with *basal cell nevus (nevoid basal cell epithelioma),* or Gorlin's Syndrome. Some pits represent early basal cell carcinomas (49). This syndrome has been reported with familial incidence in four generations (50). Palmoplantar *arsenical keratoses* are small, noninflamed, verrucous lesions that may overlie Bowen's disease or that may suggest visceral carcinomas (51, 52), especially of bronchi and bladder. Therefore, punctate keratoses require biopsy and consultation with other specialists.

Cutaneous horn (cornu cutaneum) is a reactive hyperkeratosis whose height is at least half its widest diameter (49). Lesions may underlie the base of the visible keratosis (e.g., solar kertosis [53]), seborrheic keratoses and filiform verrucae (54), both more likely to be dorsal lesions. Squamous cell carcinoma (54) and other epidermal lesions (55, 56) have been reported, as well as Kaposi's sarcoma (57). The presence of a cutaneous horn should prompt investigational biopsy.

Acanthosis nigricans involves skin changes that include hyperkeratoses. Intertriginous areas are most often affected, and of the four types (which are virtually identical histologically), the malignant form is most pronounced. Darker coloration is due to light reflection and refraction by hyperkeratotic and papillomatous changes, not melanin. In severe cases, mucosal surfaces may also be involved (58). This condition has been associated with the presence of melanoma (22) and other cancers (58-60). *Leser-Trélat* sign, associated with seborrheic keratoses, involves such changes and may suggest internal malignancies. Biopsy confirmation of acanthosis nigricans requires prompt consultation to determine the presence of visceral malignancy, or if the condition represents the endocrine form of acanthosis nigricans, there may be concomitant occurence of pituitary tumor, diabetes mellitus, Addison's disease, or the Stein-Leventhal syndrome (61).

Porokeratoses of the plaque (or Mibelli) type (62), superficial disseminated form (63), disseminated superficial actinic type (64), and punctate form (65) affect the feet. All have been associated with transformation to Bowen's disease or invasive squamous carcinoma. The forms are inherited as an autosomal dominant trait. These lesions virtually always exhibit a raised hyperkeratotic border around an atrophic, keratotic area. The Mibelli type may slowly enlarge. Punctate forms may resemble hereditary punctate keratoses. Mibelli's porokeratosis shows a keratin-filled perilesional furrow. Porokeratoses may be considered premalignant and should be removed before transformation.

Porokeratosis plantaris discreta of Steinberg and Taub (66) is different (Fig. 46.5). Considered a surface plug of an eccrine duct with underlying eccrine adenitis, it has been classified as to severity and clinical characteristics (67). The authors have not seen the plug directly related to an eccrine

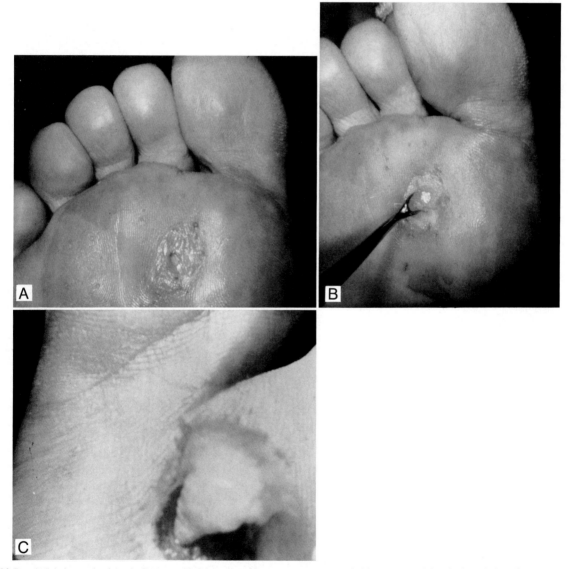

Figure 46.5. **A.** Porokeratosis plantaris discreta underlying second metatarsal head and resembling other biomechanically acquired hyperkeratoses. Treatment may involve excision of the lesion and surgical modification of underlying bone. **B.** Blunt curettage of porokeratotic lesion may expose underlying metatarsal head. These lesions bear no apparent relationships to sweat ducts. **C.** Porokeratosis plantaris discreta classified as clinical grade 3. The conical lesion has affected dermal tissues and is deep. Neuromas sometimes underlie these lesions.

duct. In a study by Potter (48), this lesion was determined to be a weight-bearing corn variant. However, like other porokeratoses, it has a cornoid lamella. A cure rate of over 90% has been claimed for lesions treated with cryotherapy and a specific strict regimen (68).

Solar (senile, actinic) keratoses occur in the sun-exposed dorsal aspects of the feet and toes. They appear in middle to later life in light-skinned persons, seemingly a result of poor protection from ultraviolet B (UVB 280-320 nm) irradiation, and may be hypertrophic, atrophic, bowenoid, acantholytic, or pigmented. The latter may be difficult to differentiate clinically from lentigo maligna (69). Solar keratoses are multiple, small, flat, reddish, scaling lesions, but they may underlie cutaneous horns (54). These can usually be treated by excisional biopsy. Given that about 20% of patients with solar keratoses develop (usually nonmetastasizing) squamous cell carcinomas (70), it is advisable to remove those seen and to consult a dermatologist if similar lesions appear elsewhere on the body or if a pedal lesion is indeed malignant. Some lesions also demonstrate *solar elastosis* underlying abnormal epidermis, unless an infiltrate has stimulated fibrosis so that damaged elastic tissue is not seen, which may be the primary manifestation of actinic damage appearing (other than in the nuchal area) as wrinkled, thin skin.

Benign Tumors of Melanocytic Origin

Keratinocyte tumors that contain melanocytes present clinical, and sometimes histological, problems in differential diagnosis from true melanocytic tumors.

Melanocytic nevus histologically designates a lesion that contains nests of nondendritic melanocytes. It may be *junctional, compound,* or *intradermal* depending on melanocyte distribution. Transitions occur between these progressive stages of nevus evolution. *Neural nevus* histologically describes a deep intradermal nevus that demonstrates spindle cells in loose collagen and that resembles neurofibroma. Nevi may be pigmented and flat, slightly elevated or papillomatous, or nonpigmented and either domelike or peduncular. Some clinicians correlate these characteristics with nevus type, but biopsy is the safest method for examination. Papillomatous forms contain little melanin and may be hyperkeratotic, resembling seborrheic keratoses. Nevus cells are designated A, B, and C on the basis of their intradermal depth. Generally nevi are small, showing regular borders, color, and texture. They begin to appear in early childhood, new ones appearing occasionally through midlife. The body shows 10 to 40 such lesions at any time. Gradually, each changes, and eventually disappears (71), leaving few in old age. *Halo nevi* demonstrate a depigmented ring around a pigmented nevus. Inflammatory forms tend to involute, whereas those without inflammation do not. *Congenital melanocytic nevi* may be of the *nongiant* or of the *giant* types. Some types within both categories may show hair growth (except the plantar *nongiant congenital acral melanocytic* type), so that hair is not a predictor of transformation to melanoma. Lesions in the giant and nongiant groups have been known to undergo malignant transformation (72, 73).

Melonychia striata represents a longitudinal hyperpigmented strip in a nail. It may be present in persons of darker complexions, but sudden appearance in light-skinned persons is immediate indication for nail avulsion and biopsy (74). The lesion may be benign nevus or a melanoma (75, 76). *Blue nevi* are intradermal melanocytic lesions that may present diagnostic problems both clinically and histologically, due to possible confusion with melanoma (77). Some blue nevi undergo malignant transformation. Rarely, a report may describe a *balloon cell nevus*, a histopathological description of an uncommon entity that may clinically appear as any of the aforementioned.

More typical epidermal melanocytes are seen in lentigines (*lentigo simplex, lentigo senilis*), in the pigmented macules of the *McCune-Albright syndrome*, in the *café-au-lait* spots of *neurofibromatosis* (1) (formerly von Recklinghausen's disease), and in *ephelides* (freckles). In some, giant melanosomes are seen. Other conditions with prominent hyperpigmentation are described in dermatology texts. Multiple lentigines may be seen in the congenital *leopard* syndrome, each letter designating a defect concurrent with the many melanocytic lesions (l = lentigines). Excisional biopsy is recommended for these small lesions.

Intraepidermal Imitators of Epidermal Malignant Tumors

Pseudocarcinomatous (pseudoepitheliomatous) hyperplasia histologically describes a benign epidermal proliferation resembling squamous cell carcinoma, seen at the edges of chronic ulcers of many types (78, 79), including basal cell carcinoma, and noted as a reaction to underlying granular cell tumors (61). It has also been seen in chronic sinus tracts of long-standing interdigital corns.

Keratoacanthomas are benign epidermal proliferations from hair follicle epidermis, which may be impossible to tell clinically or histologically (during early development) from squamous cell carcinoma. They occur as single or multiple lesions (80), one form affecting the soles (perhaps a developmental aberration in that the lesions are attributed to hair follicles) (Fig. 46.6). Some also occur subungually (81, 82) eroding underlying bone. Onset is very rapid, with full development of lesions within about 2 months. Lesions may be indolent. In some forms, lesions involute without sequelae (*self-healing epithelioma*), whereas in others involution leaves scars that may interfere with local function (80). Under the characteristic central keratin plug, the crater surface is reminiscent of an ulcer seen in some skin cancers. Patients generally seek medical attention when the lesion begins to grow, demonstrates ulceration, and acts as a "sore that won't heal."

Depending on lesion size, excisional biopsy or wedge biopsy may be indicated. Whether it is clearly keratoacanthoma or squamous cell carcinoma, foot lesions are best removed. If a lesion is malignant, its removal is necessary, but if it truly is keratoacanthoma, multiple types should be removed, if practical, to avoid scarring and interference with function. It is reported that multiple types are recurrent after surgical extirpation, but that they seem to respond well

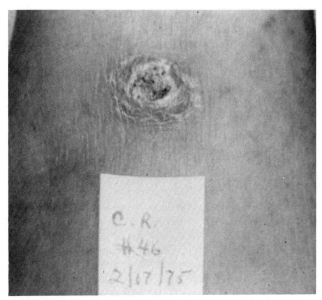

Figure 46.6. Keratoacanthoma on anterior of ankle. Rapid development and ulceration may arouse suspicion of a malignant lesion. (From Strauss H, Potter GK: Keratoacanthoma: case presentation and discussion. *J Am Coll Foot Surg* 18:72-74, 1979.)

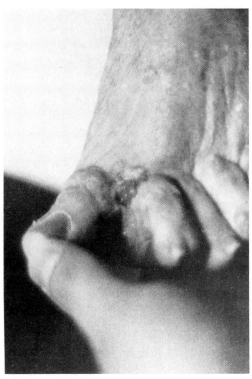

Figure 46.7. Digital basal cell carcinomas, a rare finding in the feet. Diagnosis is established by biopsy. (Courtesy of S.H. Silvers.)

to 13-*cis*-retinoic acid administered orally (83). Mechanisms are obscure but may involve effects of this synthetic vitamin A analogue on keratinization and on elements of the immune system (83). Excision of single large lesions may require grafts. Multiple keratoacanthomas on the body are frequent concomitants of *Muir-Torre syndrome* (or *Torres's syndrome*) (84-86), consisting of sebaceous tumors (adenomas, epitheliomas, hyperplasia, and nonmetastasizing carcinomas) (87) with multiple visceral malignancies involving the gastrointestinal tract (88).

Pseudomelanomatous changes may cause traumatized nevi to resemble melanoma clinically and histologically (65). Trauma includes incomplete excision of nevi that seem to "recur" rapidly. A good patient history is required as to local trauma, including recent treatment by another clinician or by the attending physician. Local evidence of recent surgery should be sought. Local excision must include a clinically normal periphery and depth, and the pathologist should be forewarned of suspicions of melanoma.

The *Spitz nevus* (*benign juvenile melanoma, spindle and epithelioid cell nevus*) is usually benign, has very little pigment, and is not limited to children. The majority occur in patients over 14 years of age (89), and about 25% occur in persons over age 30 years (90). Pedal lesions are rare (three from children have been diagnosed by Podiatric Pathology Laboratories in 11 years) but have been reported (91). They are usually small, pinkish-red, elevated, and reminiscent of pyogenic granuloma or amelantic nodular melanoma. Sometimes, dark lesions may further enhance suspicion of nodular melanoma. Histological differentiation of benign Spitz nevus from melanoma may be impossible (65, 91) so that wide excision is always indicated. A high index of suspicion, especially when a lesion is small and more locally manage-

able, is required, and excisional biopsy is warranted because true melanomas, although rare in children, do occur. Histological differentiation of benign from malignant melanocytic and other tumors is immeasurably aided by the refinement of techniques to detect cancer-specific characteristics (92-94).

Malignant Tumors of Epidermal Cell Origin

Malignant pedal epidermal tumors occasionally have been reported, but not all types seem to occur at this site. The more common epidermal cell malignancies seen in feet are described.

BASAL CELL CARCINOMA

Although considered by most clinicians to be a low-grade malignant tumor, some consider basal cell carcimona a hamartoma arising from epidermal pluripotent cells or from embryonic epidermal cell rests activated in later life (65). Adherents to this theory designate the lesion with the more benign title of *basal cell epithelioma* (65). Most lesions occur in sun-exposed skin. Occurrence in pedal skin is uncommon (Fig. 46.7). Statistics from Podiatric Pathology Laboratories over 11 years reveal one basal cell carcinoma to about 2.5 of the squamous cell type (including both the Bowen's and invasive forms). Statistical review of the 112 cases from that series shows that basal cell carcinomas were about 1.9 times more frequent in women than in men, and about 1.3 times more frequent in the left foot than in the right. The average

age of patients in the series was 73 years (range, 25 to 99 years). Occurrence is reported in the soles (95, 96), with one subungual lesion (97). A higher incidence of pedal basal cell carcinoma may occur in patients with the uncommon nevoid basal cell epithelioma (Gorlin's) syndrome, demonstrating many such tumors, pitting of the palms and soles, many systemic abnormalities (98), and sometimes other malignant tumors.

Metastatic basal cell carcinoma is uncommon, but it is reported (99) and may be extensive and life threatening. Basal cell carcinoma has occurred with cutaneous horn (56), extensive exposure to various forms of irradiation (100-102), in burn scars (103, 104), and in other hereditary and acquired skin conditions (52, 100, 105-107), some demonstrating concurrent squamous cell carcinoma. (Development of squamous cell and of basal cell carcinomas in patients with xeroderma pigmentosum has been inhibited with oral administration of 13-*cis*-retinoic acid [108]). Basal cell and squamous cell carcinomas have been seen apparently intermixed or adjoining. Some basal cell carcinomas demonstrate benign pseudoepitheliomatous hyperplasia. Therefore, biopsy from the edges of large lesions must be adequate to show whether anything other than a tumor mimic is present. Basal cell carcinomas associated with genetic defects or preexisting lesions seem to be more aggressive than others. A potentially protective role for melanin in preventing basal cell carcinomas may exist.

Basal cell carcinomas may occur in one or more clinical forms. The most frequent is the irregular and eroded *noduloulcerative* lesion (*rodent ulcer*), which begins as a small telangiectatic nodule, grows slowly, and ulcerates centrally. Borders appear pearly and rolled. Most lesions rarely cause much damage, but some may be extremely aggressive, as in the uncommon nevoid basal cell epithelioma syndrome. *Morphea-like (fibrosing)* lesions are smooth, nonulcerated, single, slightly indurated yellowish plaques that may be slightly depressed. *Superficial* types may show one or more otherwise nondescript, slightly infiltrated, and scaling reddish patches, extending peripherally. The border is a fine pearly line, and the central area may show small ulcers, scars, and crusts. It may be reminiscent of some nonneoplastic dermatoses or of *Bowen's disease*. *Fibroepithiomatous* types are small domelike lesions that may be pinkish red (as are skin fibromas) and pedunculated. *Pigmented* types resemble noduloulcerative lesions but contain more melanin and perhaps hemosiderin, thus resembling melanoma or pigmented squamous cell carcinoma. Different histological variants of basal cell carcinoma depend on the extent and direction of differentiation toward epidermal adnexa. More than one variation may be present in a given basal cell carcinoma, with no true correlation between a histological type and any clinical types.

Excisional biopsy should be performed with a clinically normal skin border, if possible. The pathologist should ascertain that all specimen edges are well clear of lesion. If not, additional surgery is indicated. Excision of large lesions may require skin grafts. In some cases consultation with a radiotherapist may benefit patients, inasmuch as basal cell carcinomas are radiosensitive. However, this may not be the approach in areas already damaged by some form of irradiation, or where an aggressive tumor has gone deep into tissues (e.g., to bone), and it may also inhibit healing. To avoid damage to peripheral and deep tissues, cryotherapy may also be used with care in selected cases. Immunotherapy and surface application of anticancer chemotherapeutics have been used, but they are experimental. Mohs surgery is not recommended for any clinician who cannot demonstrate proficiency in the surgical aspects and histopathological readings.

SQUAMOUS CELL (EPIDERMOID, PRICKLE CELL) CARCINOMA

Squamous cell carcinoma may arise anywhere on the body, including a mucous membrane (Fig. 46.8). Lesions associated with ultraviolet irradiation demonstrate a metastatic rate of about 0.5% (109). Highly metastatic forms of this cancer are associated with specific conditions (110-113), and less aggressive forms are associated with other conditions (52, 105-107). Squamous cell carcinoma is more aggressive than is basal cell carcinoma, especially if associated with preexisting lesions other than sun damage. Squamous cell carcinomas arising in heavily sun-exposed areas (other than the lip) tend to be less metastatic or locally aggressive. Aggressiveness and metastasis characterize those arising in body areas (e.g., the foot) receiving little or no solar irradiation (114). Perhaps squamous cell carcinoma is a harbinger of visceral malignancies (115, 116). Melanin may help to prevent squamous cell carcinoma in sun-exposed skin.

Unlike basal cell carcinoma, squamous cell carcinoma can occur in situ, a form called *Bowen's disease*. This constitutes a preinvasive state. Bowen's disease may arise in some chronic dermatoses (8, 9, 70, 107, 117-119). Clinically, one or more lesions may be present, especially in sun-exposed areas, appearing reddish, with sharp but irregular borders. Some crusting and scaling may be present, and the lesions may appear as large solar keratoses (although solar keratoses may demonstrate bowenoid changes). Bowen's disease seems chronic and probably remains noninvasive for many years. Statistics for transformation may be low because patients usually report these lesions as incidental findings during examination for other complaints, and excision occurs prior to transformation. In 74 cases of Bowen's disease seen over a decade at Podiatric Pathology Laboratories, women manifested the lesion 2.1 times as often as did men. Generally, Bowen's disease lesions occurred almost 1.5 times more frequently on the left foot than on the right foot. Average patient age with this lesion was 65 years (range, 25 to 92 years).

Excision should include a clinically normal periphery and depth to subcutaneous fat. Wound edges can be approximated for small lesions. The pathologist determines whether specimen edges are clear and ensures that multiple levels of the specimen were studied to determine invasion. Excision usually cures in situ lesions, but the patient will be watched for recurrences or new lesions. Because there is still dispute as to whether these lesions are harbingers of

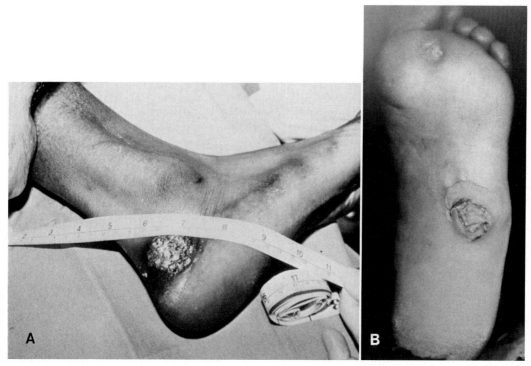

Figure 46.8. **A.** Squamous cell carcinoma. Note clinical resemblance to keratoacanthoma in Figure 46.6. **B.** Squamous cell carcinoma clinically reminiscent of recurrent plantar mosaic verruca. Diagnosis was established with biopsy.

visceral malignancies, the patient should be referred for more extensive examination.

Upon penetration of the subepidermal basement zone, the lesion is fully invasive (or infiltrative) squamous cell carcinoma. It appears as a shallow ulcer with an elevated and indurated rim, generally not showing the pearly borders of rodent ulcers nor developing as quickly as keratoacanthoma. Pigment may suggest melanoma or pigmented basal cell carcinoma. The ulcer may be crusted and impossible to differentiate clinically from the benign keratoacanthoma. Histological differentiation may also be impossible. Histopathological grading of squamous cell carcinomas is based partly on Broders' original system (percentage of differentiated cells) and partly on depth of invasion and degree of cell anaplasia. A grade 1 lesion is well differentiated and not very deep, and abnormal cells do not exceed about 25% of the total. A grade 4 lesion is poorly differentiated (quite anaplastic) and deeply invasive, and about 75% or more of the cells are abnormal. Because various parts of the same specimen can show different grades, it has been recommended that a specimen be sampled extensively by the pathologist and that the clinician be advised of the highest grade seen (most anaplastic, invasive, and abnormal tissue) and the extent of its presence (120).

An adenoid or pseudoglandular type of squamous cell has been metastatic in very few instances. Clinical appearance of the lesion is nonspecific. Occasionally, lesions may be fungating, resembling plantar mosaic verruca with overlying hyperkeratosis.

An uncommon pedal variant of squamous cell carcinoma is epithelioma cuniculatum (plantar verrucous carcinoma) (4). It may initially suggest recalcitrant plantar verruca, recurring after treatment. If a verrucous lesion is recurrent and recalcitrant to treatment over an average period for a verruca to respond, biopsy is required (121). This form of squamous carcinoma slowly enlarges to form a fungating, soft verrucous mass with deep crypts and sinuses reminiscent of rabbit warrens (cuniculatum) containing keratin and debris that become malodorous. The sinuses and crypts also become sites of chronic infection (122). The lesions can be extremely destructive, affecting underlying pedal bones and soft tissues, even reaching the dorsal tissues (123). The lesion itself is usually well-differentiated histologically but very extensive. If the lesion is not very deep (determined radiologically) or very wide, it can be widely excised and a skin graft applied (122). Extensive involvement of deep tissues and bone may require consultation for reconstructive surgery (122) or for an amputation (123, 124). This is generally not metastatic, and like other squamous cell carcinomas, it may occur in other chronic lesions. In a reported case, development of pedal verrucous carcinoma was related to a history of lead arsenate exposure (122).

A review of over a decade of statistics from Podiatric Pathology Laboratories reveals that of 205 cases of invasive squamous cell carcinoma, the lesion was almost 1.5 times more frequent in the feet of women than in those of men, and about 1.4 times more frequent in the left foot than in the right. The average age of the patients was 69 years (range, 9 to 96 years). It seems that invasive squamous cell carcinoma (more frequent than the in situ form) shares similar statistical characteristics as to location and sex prevalence. However, younger age-groups show more of the in situ form, confirming the obvious impression that it takes time before the noninvasive lesion does invade. These tumors rarely occur in childhood. Further analyses from Podiatric Pathology Laboratories reveal that plantar verrucous carcinoma constitutes about 1.5% of pedal squamous cell carcinomas.

If initial examination gave no apparent evidence of regional lymph node metastases and the history suggests sun exposure as a primary etiological factor for that particular patient, a small invasive squamous cell carcinoma may be approached essentially the same way as described for basal cell carcinomas. However, if a large lesion is present, or if multiple lesions and/or recurrent lesions occur in patients whose feet do not receive much sun exposure (or if lesions are on the sole), the patient should be referred to a diagnostic radiologist for scans or varorgans and for lymphangiography (114) in view of the greater metastatic risk. This applies also to squamous cell carcinomas that arise in chronic or preexisting lesions. Chest radiographs are also recommended for the same reason. Presence of metastatic lesions will certainly alter a treatment protocol in accordance with the worsened disease stage. Also, as for Bowen's disease, the possibility of a concurrent primary occult visceral malignant tumor with an epidermal squamous cell carcinoma remains an open question; thus referral for a work-up is important. Excision of large lesions may require grafts and reconstructive surgery. As in the case of basal cell carcinoma, Mohs surgery should not be attempted for squamous cell carcinomas by anyone not skilled in the surgical and histopathological aspects of this procedure.

EPIDERMAL ADNEXAL CARCINOMAS

Malignant sebaceous and eccrine tumors occur, as noted in a report of sebaceous carcinoma in the foot (125). They may manifest in the dorsal skin of the instep or toes, either independently or as part of Torres's syndrome (84-86). Pilar carcinomas (malignant trichilemmomas) also arise from hair follicles; they are extremely rare, and pedal cases are not yet reported. Symptoms and signs of these lesions are nonspecific. Sebaceous carcinoma would be the most likely to metastasize. On the basis of studies in other body areas, sebaceous carcinomas may manifest as a skin mass or an ulcer. They can metastasize to lymph nodes, bones, and other sites (114) and may therefore be fatal.

In contrast, malignant eccrine pedal tumors have occurred in the toes and soles (126-128). Because eccrine glands are present in all pedal skin areas, conceivably one might see *malignant* forms of *eccrine poroma*, *spiradenoma*, *clear cell hidradenoma*, or *chondroid syringoma*. These tumors do not have clinically distinct features but are known to be extensively metastatic (114) and thus dangerous. The patient must be promptly sent for an oncological consultation.

MERKEL'S CELL (TRABECULAR) CARCINOMA

Merkel's cells are sparse, scattered, intraepidermal neuroendocrine cells, whose function is obscure. Malignant, metastatic Merkel's cell skin tumors occur (129) and may be fatal (130). There are reports of these neoplasms in the lower extremities (131-134), including a primary ankle lesion (135). Statistics from Podiatric Pathology Laboratories for 11 years show one case. Symptoms and signs are not specific. The carcinoma may occur as one nodule, or may appear in multiple locales (136) or as scattered nodules (137, 138). Diagnosis of trabecular carcinoma should prompt consultation with an oncologist to evaluate for metastases and to render further systemic care as warranted.

Melanoma

Few subjects in dermatology and oncology stir as much controversy as cutaneous melanoma. The earliest description is by Hippocrates, and further case reports and discussions occurred in Europe and the United States during the nineteenth century (139-141). During this period the term *melanoma* was used, and controversy raged over whether the lesion was neoplastic. More is known today of the cell processes involved in this dangerous and potentially fatal skin cancer, as well as its prevention and treatment.

Melanoma cells are variants of the pigment-producing dendritic melanocytes of neural crest origin, becoming intraepidermal residents among basal keratinocytes. Melanocyte numbers vary in different body regions in all persons (142, 143) but not among racial groups for a body area (144). Differences lie in melanin production under similar circumstances (i.e., melanocyte activity), melanocyte and melanosome sizes, melanosome distribution to keratinocytes, intrakeratinocyte melanosome processing, and proportions of the brownish-black *eumelanins* to the reddish- and yellowish-brown sulfur-containing (cysteine) *pheomelanins*.

Racial differences are evident in melanoma incidence. These cancers occur more frequently in white persons than in black or oriental persons (145-147). In white persons, over 90% of lesions occur in sun-exposed areas (head, neck, trunk)(148). In black people, in native Americans, and in oriental people, up to 67% of lesions occur in less pigmented and less sun-exposed areas (143), for example, the sole and the subungual areas (149-153). In one study, light-skinned black people had nevi scattered over the body, whereas dark-skinned black people showed more palmoplantar nevi and few elsewhere (147). Statistics for oriental people fall between those for whites and blacks (154).

Incidence differences between the sexes are complicated by variables of sun exposure (ultraviolet irradiation), melanoma occurring about twice as often in sun-exposed lower extremities of white women as in the same areas of white men (148). At Podiatric Pathology Laboratories, of 152 cases of pedal melanoma seen over a decade, 105 were in women and 47 in men, a female to male ratio of 2.3:1 with no significant difference in occurrence of the lesions in right versus left foot. The average age of the patients was 66.6

years at diagnosis (range, 15 to 98 years). Therefore, age does not preclude occurrence of melanoma.

Sun exposure duration may be a major factor in melanoma development (155, 156) and brief, intense sunburns are implicated (157). Melanosome type, number, and distribution in plantar keratinocytes of black persons resemble those on sun-exposed white skin rather than those of sun-exposed black skin (158). Thus, protective effects of melanin in soles of black persons are equivalent to those in sun-exposed skin of white persons. Protective effects of melanin are supported by studies in the Solomon Islands where there is almost no incidence of melanoma, basal cell carcinoma, or squamous cell carcinoma in sun-exposed skin unless the skin has been depigmented because of wounds or disease (150). Thus in damaged skin, melanin is insufficient to protect generative basal keratinocyte nuclei from carcinogenesis resulting from solar radiation. This population, like other black populations, develops plantar melanomas. Whereas other mechanisms may contribute to findings in sun-exposed skin of the populations studied, the sole never receives frequent or intense ultraviolet light, unless by reflection from trod surfaces. Even then a thick plantar skin should offer additional protection. Further, wearing shoes does not affect melanoma incidence in the soles of black populations. Thus UVB irradiation (280 to 320 nm) and melanosome factors do not seem to be the only factors to explain these phenomena.

Groups most susceptible to skin cancers, including melanoma, are light-skinned persons with red or blond hair. These groups also develop more freckles (ephelides) on sun-exposed skin and produce more pheomelanins than do white persons with darker complexions and hair, as well as other groups with darker skin. Freckles demonstrate melanocytes such as those in darker persons (159). Melanocytes surrounding freckles are small, less dendritic, and less melanized. Intracytoplasmic melanosomes also differ structurally (160). Pheomelanins are shown to be mutagens (and therefore potential carcinogens) after partial photolysis by long-wave ultraviolet light at physiological pH levels and in the presence of oxygen (161), a reaction inhibited by intracellular superoxide dismutase (162). Such activity may produce carcinogens in melanocytes eventuating in melanoma (or in the other skin cancers by virtue of the normal transfer of melanin products to keratinocytes). Also, partially photolysed melanin may be unable to absorb free radicals produced by ultraviolet rays (UV) on cell lipids, permitting carcinogen accumulation. (The more common eumelanins are more protective.) Pheomelanins are soluble at alkaline (but physiological) pH levels (161) and may be inactivated. Thus biochemical factors influenced by solar radiation play a major role in melanoma development.

Genetic factors influence melanoma development. Norris (140) is now credited with the first suggestion of a familial trend in the case he described, with credibility for that genetic history given by his contemporary, Pemberton (163). More than 130 years after Norris's case, familial melanoma reappeared in the literature (164). Studies suggest heredity

as a factor in 11% of melanoma cases (165), and diagnosis of melanoma occurs about 10 years earlier in patients with familial melanoma than in the general population. Also, first-degree relatives of melanoma patients seem about twice as likely to develop cutaneous melanomas as do persons in the general population (165).

Other primary malignant neoplasms have been associated with cutaneous melanoma (166), for example, breast carcinoma (women) and small cell lung carcinoma whose Kulchitsky cells are also of neural crest origin (167). However, no association is noted between cutaneous melanoma and syndromes other than xeroderma pigmentosum (168).

Genetic defects are described in various growth phases of cutaneous melanoma (169, 170). Radial growth phase abnormalaties appear on chromosome 6 (often expressed as 6q-) but not involving the chromosome area associated with the human leukocyte antigen (HLA) system and part of the complement system. Malignant expression of human cutaneous melanomas was prevented experimentally in vivo and in vitro by the introduction of normal sixth chromosomes into melanoma cell lines (171). Vertical growth phase cells and metastatic cells show abnormalities in chromosomes 1, 6, and 7, and a translocation (t) (1;19) sometimes appears. The chromosome 1 defect may be near the Rh locus (172). Changes in the long arm of chromosome 1 (1q) are associated with development of in vitro "immortality" in various tumors. Replacement into cultured hybrid cells of intact chromosome 1 has resulted in some inhibition of tumorigenicity, and normal senescence occurs in the otherwise "immortal" cells (173).

Precursor lesions of cutaneous melanoma were originally designated *BK mole syndrome* (174) and are now called *dysplastic nevus syndrome* (DNS) (175) with BK mole syndrome as a specific subtype. Excellent clinical descriptions and histological details are available (174,176,177). However, controversy exists because some do not consider any particular lesion or lesion complex to be a melanoma precursor (178), whereas others believe that "intraepidermal melanocytic dysplasia is to cutaneous melanoma what actinic (solar) keratosis is to squamous cell carcinoma..." (179).

Some authors, in their description of clinical subtypes of in situ and invasive cutaneous melanoma (65,176,180), present another controversy. To create a unifying concept for all types, Ackerman and David (181) propose that lesion thickness correlates with prognosis and that only lesion pathogenesis may differ in various body areas and in de novo versus nevus-associated melanomas. Thus all cutaneous melanomas eventually invade and metastasize. Although Flotte and Mihm (182) agree that such classifications do not relate to prognosis, they point to clinical and biological significance of the subtypes, such as body areas in which they occur, incidence in racial groups, and length of in situ phase.

Briefly, based on biological and histological criteria, cutaneous melanomas are classified as in situ or invasive. Statistics vary as to incidence in the foot, but the pedal melanomas group may not exceed 5% of all melanomas (180).

Lentigo maligna (LM) (Hutchinson's freckle, melanosis circumscripta preblastomatosis of Dubreuilh) is the most frequent in situ form on sun-exposed skin (e.g., face) in older persons, but it is rare on lower extremities. It slowly extends peripherally and may show cleared areas, as well as shades of brown, tan, and black within irregular borders. Lesions may resemble solar keratoses or Bowen's disease (65). Within 10

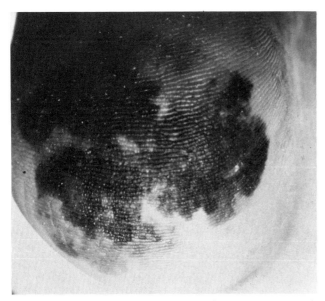

Figure 46.9. Superficial spreading (pagetoid) melanoma that arose in a congenital nevus. Note irregularity of colors, texture, and borders. Lesion was widely and deeply excised, and a graft applied.

to 15 years the lesion becomes invasive, developing a dark, indurated nodular component *(lentigo maligna melanoma [LMM])*. This form, which may account for 5% to 9% of cutaneous melanomas (65, 180), is the least common on the foot (180).

Superficial spreading melanoma (SSM) in situ (pagetoid melanoma in situ) may occur on skin, whether sun-exposed or not, and is reported in feet (181). The lesions are usually smaller than those of lentigo maligna but may show greater color variation (pinks, grays, and bluish), becoming invasive in about a year. Invasion demonstrates induration and/or papules and nodules formation *(superficial spreading melanoma or pagetoid melanoma)*. Ulceration may occur later. This form constitutes about 67% to 70% of cutaneous melanomas (65, 180) and is uncommon in the feet, occurring about twice as often as lentigo maligna types (180) (Fig. 46.9).

Acral lentiginous melanoma (ALM) in situ (palmoplantar-subungual-mucosal [PPSM, PSM]) is most commonly seen on the sole and in black patients (65,180) and is described in other pedal sites, including toes (181). It reportedly has a very short in situ growth phase, showing irregular or indefinite borders and irregular pigmentation. Nodular invasive forms supervene (ALM) and rapidly metastasize. Ulcers may occur early (in contrast to the first two forms) with invasion. *Melonychia striata*, a longitudinal ungual pigmentation, which suddenly develops with no apparent reason in a light-skinned person, is an immediate indication for nail avulsion and biopsy for suspicion of acral lentiginous melanoma (74-76). Striae occur in nails of black persons, but sudden development in a nail that did not show it before or any change (e.g., increased pigmentation and irregular eponychial pigmentation) in existing striae is a similar indication. Acral

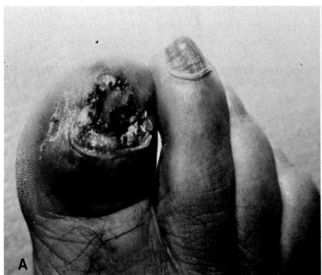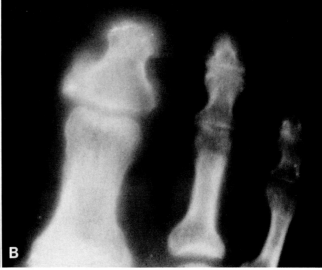

Figure 46.10. **A.** Acral-lentiginous melanoma, melanotic whitlow type. Lesion resembles chronic onychia and paronychia. Peripheral pigmentation may be confused with the postinflammatory type, and central pigmentation may be mistaken for blood. Nail bed area is amelanotic tumor. **B.** Radiograph of affected toe shows periosteal reactivity suggesting local pressure, and small lucencies suggest tumor invasion into distal phalanx.

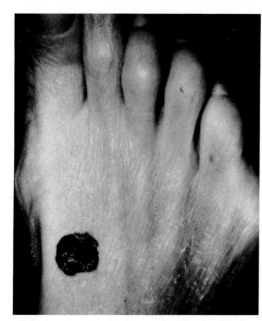

Figure 46.11. Nodular melanoma of foot that manifested as sudden changes and bleeding. Despite radical excision, metastases were found about six months later. (Courtesy of L. Rubin.)

lentiginous forms account for about 4% to 8% of cutaneous melanomas (65, 180) and may be the second most common form of a melanoma seen on the feet (180) (Fig. 46.10).

Nodular melanoma (NM) shows virtually concurrent radial and vertical growth and thus rapidly invades and metastasizes. This form is reported in the foot (183) and may occur most frequently there (180). It usually develops and enlarges rapidly as an elevated, heaped up, deeply pigmented nodule. Ulceration occurs rapidly. Nodular melanoma constitutes about 10% to 15% of cases (65, 180) (Fig. 46.11).

Nail bed or nail fold melanomas are called *melanotic whitlow of hutchinson*, or *melanotic panaris*. Melanin content may be sparse, and cases may be treated over long periods for chronic paronychial infection. The true lesion may not be discovered until it is large, ulcerated, and metastatic. Therefore a patient history of long, unsuccessful treatment for "paronychial infection" requires careful review of history and immediate biopsy.

For all forms of melanoma occurring on the foot, there are clinical mimics that can be differentiated with biopsy (148). An unusual and potentially tragic problem arises with *amelanotic melanoma*, the form with little or no pigment (possibly related to presence and activity of an endonuclease) (184) but nonetheless a melanoma. Entirely amelanotic primary cutaneous melanomas are rare (148), a testimony to the deceptively benign clinical appearance confounding proper diagnosis. Of 152 melanomas seen between 1978 and 1989 at Podiatric Pathology Laboratories, ten (6.7%) was amelanotic. Many flat or elevated lesions have some pigmentation, whether regularly or irregularly dispersed, which may not be (but may resemble) melanin. Also, dermal

nevi may lack pigment, and the dermal component of a compound nevus may lose pigment (except on the sole). In the former case, a patient may describe a fairly recently occurring, pigment-free, small, domelike dorsal pedal lesion, and the latter may show color variegation as a compound nevus enters its later stages before disappearing (71, 176).

Domelike lesions without pigment are rare in the foot (176) but not impossible. Further, as in situ melanoma progresses to invasion, invasive melanoma cell clones, forming the vertical growth phase, acquire metastatic competence, and appear different from radial growth phase cells (180). One such difference may be loss of pigment (180), so that an amelanotic pedal nodule, or a deceptively benign-appearing lightly mottled papule or a nodule of recent origin, may represent a primary or a metastatic amelanotic melanoma. Thus, a clue to such a neoplasm lies in a history of recent appearance and growth, or observation of a lesion at the site of what may have previously been thought to be a benign pigmented nevus that disappeared (suggesting dominance of an invasive amelanotic clone). There can be difficulty in histological diagnosis of amelanotic melanoma. Enzyme cytochemistry studies for tyrosinase activity (185) (diagnostic for epidermal melanocytes as producers of melanin rather than as bearers of melanin as are macrophages) and immunocytochemistry (92, 93, 186), as well as use of transmission electron microscopy, help to establish the diagnosis.

Biopsy has been another source of controversy. Not every nevus, dysplastic or otherwise, will progress to melanoma; thus excision of all pedal nevi is not considered necessary (147). Biopsy is indicated when a patient reports change in a long-standing lesion (e.g., color, size, sensation, satellite development, ulceration, recurrence locally after removal). In this context periodic examinations (semiannual to annual), including properly labeled photographs showing a ruler near the lesion(s), are of great help in determining changes in existing nevi (179) or development of new ones. Patient cooperation is vital, and patients must be advised to report changes occurring between examinations.

Ideally, suspicious lesions should undergo excisional biopsy (148, 187). Incisional biopsy for suspected melanoma has been controversial. Two studies suggested that 5-year survival rates for patients undergoing incisional biopsies were decreased significantly when compared with patients who had undergone excisions initially (188, 189), but two others found no such evidence, even with punch biopsies (190, 191). Current mainstream opinion indicates that if melanoma is suspected and excisional biopsy cannot be performed, careful incisional biopsy should be done (187). The pathologist should be notified of any such suspicions when the specimen is sent, and a telephone report can be available within a day or two. If the specimen is melanomatous and its histology is known, effective and definitive planning of surgery and overall patient care can be promptly instituted. For biopsy, the authors prefer scalpel to punch because of difficulty many clinicians may find in judging depth when using a punch. Incisional biopsy of large lesions risks sampling error. Neoplastic changes may be absent in the specimens. Lesions should be observed for suspicious change.

The pathologist will read multiple sections of specimen(s) to determine presence of melanoma (in most cases the lesion is a clinical melanoma mimic) (148), as well as its characteristics if it is present. About 35% of melanomas can be associated with a preexisting benign nevus (192). Once the characteristics are determined (thickness, invasion level, histological type, mitoses, pigmentation, perilesional immune response), they can be combined with such factors as the patient's age, sex, clinical history, familial history, lesion location and size, satellites, lymph node involvement, and other metastases. These will determine tumor grade and stage and thus patient care and prognosis. Histopathological characterization of specimens has led to fairly accurate correlation with prognosis in patients with melanoma. Some systems (193, 194) have related tumor invasion depth to prognosis.

Clark's classification (195) was more detailed but presented problems in correlating prognosis with Clark's level II because of lymph node involvement (148) and in the subjective determination of level III versus level IV (196). This does not suggest that Clark's classification has no value; however, more recently, Breslow's measurements of a primary tumor's thickness (196, 197) have been found to correlate well with prognosis. A melanoma's thickness (Breslow) is often reported with its level of invasion (Clark). Tumor thickness in the biopsy aids in determination of surgical approach to the primary lesion, including surgical margins.

The determination of surgical margins constitutes a well-known controversy. The venerable dictum of a 5-cm margin from the visible edge of a large lesion or the site of an excisional biopsy has been reviewed (148, 196, 198). It is a misinterpretation of Handley's postmortem study of a single case of late metastatic melanoma (199), in which the author recommended "about an inch" (i.e., not 5 cm), and that has no relevance to primary melanoma and does not consider other criteria presently part of an evaluation. Studies by Wong (200) led to recommendation of a 5-cm margin based on discovery of bizarre melanocytes that far from the lesion edge in some primary melanomas. Current recommendations are based on measurements of tumor thickness in a biopsy specimen, according to Breslow's technique (196, 197), as suggested by Day and Lew (201), to prevent local recurrence. For lesions under 0.85 mm in thickness in clinical stage I (148) and outside the areas of the upper *b*ack, posterolateral *a*rm, posterior and lateral *n*eck, posterior *s*calp (BANS), a margin, 1 to 1.5 cm in thickness, should avoid tumor edges and permit primary closure. For clinical stage I lesions of 0.85-mm thickness or more, a minimum of 3 cm is considered adequate. If lesion borders seem indistinct, Wood's light helps to delineate the few millimeters from the visibly pigmented area in which slight hyperpigmentation suggests abnormal melanocytes. Apparently, overall survival correlates with lesion thickness, which in turn is predictive of metastatic potential. Thus, unless satellites (visible or occult) are present, survival after excision of the primary lesion as already described has less to do with surgical margins than with the stated characteristics of the lesion itself.

In the foot and ankle area, primary closure may be difficult. Grafts may be needed there more often than elsewhere. Plastic and reconstructive surgery may be required, and the graft must be prepared and stored in saline prior to working at the tumor site (to avoid seeding tumor cells to the graft or donor site). Also, toe amputation for a subungual or other distal melanoma may be far easier and more effective for the patient than attempts to save the toe with grafts. Because superficially spreading, acral lentiginous and nodular melanomas grow relatively quickly, patients may manifest lesions exceeding 0.85 mm in thickness that are perhaps beyond clinical stage I. According to the aforementioned criteria, narrow surgical margins and saving digits are precluded. Mohs surgery is not recommended for pedal melanomas because great skill in histological analysis and surgical technique is needed.

Significance of clinical staging is illustrated by summarized studies (65). Assuming that all lesions are in clinical stage I (148), the 5-year survival rate for patients with superficial spreading melanoma is about 70%, with nodular melanoma it is about 50% to 60%, and with acral lentiginous melanoma, it is about 11% to 15%. Therefore, in the feet (183), where these three melanoma types occur, clinical type is very significant. Also, according to Ackerman and David (181), primary lesion thickness correlates with prognosis. Thus both factors are vital in pedal melanoma. Clinical type and location may determine when the disease becomes sufficiently symptomatic to warrant treatment, and lesion thickness at that time will play a major role in prognosis.

A confirmed diagnosis of pedal melanoma (i.e., even non-BANS types) requires careful regional lymph node examination and consultation with a dermatologist to determine the presence of other lesions (including dysplastic nevi) elsewhere. Consultation with a diagnostic radiologist is also necessary to arrange for soft tissue and bone scans, as well as for lymphangiography, to determine metastatic spread, although the authors of some studies doubt the value of such procedures unless there are system-associated symptoms (148). An oncologist should be involved in evaluation of disseminated melanoma because regional perfusion or other chemotherapeutic techniques may be of value, as well as surgery for other superficial or deep metastases (148), including regional lymph node dissection. A therapeutic radiologist will be needed to administer palliative irradiation for deep lesions (202).

Advances have been made in mobilizing the patient's immunological responses to melanoma (148). Injected antigens such as bacille Calmette-Guérin (BCG), purified protein derivative (PPD), *Corynebacterium parvum*, vaccinia, or use of sensitizers such as dinitrochlorobenzene (DNCB) results in nonspecific immunological response, destroying individual superficial lesions into which these materials are instilled; that is tumor cells are nonspecifically destroyed in localized overall reaction to antigen or sensitizer. For this approach to be effective the patient's immune system must be competent and uncompromised by disease or therapy. (In that context, it is interesting to note the increased incidence of dysplastic nevi in patients with Hodgkin's disease [203] and in renal transplantation patients [204], both of which involve immunosuppression.)

Current development of antibodies to specific tumor antigens enhances possibilities for systemic treatment of melanoma metastases and recurrences (92, 93) as long as tumor cells display those antigens and patients do not develop antibodies to foreign monoclonal antitumor antibody protein. Also, understanding of immune system mechanisms, coupled with recent isolation and purification of biological response modifiers (such as interleukins, colony-stimulating factors, inhibitors), may help to systemically and selectively modulate immunity to melanoma and other tumors.

Prognosis in melanoma is based on many clinical and histological features. As determined by multivariate studies (148), and discussed earlier, the major variables include tumor thickness, tumor location (non-BANS tumors have a better prognosis), and ulceration of the primary lesion, especially if it exceeds 3 mm in diameter. Lymph node metastases are a poor prognostic sign, and the more nodes involved, the worse the prognosis.

The patient's sex seems to influence prognosis. Results of various studies show that women with melanoma seem to do better than do men despite clinical stage or metastatic extent (148). This apparent advantage seems to disappear after menopause, suggesting hormonal influence. Studies by Talal and others (205, 206) in systemic lupus erythematosus indicate that in humans and in mice, females exhibit greater immune response than do males and that estrogens seem to inhibit T-suppressor (CD8 +) lymphocytes, whereas androgens suppress immunological activity that manifests clinically as disease. Thus the estrogen effect seems to be immune-response enhancement, which disappears at menopause because estrogen levels drop, permitting greater influence by the suppressive androgens although their levels have not actually risen.

Some studies propose that racial factors may play a role in prognosis of patients with melanoma. Studies by Rippey et al. (145) in South Africa and by Reintgen et al. (153) in the United States suggest that black patients have a significantly worse prognosis than do white patients when comparisons were made that included controls for many factors. Melanoma seems much more aggressive in black persons than in white persons.

In general, the future of a patient with a confirmed diagnosis of cutaneous melanoma involves vigilance by the patient, his or her family, and competent, concerned, and coordinated physicians.

Metastatic Carcinoma

Metastases of carcinomas from the viscera to skin have been documented (65), but rarely in the foot. These lesions may be initial indicators of an otherwise occult primary visceral cancer, or they may lie dormant for many years after excision of a primary carcinoma. Because epidermis is avascular, metastatic rests grow in dermis or subcutaneous tissue.

There are no distinctive symptoms or signs of metastases other than fairly recent appearance and perhaps discomfort in footwear and/or on weight bearing. In one study (207), cutaneous metastases were found to occur in under 3% of cases. For example, metastatic chondrosarcoma from a primary shoulder lesion was reported in toe skin (208-211).

Over a period of 11 years, Podiatric Pathology Laboratories recorded two pedal metastasis cases. In 25 years of experience, the senior author saw two cases (one each of carcinoma of the lung and of the kidney, the latter in a colleague's patient).

TUMORS AND TUMOR-LIKE LESIONS OF SOFT TISSUE ORIGIN

"Soft tissue" lesions are neoplasms and reactive proliferations from primarily mesodermally derived, nonosseous tissues, which also bear elements of neuroectoderm (hence the inclusion of peripheral nerve lesions). Because epidermal lesions are ectoderm, they are not in the "soft tissue" group, as are dermal lesions, inasmuch as dermal tissues are mesodermal. These lesions range from benign through malignant, and it is often difficult to decide with certainty as to the lesion's exact nature. Mesodermally derived pluripotential cells may give rise to many of the tumors, and the state of such cells (genotype) in which their maturation and/or differentiation is arrested will determine the expression of characteristics (phenotype) seen clinically and histologically.

In some cases, genetic changes have been associated with specific soft tissue tumors (212), and inheritance plays a role in others, for example, neurofibromatosis (1) (formerly von Recklinghausen's disease). Tumor nomenclature is often based on cell histogenesis, and a diagnostic difficulty lies in the multiplicity of ways in which a cell type may express itself (e.g., fibroblast vs. myofibroblast vs. leiomyocyte). Thus, enzyme cytochemistry, immunocytochemistry, and electron microscopy studies often (but not always) provide diagnostic aid when conventional light microscopy findings are not specific. *Sarcomas* are malignant soft tissue tumors.

Not all soft tissue lesions are excised; thus exact determination of general population incidence is virtually impossible. Statistics based on surgical specimens suggest that soft tissue tumors are uncommon and that the annual soft tissue sarcoma incidence is about 1.4/100,000 (213) and higher in some age-groups. Benign lesions are more common, by about 100:1 (214).

Lesions of Fibroblastic and Histiocytic Cell Origin

Fibroblasts are well defined and ubiquitous cells that produce collagen. Histiocytes are not as well defined. Tumors arising from histiocytes seem to resemble most frequently the fibroblastic tumors, but they produce little or no collagen in contrast to those in which fibroblasts are clearly identifiable. They are therefore considered with the fibroblastic group. In many of the lesions, intermediate cells, showing characteristics of more than one cell type, are also seen, for example, myofibroblasts.

REACTIVE PROLIFERATIONS

Nodular pseudosarcomatous fascitis (215) is a benign, self-limiting, infrequent lesion of obscure etiology (216-219). It occurs predominantly in the 20 to 40 year age-group, usually manifesting as a single, rapidly growing cutaneous, fascial, or intramuscular lesion with nonspecific symptoms, and it may be difficult to differentiate from fibrosarcoma. Men and women are equally affected. Lesion borders may not be clearly defined, suggesting recurrence if not completely excised. All free edges of the surgical specimen should be clear of lesion. Variants of this lesion include *ossifying* and *intravascular* types. Also known as *nodular fasciitis* or *infiltrating fasciitis*, this condition is unrelated to the plantar, eosinophilic, or necrotizing fasciitides.

Proliferative fasciitis affects men and women most often between the ages of 40 and 70 years. Its etiology is unclear. Trauma may be involved. It is a rapidly developing subcutaneous, firm, tender nodule that is not fixed to skin and presents a very serious differential diagnostic problem to pathologists because of its strong resemblance to rhabdomyosarcoma and ganglioneuroblastoma. However, immunocytochemistry studies help to establish the diagnosis. A similar lesion occurs in ischemic and necrotic areas over bony prominences in debilitated, relatively immobile patients, giving a clinical impression of neoplasm.

Fibroma of tendon sheath (tendosynovial fibroma) is considered by some to be reactive and by others to be neoplastic. Most cases occur in hands, but foot cases are reported (220). Complete excision is curative and prevents recurrence. It may histologically resemble giant cell tumor of tendon. Most cases occur in men, and antecedent trauma has been reported by some patients.

Elastofibroma (elastofibroma dorsi) is an unusual lesion that may be related to trauma (221) and most frequently is subscapular region (hence "dorsi"). It is reported elsewhere, and over an 11-year period, one case was reported by Podiatric Pathology Laboratories in a 56-year-old woman. Lesions are virtually asymptomatic (unless on weight-bearing areas), and complete excision is curative. A foot lesion was reported in a dancer, further implicating trauma (222).

Keloids represent fibrous reactions at injury sites and occur most frequently among black people (223). Familial incidence is also reported (224). The reaction involves many myofibroblasts and is thought to be related to abnormalities of capillary endothelium during granulation (225). Reaction may extend beyond the immediate trauma site and can be incapacitating (Fig. 46.12). Whereas *hypertrophic scars* may develop under similar conditions (225-227), they remain localized and eventually flatten. Mechanisms may include increased collagenization (228) and decreased collagenase activity. Glucocorticoids inhibit collagen synthesis in vitro by inhibiting assembly of its components (229), and local injections help some patients (230). Mast cells associated with these lesions (226, 227) produce tumor necrosis factor

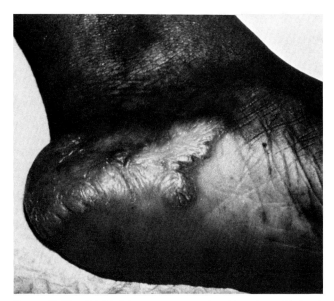

Figure 46.12. Keloid. Edges are contracted and irregular and lesion is densely fibrotic. Area may be painful on weight bearing. Edges of hypertrophic scars do not show such contractures.

(TNF-alpha) (231), a potent stimulus for fibrosis, and papillary dermal fibroblasts are far more proliferative than those of the reticular dermis (232). Elective surgery should be performed cautiously in patients who are prone to keloid formations. Keloids have been associated with fibromatoses and may be associated with peptic ulcers (233) and with enostoses.

FIBROMATOSES

Fibromatoses are benign lesions tending to infiltrative growth and suggesting malignant tumor. They are recurrent and manifest as multiple, nodular, poorly circumscribed lesions. Some types affect the feet. *Congenital generalized fibromatosis* involves subcutaneous tissues at birth (234). With no visceral involvement, subcutaneous lesions may involute during the first postnatal year. Visceral organ involvement may be fatal (235). *Fibrous hamartoma of infancy* (236) usually arises in the first year of life. The foot is not a typical site. *Juvenile hyalin fibromatosis* shows many subcutaneous nodules and begins in early infancy with flexural contractures. Distal phalangeal osteolytic lesions in fingers and toes may be seen (237). This is extremely rare and may be mistaken for neurofibromatosis. Lesions may be removed surgically. *Plantar fibromatosis (Dupuytren's disease, Ledderhose's disease)* occurs most frequently in the non-weight-bearing arch area of the foot and may manifest in childhood (Fig. 46.13). Discomfort on weight bearing may prompt investigation and surgical excision. Lesions in younger people are more cellular and may resemble fibrosarcoma (236). Lesions may adhere to skin and if symptomatic, fasciectomy is recommended (238). Plantar fibromatosis may be associated with palmar fibromatosis, penile fibromatosis (Peyronie's

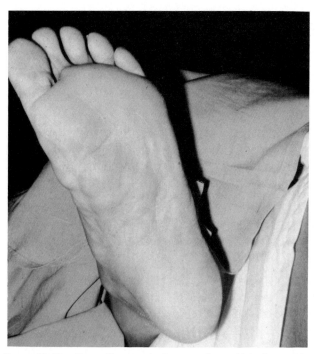

Figure 46.13. Plantar fibromatosis demonstrating multiple firm nodules in the plantar fascia. Abnormal tissue extended dorsally, making excision of the infiltrative lesions difficult.

disease), and knuckle pads on the hands, but lesions may not appear concurrently. *Knuckle pads* on the toes, with leukonychia and impaired hearing, form the *Bart-Pumphrey syndrome* (239).

Extra-abdominal desmoid (extra-abdominal musculoaponeurotic fibromatosis, well-differentiated nonmetastasizing fibrosarcoma) is a very rare foot lesion. Pedal desmoids are thought to constitute between 0.3% (240) and 1.9% (241) of all desmoids. They are reported in children and, in general, are most common in women of childbearing age. Some consider desmoid tumors to be low-grade malignancies (242). Because this lesion is infiltrative and recurrent, surgery may have to be extensive; and for large lesions, foot amputation may be necessary. Regression of desmoids is reported with use of indomethacin and ascorbic acid (243). Desmoids may also occur in *Gardner's syndrome. Infantile digital fibromatosis* is a recurrent lesion of the lesser fingers and toes (244) that may be present at birth or develop shortly thereafter. These lesions are small, periarticular, domed lesions adjacent to middle or distal interphalangeal joints, and they may regress spontaneously. Surgery is indicated for discomfort and/or interference with function. Multiple digits (fingers and/or toes) may be affected (240).

Calcifying aponeurotic fibroma (juvenile aponeurotic fibroma, Keasbey lesion), initially described as a childhood lesion (245), also occurs in adults. In one series (240), only 13% of cases were pedal. Growth is slow and diffuse (246), generally beginning early in childhood or in infancy. Older lesions are more compact, showing chondrification and calcification and occasionally ossification. Because of differences in

growth pattern and cellularity at early and later ages, there is greater tendency to postsurgical recurrence in children than in adults. Even in case of recurrences, surgery should still be limited to local excision with a clinically normal border (240).

Review of the records of Podiatric Pathology Laboratories covering 11 years reveals 1452 cases of plantar fibromatosis. Both feet were involved in 136 cases (9.4%). The average age of the patients was 45.5 years (range, 0 to 85 years). About 43.5% of cases occurred in men and 56.5% in women. Most lesions (65%) occurred in the left foot. Other fibromatoses were not reported, attesting to their relative rarity and the possibility that lesions were seen and treated by pediatricians or other physicians.

FIBROMAS

Fibromas are usually small, benign neoplasms that show collagen with special stains. Whether deep or superficial, they are usually well demarcated, and once excised with a clinically normal tissue rim, they are not recurrent. Fibromas may consist largely of fibrous tissue or may be intermixed with other elements in sufficient quantity to warrant variant names such as *angiofibroma, fibrolipoma,* and *neurofibroma.* Fibromas may manifest as individual lesions (244) or may occur with other lesions and complexes. *Koenen's periungual fibromas* on the toes are associated with *tuberous sclerosis (Bourneville's disease)*, a dominantly inherited condition. Manifestations include adenoma sebaceum lesions (angiofibromas), lumbosacral shagreen patches (seen well with Wood's light), renal angiomyolipomas in many cases (a possible source of major hemorrhage), visceral lymphangiomyomas in some cases, cardiac rhabdomyomas in some patients, and calcifying potato-shaped ("tuberous") intracranial gliomas. Mental retardation is present, and with epilepsy, the syndrome is *epiloia.* Detailed familial history is necessary, as well as consultation with other specialists. Koenen's periungual fibromas do recur.

Acquired digital fibrokeratomas may occur on fingers and toes and occasionally on palms and soles (247). In contrast to *infantile digital fibroma* (244), acquired digital fibrokeratoma occurs in adults, may demonstrate a slightly raised collarette of skin at its base, and is cured by excision.

MYXOID LESIONS

Myxoid lesions consist of a loose fibrous stroma containing gelatinous mucins and mucopolysaccharides, demonstrable with special stains. Lesions may be fluctuant. They are soft and may be difficult to detect in deep soft tissues. Symptoms are not specific. *Digital mucous cysts (cutaneous myxoid cysts)* occasionally are reported in toes (248) and may communicate with synovium of an adjacent distal interphalangeal joint (249, 250) (Fig. 46.14). Recurrence is common because excision of the cyst leaves that communication. Lesions may appear behind a toenail and alter nail growth.

Ganglionic cysts (tendosynovial cyst, synovial cyst, bursal cyst), (244) occur in articular synovial tissue or more proximally in tendon sheaths. They are fluctuant, containing the same material as cutaneous myxoid cysts (Fig. 46.15). In a series reported by Hajdu (241), of 720 such lesions, only 30 (4.2%) were pedal. They may work on a valvelike system (251), filling when their site of origin is irritated and therefore secretory. Cysts may be associated with local trauma. A re-

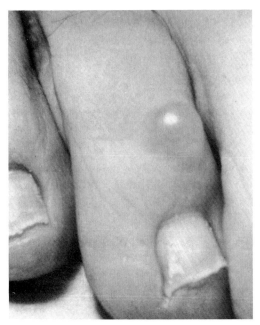

Figure 46.14. Digital mucous cyst. These lesions may involve subjacent joint tissues and may cause growth defects in the adjacent nail.

port describes a mentally retarded child with ganglia of the hands, wrists, feet, and ankles (252). During 11 years, Podiatric Pathology Laboratories recorded 6535 such lesions, 75% in women. Both feet were involved in 13.4% of cases. Slightly more lesions occurred in the right foot than in the left. A similar surgical problem exists for this lesion as for cutaneous myxoid cysts, but ganglia can sometimes be controlled by elimination or relief of biomechanical problem(s) and antiseptic aspiration followed by infiltration with a glucocorticoid. Fluid removed from this (or any) lesion should be sent for cytological examination, and the amount and physical characteristics of the fluid recorded. Ganglionic cysts may also erode local cortical bone, forming an *intraosseous ganglionic cyst* (253). Therefore, ganglionic cyst should be part of the differential diagnosis of bone cysts (254). Hajdu (241) indicates reports of such intraosseous lesions in the distal tibia, in malleoli, and in the talus. The senior author has seen one in a woman's metatarsal base. Rarely, pedal *myxomas* occur (244).

Fibrosarcoma is a fully malignant collagenous, metastatic tumor occurring at any age (240, 241). It is very uncommon in the foot, only two cases having been seen at Podiatric Pathology Laboratories over an 11-year period. Both occurred in women (46 and 48 years of age), each in the left foot. The senior author has seen one case at a large oncology center, in the dorsal aspect of the first ray of a 17-year-old woman. Statistics regarding plantar lesions may be misleading, because differential diagnosis includes other infiltrating, cellular lesions. If fibrosarcoma is confirmed, the patient must be closely examined for metastases, especially to lungs and bones. Although magnetic resonance imaging (MRI) and other radiological techniques can help to determine

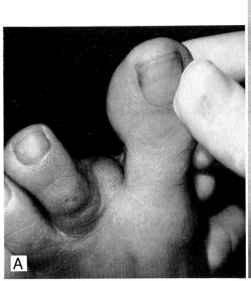
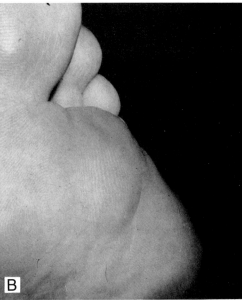

Figure 46.15. **A.** Interdigital ganglionic cyst that extended from the first metatarsal head level. **B.** Ganglionic cyst on the plantar aspect of the foot. Symptoms may be reminiscent of neuroma that may be concurrently present in the traumatized area. Clinical appearance is nonspecific.

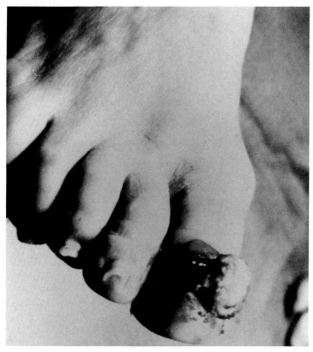

Figure 46.16. Fibrosarcoma in nail bed of hallux. This is not a common location for most pedal sarcomas. (Courtesy of S. H. Silvers, S. Weinstein, and C. Gilbert.)

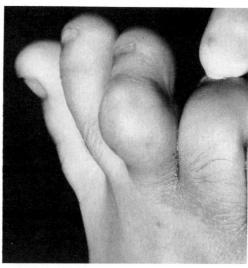

Figure 46.17. Giant cell tumor of tendon, involving third toe. In toto surgical excision included overlying skin and peripheral tissue.

extent of visible lesion, pedal tissues are compacted so that clear definition of involved tissue and blood vessels may not be as possible as in larger soft tissue compartments. A small, distal, well-differentiated lesion may require partial amputation (a digit and part of a ray) whereas larger, more proximal and/or more anaplastic lesions may require higher amputation. Plastic and reconstructive surgeons may aid in limb-saving procedures where feasible (255).

Patients require physical therapy and accommodative and functional orthoses. Also, patients must be observed for local recurrences and late metastases (Fig. 46.16).

Dermal fibrosarcomas may also occur, especially in sites of prior damage. These may (infrequently) ulcerate (256). Dermal lesions are superficial and if detected early and while small, chances for metastasis-free survival may be enhanced.

Histiocytomas are lesions caused by cells best described as facultative fibroblasts (257), and they manifest in many forms. Histiocytes may represent arrest in fibroblast development or, based on experimental findings (258, 259), a functional and morphological state (241). Benign and malignant forms exist, as do some that seem to be borderline lesions in that they may or may not act according to criteria that suggest malignancy. There are three major groups.

1. *Fibroblastic fibours*. Benign forms include sclerosing hemangioma (dermatofibroma) and some forms of xanthoma and of myxoma. Malignant forms include dermatofibrosarcoma protuberans (and its pigmented variant [240], the Bednar tumor, or pigmented

neurofibroma) and some malignant xanthomas and myxomas.
2. *Histiocytic fibrous*. Benign forms include giant cell tumor of tendon sheath, reticulohistiocytic granuloma, xanthogranuloma, pigmented villonodular synovitis, and nevoid xanthoma. Malignant forms include malignant giant cell tumor of tendon sheath, pseudosarcomatous reticulohistiocytoma, xanthomatous giant cell tumor, nevoxanthoendothelioma (juvenile xanthogranuloma), and a general category of malignant histiocytic fibrous histiocytoma.
3. *Pleomorphic fibrous*. Benign forms include atypical fibroxanthoma, as well as some other xanthomas and xanthogranulomas. Malignant forms are all in the xanthoma/xanthosarcoma group.

Histiocytic lesions occur in the dermis or deeper tissues. Borderline lesions include giant cell tumors and juvenile xanthogranuloma. *Giant cell tumors* occur in the foot (240, 244), and one study showed that of 40 lesions, 13 (32.5%) were in the ankle, foot, or toes (240) (Fig. 46.17). Many other histiocytomas are also reported in the feet (244) and have been seen at Podiatric Pathology Laboratories. Symptoms and signs are nonspecific, so that for large, deep lesions that may show evidence of bone erosion as they grow, frozen-section intraoperative diagnostic consultation may help. Giant cell tumors (the most frequent pedal histiocytoma) should be removed in toto with a clinically normal tissue rim and not taken in pieces. These tumors tend to seed locally (hence to recur) and may "pseudometastasize" to distant organs—for example, lungs—as a result of poor surgical technique and tumor manipulation, a phenomenon well recognized with giant cell tumor of bone (260, 261) and similarly presumed for the soft tissue variety because they are virtually the same except for location. They are aggressive and may enter into bone, making it impossible to tell whether the origin was intraosseous or extraosseous. A superficial dermal/subcutaneous form also is reported (262). Irradiation is not indicated because of possible recurrence in malignant form. Further, a recurrence resulting from local seeding or incomplete extirpation of the original lesion may similarly be less differentiated. Malignant forms of giant cell tumor of tendon are well recognized and are reported in the foot (241, 263).

Dermatofibrosarcoma protuberans (Darier's tumor) is a low-grade malignancy that can recur if not completely excised and that occurs in the foot (244). The authors have seen a 28-year-old woman with this lesion at the ankle, who returned 8 years after excision with another tumor at the operative site that was considered a fibrosarcoma (Fig. 46.18). It confirms recurrence and suggests that fibroblasts and histiocytes are closely related, enhancing in vitro experimental results (264) in which cultured histiocytes from dermatofibrosarcoma protuberans were seen on electron microscopic examination to assume fibroblast characteristics.

Unusual histiocytomas bear mention because of association with other conditions. *Tendon xanthomas* affect the Achilles tendon and occur in persons with elevated serum beta-lipoprotein levels, as in hyperlipoproteinemia types IIa, III, and rarely in IIB (65). Diagnosis of a lesion should prompt consultation with an internist because of potential cardiovascular sequelae. *Tuberous xanthomas* of digits, knees, elbows, and buttocks may also be present in these hyperlipoproteinemia types. *Multicentric reticulohistiocytosis* affects adults with numerous granulomatous nodules in various parts of the body that may be preceded by, or be concomitant with, polyarthritis (65) resulting from synovial granulomatous lesions (265). Severe deformity and disability may

occur as articular cartilage and underlying bone are destroyed by the granulomas. A search for skin lesions (and biopsy thereof) in the presence of a history of polyarthritis is indicated (as well as knowledge of other causes of polyarthritis). *Necrobiotic xanthogranuloma* is an unusual lesion showing subcutaneous nodules as well as plaques that may be ulcerated, telangiectatic, and atrophic. It may be accompanied by a paraproteinemia and can be a harbinger of multiple myeloma (266). The senior author has seen one case (through a colleague) with such granulomas, in the foot of a middle-aged woman who showed no other abnormalities. Such patients must be monitored for changes in serum protein levels or hematologiccal status.

Acrokeratoelastoidosis, an unusual lesion in the fibrous group, is a rare, dominantly inherited, autosomal defect of elastic tissue. Smooth, firm, shiny papules occur on palmar and plantar borders (267, 268) and may also appear along the sides of the feet and on the dorsal aspects of the fingers. These points differentiate this disorder from piezogenic papules (intradermal heel fat herniations that may undergo necrosis) in obese persons.

LESIONS RELATED TO SYNOVIAL TISSUES

Although synovial tissue is found lining the inner surfaces of joint capsules, some clinicians believe that lesions may arise outside of such well-defined areas. Perhaps they arise from less-differentiated mesenchymal cells responding to some stimulus for synovial differentiation. Because these lesions may also be associated with tendon sheaths, bursae, and fascia, the term *tendosynovial* has been offered to describe them (241).

Synovial chondromatosis (osteochondromatosis, osteochondritis

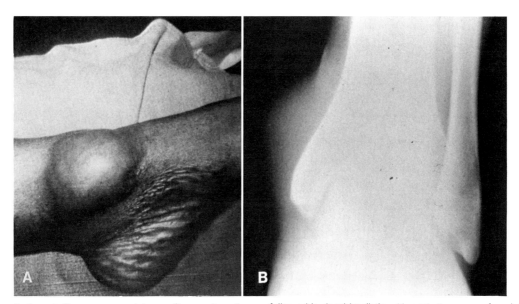

Figure 46.18.   A. Dermatofibrosarcoma protuberans (low-grade malignant fibroblastic fibrous histiocytoma) in a 28-year-old woman. Higher-grade (more anaplastic) lesion recurred locally after 8 years. Excision was followed by local irradiation. No metastases were found. **B.** Radiograph of original lesion area showing nonspecific increase in soft tissue density medially, without apparent bone involvement.

dissecans, synovial chondrometaplasia, loose bodies, joint mice, joint rice) is a rare condition that shows a predilection for large joints such as the ankle (240, 241). Most patients are adult males, and trauma has been associated with these lesions. Patients may report a growing, painful mass. It contains radiopaque globular structures, not all of which are ossified, so that on removal of the membrane and its contents, there may be many more bodies present than were seen on x-ray studies. Many metaplastic bodies are attached to synovial membrane by a pedicle that also feeds vessels to them. Detached bodies are joint mice. If left, they may damage articular cartilage. Some lesions were reported to transform to chondrosarcoma (269, 270), but whether that really developed in the metaplastic lesions proper is questioned (240).

Villonodular synovitis (pigmented villonodular synovitis) is an uncommon variant of giant cell tumor that involves joint spaces (241). Despite a title suggesting inflammation, it is neoplastic. It most frequently occurs in patients under 40 years of age. Symptoms usually have been present for a few years, including pain, joint effusion, and hemarthrosis (thus hemosiderin pigment), limited joint motion, and locking. It occurs in the same general distribution as the giant cell tumor of tendon sheath (240) and is said to differ from that lesion only by location (241). It should be differentiated clinically from true inflammatory synovitides (i.e., gout, rheumatoid arthritis, septic arthritis, traumatic synovitis, and granulomatous synovitis of tuberculosis). Foot cases are specifically mentioned by Kirby et al. (244) and Jaffe (271).

Tendosynovial sarcoma (synovial sarcoma, malignant synovioma) is a highly malignant, metastatic tumor with synovial tissue features. It is most often seen adjacent to joints rather than within them. "Tendosynovial" suggests that this neoplasm arises from mesenchymal tissues associated with joints, tendon sheaths, bursae, and fascia, as reviewed elsewhere (240, 241, 272). Histological manifestations are either monophasic (e.g., fibroblastoid, epithelioid, pseudoglandular, chordoid, and clear cell) or biphasic (glandular structures in one of the above types) (241). Immunocytochemistry studies help to establish tendosynovial sarcoma versus other malignant tumors with similar patterns, especially for the monophasic spindle cell (fibroblastoid) type. There is dispute as to whether epithelioid and clear cell tumors are of the synovial sarcoma group (240). Studies of pedal clear cell tumors have determined cytogenetic features such as those in melanoma (273). Most patients are young adults (272) (although synovial sarcoma occurs at all ages), and the foot is a common site for all types, with pedal incidence statistics from 13% to 25% (240, 241, 244, 272, 274).

Metastases occur with large tumors (> 5 cm), most frequently to lungs, lymph nodes, and bones (274). Lesions may be asymptomatic for long periods (272), or they may grow rapidly and produce symptoms. Vague symptoms of discomfort may be present with no visible mass. X-ray films may or may not show a mass (275). This is also demonstrated by a reported case of epithelioid sarcoma that manifested as reflex sympathetic dystrophy syndrome, with no other symptoms or signs until erosion of metatarsals eventually

occurred (276). A mass with calcifications may be present (275), and if there is pressure on adjacent bone, periosteal proliferative reaction may be noted. Osseous invasion may occur (Fig. 46.19). Angiography studies are helpful but not specific for diagnosis. Newer radiological techniques may help to outline visible tumor margins and locally involved structures. If biopsy shows this as a sarcoma, then amputation may be indicated (277, 278). The level depends on tumor size, location, histological type, and extent of local invasion. There also must be consultations to determine metastases, and the patient must be followed up for local recurrence and late metastases. Recently, improved survival has been due to a combination of aggressive, radical surgery, chemotherapy, and irradiation. Vascular invasion is a poor sign (277).

TUMORS AND TUMOR-LIKE CONDITIONS OF ADIPOSE TISSUE

Nonneoplastic lesions affect adipose tissues and can give an impression of tumor or can be associated with visceral tumors. *Subcutaneous nodular fat necrosis* (65) (*pancreatic panniculitis*) manifests as reddish, tender, lower extremity and pedal nodules, often accompanied by ankle arthralgias (279-281). Necrotic changes are due to serum lipase whose levels are elevated in pancreatitis and pancreatic carcinoma. Apparently elevated serum trypsin levels alter vascular permeability (281), permitting lipase to escape into the tissues. Biopsy confirmation of this condition requires prompt consultation to determine the nature and extent of pancreatic disease. X-ray studies of the affected foot/ankle area may show soft tissue calcifications representing saponification of fatty acids formed by the enzyme activity.

Lipogranulomatosis (Farber's disease) (282) is a very rare, recessively inherited sphingolipidosis showing periarticular and tendon masses especially at the wrists and ankles. Because other organs are involved, very few survive beyond the first year of life; those who do may develop flexion contractures at lesion sites.

Solitary lipogranulomas (sclerosing lipogranulomas, sclerosing panniculitis) are not inherited and may represent a proliferative fat necrosis (241). Some of these are *paraffinomas*, representing sites of injected oils and lipids during a time when oils provided the base for parenteral therapeutic agents, or (among other abused organic materials and drugs) were autoinoculated to cause the bizarre *factitial panniculitis* (283). The authors have not seen reports of this variant in the foot. *Piezogenic papules (dermatocele)* (284) represent intradermal cystic herniations of subcutaneous heel fat. Nodular herniations that may be painful are seen in obese individuals (285). They appear during weight bearing and may become necrotic. Heel-cupping orthoses control the condition. This condition should be differentiated clinically and by history from acrokeratoelastoidosis. *Dercum's disease (adiposis dolorosa)* is a rare condition that occurs as part of a syndrome that includes asthenia, depression, and psychic disturbances and affects postmenopausal women

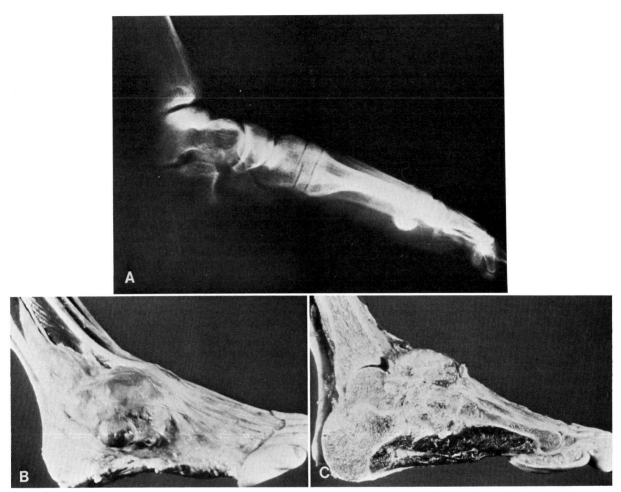

Figure 46.19. **A.** Tendosynovial sarcoma overlying and invading the talus of a 29-year-old man. Lytic area suggests invasion whereas sclerotic rim suggests pressure from expansile lesion with periosteal reaction. **B.** Skin dissected from amputation specimen of leg and foot shown in radiograph. Large mass has displaced other local structures and is pseudoencapsulated because of compression of surrounding tissues. **C.** Deeper section of same specimen shows lesion overlying and invading talus. (**A** and **C** from Potter GK, Penny TR, Walkes M: Tendosynovial sarcoma: a clinicopathologic analysis of foot cases and presentation of a case. *J Am Podiatr Assoc* 74:312-322, 1984.)

(240, 241). Painful fatty deposits occur around the ankles, knees, and elbows.

Lipomas are benign, solitary or multiple, and superficial tumors that are rare in the feet (213, 240, 241, 244). Single lesions far outnumber multiple types. Most occur in middle age and may be difficult to diagnose clinically because of slow growth, lack of symptoms, and nonspecific clinical features. They may be soft to moderately firm depending on tissues mixed in with the fat cells (Fig. 46.20). Histological variants explain these differences, for example, fibrolipoma (spindle cell lipoma, sclerosing lipoma), myxoid, pleomorphic, and myelolipoma (the latter containing hematopoietic elements). Lipomas, which may be part of the stigmata of *Gardner's syndrome* (240), have been associated with neurofibromatosis (240, 241). Lipoma fat is not metabolized as is normal fat; that is, lipomas do not decrease in size or disappear during weight loss. *Angiolipoma* is highly vascular, demonstrating a more complex branching pattern than do ordinary lipomas (286) and fewer Weibel-Palade bodies in the endothelial cells, suggesting either immature or neoplastic endothelium (286). The growths may be tender (65, 240) and painful on weight bearing. They are infiltrative, may be multiple, and may be related to trauma (240). They occur in young adults, and a nonpedal form is suspected of being more frequent in homosexual men and may be confused histologically with Kaposi's sarcoma (287).

Angiolipomas demonstrate thick vascular walls and varying amounts of smooth muscle cells. This type of lesion is often associated with tuberous sclerosis, but the authors are not aware of any cases reported in the foot. Similarly, *hibernoma*, a benign tumor of brown fat (the type seen in hibernating mammals) is not yet reported in the foot. However, records from Podiatric Pathology Laboratories do show fibroangioma and simple lipomas. *Lipoblastoma* of children's lower extremities, including the foot (244), may be present at birth (240). It is benign and may be localized and

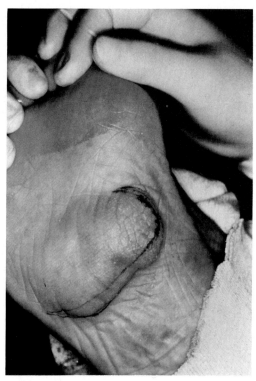

Figure 46.20. Large plantar lipoma. Tumor extirpation may, as in this case, involve excision of redundant skin. Skin lines and direction of circulation should guide excision and wound edge apposition.

superficial, or it may occur in many areas (*lipoblastomatosis*) with superficial and deep lesions. *Tendon sheath lipomas (endovaginal lipoma)* occur in the hands, feet, and in both areas concurrently (240). It affects young adults, may occur symmetrically, and is rare in the feet. It may be painful, may interfere with tendon function, and may actually cause tendon rupture. Lipomas as a group may also occur in children (288).

Liposarcoma is a malignant, metastatic, adipocytic tumor, probably the most common lower extremity sarcoma in adults (241), but it is uncommon in the feet (243). In a survey of 242 liposarcomas of which 173 were not retroperitoneal, two of the latter group (1.2%) occurred in the foot/ankle area (241). Of the total reported, those two cases constitute 0.83% of liposarcomas seen. Records of Podiatric Pathology Laboratories show one liposarcoma case (in the right foot of a 56-year-old woman) in contrast with 770 cases of simple lipoma and fibrolipoma and 10 cases of angiolipoma. Cases of primary liposarcoma in an ankle (289) and in a toe (290) are reported. It is extremely rare in children, and doubt has been cast on such diagnoses in children because of its similarity to lipoblastoma (240, 241). Whether these neoplasms arise from lipomas is also unclear. Liposarcoma occurs in middle-aged adults, and lower extremity lesions are diagnosed earlier than are retroperitoneal types. There are no specific signs or symptoms. The lesion usually lies deeper than do benign lipomas and appears as a nodular, bulging mass. In the foot, impingement on nerves may produce

symptoms. Radiographs may show a radiolucent lesion, and angiography may be of help to delineate these very vascular tumors.

Some clinicians suggest liposarcoma histology as a factor in the treatment regimen and prognosis (241). The types, increasingly anaplastic, are the well-differentiated, myxoid, fibroblastic, lipoblastic, and pleomorphic. Incompletely extirpated lesions may recur in less differentiated form, with increased metastatic tendency (240, 241). Liposarcomas are radiosensitive, so that aggressive surgery, combined with irradiation and chemotherapy, is indicated. Because the foot is so compact, amputation may be indicated (depending on the location and extent of the lesion), as well as consultation to determine metastases and to administer irradiation and chemotherapy. Long-term local care and observation must be maintained to watch for recurrence and late metastases.

LESIONS OF MUSCLE

Two types of muscle occur in the feet: smooth muscle in pedal vasculature, arrector pilorum muscles dorsally, and striated muscle on dorsal and plantar aspects of the foot.

Reactive Lesions

Proliferative myositis (myositis proliferans) is an inflammation of striated muscle that occurs in middle-aged men (241) and is virtually unknown in the foot, possibly because it has not been recognized there. Ganglion-like cells in this lesion give the impression of a malignant tumor, but they are actually histiocytes and the lesion is cured by local excision. Some lesions demonstrate osteoid formation (291). A focal form affects children and adults, manifesting as a painful, deep, fast-growing mass (292). *Polymyositis* is related to autoimmune diseases and is thought to arise from local vascular infarctions secondary to vasculitis (293), but some clinicians have seen no evidence of such vascular changes (294). It may be associated with visceral malignancies either alone or in combination with skin lesions. The latter syndrome is *dermatomyositis*. With skin involvement, incidence of visceral malignancy is higher than with polymyositis alone (294). Visceral malignancy may precede skin and muscle symptoms (295). Dystrophic calcinosis occurs in patients with dermatomyositis and is seen in x-ray studies. Patients with polymyositis must be evaluated to determine if visceral malignancy is present. For differential diagnosis the condition is also seen in anti-immune conditions that show distinct immunological findings.

Myositis ossificans (Münchmeyer's disease) is a benign reaction that may be associated with trauma to muscle. Early stages may be difficult to tell histologically from parosteal or extraosseous osteogenic sarcoma. It often occurs in young athletic adults but is reported in the age range of 9 to 84 years (240). Older lesions appear as ectopic mature bone and may show on x-ray films. If they are causing the patient distress, lesions may be excised. There is debate as to whether these lesions transform to osteogenic sarcoma (214, 240). This lesion is more apt to occur in the large, nonpedal muscles.

However, a form seen in the soft tissues of the fingers and toes is *fibroosseous pseudotumor of the digits* (296, 297). *Myositis ossificans progressiva (fibrodysplasia ossificans progressiva)* is a rare hereditary disease seen in childhood or early adulthood, with lesions in muscle and in other soft tissues (240) that eventually calcify and ossify. It is distinguished clinically from fibromatoses by the presence of shortened digits and either by missing thumbs and great toes or by deviations such as bilateral hallux valgus (298). Surgery for the malformations in a child or young adult should not be undertaken without a thorough history of onset, a familial history, and examination for other deformities.

Tumors of Striated Muscle

Rhabdomyoma is the benign tumor of striated muscle and has not, to the authors' knowledge, ever been reported in the foot. However, cardiac rhabdomyoma may be a concomitant of tuberous sclerosis, which does have pedal manifestations (Keonen's periungual fibromas). *Supernumerary muscles* in the ankle region may simulate tumors (299). The *benign triton tumor (neuromuscular hamartoma)* contains elements of striated muscle and nerve. It has been reported in association with the sciatic nerve (240) but not in the ankle/foot region. *Rhabdomyosarcoma*, a malignant striated muscle tumor, occurs in the foot (300-302). Rhabdomyosarcomas are the most common malignant soft tissue tumors of young children, adolescents, and young adults (240). These tumors are divided conveniently into the embryonal (including a number of subtypes) (240, 241) and the pleomorphic types (241). The designation "juvenile" is avoided because both major groups are seen in children and adults (241) and have occurred in feet (241).

The embryonal form is most common in young male children. Pedal lesions erode bone (240) and may be painful. They are fast-growing, deep tumors associated with locations of striated muscle (240).

Without biopsy, the tumor cannot be identified. Even with biopsy, differential diagnosis may involve special stains and immunocytochemistry studies. The tumor may arise from undifferentiated mesenchyma, because it can also be seen in areas unrelated to striated muscle. In addition to amputation, irradiation and chemotherapy are used, requiring appropriate consultations to determine such factors as clinical stage and metastatic disease. *Rhabdomyoblastoma* may actually represent a well-differentiated rhabdomyosarcoma or a rare and separate entity (241). Over a period of 11 years, Podiatric Pathology Laboratories records show two rhabdomyosarcomas, both in 37-year-old women, one in the left foot and one in the right foot.

Tumors of Smooth Muscle

Leiomyomas are benign smooth muscle tumors that may arise from superficial or deep structures (Fig. 46.21). *Pilar leiomyomas* from the arrector pili muscles of the pilosebaceous complex may be single or multiple skin lesions. They usually are tender and may be painful (303). These may be familial

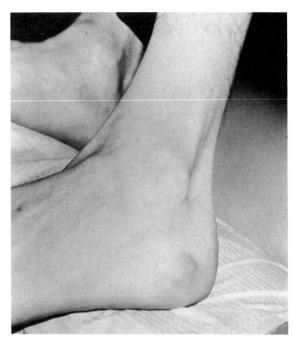

Figure 46.21. Benign leiomyoma of skin on heel. These may be painful and may arise from blood vessels in any location or from arrector pili muscles in nonplantar locations. Some may be present under digital corns, especially on the fifth toe.

and in some cases are associated with other diseases and conditions (240). They tend to develop during adolescent and early adult years. *Angioleiomyomas* usually are solitary venous lesions, are most frequent in the lower extremities of women over 40 years of age, lie subcutaneously, and are usually painful and tender (304, 305). They tend to contract to temperature changes and touch, which may account for pain. Leiomyomas of the deeper soft tissues are uncommon, and well-differentiated leiomyosarcomas may present a problem in differential diagnosis. Calcifications may occur in deep leiomyomas. Benign metastasizing leiomyomas are reported as uterine lesions (306), and intravenous leiomyomatosis originates from them (307). Such behavior by pedal lesions is not known (244), but a suggestion is that barring hormone effects on uterine tissue, leiomyomas may be a pseudometastatic lesion, requiring complete excision with surrounding clinically normal tissue, without violating the tumor. If incompletely excised, leiomyomas recur. *Smooth muscle hamartomas*, from pilar smooth muscle, have not yet been described as pedal lesions.

Leiomyosarcoma is the malignant form of smooth muscle tumor, which may also arise from pilar or venous smooth muscle and can occur in the lower extremities. A male to female ratio as high as 3:1 has been quoted (240). Superficial forms may be symptomatic (305), are usually single, small lesions, and have a better overall prognosis than do deep lesions. These may produce skin discoloration and ulceration, as well as lesion umbilication (240). Multiple superficial leiomyosarcomas suggest metastases from an occult deep tumor, which must be sought (240). Subcutaneous

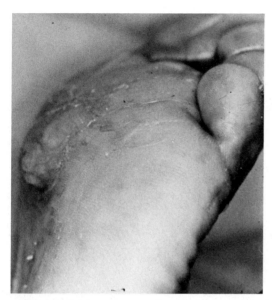

Figure 46.22. Angioleiomyosarcoma of sole. Lesion was low grade and did not invade bone. Radiograph shows poorly bordered nonspecific increase in local soft tissue density. Tumor demonstrated microcalcifications histologically. (Courtesy of M. J. Trepal.)

deeper lesions grow more quickly and to a larger size before detection, and they are painful (240). Deeper lesions are more apt to metastasize (308). Those of vascular origin may present a problem of local seeding (240) and potentially—because of extensive bleeding—iatrogenic metastasis if incisional biopsy is performed (Fig. 46.22). After radiographical evaluation (e.g., angiography, MRI) needle biopsy may decrease chances of such occurrence but with a risk of sampling error. Perhaps intraoperative frozen-section biopsy with very careful hemostasis would solve the problem. Because the lesion is infiltrative, amputation is indicated. Radiotherapy is not very promising (240) although some clinicians consider an infiltrate of eosinophils and a circulating eosinophilia with this tumor (and others) to suggest a good prognosis and response to irradiation (241). Leiomyosarcoma is reported in a chronic venous ankle ulcer (309), in the ankle without a venous problem or ulcer (310), and in the foot (302, 311).

At Podiatric Pathology Laboratories, over a period of 11 years, five leiomyosarcomas were seen, three of which occurred in women. Four of these were in the left foot. The average age of the patients was 50 years (range, 26 to 74 years). There also were 713 leiomyomas, of which 528 (74%) occurred in women, and 56 (10.6%) were bilateral. There was no significant limb preference. The average patient age was 42 years (range, 4 to 100 years). A painful, tender interdigital angioleiomyoma with calcification, chondroid metaplasia, many mast cells, and fibrosis has been reported in the fourth interdigital space of a 74-year-old diabetic woman (312). Another, in a hallux (313), was clinically considered and diagnosed as a ganglion.

Leiomyoblastoma is a very rare tumor occurring in benign and malignant forms (241). None have been reported in the pedal area.

TUMORS AND TUMOR-LIKE LESIONS OF PERIPHERAL NERVES

Conditions that may clinically simulate peripheral nerve tumors include degenerative changes (axonal degeneration, wallerian degeneration, segmental demyelinization diseases) and certain acquired and genetic hypertrophic neuropathies. Mechanisms are reviewed elsewhere (241). The most frequent reactive peripheral nerve lesion seen in the foot is *neuroma*. *Traumatic, amputation,* and *Morton's intermetatarsal* types are variants of the same lesion. That is, they are mechanisms involving (a) failure of the axonal components to find the distal pathway from which they became detached as a result of acute or chronic trauma or (b) interposed barriers such as hematomas, fibrosis, or amputation of the part (Fig. 46.23). After surgery, such lesions may develop because the severed proximal and distal ends of a nerve were not properly apposed. Axons, Schwann's cells, perineural cells, and fibroblasts become a disorganized mixture that constitutes the lesion (240, 241). These are best treated by careful excision that includes closure of the remaining sheath at the distal end of the remaining nerve tract, inasmuch as the axonal material can penetrate many tissues but not its own sheath (241).

During an 11-year period, over 14,000 neuromas have been submitted to Podiatric Pathology Laboratories, of which 81% have come from female patients. About 31% of these lesions have been bilateral. The average age of the patients is 48 years (range, 0 to 94 years). The extremely early age is explained by the rare occurrence of a *rudimentary (supernumerary) digit* that may contain neuromatous tissue (240). (Three of these have been seen at Podiatric Pathology Laboratories, all in males up to the age of 30 years). Symptoms include paresthesias distal to neuromas, Tinel's sign, and at times a palpable mass that may be tender. Neuroma is most frequent distally in the third intermetarsal space, but it may occur in any intermetatarsal space and in more than one.

Benign Tumors of Peripheral Nerve

The tumor group known as *schwannomas* includes *neurilemmomas* and *neurofibromas*. Although differences between them exist ultrastructurally (314) and clinically (age-groups and anatomical sites of the tumors) (240), they are grouped as *peripheral nerve sheath tumors*, all originating from the periaxonal cells.

Growth patterns of neurofibromas and neurilemmomas differ. Both are in the group of *collagenous schwannomas*, which also includes angioneuromas, plexiform neurofibromas, pacinian neurofibromas, and glandular, cystic, and pleomorphic schwannoma (240, 241). *Noncollagenous schwannomas* (241) include epithelioid and undifferentiated types. Some clinicians place storiform schwannomas (storiform neurofibroma, Bednar's tumor, melanotic neurofi-

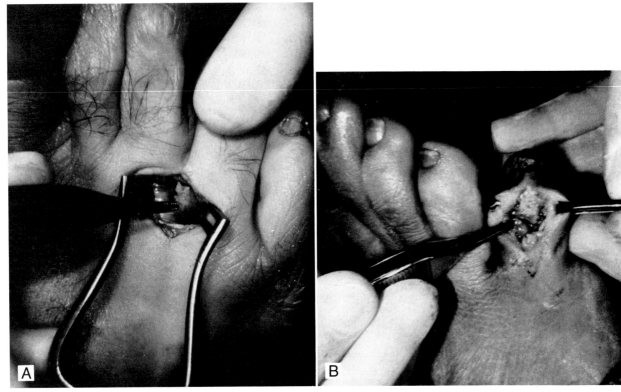

Figure 46.23. **A.** Surgical exposure of typical Morton's neuroma between third and fourth metatarsal heads. This extremely common benign lesion is considered reactive, not neoplastic. **B.** Small digital neuroma in fifth toe. These may be quite painful and may underlie digital corns, especially those on the fifth toe.

Figure 46.24. Neurilemmoma on lateral aspect of foot that manifested clinically as a neuritis. Pedal neurilemmomas are not common. (Courtesy of H. E. Confer.)

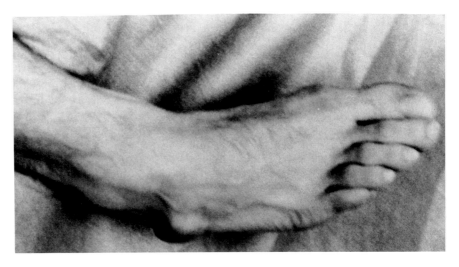

broma) in this category (241), whereas others consider it with dermatofibroma in the histiocytic group (240). Histologically, most schwannomas show *Verocay bodies* (Antoni type A or B patterns). *Ancient schwannoma* has undergone cystic degeneration and/or calcification.

Clinically, neurilemmomas are slow-growing tumors that favor the flexor surfaces of the extremities (Fig. 46.24). They occur as single lesions (65, 240) but may be multiple if as-

sociated with neurofibromatosis 1, which, in one series, occurred in 18% of cases (314). Unless large, the tumor may be painless and may fluctuate because of cystic changes (315). These tumors are not recurrent unless associated with neurofibromatosis 1. Most occur in the 20 to 50 year age-group (240), affecting both sexes about equally.

Solitary neurofibromas are usually small, superficial nodules that produce few symptoms. They are seen in a younger age-group (20 to 30 years) than are neurilemmomas, and they occur in both sexes on any part of the body. Without other stigmata or familial history, these lesions alone do not suggest neurofibromatosis 1.

Excision of the lesion is curative.

According to records from Podiatric Pathology Laboratory over an 11-year period, the ratio of pedal neurofibromas to neurilemmomas is about 3.2:1. Whereas neurilemmomas occurred almost equally among men and women, neurofibromas occurred 2.4 times more frequently in women than in men. For both lesions, a slight majority occurred in the right foot. The average age of patients with neurilemmomas was 50 years (range, 16 to 95 years), whereas for neurofibroma, the average was 54 years (range, 3 to 96 years). The very young in that group probably represent cases of neurofibromatosis 1. There were fewer multiple lesions in the neurilemmoma group (7.6%) than in the neurofibroma group (10.5%). Few pedal neurilemmomas are reported in the literature (316, 317).

Neurofibromatosis 1 (von Recklinghausen's disease, multiple neurofibromatosis), initially described in 1882 (318) as *phakomatosis*, may be accompanied by other conditions (240). Very specific criteria have been established for diagnosis, and these, as well as this condition, have been reviewed in detail elsewhere (65, 240, 241, 319). All races and both sexes are affected. The defect seems to lie in chromosome 17 (320). In addition to high risk for development of malignant changes in neurofibromas, patients with neurofibromatosis 1 have a higher incidence of unrelated secondary malignancies. Patients with this condition must receive very close follow-up by a physician. Sudden enlargement of a preexisting lesion with or without concurrent pain, or sudden development of a rapidly growing lesion, suggests malignant schwannoma, and the patient must be promptly referred for diagnostic procedures and care. In the presence of other conditions or syndromes, great care should be taken before undertaking any procedures. Patients who also have Addison's disease should not undergo even simple biopsy outside of a hospital where the patient can be carefully monitored. This also strongly suggests that a careful and detailed history is especially necessary for any patient with neurofibromatosis 1, as is concurrent care by an internist. Neurofibromas may affect many organs. Neurofibromatosis 1 occurs in about 1:3000 births, with 100% penetrance but with varying degrees of manifestation. Classical stigmata appear early in life (Fig. 46.25).

Malignant Tumors of Peripheral Nerve

Malignant tumors of peripheral nerves are *malignant schwannomas* and *malignant neurofibrosarcomas*. More recently, in recognition of other mesenchymal elements in these tumors (321-325) and the apparent pluripotent nature of Schwann's cells, the term *malignant peripheral nerve sheath tumor* has been applied. Although these are extremely rare in the feet, cases have been reported (240, 241, 326). Especially in the setting of neurofibromatosis 1, the mortality rate for these malignancies ranges between 80% (240) and 97% (241). Further

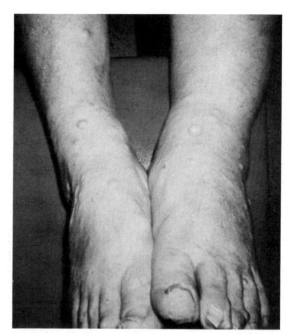

Figure 46.25. Neurofibromatosis, type 1. Multiple neurofibromas are present on the legs, feet, and toes. A café-au-lait spot is present medially on the right lower leg. Many organs may be involved. (From Potter GK, Feldman JS: Neoplasms of the peripheral nervous system. In Weber GA (ed): *Clinics in Podiatric Medicine and Surgery*. Philadelphia, WB Saunders Co, 1990, pp 141-149. Original photo courtesy of S. J. Berlin.)

complication lies in the differential diagnosis from the benign *cellular schwannoma* (327) and from other spindle cell lesions. Immunocytochemistry studies and other special techniques are helpful. For foot lesions, amputation is usually recommended (326), with frozen-section intraoperative biopsy on the proximal nerve end, to confirm clear margins in the amputation stump (326). Consultations should be arranged to seek metastases and to render appropriate systemic care, along with observation for local recurrence. It has been estimated that about 11% of these malignant peripheral nerve neoplasms may arise as a result of therapeutic or occupational irradiation (240), with a latent period of about 15 years.

Symptoms and signs may vary but rarely antedate the physical presence of a mass, and they may include paresthesias as well as other motor and sensory abnormalities (240). Pain may be present. However, symptoms and signs in the foot may arise from malignant peripheral nerve sheath tumors or from other neoplasms lying at higher levels (retroperitoneum, thigh, leg) and involving the sciatic nerve or its branches. Radiographs may demonstrate soft tissue density and osseous changes caused by pressure and invasion. Benign and malignant peripheral nerve neoplasms have demonstrated such x-ray appearances (328). MRI may help to delineate, within limits of the compact foot anatomy, size, visible borders, and the relationship of the lesion to other local structures.

At Podiatric Pathology Laboratories, there have been five

of these malignant tumors in an 11-year period, three in women and two in men. Four of these occurred in the left foot. The average age of the patients was 40 years (range, 29 to 59 years). The small percentage of patients with neurofibromatosis 1 who develop the malignant peripheral nerve sheath tumors tend to do so in the larger proximal nerves and at a much younger age than do others (240).

Malignant neuroepithelioma (peripheral neuroblastoma of adults, primitive neuroectodermal tumor) has been reported in the lower extremities (240, 241, 329), including the foot (330), where it arose as a primary intrametatarsal tumor. Another case involved the very unusual *melanocytic neuroectodermal tumor of infancy (pigmented neuroectodermal tumor of infancy, melanotic progonoma)* as a primary tumor in the fifth metatarsal of a 2-year-old boy, whose foot was subsequently amputated (331). In one report, a neuroepithelioma of the lateral popliteal nerve was the source of paresthesias, weakness, and footdrop in a 29-year-old woman, who died of metastatic disease (329).

TUMORS OF BLOOD VESSELS AND LYMPHATIC VESSELS

Blood and lymphatic vessels are made up of various cell types. However, the cells involved in tumors discussed here are of endothelial origin. Although the blood and lymphatic systems demonstrate many interconnections, their respective endothelial cells have different immunocytochemical characteristics (332). Thus their lesions, although virtually identical, are considered separately.

Benign Endothelial Tumors

Congenital hemangiomas may be localized or may involve an entire limb and/or other organs. Most of these are *capillary hemangiomas* that may be present at birth or appear shortly after. Most involute by early childhood, but the rapid early growth up to about 6 months of age may be frightening to parents (Fig. 46.26).

Patients should be referred for consultation to determine whether multiple deeper lesions are present. *Acquired tufted hemangioma* is the adult form of this lesion. *Verrucous hemangioma* lies under hyperkeratoses and may be confused with warts or *papular angiokeratoma* (240, 333), inasmuch as both occur in the lower extremities. *Cherry angiomas (De Morgan's spots, senile angiomas)* are tiny, bright red, slightly elevated papules that may appear any time after adolescence. *Nevus flammeus (nevus telangiectaticus, port-wine stain)* in the dermis consists of capillary ectasia in one or more dull-red or bluish-red patches. It may affect one limb or more and suggests the presence of other vascular malformations. These may include *arteriovenous malformations* and/or *varicosities*, as in the *Klippel-Trenaunay osteohypertrophic hemangiectasia (Parkes-Weber syndrome, hemolymphangioma)* (334, 335). Serious consequences of this syndrome include death because of "high output" cardiac failure and pulmonary embolization (336).

The senior author has followed a case of Parkes-Weber syndrome for over 20 years, in which bruits were audible over many arteriovenous malformation sites in one leg and foot. Surgical removal of defective vasculature and angiomas has been helpful in this patient and in others (337). In some foot lesions, surgical epiphysiodesis has been helpful in curtailing bone lesions (337). In other cases the condition may be controlled with elastic support (337, 338). Pedal lesions reminiscent of Kaposi's sarcoma may occur in

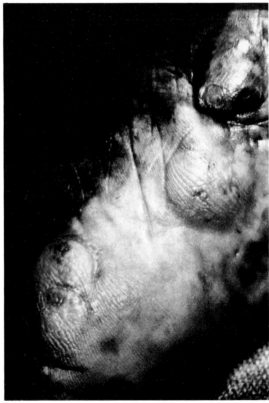

Figure 46.27. Cavernous (venous) hemangioma. Multiple swellings are present. Palpation may give the "bag of worms" impression. Angiogram reveals the tortuous vasculature. (Courtesy of E. D. McGlamry.)

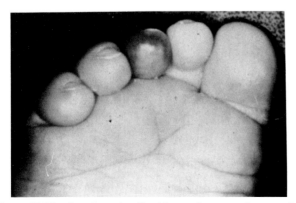

Figure 46.26. Strawberry (capillary) hemangiomas may be present at birth or shortly thereafter. Most degenerate within the first few postnatal years. Some may overlie venous hemangiomas and may be associated with Kasabach-Merritt syndrome.

patients with this syndrome, hence the designation *pseudo Kapoli's sarcoma* (65). These lesions may be painful. Rarely, capillary hemangioma with thrombocytopenia may occur in an infant. This is the *Kasabach-Merritt syndrome* (339), a consumptive coagulopathy within the lesion that can result in disseminated intravascular coagulation and hemorrhage (340). A similar syndrome occurs in adults with large or multiple venous hemangiomas (65). Whether capillary hemangiomas should be treated surgically is to be decided on the merits of a patient's condition. A vascular specialist may be consulted and angiograms obtained. Some capillary hemangiomas may overlie and connect with deeper venous hemangiomas (65, 240). The use of laser surgery has yet to be carefully explored in the treatment of these lesions.

Cavernous hemangiomas contain arterial and venous channels, are much larger and more diffuse than capillary types, and are deeper (240, 241). They may also arise in infancy and childhood. They may appear bluish if relatively superficial and may feel like a "bag of worms" (Fig. 46.27). Deeper lesions are more destructive to soft tissue and bone. Angiography examination usually delineates lesions and should be performed prior to any surgery. Routine radiographs may show calcifications in the lesion (*phleboliths*) associated with thrombi (240). Cavernous hemangiomas are also reported as hemangiomas of peripheral nerves (i.e., the posterior tibial and peroneal) (240). These lesions form part of various *multiple angiomatosis* syndromes (e.g., *blue rubber bleb*

nevus (65, 240), *Maffucci's syndrome* (*Kast-Maffucci syndrome*) (65, 240, 241), the *ataxia-telangiectasia* complex (241), von *Hippel-Lindau* retinal-cerebellar hemangiomatosis, and *Sturge-Weber* encephalotrigeminal angiomatosis) (241).

Angiokeratomas are not really vascular lesions but represent intraepidermal blood pools. All but the Fordyce type demonstrate lesions on the toes (as well as other areas) in various age-groups. The *Fabry* type represents a storage disease. *Cobb syndrome* consists of circumscriptive angiokeratomas or a nevus flammeus with a spinal angioma. Details on each of these can be obtained from texts of dermatology and dermatohistopathology (65).

Angioma serpiginosum consists of red, grouped, flat, asymptomatic, dilated capillaries, which form a netlike or macular pattern with an irregular, serpiginous border. These begin in adolescence, affecting a lower extremity, mostly in women (65).

Pyogenic granulomas (eruptive capillary hemangioma) (65, 341) are friable, easily traumatized lesions. They may therefore show inflammatory infiltrates. They usually occur as single lesions and can be excised with no recurrence. About one third of cases are associated with a history of earlier minor local trauma (240) (Fig. 46.28).

Glomus tumors (glomangioma, angioneuromyoma) arise from glomus bodies acting as vascular shunts in acral areas. Many occur as subungual lesions that may be painful and may show a reddish to reddish-purple color. They may be tiny

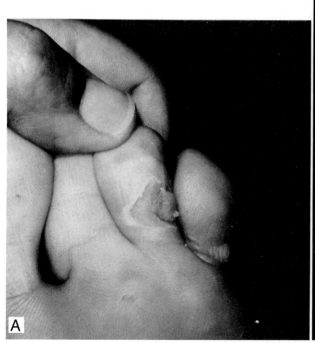
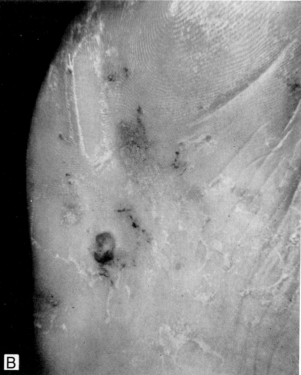

Figure 46.28. **A.** Pyogenic granuloma. Painless, pedunculated mass showed some drainage and prompted the patient to seek medical care. **B.** Pyogenic granuloma resembling amelanotic melanoma, Spitz's nevus, or Kaposi's sarcoma. Excisional biopsy established the diagnosis.

or may range up to 1 cm in size. They usually occur as single lesions and are cured by excision. In a few cases, multiple lesions have occurred (65, 241). In the very rare generalized form, a Kasabach-Merritt syndrome may be present (65). *Glomangiosarcoma* in a glomus tumor has been reported in four cases, three of which were in the lower extremity (240).

Synovial hemangiomas are extremely rare, arising in joints or tendon sheaths. There is pain, swelling, joint effusion, and hemarthrosis. Diffuse lesions are difficult to remove (240).

Hemangiopericytoma is a very rare lesion, and the authors are not aware of any reports of this lesion in the foot. However, at Podiatric Pathology Laboratories, seven cases were seen (two in men, five in women, the patients ranging in age from 34 to 75 years). It may be very difficult to predict from histological findings whether the lesion is benign or malignant; thus any patient with this lesion must be carefully observed. Perhaps all hemangiopericytomas, despite apparently innocuous histology, should be considered potentially malignant. They are metastatic, and the appropriate consultations and follow-up should be instituted. A single malignant hemangiopericytoma in a 73-year-old man was seen at Podiatric Pathology Laboratories over an 11-year period.

Lymphangiomas are uncommon. Two forms are analogous to angiokeratomas, that is, *localized lymphangioma circumscriptum*, with the papular angiokeratoma, and the more diffuse *classical lymphangioma circumscriptum* with angiokeratoma circumscriptum. These tend to be superficial. The latter form may be associated with *lymphectasia* in a limb, and the authors are aware of one such case that involved a foot (342). *Cavernous lymphangioma (cystic hygroma)* is a deep lesion that corresponds to venous hemangioma. Blood may be present in any of these lesions because of frequent communications between the lymphatic and the arterial and venous circulations, but it is not a prominent feature. Cystic hygroma in other areas of the body has been associated with various genetic defects (240, 343) and may be responsible for the edema of the hands and feet seen in *Turner's syndrome* (240). In the past decade, only 10 pedal lymphangiomas have been seen at Podiatric Pathology Laboratories, of which eight occurred in women. The average patient age was 43 years (range, 15 to 59 years). A specific mention of pedal hygroma was made in context with a muscular imbalance syndrome affecting the lateral toes (344).

During the past decade, 448 hemangiomas have been seen at Podiatric Pathology Laboratories. The female to male incidence ratio is 2.3:1, and the average patient age is 46 years, (range, 0 to 89 years). Pedal hemangiomas are mentioned in the literature (244).

Papillary endothelial hyperplasia (Masson's pseudoangiosarcoma) is an intravascular endothelial proliferation associated with a thrombus and usually follows trauma. It is not common, but it has been reported distally in the extremities (65, 240, 241). It must be very carefully differentiated from angiosarcoma and may represent an attempt at recanalization that went awry. *Telangiectasias* may occur in the feet, and the authors have seen a case of *nevus araneus (spider nevus,*

spider angioma) in the Podiatric Pathology Laboratory records. This isolated case may reflect not low incidence but rather recognition of the ectasia, and removal may not be necessary. In the foot, these nevi may arise spontaneously (65).

There is an endothelial tumor group considered by some to be of intermediate malignancy (240), called *hemangioendothelioma*. The one most apt to occur in the extremities is the very rare *spindle cell hemangioendothelioma*, which may occur at any age but is most frequent in young adult males. It has features reminiscent of cavernous hemangioma and Kaposi's sarcoma (240). The authors know of one experience with this lesion in the foot (345), mistaken for lipoma. Some clinicians may have considered this lesion an angiosarcoma; thus true incidence is unclear. *Proliferating angioendotheliomatosis* of the skin has also been described in a rapidly progressive, fatal, *neoplastic* form (*angiotropic lymphoma*) (240) and a benign *reactive* form (65). These forms cannot be distinguished histologically (65). The reactive form has been responsible for gangrene in the lower extremities (346). Whether all these entities are related is unclear.

Malignant Endothelial Tumors

The extremely rare and highly malignant endothelial tumors are *angiosarcomas*. They may arise in deep soft tissues (240, 241) or in skin and subcutaneous tissues (65). The designations lymphangiosarcoma and hemangiosarcoma relate to antecedent chronic edema (240), implicating conditions such as *Milroy's disease* (240). Angiosarcoma has arisen in long-term pedal edema secondary to filarial infestation (347) and in venous ulcers (348), as well as without these precursors (299). Of 17 cases of primary hemangiosarcoma illustrated by Hajdu by area of occurrence, five (29%) are shown in the foot/ankle region (241). These may be rapidly growing, metastatic neoplasms. Irradiation has not been very effective for angiosarcomas. Some success has been claimed for treatment of superficial lesions with a carbon dioxide laser (241). For angiosarcoma, the foot is best amputated and consultations promptly undertaken with appropriate specialists for systemic observation and care. Less-differentiated angiosarcomas require immunocytochemistry and electron microscopy examination to show endothelial cell features.

Kaposi's sarcoma (multiple idiopathic hemorrhagic sarcoma) is related to immunodeficiency. It is known to occur in patients receiving organ transplantation who are taking immunosuppressive medications (349, 350), in association with other immunosuppression diseases such as leukemia and lymphoma (351, 352), and in patients with acquired immunodeficiency syndrome (AIDS) (353). Cases in older males of eastern European and Mediterranean lineage are not as rapidly fatal (352). However, age alone is not a decisive factor in determining whether Kaposi's sarcoma is AIDS-related, inasmuch as older men may develop it after contact with infection sources (blood transfusions, homosexual partners), and some cases apparently occur spontaneously in young men who are neither homosexual nor users of intravenous drugs (354). The African form of Kaposi's sarcoma primarily affects central African males (355). Adult males may develop the condition in middle age, with skin and visceral involvement (355). The African form in children may be primarily cutaneous without rapid progression, or it may affect lymph nodes and be rapidly fatal (356).

Lesions in the non-African and non-AIDS type affecting older European men often begin in the feet as reddish to violaceous macules that may later become plaques and nodules. Because of hemosiderin deposits, lesions may assume a brownish hue. Lesions are autochthonous, not metastatic (65), and may spontaneously regress. Rarely, patients may die of hemorrhage from intestinal or pulmonary lesions (351) (Fig. 46.29). The AIDS-associated type rarely begins in the feet, but occurs there among many other sites. Biopsy will confirm the diagnosis. If AIDS is present or suspected, the patient requires consultation with an internist and testing for human immunodeficiency virus (HIV). Even a nonreactive test result may not rule out AIDS if the titer is not yet high enough to be detected by available methods; thus the test should be repeated. In this group, death may occur within 2 years of diagnosis of Kaposi's sarcoma and sooner if there is concurrent opportunistic infection. Treatment of Kaposi's sarcoma in all groups involves radiation and chemotherapy, not surgery (240), except for biopsy. In patients with AIDS, use of interferons has been of limited success in the treatment of Kaposi's sarcoma.

Without biopsy some lesions can be confused clinically with Kaposi's sarcoma, including disseminated hemangiomatosis (357), pigmented purpuric lichenoid dermatitis of Gougerot-Blum (358), acroangiodermatitis (359), arteriovenous malformation (including the rare Bluefarb-Stewart syndrome) (360, 361), and other vasculitides.

Tumors of Uncertain Histogenetic Origin

There are a few tumors in the pedal region whose origin is unclear. Even with use of special stains and electron microscopy, no particular feature identifies the cell. These tumors may be benign or malignant. *Granular cell tumor (Abrikossoff's tumor)* is uncommon and was originally thought to arise from muscle (362); thus it was called a myoblastoma. Research strongly suggests that benign and malignant forms are related to the peripheral nerve sheath tumors (363, 364). These lesions have been reported in the foot and toes (365) and may occur as single or multiple lesions affecting an area or many organs (65). In some cases histological findings do not predict biological behavior of the lesion, so that a large, fast-growing, infiltrative tumor may be potentially malignant clinically rather than histologically (365). Recurrence also suggests malignancy (241). Malignant forms are metastatic. At Podiatric Pathology Laboratories, 16 benign granular cell tumors have been seen during 11 years, predominantly in female patients, who had 11 (69%) of the lesions. There was no particular predilection for a side. Average age was 40 years (range, 9 to 61 years).

Alveolar soft part sarcoma is a very rare malignant and metastatic tumor that has been reported as occurring most frequently in the right lower extremity of women in the 20 to 40 year age-group. A few ankle region cases have been reported (366). Metastases may show up years after the primary lesion has been removed (366). Irradiation and chemotherapy have not been very successful in treating this tumor, and statements of success with these therapies are tempered with an understanding that it grows slowly (240). This may give the impression that therapy has been successful until metastases show up years later (240, 366). Although histogenesis of this lesion remains unclear, recent immunocytochemical studies suggest that alveolar soft part

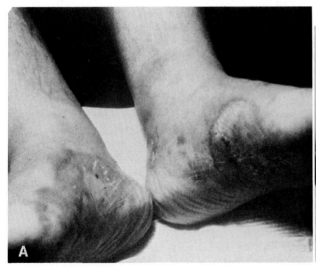
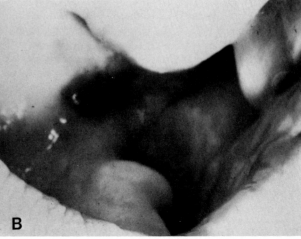

Figure 46.29. **A.** Non-AIDS Kaposi's sarcoma in a 72-year-old man. Lesions were symmetrical, well demarcated, purpuric patches. **B.** Oral nodular lesion on the upper palate of the same patient. He had a long history of gout and subsequently died of renal failure.

sarcoma may be related to muscle (367) rather than to tissues such as paragangliomas.

A single benign *mesenchymoma* was reported by Podiatric Pathology Laboratories over an 11-year span, as having occurred in the right foot of a 59-year-old woman. The definition of this tumor (benign or malignant) suggests that two or more distinctly different mesodermal elements can be identified microscopically but does not accept as one of those elements any clearly fibroblastic element or any metaplastic tissue. These are identified in earlier sections as synovial chondromatosis, myositis ossificans, plantar aponeurotic fibromatosis of Keasbey, proliferative myositis, and similar lesions.

Occasionally a diagnosis of *undifferentiated malignant tumor* may be rendered if no other distinguishing characteristics are found with special stains or electron microscopy examination. The term "tumor" is used advisedly in this context because sarcoma-like cells could represent a highly anaplastic carcinoma. This circumstance should prompt immediate consultation and search for a primary lesion elsewhere as part of patient care.

Malignant Tumors Derived From Lymph Nodes and Bone Marrow

During the course of the leukemias, lymphomas, and plasmacytomas, dermal or subcutaneous deposits of malignant cells may be found, forming nodules or plaques. In *acute myeloid leukemia*, younger patients may develop nonulcerating greenish lesions (65).

Color is due to myeloperoxidase within the granulocytes. Thus the lesion used to be called a *chloroma*. However, the color is not a uniform feature; thus the term *granulocytic sarcoma* is used. These are rare as skin lesions and may precede evidence of leukemia in the peripheral circulation (368). The *acute monocytic* and *myelomonocytic* leukemias may show similar lesions. Lesions associated with *erythroleukemia (di Guglielmo's disease)* tend to be purpuric and to ulcerate (65).

Pedal lesions associated with *multiple myeloma* (multiple lesions) or *plasmacytoma* (single lesion) are very rarely seen. Amyloidosis may occur in the myelomas.

The *non-Hodgkin's lymphomas* are far more apt to involve the skin with small intradermal or subcutaneous malignant cell nodules than does *Hodgkin's disease*, in which nodules may be present long before systemic manifestations. In the non-Hodgkin's group, the infrequent skin involvement is more apt to occur early in the disease. One case of malignant lymphoma has been reported by Podiatric Pathology Laboratories over an 11-year period, in the foot of a 67-year-old woman. Another reported case (369) involved glomus tumor-like tender, reddish-blue lesions on various toes of a 62-year-old woman, in whom an occult gastrointestinal *immunocytoma* was found, and in yet another patient, a primary lymphoma arose in ankle soft tissues (370). The other lesions have not yet been seen at Podiatric Pathology Laboratories, but the senior author has seen pedal granulocytic sarcoma.

Mycosis fungoides is a T-cell lymphoma of skin that may demonstrate a few lesions, an epidermotropic lesion that shows a predilection for lower extremities (*Woringer-Kolopp disease* [371, 372], formerly called *pagetoid reticulosis*), and a systemic form (*Sézary syndrome* [373]) that also includes abnormal circulating T-cells (*Sézary cells*), intense pruritus with erythroderma, and peripheral lymphadenopathy. In one study, skin symptoms, along with palmar and/or plantar keratoderma, preceded lymph node or skin biopsy evidence of mycosis fungoides for up to 23 years (374). More men than women were affected, by a ratio of almost 7:1374. The circulating Sézary cell is the same as the *mucosis cell* seen in the skin lesions in association with the intraepidermal *Pautrier's microabscess*. The lesions of mycosis fungoides appear psoriasiform, some showing atrophic changes. These may proceed to plaque and tumor stages, and systemic lesions may develop (65). There is some dispute relevant to the best approach to treatment (375, 376), and leukophoresis reduces skin infiltration of abnormal cells (377). A unique staging system has been developed for patient evaluation and treatment regimen (378), which also accounts for individual features of a given patient's disease presentation.

Myastocytomas are rare tumors that may localize to dermis or may be systemic. *Urticaria pigmentosa* is a localized form and is occasionally a dominantly inherited autosomal condition (379). It may arise in infancy or early childhood, consisting of brownish maculopapular lesions or nodules and plaques (380). The lesions urticate (*Darier's sign*), and there is little or no systemic involvement. Any systemic lesions tend to resolve by adolescence (380). A single nodular mass may arise in infancy. It too urticates and may form bullae. The erythrodermic (generalized) type begins in infancy with multiple soft, brownish-red skin infiltrates that urticate and may form bullae spontaneously. Bulla formation is due to exudation of fluid from local vessels dilated and made more permeable by histamine from the mast cell granules. There is systemic involvement, which may resolve. On the other hand, death, presumably resulting from histamine shock, is a possible consequence (381, 382) (Fig. 46.30).

Maculara eruptiva perstans is an extensive type arising in adult skin and demonstrating fine telangiectasias but little or no urtication. If any of these forms persist and become systemic, many organs may show mast cell infiltrates (65). Myelofibrosis may occur, with its sequelae of pancytopenia and anemia (383, 384), which may prove fatal. Dermatographism may be present. Since mast cells are usually perivascular, pruritus and flushing may occur as a vasodilatory effect of mast cell histamine and may be stimulated by heat (e.g., baths), spices, cheese, alcoholic beverages, and medications such as morphine, codeine, and aspirin. Rhinorrhea may be present, as well as epistaxis and melena. The latter two may be effects of mast cell heparin. Bone pain may be present. Myelofibrosis is more difficult to explain but may be related to the recent finding that mast cells are producers of a form of tumor necrosis factor (TNF)-alpha (231) that is a potent stimulant for fibrosis. Indeed, mast cells are prominent in keloids, hypertrophic scars, spindle cell lipo-

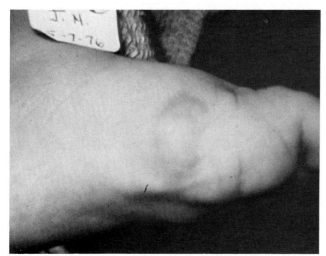

Figure 46.30. Urticaria pigmentosa (solitary mastocytoma) medially over the first metatarsophalangeal joint of a 6-month-old boy. The mother reported that it had begun as a small bump. (From Strauss H, Potter GK: Urticaria pigmentosa: case presentation and discussion. *J Am Podiatry Assoc* 67:802-804, 1977.)

mas, neurofibromas, glomus tumors, and other lesions in which fibrosis occurs.

Progressive forms of mast cell disease carry a poor prognosis, involve many systems, and may cause syncope, hypotension (because of vasodilatory effects of histamine), and tachycardia. The patient may die of vasogenic shock secondary to histamine release. In the systemic form, mast cells may be found in peripheral circulation (384, 385), a condition considered mast cell leukemia.

Two cases of urticaria pigmentosa have been reported by Podiatric Pathology Laboratories over a period of 11 years, both in 21-year-old women. Small lesions can be excised, and the patients should be observed by a physician for systemic lesions or progression to a systemic form of the disease. The senior author and a colleague reported a case in a 6-month-old child (386). Special attention is required for such pediatric patients, because they cannot accurately describe symptoms.

TUMORS AND TUMOROUS CONDITIONS OF BONE

Bone tumors are rare (214, 387), and malignant bone tumors constitute no more than about 2000 to 3000 cases per year throughout the United States (214, 387), about 0.2% in adults, but about 5% in children (214). Diagnosis is a team effort involving attending surgeon, pathologist, and radiologist. Radiological study of the lesion is equivalent to preoperative examination of a specimen in its own specific context (388). Accurate diagnosis is enhanced with consultation among these three specialists to determine the best biopsy site and technique (388). Computerized tomography (CT) scans and MRI help to delineate tumors, whereas radionuclide uptake procedures help to localize occult metastatic or synchronous tumor sites. Angiography studies are some-

times helpful. Some clinicians (214) propose that many bone tumors are identical to soft tissue lesions, but because of association with bone, they have different names. If a tumor affects bone and adjacent soft tissue, it may be difficult to determine if tumor origin was intraosseous or extraosseous.

Lesions Originating from Bone-Forming Cells

Osteoma (hyperostosis, periosteal osteoma) is a benign, expansile, nonneoplastic reactive lesion that may be pedunculated. It generally arises from intramembranous bones and may be related to trauma. Pedal forms may represent old osteochondroma (389) whose cartilaginous cap ossified or wore away. The type may be "ivory" (compact), "spongy" (trabecular) or "mixed", and usually is subungual. Symptoms and signs may include nail deformity and pain while the patient wears shoes. Ulceration of overlying skin is rare. Excision is curative. *Multiple osteomas* may occur in *Gardner's syndrome*. Over an 11-year period, Podiatric Pathology Laboratories has seen 17 such lesions, 11 of which (65%) occurred in women. The average patient age was 40.5 years (range, 9 to 87 years). *Enostoses*, benign intramedullary bone islands reminiscent of osteoid osteomas or osteoblastic metastatic carcinomas, are uncommon as single lesions. They are incidental findings. *Multiple enostoses* affect feet and may occur with *multiple enchondromatosis* and with keloid formation (390).

Osteoid osteoma (391) is a benign osteoblastic lesion with a soft tissue core (*nidus*), usually not exceeding 2 cm in diameter. It occurs in medullary or cortical bone, most frequently in males between 10 and 25 years of age. Joints may be eroded by adjacent lesions (392, 393), or growth abnormalities may occur if an epiphyseal plate is involved (390). Symptoms occur in most cases, beginning as intermittent, vague, nocturnal pain that becomes constant, boring pain. Salicylates relieve pain in many cases, which suggest influence by prostaglandins. Radiographs usually reveal a lucent nidus surrounded by a sclerotic rim. With extensive sclerosis, a nidus may not be visible, thus requiring MRI, angiography, or CT scan. Patients may limp, show muscle atrophy, and demonstrate local vasomotor defects. Slight swelling may be present over the lesion. Excision of the nidus with surrounding bone is usually curative (394). One may choose to obtain x-ray films of the excised specimen to ascertain the presence of the nidus, in hopes of avoiding recurrence (382). About 8% of osteoid osteomas occur in the feet (389). They can affect any pedal bone (394-401).

Osteoblastoma (osteogenic fibroma, spindle cell variant of giant cell tumor, giant osteoid osteoma) a benign, rapidly growing tumor that most often affects males in the 10 to 20 year age range. Local swelling and tenderness may also be present. The intermittent pain is not relieved by salicylates. Lesions are usually diaphyseal or metaphyseal and may sometimes resemble osteoid osteoma radiographically, lacking the sclerotic rim and tending to be larger. X-ray films generally reveal a lesion that, except for size, might be taken for osteoid osteoma. CT scans (402) and MRI are also helpful. On X-ray analysis the differential diagnosis between osteoid osteoma and osteoblastoma is based mainly on the size of the lesion (<2 cm vs. >2 cm, respectively) (389, 390, 400). Neither lesion may show "typical" symptoms (396). Treatment involves curettage and packing of the defect (if large, as in the tarsus). Recurrences are uncommon if surgery is assiduous. Pedal lesions constitute 5% to 10% of osteoblastomas (389, 390). Malignant change in these lesions is an unresolved question (389, 390).

Two osteoid osteomas were seen at Podiatric Pathology Laboratories over the past decade, one each in a 31-year-old man and a woman of the same age. The experience with osteoblastoma is similar, but the ages were 23 and 32, respectively. Because both types of lesion generally are resected in hospitals, the above Laboratory would not receive a quantity expressing the true incidence.

Osteogenic sarcoma (osteosarcoma) is the most common primary malignant bone tumor (second only to multiple myeloma). Its stroma produces osteoid or bone (389, 390). Primary lesions are usually solitary, but multiple synchronous or metachronous lesions may occur. Most cases occur in teenagers during the rapid growth spurt, with a male to female ratio of about 2:1 (389, 390). More cases seem to occur in urban than in rural areas (403) and in tall persons who also demonstrate high blood somatomedin levels (404). In various studies, about 2% of primary osteogenic sarcomas are pedal (389, 390), and only one toe case is documented (405). Lesion location affects prognosis; that is, tumors closer to bone surfaces have better prognoses than more central lesions (406) and may be more differentiated (407). Also, the osteogenic sarcoma type seems related to the response to irradiation and chemotherapy (408). Viral particles have been seen in some cases (409, 410), and reverse transcriptase was characterized in another (411-413). Electron microscopy has confirmed the osteoblast as the abnormal cell (414). Tumor size, location, and growth rate affect symptoms (pain and swelling) and signs (tenderness, edema, palpable mass). Athletic, teen-aged patients may be seen after local trauma. Radiographs reveal the lesion (and occasionally, pathological fracture), the degree of sclerosis varying with the type. *Codman's triangle* represents a cuff of subperiosteal new bone at the boundaries of any lesion that rapidly elevates periosteum (389, 390). It appears in radiographs of a few conditions and is not pathognomonic for osteogenic sarcoma. Chemotherapy and/or irradiation may be administered before surgery to debulk the tumor. For foot lesions, amputation is indicated. Careful search for metastases and long-term follow-up are required, including additional chemotherapy. Orthoses or prostheses and observation for local recurrences are necessary. Metastases are now treated aggressively with surgery and other means to prolong the patient's life and function (389).

Secondary osteogenic sarcomas arise, after the age of 40 years, from preexisting conditions (389, 390, 415). In osteogenic sarcomas, serum alkaline phosphatase levels are elevated, returning to normal after tumor excision. A later rise heralds recurrence and/or late (occult) metastases.

Lesions Arising from Cartilage-Forming Cells

Osteochondromas (osteocartilaginous exostoses) are the most common benign bone tumors. Various types occur (Fig. 46.31). The classical type arises from a growth plate in a long bone, forming a bony stalk facing away from the nearest joint. The cap may be smooth or bosselated and is hyaline cartilage in those that are not subungual. The lesion is more common in males than in females, and about 75% develop before age 30 years (390). There may be single lesions or *multiple cartilaginous exostoses (hereditary multiple exostosis, hereditary deforming dyschondroplasia, diaphyseal aclasis)* inherited as an autosomal dominant condition from a parent who actually manifests the condition. This type is very rare in the feet but may affect the long bones of the leg. *Subungual osteochondroma (subungual exostosis, Dupuytren's exostosis)* is common in the feet and occurs most frequently in the hallux after trauma (416). It also differs from the classical type by having a fibrocartilaginous cap. These may arise at any age and may deform overlying nail, with ensuing discomfort in shoes. They may also be the result of acute and chronic onychias and ulcerations. Excision is curative, but the subcutaneous fibrous tissue is considered perichondrial tissue; to prevent recurrence in the absence of a clear cleavage plane, the overlying nail bed should be excised also (416). Whether these are as susceptible to transformation to chondrosarcoma as are classical multiple and single types is not clear. About 3% to 5% of osteochondromas are pedal (389, 390).

Chondromas are benign cartilage anomalies, some of which may transform to sarcomas. *Solitary (central) enchondromas* are intramedullary, arising from embryonic rests derived from epiphyseal cartilage. They appear lucent on radiographs. Pain occurs after injury, but with no history of trauma, transformation to sarcoma is suspected (Fig. 46.32). Histologically, benign distal lesions may resemble chondrosarcoma, so that location and x-ray appearance are vital for the pathologist to know (388). About 3% to 7% are pedal lesions (389, 390). They are treated by curettage and cryosurgery (389), with or without bone grafts, depending on lesion size, bone involved, and cortical integrity. If chondrosarcoma is suspected, biopsy is indicated prior to definitive surgery.

Multiple enchondromatosis (Ollier's disease) is a cartilage dysplasia of endochondral bone development that can be quite deforming, can affect the feet, and carries a significant risk for transformation to chondrosarcoma (389, 390) (Fig. 46.33). *Metachondromatosis* (417) is a dominantly inherited mimic of Ollier's disease, but the lesions spontaneously regress (390), although surgery is necessary at times (418). Multiple enchondromas also occur in Maffucci's (Kast-Maffucci) syndrome (angiochondromatosis) and may affect pedal bones. Bone lesions, hemangiomas, and vascular hamartomas may not be in the same areas. Risk is high for malignant transformation of the bone lesions. Vitiligo and pigmented nevi may be present in patients with this syndrome (390).

The rare *periosteal (juxtacortical, eccentric) chondromas*, also

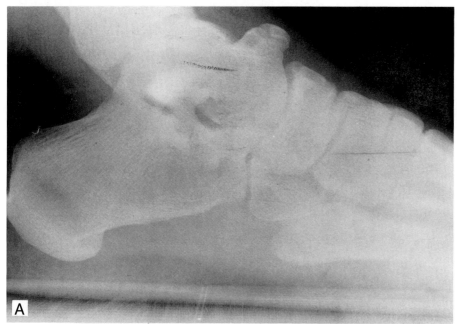

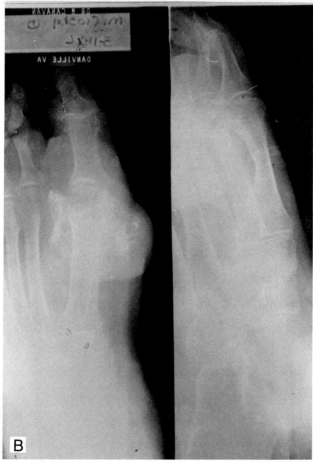

Figure 46.31. **A.** Osteochondroma of the talus. Cartilage cap overlies the visible osseous deformity and, in rare instances, may undergo malignant change. Some osteochondromas involving the talus may suggest subtalar joint coalition. **B.** Large osteochondroma of first metatarsal head and neck. Large size was of great concern. (Courtesy of M. Canavan.)

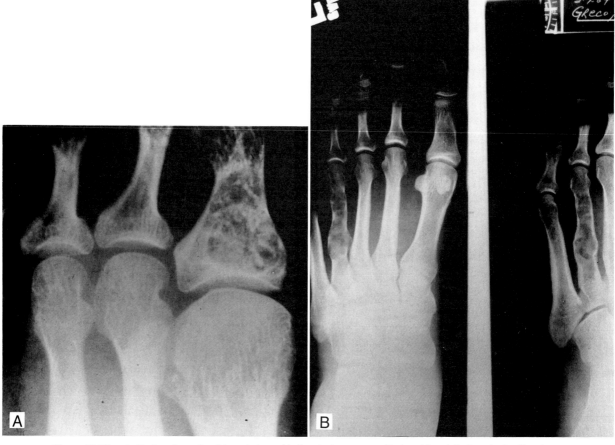

Figure 46.32. **A.** Enchondroma involving phalanx of hallux. Lesion was curetted and the defect packed with autogenous cancellous bone from the iliac crest. **B.** Extensive enchondroma, fourth metatarsal.

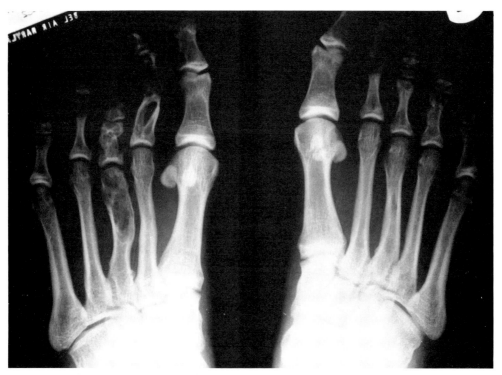

Figure 46.33. Ollier's disease (multiple enchondromatosis) involving many bones of the feet, as well as other bones. There is a high risk of malignant change, and Ollier's disease should be carefully differentiated from metachondromatosis.

called *ecchondromas*, occur subperiosteally on bone surfaces. The most common sites are hands and feet (389, 390), with about 12% as pedal lesions. Excision with a small rim of normal bone prevents recurrence. Lesion size determines need for en bloc resection or grafting. Most develop before the age of 30 years. Radiographs show sharply circumscribed lesions (388).

Chondroblastoma is a benign immature cartilage lesion that favors epiphyseal sites but may extend to metaphyses (388-390, 419). About twice as many males as females are affected, mostly in the 10 to 20 year age-group. Between 9% (389, 390) and 20.2% (419) are pedal. In a study of 499 chondroblastomas (419) 92 (18.4%) were tarsal (calcaneal or talar) and 9 (1.8%) were metatarsal. Predilection for the calcaneus and talus is noted by others (420). Secondary changes resembling aneurysmal bone cyst may occur in pedal lesions (419), and what is described as "vascular invasion" was seen in some lesions affecting flat bones (418), which may account for "pseudometastases" of some (261, 408, 421). In other cases, surgical manipulation and seeding into local blood vessels may carry cells to the lungs (389, 390). The bone lesions cause pain and sometimes effusion and swelling. X-ray examination reveals a cystic lesion in a thin shell, with fine trabeculations ("chicken-wire" calcifications). MRI helps to differentiate chondroblastoma from clear cell chondrosarcoma (388, 422). Curettage with or without cryosurgery may be curative, and the defect is packed with bone chips (388, 390). Most recurrences were observed when an aneurysmal bone cyst (or possibly an engrafted arteriovenous malformation) (390) was a concurrence, so that cryosurgery (390, 423) may provide a viable answer. Chondroblastoma is radiosensitive, but irradiation-induced sarcoma is a risk (389).

Chondromyxoid fibroma is rare and shows a predilection for lower extremities. In three independent series, about 20% occurred in pedal bones (389, 390, 424). Most develop between the ages of 10 and 20 years. In one survey (424) lesions developing between 30 and 40 years of age occurred more frequently in the foot than elsewhere. Most patients have bone pain and possibly swelling and tenderness. On x-ray film, these lesions are lucent, with well-defined sclerotic borders. Some may appear lobulated or bubbly. Foot lesions may expand the bony cortex and appear eccentric (422). Intralesional calcification is not a frequent radiographical finding but may appear histologically. Although malignant transformation of this lesion is questioned, some aggressive foot lesions (389, 425) have necessitated amputations. Lesions are best treated by en bloc resection, because curettage carries risk of recurrence. Excision of a hallux lesion, with no recurrence, has been reported (418) (Fig. 46.34). Nonpedal cases treated with irradiation have eventuated locally in malignant tumors, so that this mode of treatment is not recommended (389).

Chondrosarcoma is a malignant cartilage tumor with metastatic potential. It may show myxoid and osseous elements (Fig. 46.35). It ranks third, after multiple myeloma and osteogenic sarcoma in frequency, and is seen most often in the 40 to 60 year age-group, with a slight majority of cases

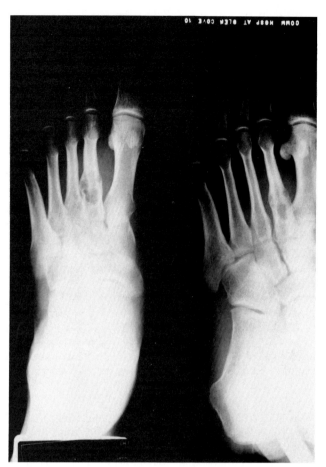

Figure 46.34. Chrondromyxoid fibroma of second metatarsal base. Lesion caused weight-bearing discomfort and was excised, followed by bone grafting. X-ray findings did not exclude other possibilities. Histological examination established diagnosis

in males (389, 390, 408) (male to female ratio, about 1.5:1). Approximately 1% to 3% occur in the feet (389, 390), including *primary* types, as well as *secondary* types that arise in pre-existing lesions. *Mesenchymal* chondrosarcomas are highly malignant, anaplastic, uncommon types that show foci of cartilaginous differentiation. *Clear cell* types have to be differentiated from chondroblastoma. Many patients with chondrosarcoma have abnormal glucose metabolism patterns (389, 426). Patients may limp, relate recent pain, and be aware of a mass. There may be a history of a preexisting lesion. On x-ray film, the tumor may be lucent or show areas of calcification. Cortices may be expanded, and pathological fracture may occur. *Central* lesions may show more calcifications than the *peripheral* or *juxtacortical* types. Angiography studies may be helpful because vascularity seems to correlate with tumor grade (i.e., the more vascular tumors are higher grade and more metastatic). MRI can help to distinguish the types, but CT scans define bone damage and areas of tumor calcification (388). For small, distal foot lesions, partial amputation may be feasible and save limb function. For larger or more proximal pedal le-

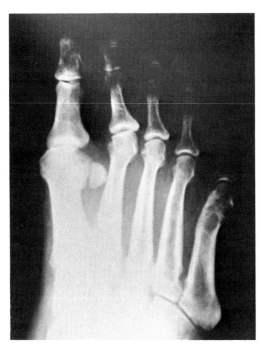

Figure 46.35. Chondrosarcoma of fifth metatarsal. These are not common pedal lesions, and x-ray findings do not reveal diagnostic specifics.

sions, higher amputation is indicated, along with consultations to seek metastases, administer therapy, and observe for recurrences or occult metastases. Whether curettage and cryosurgery might be applicable for low-grade pedal lesions is not as clear as for other body areas where it has been applied (427). Myxoid chondrosarcoma was reported in the calcaneus (428)—as was calcaneal chondrosarcoma in a setting of multiple exostoses, dermatomyositis, and mixed connective tissue disease (429)—and low-grade chondrosarcoma occurred in the second toe of a patient with multiple enchondromatosis (430).

At Podiatric Pathology Laboratories, 66 enchondromas (42 in women, 24 in men) have been seen in the past decade. A few more occurred in the left foot than in the right foot, and four cases involved more than one foot. The average age of patients was 43 years (range, 7 to 83 years). Two biopsy samples of chondrosarcoma were seen during that same period, both from males (aged 58 and 59 years) and each from a left foot.

Bone Lesions of Fibroblastic Cell or Histiocytic Cell Origin

Desmoplastic fibroma (endosteal fibroma) is a rare tumor. Both sexes are about equally affected at any age but most often between 10 and 20 years of age. It is a slow-growing, aggressive benign, intraosseous fibrous growth that on x-ray films may show indistinct borders, suggesting malignancy. Because the lesion is insidious, symptoms may consist mainly of pain and may not appear until the lesion is large. Pathological fracture may occur, and effusion can develop if the

lesion affects a joint. About 2% to 4% of these are pedal lesions (389, 390), but their overall number is very low; thus there are very few reports in the literature (431, 432). Because of the aggressiveness and recurrence of the condition, en bloc resection with bone grafting may be the best approach. Curettage may be effective in some cases. Recurrence suggests more radical surgery and perhaps partial amputation (432). *Periosteal desmoids* are related benign but aggressive lesions that have to be distinguished from the less aggressive but more infiltrative *parosteal fasciitis*.

Fibrous dysplasia of bone, which may be *monostotic* or *polyostotic*, is a nonfamilial hamartomatous fibro-osseous developmental defect that may manifest at any age. Both forms may involve the feet (about 3% of the monostotic form and up to 65% of the polyostic form) (390). Symptoms depend upon bones involved and extent of involvement. Pain and swelling may accompany pathological fracture, but no systemic manifestations are evident. In the polyostotic form, *McCune-Albright syndrome* may be present with its varied concomitants, including *myxomas* (390). The polyostotic form favors one side of the body more than another. On x-ray film, the slow-growing lesions may demonstrate lucency within a sclerotic rim, medullary cavity expansion with bone deformation, pathological fractures with signs of repair, and a ground-glass appearance if more osseous than fibrous. En bloc excision or curettage may be curative in monostotic forms. In addition to consultations, polyostotic forms require intense efforts to prevent fractures and deformity by combined surgical and nonsurgical care. In a few cases, these otherwise nontumorous lesions were reported to give rise to osteogenic sarcoma, fibrosarcoma, or chondrosarcoma, especially when the condition is polyostotic (390). A case of the monostotic type in the first metatarsal has been reported (433).

Nonossifying fibroma is a benign process that is most frequently seen between the ages of 10 and 20 years in the metaphyseal area of long bones, from which it continues to grow and become symptomatic (e.g., pathological fractures with associated pain, swelling, and disability) or undergoes repair spontaneously or perhaps after a minor injury. It is an active and proliferating form of the *fibrous cortical defect* of infants and young children (389, 390) that was not obliterated during growth. (This lesion has also been termed *metaphyseal fibrous defect*). Some consider it to be a fibrous histiocytic lesion. Symptoms depend on lesion size and whether pathological fracture occurs. Radiographs reveal lucent, eccentric lesions that may be loculated, with a sclerotic rim (390, 408) that may rarely extend along the bone shaft (389). The authors are not aware of actual foot lesions, but nonossifying fibroma has been noted in the lower tibia. If surgery is indicated, lesions may be curetted and the defect packed with bone chips. Fibrous cortical defects may be associated with tibial and femoral *osteochondritides* (434). A familial tendency has also been suggested (408). Podiatric Pathology Laboratories reported 16 nonossifying fibromas during 11 years, nine of which (56%) occurred in women. There was no apparent left/right preference. The average age of patients was 22 years (range, 9 to 39 years). One case involved lesions in both feet. (The *ossifying fibroma* is virtually always a jaw lesion [389], and the authors know of no foot cases.)

Fibrosarcoma of bone is a rare, collagen-producing, malignant, and metastatic neoplasm that some consider to be a variant of other tumors rather than an independent entity. It may arise as a *primary* or *secondary* lesion in *periosteal* or in *medullary* forms. Most that are below the knee are medullary (389), and about 2% are pedal (389, 390). Males and females are equally affected. Most cases occur between 10 and 30 years of age, but another peak occurs around the fourth decade, which may represent the secondary type (389, 390). X-ray films reveal a lucent, poorly bordered lesion. Use of MRI also is helpful. Pathologicsl fracture and pain may be present, as well as tenderness and a palpable mass, the latter more frequently with the periosteal type, which also may not be as painful as a medullary mass (389). Frozen-section biopsy may aid diagnosis, and partial amputation is indicated as a minimal procedure. Foot amputation may be indicated for large or anaplastic lesions. Consultations should occur to seek metastases and to effect follow-up.

Malignant fibrous histiocytoma of bone is extremely rare, with only one reference to a pedal (talar) lesion (389), described as well-visualized with angiography. Technetium-99 polyphosphate total body scan will reveal tumor extent, and angiography studies can aid in defining extraosseous tumor (389). Use of MRI may also be helpful. X-ray films will reveal a nonspecific lytic lesion. Pain may be present because of an intraosseous expansile lesion or a pathological fracture. These neoplasms have been associated with bone infarcts (idiopathic or in context with caisson workers), hereditary bone dysplasia, or sickle cell anemia (389, 390) so that a careful history and laboratory work-up are indicated. Foot lesions require amputation. In contrast to osteogenic sarcoma, these tumors rarely occur in children or adolescents (408). If necessary, chemotherapy and irradiation are used reoperatively to reduce tumor size and to supplement postoperative care.

Giant cell tumor of bone constitutes about 5% of bone tumors. About 3% are pedal (389, 390), and metatarsal location is a rarity (434). It is an epiphyseal lesion but may be metaphyseal. It is an aggressive lesion and is one of those considered to be pseudometastatic (259, 260, 389, 435, 436). This may be due to seeding during lesion curettage (389), or it may occur spontaneously (436), with excisable lesions of limited growth potential appearing in the lungs. Most giant cell tumors of bone occur between 20 and 40 years of age, in a male to female ratio of 3:2. Giant cell tumor of bone has been reported in context with other conditions and syndromes (437-440) (Fig. 46.36). Swelling may be present with a history of intermittent pain. Motion may be limited, especially if the lesion is adjacent to or has penetrated a joint. Acute pain and tenderness may represent pathologic fracture. Radiographs, MRI, and angiograms reveal an eccentric, small lucent lesion in mature bone. If the lesion is large, eccentricity in the small pedal bones cannot be determined. In the absence of pathological fracture an expanded bone may show a thin, perilesional sclerotic shell,

whereas with fracture the picture can suggest a malignant and invasive tumor. With a concurrent *aneurysmal bone cyst*, the lesion may appear loculated ("bubbly") on x-ray film (Fig. 46.37). If giant cell tumor of bone is suspected, an open biopsy and frozen section seem the best approach to avoid seeding the lesion in local tissue planes.

Recurrence rates are high if an aneurysmal bone cyst also is present and if curettage alone is used (389, 390, 423, 435. For metatarsal lesions, en bloc resection and bone grafting, or partial amputation if the lesion has crossed a joint and entered soft tissue, can be curative (436). In larger tarsal bones, curettage, followed by filling the defect with acrylic cement (435), postcurettage phenolization (436), or postcurettage cryosurgery (389, 390, 423, 436), after which the defect is packed with bone chips and/or struts, helps to reduce the recurrence rate. Irradiation is a contraindicated treatment for giant cell tumors because of high recurrence rates and transformation to radiation-induced fibrosarcomas or osteogenic sarcomas about 5 years after a dose exceeding 4000 rad (389, 390, 435, 436). To minimize local seeding or iatrogenic pseudometastasis, these tumors should be manipulated minimally and resected in one piece. Sometimes recurrences have appeared as higher-grade lesions than the original (including fully malignant forms), in which case more radical surgery is needed. Careful follow-up of the patients is necessary to ensure proper healing of defects and to observe for recurrence, pseudometastasis, or a missed soft tissue component, and it must include postoperative radiographs. Unfortunately, there is a very extensive list of benign and malignant lesions that demonstrate giant cells, so that careful clinical, radiological, and histopathological evaluation of the lesion is necessary in diagnosis. Because of its unpredictability, some consider the histologically benign giant cell tumor of bone to be a low-grade malignant lesion (390).

Giant cell reaction of bone (giant cell reparative granuloma) is an extremely rare lesion that shows a predilection for hands and feet (390, 408) and is similar to giant cell reparative granuloma of jawbones (389). It has been seen in the small bones of the foot (at all ages) and in the calcaneus, and it may be unicentric or multicentric (441-445). It is cured by curettage and packing (if large) of the intraosseous defect with bone chips. This condition may be a variant of giant cell tumor. As with giant cell tumor, a careful history is required and other giant cell lesions must be ruled out.

At Podiatric Pathology Laboratories, in just over a decade, 16 benign giant cell tumors of bone have been seen. Of these, 10 (63%) were in women, and 9 (57%) occurred in the right foot. The average age of the patients was 39 years (range, 12 to 75 years). In that same decade, three biopsy results showed malignant giant cell tumor, two in men. Average age was 50 years (range, 34 to 60 years).

Intraosseous Myogenic Tumors

Leiomyosarcoma very rarely occurs as a primary intramedullary bone tumor. Only two have been recorded in the foot: one talar (446) and one calcaneal (447). These have been

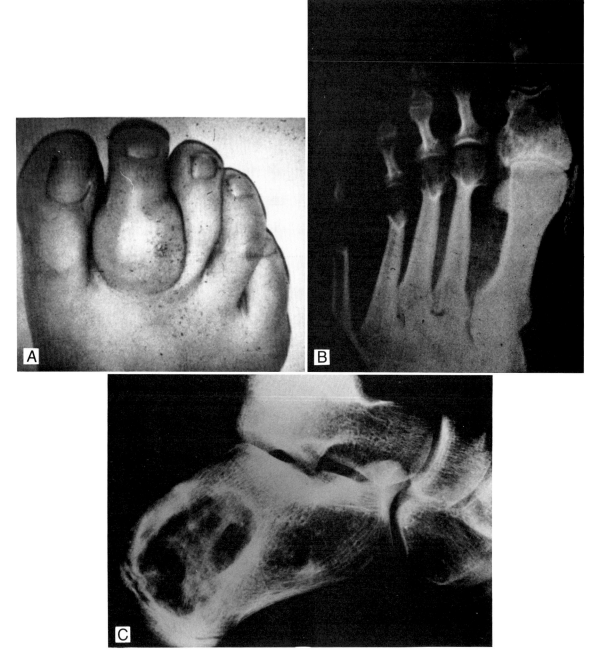

Figure 46.36. **A.** Giant cell tumor of bone in second toe. Some consider digital lesions to represent a reparative process (giant cell reaction of bone) similar to giant cell reparative granuloma of jawbones. **B.** Expansile giant cell tumor of bone in hallux, treated by curettage followed by packing with bone chips. Patients must be carefully observed for recurrences, and more radical surgical approaches may be necessary. **C.** Giant cell tumor in the calcaneus. Diagnosis was made upon excisional biopsy. Giant cell tumors may be quite aggressive and may also have a soft tissue component. A cryosurgical approach may be applicable for some pedal lesions. Giant cell tumors of bone may be associated with other lesions.

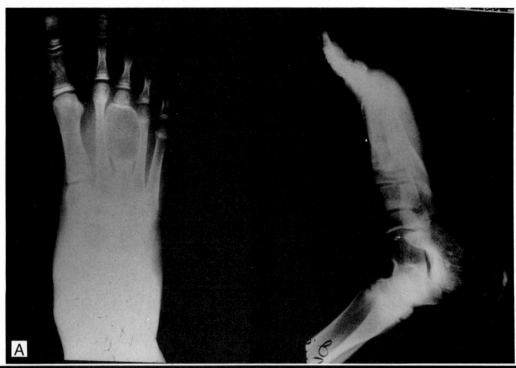

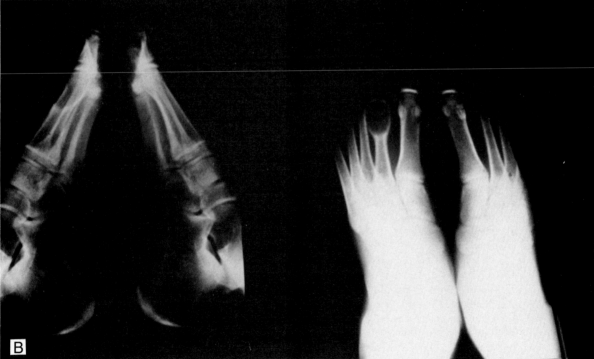

Figure 46.37. **A.** Aneurysmal bone cyst of third metatarsal in a 14-year-old female. Lesion was curetted, followed by packing of the defect with bone chips. **B.** Large, expansile, painful aneurysmal bone cyst in the second metatarsal of a 17-year-old male. Pathological fracture may occur. Other lesions may be associated with these cysts.

lytic, painful bone lesions in older persons. Electron microscopy, immunocytochemistry, and special stains are aids to diagnosis (447, 448). Intraoperative frozen section may establish the presence of a malignant spindle cell tumor, its nature clarified after amputation. Other spindle cell tumors may (rarely) occur as primary intraosseous lesions (448).

Intraosseous Vascular Tumors

Hemangiomas of bone may be solitary (390) or multiple (449). Although possible at any age, most solitary types occur between 40 and 50 years of age, foot cases constituting about 3% (390), with a slight predominance of females. *Multiple hemangiomatosis* occurs almost equally in both sexes, most often in the 10 to 20 year age-group, about 14% of cases affecting feet (390). There may be hemangiomas in other tissues, most frequently in previously mentioned syndromes. The presenting symptom may be pain resulting from an expanding intraosseous lesion or pathological fracture after local trauma. Radiographs may reveal a fusiform bone expansion with a sclerotic shell containing a lytic, loculated lesion. Angiography and MRI findings outline vascular details. Unicentric, small pedal lesions may be excised, curetted, or cauterized, with precautions for extensive intraoperative bleeding.

Disappearing bone disease (Jackson-Gorham syndrome, Gorham's disease, phantom bone disease, massive osteolysis) is a spontaneous condition affecting any bone that has hemangiomas within or adjacent to it (389). After local trauma, affected bone is apparently resorbed. It is usually seen in persons under 40 years of age (389) and shows no apparent sex predilection. Its relationship to vascular tumors in a rare syndrome associated with *hypophosphatemic rickets* (390) is unclear. In the latter syndrome, tumor extirpation relieves the osteomalacia. It is speculated that a vitamin D antagonist may be secreted by the tumors. *Solitary* pedal *lymphangiomas* are not yet reported, but tibial lesions have been seen (450). *Multiple lymphangiomas* may involve the foot, and are most likely to be seen in children. Extremely rare cases of primary *glomus tumor* in bone have been seen in terminal phalanges (389, 390). Because phalanges are so small, phalangectomy seems the choice procedure. The authors are unaware of *hemangiopericytomas* in pedal bones.

Angiosarcoma of bone (*malignant hemangioendothelioma*) is an uncommon, highly malignant tumor that may be a solitary or a multicentric lesion. Both forms are reported in the foot (389, 390, 451). Solitary forms are far more frequent and are usually diagnosed some 10 years later than are multicentric forms (389). Both sexes are about equally affected by solitary forms, but the multicentric forms occur more often in males (389). Angiosarcoma has been reported in context with chronic osteomyelitis (452), and a single lesion may represent metastasis from an occult visceral primary tumor (389). Patients may report dull, aching pain and some tenderness, as well as edema. X-ray films will demonstrate a lytic, trabeculated, or loculated—but otherwise nonspecific lesion (389, 390)—that is better defined by angiography. Foot amputation is the choice procedure, with the usual

consultations for follow-up observation and care. In one study, it was determined that the overall prognosis is better in persons with multicentric lesions than in those with solitary lesions (389). The reasons are unclear.

Adamantinoma (angioblastoma of long bones, primary epidermoid carcinoma of bone, synovial sarcoma of bone) is a highly unusual and rare neoplasm whose histogenesis is unclear. Present evidence suggests that it is a vascular neoplasm (453). Most lesions are tibial. Metatarsal lesions are reported among other sites (389), and foot lesions occur in about 1% of cases (390). Lesions occur at any age but mostly in middle-aged males. Patients usually report dull, aching pain and swelling in the tumor area. X-ray films reveal an extensive, lucent, loculated lesion. Pathological fracture may occur, and the tumor may show a prominent extraosseous component. These tumors are metastatic and aggressive and are best treated by foot amputation. Follow-up is necessary to detect recurrences, metastases, and new lesions in cases in which the neoplasm may be multicentric (389).

Kaposi's sarcoma is not restricted to skin. Whether or not it is associated with AIDS, other tissues and organs, including bones, may bear Kaposi's sarcoma lesions (389).

Aneurysmal bone cyst is considered here because it may be an arteriovenous malformation engrafted on other lesions (454). It tends to grow so quickly that it obliterates the other lesions. In one study, up to 60% of the cysts were associated with other bone lesions (390, 408). Most cases occur without sex predilection in young patients (10 to 20 years of age) (408). Foot bones may be involved in up to 10% of cases. Mild to moderate pain may be reported, especially as the lesion rapidly develops. Sudden pain may represent a pathological fracture. Limp may be present. On x-ray films, a small lytic lesion may be seen early. Later, areas resembling Codman's triangle may appear. At the "blowout" stage (408) the bone may appear expanded with no shell around the lesion. Because it usually stops growing within a few weeks, even older lesions will then develop a surrounding shell of bone, and as a result of fibrous septae and bony spicules, the late lesion may appear loculated ("bubbly"). The radiographs can suggest other lesions. Angiography may help to define the vascular malformation. In a small tubular bone, en bloc resection with bone graft will successfully cure most cases. In the tarsal bones, curettage followed by cryosurgery (389, 390, 423) will minimize recurrences. The cavity can then be packed with bone chips and/or struts. Cryosurgery has advantages as well as risks in the foot (390, 423).

Other Tumors of Bone

Paget's sarcoma is any bone sarcoma arising in the setting of *Paget's disease of bone*. The latter is a polyostotic or monostotic condition that occurs more frequently in men than in women and mostly in the 40 to 60 year age-group. Rare cases in younger and older persons are reported. The etiology is unclear, but reports of viral inclusions in osteoclasts only from Paget's disease of bone have been summarized (390) and a theory proposed (390) implicating these infected cells in abnormal destructive activity. This accounts for the lytic stage, which appears as wedgelike areas, and which stimulates reactive osteoblastic activity. Since new "woven bone" is laid down haphazardly, it is not really strong, so that stress plus continued abnormal osteoclastic activity result in laying down of thick but poorly organized bone, giving the radiographical impression of sclerosis. As this theoretical infection abates and the abnormal process slows, there is much bone deformity. In about 2% to 3% of patients, high turnover and repair may eventuate in malignant transformation, hence Paget's sarcoma. This may manifest as osteogenic sarcoma, fibrosarcoma, or chondrosarcoma (389) and can occur at any stage. In some cases, multiple myeloma has been present with Paget's disease of bone, either alone (455) or even with osteogenic sarcoma (456). Pathological fractures are common (389) and often precede development of sarcoma. Arthralgias may also occur in association with adjacent bony changes (457). Serum alkaline phosphatase levels are very high in active Paget's disease of bone but do not indicate sarcomatous change. Development of pain in an affected bone may truly herald such transformation before it is clinically obvious (389).

Urinary levels of hydroxyproline, like serum alkaline phosphatase, fluctuate with disease activity but are unrelated to malignant change. Almost any foot bone may be affected (458), but the most frequent are the calcaneus and talus (458-463). The prognosis for persons with Paget's sarcoma is not good, probably because the tumors are so vascularized that metastatic potential is high. Patients with Paget's disease of bone should be under constant care because of the presence or the possibility of polyostotic involvement, pathological fractures, and malignant transformation at any affected site.

Ewing's sarcoma is a highly malignant bone tumor that is seen most frequently before the age of 20 years in a male to female ratio of about 3:2. Some quoted studies from Africa and the United States reveal that Ewing's sarcoma is rare in the black population (389). It is the fourth most common bone tumor (390), but its histogenesis is unknown. Symptoms and signs are nonspecific (389) and may fluctuate before actual bone lesions are defined. There may be pain and swelling over the affected bone, but this too may improve for long periods (389). On x-ray films, affected bones may demonstrate nonspecific "onion skinning" and lytic lesions. Pathological fractures occur (Fig. 46.38). All foot bones have been primary tumor sites (464-471). Primary treatment for the foot is amputation, inasmuch as irradiation may impair foot function severely and result in great pain (389). Consultations to seek nonpedal sites, as well as for follow-up care, are indicated. In one study (472), primary Ewing's sarcoma was found to occur six times more frequently in the foot than in the hand. The same study determined that patients whose primary tumor was more distal had a better prognosis than those with more proximal tumors but that response of one histological type (filigree pattern) to therapy was poor at any site (472).

Lymphomas and *leukemias* very rarely arise in the foot as primary sites. The authors are not aware of any cases of *Hodgkin's disease* as a primary pedal tumor. The identifying

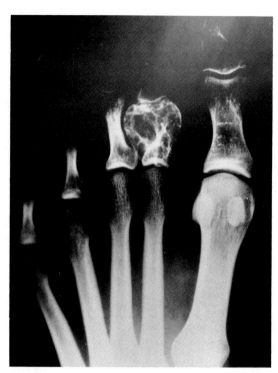

Figure 46.38. Ewing's sarcoma in the second toe. The appearance on radiograph is not specific for Ewing's sarcoma, and the diagnosis has to be made on the combination of other clinical factors and biopsy, along with the x-ray findings.

histological feature for this condition is the *Reed Sternberg* cell. The *myeloid* or *myelomonocytic leukemias* may manifest in the pedal bones as areas of rarefaction and cortical thinning, but this would be a rare occurrence. *Non-Hodgkin's lymphoma* may have a similar occurrence. The authors know of only one case of chronic lymphocytic leukemia in a toe phalanx as a primary site (473). Affected bone may be painful and tender, and unless early in these diseases when symptoms and signs are many but not necessarily specific, the patient may be debilitated, anemic, and otherwise quite ill. Details should be sought elsewhere (389, 390) with the awareness these problems are extremely rare (but possible) in the feet.

Plasma cell dyscrasias can manifest in the bones of the feet as *multiple myeloma* (388) or *solitary plasmacytoma* (474-476). The latter is very infrequent. Multiple myeloma is the most common malignant primary bone tumor (389, 390) involving feet in about 6% of cases. Most cases occur in males, usually between the ages of 40 and 70 years. Pain in one or more bones (worsened by weight bearing) is present, with bone tenderness. A monoclonal gammopathy is seen with serum protein electrophoresis, and *paraproteinemia* occurs. Proteinuria is due partly to renal damage and partly to the characteristic *Bence-Jones protein*. Also, *amyloid* is produced and is associated with development of carpal tunnel syndrome. (Whether tarsal tunnel syndrome has occurred in that context is unknown.) Other blood abnormalities include progressive anemia, erythrocyte aggregation (*rouleaux* formation), cryoglobulinemia, hypercalcemia, reversal of the albumin-globulin ratio, M-proteinemia (light chains), and high sedimentation rate. Skin lesions may include *plane normolipemic xanthoma* (65) and *necrobiotic xanthogranuloma* (65) (Fig. 46.39). Associated diseases include Paget's disease of bone, Gaucher's disease, and Fanconi's syndrome (389). Genetic factors may play a role (389). Bone lesions are lytic, and pathological fractures occur. These patients should be sent to an oncologist after biopsy confirms the diagnosis.

Eosinophilic granuloma (Langerhans' cell granulomatosis, histiocytosis-X, Taratynov's disease) is a very uncommon condition that may occur as a single lesion (*solitary* type) or as multiple lesions (*multifocal* type). Lieberman et al. (477) removed this condition from the realm of Hand-Schüller-Christian disease (a nonspecific triad rather than a true entity) and Letterer-Siwe disease (involving lymphomas with histiocytic cells and with vague infections) (477) and established it as a separate entity. The authors are aware of only one recorded pedal (tarsal) lesion, said to show a "bone within bone" appearance (478). This condition shows a *tempo phenomenon*; that is, osseous lesions may come and go with no treatment. Diagnosis is confirmed by open biopsy, and a defect can be curetted and packed if small. Larger lesions may require en bloc excision and bone grafting. Multiple lesions may require low-dose fractionated irradiation (total 300 to 600 rad). In rare cases, diabetes insipidus develops. This condition is not considered malignant even though multiple lesions may require a chemotherapeutic approach.

MISCELLANEOUS LESIONS

In addition to primary malignant soft tissue tumors in bone, benign lesions may also occur. The authors have seen *intraosseous lipoma* in the calcaneus occurring as a well-defined lytic lesion with calcifications. *Intraosseous epidermal inclusion cyst* is an extension of an overlying inclusion cyst whose growth erodes and invades bone (390). It affects the distal phalanges, may be painful, and can give a clinical and radiological impression of invasive tumor. Sinus tracts from bone may undergo *pseudoepitheliomatous hyperplasia*, as in chronic osteomyelitis. Although this condition is benign, chronic tracts may also develop *squamous cell carcinoma*. *Postirradiation sarcomas*, which may arise in bone after therapeutic or accidental exposure to cumulatively high radiation doses, are secondary sarcomas. Leukemias and some very anaplastic lesions may be among these. *Unicameral bone cysts* are not tumors, but incidental finding of a silent lytic lesion in a young person may prompt a hunt for a cancer. The lesion must be investigated. Pain suggests a fracture of the cyst wall, and a *"fallen fragment" sign* on x-ray film, CT scan, or MRI suggests a chip from an old fracture (Fig. 46.40). These may be *intraosseous synovial cysts* (389) caused by entrapment of synovial tissue into developing bone. Some contain fibro-osseous material and thus have (incorrectly) been called *cementomas*. These infrequent pedal cysts are reported (479-481) mostly in boys under the age of 10 years. Although they have been treated with curettage and packing, or with cryosurgery (a risk in a growing child in terms of epiphyseal damage), some success has been achieved by aspirating the fluid contents (which should be sent for cytological examination) and promptly injecting a glucocorticoid (390). This treatment may have to be repeated.

Hypertrophic pulmonary osteoarthropathy is a misnomer for a condition showing clubbed fingers and toes, periosteal activity with bone deposition in acral long bones, and pain in affected digits (389). Often associated with lung tumors and other lung conditions, it also occurs in some extrapulmonary benign and malignant diseases and conditions. Mechanisms involved in the digital changes are not clear.

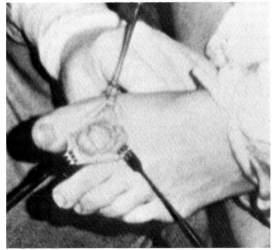

Figure 46.39. Necrobiotic xanthogranuloma in a female patient. These lesions may be associated with multiple myeloma. The patient is being monitored for paraproteinemia and other portents of multiple myeloma. (Courtesy of A. R. Iorio and C. S. Luciano.)

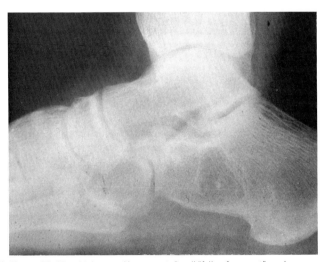

Figure 46.40. Unicameral bone cyst. Small "fallen fragment" can be seen, suggesting an old fracture.

Extraosseous bone tumors

Brief mention should be made that tumors usually considered to be of osseous or cartilaginous origin may occur as primary soft tissue lesions. These lesions are established (after careful evaluation of the patient) not to be metastatic from another occult source. Further, they are not physically related to adjacent bone. These lesions include Ewing's sarcoma (482), chondrosarcoma (483, 484), osteogenic sarcoma (241), osteoma (241), chondroma (241), osteochondroma (241), and metaplastic lesions (chondroid metaplasia, osteoid metaplasia, and myositis ossificans) (240, 241).

Metastatic Visceral Carcinomas to the Foot

Metastases to the foot are extremely rare. Although not all have been reported, a study from 1920 to 1987 revealed no more than 94 such cases reported, of which 22 were contributed by the authors of that study (485), and all of those were to bone. Bone metastases may be favored over those to soft tissue because of rich bone vascularity and sinusoids (486). Development and mechanisms of metastasis have been reviewed (209-211). Circulatory factors are involved, such as Batson's (valveless) paravertebral venous plexus (487), sluggish circulation in the lower extremities (e.g., varicose veins) (485), and links between the lymphatic and arteriovenous systems (209), as well as other cellular and biochemical influences. Mechanical factors proposed by Ewing (488) and the "seed and soil" approach of Paget (489) also are factors.

Very few malignancies metastasize to pedal skin. Metastasis to skin generally is not thought to exceed about 3% (207) and those to the lower extremity no more than about 4% (490). The authors found only five such cases (i.e., choriocarcinoma [207], chondrosarcoma [208], Merkel's cell carcinoma [491], rectal adenocarcinoma [492], and mammary adenocarcinoma [493]). Most of these are asymptomatic, and only recent development of a mass may bring a patient in for investigation. Biopsy will confirm the malignancy of the lesion but may not determine its source without special techniques. Confirmation of such a lesion demands prompt referral for a complete examination to find the primary tumor and to begin treatment. Index of suspicion and biopsy can offer patient comfortable and functional extension of life.

Metastases to bones of the foot are far more common than those to skin and soft tissue. These tend more often to be symptomatic, manifesting most frequently as lytic, painful lesions.

Pathological fractures may occur. Bone biopsy is necessary and serves the same functions as described for skin biopsy. In some cases, partial or full amputation of the foot may be indicated. Consultations should occur with diagnostic and therapeutic radiologists, a pathologist, and an oncologist to determine disease stage and therapeutic options.

Most metastases to bone are lytic; some are sclerotic. In most instances, lytic lesions are associated with carcinomas of lung, kidney, breast, thyroid, and gastrointestinal tract and with neuroblastoma. The blastic (sclerotic) lesions are most frequently associated with carcinomas of prostate, breast, bladder, and stomach. Mixed lytic/blastic lesions have been associated with carcinomas of the breast, lung, prostate, bladder and with neuroblastoma. Determinants of whether lytic, blastic, or mixtures of lesions will occur with any given tumor, are not yet clarified.

Virtually all bones of the foot have been involved by metabases from visceral cancers, but the tarsal bones (especially the calcaneus) are most frequently involved (484). Metastases to foot bones have arisen from carcinomas of the vagina (485), cervix (485, 494), endometrium (485, 495), ovary (485), bladder (485, 496), prostate gland (485, 497, 498), kidney (485, 499-504), colorectal region tissues (485, 505-508), stomach (485), lung (485, 497, 508-513), larynx (485), breast (485, 497, 514, 515), sweat gland (516), and salivary (submaxillary) gland (517). Metastases to pedal bones have also been recorded for rhabdomyosarcoma (485), osteogenic sarcoma (485), multiple myeloma (485), reticulum cell sarcoma (lymphoma) (485), leukemia (485), and malignant tumors whose origin could not be determined (485). Of interest is a lung metastasis to pedal bones (509) and a primary epithelioid sarcoma of the foot (275) that clinically manifested with symptoms and signs suggesting reflex sympathetic dystrophy. This occurrence confirms that presenting symptoms and signs of primary and metastatic tumors in the foot are nonspecific. Therefore, suspicion of a tumor, no matter how uncommon in the foot, is always a consideration. Only a properly planned and performed biopsy can confirm the nature of an otherwise nonspecific lesion that does not respond within a reasonable period to therapy for another feasible diagnostic option, as well as ensuring preparation for further surgical or other intervention if needed. Pedal metastases may appear late during malignant disease (514), may be the presenting sign of occult visceral cancer (499, 515), or may remain occult for years after a primary tumor was excised.

References

1. Berlin SJ: A laboratory review of 67,000 foot tumors and lesions. *J Am Podiatry Assoc* 74:341-347, 1984.
2. Corley E, Pueyo S, Goc B: Papillomavirus in human skin warts and their incidence in an Argentine population. *Diagn Microbiol Infect Dis* 10:93-101,1988.
3. Mroczkowski TF, McEwen C: Warts and other papillomavirus infections. *Postgrad Med* 78:91-98, 1985.
4. Aird I, Johnson HD, Lennox B: Epithelioma cuniculatum. A variety of squamous carcinoma peculiar to the foot. *Br J Surg* 42:245-250, 1954.
5. Obalek S, Glinski W, Haftek M: Comparative studies on cell-mediated immunity in patients with different warts. *Dermatologica* 161:73-83, 1980.
6. Chretien JH, Esswein JG, Garagusi VF: Decreased T cell levels in patients with warts. *Arch Dermatol* 114:213-215, 1978.
7. Ingelfinger JR, Grupe WE, Topor M: Warts in a pediatric renal transplant population. *Dermatologica* 155:7-12, 1977.
8. Prawer SE, Pass F, Vance JC: Depressed immune function in epidermodysplasia verruciformis. *Arch Dermatol* 113:495-499, 1977.
9. Yabe Y, Yasue M, Yoshino N: Viral particles in early malignant lesions. *J Invest Dermatol* 71:225-228, 1978.

10. McCarthy DJ, Montgomery R (eds): *Podiatric Dermatology* Baltimore, Williams & Wilkins, 1986.

11. Bunney MH: The treatment of plantar warts with 5-fluorouracil. *Br J Dermatol* 89:96-97, 1973.

12. Manilla GT, Hood TK, Eakin NR: Treatment of plantar warts. *Rocky Mountain Med J* 63:42, 1965.

13. Bauer DJ: Treatment of plantar warts with acyclovir. *Am J Med* 73:313-314, 1982.

14. Koenig RD, Horowitz LR: Verruca plantaris—effective treatment with bleomycin: review of the literature and case presentations. *J Foot Surg* 21:108-110, 1982.

15. Greenberg JH, Smith TL, Katz RM: Verrucae vulgaris rejection. A preliminary study of contact dermatitis and cellular immune response. *Arch Dermatol* 107:580-582, 1973.

16. Lewis HM: Topical immunotherapy of refractory warts. *Cutis* 12:863-867, 1973.

17. Lambert WC, Lambert MW, Mesa ML: Melanoacanthoma and related disorders: simulants of acral-lentiginous (P-P-S-M) melanoma. *Int J Dermatol* 26:508-510, 1987.

18. Mishima Y, Pinkus H: Benign mixed tumor of melanocytes and malpighian cells. *Arch Dermatol* 81:539-550, 1960.

19. Ronchese F: Keratoses, cancer and the sign of Leser-Trélat. *Cancer* 18:1003-1006, 1965.

20. Liddell K, White JE, Caldwell JW: Seborrheic keratoses and carcinomas of the large bowel. *Br J Dermatol* 92:449-452, 1975.

21. Lambert D, Fort M, Legoux A: Le signe de Leser-Trélat. *Ann Dermatol Venereol* 107:1035-1041, 1980.

22. Ellis DL, Kafka SP, Chow JC: Melanoma, growth factors, acanthosis nigricans, the sign of Leser-Trélat, and multiple acrochordons. A possible role for alpha-transforming growth factor in cutaneous paraneoplastic syndromes. *N Engl J Med* 317:1582-1587, 1987.

23. Kechijian P, Sadick NS, Mariglio J: Cytabarine-induced inflammation in the seborrheic keratoses of Leser-Trelat, *Ann Intern Med* 91:868-869, 1979.

24. Degos R, Civatte J: Clear-cell acanthoma: experience of 8 years. *Br J Dermatol* 83:248-254, 1970.

25. Fine RM, Chernosky ME: Clinical recognition of clear-cell acanthoma (Degos). *Arch Dermatol* 100:559-563, 1969.

26. Wilson Jones E, Wells GC: Degos' acanthoma (acanthome a cellules claires). *Arch Dermatol* 94:286-294, 1966.

27. Cramer HJ: Klarzellenakanthom (Degos) mit syringomatosen und Naevus-sebaceus-artigen Anteilen. *Dermatologica* 143:265-270, 1971.

28. Rulon DB, Helwig EB: Papillary eccrine adenoma. *ArchDermatol* 113:596-598, 1977.

29. Urmacher C, Lieberman PH: Papillary eccrine adenoma. Light-microscopic, histochemical and immunohistochemical studies. *Amer J Dermatopathol* 9:243-249, 1987.

30. Potter GK, Baldinger HG, Boxer MC: Chondroid syringoma in a toe. *Cutis* 30:339-341, 1982.

31. Pinkus H, Rogin JR, Goldman P: Eccrine poroma. *Arch Dermatol* 74:511-521, 1956.

32. Goldner R: Eccrine poromatosis. *Arch Dermatol* 101:606-608, 1970.

33. Bardach H: Hidroacanthoma simplex with in situ porocarcinoma. a case suggesting malignant transformation. *J Cutan Pathol* 5:236-248, 1978.

34. Kwittken J: Muciparous epidermal tumors. *Arch Dermatol* 109:554-555, 1974.

35. Konick L, England DM, Fain J: A, B, and H substances in syringomas. An immunohistochemical analysis of 15 cases. *Am J Clin Pathol* 89:778-783, 1988.

36. Argenyi ZB, Balogh K, Goeken JA: Immunohistochemical characterization of chondroid syringomas. *Am J Clin Pathol* 90:662-669, 1989.

37. Raab W: Talgdrusenepitheliom. *Arch Klin Exp Dermatol* 216:325-333, 1963.

38. Leonforte JF: Palmoplantare Epidermizyste. *Hautarzt* 29:657-658, 1978.

39. Delacretaz J: Keratotic basal-cell carcinoma arising from an epidermoid cyst. *J Dermatol Surg Oncol* 3:310-311, 1977.

40. Shelley WB, Wood MG: Occult Bowen's disease in keratinous cysts. *Br J Dermatol* 105:105-108, 1981.

41. McDonald LW: Carcinomatous change in cysts of skin. *Arch Dermatol* 87:208-211, 1963.

42. Brownstein MH, Arluk DJ: Proliferating trichilemmal cyst. *Cancer* 48:1207-1214, 1981.

43. Leppard BJ, Sanderson KV: The natural history of trichilemmal cysts. *Br J Dermatol* 94:379-390, 1976.

44. Brownstein MH, Wolf M, Bickowsky B: Cowden's disease. A cutaneous marker of breast cancer. *Cancer* 41:2393-2398, 1978.

45. Allen BS, Fitch MH, Smith JG Jr: Multiple hamartoma syndrome. *J Am Acad Dermatol* 2:303-308, 1980.

46. Jablonska S, Orth G, Jarzabek-Chorzelska M: Epidermodysplasia verruciformis versus disseminated verruca planae. *J Invest Dermatol* 72:114-119, 1979.

47. Gibbs RC: Alterations of palms and soles. Indicators of internal disease. *NY State J Med* 65:1220-1225, 1965.

48. Potter GK: Histopathology of clavi. *J Am Podiatry Assoc* 63:57-66, 1973.

49. Howell JB, Freeman RG: Structure and significance of the pits with their tumors in the nevoid basal cell carcinoma syndrome. *J Am Acad Dermatol* 2:224-238, 1980.

50. Totten JR: The multiple nevoid basal cell carcinoma syndrome. Report of its occurrence in four generations of a family. *Cancer* 46:1456-1462, 1980.

51. Sommers SC, McManus RG: Multiple arsenical cancers of skin and internal organs. *Cancer* 6:347-359, 1953.

52. Fierz U: Katamnestische Untersuchungen uber die Nebenwirkungen der Therapie mit anorganischem Arsen bei Hautkrankheiten. *Dermatologica* 131:41-58, 1965.

53. Bart RS, Andrade R, Kopf AW: Cutaneous horn. *Acta Derm Venereol* (Stockh) 48:507-515, 1968.

54. Cramer HJ, Kahlert G: Das Cornu cutaneum. Selbstandi ges Krankheitsbild oder klinisches Symptom? *Dermatol Wochenschr* 150:521-531, 1964.

55. Brownstein MH, Shapiro EE: Trichilemmal horn. Cutaneous horn overlying trichilemmoma. *Clin Exp Dermatol* 4:59-63, 1979.

56. Sandbank M: Basal cell carcinoma at the base of cutaneous horn (cornu cutaneum). *Arch Dermatol* 104:97-98, 1971.

57. Gibbs RC, Hyman AB: Kaposi's sarcoma at the base of cutaneous horn. *Arch Dermatol* 98:37-40, 1968.

58. Mikhail GR, Fachnie DM, Drukker BH : Generalized malignant acanthosis nigricans. *Arch Dermatol* 115:201-202, 1979.

59. Ackerman AB, Lantis LR: Acanthosis nigricans associated with Hodgkin's disease. *Arch Dermatol* 95:202-205, 1967.

60. Garrott TC: Malignant acanthosis nigricans associated with osteogenic sarcoma. *Arch Dermatol* 106:384-385, 1972.

61. Brown J, Winkelmann RK: Acanthosis nigricans: a study of 90 cases (Review). *Medicine* 47:33-51, 1968.

62. Mibelli V: Contributo allo studio della ipercheratosi dei canali suderiferi. *G Ital Mal Ven* 28:313-355, 1893.

63. Guss SB, Osbourn RA, Lutzner MA: Porokeratosis plantaris, palmaris et disseminata. *Arch Dermatol* 104:366-373, 1971.

64. Chernosky ME, Freeman RC: Disseminated superficial atinic porokeratosis (DSAP). *Arch Dermatol* 96:611-24, 1967.

65. Lever WF, Schaumburg-Lever G: *Histopathology of the skin*, ed 6. Philadelphia, JB Lippincott Co, 1983.

66. Taub J, Steinberg M: Porokeratosis plantaris discreta, previously unrecognized dermatological entity. *Int J Dermatol* 9:83-90, 1970.

67. Berlin SJ: Tumors and tumorous conditions of the foot. In McGlamry ED (ed): *Comprehensive Textbook of Foot Surgery*, vol 2. Baltimore, Williams & Wilkins, 1987.

68. Limmer BL: Cryosurgery of porokeratosis plantaris discreta. *Arch Dermatol* 115:582-583, 1979.

69. James MP, Wells GC, Whimster IW: Spreading pigmented actinic keratosis. *Br J Dermatol* 98:373-379, 1978.

70. Montgomery H, Dorffel J: Verruca senilis und Keratoma senile. *Arch Dermatol Syph* (Berlin) 166:286-296, 1932.

71. Greene MH, Clark WH Jr, Tucker MA: Acquired precursors of cutaneous malignant melanoma. The familial dysplastic nevus syndrome. *N Engl J Med* 312:91-97, 1985.

72. Kopf AW, Bart RS, Hennessey P: Congenital nevocytic nevi and malignant melanomas. *J Am Acad Dermatol* 1:123-130, 1979.

73. Rhodes AR, Sober AJ, Day CL: The malignant potential of small congenital nevocellular nevi. *J Am Acad Dermatol* 6:230-241, 1982.

74. Scher RK: Biopsy of the matrix of a nail. *J Dermatol Surg Oncol* 6:19-21, 1980.

75. Kopf AW, Waldo E: Melonychia striata. *Aus J Dermatol* 21:59-70, 1980.

76. Goldberg DJ: Melonychia striata longitudinalis: multiple benign pigmented streaks in a caucasian. *J Dermatol Surg Oncol* 12:188-189, 1986.

77. Lambert WC, Brodkin RH: Nodal and subcutaneous cellular blue nevi. A pseudometastasizing pseudomelanoma. *Arch Dermatol* 120:367-370, 1984.

78. Winer LH: Pseudoepitheliomatous hyperplasia, *Arch Dermatol Syph* 42:856-867, 1940.

79. Freeman RG: On the pathogenesis of pseudoepitheliomatous hyperplasia. *J Cutan Pathol* 1:231-237, 1974.

80. Strauss H, Potter GK: Keraoacanthoma. case presentation and discussion. *J Am Coll Foot Surg* 18:72-74, 1979.

81. Macaulay WL: Subungual keratoacanthoma. *Arch Dermatol* 112:1004-1005, 1976.

82. Stoll DM, Ackerman AB: Subungual keratoacanthoma. *Amer J Dermatopathol* 2:265-271, 1980.

83. Haydey RP, Reed ML, Dzubow LM: Treatment of keratoacanthomas with oral 13-cis-retinoic acid. *N Engl J Med* 303:560-562, 1980.

84. Torre D: Multiple sebaceous tumors. *Arch Dermatol* 98:549-551, 1968.

85. Poleksic S: Keratoacanthoma and multiple carcinomas. *Br J Dermatol* 91:461-463, 1974.

86. Stewart WM, Lauret P, Hemet J: Keratoacanthomes multiples et carcinomes visceraux syndrome de Torre. *Ann Dermatol Venereol* 104:624-626, 1977.

87. Householder MS, Zeligman I: Sebaceous neplasms associated with visceral carcinoma. *Arch Dermatol* 116:61-64, 1980.

88. Rulon DB, Helwig EB: Multiple sebaceous neoplasms of the skin. An association with multiple visceral carcinomas, especially of the colon. *Amer J Clin Pathol* 60:745-752, 1973.

89. Paniago-Pereira C, Maize JC, Ackerman AB: Nevus of large spindle and/or epithelioid cells (Spitz's nevus). *Arch Dermatol* 114:1811-1823, 1978.

90. Barr RJ, Morales V, Graham JH: Spindle cell and epithelial cell nevi (Abstract). *Arch Dermatol* 114:1833, 1978.

91. Verret JL, Schnitzler L: Melanomes de L'enfant: a propos de sept cas d'interpretation difficile. *Dermatologica* (Suppl) 11:81-86, 1980.

92. Marko O, Houghton AN, Eisinger M: Purification of human melanocytes by monoclonal antibodies combined with Percoll TM gradients. *Exp Cell Res* 142:309-315, 1982.

93. Houghton AN, Eisinger M, Albino A: Surface antigens of melanocytes and melanomas. Markers of melanocyte differentiation and melanoma subsets. *J Exp Med* 156:1755-1766, 1982.

94. Leong AS-Y, Gilham P: Silver staining of nucleolar organizer regions in malignant melanoma and melanocytic nevi. *Hum Pathol* 20:257-262, 1989.

95. Hyman AB, Michaelides P: Basal-cell epithelioma of the sole. *Arch Dermatol* 87:481-485, 1963.

96. Lewis HM, Stensaas CO, Okun MR: Basal cell epithelioma of the sole. *Arch Dermatol* 91:623-624, 1965.

97. Mikhail GR: Subungual basal cell carcinoma. *J Dermatol Surg Oncol* 11:1222-1223, 1985.

98. Southwick GJ, Schwartz RA: The basal cell nevus syndrome. Disasters occurring among a series of 36 patients. *Cancer* 44:2294-2305, 1979.

99. Safai B, Good RA: Basal cell carcinoma with metastasis. *Arch Pathol* 101:337-341, 1977.

100. Gellin GA, Kopf AW, Garfinkel L: Basal cell epithelioma. *Arch Dermatol* 91:38-45, 1965.

101. Anderson NP, Anderson HE: Development of basal cell epithelioma as a consequence of radiodermatitis. *Arch Dermatol Syph* 63:586-596, 1951.

102. Schwartz RA, Burgess GH, Milgrom H: Breast carcinoma and basal cell epitheliomas after x-ray therapy for hirsutism. *Cancer* 44:1601-1605, 1979.

103. Gaughan LJ, Bergeron JR, Mullins JF: Giant basal cell epithelioma developing in acute burn site. *Arch Dermatol* 99:594-595, 1969.

104. Margolis MH: Superficial multicentric basal cell epithelioma arising in thermal burn scar. *Arch Dermatol* 102:47-56, 1970.

105. Wechsler HL, Krugh FJ, Domonkos AN: Polydysplastic epidermolysis bullosa and development of epidermal neoplasms. *Arch Dermatol* 102:374-380, 1970.

106. Yeh S: Skin cancer in chronic arsenicism. *Hum Pathol* 4:469-85, 1973.

107. Hadida E, Marill FG, Sayag J: Xeroderma pigmentosum. *Ann Dermatol Syph* 90:467-496, 1963.

108. Kraemer KH, DiGiovanna JJ, Moshell AA: Prevention of skin cancer in xeroderma pigmentosum with the use of oral isotretinoin. *N Engl J Med* 318:1633-1637, 1988.

109. Lund HZ: How often does squamous cell carcinoma of the skin metastasize? *Arch Dermatol* 92:635-637, 1965.

110. Sedlin ED, Fleming JL: Epidermal carcinoma arising in chronic osteomyelitic foci. *J Bone Joint Surg* 45:827-837, 1963.

111. Martin H, Strong E, Spiro RH: Radiation-induced skin cancer of the head and neck. *Cancer* 25:61-71, 1970.

112. Arons AS, Lynch JB, Lewis SR: Scar tissue carcinoma. I. A clinical study with special reference to burn scar carcinoma. *Ann Surg* 161:170-188, 1965.

113. Hoxtell EO, Mandel JS, Murray SS: Incidence of skin carcinoma after renal transplantation. *Arch Dermatol* 113:436-438, 1977.

114. Haynes HA, Mead KW, Goldwyn RM: Cancers of the skin. In DeVita VT Jr, Hellman S, Rosenberg SA (eds): *Cancer, Principles and Practice of Oncology*, ed 2. Philadelphia, JB Lippincott Co, 1985, pp 1343-1369.

115. Andersen SL, Nielsen H, Raymann F: Relationship between Bowen's disease and internal malignant tumors. *Arch Dermatol* 108:367-370, 1973.

116. Callen JP, Headington J: Bowen's and non-Bowen's squamous intraepidermal neoplasia of the skin. *Arch Dermatol* 116:422-426, 1980.

117. Coskey RJ, Merhegan A: Bowen's disease associated with Porokeratosis of mibelli. *Arch Dermatol* 111:1480-1481, 1975.

118. Oberste-Lehn H, Moll B: Porokeratosis Mibelli und Stachelzellcarcinom. *Hautarzt* 19:399-403, 1968.

119. Bell ET, Rothnem TP: Xeroderma pigmentosum with carcinoma of the lower lip in two brothers aged 16 and 13 years. *Am J Cancer* 30:574-579, 1937.

120. Edmundson WF: Microscopic grading of cancer and its practical implication. *Arch Dermatol Syph* 57:141-150, 1948.

121. Neill SM, Calnan CD, Rahim GF: Carcinoma cuniculatum. *Clin Exp Dermatol* 9:309-311, 1984.

122. McCann JJ, Al-Nafussi AI: Epithelioma cuniculatum plantare. *Br J Plast Surg* 42:79-82, 1989.

123. Reingold IM, Smith BR, Graham JH: Epithelioma cuniculatum pedis, a variant of squamous cell carcinoma. *Am J Clin Pathol* 69:561-565, 1978.

124. Fugate DS, Romash MM: Carcinoma cuniculatum (verrucous carcinoma) of the foot. *Foot Ankle* 9: 257-259, 1989.

125. Kane HD, Squire MA, Callett HA: Sebaceous carcinoma of the foot. Case presentation and discussion. *J Am Podiatry Assoc* 74:120-124, 1984.

126. Teloh HA, Balkin RB, Grier JP: Metastasizing sweat gland carcinoma. *Arch Dermatol* 76:80-86, 1957.

127. Geraci TL, Jenkinson S, Janis L: Mucinous (adenocystic) sweat gland carcinoma of the great toe. *J Foot Surg* 26:520-523, 1987.

128. Kao GF, Helwig EB, Graham JH: Aggressive digital papillary adenoma and adenocarcinoma. A clinicopathological study of 57 patients, with histochemical, immunopathological and ultrastructural observations. *J Cutan Pathol* 14:129-146, 1987.

129. Tang CK, Toker C: Trabecular carcinoma of the skin. *Cancer* 42:2311-2321, 1978.

130. Sidhu JS, Mullins JD, Feiner H: Merkel cell neoplasms. *Am J Dermatopathol* 2:101-119, 1980.

131. Brucks A, Schaeg G, Mensing H: Primares Neuroendokrines Merkelzell-karzinom der Haut. *Dtsch Med Wochenschr* 114:133-137, 1989.

132. Iwafuchi M, Watanabe H., Ishihara R: A neuroendocrine (Merkel) cell carcinoma with coexisting intraepidermal squamous cell carcinoma of the skin, its growth accelerated by an extrinsic factor. *Acta Pathol J* 36:1099-1108, 1986.

133. Raaf JH, Urmacher C, Knapper WK: Trabecular (Merkel cell) carcinoma of the skin. Treatment of primary, recurrent, and metastatic disease. *Cancer* 57:178-182, 1986.

134. Doyle MA: Merkel cell carcinoma. *J Foot Surg* 25:374-377, 1986.

135. Drijkoningen M, DeWolf-Peeters C, Van Limbergen E, et al: Merkel cell tumor of the skin: an immunohistochemical study. *Hum Pathol* 17:301-307, 1986.

136. Taxy JB, Ettinger DS, Wharam MD: Primary small cell carcinoma of the skin. *Cancer* 46:2308-2311, 1980.

137. Abaci IF, Zak FG: Multicentric amyloid containing cutaneous trabecular carcinoma. *J Cutan Pathol* 6:292-303, 1979.

138. Wong SW, Dao AH, Glick AD: Trabecular carcinoma of the skin: a case report. *Hum Pathol* 12:838-840, 1981.

139. Silvers DN, Gorham JD: Observations on a melanoma by William Norris, M.D., a country practitioner of the 19th century. *Amer J Dermatopath*ol 4:421-424, 1982.

140. Norris W: Case of fungoid disease. *Edinburgh Med Surg J* 16:562-565, 1820.

141. Marmelzat WL: The first case of malignant melanoma reported in America (1837): case of melanosis by Isaac Parrish, M.D. *J Dermatol Surg Onc*ol 3:30-31, 1977.

142. Starrico RJ, Pinkus H: Quantitative and qualitative data on the pigment cells of adult human epidermis. *J Invest Dermatol* 28:33-45, 1957.

143. Fitzpatrick TB, Szabo G: The melanocytes: cytology and cytochemistry. *J Invest Dermatol* 32:197-209, 1959.

144. Quevedo WC Jr, Szabo G, Virks J: Melanocyte populations in UV-radiated human skin. *J Invest Dermatol* 45:295-298, 1965.

145. Rippey JJ, Rippey E: Epidemiology of malignant melanoma of the skin in South Africa. *S Afr Med J* 65:595-598, 1984.

146. Balch CM, Karakousis C, Mettlin C: Management of cutaneous melanoma in the United States. *Surg Gynecol Obste*t 158:311-318, 1984.

147. Coleman WP 3rd, Gately LE 3rd, Krementz AB: Nevi, lentigines, and melanoma in blacks. *Arch Dermatol* 116:548-551, 1980.

148. Mastrangelo MJ, Baker AR, Katz HR: Cutaneous melanoma. In DeVita VT Jr, Hellman S, Rosenberg SA (eds): *Cancer, Principles and Practice of Oncology*, ed 2. Philadelphia, JB Lippincott Co, 1985, pp 1371-1422.

149. Kukita A, Ishihara K: Clinical features and distribution of malignant melanoma and pigmented nevi on the soles of the feet in Japan. *J Invest Dermatol* (Suppl) 92:210S-213S, 1989.

150. Foster HM, Webb SJ: Skin cancer in the North Solomons. *Aust NZ J Surg* 58:397-401, 1988.

151. Isaacson C, Spector I: Malignant melanomas in the EuroAfrican-Malay population of South Africa. *Am J Dermatohistopatho*l 9:109-110, 1987.

152. Black WC, Wiggins C: Melanoma among southwestern American Indians. *Cancer* 55:2899-2902, 1985.

153. Reintgen DS, McCarty KM Jr, Cox E: Malignant melanoma in black American and white American populations. A comparative review. *JAMA* 248:1856-1859, 1982.

154. Collins RJ: Melanoma in the Chinese of Hong Kong. Emphasis on volar and subungual sites. *Cancer* 54:1482-1488, 1984.

155. Anaise D, Steinitz R, Ben Hur N: Solar radiation: a possible etiologic factor in malignant memanoma in Israel. *Cancer* 42:299-304, 1978.

156. Moshvitz M, Modan B: Role of sun exposure in the etiology of malignant melanoma. Epidemiologic influencs. *J Natl Cancer Inst* 51:777-779, 1973.

157. Sober AJ, Lew RA, Fitzpatrick TB: Solar exposure patterns in patients with cutaneous melanoma. *Clin Res* 27:563A, 1979.

158. Millburn PB, Sian CS, Silvers DN: The color of the skin of the palms and soles as a possible clue to the pathogenesis of acral-lentiginous melanoma. *Amer J Dermatopathol* 4:429-433, 1982.

159. Breathnach AS: Melanocyte distribution in forearm epidermis of freckled human subjects. *J Invest Dermatol* 29:253-261, 1957.

160. Breathnach AS, Wyllie LM: Electron microscopy of melanocytes and melanosomes in freckled human epidermis. *J Invest Dermatol* 42:389-394, 1964.

161. Harsanyi ZP, Post PW, Brinkmann JW: Mutagenicity of melanin from human red hair. *Experientia* 36:291-292, 1980.

162. Chedekel MR, Smith SK, Post PW: Photodestruction of pheomelanin. Role of oxygen. *Proc Natl Acad Sci USA* 75:5395-5399, 1978.

163. Pemberton O: Observations on the history, pathology and treatment of melanosis. *Midland Q J Med Sci* 1:129-166, 1857.

164. Cawley EP: Genetic aspects of malignant melanoma. *Arch Dermatol* 65:440-450, 1952.

165. Greene MH, Fraumeni JF Jr: The hereditary variant of malignant melanoma. In Clark WH, Goldman LI, Mastrangelo MJ (eds): *Human Malignant Melanoma*, New York, Grune & Stratton, 1979, pp 139-166.

166. Bellet RE, Vaisman I, Mastrangelo MJ: Multiple primary malignancies in patients with cutaneous melanoma. *Cancer* 40:1974-1981, 1977.

167. Nissenblatt MJ, WU H-V: Malignant melanoma and small-cell carcinoma of the lung. *N Engl J Med* 302:636, 1980.

168. Lynch HT, Anderson DE, Smith JL Jr: Xeroderma pigmentosum, malignant melanoma and congenital icthyosis. *Arch Dermatol* 96:625-635, 1967.

169. Balaban G, Herlyn M, Guerry D IV: Cytogenetics of human malignant melanoma and pre-malignant lesions. *Cancer Genet Cytogenet* 11:429-439, 1984.

170. Parmiter AH, Balaban G, Herlyn M: A t(1;19) chromosome translocation in 3 cases of human malignant melanoma. *Cancer Res* 46:1526-1529, 1986.

171. Trent JM, Stanbridge EJ, Heyoung L: Tumorigenicity in human melanoma cell lines controlled by introduction of human chromosome 6. *Science* 247:568-571, 1990.

172. Greene MH, Goldin LR, Clark WH Jr: Familial cutaneous malignant melanoma: autosomal dominant trait possibly linked to the Rh locus. *Proc Natl Acad Sci USA* 80:6071-6075, 1983.

173. Sugawara O, Oshimura M, Koi M: Induction of cellular senescence in immortalized cells by human chromosome. I. *Science* 247:707-710, 1990.

174. Clark WH Jr, Reimer RR, Greene M: Origin of familial melanoma from heritable melanocytic lesions—the BK mole syndrome. *Arch Dermatol* 114:732-738, 1978.

175. Kraemer KH, Greene MH, Tarome R: Dysplastic naevi and cutaneous melanoma risk. *Lancet* 2:1076-1077, 1983.

176. Clark WH Jr, Elder DE, Guerry D IV: A study of tumor progression: the precursor lesions of superficial spreading and nodular melanoma. *Hum Pathol* 15:1147-1165, 1984.

177. Barnhill RL, Roush GC, Duray PH: Correlation of histologic architecture and cytoplasmic features with nuclear atypia in atypical (dysplastic) nevomelanocytic nevi. *Hum Pathol* 21:51-58, 1990.

178. Ackerman AB, Mihara I: Dysplasia, dysplastic melanocytes, dysplastic nevi, the dysplastic nevus syndrome, and the relation between dysplastic nevi and malignant melanomas. *Hum Pathol* 16:87-91, 1985.

179. Fitzpatrick TB, Rhodes AR, Sober AJ: Prevention of melanoma by recognition of its precursors. *N Engl J Med* 302:115-116, 1985.

180. Clark WH, Elder DE, Van Horn M: The biologic forms of malignant melanoma. *Hum Pathol* 17:443-450, 1986.

181. Ackerman AB, David KM: A unifying concept of malignant melanoma: biologic aspects. *Hum Pathol* 17:438-440, 1986.

182. Flotte TJ, Mihm MC: Melanoma: the art versus the science of dermatopathology. *Hum Pathol* 17:441-442, 1986.

183. Hughes LE, Horgan K, Taylor BA: Malignant melanoma of the hand and foot: diagnosis and management. *Br J Surg* 72:811-815, 1985.

184. Lambert MW, Potter GK: A defective DNA endonuclease in melanotic but not amelanotic mouse melanomas (Abstract). *J Invest Dermatol* 8:330-331, 1983.

185. Bloch B: Das Problem der Pigmentbildung in der Haut. *Arch Dermatol Syph* (Berlin) 124:129-143, 1917.

186. Huszar M, Halkin H, Herczeg E: Use of antibodies to intermediate filaments in the diagnosis of metastatic amelanotic malignant melanoma. *Hum Pathol* 14:1006-1008, 1983.

187. Harris MN, Gumport SL: Biopsy technique for malignant melanoma. *J Dermatol Surg Oncol* 1:24-27, 1975.

188. Ironside P, Pitt TTE, Rank BK: Malignant melanoma: some aspects of pathology and prognosis. *Aus NZ J Surg* 47:70-75, 1977.

189. Rampen FHJ, Van Houten WA, Hop WCJ: Incisional procedures and prognosis in malignant melanoma. *Clin Exp Dermatol* 5:313-320, 1980.

190. Epstein E, Bragg K, Linden G: Biopsy and prognosis of malignant melanoma. *JAMA* 208:1369-1371, 1969.

191. Bagley FH, Cady B, Lee A: Changes in clinical presentation and management of malignant melanoma. *Cancer* 47:2126-2134, 1981.

192. Lopransi S, Mihm MC Jr: Clinical and pathological correlation of malignant melonoma. *J Cutan Pathol* 6:180-194, 1979.

193. Allen AC, Spitz S: Malignant melanoma—a clinicopathologic analysis of the criteria for diagnosis and prognosis. *Cancer* 6:1-45, 1953.

194. Mehnert JH, Heard JL: Staging of malignant melanoma by depth of invasion. *Am J Surg* 110:168-176, 1965.

195. Clark WH Jr, From L, Bernadino EA: The histogenesis and biologic behavior of primary human malignant melanoma of the skin. *Cancer Res* 29:705-727, 1969.

196. Breslow A: Prognosis in cutaneous melanoma: tumor thickness as a guide to treatment. In Sommers SS, Rosen PP (eds): *Pathology Annual Part 1*, vol 15. New York, Appleton-Century-Crofts, 1980, pp 1-22.

197. Breslow A: Thickness, cross-sectional area and depth of invasion in prognosis of cutaneous melanoma. *Ann Surg* 172:902-908, 1970.

198. Ackerman AB, Scheiner AM: How wide and deep is wide and deep enough? A critique of surgical practice in excisions of primary cutaneous malignant melanoma. *Hum Pathol* 14:743-744, 1983.

199. Handley WS: The pathology of melanotic growths in relation to their operative treatment. *Lancet* 1:927-1003, 1907.

200. Wong CK: A study of melanocytes in the normal skin surrounding malignant melanomata. *Dermatologica* 141:215-225, 1970.

201. Day CL Jr, Lew RA: Malignant melanoma prognostic factors. III. Surgical margins. *J Dermatol Surg Oncol* 9:797-801, 1983.

202. Hilaris BS, Raben M, Calabrese AS: Value of radiation therapy for distant metastases from malignant melanoma. *Cancer* 16:765-773, 1963.

203. Tucker MA, Misfeldt D, Coleman CN: Cutaneous malignant melanoma following Hodgkin's disease. *Ann Intern Med* 102:37-41, 1985.

204. Greene MH, Young TI, Clark WH Jr: Malignant melanoma in renal-transplant recipients. *Lancet* 1:1196-1199, 1981.

205. Talal N: Systemic lupus erythematosus, autoimmunity, sex and inheritance. *N Engl J Med* 301:838-839, 1979.

206. Talal N, Ahmed SA, Dauphinee M: Hormonal approaches to immunotherapy of autoimmune disease. In Schwartz RS, Rose NR (eds): *Autoimmunity: Experimental and Clinical Aspects.* Annals of New York Academy of Sciences, Vol 475, New York, The New York Academy of Sciences, pp 320-328, 1986.

207. Gates O: Cutaneous metastasis of malignant diseases. *Amer J Cancer* 30:718-730, 1937.

208. King DT, Gurevitch AW, Hirose FM: Multiple cutaneousmetastases of a scapular chondrosarcoma. *Arch Dermatol* 114:584-586, 1978.

209. Fidler IJ, Hart IR: Principles of cancer biology: cancer metastasis. IN: DeVita VT Jr, Hellman S, Rosenberg SA (eds): *Cancer, Principles and Practice of Oncology,* ed 2. Philadelphia, JB Lippincott Co, 1985, pp 113-125.

210. Zetter BR: The cellular basis of site-specific tumormetastasis. *N Engl J Med* 322:605-612, 1990.

211. Pauli BU, Knudson W: Tumor invasion: a consequence of destructive and compositional matrix alterations. *Hum Pathol* 19:628-639, 1988.

212. Sandberg AA, Turc-Carel C: The cytogenetics of solid tumors. relation to diagnosis, classification and pathology. *Cancer* 59:387-395, 1987.

213. Rydholm G, Berg NO: Size, site and clinical incidence of lipoma. Factors in the differential diagnosis of lipoma and sarcoma. *Acta Orthop Scand* 54:929-934, 1983.

214. Hajdu SI: *Differential diagnosis of soft tissue and bone tumors.* Philadelphia, Lea & Febiger, 1986.

215. Kleinstiver BJ, Rodriguez HA: Nodular fasciitis—a study of forty-five cases and review of the literature. *J Bone Joint Surg* 50A:1204-1212, 1968.

216. Price EB Jr, Siliphant WM, Schuman R: Nodular fasciitis, a clinicopathologic analysis of 65 cases. *Am J Clin Pathol* 35:122-136, 1961.

217. Stout AP: Pseudosarcomatous fasciitis in children. *Cancer* 14:1216-1222, 1961.

218. Hutter RVP, Stewart FW, Foote FW Jr: Fasciitis. *Cancer* 15:993-1003, 1962.

219. Soule EH: Proliferative (nodular) fasciitis. *Arch Pathol* 73:437-444, 1962.

220. Chung EB, Enzinger FM: Fibroma of tendon sheath. *Cancer* 44:1945-1954, 1979.

221. Jarvi OH, Saxen E: Elastofibroma dorsi. *Acta Pathol Microbiol Scand* 51[Suppl 144]:83-84, 1961.

222. Cross DL, Mills SE, Kulund DN: Elastofibroma arising in the foot. *Southern Med J* 77:1194-1196, 1984.

223. Onwukwe MF: Classification of keloids. A review. *J Dermatol Surg Oncol* 4:534-536, 1978.

224. Murray JC, Pollack SV, Pinnel SR: Keloids: a review. *J Am Acad Dermatol* 4:461-470, 1981.

225. Kischer CW, Thies AC, Chvapil M: Perivascular myofibroblasts and microvascular occlusion in hypertrophic scars and keloids. *Hum Pathol* 13:819-824, 1982.

226. Kischer CW, Bunce H III, Shetlar MR: Mast cell analyses in hypertrophic scars, hypertrophic scars treated with pressure and mature scars. *J Invest Dermatol* 70:355-357, 1978.

227. Asboe-Hansen G: Hypertrophic scars and keloids. *Dermatol* 120:178-184, 1960.

228. Diegelmann RF, Cohen IK, McCoy BJ: Growth kinetics and collagen synthesis in normal skin, normal scar and keloid fibroblasts in vitro. *J Cell Physiol* 98:341-346, 1979.

229. Priestley GC: Effects of corticosteroids on the growth and metabolism of fibroblasts cultured from human skin. *Br J Dermatol* 99:253-260, 1978.

230. Ketchum LD, Cohen IK, Masters FW: Hypertrophic scars and keloids. *Plast Reconstr Surg* 53:140-154, 1974.

231. Steffen M, Abboud M, Potter GK: Presence of tumour necrosis factor or a related factor in human basophil/mast cells. *Immunology* 66:445-450, 1989.

232. Harper RA, Grove G: Human skin fibroblasts derived from papillary and reticular dermis: differences in growth potential in vitro. *Science* 204:526-527, 1979.

233. Bloom D: Heredity of keloids. Review of the literature and report of a family with multiple keloids in five generations. *NY State J Med* 56:511-519, 1956.

234. Benjamin SP, Mercer RD, Hawk WA: Myofibroblastic contraction in spontaneous regression of multiple congenital mesenchymal hamartomas. *Cancer* 40:2343-2352, 1977.

235. Roggli VL, Kim HS, Hawkins E: Congenital generalized fibromatosis with visceral involvement. *Cancer* 45:954-960, 1980.

236. Reye RDK: Considerations of certain subdermal "fibromatous tumors" of infancy. *J Pathol Bacteriol* 72:149-154, 1956.

237. Puretic S, Puretic B, Fiser-Herman M: A unique form of mesenchymal dysplasia. *Br J Dermatol* 74:8-19, 1956.

238. Haedicke GJ, Sturim H: Plantar fibromatosis: an isolated disease. *Plast Reconstr Surg* 83:296-300, 1988.

239. Bart RS, Pumphrey RE: Knuckle pads, leukonychia and deafness. A dominantly inherited syndrome. *N Engl J Med* 276:202-207, 1967.

240. Enzinger FM, Weiss SW: *Soft Tissue Tumors,* ed 2. St Louis, CV Mosby Co, 1988.

241. Hajdu SI: *Pathology of soft tissue tumors.* Philadelphia, Lea & Febiger, 1979.

242. Posner MC, Shiu MH, Newsome JL: The desmoid tumor. Not a benign disease. *Arch Surg* 124:191-196, 1989.

243. Waddell WR, Gerner RE: Indomethacin and ascorbate inhibit desmoid tumors. *J Surg Oncol* 15:85-90, 1980.

244. Kirby EJ, Shereff MJ, Lewis MM: Soft-tissue tumors and tumor-like lesions of the foot. An analysis of eighty-three cases. *J Bone Joint Surg* 71A:621-626, 1989.

245. Keasbey LE: Juvenile aponeurotic fibroma (calcifying fibroma). A distinctive tumor arising in the palms and soles of young children. *Cancer* 6:338-346, 1953.

246. Weasen SR, Pelachyk JM, Bernfeld WF: Juvenile aponeurotic fibroma: a case report of a rare tumor. *Cleve Clin Q* 51:467-469, 1984.

247. Verallo VVM: Acquired digital fibrokeratomas. *Br J Dermatol* 80:730-736, 1968.

248. Gross RE: Recurring myxomatous cutaneous cysts of the fingers and toes. *Surg Gynecol Obstset* 65:289-302, 1937.

249. Newmeyer WL, Kilgore ES Jr, Graham WP III: Mucous cysts: the dorsal distal interphalangeal joint ganglion. *Plast Reconstr Surg* 53:313-315, 1974.

250. Goldman JA, Goldman L, Jaffe MS: Digital mucinous pseudocysts. *Arthritis Rheum* 20:997-1002, 1977.

251. Jayson MIV, Dixon ASJ: Valvular mechanism in juxta articular cysts. *Ann Rheum Dis* 29:415-420, 1970.

252. Sarpyener MA, Oscurumez O, Seyhan F: Multiple ganglions of tendon sheaths. A case report. *J Bone Joint Surg* 50A:985-990, 1968.

253. Hicks JD: Synovial cysts in bone. *Aust NZ J Surg* 26:138-143, 1956.

254. Sim FH, Dahlin DC: Ganglion cysts of bone. *Mayo Clin Proc* 46:484-488, 1971.

255. Steinau HU, Ehrl H, Biemer E: Reconstructive plastic surgery in soft tissue sarcomas of the extremities. *Eur J Plast Surg* 11:99-108, 1988.

256. Soule EH, Pritchard DJ: Fibrosarcoma in infants and children. A review of 110 cases. *Cancer* 40:1711-1721, 1981.

257. Ozzello L, Stout AP, Murray MR: Cultural characteristics of malignant histiocytomas and fibrous xanthomas. *Cancer* 16:331-344, 1963.

258. Hajdu SI, Fogh J: The nude mouse as a diagnostic tool in human tumor research. In Fogh J, Giovanella BC (eds): *The Nude Mouse in Experimental and Clinical Research.* New York, Academic Press, 1976.

259. Sethi J, Hirshaut Y, Hajdu SI: Growing human sarcomas in culture. *Cancer* 40:744-755, 1977.

260. Trifaud A, Chaix C: Unusual pulmonary metastases complicating giant cell tumors of bone. *Rev Chir Orthop* 61:439-442, 1975.

261. Huvos AG: "Benign" metastasis in giant cell tumor of bone. *Hum Pathol* 12:1151, 1981.

262. Gould E, Albores-Saavedra J, Rothe M: Malignant giant cell tumor of soft parts presenting as a skin tumor. *Am J Dermatopathol* 11:197-201, 1989.

263. Bliss BO, Reed RJ: Large cell sarcoma of tendon sheath. Malignant giant cell tumors of tendon sheath. *Am J Clin Pathol* 49:776-781, 1968.

264. Ozzello L, Hamels J: The histiocytic nature of dermatofibrosarcoma protuberans. Tissue culture and electron microscopic study. *Am J Clin Pathol* 65:136-148, 1976.

265. Orkin M, Goltz RW, Good RA, : A study of multicentric reticulohistiocytosis. *Arch Dermatol* 89:640-654, 1964.

266. Kossard S, Winkelmann RK: Necrobiotic xanthogranuloma with paraproteinimia. *J Am Acad Dermatol* 3:257-270, 1980.

267. Costa OG: Acrokeratoelastoidosis. *Arch Dermatol* 70:228-231, 1954.

268. Jung EG, Beil FU, Anton-Lamprecht I: Akrokeratoelastoidosis. *Hautarzt* 25:127-133, 1974.

269. Nixon JE, Frank GR, Chambers G: Synovial osteochondromatosis. With report of four cases, one showing malignant change. *US Armed Forces Med J* 11:1434-1445, 1960.

270. Goldman RL, Lichtenstein L: Synovial chondrosarcoma. *Cancer* 17:1233-1240, 1964.

271. Jaffe HL: *Tumors and Tumorous Conditions of the Bones and Joints.* Philadelphia, Lea & Febiger, 1964.

272. Potter GK, Walkes MH, Penny TR: Tendosynovial sarcoma. A clinicopathologic review of foot cases with a case report. *J Am Podiatry Assoc* 74:312-322, 1984.

273. Bridge JA, Borek D, Neff JR: Chromosomal abnormalities in clear cell sarcoma. Implications for histogenesis. *Am J Clin Pathol* 93:26-31, 1990.

274. Hajdu SI, Shiu MH, Fortner JG: Tendosynovial sarcoma. A clinicopathologic study of 136 cases. *Cancer* 39:1201-1217, 1977.

275. Craig RM, Pugh DG, Soule EH: Roentgenologic manifestations of synovial sarcoma. *Radiology* 65:837-845, 1955.

276. Summers CL, Shahi M: Epithelioid sarcoma presenting as the reflex sympathetic dystrophy syndrome. *Postgrad Med J* 63:217-220, 1987.

277. Prat J, Woodruff JM, Marcove RC: Epithelioid sarcoma. An analysis of 22 cases indicating the prognostic significance of vascular invasion and regional lymph node metastasis. *Cancer* 41:1472-1487, 1978.

278. Seale KS, Lange TA, Monson D, : Soft tissue tumors of the foot and ankle. *Foot Ankle* 9:19-27, 1988.

279. Szymanski FJ, Bluefarb SM: Nodular fat necrosis and pancreatic disease. *Arch Dermatol* 83:224-229, 1961.

280. Osborne RR: Functioning acinous cell carcinoma of the pancreas accompanied with widespread focal fat necrosis. *Arch Intern Med* 85:933-943, 1950.

281. Hughes PSH, Apisarnthanarax P, Mullins JF: Subcutaneous fat necrosis associated with pancreatic disease. *Arch Dermatol* 111:506-509, 1975.

282. Farber S: A lipid metabolic disorder: disseminated "lipogranulomatosis." A syndrome with similarity to, and important difference from, Niemann-Pick and Hand-Schuller-Christian disease. *Am J Dis Child* 84:499-500, 1952.

283. Forstrom L, Winkelmann RK: Factitial panniculitis. *Arch Dermatol* 110:747-750, 1974.

284. Shelley WB, Rawnsley HM: Painful feet due to herniation of fat. *JAMA* 205:308-309, 1968.

285. Schlappner OL, Wood MG, Gerstein W: Painful and nonpainful piezogenic pedal papules. *Arch Dermatol* 106:729-733, 1972.

286. Dixon AY, McGregor DH, Lee SH: Angiolipomas: an ultrastructural and clinicopathologic study. *Hum Pathol* 12:739-747, 1981.

287. Weldon-Linne CM, Rhone DP, Blatt D, : Angiolipomas in homosexual men. *N Engl J Med* 310:1193-1194, 1984.

288. Cristofaro RL, Maher JO 3rd: Digital lipoma of the foot in a child. A case report. *J Bone Joint Surg* 70A:128-130, 1988.

289. Wu KK: Tumor Review. Liposarcoma of the ankle. *J Foot Surg* 27:276-280, 1988.

290. Kelly PC, Shramowiat M: Liposarcoma of the foot. A case report. *J Foot Surg* 17:27-31, 1978.

291. Enzinger FM, Dulcey F: Proliferative myositis. Report of thirty-three cases. *Cancer* 20:2213, 1967.

292. Heffner RR Jr, Armbrustmacher VW, Earle KM: Focal myositis. *Cancer* 40:301-306, 1977.

293. Banker BQ, Victor M: Dermatomyositis (systemic angiopathy) of childhood. *Medicine* (Baltimore) 45:261-289, 1966.

294. Bohan A, Peter JB, Bowman RL, : A computer-assisted analysis of 153 patients with polymyositis and dermatomyositis. *Medicine* (Baltimore) 56:255-366, 1977.

295. Barnes BE: Dermatomyositis and malignancy: a review of the literature. *Ann Intern Med* 84:68-76, 1976.

296. Dupree WB, Enzinger FM: Fibro-osseous pseudotumor of the digits. *Cancer* 58:2103-2109, 1986.

297. Spjut HJ, Dorfman HG: Florid reactive periostitis of the tubular bones of the hands and feet. A benign lesion which may simulate osteosarcoma. *Am J Surg Pathol* 5:423-433, 1981.

298. Schroeder HW Jr, Zasloff M: The hand and foot malformations in fibrodysplasia ossificans progressiva. *Johns Hopkins Med J* 147:73-78, 1980.

299. Durm AW: Anomalous muscle simulating soft tissue tumors on the lower extremities. *J Bone Joint Surg* 47A:1397-1400, 1965.

300. Wu KK: Rhabdomyosarcoma of the foot. *J Foot Surg* 27:166-71, 1988.

301. Young RH, Scully RE: Alveolar rhabdomyosarcoma metastatic to the ovary. A report of two cases and a discussion of the differential diagnosis of small cell malignant tumors of the ovary. *Cancer* 64:899-904, 1989.

302. Owens JC, Shiu MH, Smith R: Soft tissue sarcomas of the hand and foot. *Cancer* 55:2010-2018, 1985.

303. Fisher WC, Helwig EB: Leiomyomas of the skin. *Arch Dermatol* 88:510-520, 1963.

304. MacDonald DM, Sanderson KV: Angioleiomyoma of the skin. *Br J Dermatol* 91:161-168, 1974.

305. Montgomery H, Winkelmann RK: Smooth-muscle tumors of the skin. *Arch Dermatol* 79:32-41, 1959.

306. Banner AS, Carrington CB, Emory WB: Efficacy of oophorectomy in lymphangioleiomyomatosis and benign metastasizing leiomyoma. *N Engl J Med* 305:204-209, 1981.

307. Timmis AD, Smallpeice C, Davies AC: Intracardiac spread of intravenous leiomyomatosis with successful surgical excision. *N Engl J Med* 303:1043-1044, 1980.

308. Fields JP, Helwig EB: Leiomyosarcoma of the skin and subcutaneous tissue. *Cancer* 47:146-169, 1981.

309. Nunnery EW Jr, Lipper S, Reddick R: Leiomyosarcoma arising in a chronic venous stasis ulcer. *Hum Pathol* 12:951-953, 1981.

310. Wu KK: Leiomyosarcoma of the foot. *J Foot Surg* 27:362-368, 1988.

311. Rifleman GT, Cronin R, Sage R: Leiomyosarcoma of the cutaneous tissue. A case occurring in the ankle and foot. *J Am Podiatr Med Assoc* 80:222-225, 1990.

312. Brenner MA, Rabinowitz AD: Interdigital angioleiomyoma. *Cutis* 34:350-353, 1986.

313. Sawada Y: Angioleiomyoma masquerading as a painful ganglion of the great toe. *Eur J Plast Surg* 11:175-177, 1988.

314. Erlandson RA, Woodruff JM: Peripheral nerve sheath tumors. An electron microscopic study of 43 cases. *Cancer* 49:273-287, 1982.

315. Stout AP: The peripheral manifestations of the specific nerve sheath tumor (neurilemoma). *Am J Cancer* 24:751-796, 1935.

316. White NB: Neurilemomas of the extremities. *J Bone Joint Surg* 49A:1605-1610, 1967.

317. Zuckerman JD, Powers B, Miller JW: Benign solitary schwannoma of the foot. A case report and review of the literature. *Clin Orthop* 228:278-280, 1988.

318. von Recklinghausen F: Uber die multiplen Fibrome der haut und ihre Beziehung zu den multiplen Neuromen. Berlin, August *Hirschwald*, 1882.

319. Potter GK, Feldman JS: Neoplasms of the peripheral nervous system. In Weber GA (ed): *Clinics in Podiatric Medicine and Surgery. Neurologic Disorders Affecting the Lower Extremity II*, Philadelphia, WB Saunders Co, 7:141-149, 1990.

320. Barker D, Wright K, Nguyen L: Gene for von Recklinghausen neurofibromatosis is in the pericentromeric region of chromosome 17. *Science* 236:1100-1102, 1987.

321. Woodruff JM, Chernick NL, Smith MC: Peripheral nerve tumors with rhabdomyosarcomatous differentiation (malignant "Triton" tumors). *Cancer* 32:426-439, 1973.

322. Woodruff JM: Peripheral nerve tumors showing glandular differentiation (glandular schwannomas). *Cancer* 37:2399-2413, 1976.

323. Masson P, Martin JF: Rhabdomyomes des nerf. *Bull Assoc Franc Etud Cancer* 27:751-767, 1938.

324. McCormick LJ, Hazard JB, Dickson JA: Malignant epithelioid neurilemoma (schwannoma). *Cancer* 7:725-728, 1954.

325. Woodruff JM: Malignant schwannoma showing heterologous tissues (complex malignant schwannoma). *Am Soc Clin Pathol* 20:14-17, 1975.

326. Giannestras NJ, Bronson JL: Malignant schwannoma of the medial plantar branch of the posterior tibial nerve (unassociated with von Recklinghausen's disease). *J Bone Joint Surg* 57A:701-703, 1975.

327. Woodruff JM, Godwin TA, Erlandson RA: Cellular schwannoma. A variety of schwannoma sometimes mistaken for a malignant tumor. *Am J Surg Pathol* 5:733-744, 1981.

328. Madewell JE, Moser RP Jr: Radiologic evaluation of soft tissue tumors. In Enzinger FM, Weiss SW: *Soft Tissue Tumors*, ed 2. St Louis, CV Mosby Co, 1988.

329. Harper PG, Pringle J, Souhami RL: Neuroepithelioma—a rare malignant peripheral nerve tumor of primitive origin: report of two new cases and a review of the literature. *Cancer* 48:2282-2287, 1981.

330. Llombart-Bosch A, Lacombe MJ, Peydro-Olaya A: Malignant peripheral neuroectodermal tumours of bone other than Askin's neoplasm: characterization of 14 new cases with immunohistochemistry and electron microscopy. *Virchows Arch* 412A:421-430, 1988.

331. Young S, Gonzalez-Crussi F: Melanocytic neuroectodermal tumor of the foot. Report of a case with multicentric origin. *Am J Clin Pathol* 84:371-378, 1985.

332. Capo V, Ozzello L, Fenoglio CM: Angiosarcomas arising in edematous extremities: immunostaining for factor VIII-related antigen and ultrastructural features. *Hum Pathol* 16:144-150, 1985.

333. Imperial R, Helwig EB: Verrucous hemangioma. *Arch Dermatol* 96:247-253, 1967.

334. Lindenauer SM: The Klippel-Trenaunay syndrome. Varicosities, hypertrophy and hemangioma with no arteriovenous fistula. *Ann Surg* 162:303-314, 1965.

335. Mullins JF, Naylor D, Redetzki J: The Klippel-Trenaunay-Weber syndrome. *Arch Dermatol* 86:202-206, 1962.

336. Cole DJ, Sood SC, Broomhead IW: Pulmonary embolism associated with hemolymphangioma of lower extremity. *Plast Reconstr Surg* 63:265-268, 1979.

337. Gloviczki P, Hollier LH, Telander RL: Surgical implications of Klippel-Trenaunay syndrome. *Ann Surg* 197:353-362, 1983.

338. Beninson J, Hurley JP: Hemolymphangioma in a neonate—a therapeutic problem-case history. *Angiology* 39:1043-1047, 1988.

339. Kasabach HH, Merritt KK: Capillary hemangioma with extensive purpura. Report of a case. *Ann J Dis Child* 59:1063-1070, 1940.

340. Lang PG, Dubin HV: Hemangioma-thrombocytopenia syndrome. *Arch Dermatol* 111:105-107, 1975.

341. Marsch WC: The ultrastructure of eruptive hemangioma ("pyogenic granuloma") (Abstract). *Cutan Pathol* 8:144-145, 1981.

342. Thelenberg G: Primer sporadishes Lymphodem mit Lymphangioma circumscriptum. *Hautarzt* 31:491-494, 1980.

343. Patil SR, Weiner C, Williamson R: Rapid chromosome analysis and prenatal diagnosis using fluid from cystic hygromas. *N Engl J Med* 317:1159-1160, 1987.

344. Mori F, Molfetta L, Recchia O: Sindrome da squilibrio muscolare delle dita esterne del piede. *Chir Piede* 9:361-367, 1985.

345. Wu KK: Spindle cell hemangioendothelioma of the foot. *J Foot Surg* 28:478-478, 1979.

346. Abulafia J, Cigorraga J, Saliva J: Angioendotheliomatosis proliferante systemica (Pfleger y Tappeiner). *Dermatol Ibero Lat Am* 11:23-40, 1969.

347. Muller R, Hajdu SI, Brennan MF: Lymphangiosarcoma associated with chronic filarial lymphedema. *Cancer* 59:179-183, 1987.

348. Dawson EK, McIntosh D: Granulation tissue sarcoma following long-standing varicose ulceration. *J R Coll Surg Edinb* 16:88-95, 1971.

349. Straehley CJ III, Santos JI, Downey DM: Kaposi's sarcoma in a renal transplant recipient. *Arch Pathol* 99:611-613, 1975.

350. Harwood AR, Asoba D, Hofstader SL: Kaposi's sarcoma in recipients of renal transplant. *Am J Med* 67:759-765, 1979.

351. Cox FH, Helwig EB: Kaposi's sarcoma (review). *Cancer* 12:289-298, 1959.

352. O'Brien PH, Brasfield RD: Kaposi's sarcoma. *Cancer* 19:1497-1502, 1966.

353. Siegal FP, Lopez C, Hammer GS: Severe acquired immunodeficiency in male homosexuals, manifested by chronic perianal ulcerative herpes simplex lesions. *N Engl J Med* 305:1439-1444, 1981.

354. Krigel RL, Friedman-Kien AE: Kaposi's sarcoma in AIDS. In DeVita VT Jr, Hellman S, Rosenberg SA (eds): *AIDS—Etiology, Diagnosis, Treatment and Prevention*. Philadelphia, JB Lippincott, 1985, pp 185-212.

355. Templeton AC: Studies in Kaposi's sarcoma. *Cancer* 30:854-867, 1972.

356. Slavin G, Cameron HM, Forbes C: Kaposi's sarcoma in east African children. *J Pathol* 100:187-199, 1970.

357. Brehmer-Andersson E, Torssander J, Tengvar M: Extensive hemangiomatosis of the extremities with the same histopathological pattern as the early lesion of Kaposi's sarcoma. *Acta Derm Venereol* (Stockh) 66:449-451, 1986.

358. Wong RC, Solomon AR, Field SI: Pigmented purpuric lichenoid dermatitis of Gougerot-Blum mimicking Kaposi's sarcoma. *Cutis* 31:406-408, 1983.

359. Secher L, Weissman K, Kobayasi T: Pseudo-Kaposi sarcoma of the feet: an electron microscopic investigation. *Acta Derm Venereol* (Stockh) 64:246-249, 1984.

360. Marshall ME, Hatfield ST, Hatfield DR: Arteriovenous malformation simulating Kaposi's sarcoma (pseudo-Kaposi's sarcoma). *Arch Dermatol* 121:99-101, 1985.

361. Alessi E, Sala F: Bluefarb-Stewart syndrome—report of a new case. *Dermatologica* 169:93-96, 1984.

362. Abrikossoff A: Uber Myome, ausgehend von der querges treiften, willkurlichen Muskultur. *Virchows Arch* [A] 260:215-233, 1926.

363. Penneys NS, Adachi K, Ziegels-Weissman J: Granular cell tumors of the skin contain myelin basic protein. *Arch Pathol Lab Med* 107:202-203, 1983.

364. Finkel G, Lane B: Granular cell variant of neurofibromatosis: ultrastructure of benign and malignant tumors. *Hum Pathol* 13:959-963, 1982.

365. Strong EW, McDivitt RW, Brasfield RD: Granular cell myoblastoma. *Cancer* 25:415-422, 1952.

366. Lieberman PH, Foote FW, Stewart FW: Alveolar soft-part sarcoma. *JAMA* 198:1047-1051, 1966.

367. Miettinen M, Ekfors T: Alveolar soft part sarcoma. Immunohistochemical evidence for muscle cell differentiation. *Am J Clin Pathol* 93:32-38, 1990.

368. Wiernik PH, Serpick AA: Granulocytic sarcoma (Chloroma). *Blood* 35:361-369, 1970.

369. Stiefel A, Hartschuh W, Dorken B: Non-Hodgkin's lymphoma of low-grade malignancy, to some extent mimicking glomus tumors. *Hautarzt* 39:384-387, 1988.

370. Travis WD, Banks PM, Reiman HM: Primary extranodal soft tissue lymphoma of the extremities. *Am J Surg Pathol* 11:359-366, 1987.

371. Woringer F, Kolopp P: Lesion erythemato-squameuse polycyclique de l'avant-bras evoluant depuis 6 ans chez un garconnet de 13 ans. *Ann Dermatol Syph* 10:945-958, 1939.

372. Oliver GF, Winkelmann RK: Unilesional mycosis fungoides: a distinct entity. *J Am Acad Dermato* 20:63-70, 1989.

373. Sezary A, Bouvrain Y: Erythrodermie avec presence de cellules monstreuses dans derm et sang circulant. *Bull Soc Franc Dermatol Syph* 45:254-260, 1938.

374. Thestrup-Pedersen K, Halkier-Sorensen L, Sogaard H: The red man syndrome. Exfoliative dermatitis of unknown etiology: a description and follow-up of 38 patients. *J Am Acad Dermatol* 18:1307-1312, 1988.

375. Desai KR, Pezner RD, Lipsett JA: Total skin electron radiation for mycosis fungoides: relationship between acute toxicities and measured dose at different anatomic sites. *Int J Radiat Oncol Biol Phys* 15:641-645, 1988.

376. Kaye FJ, Bunn PA, Steinberg SM: A randomized trial comparing combination electron-beam radiation and chemotherapy with topical therapy in the initial treatment of mycosis fungoides. *N Engl J Med* 32:1784-1790, 1989.

377. Hsu S-D: Whence the Sézary cell? *N Engl J Med* 303:1180, 1980.

378. Sausville EA, Eddy JL, Makuch RW: Histopathologic staging at initial diagnosis of mycosis fungoides and the Sézary syndrome. Definition of three distinct prognostic groups. *Ann Int Med* 109:372-382, 1988.

379. Shaw JM: Genetic aspects of urticaria pigmentosa. *Arch Dermatol* 97:137-138, 1968.

380. Klaus SN, Winkelmann RR: Course of urticaria pigmentosa in children. *Arch Dermatol* 86:68-71, 1962.

381. Yasuda T, Kukita A: A fatal case of purely cutaneous form of diffuse mastocytosis. *Proceedings of the Twelfth International Congress of Dermatology*, vol 2, Washington, DC, 1962, pp 1558-1561.

382. Allison J: Skin mastocytosis presenting as a neonatal bullous eruption. *Austr J Dermatol* 9:83-85, 1967.

383. Monheit GD, Murad T, Conrad M: Systemic mastocytosis and the mastocytosis syndrome. *J Cutan Pathol* 6:42-52, 1979.

384. Mutter RD, Tannenbaum M, Ultman JE: Systemic mast cell disease (review). *Ann Intern Med* 57:887-904, 1963.

385. Burgoon CF, Graham JH, McCaffree DL: Mast cell disease. *Arch Dermatol* 98:590-605, 1968.

386. Strauss H, Potter GK: Urticaria pigmentosa: case presentation and discussion. *J Am Podiatry Assoc* 67:802-804, 1977.

387. Mankin HJ: Current concepts in cancer. Advances in diagnosis and treatment of bone tumors. *N Engl J Med* 300:543-545, 1979.

388. Ragsdale BD, Sweet DE, Vinh TN: Radiology as gross pathology in evaluating chondroid lesions. *Hum Pathol* 20:930-951, 1989.

389. Huvos AG: *Bone Tumors. Diagnosis, Treatment and Prognosis*. Philadelphia, WB Saunders Co, 1979.

390. Mirra JM: *Bone Tumors. Diagnosis and Treatment*. Philadelphia, JB Lippincott Co, 1980.

391. Jaffe HL: "Osteoid-osteoma." A benign osteoblastic tumor composed of osteoid and atypical bone. *Arch Surg* 31:709-728, 1935.

392. Pines B, Lavine L, Grayzel DM: Osteoid osteoma: etiology and pathogenesis. Report of twelve new cases. *J Intl Coll Surg* 13:249-277, 1950.

393. Shifrin LZ, Reynolds WA: Intra-articular osteoid osteoma of the elbow. A case report. *Clin Orthop* 81:126-129, 1971.

394. Toth SP: Bone cyst, osteoid osteoma. A case report. *J Am Podiatry Assoc* 60:404-406, 1970.

395. Teeny SM, Bernstein SM: Osteoid osteoma: elements of diagnosis and treatment. *Contemp Orthop* 18:461-467, 1989.

396. Panni AS, Maiotti M, Burke J: Osteoid osteoma of the neck of the talus. *Am J Sports Med* 17:584-588, 1989.

397. Hamilos DT, Cervetti RG: Osteoid osteoma of the hallux. *J Foot Surg* 26:397-399, 1987.

398. Short LA, Mattana GW, Benton VG: Osteoid osteoma in the medial malleolus. *J Foot Surg* 27:244-247, 1988.

399. Meng Q, Watt I: Phalangeal osteoid osteoma. *Br J Radiol* 62:321-325, 1989.

400. Capanna R, Van Horn JR, Ayala A: Osteoid osteoma and osteoblastoma of the talus. A report of 40 cases. *Skeletal Radiol* 15:360-364, 1986.

401. Shader AF, Schwartzenfeld SA: Osteoid osteoma: report of a case. *J Foot Surg* 28:438-441, 1989.

402. Farmlett EJ, Magid D, Fishman EK: Osteoblastoma of the tibia: CT demonstration. *J Comput Assist Tomogr* 10:1068-1070, 1986.

403. Larsson SE, Lorentzon R: The geographic variation of the incidence of malignant primary bone tumors in Sweden. *J Bone Joint Surg* 56A:592-600, 1974.

404. McMaster JH, Scranton PE JR, Drash AL: Growth and hormone control mechanisms in osteosarcoma. Evidence for a new therapeutic approach. *Clin Orthop* 106:366-376, 1975.

405. Mirra JM, Noriaki K, Rosen G: Primary osteosarcoma of toe phalanx: first documented case. *Am J Surg Pathol* 12:300-307, 1988.

406. Shajowicz F, McGuire MH, Araujo ES: Osteosarcomas arising on the surfaces of long bones. *J Bone Joint Surg* 70A:555-564, 1988.

407. Pintado SO, Lane J, Huvos AG: Parosteal osteogenic sarcoma of bone with coexistent low- and high-grade sarcomatous components. *Hum Pathol* 20:488-491, 1989.

408. Spjut HJ, Ayala AG: Skeletal tumors in children and adolescents. *Hum Pathol* 14:628-642, 1983.

409. Hirota K: Electron-microscopic studies on bone tumors. I. Osteogenoc sarcoma (sclerosing form). *Kumamoto Med J* 12:265, 1959.

410. Hirota K: Electron-microscopic studies on bone tumors. II. Osteogenic sarcoma (sclerosing form). *Kumamoto Med J* 13:118-128, 1960.

411. Ebener U, Welte K, Chandra P: Purification and Biochemical characterization of a virus-specific reverse transcriptase from human osteosarcoma tissue. *Cancer Lett* 7:179-188, 1979.

412. Welte K, Ebener U, Chandra P: Serological characterization of a purified reverse transcriptase from osteosarcoma of a child. *Cancer Lett* 7:189-195, 1979.

413. Chandra P, Steel LK, Laube H: Immunological characterization of reverse transcriptase from human tumors: evidence for subgroup-specific interspecies antigen determinants on the reverse transcriptase molecule. In Steel LK: *Viruses in Naturally Occurring Cancers*. Cold Spring Harbor Conference on Cell Proliferation, Cold Spring Harbor Laboratory, New York, 775-791, 1980.

414. Garbe LR, Monges GM, Pellegrin EM: Ultrastructural study of osteosarcomas. *Hum Pathol* 12:891-896, 1981.

415. Tucker MA, D'Angio GJ, Boice JD Jr: Bone sarcomas linked to radiotherapy and chemotherapy in children. *N Engl J Med* 317:588-593, 1987.

416. Miller-Breslow A, Dorfman HD: Dupuytren's (subungual) exostosis. *Am J Surg Pathol* 12:368-378, 1988.

417. Maroteaux P: Metachondromatosis. *Z Kinder Heilkd* 109:246-261, 1971.

418. Dumontier C, Rigault P, Padovani JP: Cartilaginour tumors in children. *Chir Pediatr* 30:91-97, 1989.

419. Kurt A-M, Unni KK, Sim FH: Chondroblastoma of bone. *Hum Pathol* 20:965-976, 1989.

420. Bloem JL, Mulder JD: Chondroblastoma: a clinical and radiological study of 104 cases. *Skeletal Radiol* 14:1-9, 1985.

421. Huvos AG, Higinbotham NL, Marcove RC: Aggressive chondroblastoma. Review of the literature on aggressive behavior and metastases with a report of one new case. *Clin Orthop* 126:266-272, 1977.

422. Fobben ES, Dalinka MK, Schiebler ML: The magnetic resonance imaging appearance at 1.5 tesla of cartilaginous tumors involving the epiphysis. *Skeletal Radiol* 16:647-651, 1987.

423. Marcove RC, Weis LD, Vaghaiwalla MR: Cryosurgery in the treatment of giant cell tumors of bone. *Cancer* 41:957-969, 1978.

424. Zillmer DA, Dorfman HD: Chondromyxoid fibroma of bone: thirty-six cases with clinicopathologic correlation. *Hum Pathol* 20:952-964, 1989.

425. Van Horn JR, Lemmens JA: Chondromyxoid fibroma of the foot. *Acta Orthop Scand* 57:375-377, 1986.

426. Marcove RC, Shoji H, Arlen M: Altered carbohydrate metabolism in cartilaginous tumors. *Contemp Surg* 5:53-54, 1974.

427. Marcove RC, Lewis MM, Huvos AG: En bloc upper humeral interscapulothoracic resection. The Tikhoff-Linberg procedure. *Clin Orthop* 124:219-228, 1977.

428. Steiner G, Greenspan A, Jahss M: Myxoid chondrosarcoma of the os calcis: a case report. *Foot Ankle* 5:84-91, 1984.

429. Wicks IP, Fleming A: Chondrosarcoma of the calcaneum with massive soft tissue calcification in a patient with hereditary and acquired connective tissue diseases. *Ann Rheum Dis* 46:346-348, 1987.

430. Nakajima H, Ushigome S, Fukuda J: Case report 482: Chondrosarcoma (grade 1) arising from the right second toe in a patient with multiple enchondromas. *Skeletal Radiol* 17:289-292, 1988.

431. Dahlin DC, Hoover NW: Desmoplastic fibroma of bone. Report of 2 cases. *JAMA* 188:685-687, 1964.

432. Beskin JL, Haddad RJ: Desmoplastic fibroma of the first metatarsal: a case report. *Clin Orthop* 199:299-303, 1985.

433. Duncan GS: Monostotic fibrous dysplasia of the foot. *J Foot Surg* 26:301-303, 1987.

434. Hatcher CH: The pathogenesis of localized fibrous lesions in the metaphyses of long bones. *Ann Surg* 122:1016-1030, 1945.

435. Burns TP, Weiss M, Snyder M: Giant cell tumor of the metatarsal. *Foot Ankle* 8:223-226, 1988.

436. Campanacci M, Baldini N, Boriani S: Giant cell tumor of bone. *J Bone Joint Surg* 69A:106-113, 1987.

437. Selzer G, David R, Revach M: Goltz syndrome with multiple giant-cell tumor-like lesions in bones. A case report. *Ann Int Med* 80:714-717, 1974.

438. Hutter RVP, Foote FW Jr, Frazell EL: Giant cell tumors complicationg Paget's disease of bone. *Cancer* 16:1044-1056, 1963.

439. Jacobs TP, Michelsen J, Polay JS: Giant cell tumor in Paget's disease of bone. Familial and geographic clustering. *Cancer* 44:742-747, 1979.

440. Burman MS, Gardner RC, Lauter CB: Aggressive giant-cell tumor in a young female with congenital adrenal virilism (adrenogenital syndrome). Report of an unusual association of a bone neoplasm with an endocrine disorder. *Cancer* 25:1174-1177, 1970.

441. Robinson D, Hendel D, Halperin N: Multicentric giant-cell reparative granuloma. A case in the foot. *Acta Orthop Scand* 60:232-234, 1989.

442. Glass TA, Mills SE, Fechner RE: Giant cell reparative granuloma of the hands and feet. *Radiol* 149:65-68, 1983.

443. Lorenzo JC, Dorfman HD: Giant cell reparative granuloma of short tubular bones of the hands and feet. *Am J Surg Pathol* 4:551-563, 1980.

444. Picci P, Baldini N, Sudanese A: Giant cell reparative granuloma and other giant cell lesions of the bones of the hands and feet. *Skeletal Radiol* 15:415-421, 1986.

445. Wold LE, Dobyns JH, Swee RG: Giant cell reaction (giant cell reparative granuloma) of the small bones af the hands and feet. *Am J Surg Pathol* 10:491-496, 1986.

446. Trojani M, Coquet M, Peres P: Leiomyosarcome primitif de l'os. One observation avec etude ultrastructurate et revue deal litterature. *Semin Hop Paris* 59:1179-1183, 1983.

447. Marymont JV, Clanton TO: Leiomyosarcoma of the os calcis. *Foot Ankle* 10:239-242, 1990.

448. Wang T-Y, Erlandson RA, Marcove RC: Primary leiomyosarcoma of bone. *Arch Pathol Lab Med* 104:100-104, 1980.

449. Lidholm SO, Lindbom A, Spjut HJ: Multiple capillary hemangiomas of the bones of the foot. *Acta Pathol Microbiol Scand* 51:9-16, 1961.

450. Bullough PG, Goodfellow JW: Solitary lymphangioma of bone. A case report. *J Bone Joint Surg* 58A:418-941, 1976.

451. Castillo M, Tehranzadeh J, Ghandur-Mnaymneh L: Hemangiosarcoma of the left foot and tibia: case report. *Foot Ankle* 9:49-53, 1988.

452. Olmi R, Rubbini L: Hemangiosarcoma developed in a chronic osteomyelitis of the tibia. *Chir Organi Mov* 61:765-768, 1975.

453. Llombart-Bosch A, Ortuno-Pacheco G: Ultrastructural findings supporting the angioblastic nature of the so-called adamantinoma of the tibia. *Histopathol* 2:189-200, 1978.

454. Biesecker JL, Marcove RC, Huvos AG: Aneurysmal bone cysts: a clinicopathologic study of 66 cases. *Cancer* 26:615-625, 1970.

455. Scurr JA: Myeloma occurring in Paget's disease. *Proc R Soc Med* 65:725, 1972.

456. Grader J, Moynihan JW: Multiple myeloma and osteogenic sarcoma in a patient with Paget's disease. *JAMA* 176:685-687, 1961.

457. Winfield J, Stamp TC: Bone and joint symptoms in Paget's disease. *Ann Rheum Dis* 43:769-773, 1984.

458. Claustre J, Blotman F, Simon L: Foot involvement in Paget's disease of bone. *Rev Rhum Mal Osteoartic* 43:45-49, 1976.

459. Barbieri L: On 2 rare diseases of the heel: bone cysts and Paget's disease. *Minerva Ortop* 20:328-332, 1969.

460. Rubin RP, Adler JJ, Adler DP: Paget's disease of the calcaneus. *J Am Podiatry Assoc* 73:267-267, 1983.

461. Meunier PJ, Salson C, Delmas PD: Skeletal distribution and biological markers of Paget's disease. *Rev Prat* 39:1125-1128, 1989.

462. Heuck F, Buck J: Rare localization of Paget's osteodystrophia deformans in the skeleton. *Radiologe* 24:422-427, 1984.

463. Brackenridge CJ: A statistical study of sarcoma complicating Paget's disease of bone in three countries. *Br J Cancer* 40:194-200, 1979.

464. Sandrasagra FA: Ewing's sarcoma of a metatarsal bone. *Ceylon Med J* 18:58-61, 1973.

465. Dunn EJ, Yuska KH, Judge DM: Ewing's sarcoma of the great toe. A case report. *Clin Orthop* 116:203-208, 1976.

466. Levin NB: Ewing's sarcoma of the calcaneus. *J Foot Surg* 19:127-129, 1980.

467. Chen KT, McGann PD, Flam MS: Ewing's sarcoma of the phalangeal bone. *J Surg Oncol* 22:92-94, 1983.

468. Reinus WR, Gilula LA, Shirley SK: Radiographic appearance of Ewing sarcoma of the hands and feet: report from the Intergroup Ewing Sarcoma Study. *AJR* 144:331-336, 1985.

469. Isobe H, Enomoto K, Morioka E: A case of Ewing's sarcoma treated successfully by combination chemotherapy consisting of high-dose methotrexate, aclacinomycin-A and vindesine. *Gan To Kagaku Ryoho* 14:2969-2972, 1987.

470. Wu KK: Ewing's sarcoma of the foot. *J Foot Surg* 28:166-170, 1989.

471. Leeson MC, Smith MJ: Ewing's sarcoma of the foot. *Foot Ankle* 10:147-151, 1989.

472. Kissane JM, Askin FB, Foulkes M: Ewing's sarcoma of bone: clinicopathologic aspects of 303 cases from the intergroup Ewing's Sarcoma Study. *Hum Pathol* 14:773-779, 1989.

473. Silverman EM, Reznick HA, Wolf BA: Chronic lymphocytic leukemia presenting in the marrow of a phalanx. *J Foot Surg* 28:151-153, 1989.

474. Sprinkle RL III, Santangelo L, DeUgarte R: Solitary plasmacytoma of bone in the calcaneus. *J Am Podiatr Med Assoc* 78:636-642, 1988.

475. Burkus JK, Bonatus TJ: Solitary plasmacytoma of the cuboid. *Foot Ankle* 8:344-349, 1988.

476. Burke WA, Merritt CC, Briggaman RA: Disseminated extramedullary plasmacytomas. *J Amer Acad Dermatol* 14(2, Part 2):335-339, 1986.

477. Lieberman PH, Jones CR, Dargeon HWK: A reappraisal of eosinophilic granuloma of bone, Hand-Schuller-Christian syndrome and Letterer-Siwe syndrome. *Medicine* 48:375-400, 1969.

478. Li JM: Some problems concerning the radiologic diagnosis of eosinophilic granuloma of the bone. *Chung Hua Fang Ske Hsueh Tsa Chih* 23:168-169, 1969.

479. Chieppa WA, Shinder M: Unicameral bone cyst of the talus. *J Am Podiatr Med Assoc* 79:441-446, 1989.

480. Martin SJ, Schiller JE: Unicameral bone cyst of the second metatarsal with pathologic fracture. *J Am Podiatr Med Assoc* 77:143-147, 1987.

481. Gordon SL, Denton JR, McCann PD: Unicameral bone cyst of the talus. *Clin Orthop* 215:201-205, 1987.

482. Peters MS, Reiman HM, Muller SA: Cutaneous extraskeletal Ewing's sarcoma. *J Cutan Pathol* 12:476-485, 1985.

483. Englert TP, Kahn MR, Bushkoff SH: Mandibular metastasis of an extraskeletal myxoid chondrosarcoma arising in the plantar surface of the foot. Report of a case. *J Oral Surg* 36:401-405, 1978.

484. Amir D, Amir G, Mogle P: Extraskeletal soft-tissue chondrosarcoma. Case report and review of the literature. *Clin Orthop* 198:219-223, 1985.

485. Libson E, Bloom RA, Husband JE: Metastatic tumours of bones of the hand and foot. A comparative review and report of 43 additional cases. *Skeletal Radiol* 16:387-392, 1987.

486. Bullough PG, Vigorita VJ: *Atlas of Orthopaedic Pathology with Clinical and Radiologic Correlations*. Philadelphia, JB Lippincott Co, 1984, pp 13.20-13.21.

487. Batson OV: The function of the vertebral veins and their role in the spread of metastases. *Ann Surg* 112:138-149, 1940.

488. Ewing J: *A Treatise on Tumors*, ed 3. Philadelphia, WB Saunders Co, 1928.

489. Paget S: The distribution of secondary growths in cancer of the breast. *Lancet* 1:571-573, 1989.

490. Brownstein MH, Helwig EG: Patterns of cutaneous metastasis. *Arch Dermatol* 105:862-868, 1972.

491. Watson CW, Friedman KJ: Cytology of metastatic neuroendocrine (Merkel-cell) carcinoma in pleural fluid. A case report. *Acta Cytol* 29:397-402, 1985.

492. Reingold IM: Cutaneous metastases from internal cancer. *Cancer* 19:162-168, 1966.

493. Ingram JT: Carcinoma erysipelodes and carcinoma telangiectaticum. *Arch Dermatol* 77:227-231, 1958.

494. Adamietz IA, Emminger A, Unverferth D: Unusual site of misinterpreted bone metastases in irradiated stage IIb cervix cancer. *Geburtshilfe Frauenheilkd* 49:682-684, 1989.

495. Zorzi R, Pescatori E: Metastasis of endometrial carcinoma to the tarsus. *Chir Organi* 68:727-730, 1982.

496. Dumontet C, Tebib J, Noel E: Tarsal bone metastasis of bladder carcinoma. *Ann Radiol* (Paris) 30:65-66, 1987.

497. Francis KC: Tumors and infections of the foot. In Giannestras NJ (ed): *Foot Disorders. Medical and Surgical Management*. Philadelphia, Lea & Febiger, 1967, p 471.

498. Farina R, Filho AP, de Souza CA: Metastase rara de adenocarcinoma de prostata. *Rev Assoc Med Brasil* 23:21-22, 1977.

499. Andreasi A, Danda F, Visona A: Rare case of bony metastasis of an asymptomatic renal cell carcinoma to a toe. *Chir Organi* 67:123-129, 1981.

500. Barnett LS, Morris JM: Metastases of renal-cell carcinoma simultaneously to a finger and a toe. A case report. *J Bone Joint Surg* 51A:772-774, 1969.

501. Anderson EE, Leitner WA, Boyarsky S: Renal-cell carcinoma metastatic to great toe. *J Bone Joint Surg* 50A:997-998, 1968.

502. Bright M, Unlkie JR: Carcinoma metastasis to talus and metatarsals. *JAMA* 210:1592, 1969.

503. Gall RJ, Sim FH, Pritchard DJ: Metastatic tumors to the bones of the foot. *Cancer* 37:1492-1495, 1976.

504. Goldman FD, Dayton PD, Hanson CJ: Renal cell carcinoma and osseous metastases. Case report and literature review. *J Am Podiatr Med Assoc* 79:618-625, 1989.

505. Cayla J, Rondier J, Forest M: Bone metastases of colonic and rectal neoplasms. Apropos of 11 cases. *Semin Hop Paris* 51:507-518, 1975.

506. Ihle PM, McBeath AA: Bone metastases from colonic carcinoma. *J Bone Joint Surg* 55A:398-399, 1973.

507. Harkonen M, Olin PE: Rectal carcinoma metastasizing to a toe. *Act Med Scand* 207:235-236, 1980.

508. Sworn MJ, Buchanan R, Moynihan FJ: Rectal carcinoma presenting as massive metastatic involvement of foot bones. *Br Med J* 2:98-99, 1978.

509. Ameratunga R, Daly M, Caughey DE: Metastatic malignancy associated with reflex sympathetic dystrophy. *J Rheumatol* 16:406-407, 1989.

510. Ghandur-Mnaymneh L, Mnaymneh W: Solitary bony metastasis to the foot with long survival following amputation. *Clin Orthop* 166:117-120, 1982.

511. Paul GR, Leach RE, Beetham WP: Pulmonary carcinoma metastasis to great toe. *JAMA* 208:2163-2164, 1969.

512. Mathiesen B, Hejgaard N: Lungekarcinommetastaser til foden. En sjaelden arsag til fodsmerter. *Ugeskr Laeger* 142:1223-1224, 1980.

513. Mulvey RB: Peripheral bone metastases. *Ther Nucl Med* 91:155-160, 1969.

514. Liszka G, Peter Z, Herics I: Rare localization of bone metastases by patients with primary mamma carcinoma. *May Traumatol Orthop Helyreallito Sebesz* 23:64-69, 1980.

515. Rosen A, Halperin N, Halevi A: A rare metastasis from breast adenocarcinoma to the big toe. *Orthop Rev* 14:429-431, 1985.

516. Morrissey K, Ward MD, Stadecker MJ: Metastatic sweat gland carcinoma in an adolescent. A case report. *Foot Ankle* 9:96-100, 1988.

517. Weitzner S: Adenoid cystic carcinoma of submaxillary gland metastatic to great toe. *Ann Surg* 41:655-658, 1975.

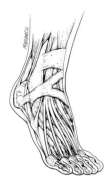

CHAPTER 47

Congenital Deformities of the Forefoot

James L. Bouchard, D.P.M.

The purpose of this chapter is to discuss congenital anomalies involving the foot. Emphasis is on the clinical evaluation and treatment of the more common congenital anomalies rather than the genetic considerations. The highlights of this chapter include the following: congenital underlapping (varus) toe; congenital overriding fifth toe; valgus deformity of the distal phalanx (hallux abductus interphalangeus); polydactyly; polymetatarsia; syndactyly; macrodactyly; brachymetatarsia; and miscellaneous other congenital deformities.

CONGENITAL UNDERLAPPING TOE

Definition

Congenital underlapping (varus) toe is a general term used to describe a common congenital occurrence in which one or more of the lesser toes deviate medially under the adjacent toe. Anatomically the toe in this condition is plantarflexed, medially deviated, and shows a varus rotation, usually at the level of the distal interphalangeal joint. In the more severe deformity both the distal and proximal interphalangeal joints may be involved. These deformities may involve any of the lesser toes and often occur bilaterally (Figs. 47.1 and 47.2).

Historical Review

Historically, the literature is sparse for such a common congenital deformity. Trethowan (1) described the congenital underlapping or varus toe as a congenital form of hammer toe. Sweetnam (2) used the term *congenital curly toe* to describe the condition. Sweetnam also observed that the con-

genital curly toe tends to worsen with growth and does not correct spontaneously.

Etiology

The exact cause of congenital underlapping toes (varus toes) is uncertain. Some authors suggest the condition is caused by hypoplasia of the intrinsic muscles of the affected toe (2, 3).

Gamble and Yale (4) suggested that underlapping toes are caused by ligamentous restrictions present at birth that usually respond to conservative splinting of the infant's toe with adhesive tape.

In Yale's observation (5), the feet of many children and adults were characterized by a hypermobile deformity of the lesser toes that leads to the formation of underlapping and overlapping digits.

The deformity may also be acquired because of abnormal foot type aggravated by foot gear. Common forms of digital deformities that tend to be acquired include mallet toes, claw toes, and hammer toes, which are described elsewhere in this textbook.

Clinical Presentation

Congenital underlapping or varus toe is usually a bilateral and symmetrical deformity. This condition has a high familial incidence and usually becomes exaggerated with growth and development (3). Figure 47.3 depicts the case of a 7-year-old boy with painful bilateral overlapping third

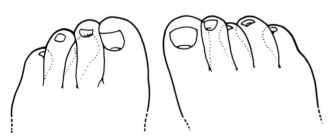

Figure 47.1. Congenital underlapping (varus) toes.

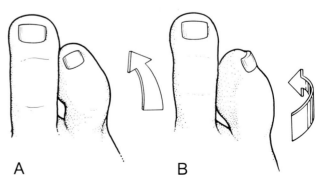

Figure 47.2. Congenital underlapping (varus) fifth toe. **A.** Adductus type rotated fifth toe. **B.** Adductovarus type rotated fifth toe.

and fourth digits corrected by arthroplasty of the head of the middle phalanges. The surgical correction of varus toes is commonly performed in conjunction with a skin plasty to help derotate the digit. The amount of deformity will determine not only the amount of bone to be resected but the size of the skin wedge to be removed.

Treatment

The treatment of congenital underlapping toes varies with the degree of deformity as it relates to the biomechanics of the foot, age of the patient, and the symptoms. According to Tachdjian (3), if the deformity is mild and there is no impingement of the curly toe on the adjacent toe, then the condition may be ignored and no treatment is necessary. Disabling symptoms are more likely to occur later in life when the underlapping toe develops symptoms because of shoe pressure. This is particularly true for women who wear high-heeled shoes.

The treatment of the congenital underlapping or varus toe may be divided into conservative and surgical treatment. Most authors agree that early recognition of the deformity and appropriate treatment are essential in obtaining the maximum correction.

The success of conservative care of these deformities depends on the proper foot gear to provide sufficient room for function of the deformed toes (5). The use of orthodigital corrective or accommodative devices has been advocated in allowing for maximum function within the limits of the deformity (6). Budin (7), Polokoff (8), Whitney (9), McGlamry and Kitting (10), Rosoff (11), Roven (12), and others have demonstrated the importance of orthodigital corrective forces as a conservative approach to this deformity. Turner (13), in a retrospective review of 24 children (44 toes), demonstrated improvement with strapping of curly toes in 68% of the cases while strapping was maintained. A significant loss of correction was found when strapping was discontinued. He concluded that strapping was of little benefit in the treatment of persistent curly toe deformity. In the severe deformity, he recommended surgical correction at a young age in order to prevent symptoms later in life. Marr (14) described the use of toe buttressing using silicone rubber filler under and between the toes as a wedge to help straighten toes and to aid in the propulsive phase of gait. The buttress also helps to straighten flexible digital deformities, relieving pain associated with shoe pressure.

The surgical treatment of these deformities consists of a combination of surgical intervention and digital splinting to maintain correction. The surgical treatment may include many techniques such as tendon Z-plasty, extensor tendon lengthening, tendon transfers, tenotomy, tenectomy, capsulotomy, arthroplasty, syndactylization, partial phalangectomy, or middle phalangectomy of the involved digits (5).

A common and an effective surgical correction of underlapping or varus fifth toe consists of arthroplasty of the proximal interphalangeal joint or partial phalangectomy using two semielliptical oblique skin incisions. This procedure is diagrammatically illustrated in Figure 47.4. Middle phalangectomy combined with skin plasty is an effective surgical procedure for correction of the elongated underlapping digit. Friend (15) described the surgical correction as a procedure that is not technically difficult and may readily be performed on an outpatient basis.

In children, Kelikian (16) recommends syndactylization of the curly toe to the medial side of the adjacent toe. In adults, he recommends partial phalangectomy with surgical syndactylization of the adjacent toe.

Other authors have described tendon transfers of the flexor digitorum longus tendon of the curly toe to the dorsal and lateral aspect of the extensor hood (17, 18).

In the long-standing underlapping or varus toe, bony involvement of the proximal interphalangeal joint, middle phalanx, and distal phalanx is usually evident. This deformity requires a surgical approach that provides exposure to the dorsal, lateral, and plantar aspect of the toe. McGlamry (19) and Korn (20) described a lazy-S approach for correction of the painful underlapping fifth digit. The lazy-S incisional approach has been used with success when the deformity involves multiple levels at the proximal, middle, and distal phalanges of the fifth digit.

VALGUS DEFORMITY OF THE DISTAL PHALANX OF THE HALLUX

Definition

Valgus deformity of the distal phalanx of the hallux is a relatively common congenital deformity. The condition can be defined anatomically as a valgus or lateral deviation deformity of the distal phalanx of the great toe. Other authors have described the deformity as hallux abductus interphalangeus or ungual phalanx valgus (3) (Fig. 47.5).

Historical Review

Historically, valgus deformity of the distal phalanx (hallux abductus interphalangeus) is commonly seen in mature feet. This deformity is less evident in infants and young children. Gillett (21) conducted a survey in 1978 comparing the incidence of ungual phalanx valgus (hallux abductus interphalangeus) among neonates with a random sample of adult females. His findings indicate that the presence of a valgus

Figure 47.3. Surgical correction of congenital underlapping (varus) toes third and fourth toes. **A.** Preoperative right foot. **B.** Postoperative right foot. **C.** Preoperative left foot. **D.** Postoperative left foot. **E.** Preoperative radiograph of left foot. **F.** Preoperative radiograph of right foot. **G.** Postoperative film at 2 weeks after surgical correction. **H.** Postoperative films of both feet, at 2½ years. **I.** Postoperative long-lasting clinical correction of curly toe deformity at 2½ years.

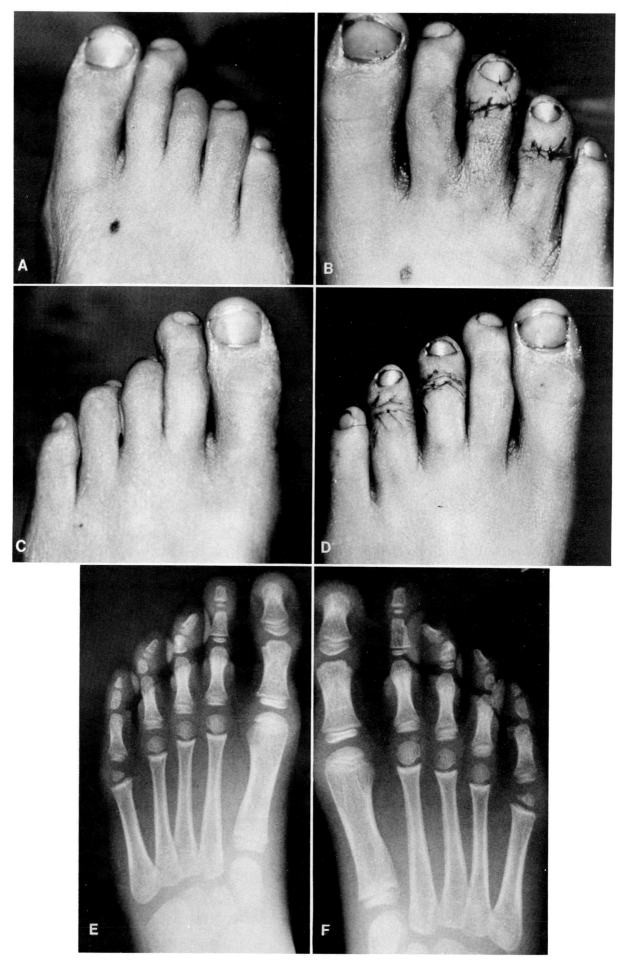

Figure 47.3. A-F.

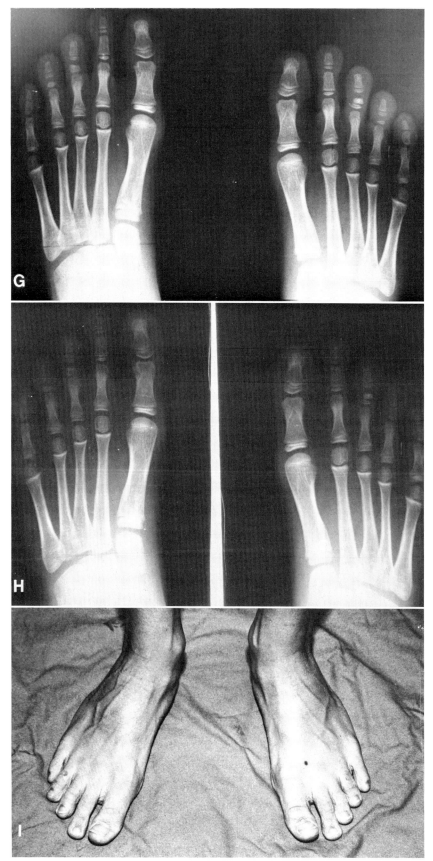

Figure 47.3. G-I.

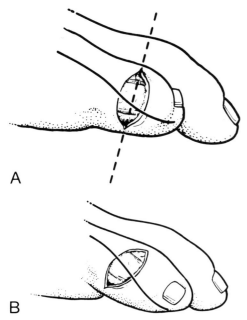

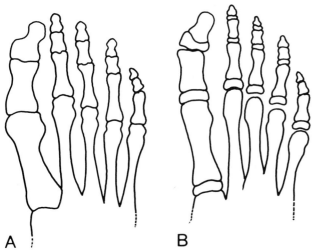

Figure 47.4. Diagrams demonstrating placement of skin wedges in surgical correction of underlapping or varus fifth toe. **A.** Adductus type rotated fifth toe. **B.** Adductovarus type rotated fifth toe.

Figure 47.5. Illustration of valgus deformity of distal phalanx of hallux in adult foot **(A)** and in pediatric foot **(B)**. (Modified from Tachdjian MD (ed): *Pediatric Orthopedics*, vol 2. Philadelphia, WB Saunders, 1972, p 1427.)

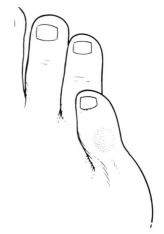

Figure 47.6. Diagram of congenital overlapping fifth toe with hyperextension and adduction of the overlapping toe across the adjacent toe.

with certain foot types accounts for the higher incidence of the deformity in the adult population.

Etiology

The exact cause of a valgus deformity of the distal phalanx is unknown. Several authors suggest the deformity may result from asymmetrical overgrowth of the medial portion of the epiphysis of the distal phalanx of the great toe (3, 21).

Treatment

The treatment of a valgus deformity of the distal phalanx of the hallux depends on many factors, including the age of the patient, the degree of deformity, and the symptoms. In the pediatric patient, according to Tachdjian (3), "If symptoms warrant treatment, the bony protuberance is excised and growth of the medial half of the growth plate is arrested. In the skeletally mature foot, the interphalangeal joint of the great toe is fused in correct alignment following partial excision of the hypertrophied medial portion of the epiphysis." Other surgical considerations include a closing wedge osteotomy to realign the phalanx (3, 21). The use of the Akin osteotomy for correction of hallux abductus interphalangeus is discussed elsewhere in this textbook.

CONGENITAL OVERLAPPING TOES

Definition

Congenital overlapping toe is a general term to describe a common congenital occurrence in which one toe lies on the dorsal aspect of an adjacent toe. Other authors have described this condition when it affects the fifth toe as congenital digitus minimus varus or congenital dorsal overriding of the fifth toe (3). The condition may affect any toe; however, fifth toe overlapping of the fourth toe is the most common. Overlapping of the second toe over the great toe

deformity of the distal phalanx of the hallux (ungual phalanx valgus) in neonates is uncommon (9%) whereas more than one half of the adults examined exhibited the deformity. Gillett's findings suggest that a valgus deformity of the hallux (hallux abductus interphalangeus) may be congenital; however, more often the deformity is acquired because of foot gear and foot type, which may predispose the distal phalanx to deforming stress during early childhood development. Gillett suggests that this stress from foot gear

is the second most common congenital overlapping toe deformity and is described elsewhere in this text. Anatomically, the deformity occurs as hyperextension and adduction of the overlapping toe across the adjacent toe (Fig. 47.6).

Historical Review

Lapidus (22) in 1942 and Lantzounis (23) in 1940 suggested that overlapping toes may be a hereditary condition and described various tendon transplantation procedures to correct the overlapping fifth toe deformity.

Numerous surgical procedures have been described in the literature for the correction of overlapping toes. Kelikian (24) and Tachdjian (3) provide rather detailed reviews of the literature, outlining the various surgical procedures that range from simple, but often unreliable, soft tissue procedures to the once common surgical treatment of amputation of the digit.

Clinical Presentation

Congenital dorsal overriding fifth toe is a common familial deformity. This condition is usually bilateral and can cause pain and disability as the result of shoe pressure and irritation. In this condition the fifth toe is hyperextended and adducted, lying on the dorsal aspect of the fourth toe. The capsule of the metatarsophalangeal joint is contracted on the dorsomedial aspect, causing the toe to be displaced dorsomedially. Secondary shortening of the extensor tendon and skin on the dorsal aspect of the fifth toe, with rotation of the fifth toe about its longitudinal axis, is characteristic. The resulting irritation by shoe pressure often causes disability requiring surgical correction of the deformity.

Treatment

Most authors agree that conservative treatment of the overlapping fifth toe in the infant and young child is indicated;

Figure 47.7. Diagram of surgical correction of congenital overlapping fifth toe. **A.** Placement of retraction sutures in fourth and fifth toes. **B.** Placement of vertical and horizontal interdigital web space skin incisions. **C.** Excision of triangular patches of skin. **D.** Capsular incisions at both joint levels. **E.** Resection of proximal phalanx. **F.** Final skin closure. (Modified from Tachdjian MD (ed): *Pediatric Orthopedics*, vol 2. Philadelphia, WB Saunders, 1972, pp 1418-1419.)

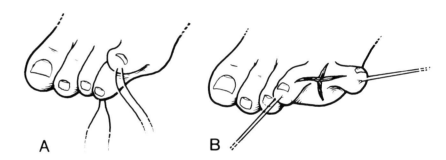

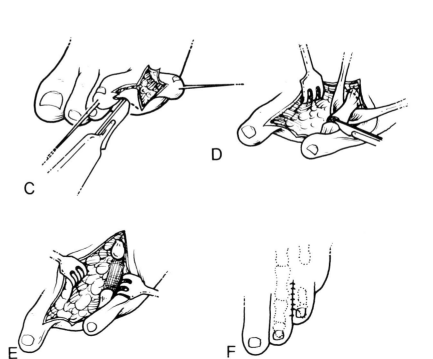

however, the results are varied and usually do not maintain correction of the deformity. Giannestras (25) described the use of adhesive tape splinting that is changed daily by the parents as a conservative method of treatment in the infant and younger child. Many conservative methods of treatment of overlapping and underlapping toes are modifications of the elastic toe slings described by Budin (7).

Jordan and Caselli (26) described a simple and effective modification of the Giannestras adhesive splint for correction of the overlapping and underlapping digit in the pediatric patient. Although their method using one-half inch cohesive gauze, flexible collodion, and tincture of benzoin compound is not new, it permits the maintenance of corrective forces to the digit for an extended period of time.

As mentioned previously, many procedures have been used in attempting surgical correction of the overlapping fifth toe. Tachdjian (3) recommends the procedure outlined by McFarland (1950) and Scrase (1954), which was described and illustrated by Kelikian (24) in 1965. The operative technique is described in detail by Tachdjian as follows (Fig. 47.7).

Attention is directed to the fourth and fifth toes where retraction sutures are passed through the ends of each toe to allow retraction and exposure of the interdigital web space (Fig. 47.7A). One incision is placed vertically running dorsal to plantar to bisect the interdigital web space between the adjacent toes. Second and third skin incisions are placed horizontally to the first incision, one from the lateral aspect of the fourth toe and the other from the medial aspect of the fifth toe crossing the vertical incision in the web space (Fig. 47.7B). The triangular patches of skin are excised, providing excellent exposure to the deeper subcutaneous structures while preserving the neurovascular status to the toes (Fig. 47.7C). Dissection is then extended proximally along the course of the long extensor tendon isolating the proximal phalanx through incisions in the joint capsules at the level of the metatarsophalangeal joint and proximal interphalangeal joint (Fig. 47.7D). The proximal phalanx is then excised (Fig. 47.7E), and the remaining long extensor tendon is transferred to the fifth metatarsal head. The skin incisions are sutured together, bringing the toes together in a corrected position (Fig. 47.7F). The foot is immobilized in a below-knee walking cast, with the toes held in their corrected position with bandaging for 4 weeks.

Another common and rather successful procedure for correction of the overlapping fifth toe is the Butler procedure recommended by Cockin (27) as a simple and safe procedure capable of full correction of the deformity. The Butler procedure for correction of overlapping fifth toe, which is also described by Tachdjian (3), is performed through a dorsal racquet-shaped incision with an arm extending to the plantar aspect of the fifth metatarsophalangeal joint. A dorsomedial capsulotomy and Z-plasty extensor tendon lengthening or tenotomy are performed, exposing the fifth metatarsal head. Any plantar adhesions of the capsule are released, and the fifth toe alignment is corrected. The mechanics of correction of the overlapping fifth toe is diagrammatically illustrated in Figure 47.8.

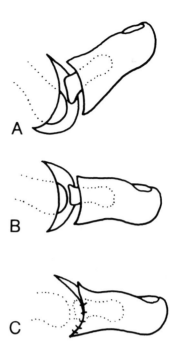

Figure 47.8. Diagrammatic illustration of mechanics of correction of overlapping fifth toe. **A.** Release of dorsal contracted structures. **B.** Release of plantar adhesions. **C.** Final skin closure with corrected alignment of deformity without tension. (Modified from Cockin J: Butler's operation for an overriding fifth toe. *J Bone Joint Surg* 50B:78-80, 1968.)

Cockin reported good results in 90% of the patients, fair in 6%, and poor in only 3%. Care must be taken by the surgeon during dissection to avoid vascular compromise to the toe. Many modifications of these procedures have been used in the surgical correction of the overlapping fifth toe. Procedures involving arthroplasty of the proximal interphalangeal joint, Z-plasty extensor tendon lengthening, metatarsophalangeal joint releases, and excision of plantar wedges of skin have proved to be the most effective and successful in the correction of this deformity. The importance and effectiveness of combining release procedures with the corrective forces of plantar skin wedges are demonstrated in Figures. 47.9 to 47.11.

SYNDACTYLY

Definition

Syndactyly is a congenital anomaly characterized by persistent webbing between adjacent digits. Most of the literature describes syndactyly involving the hands, which is not only a cosmetic problem but can be a severe functional problem. Syndactyly of the toes usually is not a functional problem but rather a cosmetic concern, with possible psychological effects.

Many authors have classified syndactyly as an inheritable or a developmental webbing of the digits (28). Davis and German (29) further divided syndactyly into four major categories as follows: (*a*) incomplete, when the webbing be-

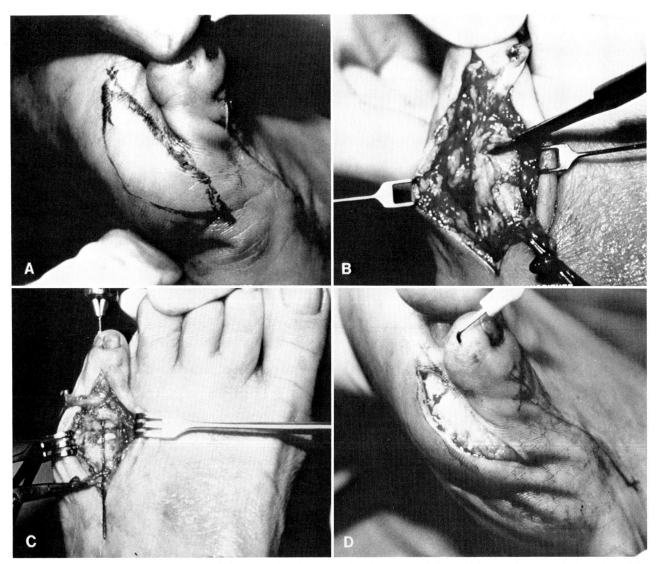

Figure 47.9. Surgical correction of overlapping fifth toe. **A.** Arthroplasty of the proximal interphalangeal joint. **B.** Z-plasty extensor tendon length-ening. **C.** Metatarsophalangeal joint capsulotomy and release. **D.** Excision of planar wedge of skin to correct soft tissue deformity.

tween two digits does not extend to the distal aspect of the digits, (*b*) complete, when the webbing extends to the distal ends of the digits, (*c*) simple, when the phalanges are not involved, and (*d*) complicated, when the phalanges are involved and are abnormal.

Etiology

Congenital syndactyly is described by most authors as a her-itable deformity or as a developmental defect occurring be-tween the sixth and eighth weeks of fetal life. Embryolog-ically, the limb buds appear during the fourth week, with a connecting band of tissue between each digit developing around the fifth week. At this time the digits are all webbed,

and during the seventh to eighth week rapid growth occurs because the digits grow much more rapidly than the inter-digital webbing. Most investigators agree that rapid arrest of normal embryological development at this time will lead to syndactyly. The exact cause of the arrested development is unknown (28, 30, 31).

Figure 47.12 illustrates the development of limb buds between the fifth and eighth weeks of fetal development (32).

In normal development the webbing between the second and third toes is the last to disappear, and those toes are considered to be the most sensitive digits to any arrest in development. This may explain why syndactyly involving the second and third toes is the most frequent type of the abnormality found in the foot (29).

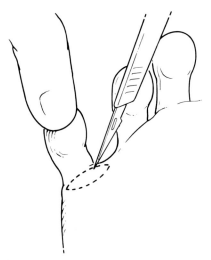

Figure 47.10. Placement of plantar skin wedge.

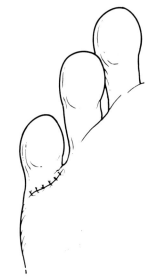

Figure 47.11. Closure of plantar skin wedge with correction of deformity.

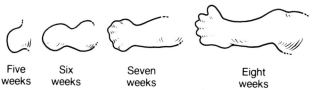

Five   Six   Seven   Eight
weeks   weeks   weeks   weeks

Figure 47.12. Development of lower extremity limb buds between fifth and eighth weeks of fetal development. (Modified from Arey SB: *Developmental Anatomy—a Textbook and Laboratory Manual of Embryology*, ed 7. Philadelphia, WB Saunders, 1966, p 210.)

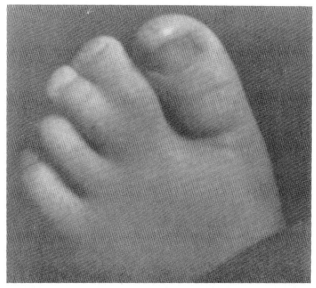

Figure 47.13. Preoperative photograph of left foot with syndactyly of second and third digits. (From Coleman WB, Kissel CG, Sterling HD Jr: Syndactylism and its surgical repair. *J Am Podiatry Assoc* 71:547, 1981.)

Clinical Presentation

The patient usually views syndactyly of the toes as a cosmetic concern rather than a functional problem. Most authors, including Gates (33) and Malhorta and Riffe (34), agree that the most frequent syndactylism of the foot occurs between the second and third toes. Davis and German (29) investigated 50 cases of syndactyly involving the hands and feet and found that syndactyly of the toes alone occurred in 11 cases (22%), with most of these cases involving the second and third toes.

Syndactyly of the hand has been associated with many other abnormalities, including syndactyly of the feet, cleft palate, Apert's syndrome, Poland's syndrome, brachydactylia, polysyndactyly, talipes equinovarus, dysplasia of the long bones, and many others (35).

Most authors agree that the incidence of syndactyly varies from 1/1000 to 1/3000 live births. MacCollum (36) stated that syndactyly of the fingers and toes occurs in 1/2000 to 1/2500 live births. Most authors indicate a higher incidence of syndactyly in male patients. Barsky (37) reported a male incidence of syndactyly of 56%, whereas Davis and German (29) reported 68%, and Nylen (38) reported an incidence of 84%. Bunnell (39) reported that bilateral syndactyly occurs with an incidence of 50%. Similarly, Skoog (40) reported an incidence of bilateral syndactyly of 36%.

Treatment

Surgical correction of syndactyly can be a major challenge to the surgeon. Although syndactyly of the toes is usually asymmetrical and creates no functional problems, the emotional and psychological problems can be of great concern.

Coleman and associates (28) present a case of syndactyly of the second and third toes. They discuss in detail the problems encountered in surgical desyndactylization, as well as the goals of surgical intervention, as follows:

Figure 47.14. Surgical correction of syndactyly. **A.** Syndactyly of second and third digits. **B.** Proposed skin incisions drawn on dorsum of syndactylized toes with two triangular flaps medially and three laterally. Placement of needles from dorsal to plantar to ensure proper interposition of skin flaps. **C.** Proposed skin incisions drawn on plantar of syndactylized toes. **D.** With scalpel in zigzag pattern, dorsal incision is made along solid lines and plantar incision is made along broken lines. **E.** Suturing of dorsal and plantar skin flaps in corrected desyndactylized position. (Modified from Coleman WB, Kissel CG, Sterling HD Jr: Syndactylism and its surgical repair. *J Am Podiatry Assoc* 71:547-548, 1981.)

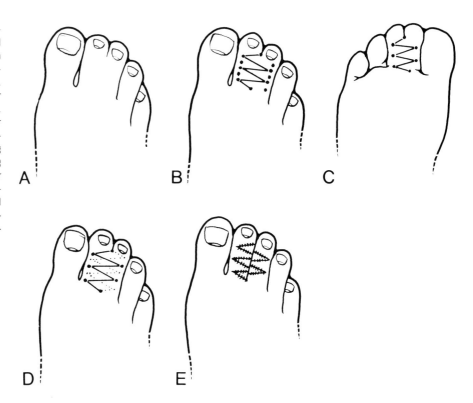

The goals of surgical desyndactylization of simple incomplete syndactyly are threefold: 1) To provide adequate coverage of adjacent surfaces of the fingers or toes, 2) To prevent flexion contracture as a result of the cicatrization process, and 3) To form a commissure or groove at the base of the digits. All three goals must be achieved in order to prevent recurrence or unacceptable results."

Coleman and associates (28) also described elective surgery to correct syndactylized second and third toes bilaterally in a 4½-year-old white male as follows (Figs. 47.13 and 47.14A).

With the use of general anesthesia and a pneumatic tourniquet attention is directed to the right foot. A skin scribe is used to draw the proposed skin incisions on the dorsum of the syndactylized toes in such a way as to create two triangular flaps medially and three laterally (Fig. 47.14B). At the bases of each triangle, as well as at the most proximal and most distal aspects of the incision line, 27-gauge needles are placed from the dorsal to the plantar aspect of the syndactylized toes. This provides proper positioning for the apices of the plantar incision, which are correspondingly marked with the skin scribe (Fig. 47.14 B and C). A scalpel is used in a zigzag pattern to make dorsal and plantar incisions (Fig. 47.14D). Skin flaps are undermined with the scalpel, and the toes are carefully separated along tissue planes, using great care to preserve the neurovascular status of the toes. Following hemostasis and flushing of the wound with sterile saline solution, the dorsal and plantar skin flaps are apposed and sutured into place using apical sutures of 5-0 Vicryl simple interrupted sutures (Fig. 47.14E). The same skin plasty and desyndactylization were performed on the left foot. Total primary closure at the base of the second toe on the left foot was not possible, and this small defect was left to granulate in. Figures 47.15 and 47.16 demonstrate excellent postoperative results at 3 months.

The major surgical complications following desyndactylization have been inadequate skin coverage and secondary digital contracture caused by scar formation. Most authors agree that the zigzag or modified Z-plasty procedures have helped to minimize these complications. Weinstock and associates (41) have more recently described a desyndactylization that they report to be surgically less complicated and technically easier to perform. The surgical procedure is outlined as follows (Fig. 47.17).

The surgical approach is through a linear longitudinal incision placed midway through the syndactylized skin extending dorsally to plantarly. To create a normal web space the dorsal incision extends more proximally than does the plantar incision. The vascular structures are preserved during dissection and hemostasis obtained by clamping and coagulating all bleeders (Fig. 47.17B).

Following interdigital dissection and separation of the syndactylized digits, a template (Fig. 47.17 *a* to *d*) is fabricated from sterile paper that approximates the size necessary for a full-thickness graft to fill the surgical defect between the adjacent digits (Fig. 47.17 a_1 to d_1).

The full-thickness graft is then obtained from the lateral aspect of the foot just inferior to the lateral malleolus. The dorsomedial aspect of the foot or other areas of skin redundancy may also be used as donor sites (Fig. 47.17D). With the use of the template to determine the exact size of the graft, the full-thickness graft is obtained through two semielliptical incisions and kept moist in normal saline so-

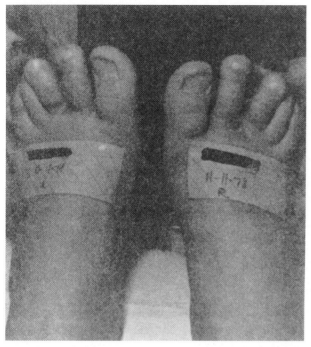

Figure 47.15. Dorsal view, 3 months after surgery. (From Coleman WB, Kissel CG, Sterling HD Jr: Syndactylism and its surgical repair. *J Am Podiatry Assoc* 71:549, 1981.)

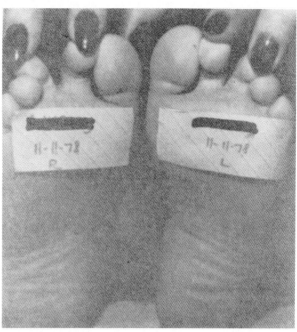

Figure 47.16. Plantar view, 3 months after surgery. (From Coleman WB, Kissel CG, Sterling HD Jr: Syndactylism and its surgical repair. *J Am Podiatry Assoc* 71:549, 1981.)

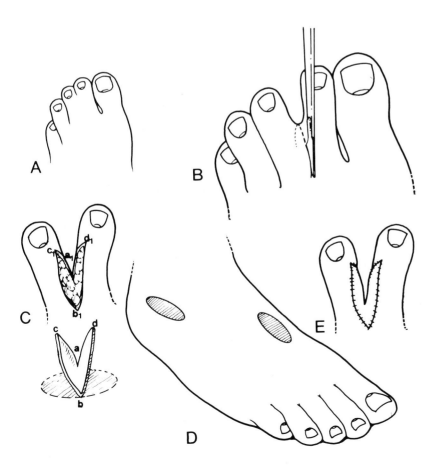

Figure 47.17. Surgical modification of desyndactylization. **A.** Syndactyly of second and third digits. **B.** Placement of linear longitudinal incision extending dorsally to plantarly midway through syndactylized skin. **C.** Fabrication of sterile paper template to approximate size of full-thickness skin graft to fill surgical defect between adjacent digits. **D.** Potential full-thickness skin graft donor sites. **E.** Final closure of full-thickness skin graft into skin defect between desyndactylized digits. (Modified from Weinstock RE, Bass SJ, Farmer MA: Desyndactylization—a new modification. *J Am Podiatry Assoc* 74:458-461, 1984.)

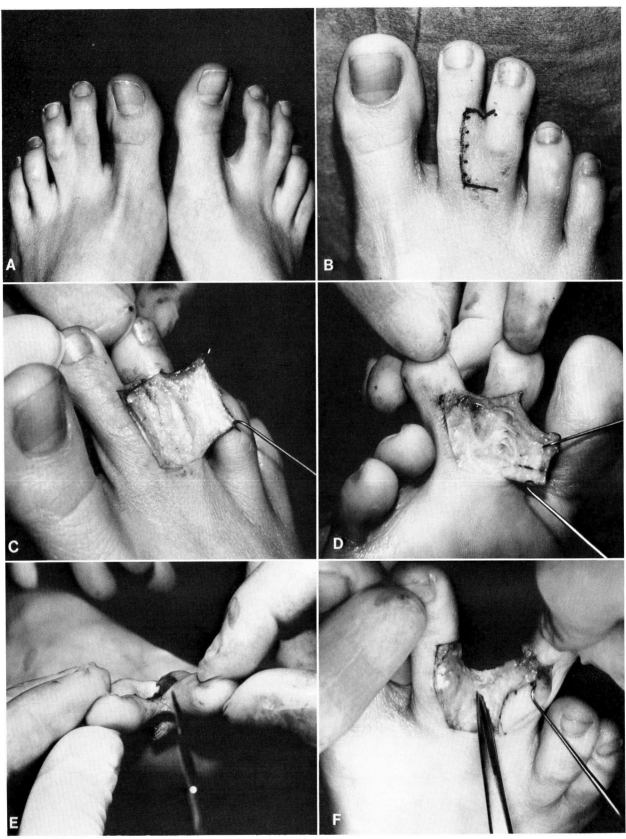

Figure 47.18. Surgical correction of bilateral incomplete simple syndactyly type 1 of the second and third toes. **A.** Preoperative appearance of deformity. **B.** Marking of the dorsal skin flap with base of flap on third toe dorsally. **C.** Careful dissection and retraction of dermal-superficial fascial junction preserving the neurovascular structures. **D.** Dissection and retraction of plantar skin flap with base of flap on second toe plantarly. **E.** Web space incision. **F.** Careful blunt dissection of web space to preserve neurovascular supply to the toes. **G.** Positioning of the plantar skin flap on second toe. Note the triangular defect at the base of the web space. **H.** Positioning of the dorsal skin flap on the third toe. **I.** Immediate postoperative result, with defect of the web space covered by a proximally based rotational skin flap from dorsum of foot. **J.** Immediate plantar postoperative result, with skin flap sutured with 6-0 nylon suture. (Courtesy of A. L. Jimenez.)

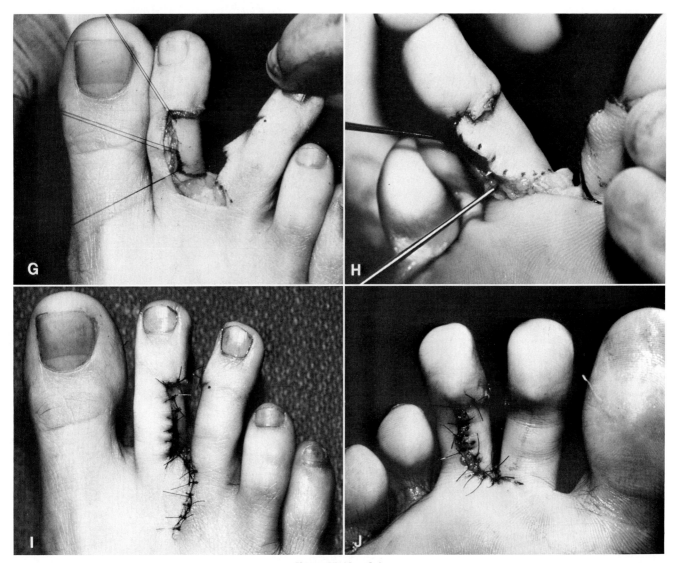

Figure 47.18.   G-J.

lution. The donor site is reapproximated in a plastic fashion.

The full-thickness skin graft is placed into the skin defect between the desyndactylized digits. With use of simple interrupted sutures of 5-0 monofilament nylon, the suturing of the flap begins with one suture placed dorsally and a second plantarly. The skin graft is sutured in place radiating outward from the central suture and alternating dorsal to plantar to ensure more even tension on the skin graft. The ends of each suture are kept long to provide for easier retraction and better visualization of the graft site. Before final closure the excess skin is trimmed from the graft tips, which are carefully sutured in place, avoiding excessive tension on the skin flap (Fig. 47.17E).

Castellano (42) describes a case of syndactyly involving the second and third toes corrected with the use of combined dorsal and plantar skin flaps. With careful planning, pri-

mary closure of the skin and flaps may be obtained, and skin grafting is usually unnecessary (Fig. 47.18).

Morreale and associates (43) present a case of complicated incomplete syndactylism corrected by desyndactylization without using skin grafts. The surgical method creates a commissure using a dorsal V-flap skin incision with the base proximal to form a web space. The web is divided plantarly, and the apex forms the commissure as it is brought plantarly. This technique works especially well in syndactylism of the fourth and fifth digits when supernumerary bones are surgically removed.

Rosen and associates (44) present a case of synpolydactyly, which is a form of syndactyly associated with duplication of a portion or an entire digit. This condition usually involves the fourth and fifth toes. An alternative procedure is shown in Figure 47.19, which demonstrates surgical desyndactyli-

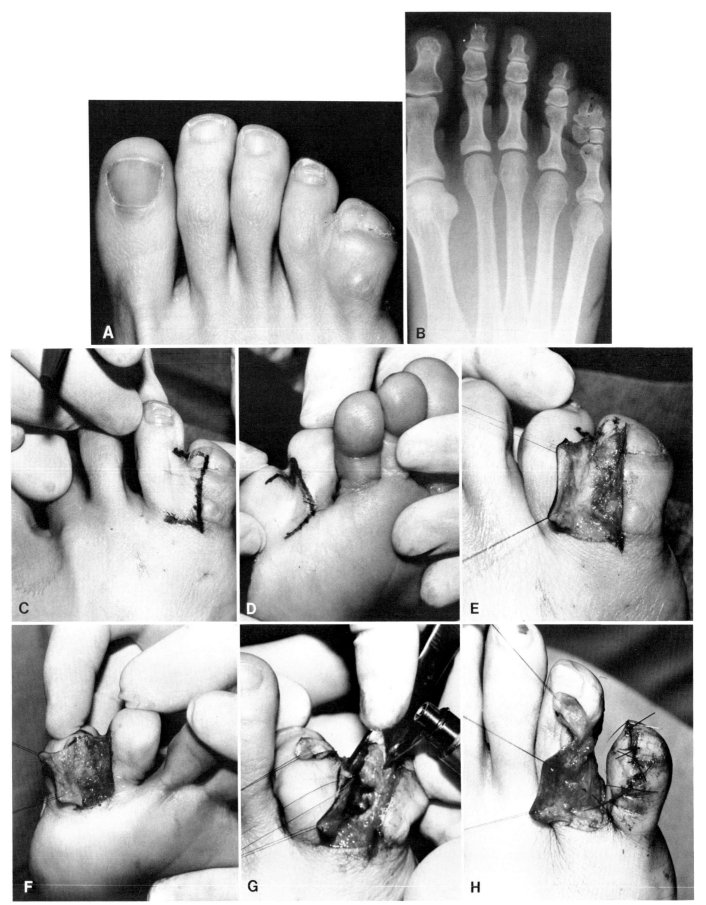

Figure 47.19.   A-H.

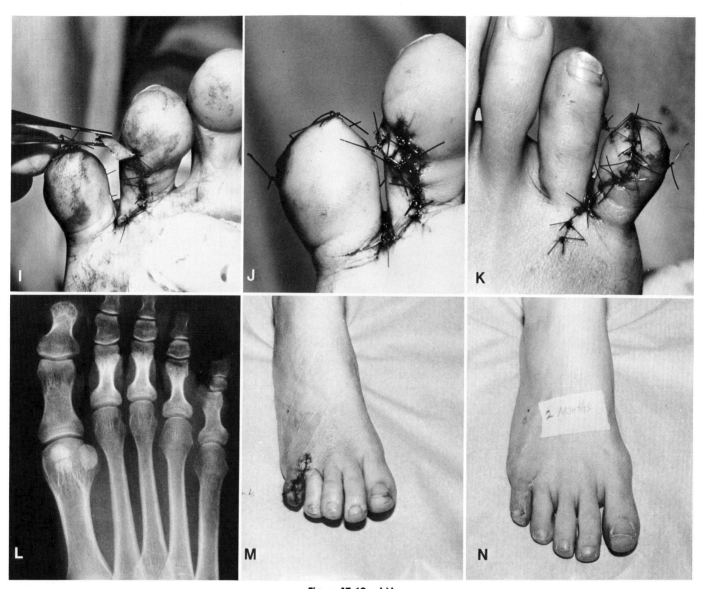

Figure 47.19.   I-N.

Figure 47.19.   Surgical correction of complicated complete syndactyly, or type 2 syndactyly, involving the fourth and fifth toes. **A.** Preoperative clinical appearance of the deformity. **B.** Radiographs demonstrating complete duplication of the middle and distal phalanges of the fifth digit. **C.** Skin marking for dorsal skin flap with base of flap on fourth digit dorsally. **D.** Skin marking for plantar dorsal skin flap with base of flap on fifth toe plantarly. **E.** Dissection and retraction of dorsal skin flap to provide skin coverage on lateral aspect of desyndactylized fourth digit. Note redundant nail tissue removed from dorsal lateral aspect of skin flap. **F.** Dissection and rotation of plantar skin flap to provide skin coverage of medial aspect of desyndactylized fifth toe. **G.** Resection of accessory middle and distal phalanges with power instrumentation. **H.** Skin closure of plantar skin flap with 6-0 nylon suture to cover medial wound defect, fifth toe. **I.** Skin closure of dorsal skin flap with 6-0 nylon suture to cover lateral wound defect, fourth toe. **J.** Final skin closure following desyndactylization, plantar aspect. **K.** Final skin closure following desyndactylization, dorsal aspect. Note proximally based rotational skin flap to lose dorsal defect at web space. **L.** Postoperative film following desyndactylization and resection of accessory middle and distal phalanges. **M.** Desyndactylization, dorsal view, 2 weeks after surgery. **N.** Postoperative desyndactylization, dorsal view, at 2 months. (Courtesy of M. Niknafs.)

zation of a complicated complete syndactyly or type 2 syndactyly involving the fourth and fifth toes.

POLYDACTYLY

Definition

Polydactyly, one of the most common congenital anomalies, is characterized by the presence of an accessory, supernumerary, or extra digit. It can occur in a rudimentary form as a hypoplastic digit devoid of osseous structure or as a complete duplication of a fully developed digit or digits. The condition has many variations as to location, morphology, and association with polymetatarsia and other inherited conditions (45).

Historical Review

Polydactyly was classified by Temtamy and McKusick (46) in terms of whether a case of polydactyly was part of a syndrome (syndromatic) or an isolated deformity (nonsyndromatic). They further divided polydactyly into the categories of syndromatic and nonsyndromatic according to the anatomical location of the supernumerary or accessory digits as either preaxial or postaxial (Fig. 47.20).

Postaxial Polydactyly

Postaxial polydactyly (fifth digit duplication) was further classified by Temtamy and McKusick into types A and B. Type A refers to a true postaxial polydactyly characterized by a fully developed accessory digit that articulates with either the fifth metacarpal or metatarsal or with a duplicated fifth metacarpal or metatarsal. Type B refers to postaxial polydactyly characterized by an accessory digit devoid of osseous tissue, which represents a vestigial or rudimentary digit (Fig. 47.20).

Polydactyly may be present in a variety of forms, ranging from a rudimentary hypoplastic digit devoid of osseous structure to a fully developed accessory digit with complete duplication. Temtamy and McKusick's classification of poly-

dactyly into types A and B (46) fails to classify the wide range of intermediate forms of polydactyly between a rudimentary digit devoid of osseous structure and a completely duplicated digit. Venn-Watson (47) further divided postaxial polydactyly into five specific morphological patterns based on the degree of metatarsal duplication, from the least differentiated to the most differentiated as follows: soft tissue duplication, wide metatarsal head, T-metatarsal, Y-metatarsal, and complete duplication (Fig. 47.21).

Preaxial Polydactyly

Preaxial polydactyly (first digit duplication) involving the foot is rare and not well documented compared with preaxial polydactyly of the hand, which is more common. Temtamy and McKusick (46) classified four types of preaxial polydactyly of the hand: type 1, polydactyly of the first digit; type 2, polydactyly of a triphalangeal first digit; type 3, polydactyly of the second digit; and type 4, polysyndactyly.

Preaxial polydactyly of the metatarsals and toes is not well documented, and the four types of preaxial polydactyly are more commonly used in describing polydactyly of the hand. Many authors consider this classification less applicable to polydactyly of the foot (46, 47).

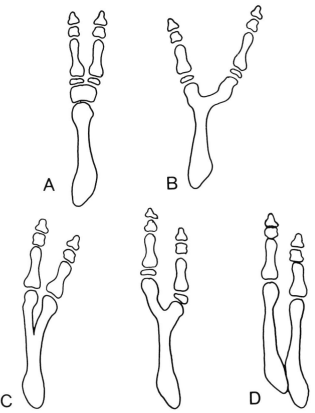

Figure 47.21. Venn-Watson classification of postaxial polydactyly. **A.** Wide metatarsal head. **B.** T-metatarsal. **C.** Y-metatarsal. **D.** Complete duplication. (Modified from Venn-Watson EA: Problems in polydactyly of the foot. *Orthop Clin North Am* 7:909, 1976.)

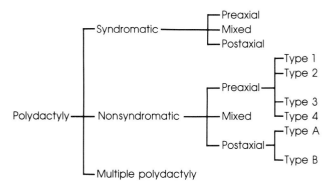

Figure 47.20. Classification of polydactyly. (Modified from Temtamy SA, McKusick VA: Synopsis of hand malformations with particular emphasis on genetic factors. *Birth Defects* 3:125, 1969.)

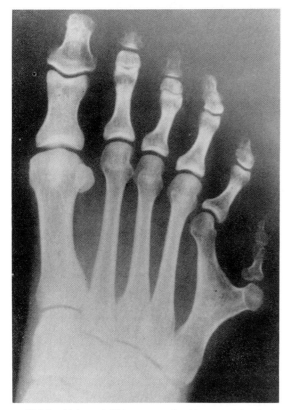

Figure 47.22. Y-shaped fifth metatarsal with postaxial polydactyly. (From Knecht JG: Polydactyly of the foot. *J Foot Surg* 22:24, 1983.)

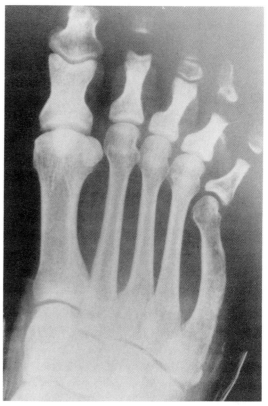

Figure 47.23. Postoperative x-ray film of surgical correction of Y-shaped fifth metatarsal with postaxial polydactyly. (From Knecht JG: Polydactyly of the foot. *J Foot Surg* 22:26, 1983.)

Etiology

Because polydactyly is genetically heterogenous, the primary cause of polydactyly appears to be genetic. Most authors suggest that the different types of polydactyly represent distinct genetic entities (48, 49). Castilla (50), Woolf and Myrianthopoulous (51), and Milles (48) described distinct differences of the inheritance patterns between types A and B postaxial polydactyly. Temtamy and McKusick (30) suggest that types A and B polydactyly represent completely different genetic entities inherited as irregular autosomal dominant traits. Castilla (50) determined that postaxial type A polydactyly occurs most commonly in the foot, and postaxial type B polydactyly more commonly involves the hand.

TREATMENT

The treatment of polydactyly varies with the degree and type of deformity. Despite the wide variety and types of polydactyly most authors agree that in the patient with symptoms the primary treatment for polydactyly is surgical removal. Each case should be carefully evaluated as to function, cosmetic effect, and effect on type of foot gear.

Knecht (52) presented two cases of polydactyly involving three types. One patient had postaxial polydactyly of the right foot with a Y-shaped fifth metatarsal, as illustrated in

the preoperative (Fig. 47.22) and the postoperative x-ray films (Fig. 47.23). In addition, this patient had postaxial polydactyly involving a wide fifth metatarsal head of the left foot. Figure 47.24 demonstrates the preoperative appearance of the deformity, and Figure 47.25 depicts the surgical correction. Figure 47.26A demonstrates the preoperative x-ray film of a patient with incomplete syndactyly-polydactyly of the fifth toe. The postoperative x-ray films are demonstrated in Figure 47.26B.

Green and associates (53) presented a case of polydactyly outlining in detail the surgical considerations, surgical plan, and postoperative considerations for correction of the more common condition of postaxial polydactyly (Fig. 47.27).

SURGICAL CONSIDERATIONS

One of the main surgical considerations in the treatment of polydactyly is to remove anomalous structures so that the appearance of the foot will be as near normal as possible. Skin incisions must be planned to leave skin borders of equal length and shape to promote plastic skin closure without skin redundancy or dermal tags. The skin incision should be planned to prevent the formation of the scar over pressure areas, particularly avoiding bony prominences. In polydactyly and polymetatarsia of the fifth toe and fifth meta-

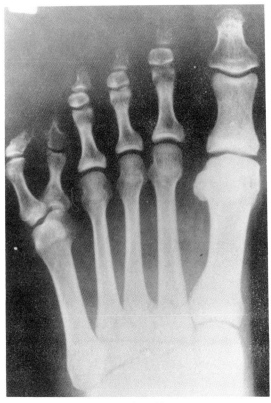

Figure 47.24. Preoperative x-ray film of foot, with postaxial polydactyly with wide fifth metatarsal head. (From Knecht JG: Polydactyly of the foot. *J Foot Surg* 22:24, 1983.)

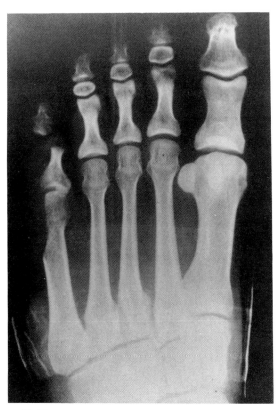

Figure 47.25. Postoperative x-ray film following surgical correction of postaxial polydactyly with wide fifth metatarsal head. (From Knecht JG: Polydactyly of the foot. *J Foot Surg* 22:26, 1983.)

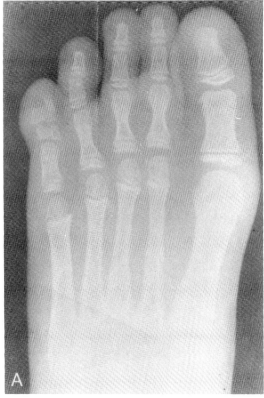

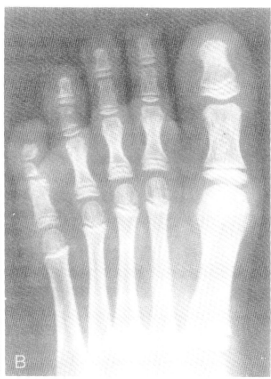

Figure 47.26. **A.** Preoperative x-ray film of foot with incomplete syndactyly-polydactyly of fifth toe. **B.** Postoperative x-ray film of surgical correction of syndactyly-polydactyly of fifth toe. (From Knecht JG: Polydactyly of the foot. *J Foot Surg* 22:27, 1983.)

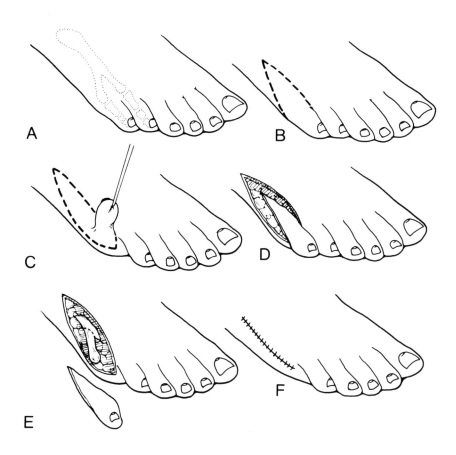

Figure 47.27. Surgical correction of polydactylism with Y-shaped fifth metatarsal and extra sixth digit. **A.** Diagram of clinical appearance of deformity. **B.** Placement of dorsal and plantar skin incision equal in length. **C.** Reflecting of sixth toe, demonstrating proposed skin incisions in web space. **D.** Deepening of skin incisions and soft tissue dissection to underlying bone. **E.** Proposed resection of sixth metatarsal and sixth toe. **F.** Final skin closure and correction of polydactylism. (Modified from Green DR, Ruch JA, Butlin WE: Polydactylism repair. *J Am Podiatry Assoc* 66:304-309, 1976.)

tarsal it is important not only to preserve the vascular supply to the fifth toe but also to allow thick dermal tissue closure over the lateral aspect of the fifth metatarsal when removing bone (Fig. 47.27A). It is also important to transect bone at its junction, avoiding the complication of cortical splitting. Attention to careful surgical dissection and preservation and repair of the periosteal tissue over the denuded bone will help in preventing regeneration.

SURGICAL PLAN

The surgical approach to correction of polydactyly of the fifth digit is through an initial skin incision extending through the dermis from the medial plantar aspect of the fifth web space dorsally to the fifth intermetatarsal space. The second incision is horizontal extending from the medial plantar fat pad in the web space to the sixth metatarsal head. The second incision should be equal in length to the initial incision. The initial incision should then be extended proximally to the lateral border of the base of the fifth metatarsal, whereas the second incision should be extended proximally to connect with the original incision so as to equal in length the extension of the original incision (Fig. 47.27B). To ensure preservation of the lateral vasculature to the fifth toe the medial dermal tissue is undermined approximately 3 mm (Fig. 47.27C).

The incisions are deepened to the dorsolateral aspect of the sixth metatarsal bone, and the soft tissue is dissected

from the underlying bone (Fig. 47.27D). The extensor to the sixth toe is transected at the level of the metatarsal shaft. The periosteum of the anomalous metatarsal is incised dorsally and reflected, identifying the junction of the fifth metatarsal and the anomalous sixth metatarsal. The sixth metatarsal is removed flush with the fifth metatarsal with an oscillating power saw to prevent cortical splitting (Fig. 47.27E). The redundant metatarsal shaft is dissected free from the surrounding tissues and excised in toto. The flexor tendon of the sixth toe is incised at the level of the base of the proximal phalanx. Thus the toe and the proximal, middle, and distal phalanx are removed as a unit (Fig. 47.27E). All redundant tissue is excised followed by closure of the periosteal tissue over the denuded bone. The cutaneous tissue is approximated, and any redundant subcutaneous tissue is excised before final skin closure. If the incisions have been made correctly, (*a*) the two skin margins will be of equal length and shape, (*b*) the lateral aspect of the fifth metatarsal will be covered with thick dermal tissue originally located beneath the sixth metatarsal head, and (*c*) the final scar will be distal and dorsal to the fifth metatarsal head and shaft and therefore away from any area of potential pressure. The subcutaneous tissue is closed with 3-0 absorbable continuous interlocking suture. The skin is closed with multiple 6-0 nonabsorbable simple interrupted sutures (Fig. 47.27F). Postoperative ambulation is allowed in a surgical shoe as tolerated on the second postoperative day. Skin sutures are removed 14 days after surgery. Usually the patient

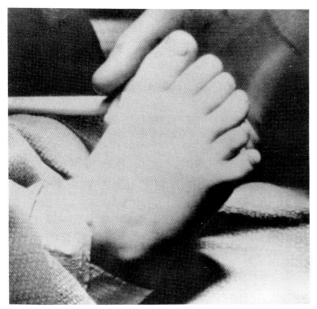

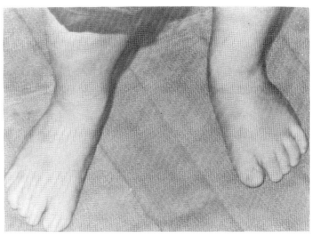

Figure 47.29. Clinical appearance 6 months after surgical correction of polydactyly. (From Green DR, Ruch JA, Butlin WE: Polydactylism repair. *J Am Podiatry Assoc* 66:308, 1976.)

Figure 47.28. Preoperative clinical appearance of case of polydactyly. (From Green DR, Ruch JA, Butlin WE: Polydactylism repair. *J Am Podiatry Assoc* 66:304, 1976.)

Figure 47.30. Brachymetatarsia affecting the fourth metatarsal and associated digit. (From McGlamry ED, Cooper CT: Brachymetatarsia: a surgical treatment. *J Am Podiatry Assoc* 59:259, 1969.)

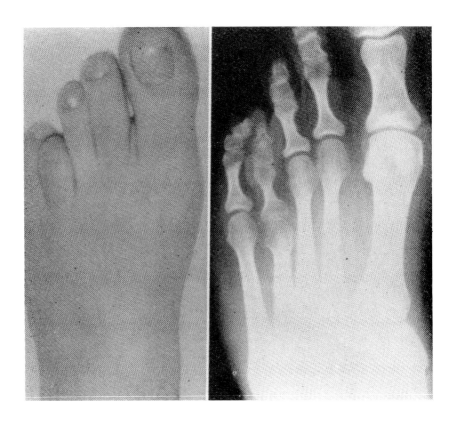

returns to a closed shoe in 3 to 4 weeks following surgery. Figure 47.28 demonstrates the preoperative clinical appearance of a patient with polydactyly and polymetatarsia. The postoperative result is demonstrated in Figure 47.29.

BRACHYMETATARSIA

Definition

Brachymetatarsia is a hereditary anomaly characterized by premature closure of the epiphyseal plate of one or more metatarsals. This condition most commonly affects the fourth metatarsal, but it can affect any or multiple metatarsals (Figs. 47.30 and 47.31). Brachymetatarsia may be present unilaterally or more commonly bilaterally. The condition has also been described as a short metatarsal or as a hypoplastic metatarsal. Brachymetatarsia can be a congenitally, developmentally, surgically, or traumatically induced deformity (54).

Historical Review

Historically, brachymetatarsia may be idiopathic or can be associated with congenital anomalies, Down's syndrome, Albright's hereditary osteodystrophy, osteodystrophy, diastrophic dwarfism, multiple epiphyseal dysplasia, myositis ossificans, Turner's syndrome, pseudohypoparathyroidism, pseudo-pseudohypoparathyroidism, and poliomyelitis. In poliomyelitis, the shortened fourth metatarsals were pri-

marily asymmetrical, involving only the paralyzed limb (55). The correlation between these medical disorders and brachymetatarsia is not clearly understood. Kite (56) states that "the shortening is due to premature fusion of the epiphyseal line at the distal end of the metatarsal and occurs most often in the fourth metatarsal." McGlamry and Cooper (57) add that "a short metatarsal segment may result in over-

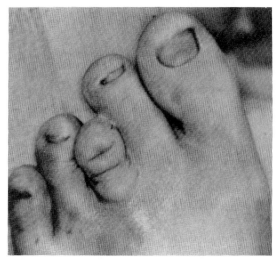

Figure 47.31. Brachymetatarsia affecting third metatarsal and associated digit. (From Jimenez AL: Brachymetatarsia: a study in surgical planning. *J Am Podiatry Assoc* 69:246, 1979.)

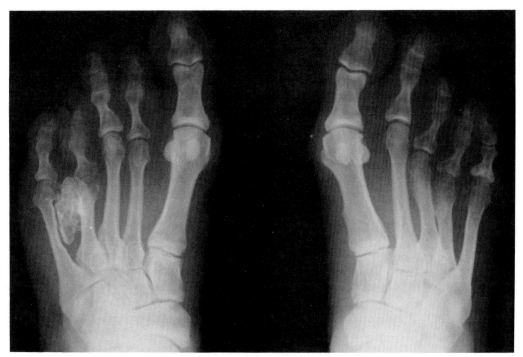

Figure 47.32. X-ray film of unusual case of brachymetatarsia of third and fourth metatarsals of right foot and shortening of second and fourth metatarsals of left foot. Note osseous growth on left foot that was found to be benign after removal. (Courtesy of Henry A. McAninch.)

loading adjacent metatarsals which then react as long metatarsals." Inman (58) concurs: "It results in excessive loading of the adjacent segments with consequent plantar callus."

Although the fourth metatarsal is most commonly short, occasionally brachymetatarsia may involve two or more metatarsals. When the condition affects more than one metatarsal, it is known as brachymetapody (Fig 47.32).

Brachymetatarsia of the third and fourth metatarsals is frequently the result of pseudohypoparathyroidism or chromosomal abnormalities of the trisomy 21 pattern. Also, it is possible that a neurotrophic disorder or injury to the distal epiphysis could cause early union of the epiphyseal plate, causing cessation of metatarsal growth (59). Yale (60) reports on the common early union of epiphyses resulting from the accumulation of x-ray exposure.

Etiology

Most authors suggest that brachymetatarsia may be produced by premature closure of the epiphysis of a metatarsal. The exact cause of early epiphyseal closure of the metatarsal is unknown (54, 60). Brachymetatarsia may be congenital, developmental, postsurgical, or posttraumatic (54, 61, 62). It can be associated with many conditions.

Clinical Presentation

Brachymetatarsia is usually not seen at birth but becomes clinically evident in children between the ages of 4 and 15 years. It is more common in females with a female to male ratio of 25 : 1 (63, 64). The premature closure of the epiphysis results in early union and cessation of metatarsal growth. The result of an abnormally short metatarsal is both clinically and radiographically evident as a short metatarsal with an associated shortened and contracted toe (60, 61). The final diagnosis is confirmed by radiographical examination.

The signs and symptoms vary with the degree of deformity, age, and sex of the patient. In the younger patient, especially in females, the major concern may be cosmetic or psychological. Self-consciousness and concern over the appearance of the deformity can be a major psychological problem when the patient wears open-toed shoes or goes barefoot. The older patient experiences pain more often because the deformity causes excessive loading of the adjacent metatarsals, with associated plantar callus formation or metatarsalgia. These symptoms are more common in the obese patient or in the patient who has long periods of standing, lifting, or walking. In addition to plantar callus under adjacent metatarsals, the shortness of the metatarsal can cause overlapping of the associated toe of the short metatarsal on an adjacent toe. Over a period of time this overlapping can cause soft tissue changes resulting in contracture of the extensor tendons, flexor tendons, and skin. The resulting deformity can cause pain and discomfort when the individual wears foot gear (Fig. 47.33). The floating toe syndrome is characteristic of brachymetatarsia as the unstable digit is shortened and contracted over the short-

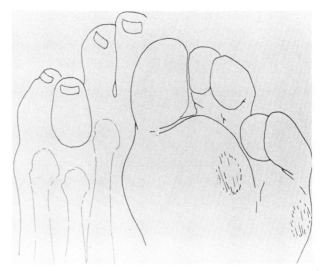

Figure 47.33. Illustration demonstrating effects of shortened metatarsal on adjacent toes, causing painful plantar callus. (From McGlamry ED, Cooper CT: Brachymetatarsia: a surgical treatment. *J Am Podiatry Assoc* 59:259, 1969.)

ened metatarsal. The resultant instability affects gait and the ability of the digit to purchase the ground, creating the resultant floating toe appearance.

Conservative Treatment

The treatment of brachymetatarsia may vary with the degree of metatarsal shortening, symptoms, age, and activity of the patient. Essentially the treatment may be divided into conservative care and surgical correction. Conservative care consists of palliative care or the use of orthotic or accommodative devices in the shoe to redistribute stresses so that they will be removed from the adjacent metatarsal heads. Conservative treatment will not solve the cosmetic, psychological, or underlying anatomical and structural problems of the deformity.

Soft Tissue Correction

Soft tissue correction associated with a shortened metatarsal must be carefully achieved. Various soft tissue techniques include V-Y skin plasty (Fig. 47.34) to correct skin contractures. Typically, the long extensor is lengthened by open Z-plasty or slide Z-plasty lengthening. The short extensor in most cases is sectioned. The dorsally displaced digit cannot be positioned without appropriate capsulotomy of the metatarsophalangeal joint, including dorsal, medial, and lateral releases of the capsule. To allow metatarsal lengthening, the deep transverse intermetatarsal ligament is sectioned to distally lengthen the metatarsal and the associated digit. Great care, with use of atraumatic technique and anatomical dissection, is necessary to ensure preservation of neurovascular structures.

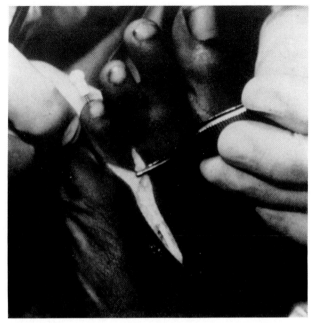

Figure 47.34. V-Y skin plasty was necessary to reduce skin tension in contracted fourth digit. (From McGlamry ED, Fenton CF III: Brachymetatarsia: a case report. *J Am Podiatry Assoc* 73:76, 1983.)

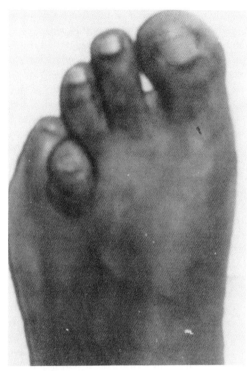

Figure 47.35. Preoperative clinical appearance of brachymetatarsia with associated contracted fourth toe. (From McGlamry ED, Fenton CF III: Brachymetatarsia: a case report. *J Am Podiatry Assoc* 73:76, 1983.)

Osseous Correction

The goal of the osseous component of brachymetatarsia surgery is to help restore a more normal metatarsal parabola. Historically, the objective has been accomplished by either lengthening or plantarflexing the involved metatarsal or shortening or dorsiflexing the adjacent metatarsal(s). In more severe instances, a panmetatarsal head resection with associated arthrodesis of the proximal phalanges of the second, third, and fourth digits, combined with total implant arthroplasty of the first metatarsophalangeal joint, has provided a desirable postoperative result.

Martin and Kalish (65) classify lengthening procedures for the treatment of brachymetatarsia into four major groups as follows:

1. Single metatarsal osteotomy with bone graft
2. Combined lengthening and shortening metatarsal osteotomies with bone graft
3. Metatarsal osteotomy with insertion of synthetic implant
4. Slide lengthening metatarsal osteotomies with/without bone grafting.

SINGLE METATARSAL OSTEOTOMY WITH BONE GRAFT

Many different surgical alternatives have been presented and discussed previously in the treatment of brachymetatarsia. The surgical correction of brachymetatarsia includes a combination of soft tissue and osseous correction tech-

niques. McGlamry and Cooper (57) described a surgical correction of brachymetatarsia using an autogenous cylindrical bone graft from the calcaneus as a metatarsal neck graft in an 18-year-old female patient. They recommend an inlaid autogenous or homologous bone graft as the preferred method of lengthening a short metatarsal. Jimenez (66) and McGlamry and Fenton (67) described separate cases of brachymetatarsia that were surgically corrected using an autogenous inlaid bone graft, providing not only a good cosmetic result but an excellent functional result. A description of the procedure, as performed on a 12-year-old female (67), follows.

The patient complained of a painful shortened fourth toe of the left foot, which had stopped growing. The examination revealed a cleft beneath the fourth metatarsal with a markedly contracted fourth toe (Fig. 47.35). Radiographical examination confirmed the diagnosis of brachymetatarsia with complete and premature closure of the epiphyseal plate of the fourth metatarsal (Fig. 47.36).

A 3-cm incision was placed over the upper third of the tibia, medial to the tibial crest, to obtain an autogenous bone graft. The incision was deepened to the level of the periosteum, which was incised and reflected. With use of an oscillating bone saw a 25-mm autogenous bone graft was obtained.

Attention was then directed to the dorsal aspect of the left foot where a 6-cm linear longitudinal incision was placed over the fourth metatarsal. The incision began at the mid-diaphysis and extended distally to the web space of the fourth and fifth toes. The contracted tendon of the extensor digitorum longus to the fourth toe was identified and a Z-plasty tendon lengthening performed. Dissection was continued deeper to the level of the periosteum of the fourth metatarsal, which was incised and reflected. The fourth metatarsal was divided at the distal third of the shaft with use of an oscillating saw. To provide distal distraction of the digit a 0.045-inch Kirschner wire (K-wire) was driven into the metatarsal head and through the base of the proximal phalanx distally through the distal aspect of the digit. With the autogenous bone graft in proper position, the K-wire was driven proximally through a predrilled canal in the bone graft and subsequently into the proximal portion of the metatarsal shaft. Extreme care was taken to avoid trauma and stretching of the digit and adjacent soft tissues. Intraoperative radiographs revealed adequate alignment (Fig. 47.37).

The periosteum was closed with 3-0 absorbable interlocking continuous sutures. The extensor tendon was repositioned in a corrected and lengthened position and repaired with 3-0 absorbable simple sutures. The subcutaneous tissue was closed with interlocking continuous absorbable sutures. In this case the skin over the fourth metatarsophalangeal joint appeared tight dorsally, which required a V-Y skin plasty to reduce the tension dorsally on the digit (Fig. 47.34). Final skin closure was accomplished in a plastic fashion using a 5-0 or 6-0 absorbable suture.

After surgery the patient abstained from weight bearing for 2½ months, at which time the cast was removed. Postoperative radiographs at 4 months revealed excellent healing (Fig. 47.38). Figure 47.39 shows a long-term postoperative radiograph at 15 months demonstrating excellent correction and lengthening of the shortened fourth metatarsal.

COMBINED LENGTHENING AND SHORTENING METATARSAL OSTEOTOMIES

Handelman and associates (68) describe a modification for restoring metatarsal length using a lengthening allogeneic bone graft of the fourth metatarsal, combined with shortening osteotomies of the adjacent third and fifth metatarsals, establishing good alignment and restoration of the normal metatarsal parabola. Hosokawa and Susuki (69) describe bilateral brachymetatarsia of the first and fourth metatarsals. In this case, the surgeons chose not to lengthen the first metatarsal but to shorten the metatarsals involving the second and third metatarsals, using an allogenic bone graft taken from a section of the fourth metatarsal.

Chairman and associates (70) describe a correction of

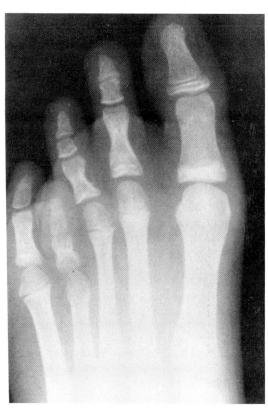

Figure 47.36. Preoperative x-ray film reveals short fourth metatarsal with complete closure of epiphyseal plate. (From McGlamry ED, Fenton CF III: Brachymetatarsia: a case report. *J Am Podiatry Assoc* 73:76, 1983.)

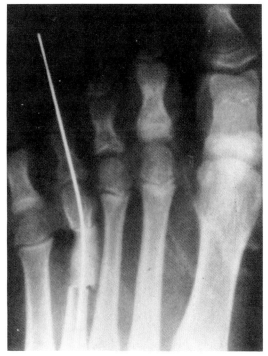

Figure 47.37. Intraoperative x-ray film reveals bone graft held in place with K-wire, with adequate alignment of metatarsal parabola. (From McGlamry ED, Fenton CF III: Brachymetatarsia: a case report. *J Am Podiatry Assoc* 73:76, 1983.)

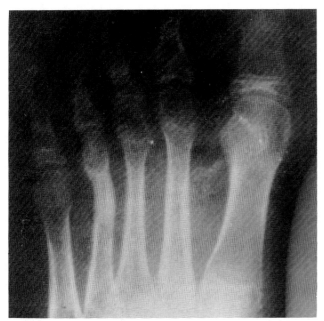

Figure 47.38. X-ray film appearance 4 months after surgery. (From McGlamry ED, Fenton CF III: Brachymetatarsia: a case report. *J Am Podiatry Assoc* 73:77, 1983.)

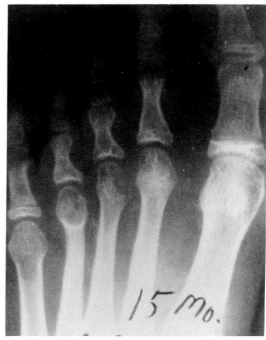

Figure 47.39. X-ray film appearance 15 months after surgery demonstrating that graft has been fully incorporated, with restoration of metatarsal length. (From McGlamry ED, Fenton CF III: Brachymetatarsia: a case report. *J Am Podiatry Assoc* 73:77, 1983.)

brachymetatarsia using transplantation of a portion of the fifth metatarsal shaft and head to the shortened fourth metatarsal. The results provided better alignment of the fourth digit following surgery.

METATARSAL OSTEOTOMY WITH INSERTION OF SYNTHETIC IMPLANT

Page and associates (71) present a unique case involving brachymetatarsia involving the fourth metatarsal combined with familial absence of the middle phalanges. In this case, a double-stemmed prosthetic joint was used as a spacer in lengthening the shortened digit. In most cases, joint implants serve simply as a spacer and not a functional correction to a structural deformity such as brachymetatarsia.

Yonenobu and associates (72) describe elongation of a shortened metatarsal bone using intercalar implantation with a ceramic implant in two patients with brachymetatarsia. They conclude that the ceramic implant can be a useful substitute for a bone graft because of its strength and biocompatibility.

SLIDE LENGTHENING METATARSAL OSTEOTOMIES

Tabak and associates (73) present a case of brachymetatarsia of the second metatarsal corrected surgically using a metatarsal slide lengthening procedure without bone grafting. This procedure is a modification of the Giannestras step-down procedure.

Martin and Kalish (65) describe a two-stage surgical technique for correction of brachymetatarsia, which corrects the

obvious structural deformity as well as the soft tissue contractures associated with this deformity. The technique described includes the use of an external fixator, which provides gradual distraction of the metatarsal segments following osteotomy. Over a period of 3 or 4 weeks, the desired length is obtained, and the second stage of the surgery, incorporating the bone graft and internal fixation, is performed.

Marcinko and associates (74) describe a modification of the Giannestras step-down osteotomy to lengthen a posttraumatic case of brachymetatarsia. In this case, after elongation, the osteotomy is reduced with two parallel K-wires fixating the metatarsal transversely. Bone grafting was not used in this case. Slide lengthening without bone graft should be reserved for a mild to moderate deformity not requiring excessive lengthening.

Martin and Kalish (65) describe the two-stage surgical technique for correction of brachymetatarsia as follows.

First Stage

The purpose of the first stage is to effectively prepare the involved metatarsal for lengthening by mobilizing periarticular soft tissues, including vital neurovascular structures. Soft tissue releases are performed through a dorsal incision extended from the midshaft of the metatarsal to the base of the proximal phalanx. The extensor digitorum brevis muscle is identified and transected along with a dorsal, medial, and lateral capsulotomy. The extensor digitorum longus is not lengthened surgically at this time because of possible fibrosis and scarring that may result from the other procedures.

Attention is then directed to the proximal phalanx for insertion of the external fixation device. After adequate exposure of the proximal phalangeal base and shaft of the metatarsal, a 2.7-mm self-tapping pin is inserted into both segments. Once the external frame of the external fixation device is slipped into place and locked over the two pins, several millimeters of traction are added before final closure. Approximately 1.5 mm distraction is applied every day for approximately 2 weeks to ensure adequate soft tissue lengthening without compromising the neurovascular supply. The patient receives careful postoperative follow-up with frequent dressing changes, uses crutches, and observes strict abstinence from weight bearing.

Second Stage

The purpose of the second stage is to effectively lengthen the shortened metatarsal to the desired length once adequate soft tissue lengthening has been obtained. Usually the second stage is performed approximately 3 weeks following the first procedure. The same dorsal skin incision is used, and the external fixation device and pins are removed. The increase in soft tissue lengthening and mobility is dramatically apparent at this time. The extensor digitorum longus is identified and lengthened in an open Z-plasty or slide lengthening fashion. The metatarsophalangeal joint is exposed, and the deep transverse intermetatarsal ligaments are incised to enable final adequate lengthening. At this time, a decision is made concerning which type of metatarsal lengthening will be most appropriate. In most cases, a slide lengthening of the metatarsal with internal fixation using 2.0-mm cortical screws will provide adequate fixation and lengthening. In severe cases, a slide lengthening may be inadequate because the thickness of the shaft of the metatarsal is significantly reduced as the metatarsal is advanced distally, making it highly unstable and prone to fracture. In these cases, the traditional inlaid bone graft is more suitable to ensure adequate lengthening of the metatarsal. Martin

and Kalish (65) described a modified Z-type osteotomy fixated with 2.0-mm screw to achieve greater lengthening and bone to bone contact (Fig. 47.40 A-O). The metatarsal defect, which is left proximally after sliding the metatarsal, is filled with a corticocancellous inlay bone graft fixated with an additional 2.0-mm screw. After surgery, the patient abstains from weight bearing in a below-knee cast and uses crutches for approximately 6 to 10 weeks until there is radiographical evidence of osseous union. Following cast removal, a gradual return to weight bearing will prevent failure or disruption of the bone graft. Usually at the fourteenth to the sixteenth postoperative week, the patient may return to full weight bearing upon evidence of radiographical bone healing.

Results and Discussion

The results of using an autogenous bone graft for the surgical correction of brachymetatarsia have been consistently good in providing an anatomical and functional correction cosmetically acceptable to most patients. When using a bone graft, the surgeon must determine whether to use an autogenous or a homologous bone graft. The autogenous bone graft results in more rapid healing of the graft site; however, it requires a separate incision and procedure for obtaining the graft.

Complications

The inherit potential complications associated with bone grafting techniques are described in detail elsewhere in this text. Complications in correction of brachymetatarsia may include delay of incorporation of the graft, resorption and collapse of the graft site, and painful delayed union or nonunion. Another devastating complication in brachymetatarsia surgery is too aggressive lengthening of the metatarsal with resultant vascular compromise. If excessive distraction is continued for a long period of time, the vessels become constricted, limiting the amount of blood flow to the digit, which may lead to irreversible gangrenous changes. The technique described by Martin and Kalish (65) using a two-

Figure 47.40. Two-stage surgical correction for brachymetatarsia. *A, 1* and *2.* Congenital form of brachymetatarsia with shortened fourth metatarsal and associated forefoot imbalance. **B.** Floating toe syndrome associated with congenital brachymetatarsia of the fourth metatarsal. **C.** Incision marking for surgical correction of brachymetatarsia, extending from the proximal portion of the metatarsal to the metatarsophalangeal joint. **D.** First-stage correction of brachymetatarsia using two separate incisions for placement of external fixation device utilized 2.7-mm self-tapping pins. **E.** Synthes-mini external device with two 2.7-mm self-tapping pins and external frame that slides over the two pins and locks into place with appropriate distraction tension. **F.** Final placement of external fixation device before application of surgical dressing. Note the circular knob in center of the device is adjusted with gradual distraction of the soft tissues. **G.** Application of surgical dressing with careful padding around the fixation device to avoid irritation of the surgical wound. **H.** Postoperative

radiograph at 2 weeks, demonstrating positioning of the external fixator and distraction of the soft tissues in preparation for bone lengthening and grafting. **I.** The extensor digitorum longus tendon to the associated toe is lengthened as part of the second-stage surgery. **J.** Positioning of the frontal plane Z-osteotomy using bone model. **K.** Internal fixation of slide lengthening of the metatarsal, utilizing 2.0-mm cortical screw delivered from a dorsal to plantar position before placement of bone graft proximally. **L.** Placement of allogeneic bone graft in the proximal defect following slide lengthening of metatarsal. Note the graft is fixated with a second 2.0-mm cortical screw in a dorsal to plantar position. **M.** Postoperative radiograph at 6 weeks, demonstrating increase in length of the fourth metatarsal with two 2.0-mm cortical internal fixation screws. **N.** Postoperative radiograph at 12 weeks demonstrating signs of early bone healing. **O.** Postoperative radiograph at 5 months demonstrating complete osseous healing, with correction of the deformity. (Courtesy of D.E. Martin and S.R. Kalish.)

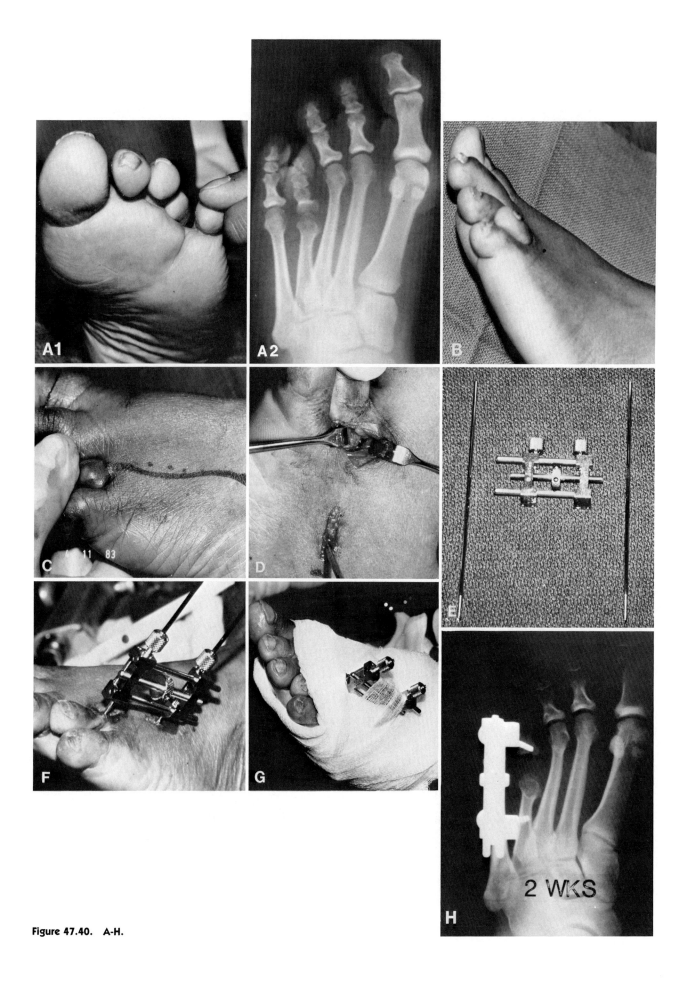

Figure 47.40. A-H.

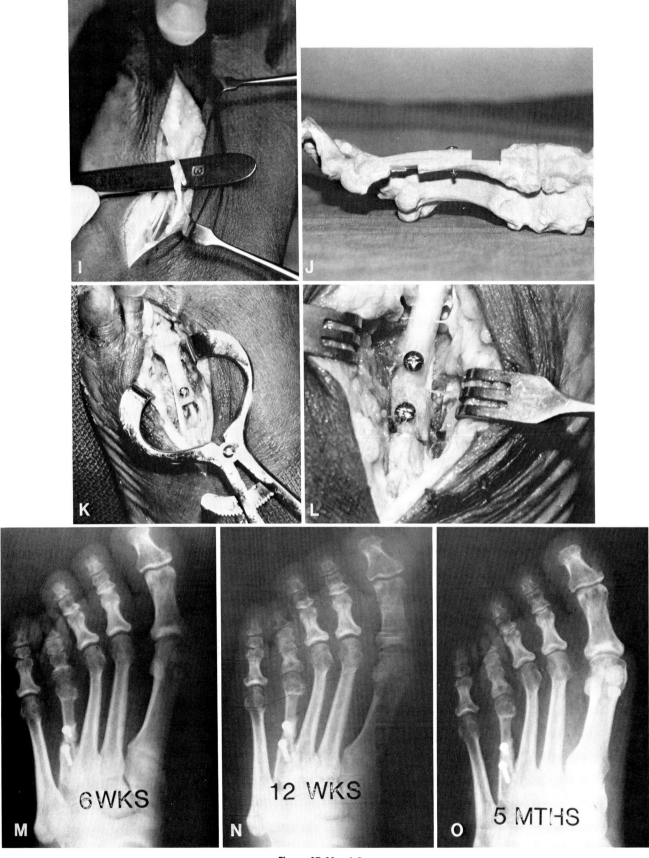

Figure 47.40. I-O.

stage approach helps prevent vascular compromise by mobilizing periarticular soft tissues, including the neurovascular structures.

Another complication, frequently undiagnosed postoperatively, is lesser metatarsophalangeal joint limitus deformity. Excessive lengthening of the metatarsal frequently causes jamming of the metatarsophalangeal joint, with development of lesser metatarsophalangeal joint limitus. This may be prevented by careful preoperative determination of the amount of desired lengthening. Fibrosis and scarring around the metatarsophalangeal joint also may be a cause of restriction of motion and metatarsophalangeal joint limitus. In the hands of the skilled and experience surgeon, brachymetatarsia is a deformity that may be successfully corrected giving the patient not only a cosmetically acceptable result but a good functional result.

MACRODACTYLY

Definition

Macrodactyly is a rare congenital deformity characterized as an overdevelopment of one or more fingers or toes. This condition has also been described as localized gigantism, localized hypertrophy, megalodactyly, and megalodactylia.

Historical Review

Historically, the literature review of macrodactyly relates primarily to macrodactyly of the hands. Barsky (75), in a literature review over the past 180 years, noted 64 cases of macrodactyly. All these cases involved the hand except one that involved the foot. In contrast, Moore (76) and Khanna and associates (77) reported 25 cases of macrodactyly since 1970 that involved the foot and only five cases involving the hand.

Peridive and associates (78) presented a thorough review of the literature, as well as a very rare and severe case of bilateral asymmetrical progressive macrodactyly of the foot. They noted 143 cases of macrodactyly, 38 involving the foot. In the same review, one other case of bilateral asymmetrical macrodactyly of the feet was also reported.

Clinical Presentation

Macrodactyly is a rare deformity present at birth that usually does not become clinically apparent as a grotesque problem until neonatal development. Macrodactyly involves the hands more often than the feet and usually occurs unilaterally, affecting one or more of the digits. The usual presentation is unilateral, multiple digital involvement more commonly affecting one or more of the first, second, or third digits. When more than one digit is involved, they are almost always adjacent. Macrodactyly of the fourth and fifth digits and bilateral cases are extremely rare. A familial history or association with other congenital anomalies is also rare (77). More males have been affected than females by a ratio of 7:5 (75, 79). Barsky (75) recognized two types of macro-

dactyly, the static deformity and the progressive deformity. Other investigators, including Khanna and associates (77), described differences in the clinical presentation of these two types of macrodactyly.

STATIC DEFORMITY

The static deformity is the most common type of macrodactyly present at birth, characterized as an enlarged digit or digits, with a growth rate of the enlarged digit that is proportionate to the growth rate of the patient. Single-digit involvement is more common in the static deformity.

PROGRESSIVE DEFORMITY

The progressive deformity is the much less common type of macrodactyly. It is present at birth and is characterized by a disproportionate growth rate of the enlarged digit or digits until puberty. The progressive deformity, in contrast to the static deformity, is characterized by involvement of multiple digits with hypertrophy proximal to the digits involving the metatarsal and soft tissue (78) (Figs. 47.41 and 47.42).

Etiology

The cause of macrodactyly is uncertain. Many authors suggest the hypertrophy of macrodactyly is related to neurofibromatosis or to congenital hyperplasia of lymphatic and adipose tissue. Presumably the condition is caused by excessive abnormal growth of embryonic tissues of the involved digit (78, 80). Rarely is there a family history of macrodactyly, which suggests that heredity does not play a

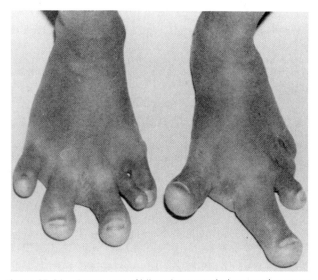

Figure 47.41. *Severe case of bilateral asymmetrical progressive macrodactyly in 7-year-old female. In left foot there is involvement of middle three digits, and in right foot outer three digits are involved. (From Perdive RL, Mason WH, Bernard TN: Macrodactyly: a rare malformation. J Am Podiatry Assoc 69:659, 1979.)*

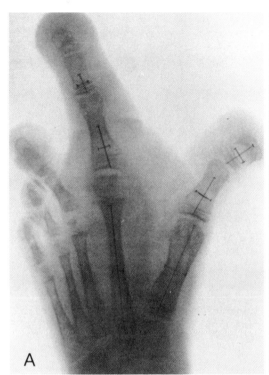
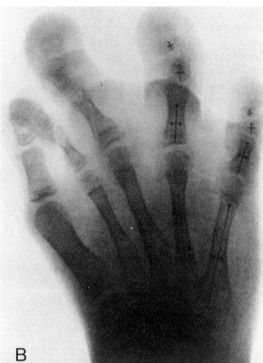

Figure 47.42.   **A.** X-ray film of left foot, demonstrating osseous enlargement of middle three digits. **B.** X-ray film of right foot, demonstrating osseous enlargement of lateral three digits. (From Perdive RL, Mason WH, Bernard TN: Macrodactyly: a rare malformation. *J Am Podiatry Assoc* 69:660, 1979.)

part in this deformity (77). Capel (81) reported macrodactyly to be almost always unilateral and rarely associated with other congenital anomalies.

Treatment

The treatment of macrodactyly is usually surgical and depends on the age, type, and degree of deformity. The usual surgical treatment is amputation; however, occasionally a plastic procedure to reduce the size of the affected digit is preferable in maintaining function. Tsuge (82) describes a multiple stage operation for digital reduction that is suitable for toes (Fig. 47.43).

DeValentine and associates (83) described a two-stage surgical correction for progressive macrodactyly in a 47-year-old female who complained of progressive enlargement of her left foot since birth with associated numbness, shooting pains, and difficulty wearing shoes (Figs. 47.44 and 47.45).

The first-stage surgical correction in this case included resection of the plantar exostosis and excision of the enlarging dorsal soft tissue mass. The large mass of the heterotrophic bone projecting plantarly from several tarsal bones is resected through a lateral plantar incision. Three separate fibrolipomatous masses, approximately 2.5 cm in diameter, were excised through a dorsal curvilinear incision.

The second-stage surgical correction included reduction of the enlarged digits and was performed approximately 5 months later. The objective of the second-stage surgical cor-

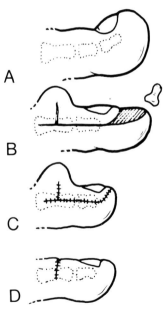

Figure 47.43.   Surgical reduction of macrodactyly of toe. **A.** Deformity with enlargement of bone and soft tissues. **B.** Portion of middle and distal phalanx is excised with proximal retraction of dorsal flap, including nail, to shortened position. **C.** Excision of distal aspect of toe with partial excision of nail. **D.** Excision of redundant skin dorsally with plastic skin closure in corrected position. (Modified from Tsuge K: Treatment of macrodactyly. *Plast Reconstr Surg* 39:590, 1967.)

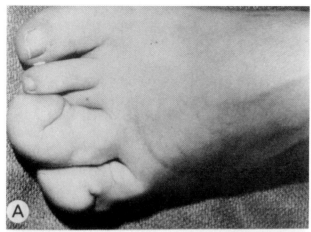

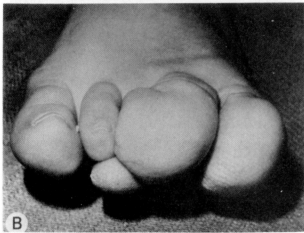

Figure 47.44. Preoperative clinical appearance of left foot, demonstrating grossly enlarged fourth and fifth toes. **A.** Dorsoplantar view of foot. **B.** View from distal aspect of toes. (From DeValentine S, Scurran BL, Tuerk D, Karlin J: Macrodactyly of the lower extremity. *J Am Podiatry Assoc* 71:177, 1981.)

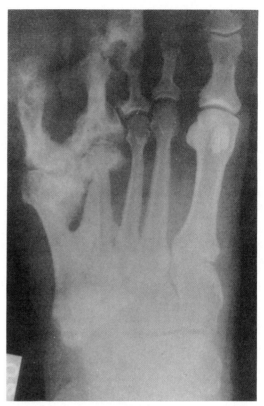

Figure 47.45. X-ray film demonstrating massive bony overgrowth of fourth and fifth metatarsals and associated digits. (From DeValentine S, Scurran BL, Tuerk D, Karlin J: Macrodactyly of the lower extremity. *J Am Podiatry Assoc* 71:177, 1981.)

rection was to decrease the length and girth of the enlarged digit. The entire nail and nail matrix were removed, followed by a linear incision over the dorsal aspect of the digit, creating a long plantar flap. The underlying phalanges were exposed and in this case were found to be fused into a solid mass of deformed bone. The deformed phalanges were resected approximately midshaft and narrowed to accommodate the future reduction of the digit. Thus the distal aspect of the enlarged toe and nail, with remaining plantar skin flap, were removed and defatted to reduce the size of the digit. The extensor and flexor tendons were retracted distally and resected, followed by defatting of the medial and lateral full-thickness skin flaps. Before final skin closure, all bleeding was controlled with digital vessels ligated at the digital portion of the skin flap. The skin incision was closed with 5-0 nonabsorbable, simple interrupted sutures. After surgery, the patient abstained from weight bearing for 1 to 2 weeks, and the postoperative course was uneventful (84) (Fig. 47.46).

Cavaliere and McElgun (84) presented a rare case of macrodactyly and hemihypertrophy that not only provided a good cosmetic result but maintained a postoperative functional result. The importance of staging the surgery in severe combined deformities is noted. Boberg and co-workers (85) present a case of macrodactyly in which the patient's chief complaint was excessive length of the toe. In this case the resection of the distal end of the toe proved to be a simple procedure, with little postoperative morbidity, as an alternative to the conventional defattening and shortening procedures, which may be prone to dehiscence, prolonged edema, sensory loss, vascular compromise, and prolonged disability.

Results and Discussion

Congenital macrodactyly involving the foot is a rare disorder that has not been well recognized and documented because it usually does not become clinically apparent until later development. The surgical treatment depends on the type and degree of deformity. The defatting and shortening procedures presented are an alternative to the more common practice of partial or complete amputation of the involved digit. The surgeon must evaluate each case on an individual basis to achieve the best result.

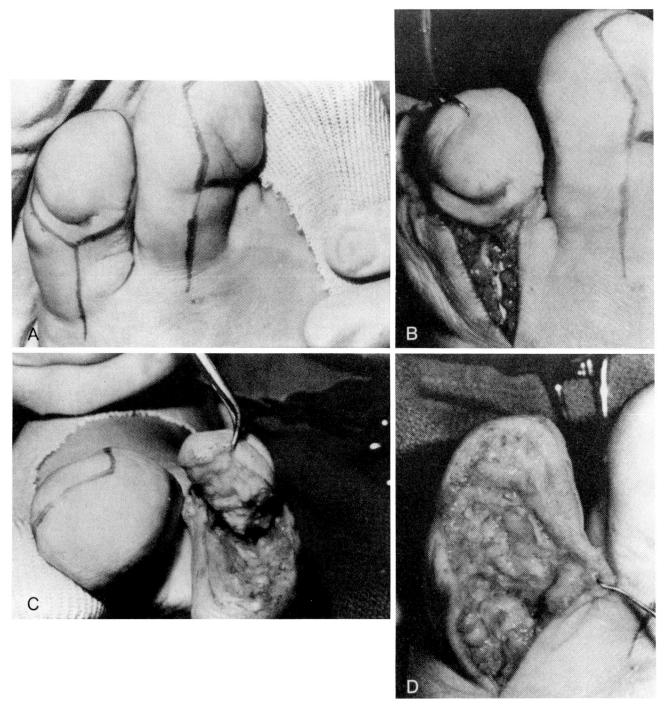

Figure 47.46. Surgical technique and defatting procedures for correction of macrodactyly of the fourth and fifth digits. **A.** Proposed skin incisions. **B.** Creation of plantar skin flap as distal toe and nail matrix are freed dorsally. **C.** Removal of distal toe and nail matrix with remaining plantar skin flap. **D.** Appearance of skin flap before defatting procedures. **E.** Skin flap after defatting procedures. **F.** Completion of defatting procedures in fourth and fifth toes. **G.** Revision of skin flaps and final skin closure. **H.** Clinical appearance of foot 3 months after surgery. (From DeValentine S, Scurran BL, Tuerk D, Karlin J: Macrodactyly of the lower extremity. *J Am Podiatry Assoc* 71:178, 1981.)

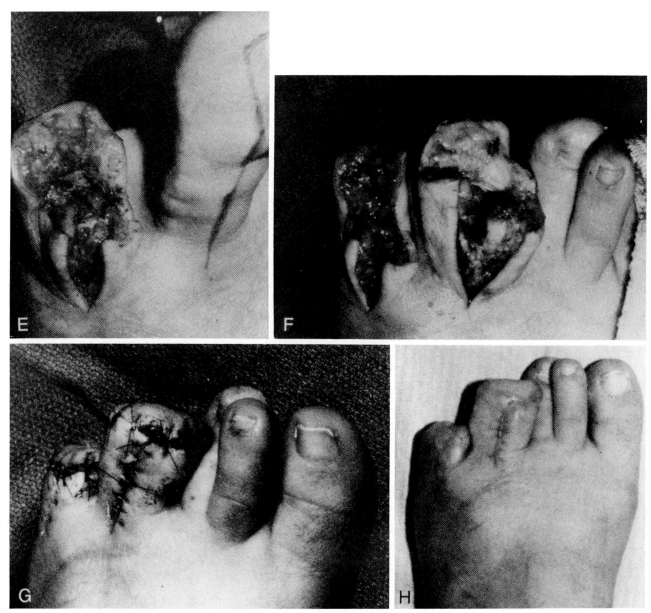

Figure 47.46. E-H.

MISCELLANEOUS CONGENITAL DEFORMITIES

Many other miscellaneous congenital deformities involving the foot are considered to be rare and are beyond the scope of this chapter. Two interesting congenital deformities that may involve the foot include congenital hemihypertrophy and cleft foot or lobster foot.

Congenital Hemihypertrophy

DEFINITION

Congenital hemihypertrophy is a rare miscellaneous congenital deformity characterized by an asymmetrical development of two lateral halves of the body. More commonly this condition involves the upper and lower extremities or a part of an extremity. Slight differences in the size and development of two lateral halves of the body are a common and normal finding and usually do not interfere with function. The more noticeable and severe differences in development of lateral halves of the body are not only a cosmetic problem but also may severely limit or compromise the function of the individual (86).

ETIOLOGY

The exact cause of congenital hemihypertrophy is unknown. Many authors suggest it may be caused by increased blood supply to one side of the body or be secondary to an abnormality of the primary development of the circulation system. Some investigators believe neurofibromatosis may produce a similar appearance as seen in macrodactyly. Occasionally an arteriovenous fistula may be the cause of hemihypertrophy. The possibility of malignancy should be investigated, especially in the presence of pain and a rapid change in the size and development of an extremity (3, 86-88).

TREATMENT

The surgical treatment of congenital hemihypertrophy varies with the degree of deformity, age of the patient, and interference of the deformity with normal function. In most cases of congenital hemihypertrophy, when the deformity interferes with normal function, the size of the hypertrophied part must be reduced by surgical procedures on both the bone and soft tissues. When possible the cause of the hemihypertrophy should be identified and eliminated to prevent recurrence of the deformity. Examples include a case of hemihypertrophy caused by a malignancy, multiple neurofibromas, or an arteriovenous fistula (86). Estersohn and associates (87) described a rare case involving a congenital hypertrophic abductor digiti minimi muscle of the right foot. There was also slight abnormality and mild hypertrophy of the third and fourth plantar interosseous muscles, which was asymptomatic and did not require surgical correction. Excision of the entire hypertrophic muscle in this case provided complete relief and allowed the patient to wear normal foot gear.

CLINICAL PRESENTATION

One case involved a 13-year-old female with congenital hemihypertrophy of the left lower extremity and left foot. The condition was present at birth but did not become a severe functional problem until later development during adolescence. In this case, as well as in most instances, the size of the hypertrophied part was modified and reduced by both osseous and soft tissue procedures (Figs. 47.47 to

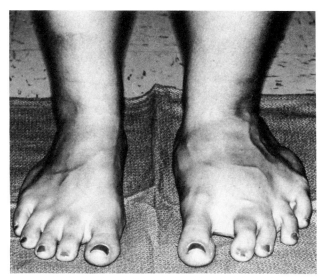

Figure 47.47. Preoperative clinical appearance of hemihypertrophy of left foot in 13-year-old female.

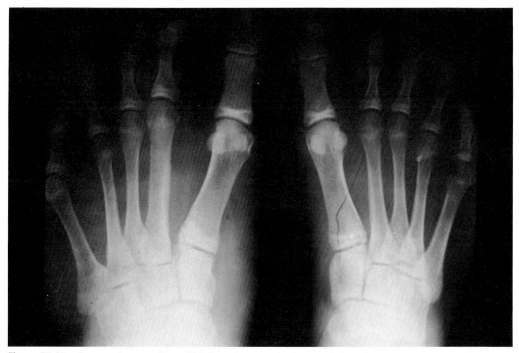

Figure 47.48. Preoperative x-ray films of left foot demonstrating increased size of osseous structures and splaying of first and fifth metatarsals compared with normal x-ray film of right foot.

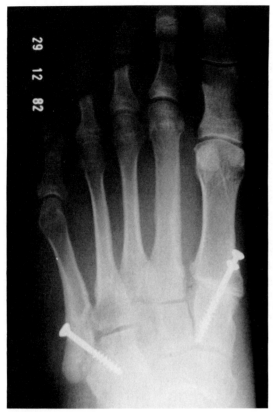

Figure 47.49. Postoperative x-ray film demonstrating internal screw fixation.

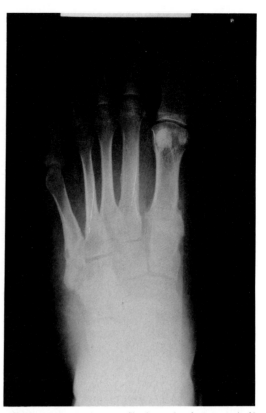

Figure 47.50. Postoperative x-ray film 9 months after removal of internal fixation screws, demonstrating osseous correction of splaying of first and fifth metatarsals.

47.52). Figure 47.47 demonstrates the preoperative clinical appearance of the left foot. Note the increased size, splaying, and separation of the first and second digits in comparison with the normal right foot. Figure 47.48 demonstrates the preoperative x-ray film of the left foot, showing increased size of the osseous structures and splaying of the first and fifth metatarsals in comparison with the normal findings on the right foot radiograph.

The soft tissue reduction procedures in this case included excision of portions of hypertrophied muscle of the abductor hallucis and portions of the abductor digiti quinti muscle followed by skin plasty. The osseous procedures in this case included a Lapidus fusion of the first metatarsocuneiform joint, with abductory wedge and abductory fusion of the fifth metatarsal-cuboid joint. This provided stability and correction of the forefoot splaying.

Figure 47.49 shows a postoperative radiograph demonstrating the use of internal fixation screws in correcting the osseous deformity and splaying of the first and fifth metatarsals. An alternative surgical consideration may include complete resection of the fifth metatarsal and digit. Figure 47.50, a postoperative x-ray film at 9 months after the removal of internal fixation screws, demonstrates a more normal radiographic appearance of the foot. Figure 47.51 demonstrates the postoperative clinical appearance of the left foot at 18 months, revealing a more normal appearance,

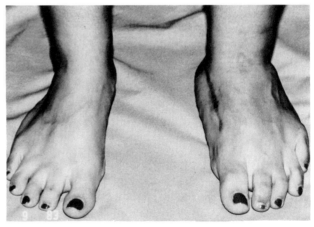

Figure 47.51. Postoperative clinical appearance at 18 months, demonstrating not only good cosmetic result but improved functional result.

with not only a good cosmetic result but an improved functional result. Figure 47.52A demonstrates a 7-year postoperative follow-up result. Note the absence of splaying of the forefoot and the decrease in the separation between the first and second digits (Fig. 47.52B)

The results of surgical correction of hemihypertrophy depend on the severity and degree of deformity. Appro-

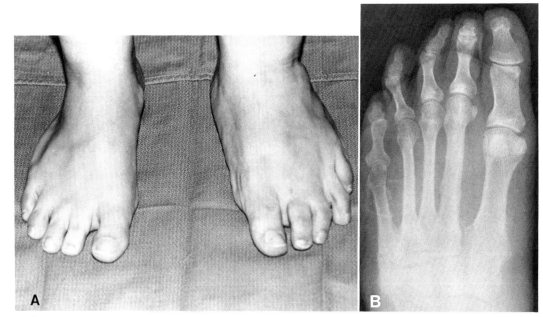

Figure 47.52. Seven years after surgery, clinical appearance **(A)** demonstrating maintenance of excellent cosmetic and functional result and radiograph **(B)** showing correction of the deformity.

priate evaluation of foot function and establishing as near a normal functional result are essential in obtaining optimal results. Overall the results in this case were good both from a cosmetic and a functional viewpoint.

Cleft Foot

DEFINITION

Cleft foot is a general term to describe a rather rare congenital anomaly that usually involves congenital absence of part of the foot, characterized by a cleft or division in the middle of the foot. Cleft foot has also been described as a lobster foot or claw foot because of its clinical appearance.

ETIOLOGY

Barsky (89) classified two types of cleft hand, one type as atypical that involved a unilateral deformity without associated cleft foot or evidence of familial involvement. The second type of cleft hand is described as typical, involving bilateral cleft hand deformities often associated with bilateral cleft foot, with a strong familial history of deformity. Lepow and associates (90) described a case of atypical unilateral cleft foot deformity involving a 31-year-old female in which surgical intervention provided symptomatic relief, enabling pain-free ambulation.

CLINICAL PRESENTATION

In the cleft foot deformity usually one or more of the middle metatarsals and toes are absent in the deformity, giving an unsightly appearance of a lobster claw. Often the cleft or division of the forefoot may extend to the tarsal bones. Frequently the cleft foot deformity is associated with cleft lip and palate, syndactyly, polydactyly, and deafness. Cleft foot is not only a cosmetic problem but often a functional problem in the fitting of foot gear and normal ambulation. The deformity may vary greatly in degree and type of deformity. Usually the first and fifth metatarsals and toes are present, and the middle metatarsals and toes are absent (3, 88, 91-93).

Figure 47.53 demonstrates a case of cleft foot treated by a podiatrist in the north Georgia mountains. The difficulty in wearing foot gear and in normal ambulation can be appreciated in Figure 47.54. Figure 47.55 shows the osseous changes and absence of the middle metatarsals and toes, causing a cleft or division in the middle of the foot.

Figure 47.56 demonstrates the preoperative radiograph of a cousin of the previously described case of bilateral cleft foot. This patient had pain, difficulty wearing shoes, and difficulty ambulating. Surgical procedures performed for correction of this deformity included removal of osseous structures, closing wedge osteotomy of the first metatarsal, and plastic closure. The postoperative x-ray film (Fig. 47.57) shows a more normal appearance.

The results of cleft foot surgery depend on many factors, including the degree and severity of the deformity and the expected results. Most investigators agree that the primary goal of surgery on the cleft foot is to improve foot function, rather than correction for cosmetic reasons only. Sumiya and Onizuka (94) describe a 7-year survey of a new cleft foot repair procedure using a double-pedicled flap from the cleft area to make a wide third toe that is later divided into

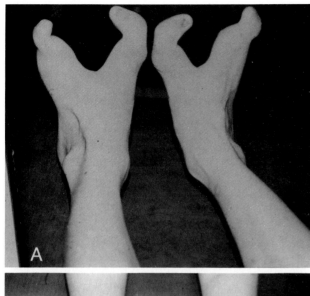

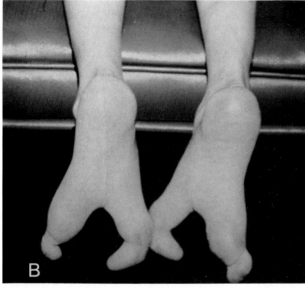

Figure 47.53. Clinical appearance of bilateral cleft foot (lobster foot). **A.** Dorsal view. **B.** Plantar view. (Courtesy of J. E. Williams.)

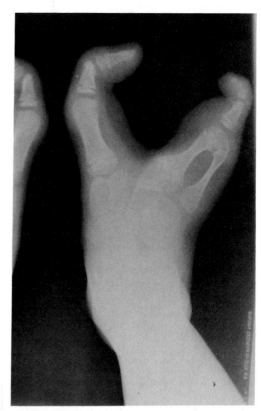

Figure 47.55. X-ray film of cleft foot demonstrating osseous changes and absence of middle metatarsals and toes. (Courtesy of J. E. Williams.)

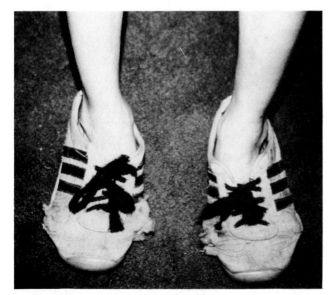

Figure 47.54. Difficulty in normal ambulation and wearing foot gear. (Courtesy of J. E. Williams.)

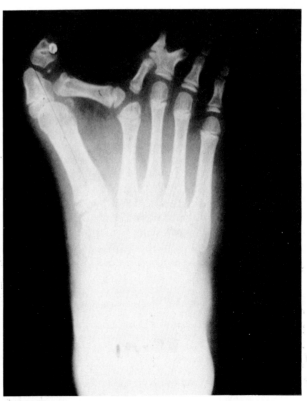

Figure 47.56. Preoperative x-ray film of cousin of patient in Figure 47.47. (Courtesy of J. E. Williams.)

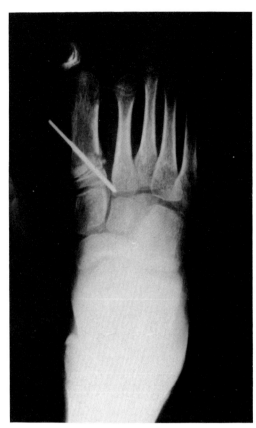

Figure 47.57. Postoperative x-ray film demonstrating removal of osseous structures and closing wedge osteotomy of first metatarsal with a more normal appearance. (Courtesy of J. E. Williams.)

two new toes. In addition, the fifth toe is divided into a fourth and fifth toe, along with surgical straightening of the great toe. The overall results demonstrate a significant improvement in cosmetic appearance and function. According to these clinicians, the newly formed toes, if corrected before the child is weight bearing, help to prevent the progression of the deformity and the formation of the pincerlike deformities characteristic of cleft foot (lobster foot). Coleman and Aronovitz (95) present a two-stage correction of cleft foot in a 7-year-old white male with congenital cleft foot deformity. The purpose of the first stage was to reduce the overall width of the cleft foot deformity, followed by the second stage with the purpose of correcting the digital deformities and performing desyndactylizations. The case presented demonstrates one of the many different strategical surgical approaches to this complex deformity.

References

1. Trethowan WH: The treatment of hammertoe. *Lancet* 1:1257-1312, 1925.
2. Sweetnam R: Congenital curly toes. An investigation into the value of treatment. *Lancet* 2:398, 1958.
3. Tachdjian MO (ed): *Pediatric Orthopedics*. Philadelphia, WB Saunders, 1972, pp 1415-1416, 1417-1422, 1427, 1514-1515.
4. Gamble FO, Yale I: *Clinical Foot Roentgenology: An Illustrated Handbook.* Baltimore, Williams & Wilkins, 1966, p 204.
5. Yale I: *Podiatric Medicine.* Baltimore, Williams & Wilkins, 1974, pp 232-233.
6. Weinstein F (ed): *Principles and Practice of Podiatry.* Philadelphia, Lea & Febiger, 1968, p 268.
7. Budin H: Pain in the great toe joint. *J Exp Podiatry* 1:45, 1940.
8. Polokoff M: Removable shield for lesions about head of fifth metatarsal. *J Am Podiatry Assoc* 57:566-568, 1967.
9. Whitney AK: Urethane mould therapy. *N Engl J Podiatry* 42:17, 1963.
10. McGlamry ED, Kitting R: Postoperative urethane molds. *J Am Podiatry Assoc* 58:169-175, 1968.
11. Rosoff S: Fabrication of orthotic devices with the use of silicone gel. *J Am Podiatry Assoc* 60:313-321, 1970.
12. Roven MD: A traction sling to affect an overlapping fifth toe. *J Am Podiatry Assoc* 49:396, 1959.
13. Turner PL: Strapping of curly toes in children. *NZ J Surg* 57:467-470, 1987.
14. Marr SJ: Toe buttressing for forefoot problems. *J Am Podiatry Assoc* 74:136-140, 1984.
15. Friend G: Correction of elongated underlapping lesser toes by middle phalangectomy and skin plasty. *J Foot Surg* 23:470-476, 1984.
16. Kelikian H: *Hallux Valgus, Allied Deformities of the Forefoot, and Metatarsalgia.* Philadelphia, WB Saunders, 1965, p 330.
17. Sharrard WJW: The surgery of deformed toes in children. *Br J Clin Pract* 17:263, 1963.
18. Taylor RG: The treatment of claw toes by multiple transfers of flexor with extensor tendons. *J Bone Joint Surg* 33B:539, 1951.
19. McGlamry ED: Approaches to digital surgery. A new 16 mm color sound motion picture film from APA. *J Am Podiatry Assoc* 68:358, 1978.
20. Korn SH: The lazy S approach for correction of painful underlapping fifth digit. *J Am Podiatry Assoc* 70:30-33, 1980.
21. Gillett HG: Ungual phalanx valgus. *J Am Podiatry Assoc* 68:83-85, 1978.
22. Lapidus PC: Transplantation of the extensor tendon for correction of the overlapping fifth toe. *J Bone Joint Surg* 24:555, 1942.
23. Lantzounis LA: Congenital subluxation of the fifth toe and its correction by a periosteocapsuloplasty and tendon transplantation. *J Bone Joint Surg* 22:147, 1940.
24. Kelikian: *Hallux Valgus, Allied Deformities of the Forefoot, and Metatarsalgia.* Philadelphia, WB Saunders, 1965, pp 327-330.
25. Giannestras NJ: *Foot Disorders—Medical and Surgical Management.* Philadelphia, Lea & Febiger, 1967, pp 94-96.
26. Jordan RP, Caselli MA: Overlapping deformity of the digits in the pediatric patient—a conservative approach to treatment. *J Am Podiatry Assoc* 68:503-505, 1978.
27. Cockin J: Butler's operation for an overriding fifth toe. *J Bone Joint Surg* 50B:78-80, 1968.
28. Coleman WB, Kissel CG, Sterling HD Jr: Syndactylism and its surgical repair. *J Am Podiatry Assoc* 71:545-549, 1981.
29. Davis JS, German WJ: Syndactylism (coherence of the fingers or toes). *Arch Surg* 21:32, 1930.
30. Temtamy SA, McKusick VA: The genetics of hand malformations, *Birth Defects* 14:364, 1978.
31. Losch GM, Duncker HR: Anatomy and surgical treatment of syndactylism. *Plast Reconstr Surg* 50:167, 1972.
32. Arey SB: *Developmental Anatomy—A Textbook and Laboratory Manual of Embryology,* ed 7. Philadelphia, WB Saunders, 1966, p 210.
33. Gates (cited in Barsky AJ): *Congenital Anomalies of the Hand and Their Surgical Treatment.* Springfield, IL, Charles C Thomas, 1959.
34. Malhorta KC, Riffe DC: Syndactyly and clinodactyly within an Indian family. *J Hered* 54:219, 1963.
35. Wyard GE, Thompson WW, Eilers VE: Syndactylism. *Minn Med* 61:177, 1978.
36. MacCollum DW: Clinical surgery—webbed fingers. *Surg Gynecol Obstet* 71:782, 1940.
37. Barsky AJ: Congenital anomalies of the hand. *J Bone Joint Surg* 33:35, 1951.
38. Nylen B: A report on the repair of congenital finger syndactyly. *Acta Chir Scand* 113:310, 1957.
39. Bunnell S: *Surgery of the Hand,* ed 2. Philadelphia, JB Lippincott, 1948.

40. Skoog T: Syndactyly. *Acta Chir Scand* 130:537, 1965.
41. Weinstock RE, Bass SJ, Farmer MA: Desyndactylization—a new modification. *J Am Podiatry Assoc* 74:458-461, 1984.
42. Castellano BD: Surgical repair of congenitally syndactylized toes. In DiNapoli DR (ed): *Reconstructive Surgery of the Foot and Leg, Update '90.* Tucker, GA, Podiatry Institute Publishing Co, 1990, pp 72-76.
43. Morreale PF, Carrozza LP, Byrnes MF: A complicated incomplete syndactylism. *J Foot Surg* 27:428-432, 1988.
44. Rosen RC, Anania WC, Weinblatt MA, Klein R: Synpolydactyly—a case report and literature review. *J Am Podiatry Assoc* 75:540-544, 1985.
45. Christensen JC, Leff FB, Lepow GM, Schwartz RI, Colon PA, Arminio ST, Nixon P, Segel D: Congenital polydactyly and polymetatarsalgia: classification, genetics and surgical correction. *J Foot Surg* 20:151-158, 1981.
46. Temtamy SA, McKusick VA: Synopsis of hand malformations with particular emphasis on genetic factors. *Birth Defects* 3:125, 1969.
47. Venn-Watson EA: Problems in polydactyly of the foot. *Orthop Clin North Am* 7:909, 1976.
48. Milles BL: The inheritance of human skeletal anomalies. *J Hered* 19:28, 1928.
49. DeMarinis F, Sobbota A: On the inheritance and development of preaxial and postaxial types of polydactyly. *Acta Genet (Basel)* 7:215, 1957.
50. Castilla E: Polydactyla, a genetic study in South America. *Am J Hum Genet* 25:405, 1973.
51. Woolf CM, Myrianthopoulous NC: Polydactyly in American Negroes and whites. *Am J Hum Genet* 25:347, 1973.
52. Knecht JG: Polydactyly of the foot. *J Foot Surg* 22:23-28, 1983.
53. Green DR, Ruch JA, Butlin WE: Polydactylism repair. *J Am Podiatry Assoc* 66:304-309, 1976.
54. Biggs EW, Brahm TB, Efron BL: Surgical correction of congenital hypoplastic metatarsals. *J Am Podiatry Assoc* 69:241-244, 1979.
55. Greenfield GB: *Radiology of Bone Diseases,* ed 2. Philadelphia, JB Lippincott, 1975, p 285.
56. Kite JH: *The Clubfoot.* New York, Grune & Stratton, 1964, p 156.
57. McGlamry ED, Cooper CT: Brachymetatarsia: a surgical treatment. *J Am Podiatry Assoc* 59:259, 1969.
58. Inman VT (ed): *DuVries' Surgery of the Foot,* ed 3. St Louis, CV Mosby, 1973, p 74.
59. Gamble FO, Yale I: *Clinical Foot Roentgenology,* ed 2. Baltimore, Robert E Krieger, 1975, p 237.
60. Yale I: *Podiatric Medicine.* Baltimore, Williams & Wilkins, 1974, p 218.
61. Page JC, Dockery GL, Vance CE: Brachymetatarsia with brachymesodactyly. *J Foot Surg* 22:104-107, 1983.
62. Scheimer DE, Chamas CE: Brachymetatarsia: a review and case study. *J Foot Surg* 22:257-262, 1983.
63. Mah KS, Beegle TR, Falknor DW: A correction for short fourth metatarsal. *J Am Podiatry Assoc* 73:196-200, 1983.
64. Urano V, Kobayashi A: Bone-lengthening for shortness of the fourth toe. *J Bone Joint Surg* 60A:91, 1978.
65. Martin DE, Kalish SR: Brachymetatarsia: recent advances in surgical technique. *Reconstructive Surgery of the Foot and Leg—90.* Tucker, GA, Podiatric Education and Research Institute, 1990, pp 193-198.
66. Jimenez AL: Brachymetatarsia: a study in surgical planning. *J Am Podiatry Assoc* 69:245-251, 1979.
67. McGlamry ED, Fenton CF III: Brachymetatarsia: a case report. *J Am Podiatry Assoc* 73:76-78, 1983.
68. Handelman RB, Perlman MD, Coleman WB: Brachymetatarsia: a review and case report. *J Am Podiatry Assoc* 76:413-416, 1986.
69. Hosokawa K, Susuki T: Treatment of multiple brachymetatarsia: a case report. *Brit J Plast Surg* 40:423-426, 1987.
70. Chairman EL, Dallalio AE, Mandracchia VJ: Brachymetatarsia IV. A different surgical approach. *J Foot Surg* 24:361-363, 1985.
71. Page JC, Dockery GL, Vance CE: Brachymetatarsia with brachymesodactyly. *J Foot Surg* 22:104-107, 1983.
72. Yonenobu K, Takaoka K, Tsuyuguchi Y, Ono K, Tada K: Elongation of brachymetatarsy with ceramic implant: a roentgenographic evaluation of its utility. *J Biomed Mater Res* 20:1249-1256, 1986.
73. Tabak B, Lefkowitz H, Steiner I: Metatarsal-slide lengthening without bone grafting. *J Foot Surg* 25:50-53, 1986.
74. Marcinko D, Rappaport M, Gordon S: Post-traumatic brachymetatarsia. *J Foot Surg* 23:451, 1984.
75. Barsky AJ: Macrodactyly. *J Bone Joint Surg* 49:1255, 1967.
76. Moore BH: Macrodactyly and associated peripheral nerve changes. *J Bone Joint Surg* 24:617, 1942.
77. Khanna N, Gupta S, Knanna S, Tripathi F: Macrodactyly. *Hand* 7:215, 1975.
78. Perdive RL, Mason WH, Bernard TN: Macrodactyly: a rare malformation. *J Am Podiatry Assoc* 69:657-664, 1979.
79. Rechnagel K: Megalodactylism. *Acta Orthop Scand* 38:57, 1967.
80. Winestine F: Relationship of von Recklinghausen's disease (multiple neurofibromatosis) to giant growth and blastomatosis. *J Cancer Res Clin Oncol* 8:409, 1924.
81. Capel EH: Macrodactyly, with report of a case. *J Anat* G9:528, 1935.
82. Tsuge K: Treatment of macrodactyly. *Plast Reconstr Surg* 39:590, 1967.
83. DeValentine S, Scurran BL, Tuerk D, Karlin J: Macrodactyly of the lower extremity. *J Am Podiatry Assoc* 71:174-180, 1981.
84. Cavaliere RG, McElgun TM: Macrodactyly and hemihypertrophy: a new surgical procedure. *J Foot Surg* 27:226-235, 1988.
85. Boberg JS, Yu GV, Xenos D: Macrodactyly—a case report. *J Am Podiatry Assoc* 75:41-45, 1985.
86. Raney RB Sr, Brashear HR Jr: *Shand's Handbook of Orthopaedic Surgery,* ed 10. St Louis, CV Mosby, 1986, p 49.
87. Estersohn HS, Agins SW, Ridenour J: Congenital hypertrophy of an intrinsic muscle of the foot. *J Foot Surg* 26:501-503, 1987.
88. Edmonson AS, Crenshaw AH (eds): *Campbell's Operative Orthopaedics,* ed 6, vol 2. St Louis, CV Mosby, 1980, pp 1748-1749.
89. Barsky AJ: Cleft hand: classification, incidence and treatment. *J Bone Joint Surg* 46A:1707, 1964.
90. Lepow GM, Kuritz HM, Gomes DR, Stahl WE: Congenital claw foot deformity—a case presentation. *J Am Podiatry Assoc* 65:349-352, 1977.
91. Raney RB Sr, Brashear HR Jr: *Shand's Handbook of Orthopaedic Surgery,* ed 10. St Louis, CV Mosby, 1986, p 48.
92. Inmann VT (ed): *DuVries' Surgery of the Foot,* ed 3. St Louis, CV Mosby, 1973, pp 110-112.
93. Tachdjian MO (ed): *Pediatric Orthopedics,* vol 2. Philadelphia, WB Saunders, 1972, pp 1376-1377.
94. Sumiya N, Onizuka T: Seven years survey of our new cleft foot repair. *Plast Reconstr Surg* 65:447-459, 1980.
95. Coleman WB, Aronovitz DC: Surgical management of cleft foot deformity. *J Foot Surg* 27:497-502, 1988.

ADDITIONAL REFERENCES

Askins G, Ger E: Congenital constriction band syndrome. *J Pediatr Orthop* 8:461-466, 1988.
Baraitser M: Recessively inherited brachydactyly type C. *J Med Genet* 20:128-129, 1983.
Baran R, Juhlin L: Bone dependent nail formation. *Br J Dermatol* 114:371-375, 1986.
Baruchin AM, Herold ZH, Shmueli G, Lupo L: Macrodystophia lipomatosa of the foot. *J Pediatr Surg* 23:192-194, 1988.
Beck RB, Brudno DS, Rosenbaum KN: Bilateral absence of the ulna in twins as a manifestation of the split hand-split foot deformity. *Am J Perinatol* 6:1-3, 1989.
Behr JT, Kohli KK, Millar EA: Giant dermoid associated with foot duplication—a case report. *J Pediatr Orthop* 6:486-488, 1986.
Bernhardt DB: Prenatal and postnatal growth. *Phys Ther* 68:1831-1839, 1988.
Bhat BV, Ashok BA, Puri RK: Lobster claw hand and foot deformity in a family. *Ind Pediatr* 24:675-677, 1987.
Blauth W, Olason AT: Classification of polydactyly of the hands and feet. *Arch Orthop Trauma Surg* 107:334-344, 1988.
Bujdoso G, Lenz W: Monodactylous splithand-splitfoot—a malformation occurring in three distinct genetic types. *Eur J Pediatr* 133:207-215, 1980.
Calver D, Keast-Butler J, Taylor D: The extra digit—a pointer to the eye? *Trans Ophthal Soc UK* 101:35-38, 1981.
Can'un S: Absent tibiae. *Clin Genet* 25:182-186, 1984.
Carnevale A, Herandez M, Castillo VD, Torres P: A new syndrome of triphalangeal thumbs and brachy-ectrodactyly. *Clin Genet* 18:244-252, 1980.

Castle D: Trisomy 18 syndrome with cleft foot. *J Med Genet* 25:568-570, 1988.

Clark CD: The intrauterine position and deformities of the lower extremity. *J Am Podiatry Assoc* 71:145-153, 1981.

Cooks RG: A new nail dysplasia syndrome. *Clin Genet* 27:85-91, 1985.

Crossan JF, Wynne-Davies R: Research for genetic and environmental factors in orthopedic diseases. *Clin Orthop* 210:97-105, 1986.

Cybulski JS: Brachydactyly, a possible inherited anomaly at prehistoric Prince Rupert harbour. *Am J Phys Anthropol* 76:363-376, 1988.

Czeizel A: Familial combination of brachydactyly. *Eur J Pediatr* 149:117-199, 1989.

Dabdoub W, Short L, Lindholm J, Gudas CJ: Aphalangia, adactylia, anterior cavus and limb length inequality—a case report. *J Am Podiatry Assoc* 76:441-447, 1983.

Danielsson LG: Resection for macrodactylism of toes. *Acta Orthop Scand* 57:560-562, 1986.

Dell PC, Sheppard JE: Deformities of the great toe in Apert's syndrome. *Clin Orthop* 157:113-118, 1981.

De Laurenzi V: Macrodatillia del medio. *Gior Med Mil* 112:401, 1962.

Dooley JL, Niehaus LP: Preaxial polydactyly. *J Foot Surg* 24:122-126, 1985.

Entin MA: Reconstruction of congenital aplasia of digits. *Surg Clin North Am* 61:407-422, 1981.

Etches PC, Stewart AR, Ives EJ: Familial congenital amputations. *J Pediatr* 101:448-449, 1982.

Fiedler BS, De Smet AA, Kling TF, Fisher DR: Foot deformity in hereditary onycho-osteodysplasia. *J Can Assoc Radiol* 38:305-308, 1987.

Freire-Maia N: Mohr-Wriedt (A2) brachydactyly. *Hum Hered* 30:225-231, 1980.

Fujimoto A, Smolensky LS, Wilson MG: Brachydactyly with major involvement of proximal phalanges. *Clin Gen* 21:107-111, 1982.

Gadegene WM: Poly-syndactyly. *J Hand Surg [Brit]* 9:149-150, 1984.

Giorgini RJ, Aquino JM: Surgical approach to polydactyly. *J Foot Surg* 23:221-225, 1984.

Gorlin RJ: Apert syndrome with polysyndactyly of the feet. *Am J Med Genet* 32:557, 1989.

Graham JM, Higginbottom MC, Smith DW: Preaxial polydactyly of the foot associated with early amnion rupture: evidence for mechanical teratogenesis? *J Pediatr* 98:943-945, 1981.

Graudal N: The pattern of shortened hand and foot bones. *ROFO* 148:460-462, 1988.

Halal F: The hand-foot-genital (hand-foot-uterus) syndrome: family report and update. *Am J Med Genet* 30:793-803, 1988.

Hall JG, Pallister PD, Clarren SK, Beckwith JB, Wiglesworth FW, Fraser FC, Cho S, Benke PJ, Reed SD: Congenital hypothalamic hamartoblastoma, hypopituitarism, imperforate anus, and postaxial polydactyly—a new syndrome? I. Clinical, causal and pathogenetic considerations. *Am J Med Genet* 7:47-74, 1980.

Harrison RB, Keats TE: Epiphyseal clefts. *Skeletal Radiol* 5:23-27, 1980.

Hecht JT, Scott CI: Limb deficiency syndrome in half sibs. *Clin Genet* 20:432-437, 1981.

Hentz VR: Congenital anomalies—looking ahead. *Clin Plastic Surg* 13:175-189, 1986.

Hernandez A, Garcia-Esquivel L, Reynoso MC, Fragoso R, Enriquez-Guerra MA, Nazara Z, Anzar MB, Cantu JM: Cortical blindness, growth and psychomotor retardation and postaxial polydactyly: a probably distinct autosomal recessive syndrome. *Clin Genet* 28:251-254, 1984.

Hoffmann EB, Rehder H, Langenbeck U: Skeletal anomalies in trisomy 21 as an example of amplified developmental instability in chromosome disorders: a histological study of the feet of 21 mid-trimester fetuses with trisomy 21. *Am J Med Genet* 29:155-160, 1988.

Hogh J: Foot deformities. *Int Orthop* 9:135-138, 1985.

Hoon A: Familial limb deficiency. *Clin Genet* 34:141-142, 1988.

Hootnick DR: Congenital tibial aplasia. *Teratology* 27:169-179,1983.

Horowitz M, Gerstman M, Harding P: Familial brachymetacarpalia—pseudo pseudo-hypoparathyroidism? *NZ Med J* 95:810-811, 1982.

Iida H, Shikata J, Yamamuro T, Takede N, Ueba Y: A pedigree of cervical stenosis, brachydactyly, syndactyly and hyperopia. *Clin Orthop* 247:80-86, 1989.

Izumikawa Y, Naritomi K, Ikema S, Goya Y, Shiroma N, Yoshida K, Yara A, Hirayama K: Apert syndrome with partial polysyndactyly: a proposal on the classification of acrocephalosyndactyly. *Jpn J Hum Genet* 33:487-492, 1988.

Jeanty P: In utero sonographic detection. *J Ultrasound Med* 4:595-601, 1985.

Kalen V, Burwell DS, Omer GE: Macrodactyly of the hands and feet. *J Pediatr Orthop* 8:311-315, 1988.

Kameyana Y: Pathogenetic correlations. *Prog Clin Biol Res* 163C:105109, 1985.

Keppen LD, Rennert OM: Silver-Russell syndrome with absence digits and syndactylism of the fingers. *Clin Genet* 24:453-455, 1983.

Kerel D: Macrodactyly. *J Hand Surg* 12:610-614, 1987.

Kleiner BC, Holmes LB: Brief clinical report: hallux varus and preaxial in brothers. *Am J Med Genet* 6:113-117, 1980.

Kopy's'c Z: The Saethre-Chotzen syndrome with partial bifid of the distal. *Hum Genet* 56:195-204, 1980.

Kucheria K: An Indian family. *Clin Genet* 20:36-39, 1981.

Kucheria K, Kenue RK, Taneja N: An Indian family with postaxial polydactyly in four generations. *Clin Genet* 20:36-39, 1981.

Kumar K, Kumar D, Gadegone WM, Kapahtia NK: Macrodactyly of the hand and foot. *Int Orthop* 9:259-264, 1985.

Kumar P: Median cleft lip with bimanual hexadactyly. *J Craniomaxillofac Surg* 16:243-244, 1988.

Learman Y, Katznelson MB, Bonne-Tamir B, Engel J, Hertz M, Goodman RM: Symphalangism with multiple anomalies of the hands and feet: a new genetic trait. *Am J Med Genet* 10:245-255, 1981.

Majewski F, Kuster W, Haar B, Goecke T: Aplasia of tibia with split-hand/split foot deformity, report of six families with 35 cases and considerations about variability and penetrance. *Hum Genet* 70:136-147, 1985.

Marlob P: Familial opposable triphalangeal thumbs. *J Med Genet* 22:78-80, 1985.

Maroteaux P: Apparent Apert syndrome with polydactyly. *Am J Med Genet* 28:153-158, 1987.

Masada K, Tsuyuguchi Y, Kawabata H, Kawai H, Tada K, Ono K: Terminal limb congenital malformations: analysis of 523 cases. *J Pediatr Orthop* 6:340-345, 1986.

Masada K, Tsuyuguchi Y, Kawabata H, Ono K: Treatment of preaxial polydactyly of the foot. *Plast Reconstr Surg* 76:251-258, 1987.

Mathews JL: Familial brachydactyly. *J Rheumatol* 10:819-822, 1983.

Mattei JF: Syndrome of polydactyly, cleft lip. *J Med Genet* 20:433-435, 1983.

Matthews S, Farnish S, Young ID: Distal symphalangism with involvement of the thumbs and great toes. *Clin Genet* 32:375-378, 1987.

May JW, Smith RJ, Peimer CA: Toe to hand free tissue transfer for thumb construction with multiple digit aplasia. *Plast Reconst Surg* 67:205-213, 1981.

McCormack MK, McCormack PJC, Lee M: Autosomal-dominant inheritance of distal arthrogryposis. *Am J Med Genet* 6:163-169, 1980.

McDonough MW: Fetal position as a cause of right and left sided foot and leg disorders. *J Am Podiatry Assoc* 71:65-68, 1981.

Meals RA: Hallux to hand transfer. *JAMA* 249:72-73, 1983.

Meiselman SA: Brachydactyly. *Clin Genet* 35:261-267, 1989.

Meltzer RM: Polydactyly. *Clin Podiatr Med Surg* 4:57-62, 1987.

Merlob P, Grunebaum M: Type II syndactyly or synpolydactyly. *J Med Genet* 23:237-241, 1986.

Merlob P, Levy Y, Shuper A: Postaxial polydactyly in association with neurofibromatosis. *Clin Genet* 32:202-205, 1987.

Mick TJ, Schultz GD: Atypical brachydactyly. *J Manipulative Physiol Ther* 12:131-134, 1989.

Mickleson KN: Developmental delay. *J Clin Dysmorphol* 1:21-23, 1983.

Mishalanie MA, Dockery GL: Spina bifida and its effect on the lower extremities. *J Am Podiatry Assoc* 70:84-88, 1980.

Miura T: Polydactyly in Japan. *Handchirugie* 12:39-46, 1980.

Miura T: Congenital hand anomalies. *Hand* 13:267-270, 1981.

Miura T: Congenital familial hypopostic thumb. *J Hand Surg* 9:420-422, 1984.

Miura T: Polydactyly. *J Hand Surg* 12:474-476, 1987.

Mollica F, Li Volti S, Guarneri B: New syndrome: exostoses, anetoderma, brachydactyly. *Am J Med Genet* 19:665-667, 1984.

Morris EW: Varus fifth toe. *J Bone Joint Surg* 64A:99-100, 1982.

Neil MJ, Conacher C: Bilateral delta phalanx of the proximal phalanges of the great toes: a report on an affected family. *J Bone Joint Surg* 66B:77-80, 1984.

Nogami H: Polydactyly and polydactyly of the fifth toe. *Clin Orthop* 204:261-265, 1986.

Notari MA, Mittler BE: A study of the incidence of pedal pathology in children. *J Am Podiatry Assoc* 78:518-521, 1988.

O'Flanagan SJ, Moran V, Colville J: Brief report—congenital macrodactyly. *Indian J Med Sci* 156:151-153, 1987.

Ofodile FA: Macrodactyly in blacks. *J Hand Surg* 7:566-568, 1982.

Olason AT, Dohler JR: Delta formation in foot polydactyly. *Arch Orthop Trauma Surg* 107:348-353, 1988.

Osebold WR, Remondini DJ, Lester EL, Spranger JW, Opitz JM: An autosomal dominant syndrome of short stature with mesomelic shortness of limbs, abnormal carpal and tarsal bones, hypoplastic middle phalanges and bipartite calcanei. *Am J Med Genet* 22:791-809, 1985.

Pearn J, Bloch CE, Nelson MM: Macrodactyly simplex congenita—a case series and considerations of differential diagnosis and aetiology. *S Afr Med J* 70:755-758, 1986.

Pfeiffer RA: Aplasia of the thumbs and great toes. *Ann Genet* 31:241-243, 1988.

Phelps DA, Grogan DP: Polydactyly of the foot. *J Pediatr Orthop* 5:446-451, 1985.

Pilarski RT: Karsch-Neugebauer syndrome. *Clin Genet* 27:97-101, 1985.

Pirnar T, Balci S, Caglar M: Short-rib-polydactyly syndrome. *Turk J Pediatr* 24:175-182, 1982.

Pitt P: A new brachydactyly syndrome. *J Med Genet* 22:202-204, 1985.

Plotkin S: In utero fetal lower extremity examination by diagnostic ultrasound. *J Am Podiatr Med Assoc* 78:287-291, 1988.

Qazi QH, Nangia BS: Abnormal distal phalanges and nails, deafness, mental retardation, and seizure disorder: a new familial syndrome. *J Pediatr* 104:391-394, 1984.

Rao GSS, James JH: Artificial syndactylisation for congenital crossed toes. *Br J Plast Surg* 40:502-504, 1987.

Reynolds JF: Familial Hirschsprung's disease. *Pediatrics* 71:246-249, 1983.

Reynolds JF: Preaxial polydactyly type 4. *Clin Genet* 25:267-272, 1984.

Richards HMS, Golimbu C, Greco MA, Genieser NB, Mitnick J, Golimbu M: Hydrometrocolpos and polydactyly. *Urology* 15:53-55, 1980.

Robertson WW Jr: The bifid great toe: a surgical approach. *J Pediatr Orthop* 7:25-28, 1987.

Robinow M: Syndactyly type 5. *J Med Genet* 11:475-482, 1982.

Roubicek M: Syndrome of polydactyly. *Am J Med Genet* 20:205-206, 1985.

Ruprecht A, Chaney SA, Shokeir MHK: Ectodermal dysplasia associated with cleft palate and lobster claw deformity of hands and feet. *J Can Dent Assoc* 2:147-149, 1986.

Sanchez AJ, Kamal B: Macrodactyly in the foot. *Ann Acad Med* 10:442-444, 1981.

Sanchis A, Cervero L, Martinez A, Valverde C: Duplication of hands and feet, multiple joint dislocations, absence of corpus callosum and hypsarrhythmia: acrocallosal syndrome? *Am J Med Genet* 20:123-130, 1985.

Sandomenico C: Mesomelic dysplasia. *Pediatr Radiol* 13:47-50, 1983.

Schantz K, Rasmussen F: Thiemann's finger or toe disease—follow up of seven cases. *Acta Orthop Scand* 57:91-93, 1986.

Schinzel A, Schmid W: Hallux duplication, postaxial polydactyly, absence of the corpus callosum, severe mental retardation, and additional anomalies in two unrelated patient: a new syndrome. *Am J Med Genet* 6:241-249, 1980.

Schroeder HW Jr, Zasloff M: The hand and foot malformations in fibrodysplasia ossificans progressiva. *Johns Hopkins Med J* 147:73-78, 1980.

Shiota K: Holoprosencephaly. *J Med Genet* 25:502-503, 1988.

Siegel IM: Foot deformity. *Arch Neurol* 40:589, 1983.

Smith JC: A new recessive syndrome. *J Med Genet* 26:339-342, 1989.

Sonoga AL, Guttmann GG: Pedal polydactyly—a case report. *J Am Podiatr Med Assoc* 79:454-458, 1989.

Spranger M: Anomalous inheritance in a kindred with split hand. *Eur J Pediatr* 147:202-205, 1988.

Sprinkle RLB, Morales LM, Grochowski E, Licudine F: Postaxial polydactylism and subsequent surgical correction. *J Am Podiatry Med Assoc* 78:512-517, 1988.

Swanson AB: A classification for congenital limb malformation. 8:693-702, 1983.

Tax HR: A podiatric presentation of diastematomyelia. *J Am Podiatry Assoc* 72:337-341, 1982.

Tozzi MA: Postaxial polydactyly with polymetatarsia. *J Am Podiatry Assoc* 71:374-379, 1981.

Turra S, Frizziero P, Cagnoni G, Jacopetti T: Macrodactyly of the foot associated with plexiform neurofibroma of the medial plantar nerve. *J Pediatr Orthop* 6:489-492, 1986.

Varadi V, Szabo L, Papp Z: Syndrome of polydactyly, cleft lip/palate or lingual lump, and psychomotor retardation. *J Med Genet* 17:119-122, 1980.

Ventruto V, Theo G, Celona A, Fioretti G, Pagano L, Stable M, Cavaliete ML: A and B postaxial polydactyly in two members of the same family. *Clin Genet* 18:342-347, 1980.

Verp MS: Urinary tract abnormalities in hand-foot-genital syndrome. *Am J Med Genet* 32:555, 1989.

Viljoen DL, Beighton P: The split-hand and split-foot anomaly in a central African negro population. *Am J Med Genet* 19:545-552, 1984.

Wallis CE: Ectrodactyly. *Clin Genet* 34:252-257, 1988.

Walpole IR, Hockey A: Syndrome of imperforate anus, abnormalities of hands and feet, satyr ears and sensorineural deafness. *J Pediatr* 100:250-252, 1982.

Weber RB: Surgical criteria for correcting the overlapping fifth toe. *J Foot Surg* 21:30-33, 1982.

Wein BK, Cowell HR: Genetic considerations of foot anomalies in office practice. *Foot Ankle* 2:185-189, 1982.

Widhe T, Aaro S, Elmstedt E: Foot deformities in the newborn— incidence and prognosis. *Acta Orthop Scand* 59:176-179, 1988.

Wiedemann HR: Brief clinical report. *Am J Med Genet* 14:467-471, 1983.

Wiedemann HR, Burgio GR, Aldenhoff P, Kunze J, Kaufmann HJ, Schirg E: The proteus syndrome. *Eur J Pediatr* 140:5-12, 1983.

Wilson WG, Greer KE, Martof AB, McIlhenny J, Hatter DL: "New" ectodermal dysplasia syndrome with distinctive facial appearance and preaxial polydactyly of feet. *Am J Med Genet* 34:227-229, 1989.

Wong HB: Genetic aspects of foot deformities. *J Singapore Paediatr Soc* 29:13-23, 1987.

Yunis E, Varon H: Cleidocranial dysostosis, severe micrognathism, bilateral absence of thumbs and first metatarsal bone, and distal aphalangia. *Am J Dis Child* 134:649-653, 1980.

Zhen-fan L, He-ming W, Shu-sheng Z: Hereditary polydactylic dwarfism syndrome. *Chin Med J [Engl]* 100:124-126, 1987.

Zlotogora J: Is there an autosomal recessive form? *J Med Genet* 26:138-140, 1989.

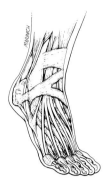

CHAPTER **48**

Bone Grafting

Kieran T. Mahan, M.S., D.P.M., F.A.C.F.S.

The use of transplantable tissues in lower extremity surgery is widespread. The most frequently transplanted tissue is bone. The history of bone grafting dates back to at least 1682, when Job-Van Meekeren transplanted a dog's cranium to a soldier's skull. Two years later the soldier requested that the transplant be removed for religious reasons, although by that time the graft had healed (1). In 1820 the first recorded autogenous bone transplant was performed by Von Walther (1). The early 1900s marked a time of increased interest in bone grafting, spurred by biological investigations and increasing clinical reports. Phemister (2) reported in 1914 that success in bone grafting depended on perfect hemostasis, asepsis, and coaptation of parts. During this same period Axhausen (3) contributed a great deal to the understanding of bone transplantation. Fixation was crude, and stabilization was by means of peg grafting or wire loops. As early as 1923 Albee (4) reported on more than 3000 bone grafts. This work contributed significantly to an increase in bone transplantation. An extensive historical review of this period is provided by Chase and Herndon (5). The next leap in the development of bone grafting occurred with advances in metallurgy and internal fixation by Lane, Danis (6), and later the AO group.

The last decade has seen a dramatic increase in the use of new bone-grafting techniques. This has included the widespread use of allogeneic bone and the refinement of microvascular techniques for free tissue transfers. As the numbers and types and indications for bone grafting increase in lower extremity reconstructive surgery, it becomes even more important to understand bone graft materials and the biological basis behind grafting.

TERMINOLOGY

The distinction must be made between transplantation and implantation. Transplantation implies the transfer of viable tissue that will continue to thrive in the new environment of the host bone. Bone implantation describes the transfer of nonliving tissue, such as freeze-dried bone (7). A time element can also be involved in the determination of transplanted versus implanted bone. After autogenous bone is removed from the donor site, there is a limited time period during which the cells will maintain their viability. After the cells have lost their viability, autogenous bone becomes an implant material.

A variety of different bone graft materials is available.

Table 48.1.
Bone Graft Material Terminology

Old	New	Donor
Autograft	Isograft	Same individual
Isograft	Isograft	Identical twin
Homograft	Allograft	Same species (live)
Homoimplant	Alloimplant	Same species (dead)
Heterograft	Xenograft	Different species

The most useful nomenclature for these materials is based on an immunological classification system (Table 48.1) (8).

INDICATIONS

Bone grafting serves three principal functions: osteogenesis, immobilization, and replacement. Grafts can serve both an active function (stimulation or induction of osteogenesis) and a passive function (osteoconduction, a scaffold effect for ingrowth from the host). More specific functions (9) (Fig. 48.1) include the following:

1. Treatment of delayed unions, nonunions, and pseudoarthroses. This includes provision of viable cells to assist osteogenesis, as well as establishment of an adequate bone stock for fixation and allowing for correction of deformity.
2. Augmentation of defects. Bone grafting is useful for packing of defects created by trauma or the resection of tumors or cysts.
3. Facilitation of arthrodesis by bridging of joints.
4. Bone block to limit excessive or inappropriate motion.
5. Reconstructive procedures. Examples of this in the lower extremity include lengthening of the lateral column of the foot and other opening wedge osteotomies. Repair of brachymetatarsia by grafting is another example.
6. Autogenous grafting as part of treatment for osteomyelitis.

In addition to the foregoing, there are numerous other situations in which bone grafting is used in the lower extremity. In each of these situations use is made of one or more of the three functions of the graft. Selection of the proper bone graft material is dependent on which function of the graft is of prime importance. For example, in an atrophic nonunion of the first metatarsal, osteogenesis is the

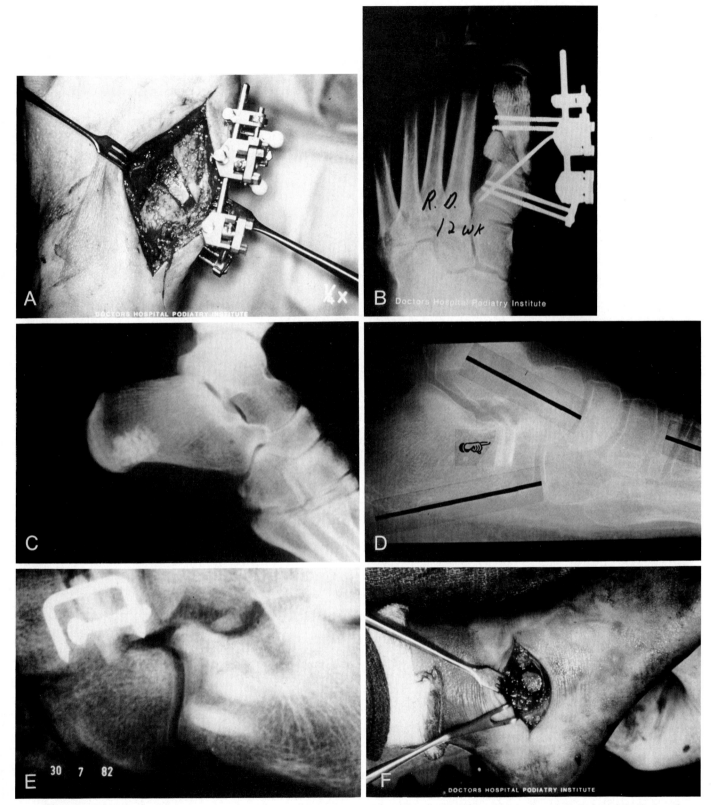

Figure 48.1. **A.** Clinical photograph of bone graft repair of first metatarsal nonunion with external fixation. **B.** Dorsoplantar radiograph of same patient 12 weeks postoperatively. **C.** Calcaneal cyst packed with allogeneic bone chips. **D.** Ten weeks' postoperative radiograph showing allogeneic rib used for Evans lateral column lengthening. **E.** Bone graft facilitation of arthrodesis: naviculocuneiform fusion with interpositional graft. Note that Evans osteotomy of calcaneus with bone graft has also been performed. **F.** Green-Grice extra-articular arthrodesis of subtalar joint with graft.

most important consideration and autogenous cancellous bone is the most useful material. The requirements of the specific grafting situation dictate the type of material that should be used.

MATERIALS

At one time the surgeon's only choice was whether to use cancellous or cortical autogenous bone. Although that decision is still important, the surgeon now has many other choices available. To make these decisions intelligently, the surgeon must have an understanding of the physical and biological properties of each material.

Cortical Versus Cancellous Bone

The characteristics of cortical and cancellous bone are quite different and present a distinct choice to the surgeon. The dense compact structure of cortical bone is useful because it provides a stable graft that can be fixated to surrounding host bone by conventional fixation techniques. Before the widespread use of internal fixation techniques, cortical bone was the only means available to provide stability for the graft-host junction. These inlay and onlay techniques provided gross stability without rigidity. Interestingly enough, Malinin and associates (10) have published work showing a possible new use for cortical bone as a fixation material. In experimental work on dog fractures they used freeze-dried allogeneic cortical bone plates as compression devices. Although this work showed promising results, it is much too soon to determine whether cortical bone plates will have any advantages over metallic internal fixation devices.

The dense structure of cortical bone results in the transplantation of few viable cells. The incorporation process of cortical bone is slow. Consequently, the use of cortical grafts has lost popularity and is limited to a few specific indications.

Cancellous bone is a honeycomb structure of much less density than cortical bone. Transplantation of autogenous cancellous bone results in the transfer of many more viable cells than is the case with cortical bone. Although cortical bone is useful for stability, cancellous bone is too fragile to provide any significant stability. The primary advantage of cancellous bone is its facilitation of osteogenesis.

With autogenous cancellous bone this is achieved by three mechanisms:

1. *Osteogenesis*. Transfer of viable osteoprogenitor cells causing new bone growth (11).
2. *Osteoconduction*. The honeycomb structure of cancellous bone allows for permeation of nutrients to enable cell survival and provides an ideal structure for the ingrowth of new vessels and for "creeping substitution" of new bone (12) (Fig. 48.2).
3. *Osteoinduction*. The bone morphogenetic protein described by Urist (13) induces the formation of new bone (Fig. 48.3). This process involves "recruitment" of mesenchymal cells to a developmental pathway leading to osteoprogenitor cell formation rather than fibrous tissue.

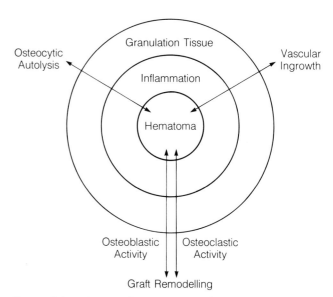

Figure 48.2. *Diagrammatic representation of bone graft healing beginning with initial phases of hematoma, inflammation, and granulation tissue. This is modified by resorption of necrotic bone and replacement with new bone, processes that occur simultaneously. Feedback mechanism for control of graft remodeling is biomechanical stress on graft.*

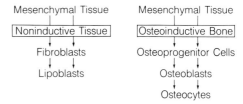

Figure 48.3. *Diagrammatic representation of osteoinduction with recruitment of new osteoblasts from mesenchymal tissue.*

Cancellous bone is incorporated more rapidly than cortical bone.

Frequently neither cortical nor cancellous bone is the ideal bone graft structure because what one lacks in osteogenic potential, the other lacks in mechanical stability. Corticocancellous grafts combine the stability of the cortical graft with the osteogenic capability of the cancellous bone. Iliac crest grafts are an excellent example of such a combination. The thin cortical shell of the iliac crest provides material through which fixation can be securely attached. The interior cancellous structure promotes rapid healing.

GRAFT SOURCE

As noted in Table 48.2, there are various sources of bone other than the patient's own bone. Boyne (14) described four criteria that should apply regardless of the type of material used:

1. The graft material must be immunologically acceptable to the host.
2. The graft should assist osteogenesis, either actively or passively.

Table 48.2.
Xenograft Materials

Material[a]	Preparation	Comments	Reference[a]
Frozen calf bone	−40° C frozen storage	Inferior	Kingma, 1960
Boplant	Freeze-dried	Discontinued	Bassett & Creighton, 1962
Ox bone	Decalcified	Discontinued	Senn, 1889
Os purum	KOH, acetone	Discontinued	Orell, 1937
Anorganic bone	Ethylenediamine	Slow absorption	Williams & Irvine, 1954
		No bone induction	
Oswestry	Hydrogen peroxide, ethylenediamine	Not available	Roaf & Hancox, 1961
Kiel bone	Hydrogen peroxide-maceration	Unacceptable in spinal fusions	McMurray, 1982
Kiel bone—autologous	Cancellous Kiel prepared as above	Excellent results	Salama, 1983
marrow	Combine with autologous marrow		

[a] Materials and references from Salama R: Xenogeneic bone grafting in humans. *Clin Orthop* 174:113-121, 1983.

3. The graft must provide support for the osseous structure during the healing phase.
4. The graft material must be such that it will be replaced by new bone.

AUTOGENOUS BONE

Autogenous bone has been, and continues to be, the material of choice for most situations. The clear advantages include: (*a*) viable cells (the amount depending on whether cortical or cancellous bone is used) and (*b*) immunological compatibility with the host tissue. In situations in which osteogenesis and vascularity are of prime importance, autogenous bone is the material of choice. There are many sources of autogenous bone, each offering different ratios of cortical to cancellous bone (Table 48.3).

The advantages of autogenous bone are not achieved without cost. The procurement of autogenous bone graft material entails the following:

1. Creation of a stress point in the donor site with the possibility of prolonged immobilization or fracture through the site.
2. The additional surgical procedure prolongs surgical and anesthesia time. This increases the risk of surgical complications such as infection, dehiscence, and hematoma.
3. There may be an insufficient quantity of donor bone that can be removed safely.
4. The additional surgical site creates increased postoperative pain and limitations and results in an additional surgical scar.

FREE VASCULARIZED GRAFT

A specialized type of autogenous graft is the free vascularized bone graft. This procedure is based on microsurgical technique (15-19). The process involves removal of a segment of bone with its nutrient artery and veins. The graft is then placed in the recipient site, and the nutrient vessels are reanastomosed (Fig. 48.4). It is possible to transfer not only bone but also overlying muscle and soft tissue to cover major defects. The fibula, rib, and iliac crest have all been used with some success.

Table 48.3.
Preparation of Demineralized Allogeneic Bone

1. Human long bone and calvaria cut into small pieces
2. Chloroform-methanol (1 : 1) 6 hours at room temperature
3. Partial and total demineralization with 0.6 HCL, 4° C
4. 8M liCl treatment at 2° C, 24 hours
5. H_2O treatment at 55° C, 24 hours
6. 0.1M phosphate buffer pH 7.4 containing antibiotics, 3mM IAM, 10mM NaN3, incubating at 37° C for 4 days
7. Lyophilization
8. Sterilization with ethylene oxide

Iwata H, et al.: Chemosterilized autolyzed antigen-extracted allogeneic (AAA) bone matrix gelatin for repair of defects from excision of benign bone tumors: A preliminary report. *Clin Orthop* 154:150, 1981.

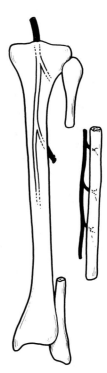

Figure 48.4.   Diagram of free fibular bone graft with nutrient vessels.

Table 48.4.
Donor Sites for Autogenous Bone

Iliac crest—anterior
       —posterior
Greater trochanter
Rib
Tibial metaphysis (proximal and distal)
Calcaneus
Fibula

The technique is useful because, by ensuring the continual circulation to the graft, the healing process is simplified from graft incorporation with creeping substitution to simple fracture healing. Incorporation of the graft is much more rapid with this technique, and it has the advantage of being a one-stage procedure.

Reconstruction of traumatic injuries has been a tremendous stimulus for work with vascularized bone grafts. Nusbickel et al. reviewed vascularized autograft techniques for reconstructing lower extremities following trauma (20). Of the three most common vascularized grafts, the rib is not commonly used in the lower extremities because of its shape and small bone mass. The iliac crest has a maximum length of 10 cm and a curved corticocancellous structure.

Stevenson et al. described the use of a circumflex iliac artery osteocutaneous flap for reconstruction of a heel defect in a young girl (21). Salibian et al. also described the use of iliac vascularized grafts in the lower extremity. They reported an average time to osseous union of 8.8 months, as compared to 4 months in the upper extremity (22). The iliac crest has a larger cross-sectional area than the fibula and may be better suited for end-to-end healing.

The fibula can be used as a vascularized graft on the basis of its peroneal artery blood supply. Because of its length and strength, it is the most common vascularized graft in the lower extremities. De Boer and Wood reviewed 62 patients who had vascularized fibular transfers (23). They reported a 25% incidence of fractures of the graft at an average of 8 months postoperatively. This compares quite favorably with the incidence in avascular cortical grafts. Hypertrophy of the fibula was not uncommon and occurred more often in mechanically loaded extremities. De Boer and Wood concluded that vascularized fibular grafts should be protected during the first year.

Jones et al. modified the free fibular graft by performing an osteotomy just distal to the entry of the nutrient artery (24). This allows a double-barrel graft when the two pieces are folded on each other. A cuff of the flexor hallucis longus and tibialis posterior is maintained to preserve the periosteal blood supply to the fibula.

BONE BANKING

The hazards and risks associated with autogenous bone grafts are well known. The desire to have a suitable alternative to autogenous bone has been expressed by authors for many years, but Inclan (25), in 1942, was the first to report on efforts in this area. There are three alternatives: xenogeneic bone, allogeneic bone, and synthetic alloimplants.

The goal of a bone bank is to (a) provide sterile bone with (b) minimal antigenicity and (c) maximum osteogenic potential. These three requirements are paramount in the consideration of selection and preparation of materials.

Xenografts

The search for a substitute for autogenous bone has been a long one. The use of animal bone is an intriguing prospect because it would solve the problem of bone availability. Meekeren performed the first bone graft in 1682, when he used canine bone to fill a skull defect (1). Various other materials have been used, including cow horns, ivory tusks, and bovine bone (with or without autologous marrow) (1) (Table 48.2).

Because of the unique problems of using animal bone, various sterilizing techniques have been attempted without success. These techniques have included boiling, deproteinization with ethylenediamine, thimerosal, and irradiation (1, 26, 27). Each of these techniques produced bone that was unsatisfactory for mechanical, immunological, or osteogenic reasons.

In the 1950s thousands of frozen calf bone transplantations were performed in the Netherlands. Initial results appeared encouraging, but later studies demonstrated that this type of bone elicits a foreign body reaction that may actually inhibit osteogenesis. The two most common commercial forms of bovine xenograft material were Boplant and Kiel bone. Boplant was a freeze-dried form of calf bone introduced by Bassett and Creighton (28). Long-term clinical studies demonstrated disappointing results (29). Kiel bone is prepared from freshly killed calves. The bone is extracted with hydrogen peroxide, treated with fat solvents, dried with acetone, and gas sterilized with ethylene oxide. This form is still available, although McMurray (30) has demonstrated that it is an unacceptable material in spinal fusions. Histological studies did not demonstrate any autogenous bone invasion of the Kiel bone graft in McMurray's study. Salama (26) reported on 98 patients in whom Kiel bone was combined with autogenous red marrow. He reported excellent results because of the osteogenic property of the marrow.

At the present time there are no xenograft materials that can be recommended for general use.

Allografts and Alloimplants

In contrast to the failure of xenogeneic bone, allogeneic bone has been successfully used on a widespread basis (31) (Fig. 48.5). The two most important considerations in the use of allogeneic bone are immunological compatibility and sterility (32, 33). For this reason, the use of allografts (live bone) is unusual. Alloimplants are portions of allogeneic bone (dead) that have undergone treatment to reduce antigenicity and ensure sterility. The three basic processes for

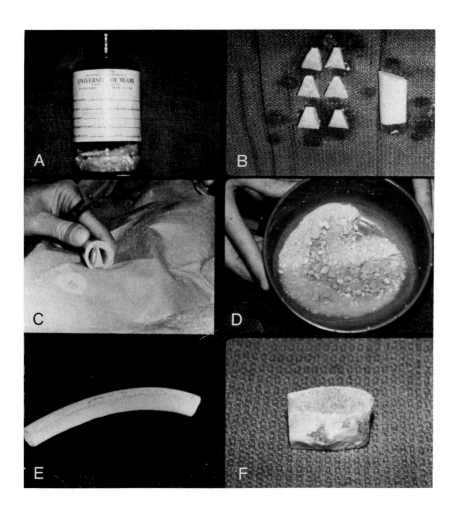

Figure 48.5. Allogeneic freeze-dried bone is available in variety of forms with different proportions of cortical and cancellous bone. **A.** Bone is stored in vacuum-packed glass bottles. **B.** Cortical struts of bone prepared from tibial shaft cortical segments. **C.** Cross section of allogeneic femur. **D.** Cancellous chips. **E.** Section of allogeneic rib. **F.** Allogeneic iliac crest: note three sides of cortical bone with cancellous interior.

modification are freezing, freeze-drying, and decalcification.

Freezing of allogeneic bone has been accomplished at a variety of different temperatures; however, a temperature of -70° C or below should be used to retard enzymatic degradation (13).Liquid nitrogen storage (-196° C), although the most expensive form of freezing, may be the most effective (34). Deep-freezing of allograft bone has a minimal effect on the biomechanical properties of the bone (35). Freezing, however, presents problems with respect to storage and transfer of the bone. Freezing of bone is generally thought to be less effective than freeze-drying in reducing antigenicity (36, 37).

The most common technique for preparing allograft bone is freeze-drying, or lyophilization. The main advantage of this technique is that it allows bone to be stored indefinitely as long as the vacuum is present. Freeze-drying also reduces antigenicity (37). The biomechanical properties of allograft bone are adversely affected by freeze-drying: torsional and bending strength are significantly decreased. Compressive and tensile strength are not seriously affected (35). The development of tissue banks, such as the United States Navy and regional tissue banks, have popularized the use of the freeze-dried allograft by facilitating its availability.

Preparation of the graft must, first of all, prevent the transmission of disease (32, 34, 36). The issue of sterility has become more apparent since the report that the human immunodeficiency virus (HIV) may reside in bone (38). Transmission of HIV with a bone allograft has been reported (39). Buck et al. speculate that freezing may reduce the viral load in bone, thus contributing to the low rate of transmission of HIV by bone allograft (38). One study reports that, with proper precautions, the chance of using a bone allograft from an infected donor is less than one in a million (40). Sterile bone can be procured by careful preparation during donor selection, excision of the graft, and treatment and storage of the graft. Selection of appropriate donors is based on medical guidelines developed by the American Association of Tissue Banks (41). Potential donors must be free from infection, malignant disease, potentially transmissible diseases of unknown etiology, a history of syphilis, malaria, leprosy, tuberculosis, or viral hepatitis, severe trauma, poisoning, drug overdose, or steroid use that might have masked infection (42). Serological tests, an autopsy, and blood and tissue bacteriological cultures are performed to ensure that there is the least possible risk of transmission of disease (43).

There are two principal methods of achieving sterile donor bone from cadavers: (*a*) procurement under sterile con-

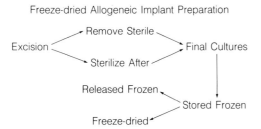

Figure 48.6. Diagram illustrating flow scheme for preparation of allogeneic bone by University of Miami technique.

ditions and (*b*) sterilization of the bone after procurement. The United States Navy Tissue Bank and the University of Miami Tissue Bank remove bone under sterile conditions (e.g., sterile preparation and draping) (36, 44). Bacteriological cultures are taken from the bone immediately after excision and just before storage. The bone is placed in a sterile glass container, aseptically sealed, and usually frozen to -80° C. After completion of the bacteriological studies, the bone is either released for use in the frozen state or, more commonly, freeze-dried (Fig. 48.6).

The freeze-drying cycle reduces the moisture content of the bone to 5° or less. The graft can then be stored in this state at room temperature almost indefinitely. It is reconstituted with an intravenous sterile saline infusion set 18 to 24 hours before use. Reconstitution is most important for cortical allografts to facilitate the shaping of the graft. Tomford and associates (45) have reported that the clinical infection rate with allograft bone prepared by this technique compares quite favorably with the infection rate associated with the use of autogenous bone. An altogether different scenario exists with massive allografts, such as those performed for the management of bone tumors. Ford et al. identified a 11.7% infection rate in these patients, with gram-positive organisms being the most common cause (46). Thirty-six percent were due to *Staphylococcus epidermidis*. The reasons for this high rate are speculative but may include the lack of defense mechanisms available to the graft or the possibility that these infections are a symptom of rejection of the graft. In either event, in this subset of patients with massive allografts infection is a disastrous complication, with more than 80% of the infected grafts going on to graft resection or amputation.

A second technique for procuring sterile cadaver bone involves removal of the bone under clean, but not necessarily sterile, conditions and sterilization of the bone with an exogenous agent. The advantage of this technique is that it simplifies procurement while increasing the number of potential donors. Numerous agents have been used in the past to sterilize bone. Of these techniques, irradiation, boiling, autoclaving, beta-propiolactone, antibiotic powders and solutions, and benzalkonium all slow the rate of incorporation of the graft by negating the bone morphogenetic protein (47). The Neuroskeletal Transplantation Laboratory in San Jose, CA, uses ethylene oxide for gaseous sterilization of allogeneic bone. Prolo and associates (47) have

demonstrated that freeze-drying for more than 72 hours reduces ethylene oxide and its reaction products to acceptable levels (48). They report more than 2000 implantations of tissue sterilized by this technique without any infections (47).

The physical properties of bone grafts may be altered by radiation (49). Doses of greater than 3 megarads weaken the breaking strength of bone. Doses of less than 3 megarads, when combined with freeze-drying, also weaken the graft. The clinical importance of this depends to a large extent on the need for structural support at the recipient site. Given the concern of the potential for transmission of human immunodeficiency virus or slow viruses, sterility achieved through irradiation must be considered.

Allogeneic bone prepared by aseptic procurement (e.g., University of Miami bone) or by ethylene oxide sterilization (Neuroskeletal Transplantation Laboratory) has been used extensively by podiatric surgeons with excellent results. In general, this mineralized allogeneic bone functions best as a spacer for osteoconduction in orthotopic sites such as the calcaneus (50-52). In a review of 200 allogeneic implants used at Doctors Hospital, Tucker, GA, most were used for reconstructive osteotomies of the calcaneus or for the packing of cysts.

Demineralized Allogeneic Bone

Another form of allogeneic bone is the autolyzed antigen-extracted allogeneic (AAA) bone developed by Urist (53-57). In contrast to freeze-dried Miami bone, the AAA bone is demineralized. The principle behind the grafting of demineralized bone is to use bone-morphogenetic protein to induce new bone formation (57). Preparation of demineralized bone differs significantly from that of mineralized allogeneic bone (58) (Table 48.3). Urist (55) insists that long cortical bone must be used. Cancellous bone or iliac crest is not sufficiently inductive and may be highly antigenic (55, 59). After demineralization, the bone is sterilized either chemically with ethylene oxide (58) or by irradiation (60). Clinical studies of the use of demineralized bone implants in maxillofacial surgery have demonstrated several advantages of this technique (59, 61).

These advantages include easy fashioning to a desired shape, rapid healing of defects, and reduced graft resorption. Demineralized bone has been used largely for treatment of craniofacial defects and defects created by the excision of tumors. Its use in nonunions and in weight-bearing areas is experimental at this point. Further research on the mechanism of induction and the subsequent healing process may make this technique more useful clinically (62-66).

Johnson et al. have reported the successful use of human bone morphogenetic protein implants and internal fixation to treat intractable femoral nonunions (67). Schmitz and Hollinger have described the successful use of a biodegradable copolymer of polylactide-polyglycolide combined with allogeneic demineralized freeze-dried bone as an osteoinductive implant (68). This combination of materials provided some stability to the implant. Further work in the area of osteoinduction may produce new materials for surgeons to use in place of conventional autogenous bone grafts.

Callus Distraction

The concept of callus distraction involves a technique of slow distraction of callus following submetaphyseal corticotomy. The technique is beyond the scope of this chapter but is mentioned here because it is an alternative to bone grafting for long bone lengthening. There are significant sequelae associated with the procedure, but the technique has increasing indications in lower extremity surgery (69).

Osteoarticular Allografts

In addition to the forms of allograft bone already described, entire joints can be implanted in the form of osteoarticular allografts (70-72). The osteoarticular allografts generally consist of the articular side of a joint with a portion of attached shaft. The primary indication for this procedure has been for joint excisions performed in the treatment of aggressive benign or low-grade malignant tumors. The primary site has been the knee, where the procedure is used as an alternative to amputation or shortening fusion. Mankin and associates reviewed a series of 100 osteoarticular allografts and reported 64.5% good or excellent results (71).

The technical problems associated with osteoarticular allografts include (*a*) preservation of cartilage, (*b*) minimization of the immune response, (*c*) ensuring of sterility, and (*d*) creation of an osseous stable environment. These issues are central to noncartilaginous grafts as well, with the exception of the preservation of cartilage. The donor-selection criteria are identical to those described previously, with the additional constraints that bone procurement should occur within 12 to 15 hours of death and the donor should be between 15 and 45 years of age. After sterile procurement, cartilaginous surfaces are treated for at least 1 hour with 10% glycerol to preserve articular cartilage viability. The graft is then slowly frozen to -80° C. When ready for use, the graft is rapidly thawed in Ringers' lactate solution at 45° C. Additional factors that may be important in successful cartilage implantation include an osseous component more than 1 cm thick, stability of the graft-host junction, and a rectus alignment of the joint.

An additional concern with osteoarticular allografts is the immune response. There is no doubt that there is a host immune response directed at the allograft implant. The significance of that response to the failure rate in osteoarticular allografts is not known. What is known is that while freezing or immunosuppression does serve to decrease the immune response to an allograft, only fresh autografts appear to function satisfactorily for a prolonged period of time (73). Subchondral bone failure, with a loss of mechanical integrity, has been the ultimate result in osteoarticular allograft surgery. Even after successful incorporation, long-term joint degeneration may occur (74-75).

The future of osteoarticular allografts is cautiously optimistic. Greater success for these grafts will depend on solution of the immune and incorporation problems that occur with these implants.

Alloplastic Materials

Several materials, including plaster of Paris (76), polyvinyl alcohol sponge (77), tantalum mesh (78), and hydroxyapatite implant (79), have been used in the past as alloplastic filling materials. Coralline hydroxyapatite appears to be the most promising of these unproven materials because of its mechanical strength, biocompatibility, biodegradation, and adequate pore size for vascular ingrowth (80-81). The brittle ceramic nature of these calcium phosphate biomaterials (hydroxyapatite and tricalcium phosphate) makes them unsuitable as structural substitutes for cortical bone. As packing material for bone cysts or beneath articular surfaces in comminuted fractures, these substitute materials may be quite acceptable (82). Their principal property is as an excellent osteoconductive scaffold for bone ingrowth (83).

Composite Grafting

The composite graft is simply a combination of two different graft materials. Most commonly the term refers to a combination of autogenous cancellous bone with allogeneic cortical bone. The purpose of this composite is to combine the high osteogenic potential of autogenous cancellous bone with the high osteoinductive property of allogeneic bone (Fig 48.7). It is a practical solution, particularly in areas where large amounts of graft material are required. In animal models it has been demonstrated that autogenous bone accelerates the healing of allogeneic cortical grafts (84). The concept of the composite graft has been extended to other materials, such as the combination of autogenous cancellous bone or marrow with xenogeneic bone (26) or coralline hydroxyapatite (80), with promising results. Nade (85) advocates the use of autogenous marrow as a composite substance along with decalcified "bank bone." Composite grafting can be quite useful in foot surgery. The surgeon can use an allogeneic graft for structural support and inductive effect and add the osteogenic effect of autogenous bone procured from the calcaneus. Many times this technique eliminates the necessity for tibial or iliac crest grafts with their accompanying morbidity.

SURGICAL MANAGEMENT OF BONE GRAFTS

It is well recognized that it is important to prepare a healthy host bed for the graft. However, it is equally important to obtain the donor bone in such a way as to minimize the trauma to the graft and maximize the number of viable cells. This is accomplished by (*a*) removing the graft with minimal trauma, (*b*) storing the graft in a solution that is supportive of the surviving cells, and (*c*) minimizing the amount of time that the graft is out of the body.

The effect of surgical trauma to the graft is well documented. High-pressure drilling with insufficient irrigation

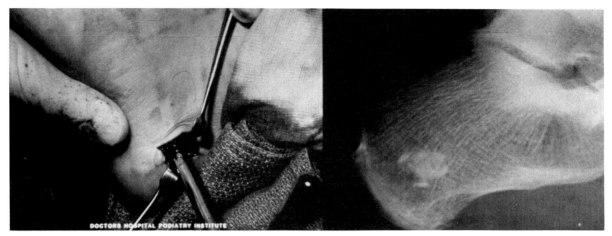

Figure 48.7. Composite grafts in foot can be fashioned from small amounts of autogenous cancellous bone from calcaneus. Small trephine can be used for procurement, and defect in calcaneus can be packed with allogeneic bone.

causes delayed healing (86). Even under ideal conditions, surgical trauma results in a necrotic border of 0.4 mm (87). Although this finding is more important at the host site, clearly the necrotic border decreases the number of viable cells transferred in the graft. Recommendations to minimize surgical trauma to the graft include (*a*) thorough irrigation and cooling during cutting of the bone (88), (*b*) use of only sharpened drills, saws, and osteotomes (89), and (*c*) avoidance of excessive total speed above 1500 revolutions per minute (90). Ferguson and associates (91) demonstrated that a graft cut with an osteotome functioned better than one cut with a high-speed saw. Albrektsson (92) studied bone graft healing under varying amounts of surgical trauma. He found that revascularization occurred more rapidly with minimal trauma and that subsequent bone remodeling also began earlier.

Another interesting technique for minimizing trauma to the graft and increasing graft viability is the "preformed graft." Albrektsson and associates (93) devised a two-step procedure for procuring an autologous graft. Step one is the insertion of a titanium mold of the desired shape into the donor bone. After a suitable period of time to allow for bone healing and vascular adaptation, the graft is removed. These grafts have a more marrow-dominated circulation that revascularizes more quickly and heals more rapidly. This technique is somewhat similar to the "delay" process used for flaps in plastic surgery. Albrektsson demonstrated that this technique decreases cell necrosis after removal of the graft and increases the number of vessels communicating between the marrow space and the bone tissue. The necessity for two surgical procedures and the time interval involved for the delay make this technique impractical in most situations.

Once an autologous graft is removed, there is often a period of time during which the graft must be stored before implantation. This may vary anywhere from minutes to hours. Gray and Elves (94) have demonstrated that there are important guidelines for temporary storage of the graft:

(*a*) antibiotic powders or sprays inhibit osteogenesis, (*b*) antibiotic solutions for irrigation do not appear to inhibit osteogenesis, (*c*) storage in saline solution is detrimental to the graft, whereas exposure to moist air for a similar period is not harmful, and (*d*) tissue culture medium preserves the osteogenic potential of the graft and, under certain circumstances, enhances it. Gray and Elves (94) recommend short-term storage of the graft in a closed container covered with a moistened saline sponge, without immersion (Fig. 48.8).

In the event of inadvertent contamination of a graft, mechanical cleansing is the most important factor in preventing infection. Saline solution, povidone iodine, and cefazolin have been reported by Cruz and associates to be equally effective (95). Clearly, the amount of time between removal of the graft and transplantation into the host site should be minimized. This time interval can be minimized by having two surgical teams available so that there can be optimum timing and coordination between the graft and host procedures.

As with any other surgery, atraumatic technique is important in the handling of the graft and the host tissues. Hemostasis is also critical to prevent hematoma and dehiscence. Microfibrillar collagen, an exogenous hemostatic agent, should be used with caution because it has been demonstrated to impede bone healing (96).

Many surgeons have placed drill holes in cortical grafts to accelerate revascularization. This fenestration of the graft has been demonstrated to be inconsequential to the mechanical strength of the graft; that is, it does not create any significant weakness (12) except in large osteoarticular allografts, where fenestration may create stress risers.

Drill holes placed perpendicular to the long axis of the graft segment have not been proved to accelerate healing in autografts. Drill holes parallel to the long axis of the graft segment may be more beneficial by facilitating osteoconduction in cortical grafts. Fenestration of lyophilized allografts has been demonstrated to accelerate graft repair (97) (Fig. 48.9).

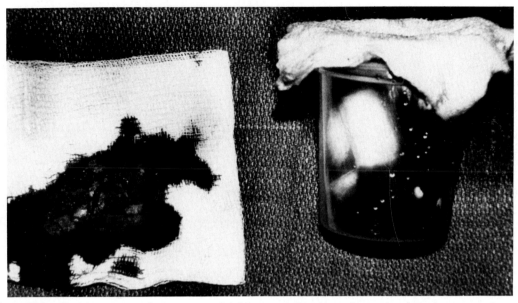

Figure 48.8. Short-term storage of autogenous graft is best accomplished in sterile container covered with moist sponge.

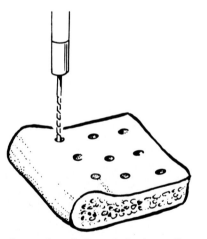

Figure 48.9. Fenestration of allogeneic implants will accelerate graft repair.

Another important consideration is the use of prophylactic antibiotics. As with any other procedure, the risks must be weighed against the potential benefits. In traumatic situations, or in situations involving elective use of allogeneic bone graft material, the administration of prophylactic antibiotics in an appropriate and timely manner can probably be justified. Development of postsurgical osteomyelitis would be a devastating complication. In the author's own use of prophylactic antibiotics, he generally prefers use of a first-generation cephalosporin such as cefazolin, beginning in the operating room 30 minutes before inflation of the tourniquet and continuing for no more than 24 hours.

TECHNIQUE FOR HARVESTING OF GRAFTS

Radiographs of potential donor sites should be reviewed before surgery to rule out anatomical variations or intrinsic disease.

Iliac Crest

The iliac crest provides a good source of cancellous bone in quantities that are more than ample for foot surgery. Corticocancellous grafts can be obtained with one to three sides of cortical bone.

A number of surgical techniques are available for procurement of iliac crest bone (Fig. 48.10). The patient's position on the table may also determine the surgical approach: a prone patient gives access to the posterior superior iliac spine. A 5 cm incision beginning 1 to 2 cm posterior to the anterior superior spine provides sufficient exposure for most grafts needed for foot surgery. Careful attention must be paid to avoid the lateral femoral cutaneous nerve during dissection. After dissection down to bone, the periosteum is reflected and a window is created on the lateral side of the ilium (98). Cancellous bone can be removed with a curette or a gouge. The window can then be replaced or used for its cortical bone content in the graft (Fig. 48.11). Other techniques can be used, including (*a*) a sagittal split of the crest that is then rewired after removal of the graft or (*b*) removal of the crest with the graft followed by separation of the two and then rewiring of the crest (99).

The need for certain precautions should be noted. The epiphysis of the iliac crest is open until the age of 20 to 25 and should be carefully avoided. Profuse bleeding may occur with this procedure. Laurie and associates (99) report an average blood loss of 750 to 1000 ml intraoperatively

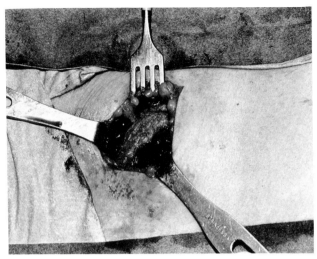

Figure 48.10. Exposure of iliac crest. Lateral cortical surface can be windowed for procurement of cancellous bone with bone curets.

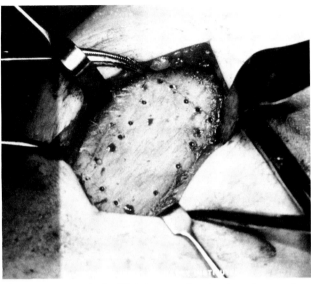

Figure 48.12. Multiple drill holes to outline the donor bone graft are particularly helpful in tibia.

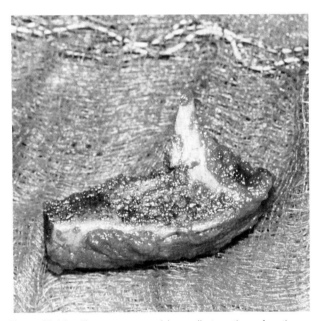

Figure 48.11. Iliac crest can provide excellent portions of corticocancellous bone.

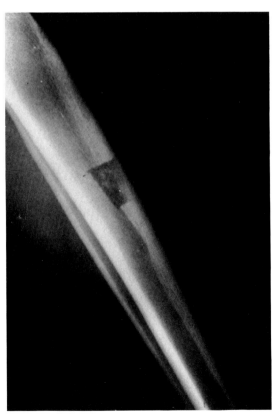

Figure 48.13. Bone grafts procured from tibial shaft provide less cancellous bone and carry greater structural risks.

and postoperatively. Suction drainage, good wound closure, and exogenous hemostatic agents can decrease the risk of hematoma and wound-healing problems.

Laurie and associates (99) reported on donor site morbidity at the iliac crest and noted the following: (*a*) patients had an average of 6 weeks of pain, with 10% of the patients reporting pain 2 years after the surgery; (*b*) 8.3% of the patients reported hypesthesia/anesthesia in the thigh; (*c*) incisions directly over the crest have a higher rate of wound breakdown, and (*d*) bone irregularity of the crest was common postoperatively (30%), especially after sagittal splitting of the crest.

The iliac crest provides a high quality and volume of cancellous bone but the procedure requires meticulous attention to regional anatomy, wound closure, and hemostasis. The pain and potential complications associated with this procedure must be carefully weighed before one elects to use autogenous bone from this area.

Tibia

Grafts from the proximal tibial metaphysis provide good cancellous bone, as well as an excellent source of cortical bone. An oblique anteromedial or anterolateral incision is made without extension over the crest. The periosteum is incised and reflected. Drill holes are placed to outline the size of the graft in order to prevent the formation of stress risers in the donor site. The graft is removed by power instrumentation to prevent splitting or shattering of the bone (Fig. 48.12). Cancellous bone can then be removed with a curette. Mears (100) states that a sphere of bone 40 mm in diameter can be safely removed from the tibial metaphysis. If only cancellous bone is needed, a small window is made through the cortical surface and the graft is removed with a curette. Careful closure of the periosteum is followed by routine closure of other tissues. The graft is taken from the limb ipsilateral to the host site to avoid compromising both limbs at the same time. The limb is protected until radiographic evidence of healing has been demonstrated. Excessive decortication must be avoided (Fig. 48.13). Fractures through the donor site can occur, and these can be extremely debilitating.

The distal tibial metaphysis is also a potential donor site. Small corticocancellous sections of bone can be removed,

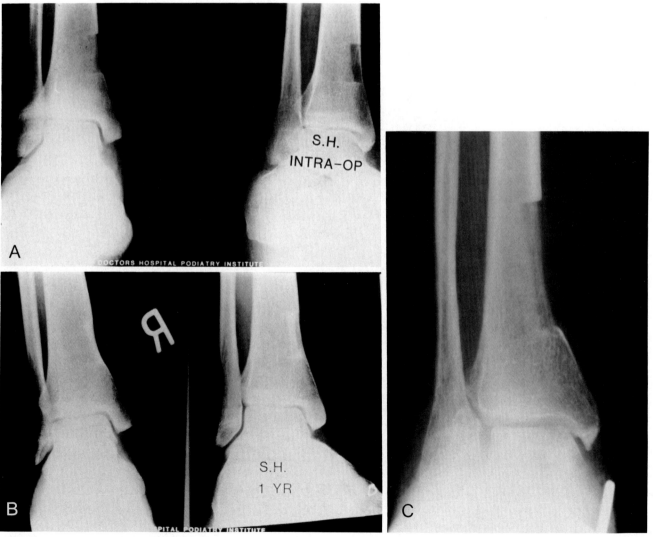

Figure 48.14. Radiographs of graft donor site from medial aspect of distal tibial metaphysis. **A.** Intraoperative radiographs showing proper resection of bone. **B.** Postoperative views 1 year later showing filling-in of donor site of same patient. **C.** Excessive decortication of tibia.

most readily from the medial side (Fig. 48.14). Care must be taken both proximally and distally to avoid excessive bone removal near the joint surface.

Fibula

The fibula is a good source of corticocancellous bone and is ideally suited for metatarsal grafts and other areas where both cortical and cancellous bone are required. Two precautions should be observed: (*a*) avoidance of the peroneal nerve and (*b*) maintenance of the stability of the ankle mortise by preservation of the lower third of the fibula (Fig. 48.15). An ankle valgus can result after overly aggressive resection of the fibula. The distal tip of the fibula contains cancellous bone, but the shaft of the fibula consists largely of cortical bone.

A posterolateral approach is used for exposure of the middle third of the fibula. The peroneal nerves can be reflected anteriorly. The graft is then cut with a power saw after the periosteum is reflected. The nutrient artery may have to be ligated. In some situations it may be possible to split the middle third of the fibula sagittally and use only one half of the bone. After removal of the graft, the peri-

osteum is reapproximated. Sometimes this will result in full regeneration of the fibula.

Calcaneus

Many situations require only a small amount of cancellous bone. In these cases the calcaneus can often provide an adequate volume of high-quality cancellous bone. This can be procured in one of two ways. A hand trephine can be inserted through a small incision on the lateral side of the calcaneus. One or two passes with the trephine can secure enough cancellous bone for a small composite graft or to augment other autogenous bone.

Alternatively, a somewhat larger lateral incision can be made on the calcaneus posterior to the neutral triangle and above the plantar condyles (Fig. 48.16). The incision is placed to avoid the sural nerve and is deepened by layers to bone. Drill holes are made to outline a cortical window, which is then removed with a power saw. If the cortical bone is not needed for the graft, it is replaced on the lateral side of the calcaneus and covered with periosteum. The defect can be packed with allogeneic freeze-dried cancellous chips if necessary.

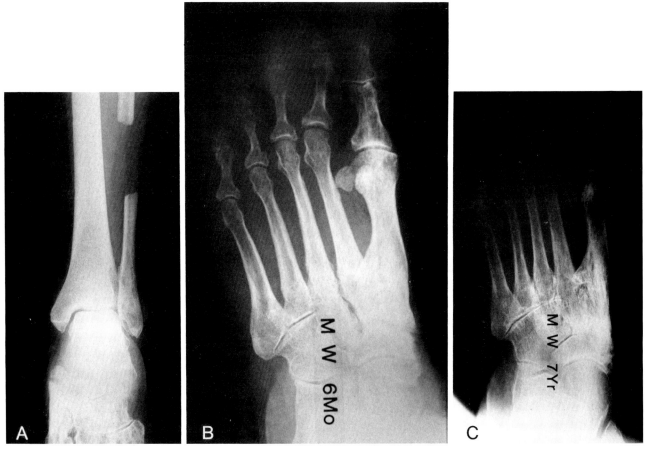

Figure 48.15.   **A.** Radiograph of fibular donor site 6 months postoperatively. Ankle mortise has been preserved. **B.** Inlay bone graft of fibula in navicular, cuneiform, and first metatarsal at 6 months. **C.** Same as **B** at 7 years.

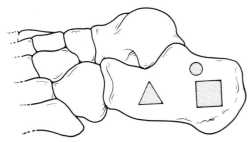

Figure 48.16. Diagram of lateral aspect of calcaneus. Important considerations include protection of neutral triangle (shaded triangle) and calcaneofibular ligament attachment to calcaneus (shaded circle), as well as the plantar condyles and Achilles tendon insertion. Cancellous bone can be safely removed from shaded square area. Corticocancellous bone can be procured from the dorsolateral surface of the calcaneus.

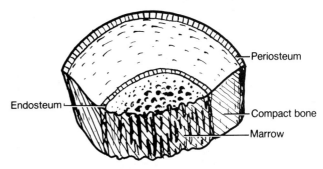

Figure 48.17. Periosteal tissue on graft can account for up to 30% of new bone formed by graft.

After bone is procured from the calcaneus, the limb must be protected, with no weight bearing until there is evidence of healing. The time required for healing of the donor site will vary with the amount of bone removed. Medial approaches to the calcaneus should be avoided when possible to avoid postoperative fibrosis resulting in a tarsal tunnel syndrome. Clearly, removal of bone from any donor site weakens that bone and the risks involved with procurement should be weighed against the possible benefits of using autogenous bone rather than allogeneic bone.

Other Sources

Autogenous bone from the foot can also be obtained from the medial side of the first metatarsal head and lateral fifth metatarsal tuberosity (101). Possible donor sources are limited only by the need to preserve function in the donor bone and the requirements of the recipient area (102).

BONE GRAFT HEALING

General Considerations

The process of survival and incorporation of a bone graft consists of a complex temporal and spatial relationship. Among several processes, the following are important: (*a*) differentiation of osteoprogenitor cells and subsequent osteoblast proliferation, (*b*) vascular ingrowth, (*c*) osteoinduction, (*d*) osteoconduction, and (*e*) biomechanical remodeling of the graft. The time required for graft repair depends on a multitude of factors, including graft material, host tissue, mechanical stability, and various other environmental factors.

Several processes and terms must be discussed, including creeping substitution, osteoconduction, osteoinduction, and the relative contribution of different graft and host tissues to the repair process. The term *creeping substitution* is a translation from the German phrase *schleichender Ersatz* used by Axhausen (3). Axhausen's concept was that the necrotic graft material was invaded and replaced by new tissue. Burchardt and Enneking (1), in 1978, redefined creeping sub-

stitution as the temporal and spatial repair activities whereby new viable bone replaces necrotic bone. The exact contribution of host and graft tissue has not been defined in this process. Osteoconduction is the means by which creeping substitution can take place. The term refers to the "scaffolding" effect of the bone graft that acts as a conduit for migration of viable cells. Cancellous allografts are particularly effective in providing the osteoconductive pathways necessary for graft healing.

Osteoinduction is an interesting phenomenon reported by Urist and associates (54), who describe a bone morphogenetic protein or inductor substance that is present in bone matrix. This inductor substance causes nonosseous tissue to become osteogenic in the presence of a favorable environment. It is well accepted that bone induction occurs. The mechanism of possible inductor substances and clinical significance has yet to be defined. Nade and Burwell (59) have reported that decalcified iliac crest is only weakly inductive, whereas Urist and Dawson (55) have stated that decalcified diaphyseal cortical bone is strongly inductive.

Axhausen (103) proposed that osteogenesis after autogenous bone grafting occurs in two phases. Phase 1 is a graft-dependent process that produces the majority of the osteogenesis that occurs within the first 4 weeks. Phase 2 occurs after the initial 4- to 8-week period and is a host-dependent process. Gray and Elves (104) analyzed the relative contributions to osteogenesis during the phase 1 process and concluded that (*a*) endosteal and marrow stroma graft cells account for more than 50% of the bone formation, (*b*) periosteal cells contribute about 30%, (*c*) osteocytes contribute 10%, and (*d*) free hemopoietic cells make no significant contribution (Fig. 48.17).

Autograft Healing

The initial phase of autograft healing is similar to other types of wound healing. The first week consists of establishment of hemostasis and inflammatory cell infiltration. Vital vascular budding occurs. The second week is dominated by fibrous granulation tissue formation and by necrosis of graft osteocytes (1). This process is similar for both cortical and cancellous bone. However, major differences exist between cortical and cancellous grafts.

Cortical Versus Cancellous Autograft Healing

In cortical graft healing, vascular penetration does not occur until the sixth day. Because of its structure, vascular penetration takes twice as long in cortical bone as in cancellous bone. Second, cortical graft healing begins with osteoclastic resorptive activity, which continues until the graft-host junction is consolidated (105). At that time osteoblastic activity begins. Cortical grafts are incompletely repaired; they remain mixtures of necrotic material and viable new bone. Because of the initial osteoclastic activity, cortical grafts initially lose 40% of their strength from 6 weeks to 6 months and become less radiodense (106). The duration of this osteoclastic phase explains why most fatigue fractures occur at between 6 and 18 months. The knowledge that the graft is weakened over time is important to the surgeon in determining how long a graft must be protected (Fig. 48.18).

Conversely, in cancellous bone vascularization begins within hours of grafting. Osteogenesis proceeds with a resulting increase in radiodensity and mechanical strength of the graft. Eventually the entire cancellous graft is replaced by new bone (106).

There are three prerequisites for graft healing: mechanical stability, vascularization of the graft bed, and close contact between the graft and its host environment (11). As long as shearing forces exist at the graft-host junction, revascularization of the graft and its subsequent healing will

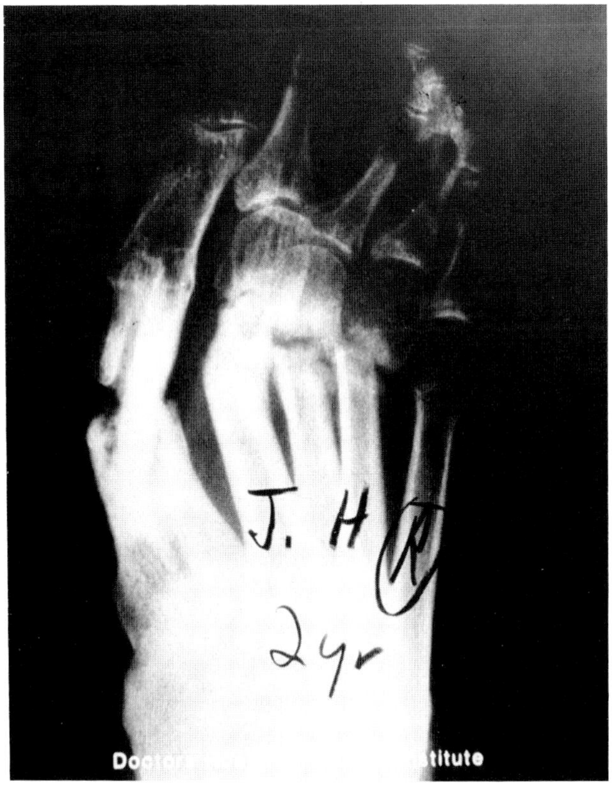

Figure 48.18. Failure of pure cortical graft at 24 months. Slow incorporation of compact bone means that these types of grafts must be protected for a prolonged period of time.

not take place. Mechanical stability, important for fracture healing, is essential for graft healing to occur. Similarly, osteogenesis and incorporation of the graft are dependent on the nutritional support of the graft bed vascular supply and the surrounding host tissues. Surgical manipulation of the graft and the host bed by the surgeon is designed to ensure that these three prerequisites for healing are protected.

Allogeneic Graft Healing

No discussion of allogeneic bone is complete without a consideration of bone antigenicity. Fresh allografts elicit both a cell-mediated immune response and a humoral response of antibody production (1). Frozen allogeneic bone elicits the same response as measured by leukocyte migration, donor skin graft rejection time, and humoral cytotoxic antibody titers. Blocking antibodies are delivered in response to both forms of allogeneic bone (107). The blocking antibodies enhance survival of the graft by affixing to the immunogenic cells, neutralizing their stimulating effect. Because the donor cells of a frozen alloimplant do not survive anyway, the immunological response becomes important primarily in terms of local tissue reaction and destruction of the osteoinductive property of bone. Studies using rat and canine models have suggested that histocompatibility typing may be advantageous when frozen allograft bone is used (108). This potential antigenicity associated with frozen bone is one of the reasons that it has not been popular in podiatric surgery.

In freeze-dried bone antigenicity is reduced because of the lyophilization process. The actual clinical significance of this antigenicity is unknown, partly because of the multitude of different models and variables that have been tested and measured (37). Further research in immunology and bone graft healing will help surgeons to delineate the proper role of allogeneic freeze-dried bone.

Grafting Techniques

Early grafting techniques were designed to provide not only osteogenesis but also stabilization of the graft. This necessitated the use of cortical grafts to provide that stability. With the advent of modern fixation materials and devices, the osteogenic power of cancellous bone can be used more efficiently.

Historically, the cortical onlay graft was a popular technique for the repair of nonunions. The graft may be single, double, or multiple (barrel stave) strips. Phemister described a modification of the onlay graft where the graft is placed subperiosteally without fixation. This technique is inferior to other techniques in both osteogenesis and mechanical stability (Fig. 48.19). Other graft techniques used for stability include peg grafting and inlay grafting (109, 110) (Fig. 48.20). A useful modification is the peg-in-hole technique of grafting (Fig. 48.21). This provides both some mechanical stability and an increased surface area for vascular ingrowth. This technique can be used for interpositional metatarsal

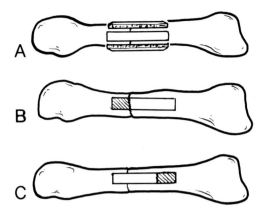

Figure 48.19. Traditional bone grafting techniques include Phemister onlay technique (**A**), and sliding inlay graft (**B** and **C**). These techniques provide crude stability without rigidity.

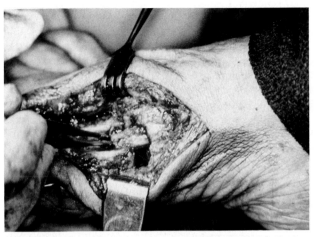

Figure 48.20. Inlay grafting technique supplemented with Kirschner wire fixation.

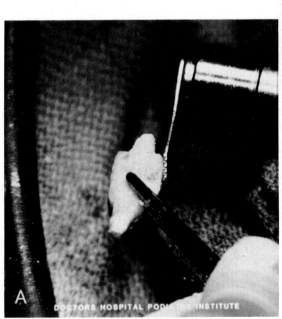

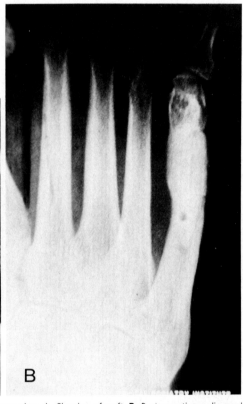

Figure 48.21. Pegged autogenous tibial graft provides stability and increased host-graft interface for more rapid healing in this metatarsal nonunion. **A.** Shaping of graft. **B.** Postoperative radiograph demonstrates rapid consolidation around pegs.

grafts and in other areas of the foot. It is generally combined with additional fixation, such as Kirschner wire (K-wire) stabilization or tension band plating.

A specialized bone-grafting method is the so-called Papineau technique, or open cancellous bone grafting. It is used for the treatment of chronic osteomyelitis and infected nonunions. Rhinelander (111, 112) described the technique and demonstrated experimentally the rapid revascularization of

the cancellous grafts. Papineau (113) helped popularize the technique, which involves three steps: (*a*) excision of necrotic bone, (*b*) cancellous bone grafting, and (*c*) skin coverage (114).

The first step consists of excision of necrotic bone and soft tissue. When the procedure is performed for a septic nonunion, the bone ends are stabilized, usually with external fixation (115). The wound is then fully packed, and the dressing is changed every other day until the entire wound is covered with granulation tissue. After the entire wound is covered with a healthy layer of granulation tissue the second step of cancellous grafting can be performed (116, 117). Small pieces (0.5 × 0.5 × 0.5 cm) of autogenous cancellous bone are packed into the bone cavity until it is heaped above the level of the bone surface. The superficial layer of the graft dies and the remainder is revascularized from the surrounding granulation tissue. The graft is covered with petrolatum gauze to prevent desiccation or else is kept continuously moist. The third step in the technique is skin coverage. If the defect is small, this may be allowed to occur spontaneously. In a large defect, skin grafting can be performed after granulation tissue completely covers the graft. This may be in 2 to 4 months. Alternative methods of skin coverage, including local flaps and muscle or myocutaneous flaps, may be required in specific situations.

Mears (100) emphasizes the importance of keeping the graft continuously moist, often for a period of several months, until the wound is ready for skin coverage. He reports that, even with rigorous technique, approximately 20% of these patients have periodic drainage and ejection of small bone fragments. For this reason, muscle flaps are now often used in place of open cancellous grafting. This technique has the advantage of providing immediate coverage of exposed bone.

Evaluation of Healing

Once the graft is in place, postoperative management decisions must be based on the speed of union of the graft with the host. In the lower extremity the decision as to when to allow unprotected weight bearing is particularly crucial. This decision can be based on several types of information: clinical findings, conventional radiographs, technetium scans, tomograms, fluoroscopy, and/or computed tomography (CT) scans.

Reduction of edema and discomfort is an excellent clinical sign of healing. However, clinical signs are accurate mainly as a means of diagnosis by exclusion. Absence of induration indicates that there probably is no unstability. This does not mean, however, that the graft is sufficiently strong to withstand weight bearing.

Conventional radiographs, with three to four views, should be taken at appropriate intervals, such as every 6 weeks or whenever a change in management is to be made. Attention is focused on two sites: the graft-host junction and the internal fixation devices. Consolidation at the graft-host junction indicates active graft incorporation. A gradual blurring of cortical margins occurs, with eventual crossing of the trabeculation pattern across the graft-host junction (Fig. 48.22). As discussed in the section on graft healing, cancellous grafts will initially appear more radiodense whereas cortical grafts will initially appear more radiolucent. Early

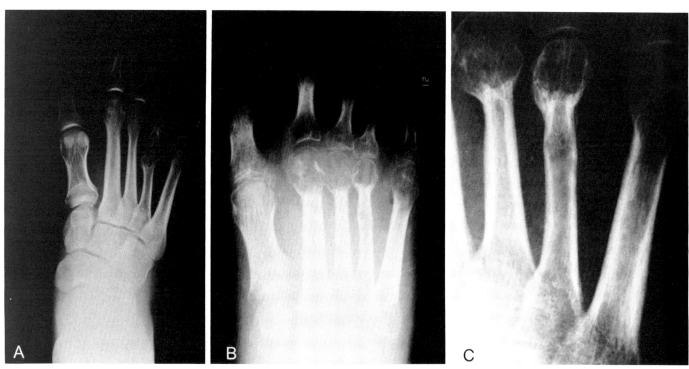

Figure 48.22. **A.** Preoperative radiograph of 17-year-old patient with brachymetatarsia of first and fourth metatarsals. **B.** Twelve weeks' postoperative radiograph demonstrates visible graft-host junctions of this autogenous graft with moderate consolidation. **C.** Five months' postoperative radiograph demonstrates complete consolidation of graft.

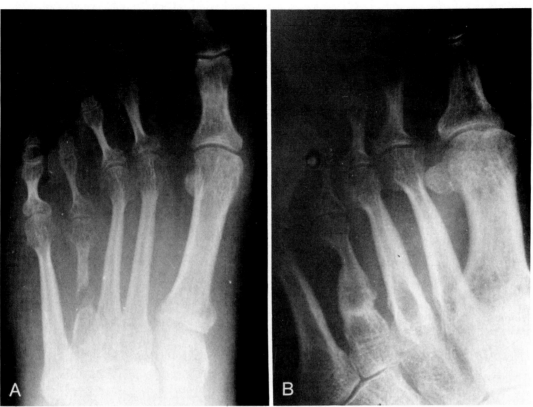

Figure 48.23. **A.** Six months' postoperative view of fourth metatarsal allogeneic implant for brachymetatarsia shows obvious dissolution of implant. **B.** Same patient 6 months after repair with autogenous iliac crest. Radiograph reveals total consolidation.

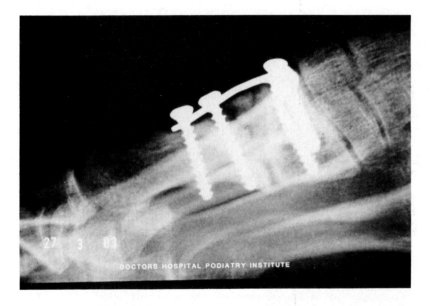

Figure 48.27. Fourteen-year follow-up of graft lengthening for treatment of brachymetatarsia. Arrow shows area of bone remodeling in response to weight-bearing stress.

changes on radiographs are few, although an impending disaster may be signaled by sclerosis or dissolution of the graft (Fig. 48.23). Attention must also be focused on the fixation device. If the fixation device or, worse yet, the graft moves, it is indicative of an unstable situation caused by poor fixation technique, inappropriate materials or techniques, or poor patient compliance. As discussed earlier, graft healing cannot occur until mechanical stabilization of the graft-host junction is complete. Lifting of the plate, a screw backing out, or a sudden bend in a K-wire may signal the need for additional external support to the graft (e.g., a cast) (Fig. 48.24).

Tomograms and CT scans are useful, particularly when a selected area of the graft is in question. Fluoroscopy is most useful to confirm motion in a suspected nonunion. Intraosseous phlebography can be used in large bones.

Technetium scans have been advocated as the most useful technique for assessing early viability of the graft (118). This has more practical use in large grafts.

Although all of these techniques can be useful, they all have limitations. Evaluation of graft healing in the small bones of the foot is particularly troublesome because of the difficulty of producing a useful image of such a small graft-host junction. Unfortunately areas such as the metatarsal are both the most difficult to image and a difficult area to heal. Clinical experience and conventional radiographs continue to be the most useful tools in evaluating graft healing in the foot.

Complications

The most common complication of bone grafting is failure of the graft to heal. Most studies indicate a failure rate of 15% to 20% (1). The two primary causes of graft failure are inadequate mechanical stabilization and inappropriate selection of graft material.

Selection of the proper graft material requires a careful balance between the need for the rigidity afforded by cortical bone and the need for the rapid incorporation of can-cellous bone. A graft consisting solely of cortical bone may require a long period of time for full incorporation. A graft consisting of only cancellous bone has little mechanical strength and is difficult to stabilize without causing compression and deformation of the graft (Fig. 48.25).

Inadequate fixation and weight bearing can rapidly destroy a graft (*a*) by delivering an unacceptable mechanical load through the graft, causing deformation (Fig. 48.26), and (*b*) through the production of shearing forces at the graft-host junction, causing interruption of vascular budding.

Treatment for a failed graft is based on the cause of the failure. Certain principles become even more paramount when one is dealing with a failed graft. Autogenous bone should be used after failure of a first graft. At that point any disadvantages associated with autogenous grafting are outweighed by the potential failure of other types of grafts. In addition, careful planning is necessary to achieve maximum mechanical stabilization of the graft. Soft tissue structures must be carefully preserved. Vascularity and stability become the cornerstones for repair of a failed graft.

Other complications associated with bone grafting include graft resorption, infection, hematoma, and other wound complications (Fig. 48.27). In the author's experience the infection rate is no higher for allogeneic bone than for autogenous bone. In clean elective surgery, infection of a graft is uncommon. Graft resorption is generally caused by premature excessive compression on the graft, such as weight

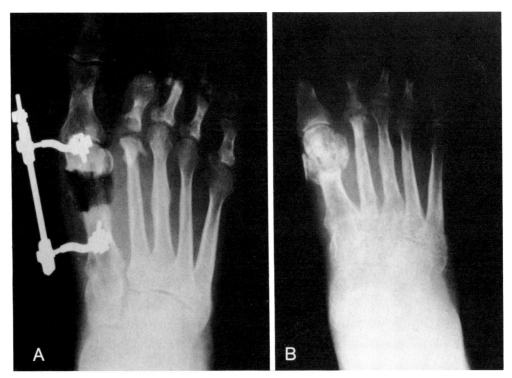

Figure 48.25. **A.** Autogenous iliac crest graft for repair of nonunion of first metatarsal. **B.** Inadequate cortical portion of graft resulted in compression of graft and loss of length.

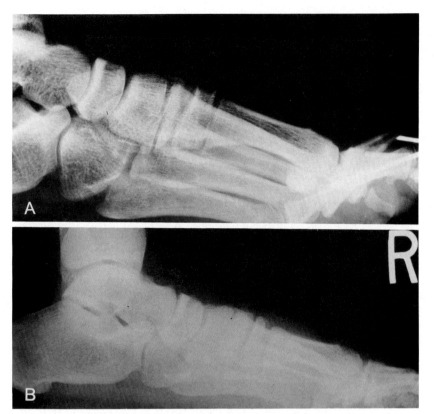

Figure 48.26. **A.** Opening wedge plantarflexory osteotomy of first metatarsal with cortical allogeneic implant. **B.** Resorption of implant secondary to early weight bearing. Note soft tissue swelling and dorsiflexion of first metatarsal.

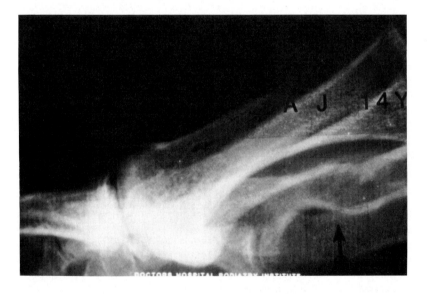

Figure 48.27. Fourteen-year follow-up of graft lengthening for treatment of brachymetatarsia. Arrow shows area of bone remodeling in response to weight-bearing stress.

bearing, or excessive use of cancellous bone in an area that requires greater support.

DISCUSSION

Although particulars concerning bone grafting in specific situations will be discussed under each of the appropriate headings, some general observations concerning materials and fixation are in order. In reviewing 200 bone grafts performed at Doctors Hospital/Northlake Regional Medical Center, Tucker, GA, graft failure could be broken down into two major areas: inappropriate selection of bone graft material and inadequate fixation.

With the availability of good-quality allogeneic bone, the indications for its use have expanded. Certainly, the most successful use of allogeneic bone continues to be as a packing material for defects in orthotopic locations such as the calcaneus (31). Other reconstructive procedures on the calcaneus, such as the Silver and Evans calcaneal osteotomies or the Grice extra-articular arthrodesis, are also good applications for an appropriate allogeneic graft. Calcaneal osteotomies with insertion of a graft and excision of bone cysts with packing of the defect accounted for more than 50% of the indications for grafting in the author's recent review. Because of the frequency of these types of procedures, allogeneic bone accounts for close to 75% of the graft material used at Doctors Hospital/Northlake Regional Medical Center. In this series there were no nonunions when allogeneic bone was used in these situations. Consequently, in the previously mentioned applications, allogeneic bone is as suitable as autogenous bone and in many situations may be preferable because of the lack of a donor site and the morbidity that accompanies harvesting of the graft.

There are additional situations in which allogeneic bone can be used, such as the packing of defects in comminuted fractures of the foot. Another acceptable method of using allogeneic bone is as the cortical portion of a composite graft along with the autogenous cancellous bone. Brachymetatarsia repair can also be accomplished with allogeneic bone.

Autogenous bone is the preferred material for repair of nonunions, and its use is essential in avascular nonunions. This includes nonunions from both traumatic and surgical fractures, as well as failed arthrodesis. In hypervascular nonunions the decision is less clear because the cause is mechanical rather than biological in nature. Because of the debilitating nature of these conditions, however, the advantages of using autogenous bone generally outweigh the risks. At the minimum, a composite graft of allogeneic cortical bone and autogenous cancellous bone should probably be considered.

Open nonunions and fractures also require autogenous bone for both promotion of vascular ingrowth and stimulation of granulation tissue.

Autogenous bone should be used whenever there is some question as to the biological potential of the host tissue. When rapidity of fusion is important, as in arthrodeses of joints, autogenous bone is also preferred.

Regardless of the type of bone used, corticocancellous grafts are the most useful type in the foot and leg. They combine the mechanical strength of cortical bone with the porosity of cancellous bone for vascular ingrowth. Cancellous bone is useful for the packing of defects and for composite grafts. Fenestrated cortical bone can be used for opening wedge osteotomies of the calcaneus or other orthotopic locations. It should be remembered that only cortical allogeneic bone has significant inductive potential. Therefore the use of cancellous allogeneic bone in areas that are nonorthotopic is not advisable.

Fixation of bone grafts is most easily accomplished in areas where there is some intrinsic stability, such as with lengthening osteotomies. For example, in opening wedge calcaneal osteotomies fixation often is not required because of the compression on the graft generated by the tension on surrounding soft tissues. Depending on the size and design of the graft, this inherent compression can provide enough stability (along with the external support of a cast) for the critical revascularization process. Similarly, in repair of brachymetatarsia the length added to the metatarsal by the graft generates sufficient compression to provide some stability. This can be supplemented by axial K-wire fixation to prevent shifting of the graft or by a quarter tubular plate for rigidity.

In nonunions, arthrodeses, and mechanically unstable areas, the stability of the fixation will determine the success of the graft. This is particularly true of the medial column because of its mobile character. The first and fifth metatarsals have osseous buttressing from adjacent metatarsals on only one side. Lack of inherent stability in an area makes rigid internal fixation the key to successful grafting.

SUMMARY

The spectrum of useful bone graft materials and substitutes will continue to expand as knowledge of the biological processes involved in graft healing continues to grow. Knowledge of the available materials and their properties will enable the surgeon to exploit each material to its best advantage.

Regardless of the material selected, successful graft incorporation will not occur unless there is mechanical stability of the graft-host junction, a vascular graft bed, and close contact between the host and its environment.

References

1. Burchardt H, Enneking WF: Transplantation of bone. *Surg Clin North Am* 58:403-427, 1978.
2. Phemister DB: The fate of transplanted bone and regenerative power of its various constituents. *Surg Gynecol Obstet* 19:303-333, 1914.
3. Axhausen G: Die patologisch-anatomischen Grundlagen der Lehre von frein Knochentransplantation beim Menschen und beim tier. *Med Klin* 2:23, 1908. (Cited by Albrektsson T: Repair of bone grafts. *Scand J Plast Reconstr Surg* 14:1-12, 1980.)
4. Albee FH: Fundamentals in bone transplantation: experiences in three thousand bone graft operations. *JAMA* 81:1429-1432, 1923.
5. Chase SW, Herndon CH: The fate of autogenous and homogenous bone grafts: a historical review. *J Bone Joint Surg* 37A:809-841, 1955.
6. Danis R: *Theorie et Pratique de l'Ostosynthese*. Paris, Masson & Cie, 1949, p 3. Translation by Perren SM: The aims of osteosynthesis. *Clin Orthop* 138:23-25, 1979.
7. Boyne PJ: Implants and transplants: review of recent research in this area of oral surgery. *J Am Dent Assoc* 87:1074-1080, 1973.
8. Snell GO: The terminology of tissue transplantation. *Transplantation* 2:655-657, 1964.
9. Edmonson AS: Surgical techniques. In Edmonson AS, Crenshaw AH (eds): *Campbell's Operative Orthopaedics*, ed 6, vol 1. St Louis, CV Mosby, 1980, p 20.
10. Malinin T, Latta L, Wagner J, Brown M: Healing of fractures with freeze-dried cortical bone plates. *Clin Orthop* 190:281-286, 1984.
11. Van der Werken C, Marti R: Bone transplantations. *Injury* 13:271-278, 1982.
12. Burchardt H, Busbee GA, Ennekin WF: Repair of experimental autologous grafts of cortical bone. *J Bone Joint Surg* 57A:814-819, 1975.
13. Urist M: Bone transplants and implants. In Urist M (ed): *Fundamental and Clinical Bone Physiology*. Philadelphia, JB Lippincott, 1980, p 365.
14. Boyne PJ: Methods of osseous reconstruction of the mandible following surgical resection. *J Biomed Mater Res* 7:195-204, 1973.

15. Weiland AJ, Moore JR, Daniel RK: Vascularized bone autografts: experience with 41 cases. *Clin Orthop* 174:87-95, 1983.

16. Weiland AJ: Current concepts review: vascularized free bone transplants. *J Bone Joint Surg* 63A:166-169, 1981.

17. Berggren AM, Weiland AJ, Dorfman H: Free vascularized bone grafts: factors affecting their survival and ability to heal to recipient bone defects. *Plast Reconstr Surg* 69:19-29, 1982.

18. Puckett CL, Hurvitz JS, Metzler MH, Silver D: Bone formation by revascularized periosteal and bone grafts, compared with traditional bone grafts. *Plast Reconstr Surg* 64:361-365, 1979.

19. Taylor GI: Microvascular free bone transfer: a clinical technique. *Orthop Clin North Am* 8:425-447, 1977.

20. Nusbickel F, Dell P, McAndrew M, Moore M: Vascularized autografts for reconstruction of skeletal defects following lower extremity trauma. *Clin Orthop* 243:65-70, 1989.

21. Stevenson TR, Greener TL, King TF: Heel reconstruction with the deep circumflex iliac artery osteocutaneous flap. *Plast Reconstr Surg* 79:982-986, 1987.

22. Salibian A, Anzel S, Salyer W: Transfer of vascularized grafts of iliac bone to the extremities. *J Bone Joint Surg* 69A:1319-1327, 1987.

23. DeBoer H, Wood M: Bone changes in the vascularized fibular graft. *J Bone Joint Surg* 71B:374-378, 1989.

24. Jones NF, Swartz W, Mears D, Jupiter J, Grossman A: The "double barrel" free vascularized fibular bone graft. *Plast Reconstr Surg* 81:378-385, 1988.

25. Inclan A: The use of preserved bone graft in orthopaedic surgery. *J Bone Joint Surg* 24:81-96, 1942.

26. Salama R: Xenogeneic bone grafting in humans. *Clin Orthop* 174:113-121, 1983.

27. Longacre JJ, Converse JM, Knize DM: Transplantation of bone. In Converse J (ed): *Reconstructive Plastic Surgery*, ed 2, vol 1. Philadelphia, WB Saunders, 1977, p 313.

28. Bassett CL, Creighton DKJ: A comparison of host response to cortical autografts and process calf heterografts. *J Bone Joint Surg* 44A:842, 1962.

29. Pieron AP, Bigelow D, Hamonic M: Grafting with Boplant: results in thirty-three cases. *J Bone Joint Surg* 50B:364, 1968.

30. McMurray GN: The evaluation of Kiel bone in spinal fusions. *J Bone Joint Surg* 64B:101-104, 1982.

31. Miller F, Sussman MD, Stamp WG: The use of bone allograft: a survey of current practice. *J Pediatr Orthop* 4:353-355, 1984.

32. Friedlander GE: Current concepts review: bone banking. *J Bone Joint Surg* 64A:307-311, 1982.

33. Jonck LM: Allogeneic bone transplantation. Part I. A review of the status of allogenic bone banks. *S Afr Med J* 60:428-430, 1981.

34. Tomford WW, Doppelt SH, Mankin HJ, Friedlander GE: 1983 bone bank procedures. *Clin Orthop* 174:15-21, 1983.

35. Pelker RR, Friedlander GE, Markham TC: Biomechanical properties of bone allografts. *Clin Orthop* 174:54-57, 1983.

36. Malinin TI, Thomson CB, Brown MD: Freeze-dried tissue allografts in surgery. In Karow AM, Pegg DE (eds): *Organ Preservation for Transplantation*, ed 2. New York, Marcel Dekker, 1981, p 677.

37. Turner DW, Mellonig JT: Antigenicity of freeze-dried bone allograft in periodontal osseous defects. *J Periodont Res* 16:89-99, 1981.

38. Buck B, Resnick L, Shah S, Malinin T: Human immunodeficiency virus cultured from bone. *Clin Orthop* 251:249-253, 1990.

39. Transmission of HIV through bone transplantation: Case report and public health recommendations. *MMWR* 37:597, 1988.

40. Buck B, Malinin T, Brown M: Bone transplantation and human immunodeficiency virus: an estimate of risk of acquired immunodeficiency syndrome (AIDS). *Clin Orthop* 240:129, 1989.

41. American Association of Tissue Banks: Provisional guidelines for cell, tissue and organ preservation. *Am Assoc Tissue Banks Newsletter* 4:25-43, 1980.

42. Malinin TI: University of Miami Tissue Bank: collection of postmortem tissues for clinical use and laboratory investigation. *Transplant Proc* 8(suppl):53-58, 1976.

43. Friedlander GE, Mankin HJ: Bone banking: current methods and suggested guidelines. In Murray D (ed): *AAOS Instructional Course Lecture Series*. St Louis, CV Mosby, 1981, p 36.

44. Bright RW, Friedlander GE, Sell KW: Tissue banking: the United States Navy tissue bank. *Milit Med* 142:503-510, 1977.

45. Tomford WW, Starkweather RJ, Goldman MH: A study of the clinical incidence of infection in the use of banked allograft bone. *J Bone Joint Surg* 63A:244-248, 1981.

46. Lord CF, Gebhardt M, Tomford W, Mankin HJ: Infection in bone allografts. *J Bone Joint Surg* 70A:369-376, 1988.

47. Prolo DJ, Pedrotti PW, White DH: Ethylene oxide sterilization of bone, dura mater, and fascia lata for human transplantation. *Neurosurgery* 6:529-539, 1980.

48. Cloward RB: Gas-sterilized cadaver bone grafts for spinal fusion operations: a simplified bone bank. *Spine* 5:4-10, 1980.

49. Pelker R, Friedlander G: Biomechanical aspects of bone autografts and allografts. *Orthop Clinic North Am* 18:235-239, 1987.

50. Chaney SL, Karp NE: The use of freeze-dried bone allografts: a review of the literature with special emphasis on their use in treatment of solitary bone cysts. *J Foot Surg* 20:41-43, 1981.

51. Spence KF, Bright RW, Fitzgerald SP, Sell KW: Solitary unicameral bone cyst: treatment with freeze-dried crushed cortical-bone allograft: a review of 141 cases. *J Bone Joint Surg* 58A:636-641, 1976.

52. Rinaldi FT: The use of human cadaver homologous bone graft in foot surgery. *J Foot Surg* 22:165-169, 1983.

53. Urist MR: Bone: formation by autoinduction. *Science* 150:893-899, 1965.

54. Urist MR, Silverman BF, Buring K: The bone induction principle. *Clin Orthop* 53:143-283, 1967.

55. Uris M, Dawson E: Intertransverse process fusion with the aid of chemosterilized autolyzed antigen-extracted allogeneic (AAA) bone. *Clin Orthop* 154:97-113, 1981.

56. Urist MR, Sato K, Brownell AG, Malinin TI, Lietze A, Huo Y-K, Prolo DJ, Okund S, Finerman GAM, DeLange RJ: Human bone morphogenetic protein (LBMP). *Proc Soc Exp Biol Med* 173:194-199, 1983.

57. Urist MR, DeLange RJ, Finerman GAM: Bone cell differentiation and growth factors. *Science* 220:680-685, 1983.

58. Iwata H, Hanamura H, Kaneko M, Yasahura N, Terashima Y, Kajino G, Ida K, Mabuchi Y, Nakagawa M: Chemosterilized autolyzed antigen-extracted allogeneic (AAA) bone matrix gelatin for repair of defects from excision of benign bone tumors: a preliminary report. *Clin Orthop* 154:150-155, 1981.

59. Nade S, Burwell RG: Decalcified bone as a substrate for osteogenesis: an appraisal of the interrelation of bone and marrow in combined grafts. *J Bone Joint Surg* 59B:189-196, 1977.

60. Mulliken JB, Glowacki J, Kaban LB, Folkman J, Murray JE: Use of demineralized allogeneic bone implants for the correction of maxillo-craniofacial deformities. *Ann Surg* 194:366-372, 1981.

61. Glowacki J, Murray JE, Kaban LB, Folkman J, Mulliken JB: Application of the biological principle of induced osteogenesis for craniofacial defects. *Lancet* 8227:959-963, 1981.

62. Glowacki J, Altobelli D, Mulliken JB: Fate of mineralized and demineralized osseous implants in cranial defects. *Calcif Tissue Int* 33:71-76, 1981.

63. Harakas NK: Demineralized bone-matrix-induced osteogenesis. *Clin Orthop* 188:239-251, 1984.

64. Lindholm TS, Urist MR: A quantitative analysis of new bone formation by induction in compositive grafts of bone marrow and bone matrix. *Clin Orthop* 150:288-300, 1980.

65. Nade S: Osteogenesis after bone and bone marrow transplantation. II. The initial cellular events following transplantation of decalcified allografts of cancellous bone. *Acta Orthop Scand* 48:572-579, 1977.

66. Takagi K, Urist M: The reaction of the dura to bone morphogenetic protein (BMP) in repair of skull defects. *Ann Surg* 196:100-109, 1982.

67. Johnson E, Urist M, Finerman G: Bone morphogenetic protein augmentation grafting of resistant femoral nonunions. *Clin Orthop* 230:257-265, 1988.

68. Schmitz J, Hollinger J: A preliminary study of the osteogenic potential of a biodegradable alloplastic-osteoinductive alloimplant. *Clin Orthop* 237:245-255, 1988.

69. DeBastiani G, Aldegheri R, Renzi-Brivio L, Trivella G: Limb lengthening by callus distraction (callotasis). *J Pediatr Orthop* 7:129-134, 1987.

70. Mankin HJ, Doppelt SH, Sullivan TR, Tomford WW: Osteoarticular and intercalary allograft transplantation in the management of malignant tumors of bone. *Cancer* 50:613-630, 1982.

71. Mankin HJ, Doppelt S, Tomford W: Clinical experience with allograft implantation: the first ten years. *Clin Orthop* 174:69-86, 1983.

72. de Santos LA, Murray JA, Parrish FP, Wallace S, Finkelstein JB, Spjut HJ, Ayala AG, Terry AF: Radiographic aspects of massive bone osteoarticular allograft transplantation. *Radiology* 128:635-641, 1978.

73. Goldberg V, Herndon C, Lance E: Biology of Osteoarticular allografts. In: Aebri M, Regazzoni P (eds): *Bone Transplantation*. Heidelberg, Springer-Verlag, 1989, pp 51-58.

74. Friedlander GE: Immune responses to osteochondral allografts. *Clin Orthop* 174:56-68, 1983.

75. Goldberg VM, Heiple KG: Experimental hemijoint and whole joint transplantation. *Clin Orthop* 174:43-53, 1983.

76. Calhoun NR, Neiders ME, Greene GW: Effects of plaster-of-Paris implants in surgical defects of mandibular alveolar process of dogs. *J Oral Surg* 25:122-128, 1967.

77. Lewis-Epstein J: Use of polyvinyl alcohol sponge in alveoplasty: a preliminary report. *J Oral Surg* 18:453-460, 1960.

78. Holland DJ: Alveoplasty with tantalum mesh. *J Prosthet Dent* 3:354-357, 1953.

79. Holmes RE: Bone regeneration within a coralline hydroxyapatite implant. *Plast Reconstr Surg* 63:626-633, 1979.

80. Finn RA, Bell WH, Brammer JA: Interpositional "grafting" with autogenous bone and coralline hydroxyapatite. *J Maxillofac Surg* 8:217-227, 1980.

81. Holmes RM, Mooney V, Bucholz R, Tencer A: A coralline hydroxyapatite bone graft substitute: preliminary report. *Clin Orthop* 188:252-262, 1984.

82. Bucholz R, Carlton A, Holmes R: Hydroxyapatite and tricalcium phosphate bone graft substitutes. *Orthop Clin North Am* 18:323-334, 1987.

83. Bucholz R: Clinical experience with bone graft substitutes. *J Orthop Trauma* 1:260-262, 1987.

84. Bacher JD, Schmidt RE: Effects of autogenous cancellous bone on healing of homogenous cortical bone grafts. *J Small Anim Pract* 21:235-245, 1980.

85. Nade S: A reappraisal of bone-graft surgery. *Acta Orthop Scand* 51:189-194, 1980.

86. Branemark P-I, Breine U, Adell R, Hansson BO, Lindstrom J, Ohlsson A: Intra-osseous anchorage of dental prostheses. I. Experimental studies. *Scand J Plast Reconstr Surg* 3:81-100, 1969.

87. Albrektsson T, Albrektsson B: Microcirculation in a grafted bone. *Acta Orthop Scand* 49:1-7, 1978.

88. Jacobs R, Ray R: The effect of heat on bone healing. *Arch Surg* 104:687-691, 1972.

89. Peyton FA: Temperature rise and cutting efficiency of rotating instruments. *NY State Dent J* 18:439-450, 1952.

90. Jacobs CH: Fundamental investigations of the bone cutting process. *Bull Hosp Joint Dis* 38:4, 1977.

91. Ferguson A Jr, Laing P, Grebner M, Mandancy L: Study of revascularization of autogenous cortical bone grafts in rabbits using radiophosphorus. *Arch Surg* 78:551-555, 1959.

92. Albrektsson T: The healing of autologous bone grafts after varying degrees of surgical trauma. *J Bone Joint Surg* 62B:403-410, 1980.

93. Albrektsson T, Branemark PI, Eriksson A, Lindstrom J: The preformed autologous bone graft: an experimental study in the rabbit. *Scand J Plast Reconst Surg* 12:215-224, 1978.

94. Gray JC, Elves MW: Osteogenesis in bone grafts after short-term storage and topical antibiotic treatment: an experimental study in rats. *J Bone Joint Surg* 63B:441-445, 1981.

95. Cruz NI, Cestero HJ, Cora ML: Management of contaminated bone grafts. *Plast Reconstr Surg* 68:411-414, 1981.

96. Dachners L, Jacobs R, Kliethermes J, Wetze L, Rhoades C: A comparison of grafting materials in experimental bone grafts. *Orthopedics* 7:984-988, 1984.

97. Tarsoly E, Ostrowski K, Moskalewski S, Lojek T, Kurnatowski W, Krompecher S: Incorporation of lyophilized and radiosterilized perforated and unperforated bone grafts in dogs. *Acta Chir Acad Sci Hung* 10:55-63, 1969.

98. Mrazik J, Amato CM, Leban S, Mashberg A: The ilium as a source of autogenous bone for grafting: clinical considerations. *J Oral Surg* 38:29-32, 1980.

99. Laurie SW, Kaban LB, Mulliken JB, Murray JE: Donor-site morbidity after harvesting rib and iliac bone. *Plast Reconstr Surg* 73:933-938, 1984.

100. Mears D: Non-unions, infected non-unions, and arthrodeses. In Mears D (ed): *External Skeletal Fixation*. Baltimore, William & Wilkins, 1982, pp 107-121.

101. Beronio JP: One approach to a viable method of obtaining cancellous bone for grafting. *J Foot Surg* 22:240-242, 1983.

102. McGlamry ED, Miller IH: A review of the current status of bone grafting. *J Am Podiatry Assoc* 67:42-55, 1977.

103. Axhausen W: The osteogenetic phases of regeneration of bone. *J Bone Joint Surg* 38A:593-600, 1956.

104. Gray JC, Elves MW: Early osteogenesis in compact bone isografts: a quantitative study of the contributions of the different graft cells. *Calcif Tissue Int* 29:225-237, 1979.

105. Smith TF: Bone graft physiology: survival and incorporation of the graft. *J Am Podiatry Assoc* 73:70-74, 1983.

106. Burchardt H: The biology of bone graft repair. *Clin Orthop* 174:28-42, 1983.

107. Brown KL, Cruess RL: Bone and cartilage transplantation in orthopaedic surgery. *J Bone Joint Surg* 64A:270-279, 1982.

108. Bos GD, Goldberg VM, Powell AE, Heiple KG, Zika JM: The effect of histocompatibility matching on canine frozen bone allografts. *J Bone Joint Surg* 65A:89-96, 1983.

109. Jones RO: Reverse inlay bone graft for non-union of a lesser metatarsal. *J Am Podiatry Assoc* 74:265-267, 1984.

110. McGlamry ED, Cooper CT: Brachymetatarsia: a surgical treatment. *J Am Podiatry Assoc* 59:259-264, 1969.

111. Rhinelander FW: Minimal internal fixation of tibial fractures. *Clin Orthop* 107:188-220, 1975.

112. Rhinelander FW: Tibial blood supply in relation to fracture healing. *Clin Orthop* 105:34-81, 1981.

113. Papineau LJ: L'excision-greffe avec fermeture retardee deliberee dans l'osteomyelite chronique. *Nouv Presse Med* 2:2753-2755, 1973.

114. Cabanela ME: Open cancellous bone grafting of infected bone defects. *Orthop Clin North Am* 15:427-440, 1984.

115. Vidal J, Buscayret C, Connes H, Melka J, Orst G: Guidelines for treatment of open fractures and infected pseudoarthroses by external fixation. *Clin Orthop* 180:83-95, 1983.

116. Graelner JE, Quinn WB, Areson DJ: The use of the Papineau bone-grafting technique in salvage of the infected total joint implant. *J Foot Surg* 22:339-345, 1983.

117. Green SA, Dlabal TA: The open bone graft for septic nonunion. *Clin Orthop* 180:117-124, 1983.

118. Stevenson JS, Bright RW, Dunson GL, Nelson FR: Technetium-99m phosphate bone imaging: a method of assessing bone graft healing. *Radiology* 110:391-394, 1974.

Additional References

Albrektsson T: Repair of bone grafts: a vital microscopic and histological investigation in the rabbit. *Scand J Plast Reconstr Surg* 14:1-12, 1980.

Burchardt H: Biology of cortical bone graft incorporation. In Aebi M, Regazzoni P (eds): *Bone Transplantation*. Heidelberg, Springer-Verlag, 1989, pp 23-28.

Chacha PB: Vascularised pedicular bone grafts. *Int Orthop* 8:117-138, 1984.

DeBoer HH: The history of bone grafts. *Clin Orthop* 226:292-298, 1988.

Enneking WF, Eady JL, Burchardt H: Autogenous cortical bone grafts in the reconstruction of segmental skeletal defects. *J Bone Joint Surg* 62A:1039-1058, 1980.

Friedlander GE: U.S. Navy tissue bank. *J Am Podiatry Assoc* 67:38-41, 1977.

Friedlander G: Current Concepts Review: bone grafts: The basic science rationale for clinical applications. *J Bone Joint Surg* 69A:786-790, 1987.

Glidear J: Bone grafts: a review of the literature. *J Foot Surg* 16:146, 1977.

Griffin DJ: The effect of power instrumentation on bone healing. *J Foot Surg* 20:81-83, 1981.

Heiple KG, Chase SW, Herndon CH: A comparative study of the healing process following different types of bone transplantation. *J Bone Joint Surg* 45A:1593-1616, 1963.

Homminga G, Van der Linden T, Terwindt-Rowenhorst, E, Drukker J: Repair of articular defects by perichondrial grafts. *Acta Orthop Scand* 60:326-329, 1989.

McCarthy D, Hutchinson B: Autologous bone grafting in podiatric surgery. *J Am Podiatr Med Assoc* 78:217-226, 1988.

McCarthy D, Hutchinson B: Homologous and heterogenous bone grafting in podiatric surgery. *J Am Podiatr Med Assoc* 79:175-181, 1989.

Muller ME, Allgower M, Schneider R, Willenegger H: *Manual of Osteosynthesis, AO Technique*. New York, Springer-Verlag, 1978.

Nade S: Clinical implications of cell function in osteogenesis: a reappraisal of bone-graft surgery. *Ann R Coll Surg Engl* 61:189-194, 1979.

Pearson GE, Freeman E: The composite graft: autogenous cancellous bone and marrow combined with freeze-dried bone allograft in the treatment of periodontal osseous defects. *Ontario Dentist* 56:10-13, 1980.

Ray RD: Bone grafts and bone implants. *Otolaryngol Clin North Am* 5:389-398, 1972.

Schneekboth D, Gronen W, Lichty T: Human cadaveric bone implants. *J Am Podiatr Med Assoc* 79:77-81, 1989.

Shapoff CA, Bowers GM, Levy B, Mellonig JT, Yukna RA: The effect of particle size on the osteogenic activity of composite grafts of allogeneic freeze-dried bone and autogenous marrow. *J Periodontol* 51:625-630, 1980.

Simmons DJ, Bratberg JJ, Lesker PA, Aab L: What is the best time of day to schedule a bone graft operation? *Clin Orthop* 116:229-239, 1976.

Urist MR: *Fundamental and Clinical Bone Physiology*. Philadelphia, JB Lippincott, 1981.

Waris P, Penttinen R, Slatis P, Karaharju E, Aalto K: Biochemical changes in bone grafts stabilized with rigid plates. I. Cancellous grafts. *Acta Orthop Scand* 52:257-264, 1981.

Waris P, Penttinen R, Slatis P, Karaharju E, Joukainen J: Biochemical changes in bone grafts stabilized with rigid plates. II. Cortical grafts. *Acta Orthop Scand* 52:265-272, 1981.

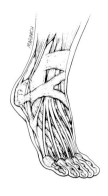

CHAPTER 49

Plastic Surgery and Skin Grafting

Kieran T. Mahan, M.S., D.P.M., F.A.C.F.S.

Plastic surgery involves the manipulation of skin and soft tissues to produce a fine cosmetic result or coverage over a wound. The topic is broad, but plastic surgery includes such techniques as specialized procedures for excision of skin lesions and wound closure, skin plasties such as V-Y and Z-plasties, skin grafting, and the various types of flaps. In the lower extremity, the primary concerns are twofold: (*a*) production of a fine cosmetic result after reconstructive surgery and (*b*) wound coverage for defects caused by trauma, disease processes, or postoperative complications.

SKIN INCISION

Seven times turn your knife in your hand,
Ere you cut the skin of a fellow man.
—*Gillies.*

The final scar that results after a surgical procedure is an everlasting reminder to the patient of the surgeon's degree of competence. There are many factors involved in the final scar result (Table 49.1). Some of these factors are not within the surgeon's control. These include such influences as the region of the body and the age and skin type of the patient. Whereas sternal scars tend to hypertrophy, scars in hairless areas such as the palms of the hands and soles of the feet tend to be less noticeable and thinner. Children and adolescents heal rapidly but tend to form scars that are more often hypertrophied and erythematous. Patients with thick oily skin may form scars that are depressed and noticeable (1).

Factors that the surgeon can control with regard to the final scar are related to incision placement and design, surgical technique, and closure by the appropriate suture material and technique. The factors involved in the skin incision are probably most often neglected by the surgeon. These considerations include the course, depth, angle, and length of the wound (2). An incision coursing parallel to the skin tension lines will heal with minimal scarring, whereas an incision perpendicular to the skin tension lines will tend to hypertrophy. A long uninterrupted skin incision will have more tendency to contract, whereas multiple smaller inci-

sions benefit from the elasticity of interposed skin that somewhat limits detrimental tension forces.

Incision design has traditionally been based more on the surgeon's convenience than on surgical principle. One of the best examples of this phenomenon is the transverse anterior incision described by Charnley (3) for ankle fusion. This incision violated tendons, arteries, veins, and nerves as the price for ideal exposure of the ankle.

With all this in mind, the following criteria should ideally be used to design an incision: (*a*) parallel to the relaxed skin tension lines, (*b*) adequate length and direction for exposure, and (*c*) avoidance of neurovascular structures.

SKIN LINES

If one looks at the plantar aspect of the foot, a variety of different skin creases and lines can be appreciated, each one oriented in a different direction from the others. Which lines should one follow with the surgical incision? The multitude of possibilities can make this quite confusing.

To understand the subject better, it is necessary to review the history of skin lines. In 1834 Dupuytren (4) observed that lines of tension are formed on the body. His interest was stimulated by a suicide in which round puncture wounds from an awl formed flat wounds much like a knife. After further research on cadavers, Dupuytren concluded that this phenomenon was the result of fiber alignment.

In 1861 Langer (5) published his paper on the lines of skin tension. This work was based on observations made on cadavers with multiple 2 mm awl punches. He thought that

To provide more consistent organization, many figures pertaining to plastic surgery and skin grafting have been taken from Miller SJ: Surgical principles. In McGlamry ED (ed): *Fundamentals of Foot Surgery.* Baltimore, Williams & Wilkins, 1987, p 174-197. Appreciation is expressed to the original author, Stephen J. Miller, D.P.M., for allowing us to freely use his material.

Table 49.1.
Factors in Scar Prognosis in the Lower Extremity

Factors	Effects
Age	Young patients may hypertrophy
Race	Blacks more likely to hypertrophy
	Among whites: blondes have finer scarring than brunettes
Body region	Foot and leg heal well; related to wound tension
Wound course and pattern	(See "Tension")
Wound length	Multiple small incisions heal better than one long uninterrupted incision
Tension	Tension hypertrophies a scar
Skin tension lines	Parallel lines give fine scars, antitension lines hypertrophy

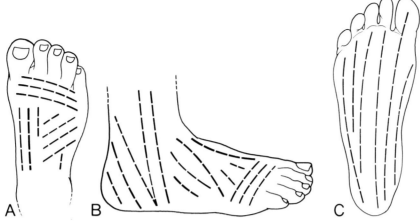

Figure 49.1. Lines of tension on the foot as conceived by Langer.

the lines of tension were in the direction of muscle pull (Fig. 49.1). Kocher (6), in 1892, was the first to recognize the surgical importance of Langer's lines and later described a set of incisions designed to parallel these lines. Although Langer's lines have historical importance, they have very little relevance to surgery on a living patient.

Cox (7) investigated the tension lines in 28 fresh cadavers by making multiple round punctures. Although his technique was similar to Langer's, he arrived at a set of lines that differed in various regions, including the foot (Fig. 49.2). These lines are valid only for individuals of average build. Cox reported that the pattern of tension lines varies with body configuration because of differences in body curvature and shape.

Both Langer's lines and Cox's cleavage lines have been used by surgeons as guidelines for surgical incisions. This becomes a problem because the two sets of lines differ and no set of lines can be valid for all body types or age groups.

Borges and Alexander (8) described skin lines as "relaxed skin tension lines" (RSTLs). How are the RSTLs important? Tension is the force that causes scars to widen or hypertrophy. In most areas of the body there is tension in many different directions, but the tension is greatest in the direction of the RSTLs (Fig. 49.3). An incision made perpendicular to the RSTLs will gap widely, whereas an incision made parallel to the RSTLs will remain approximated (Fig. 49.4). The RSTLs are created by the directional pull of structures underlying the relaxed skin. Structures that exert some pull include underlying muscles, as well as bone, tendons, and other anatomical features that protrude and cause a tenting effect of the skin.

Gardner and Raybuck (9) described the development of "cleavage lines" in the fetus. They noted that, even at 28 mm (crown-rump length), the pattern of RSTLs may be present in the foot and lower leg. Usually, cleavage lines appear by the 50 mm length. Cleavage lines in the extremities undergo significant pattern changes during development. The lines initially are parallel to the long axis of the extremity. Later, at the 240 mm stage, the lines become

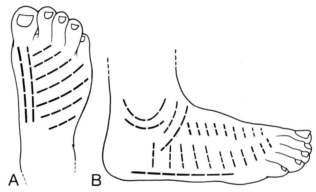

Figure 49.2. Lines of tension on the foot as conceived by Cox.

perpendicular to the long axis of the extremity. The RSTLs are actually imaginary. There is no set number of lines or space between them (8, 10).

The RSTLs are important for the direction that they convey rather than the location of the lines themselves. It is important to realize that the tension along the RSTLs is constant, even during sleep. The RSTLs are also constant while the affected part is in a cast. Therefore, even if an incision line will be immobilized in a cast for an extended period of time, the RSTLs are still quite important.

Courtiss and associates (11) discuss three factors that are significant in incision placement: (a) bands run between the skin and fascia in a plane perpendicular to the long axis of the muscles, (b) in all incisions the orientation of dermal collagen is perpendicular to the long axis of the muscles, and (c) the orientation of collagen in a scar is parallel to the long direction of the scar, regardless of where the scar is placed. Optimal healing can be produced by ensuring that the collagen of the scar forms parallel to the adjacent dermal collagen. Although Courtiss and associates were discussing incision placement in the wrinkle lines, their discussion also applies to the RSTLs.

To find the RSTLs, one simply relaxes the skin in an area

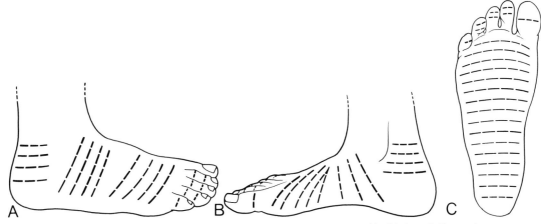

Figure 49.3.   Relaxed skin tension lines of the foot. **A.** Lateral view. **B.** Medial view. **C.** Plantar view.

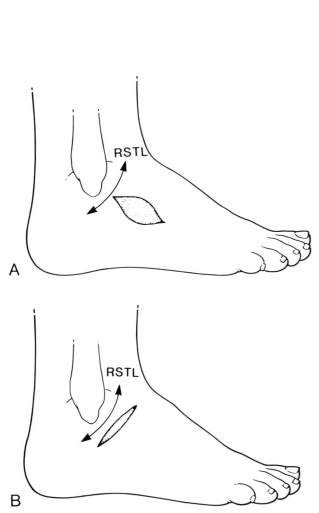

Figure 49.4.   A. An incision placed perpendicular to the RSTL gaps. **B.** An incision placed parallel to the RSTL coapts easily.

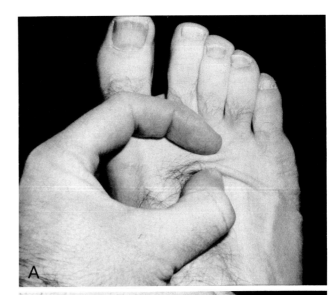

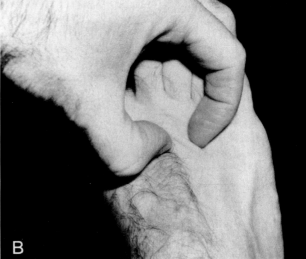

Figure 49.5.   A. Pinching the skin in line with the RSTL gives rise to a regularly shaped furrow. **B.** Pinching the skin perpendicular to the RSTL demonstrates limited skin mobility.

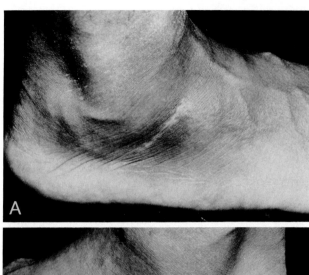

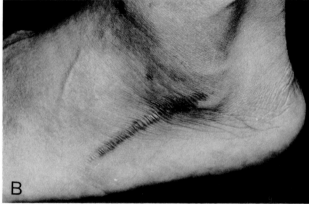

Figure 49.6. **A.** Four months' postoperative view of an oblique incision for an Evans calcaneal osteotomy demonstrates a fine line scar. **B.** Nine months' postoperative view of a linear scar in the same patient, contralateral foot, demonstrates the hypertrophy that occurs when RSTLs are violated.

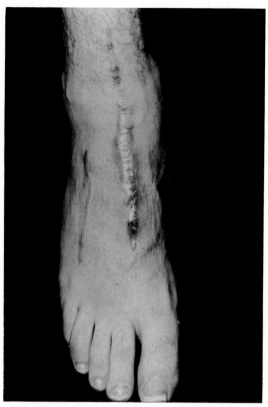

Figure 49.7. Linear antitension incision across the ankle joint hypertrophied after excessive early mobilization of the ankle.

by passive manipulation or by muscle movement. By pronating the foot, one finds that the RSTLs over the sinus tarsi are oblique in nature. Similarly, with flexion and extension of the toes, it becomes apparent that the RSTLs are transverse on the dorsal metatarsophalangeal joint (MPJ) and the plantar surface of the foot. In areas where there is little motion the RSTLs can be found by pinching the skin over the area. This will form furrows or ridges in the skin. Pinching the skin in line with the RSTLs gives rise to a regularly shaped furrow. Pinching oblique to the direction of the RSTLs gives rise to an S-shaped pattern (Fig. 49.5). A pinch of the skin opposite the direction of the RSTLs demonstrates limited skin mobility perpendicular to the RSTLs.

In certain areas the incision can be made parallel to the RSTLs without much difficulty. An example of this is the oblique incision for the Evans calcaneal osteotomy (Fig. 49.6). Difficulty arises when the RSTLs are transverse, but the required surgical exposure is longitudinal. An example of this is the surgical exposure for plantar fibromatosis. The RSTLs are transverse on the plantar aspect of the foot, but an incision parallel to the RSTLs would not give sufficient

exposure for excision of the fibromatosis. Because of this, most surgeons perform a linear or S-shaped incision that can be characterized as an antitension line (ATL). Antitension incisions have an increased tendency to hypertrophy and contract because they are perpendicular to the RSTLs (Fig. 49.7).

An alternative is the zigzag ATL line incision (Fig. 49.8). This incision provides the required exposure in a longitudinal direction while placing a major portion of the incision in line with the RSTLs. Curtin (12) and Burns and Harvey (13) have described slightly different zigzag incisions for excision of plantar fibromatosis.

Surgical approaches to other areas can also be modified to make use of the RSTLs. An example of this is the approach for the excision of a Morton's neuroma. The traditional approaches are most commonly the dorsal linear and plantar linear incisions (14). Both of these incisions violate the transverse RSTLs. Burns and Stewart (15) reported on preliminary results with a transverse plantar approach distal to the weight-bearing area. For purposes of this discussion, the importance of the approach is that it follows the RSTLs while still providing adequate surgical exposure.

Other approaches have also been modified to follow the RSTLs. Evans's (16) approach for his anterior calcaneal osteotomy was originally described as a linear incision running along the lateral border of the calcaneus. This approach has

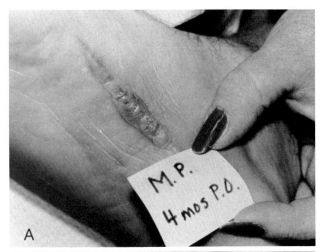

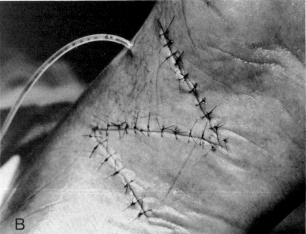

Figure 49.8. A. Antitension line incision results in hypertrophy of a linear scar for excision of plantar fibromatosis. **B.** Zigzag antitension line incision provides linear exposure for excision of plantar fibromatosis while placing the major portion of the incision in line with RSTL.

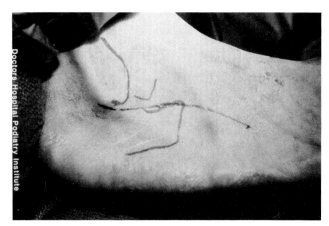

Figure 49.9. Mapping out the incision, as well as important vital structures, can be performed with a skin marker.

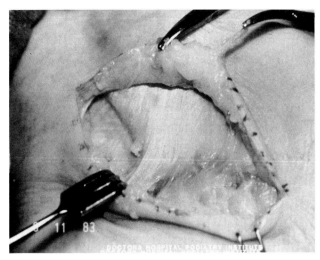

Figure 49.10. A curved medial arch incision demonstrates the ease of retraction of the convex side of the incision and the immobility of the concave portion of the incision.

been modified, and the author (17) uses an oblique incision in the RSTLs extending from distal superior (over the anterior beak of the calcaneus) to proximal inferior (inferior to the lateral plantar border of the calcaneus) (Fig. 49.6).

EXECUTION OF THE SURGICAL INCISION

Proper planning of the surgical incision can both facilitate the operation and create a more desirable cosmetic result. The use of a skin marker is a good way to begin the incision. This allows the surgeon to map out important vital structures that he or she wishes to avoid (e.g., sural nerve), as well as the boundaries of the area he or she wishes to expose, before drawing the actual incision (Fig. 49.9). This gives the surgeon a good opportunity to visualize the incision before actually performing the cut. A poorly placed incision can turn a routine procedure into a prolonged struggle. Taking time to plan the incision usually results in a procedure that goes much more smoothly. The skin marker can also be

used to facilitate closure. Crosshatches can be drawn across the incision before the start of the procedure to allow accurate reapproximation at the time of closure. This is particularly helpful for curved incisions.

The shape of the incision must be carefully planned. Wherever possible, the incisions should be designed to parallel the RSTLs. However, there are other considerations. Neurovascular structures are best avoided by incisions that parallel them. In the foot this would result in incisions that are longitudinal and do not parallel the RSTLs. A curved incision presents special considerations. The curve creates a convex side and a concave side to the incision. The convex side can be retracted easily, whereas the concave side of the incision has very little mobility. Consequently, a curved incision for a medial arch approach must be placed high enough to reach all the superior structures (e.g., tibialis anterior) without excessive retraction of the concave side of the wound (Fig. 49.10).

The choice of blade size for the surgical knife is a matter of individual preference. In small areas of the foot the No. 15 blade is preferred to the No. 10 blade. The No. 15 blade should be held like a pencil for best use of the cutting edge. The No. 10 blade is larger and best used around the ankles. It must be held in a more horizontal position to place the cutting edge of the blade along the incision. There is apparently no justification for the "first knife for skin, second knife for deep" technique. Although most surgeons still do this out of habit, it has been demonstrated that the first knife is not contaminated simply by its incision through skin (18).

The first incision is made through the epidermis and a portion of the dermis. This controlled-depth incision prevents the surgeon from lacerating underlying vessels. The second incision penetrates through the remainder of the dermis, allowing underlying vessels to be visualized for ligation. This incision technique is actually as much a key to hemostasis as is epinephrine or a tourniquet. The slash-to-fascia approach used by many surgeons results in many small vessels that are never properly ligated. These patients demonstrate both ecchymosis and greater edema postoperatively.

The knife blade must be oriented perpendicular to the skin, regardless of any curves or other topographical irregularities of the skin surface. This very basic technique is quite influential in the outcome of the procedure. Scarring

is a function of dermal injury. A scived incision makes an oblique cut through the dermis, creating a longer scar through this tissue layer. This does two things: (*a*) with a greater injury in the dermis, the scar is more likely to hypertrophy, and (*b*) with creation of an irregular surface, the scar is also more likely to be noticeable (Fig. 49.11).

INCISIONAL APPROACHES

Aside from the principles of skin mechanics, the key consideration is that the incisional approach should be based on a sound knowledge of the anatomy plus an assessment of the pathological condition in the area of surgery. Incisions must be planned and tailored to the individual patient's needs. Incisional names have little value when there is a failure to study the local anatomy.

Several other principles are involved in the planning and execution of surgical incisions: (*a*) anatomical landmarks, including vital structures, should be identified and marked or noted before the incision is initiated; (*b*) tension on the healing incision must be avoided; (*c*) there should be adequate easy access to all the structures involved; (*d*) the incision should be long enough to avoid excess traction on the wound margins, and it should be recalled that skin heals from side to side and not end to end; (*e*) vital nerves and blood vessels should be identified and preserved or protected if possible to avoid vascular disruption and nerve damage; (*f*) excess manipulation and damage to the deeper tissues must be avoided by following the lines of cleavage and planes of fascia; and (*g*) scars over bony prominences or weight-bearing surface points should be avoided.

ANATOMICAL APPROACHES

Toes

As in the fingers, the blood supply to the toes is provided through four vascular complexes situated roughly at each of the four digital corners. These vessels end in an anastomotic complex within the digital pulp. Longitudinal incisions across dorsal or plantar creases should be made only with plans for their contracture. Lateral or medial incisions

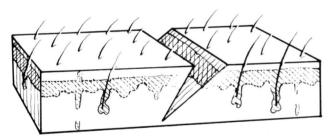

Figure 49.11. Illustration of the effect of a scived incision. Note that injury to the dermis is greater with a scived incision.

Figure 49.12. Some incisional approaches to toes.

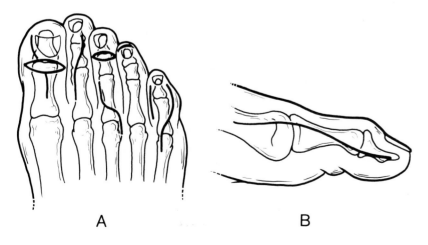

A   B

will heal well, allowing the scar to bend. Transverse and oblique incisions heal nicely, whether or not they are double elliptical. However, care must be taken not to transect both dorsal neurovascular bundles within the digit. Long curvilinear incisions are especially applicable to the first and fifth toes. These will be described in detail in later chapters. Dorsal toe incisions will interrupt the dorsal venous circle of the superficial venous network, and these vessels should be occluded for hemostasis. The distal pulp is quite vascular and may be incised to the bone for approaches in this area (Fig. 49.12).

First Metatarsophalangeal Joint

Only the dorsal and medial surfaces are available for approaches to the first metatarsophalangeal joint. Rarely is the plantar surface violated. Most approaches involve longitudinal incisions directed either dorsally, dorsomedially, or medially across the joint. Curves should be incorporated when possible, and an incision at the junction of the plantar and dorsal skin will yield a very fine scar. Care should be taken to avoid severance or entrapment of the neurovascular structures, especially dorsomedially and plantarmedially. For hallux valgus correction the incision can be made to

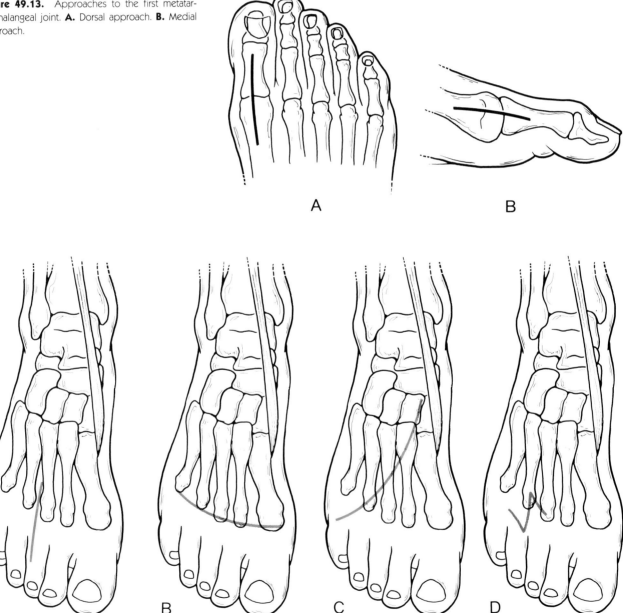

Figure 49.13. Approaches to the first metatarsophalangeal joint. **A.** Dorsal approach. **B.** Medial approach.

Figure 49.14. Some dorsal approaches to the forefoot. **A.** Neurectomy—McKeever, 1952; Kitting and McGlamry, 1973. **B.** MP joint resection—Clayton, 1963. **C.** Hibbs' tendosuspension. **D.** Z-plasty for MP joint release.

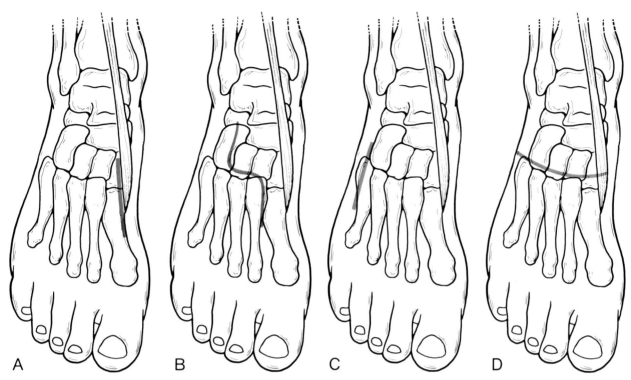

Figure 49.15.   Some midfoot incisions. **A.** First metatarsocuneiform articulation. **B.** Midfoot lazy-S approach. **C.** Access to fifth metatarsal base. **D.** Midfoot capsular release.

curve along the dorsomedial lines of the deformity. No incision should be made directly over the tendon of the extensor hallucis longus (Fig. 49.13).

Lesser Metatarsophalangeal Joints

The pliability of the dorsal skin can usually accommodate longitudinal incisions about the lesser metatarsophalangeal joints. A lazy S incision will help allow for scar contracture. However, when there are severe digital dorsal contractures or previous scars, Z-plasties may be necessary to lengthen the skin when the toes are straightened. For entering the intermetatarsal spaces, the incisions should be somewhat curvilinear, especially when more than one space is to be entered through the same incision. All three lateral intermetatarsal spaces can be entered through one well-planned, lazy C or lazy S incision (Fig. 49.14). If individual longitudinal incisions are used, they should be no less than 1 cm apart to respect blood supply to the intervening skin. A single transverse dorsal incision may be used when there is no evidence of vascular disease, as long as the underlying longitudinal structures are respected.

Dorsal Midfoot

Longitudinal incisions are also well tolerated in the dorsal midfoot because of limited skin movement and tension (Fig. 49.15). Transverse incisions across the foot can be used when necessary, however, provided that, once through the

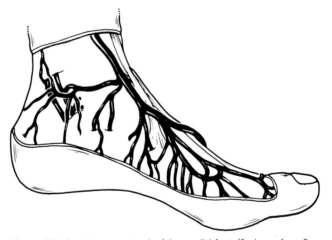

Figure 49.16.   Venous network of the medial foot. (Redrawn from Sarrafian SK: *Anatomy of the Foot and Ankle.* Philadelphia, JB Lippincott, 1983.)

dermis, the nerves and larger blood vessels are identified, retracted, and protected as much as possible. The superficial dorsal venous network imposes a generous supply of vessels to negotiate. Care must be taken in this area not to damage extensor tendons, superficial peroneal nerve branches, the marginal veins, and the dorsal venous arch (unless necessary), as well as the dorsalis pedis and deep peroneal neurovascular bundle. Other arteries encountered on the dorsum of the foot include the anterior peroneal (when pres-

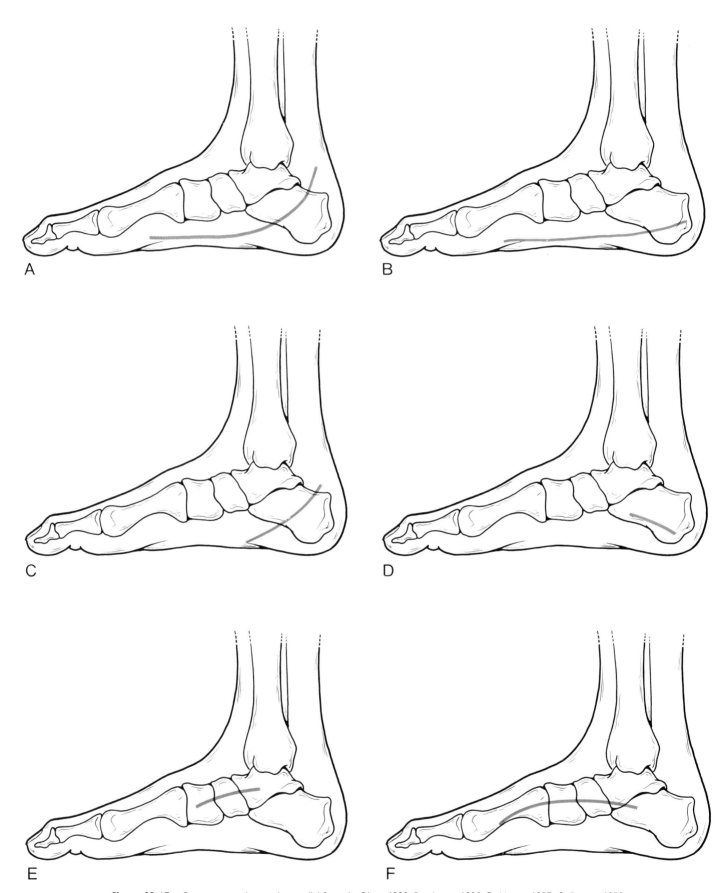

Figure 49.17. Some approaches to the medial foot. **A.** Ober, 1920; Brockman, 1930. **B.** Henry, 1957. **C.** Dwyer, 1959. **D.** DuVries, 1965. **E** and **F.** Access for medial arch reconstruction.

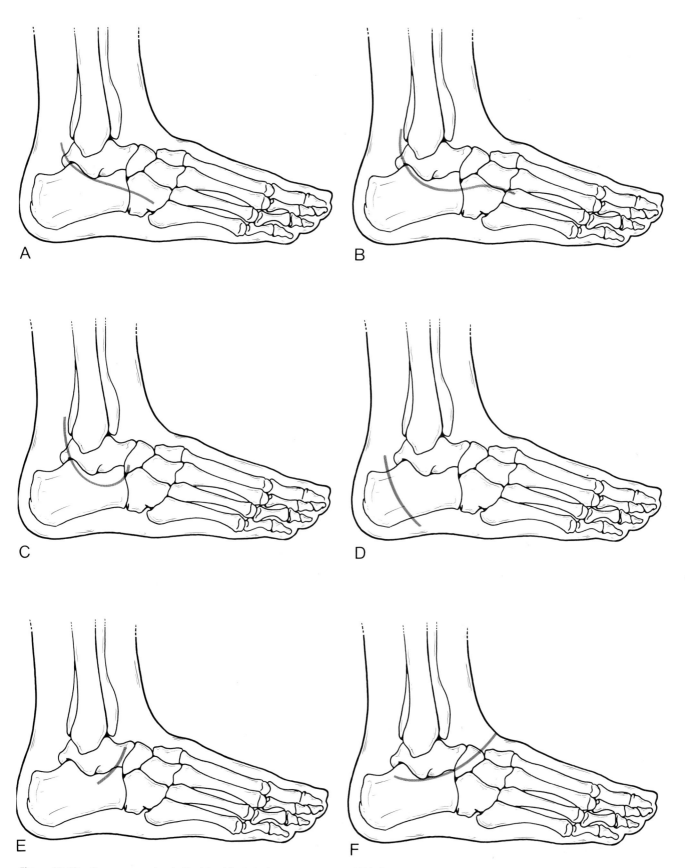

Figure 49.18. Some approaches to the lateral foot. **A.** Access to posterior facet of subtalar joint. **B.** Approach to subtalar and calcaneocuboid joint. **C.** Kocher's approach, 1911. **D.** Dwyer, 1959; Banks and Laufman, 1953. **E.** Approach to the sinus tarsi. Grice, 1952; Westin and Hall, 1957. **F.** Ollier incision, 1891.

ent), the arcuate with its branches, and the lateral tarsal arteries. The inferior extensor retinaculum should be respected and repaired if severed.

Medial Foot

Vital structures in the medial part of the foot include the medial marginal vein, the dorsalis pedis artery, and the posterior tibial neurovascular plexus, as well as the anterior and posterior tibial tendons. The venous network is quite intricate, requiring a working knowledge of its design (Fig. 49.16). The inferomedial band of the inferior extensor retinaculum should be identified and repaired when severed (Fig. 49.17).

Lateral Foot

Approaches in the lateral foot should avoid the intermediate and lateral (sural) dorsal cutaneous nerves and preserve the lateral marginal vein when possible (Fig. 49.18). The perforating or anterior peroneal artery and lateral tarsal arteries are quite anomalous in this area and are frequently encountered, as are the peroneal tendons and the tendons of extensor digitorum longus. As in the medial side of the foot, there is a generous plexus of veins carrying blood in a plantar to dorsal direction (Fig. 49.19).

Medial and Lateral Heel

More arteries supply the skin of the medial heel than the lateral heel. The medial calcaneal arterial branches arise mostly from the lateral calcaneal artery, although one may arise from the posterior tibial artery. When one is cutting along the medial rearfoot (as in heel spur surgery), care must be taken not to initiate a tarsal tunnel syndrome. Also, when this approach is used it is almost impossible to avoid severing the medial calcaneal nerve and muscular branches of the lateral plantar nerve. These nerves should be preserved, and their severance can lead to stump neuromas and painful scar formation. When the laciniate ligament is

violated in this area, the contents of each compartment of the tibiotalocalcaneal tunnel must be clearly identified and protected. The arteries that supply the skin of the lateral surface of the heel arise from the posterior peroneal artery above and the lateral tarsal artery below. Vital structures coursing in the area include the short saphenous vein, the sural nerve, and the peroneal tendons, the latter two of which can be palpated. The calcaneofibular ligament must be identified when encountered and repaired if cut.

Plantar Approaches

Incisions directly over the weight-bearing metatarsal heads and plantar heel are generally contraindicated in foot surgery. However, painful plantar metatarsal head lesions can be excised without leaving a painful scar if the incision is closed carefully and no weight bearing is allowed for 3 weeks. A transverse incision distal to the metatarsal heads can be used for neurectomies (Fig. 49.20), but this makes for difficult access to panmetatarsal head resection (Fig. 49.21). Although dorsal approaches for the latter make the osteotomies less awkward, a double elliptical transverse plantar incision at the level of the metatarsal heads has three advantages: *(a)* immediate access to the bones with minimal dissection, *(b)* drawing of the anteriorly displaced fat pad proximally into a weight-bearing position, and *(c)* location of the scar where there are no weight-bearing bony prom-

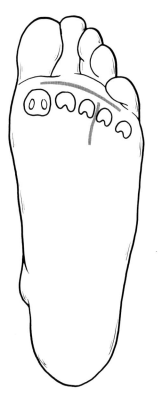

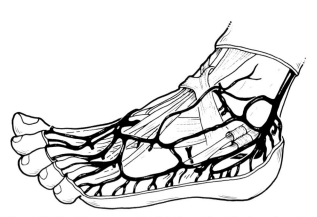

Figure 49.19. Venous network of the lateral foot. (Redrawn from Sarrafian SK: *Anatomy of the Foot and Ankle.* Philadelphia, JB Lippincott, 1983.)

Figure 49.20. Plantar approaches for neurectomy. Transverse incision—Hoffman, 1911; Nissen, 1948; Burns and Stewart, 1982. Longitudinal incision—Hoadley, 1893; Betts, 1940; Mulder, 1951.

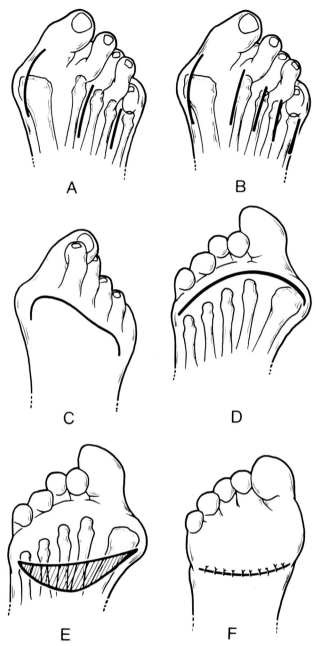

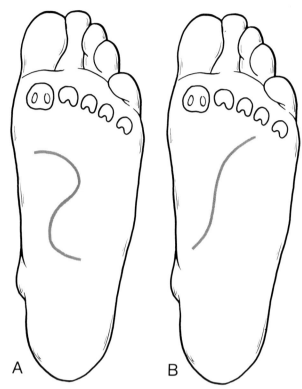

Figure 49.22. Approaches for plantar fibromatosis. **A.** Curtin, 1965. **B.** Burns and Harvey, 1983.

Figure 49.21. Approaches for panmetatarsal head resection. **A.** Three-incision dorsal longitudinal approach. **B.** Five incisional dorsal longitudinal approach. **C.** Dorsal transverse approach. **D.** Plantar transverse approach. **E.** Plantar elliptical approach. **F.** Closure of the plantar ellipse draws the fat pad proximally. (Redrawn from Hodor L, Dobbs BM: Pan-metatarsal head resection; a review and new approach. *J Am Podiatry Assoc* 73:287-292, 1983.)

inences. Incisions meticulously placed between the metatarsal heads have been successfully used for removal of Morton's neuroma. With careful surgical technique, many disorders can be approached safely through plantar incisions because the plantar skin is as well vascularized as the skin of the scalp.

Adequate incisions for entering the non-weight-bearing longitudinal arch area, especially with reference to access to the plantar fascia for resection of plantar fibromatosis, were reviewed by Curtin (12) and by Burns and Harvey (13). Using infrared photography, Curtin demonstrated that the standard longitudinal arch incision violates most of the arterial supply to the skin beneath this area. These authors used curvilinear incisions as shown in Figure 49.22 for good access to most of the plantar fascia without endangering local circulation.

Posterior Heel

Access to the posterior calcaneus and Achilles tendon insertion should be gained, with the patient in the prone position, through either a longitudinal or a transverse incision. Central incisions across the most prominent posterior heel are best avoided to prevent future shoe irritation from the counter area. Even though a transverse incision will more correctly follow the creases of relaxation, this incision should be made only above the level of the heel counter with the following exception: When deep access to plantar structures is necessary, then a low transverse incision will allow the heel pad to be flapped inferiorly. The split-heel incision is discouraged. The medial or lateral surface of the calcaneus can be adequately exposed through curved incisions close to the posterior heel (Fig. 49.23).

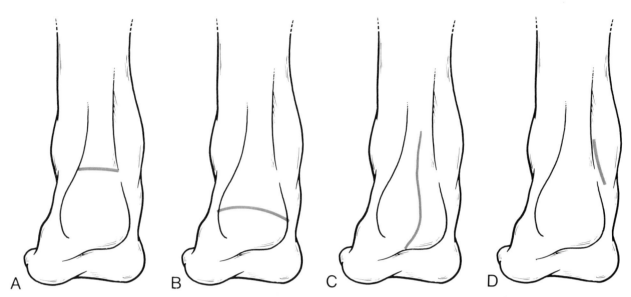

Figure 49.23. Some approaches to the posterior heel. **A.** Fowler and Philip, 1945. **B.** Banks and Laufman, 1953. **C.** Gaenslen, 1931; Pridie, 1946. **D.** Zadek, 1939.

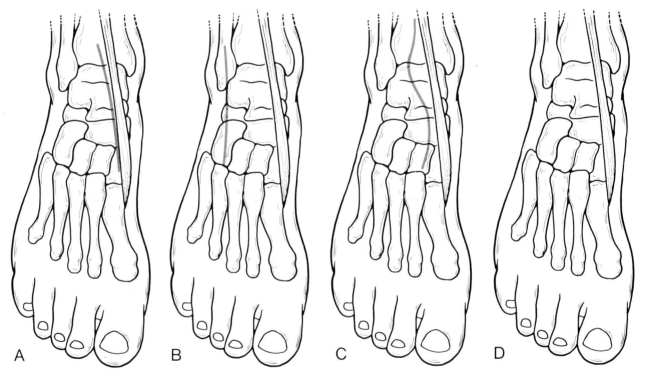

Figure 49.24. Approaches to the anterior ankle. **A.** Anteromedial—Nicola, 1945; Colonna and Ralston, 1951. **B.** Anterolateral—Colonna and Ralston, 1951; Boyd, 1971.

Anterior Ankle

The two basic approaches to the anterior ankle are antero-medial, between the tendons of the extensor hallucis longus and the extensor digitorum longus, and anterolateral, immediately in front of the anterior edge of the fibula (Fig. 49.24). Either incision should be curved to allow for scar contracture. Because of the friability of the skin in this area, prolonged retraction and flaps should be avoided. Care must be taken to preserve the superficial peroneal nerve and its branches plus the long saphenous vein in the immediate area. The anterior tibial neurovascular bundle is best dissected free but kept together as one group still joined to the underlying tissues. It can then be retracted from side to side as a unit for maximum protection. This is especially im-

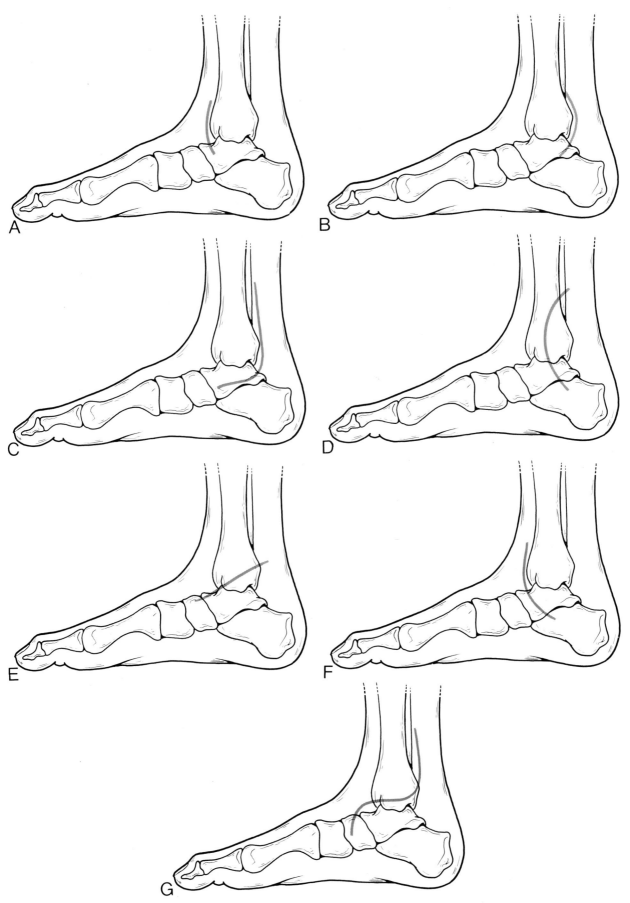

Figure 49.25. Approaches to the medial ankle. **A.** Simple medial—DuVries, 1973. **B.** Posteromedial—Jergesen, 1959. **C.** To posterior tibia—Broomhead, 1932. **D.** Colonna and Ralston, 1951. **E.** Koenig and Schaefer, 1929. **F.** Anteromedial—Jergesen, 1959. **G.** Couvelaire, 1938.

portant when a midline anterior approach to the ankle is selected. The transverse crural and cruciate crural ligaments should be repaired after they are divided.

Medial Ankle

The principles applied to incisional approaches in the medial ankle involve adequate joint access while protecting and manipulating the laciniate compartment tendons and the posterior tibial neurovascular bundle. When these structures cannot be gently retracted posteriorly, they should be mobilized and reflected anteriorly, especially if combined access to the ankle and subtalar joint is anticipated. Both the middle and anterior facets of the subtalar joint can be approached medially (Fig. 49.25).

The incision may curve around the posterior aspect of the medial malleolus or anteriorly directly across the bony prominence. When the tissue is reflected, dissection must first be carried directly down through the subcutaneous tissue. A curved transverse incision is acceptable, but it is better made parallel to the posterior tibial vessels when they must be crossed. Multiple arterial branches of the medial malleolar rete are found in this region. It is an anastomotic network supplied from two principal sources— the anterior medial malleolar artery arising from the dorsalis pedis artery and the posterior medial malleolar artery arising from the posterior tibial artery.

Lateral Ankle

The lateral malleolar area is commonly entered for fracture repair, subtalar joint access, and ankle joint surgery, including ligamentous repair or reconstruction. Vital structures in the immediate area are the sural nerve, the peroneal tendons, and the joint ligaments. A variety of curved longitudinal incisions can be used if both anatomical landmarks and vital structures are kept in mind, whether one is entering posterolaterally or anterolaterally. Again, dissection must be carried down through subcutaneous tissue before the skin is reflected. Arterial branches of the lateral malleolar rete may be encountered here. Also, the anterior lateral malleolar artery from the dorsalis pedis is found in this area, as it contributes to the perimalleolar transverse and sagittal arterial loops. A transverse incision in the ankle flexion creases provides good exposure to the subtalar joint and sinus tarsi, but the intermediate dorsal cutaneous nerve must not be damaged (Fig. 49.26).

Posterior Ankle and Triceps Surae

The tendoachillis or gastrocnemius aponeurosis can be approached posteriorly through a longitudinal medial, lateral, or central incision. However, a longitudinal incision placed somewhat medially will make the scar less obvious and, at the same time, help one avoid the sural nerve. Transverse incisions are acceptable because they are at right angles to the direction of pull of the underlying muscles. However,

exposure across the wound is not always adequate for lengthenings (Fig. 49.27).

Access to the posterior ankle and subtalar joint requires Z-plasty division of the tendoachillis and dissection through the crural fascia, as well as the adipose tissue in Kager's triangle. The posterior branch of the peroneal artery with its veins and the smaller medial posteromedial and lateral calcaneal arteries may be encountered in this area. The posterior tibial nerve and artery should be identified and protected as they run along the medial border of the incision. As dissection is continued deeper into the wound, the musculotendinous flexor hallucis longus will be found to course across the posterior process of the talus and disappear beneath the sustentaculum tali. It can easily be transected inadvertently if a capsulotomy has to be performed. The periarticular fat in this area can make visualization difficult. A comprehensive posterior approach to the medial, lateral, and posterior parts of the rearfoot and ankle was devised by Crawford (19) for extensive procedures, such as clubfoot release (Fig. 49.28)

When one is dealing with incisions and surgical approaches, it is obvious that local circulation is as important as skin mechanics. Although the location of major arteries is well detailed in anatomy textbooks, little is known about the fine circulation beneath the skin of the lower extremity. There is a definite need for studies such as that of Curtin if these patterns in each anatomical area are to be understood. Only then will the knowledge necessary for making intelligent incisions be complete and available.

SKIN CLOSURE

The techniques and materials used for skin closure will be covered in a separate chapter. Certain general principles should be mentioned in this context as they relate to the goal of a fine-line scar. Tissue must be handled gently. Forceps and other instruments should not be used to crush the skin. Layers must be reapproximated anatomically. Closure of the deep and superficial fascia is as important to the final cosmetic result as is closure of the skin.

Skillful closure of deep layers removes tension that otherwise would be transferred to the skin. Ideally, the material used for closure should be the least reactive. The size (gauge) of the material that is used should be sufficient to remove the tension on that layer while holding the tissue in approximation.

Subcuticular closure with a fine-gauge absorbable suture provides a fine cosmetic result. The technique is really an intradermal stitch. Special needles such as the Dexon SBE-4 are specially sharpened needles that are particularly helpful for performing the subcuticular stitch.

Dog-Ear Repair

Dog-ear is the term used to describe the bunched-up tissue that may develop during wound closure. Frequently this is noted during the repair of a complex laceration with soft

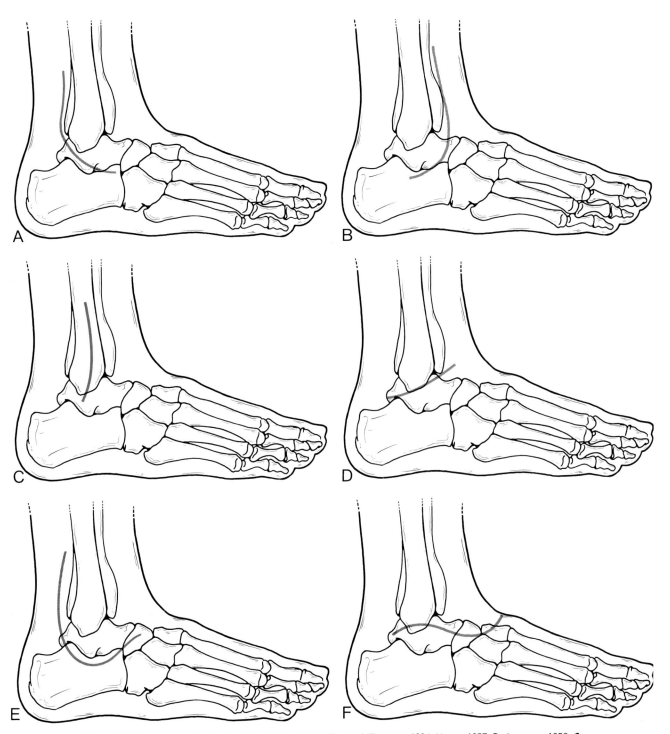

Figure 49.26.   Approaches to the lateral ankle. **A.** Gatellier and Chastang, 1924; Henry, 1957. **B.** Jergesen, 1959. **C.** McLaughlin and Ryder, 1929. **D.** Ollier, 1891. **E.** Kocher, 1911. **F.** Sutherland and Rowe, 1946.

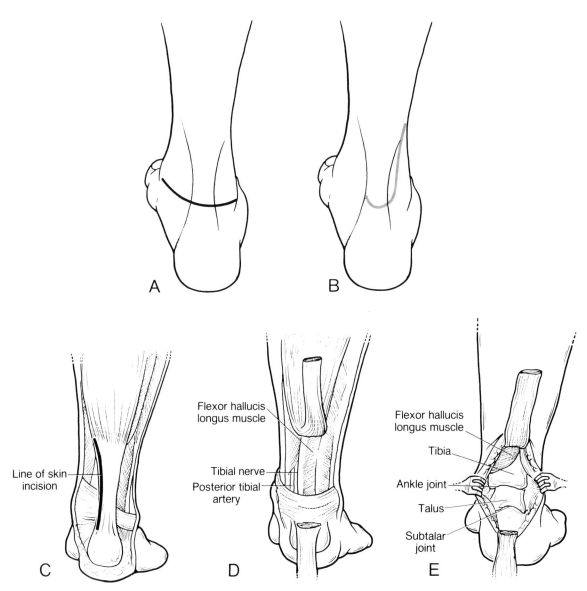

Figure 49.27. Posterior approaches to the triceps surae, ankle, and subtalar joint. **A.** Transverse approach. **B.** J approach—Picot, 1923. **C.** Longitudinal approach, medially placed. **D.** Reflecting the Achilles tendon. **E.** Visualizing the posterior ankle and subtalar joints.

tissue loss or after excision of a skin lesion. It can also be the result of an improper suturing technique. Uneven advancement of the needle during closure results in an excess of tissue on one side of the incision at the end of the incision line. This dog-ear is a bunched-up portion of tissue that is cosmetically displeasing. It can be either everted or inverted.

Many dog-ears will flatten with time. A large dog-ear will not flatten significantly and should be removed at the time of surgery. Treatment consists of equalizing the two remaining arms of the incision, usually by excising a wedge of tissue. Borges (20) discusses numerous techniques that can be used to repair the dog-ear and emphasizes that, when possible, the wedge of tissue should be excised in line with the RSTLs (Fig. 49.29).

WOUND COVERAGE TECHNIQUES

Open wounds must be provided with coverage. There is an ever-increasing number of coverage techniques available. These include direct closure, skin grafting, flaps (including musculocutaneous and free flaps), artificial skin, cultured cells, amnion, and xenografts. Amnion, artificial skin, and xenografts provide temporary coverage. Skin grafts, flaps, and cultured cells provide permanent coverage.

The skin is the human being's greatest protection against the bacterial environment. Krizek and Robson (21) have demonstrated that the presence of bacterial growth in a wound is less important as a predictor of infection than is the level of bacterial contamination. They demonstrated that the presence of 10^5 bacteria represents a significant level of bacterial contamination indicative of infection. Tempo-

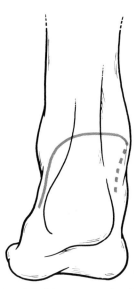

Figure 49.28. Cincinnati incision—comprehensive approach to the posterior ankle and associated structures (Crawford, 1982).

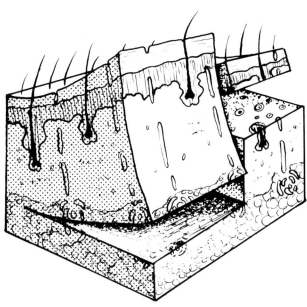

Figure 49.30. Full-thickness cut of a skin graft involves superficial fascia; partial-thickness cut is through a portion of the dermis.

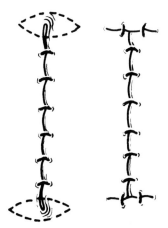

Figure 49.29. Diagram illustrating the excision of dog ears in line with the RSTLs. (Redrawn from Borges A: Dog-ear repair. *Plast Reconstr Surg* 69:707-713, 1982.)

rary wound coverage functions to reduce the level of bacterial contamination and to allow host defenses to act more effectively. Reduction of the level of bacterial contamination through proper local wound care is vital before permanent coverage of the wound with a graft or flap. In one study of 50 open wounds judged ready for skin grafting by clinical appearance, the graft success was 94% in those wounds with fewer than 10^5 bacteria per gram of tissue and only 19% in those wounds with more than 10^5 bacteria per gram of tissue (22).

Proper local care, including mechanical and surgical debridement, topical medicaments (antibiotics, enzymatic agents), and appropriate dressing materials, is the first step in achieving wound closure. Krizek and Robson's (21) tech-

nique of quantitative bacteriology provides the surgeon with an objective indication of when a wound is ready for coverage, rather than the subjective clinical wound appearance. In addition to the amount of bacteria present in a wound, the type of bacteria that are present is also important. Two organisms are particularly destructive to a skin graft: *Streptococcus pyogenes* and *Pseudomonas pyocyanea* (23). Systemic antibiotic therapy may be appropriate in certain situations; however, local care of the wound is far more important in eliminating local infection. Once a wound is clean, free of infection and necrotic material, and has a good base of granulation tissue, it should be grafted without delay.

SKIN GRAFTS

A free skin graft is completely detached from the body during its transfer from donor to recipient site. Its subsequent nourishment is derived from its attachment and new vascular connections at the recipient site. The skin graft is a segment of epidermis and dermis. The characteristics of the graft depend on the thickness of the dermis associated with the graft and the region of the body from which the graft is harvested. Skin grafts can be classified as autografts (transfer within the same individual), allografts (transfer to a different individual of the same species), isografts (from an identical twin), and xenografts (from a different species) (24). Allograft skin from a cadaver will initially take and survive, but its survival is brief and is terminated by a rejection episode. Xenografts never take and function only as a biological dressing. Grafts can also be classified as partial-thickness (split-thickness) or full-thickness, depending on whether all of the dermis (full-thickness) or only a portion of it (split-thickness) is taken with the graft (Fig. 49.30).

Indications

Skin grafts provide a useful permanent coverage in a variety of situations. They are technically simple to perform and carry less risks than other more complicated types of wound coverage. Skin grafts can be applied to almost any area of the body where there is sufficient vascularity in the wound to support a base of granulation tissue. Certain areas, such as bare bone, tendon, cartilage, and nerve, will not support a graft (25). Skin grafts that overlie small avascular areas may heal by a process of *bridging* from surrounding vascular tissue (23). Bone that is covered with periosteum or tendon covered with paratenon may support a graft. Skin grafts can be quite durable when applied over a good vascular bed with underlying soft tissue. In the lower extremity skin grafts are commonly used for coverage of burns, ulcerations, traumatic loss of soft tissue, secondary defects from flap donor sites, and defects created by excision of large masses.

Split-thickness skin grafts are used more commonly than full-thickness skin grafts. They are generally thought of as being of three types: thin, intermediate, and thick, depending on how much of the dermis is taken with the graft (Fig. 49.31). Thin grafts are 0.008 to 0.012 inch thick. These grafts are quite translucent and take quite readily but contract a great deal. Intermediate split-thickness skin grafts are 0.012 to 0.016 inch thick. These grafts contain a thicker portion of dermis than the thin grafts, which means that they are more durable and contract less but do not heal quite as readily. Thick split-thickness skin grafts are 0.016 to 0.020 inch thick (26). The thick graft contains more dermis than the intermediate graft, and therefore it is more durable, contracts less, and has more of the properties of normal skin. The thick graft requires greater nourishment immediately and has a much greater chance of failure. Often the intermediate split-thickness skin graft is the best choice because it provides adequate, durable coverage and takes readily.

In general, split-thickness skin grafts have more smaller-caliber blood vessels that contact the recipient site than do full-thickness grafts. This helps to account for the "easier take" of split-thickness grafts as compared with full-thickness grafts. Depending on the thickness of the graft, split-thickness grafts generally do not have sebaceous gland function, have little or no hair, and have minimal sweat gland function. Pigmentation is usually different than the surrounding recipient tissue, depending on where the graft was taken. Varying amounts of sensation may return after 1 to 2 years. Donor sites for split-thickness grafts have more epithelial structures remaining in the dermis and, therefore, heal more rapidly than donor sites for full-thickness skin grafts. There is also much less contraction at the donor site of a split-thickness skin graft. At the recipient site, the thinner the graft, the greater the secondary contracture.

Full-thickness skin grafts contain all of the epidermis and dermis. No superficial fascia or fat is transferred with the graft. The full-thickness graft provides thick wound coverage that contracts very little at the recipient site. Because it contains all elements of the dermis, it most closely mimics normal skin, including sweat and sebaceous function. The process of graft take is more tenuous with a full-thickness graft and limits the situations in which it can be used. In addition, a great deal of contraction occurs at the donor site (up to 70%), which usually must be closed either by direct closure or by a split-thickness skin graft.

Each type of skin graft has specific properties that dictate where it is most readily used. When choosing the type of graft material, the surgeon must consider many factors, including the function of the recipient area, the condition of the recipient bed, and cosmetics. Recipient sites that are subjected to a great deal of irritation, such as weight-bearing areas of the foot or areas that rub in a shoe (e.g., the posterior heel), require thicker coverage. Recipient beds of questionable condition or vascularity are better treated with thinner grafts that take more easily. The cosmetics of both the recipient and donor sites must also be considered, particularly in a young female patient. Taking the graft from a hidden area is often an important part of the overall success of the procedure from the patient's point of view.

Technical Considerations

INSTRUMENTATION FOR HARVESTING

Cutting a skin graft of even thickness requires fine instrumentation, good assistance, and an experienced surgeon. Grafts can be cut with either hand or power instruments. The Blair and Humby knives are the more common hand knives. The Humby knife consists of a knife blade and an adjustable roller to control the thickness of the graft. This technique requires more experience than power instrumentation. Large sheets of skin, however, can be more easily obtained with the hand instrument. Small grafts can be obtained by hand with the use of a razor blade (26). Power instruments include units driven by electricity, gas, or bat-

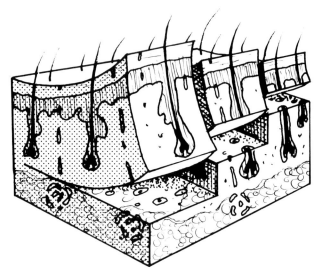

Figure 49.31. Split-thickness skin grafts can be classified as thick, intermediate, or thin, depending on the percentage of dermis taken with epidermis in the graft.

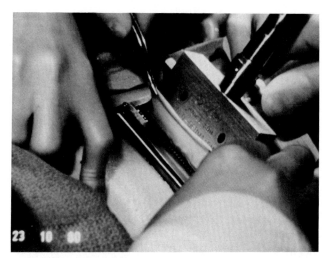

Figure 49.32. An electric dermatome is most commonly used for obtaining split-thickness skin grafts.

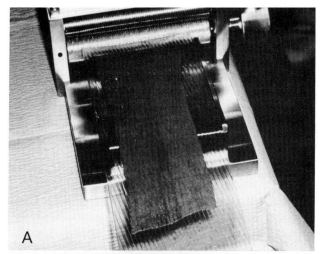

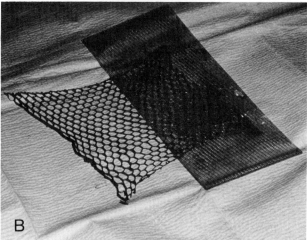

Figure 49.33. A meshing device can expand grafts to cover larger areas, as well as allow for drainage. **A.** Graft inserted for meshing. **B.** Meshed graft.

tery. The electrical or gas-powered dermatome is the most popular device. It can rapidly harvest a large graft of uniform width and thickness. The thickness of the graft can be adjusted by a calibrating device on the head of the instrument.

The technique for harvesting a split-thickness skin graft begins with lubrication of the skin and dermatome with either saline solution or sterile mineral oil. The skin is then stabilized by the assistant with two sterile tongue blades. This is particularly important in areas of uneven contour, such as the buttocks. Failure to stabilize the skin will result in a graft of irregular thickness. Firm and, most important, even pressure is maintained on the dermatome during the harvesting procedure. The dermatome must be advanced slowly. As the graft comes out of the dermatome, an assistant holds it with two atraumatic pick-ups (Fig. 49.32). After the graft has been harvested, it should be inspected for uniformity of thickness. This can be determined in two ways: by the translucency of the graft and by the vascular pattern at the donor site. The more translucent the graft, the thinner it must be. A donor site that shows many fine, small, blood vessels is associated with a thin split-thickness graft, whereas a donor site that shows fewer, larger vessels is seen after harvesting of a thick split-thickness skin graft. After harvesting the graft is then put aside on a piece of moist saline gauze until it is used.

Another useful piece of equipment is the graft mesher. This device takes a split-thickness graft and meshes it uniformly to produce a graft with a uniform fishnet appearance (Fig. 49.33). This has two important uses: (*a*) it expands the graft, allowing it to cover a much greater surface area, and (*b*) it allows drainage to flow from beneath the graft, preventing hematoma and allowing earlier coverage in contaminated wounds (27). After the initial take of the graft, the interposed spaces heal by epithelial migration from the surrounding graft. This can sometimes give rise to an uneven appearance.

APPLICATION OF THE GRAFT

Before application of the graft, the wound must be properly prepared. This consists of sharp debridement of the wound edges and curettage of the base of the wound to remove excessive fibrous tissue. The wound should be thoroughly irrigated during the debridement process. The debridement usually initiates some hemorrhage that must be controlled before the graft can be laid in place. Hemostasis can be achieved in a number of ways, including cauterization or ligation of large vessels, application of gauze soaked in local anesthetic with epinephrine 1:100,000, or application of a topical hemostatic agent such as topical thrombin. Once harvested, the graft can be either meshed, pie-crusted, or applied intact. Meshing allows the graft to be used to cover a larger area. The expansion can be increased by increasing the distance between the stands of the mesh. This is particularly important in the treatment of large burns. Pie-crusting allows the surgeon to get a smaller amount of expansion and drainage out of the graft than by meshing. The technique for pie-crusting involves application of the graft (dermis side down) to a hard surface, such as the flat portion of an inverted metal bowl. A scalpel blade is then used to make small cuts in the graft (Fig. 49.34).

For the graft to survive, it must be in intimate contact with the recipient tissue. This means that it must be applied in such a way that all portions of the graft are in contact with the underlying wound. A rolled gauze sponge or a cotton-tipped applicator is used to remove any excess fluid beneath the graft. The graft is trimmed to the appropriate size, but it is allowed to overlap the edge of the wound. One way to facilitate the trimming of the graft is to use an impression of the wound against the graft to estimate the size that is needed. A skin marker is used to outline the wound. The graft is then placed against the outline, thus marking the graft itself. The graft is trimmed to the appropriate size and then sutured into place with fine-gauge suture material.

After application of the graft, it must be fixed in place to resist shearing forces that can disrupt revascularization and to prevent the accumulation of underlying fluid. Pressure dressings are commonly used to maximize contact between the graft and its host. The stent tie-over dressing is very useful in this regard, although it is not mandatory. It consists of cotton balls or fluffed gauze held in place with sutures tied over the fluff (Fig. 49.35). A variation on the technique is the use of gauze dressing that is cut to shape several thicknesses deep. Peacock (28) also describes this technique and mentions moistening of the gauze before application. Sutures are then tied over the gauze from surrounding dental rubber bands (Fig. 49.36). Regardless of the type of pressure dressing that is used, one must be careful that excessive pressure is not applied to the graft. Excessive pressure will shut down vascular channels, causing death of the graft by ischemia. The limb must also be immobilized in a cast or a posterior splint to prevent the shearing forces from disrupting the connections of the vascular networks of the graft and recipient tissues.

STORAGE OF EXCESS GRAFT

It is usually a good idea to take a graft slightly larger than the anticipated need. This ensures that there will be a proper-sized graft, even if the surgeon errs in estimation of the dimensions. This also allows the surgeon to store some excess graft material in case of failure of a portion of the original graft. The material to be stored should be wrapped in a moist saline sponge and placed in a sterile cup. The

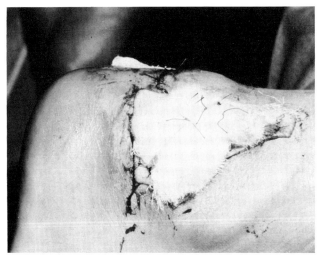

Figure 49.35. Traditional stent dressing for compression over a graft.

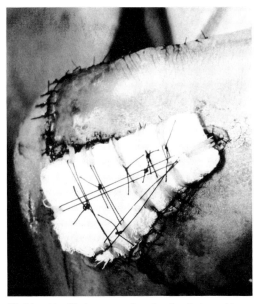

Figure 49.36. Modified compression dressing that provides a uniform compressive surface.

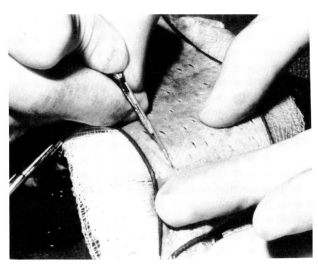

Figure 49.34. Pie-crusting technique for graft preparation.

graft is then refrigerated at 0^0 to 5^0 C. A constant temperature is important for survival of the stored graft. This material can be used up to 21 days after storage. Peacock (28) states, however, that after 3 or 4 days the rate of success of refrigerated grafts falls precipitously. Grafts may also be stored at the original donor site, where the diffusion of nutrients and waste products can occur.

POSTOPERATIVE CARE

There is a natural tendency to want to view the graft as often as possible as a form of self-reassurance. Unfortunately, the more one disturbs the graft, the more likely it is to fail. It is best to leave the immediate postoperative dressing in place for 3 to 4 days. The dressing change must be performed carefully to prevent disruption of the graft-host interface. The wound is carefully inspected for hematomas, seromas, and any irregularity of the graft. If any underlying fluid accumulation is seen, then it must be drained immediately. A No. 11 blade or a fine-gauge needle is used to puncture the space and drain the fluid. By the third day the graft should be "pinking up." If any areas are frankly necrotic, they should be removed and replaced with the refrigerated graft material. A compression dressing is carefully reapplied to maintain graft-host contact. Maintenance of compression over the graft site for several months with elastic bandages is an important adjunct to therapy.

DONOR SITES

There are numerous potential donor sites available for skin grafts. Most commonly, split-thickness skin grafts are taken from the thigh because of its broad, flat surface. Split-thickness skin grafts can also be taken from the buttock area. Although procurement of the graft is more difficult from the curved surface of the buttock, the buttock has the advantage of being hidden from view. Therefore, for some patients the buttock is the preferable donor site.

After the skin graft is harvested the donor site often becomes a secondary concern. However, proper wound management is just as important for the donor site as it is for the recipient site. Infiltration of the donor site with bupivacaine and epinephrine 1:200,000 provides long-acting anesthesia and controls excessive bleeding. Topical thrombin may be applied to the donor site to control bleeding. Application of pressure to the donor site for 5 minutes will also aid in the control of excess bleeding.

There are basically two schools of thought concerning the type of dressing that should be applied to the donor site. The most common technique has been to use a dry dressing of one or two thicknesses of gauze and let the wound dry (23, 25, 26). This technique is usually quite painful because the regenerating epithelium is torn off as the dried dressing is changed. More recent reports have suggested that there are several advantages to the use of an occlusive, vapor-permeable, polyurethane film as a dressing material (29, 30) (Fig. 49.37). Epidermal regeneration occurs best in a moist

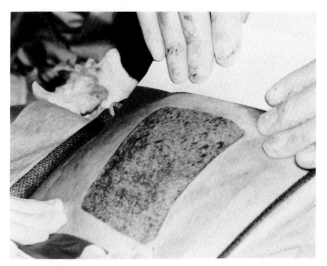

Figure 49.37. Polyurethane film dressing for the donor site promotes rapid regeneration of epithelium.

environment, such as is provided by an occlusive dressing (31). Most important, patients have much less pain during the healing process and at the dressing change when a dressing such as Op-Site is used. This transparent, occlusive dressing is applied easily at the time of surgery and is usually maintained under a compression dressing for the first 24 hours. The Op-Site dressing can be left in place until the wound is healed. If hematoma or seroma occurs, it can be drained from a puncture through the dressing. The puncture is then covered with another piece of Op-Site.

Specialized Techniques

Some specialized techniques of grafting include mesh grafting, pinch grafting, and dermal overgrafting. Both mesh grafting and pinch grafting are used in situations where a large area of wound must be covered with a limited amount of graft material. The mesh graft, which has been discussed previously, is most useful in this situation. The pinch or postage stamp grafting technique involves harvest of a series of small grafts, with space left between them to be filled in from surrounding tissue. This technique is not nearly as efficient for this purpose as mesh grafting.

Dermal overlay grafting is a technique for situations in which a full-thickness graft is needed but the recipient wound is not capable of supporting such a graft. First, a very thin split-thickness skin graft is taken from the donor site; this removes the epidermis. The dermatome is then passed through the dermis, which is removed and placed, superficial side down, on the recipient site. Placing the superficial side down allows more vessels to come in contact with the recipient bed. The thin split-thickness graft is then replaced over the donor site, and both recipient and donor sites are managed in the usual manner. After 1 week either an additional dermal graft or a split-thickness skin graft may be applied to the original dermal graft (26).

Figure 49.38. Early stages of graft healing. **A.** Plasmatic stage with diffusion across liquid layer. **B.** Film anchorage of a graft. **C.** Early vascular budding. **D.** Link-up of vascular buds from graft and host. (Redrawn from McGregor I: *Fundamental Techniques of Plastic Surgery*, ed 7. New York, Churchill Livingstone, 1980, p 58.)

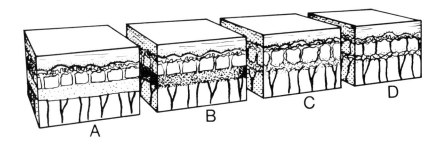

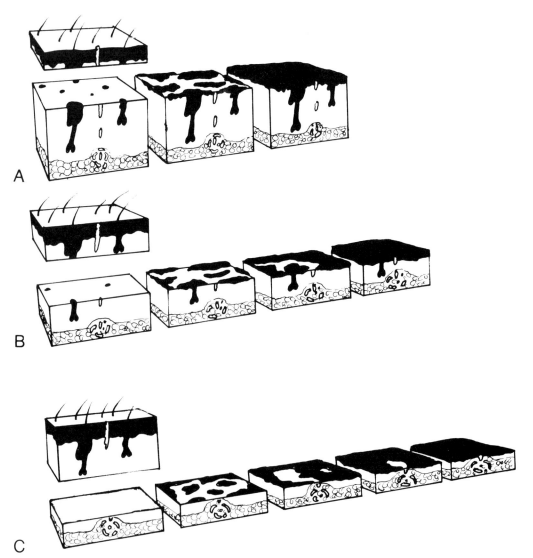

Figure 49.39. Healing of donor sites will vary, depending on the thickness of graft and the number of epithelial structures remaining. **A.** Thin split-thickness donor site. **B.** Intermediate-thickness split-thickness donor site. **C.** Thick split-thickness donor site demonstrates slowest healing. (Redrawn from McGregor I: *Fundamental Techniques of Plastic Surgery*, ed 7. New York, Churchill Livingstone, 1980, p 80.)

GRAFT AND DONOR HEALING

There are three basic stages of graft healing: plasmatic stage, inosculation, and reorganization and reinnervation. For these events to occur, there must be complete contact between the graft and a suitable recipient bed.

The healing process begins with the plasmatic stage. A fibrin layer is formed between the graft and the wound bed, allowing a diffusion process to occur between them. This fibrin layer serves as an anchor so that sufficient nourishment can pass from the wound to the graft to promote survival of the graft (25). During this process many transplanted cells die, much the same as occurs with a bone graft (Fig. 49.38). Most likely it is the surface layers of keratinized cells that do not survive this process. It is probably the stratum germinativum cells of the epidermis that are most important in promoting the rejuvenation of the graft (28). The plasmatic stage lasts approximately 24 to 48 hours.

The second stage of graft healing is inosculation of blood vessels, which occurs through the fibrin layer between the graft and the wound bed. At approximately 48 hours the graft begins to "pink up" because of the re-establishment of circulation. It is believed that re-establishment of the vascular connections occurs from vascular buds from the wound, which grow into the arteries and veins of the graft (1). Lymphatic drainage develops by the fourth or fifth day.

The process of reorganization and reinnervation occurs during the months after grafting. This period is dominated by connective tissue reorganization, the regulation of inflow and outflow, and the reinnervation of the graft. Reinnervation is variable and may take as long as 1 to 2 years (32, 33).

The healing of the donor site is similar to that of a superficial burn. Epithelialization occurs from the remaining epithelial structures, such as sebaceous and sweat glands and hair follicles. The thickness of the harvested graft determines the type and amount of epithelial structures that are left at the donor site to aid in healing. A donor site for a thin split-thickness skin graft will heal in 7 to 9 days, whereas it takes a donor site for a thick split-thickness skin graft 14 days or longer to heal (23) (Fig. 49.39). If there are no sebaceous or sweat glands and no hair follicles, then the donor site must granulate in and heal from the surrounding wound margin.

FULL-THICKNESS SKIN GRAFTS

Most of this discussion has concerned the split-thickness skin graft because that is the technique that is more commonly used. There are some unique considerations for full-thickness skin grafting. The indications for full-thickness grafts include weight-bearing areas and areas where the greater flexibility of the full-thickness skin graft is desirable.

The size and shape of the necessary graft are marked on a sterile pattern (gauze is most useful). The pattern is then traced over the donor site, and the skin is removed sharply. Sometimes the graft shape can be incorporated into two semielliptical incisions to facilitate direct closure of the donor site (Fig. 49.40). The skin is dissected to below the level

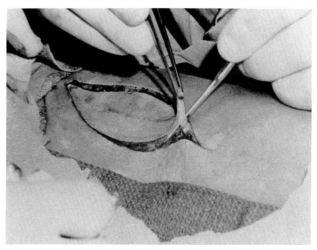

Figure 49.40. Outline for removal of full-thickness skin graft and direct closure of the defect.

of the dermis, but subcutaneous tissue is left in the wound. Any fat that has been taken with the graft is then removed with a sharp iris or Metzenbaum scissors. The graft is laid in place and covered with a pressure dressing. The donor site is then either closed directly or covered with a split-thickness skin graft.

Potential donor sites for full-thickness skin grafts include the inguinal area, the popliteal fossa, and, for small grafts, the skin over the sinus tarsi, the medial arch, or plantarly just distal to the metatarsals in the plantar fat pad.

COMPLICATIONS

Contact between the graft and the host bed is absolutely essential for survival of the graft. Anything that interferes with that relationship will cause the graft to fail (Fig. 49.41). Factors that can cause failure include accumulation of fluid beneath the graft, movement across the graft-host interface, and excessive tension on the graft.

The most common complication is the development of a seroma beneath the graft (Fig. 49.42). This is particularly common in grafts over a concave surface or after removal of a pressure dressing (23). Treatment is initiated by aspiration of the fluid in the seroma, treatment of any contraction that has occurred across the concave surface, and reapplication of a pressure dressing. If the seroma has been present for several days, it may be necessary to curet the base of the wound to remove epithelium before application of a fresh or stored skin graft.

Infection can also be a devastating complication. In particular, *Streptococcus pyogenes* can totally destroy a graft because of its fibrinolysin, which disrupts the normal fibrin bonding between the graft and the host. *S. pyogenes* is so devastating that it can make the graft appear to dissolve. In certain situations infection will cause total loss of the graft, although there are instances in which infection will be limited to a portion of the graft where it can be treated locally.

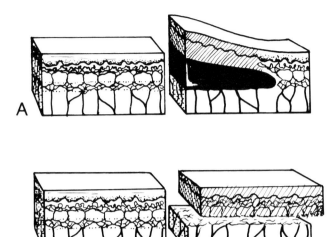

Figure 49.41. Forces that disrupt the link-up of vascular buds from the graft and host can result in failure of a graft. **A.** Hematoma or seroma presents a mechanical barrier to the link-up. **B.** Shearing forces make link-up impossible because of excessive motion. (Redrawn from McGregor I: *Fundamental Techniques of Plastic Surgery*, ed 7. New York, Churchill Livingstone, 1980, p 61.)

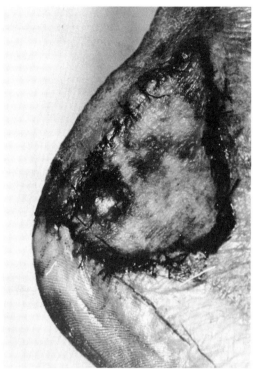

Figure 49.42. Seroma beneath a graft 5 days postoperatively at the second dressing change. The initial dressing was adequate but was changed too early.

As noted by Teh (34), the number of organisms present in the wound at the time of grafting is less important than the types of organisms that are present. The destruction of fibrin by certain bacteria is the key element in the failure of the graft. Fibrin is important not only as the adherent that makes revascularization possible but also for its antibacterial properties, primarily the enhancement of phagocytosis (34).

Necrosis of the graft because of fluid, infection, or movement must be treated first by removal of the necrotic tissue. The wound can then be either allowed to granulate in from surrounding tissue or recovered with fresh graft, stored autograft, or allograft.

ALTERNATIVE SKIN COVERAGE

There are various types of wound coverage in addition to grafts and flaps. These include human extraembryonic membranes (amnion), artificial skin, cultured epidermal cells, xenografts, and a number of new dressing materials. Amnion, xenografts, and the occlusive dressing materials are designed to provide temporary coverage, eventually to be replaced by a skin graft or epithelialization from surrounding tissue. Amnion is a useful dressing that appears to promote wound healing through macrophage activation, which then stimulates endothelial proliferation (35).

Porcine xenografts have been used for temporary wound coverage in many different situations (36-39). They appear to be most useful in reducing bacterial contamination of wounds populated by gram positive organisms, but are of limited use in wounds contaminated with gram-negative organisms (39).

A variety of bio-occlusive dressing materials are also available. These dressings have found application in certain specific situations, such as the donor sites for split-thickness skin grafts. These dressings act by producing a moist environment that encourages epithelialization, although the rate of increase of tensile strength of the wound may be delayed (40). Geliperm is a gelatin film that is permeable to wound secretions but impermeable to bacteria.

A physiologically acceptable bilayer artificial skin has been developed; at present it is a temporary dressing since it must be covered with a very thin split-thickness skin graft. The skin consists of a temporary silicone epidermis and a porous collagen-chondroitin sulfate fibrillar dermis (41). It has been used to cover large burn wounds. The advantage of this technique is that it encourages formation of a new dermis over the scaffold provided by the artificial dermis. The silicone covering is then removed anywhere between 7 and 46 days, and the wound is covered with a thin (0.002 inch thick) autologous meshed graft of epithelium.

Autologous cultured epithelium is the newest technique for wound coverage. It is a dramatic advancement for patients with large burns when there is insufficient autogenous skin available for grafting (42-44). This technique allows a small skin sample the size of a biopsy specimen to be cultured to provide thin coverage over a wide area. A biopsy specimen of 2 cm × 2 cm can be expanded in surface area by a factor of 10,000 in 3 to 4 weeks (42). During the period of time when the grafts are growing in culture the wounds can be covered with human allograft.

Skin Flaps

Skin flaps are distinct from skin grafts because they retain their vascular attachments, including arterial, capillary, and venous structures. The mainstay of skin coverage continues to be skin grafting, because of its simplicity and its lower morbidity as compared with flaps (Fig. 49.43). In many situations, however, a graft does not provide adequate coverage. Over the past decade advances in microsurgical techniques have led to the development and refinement of the free flap, which has opened new horizons in wound coverage.

Specific indications for skin flaps include (*a*) coverage of areas with poor vascularity (e.g., bare bone or tendon), (*b*) reconstruction for full thickness, (*c*) padding over bony prominences, (*d*) coverage of areas requiring an operation at a later date, and (*e*) restoration of sensation to an area may be possible if a flap is transferred with its nerve supply.

The word *flap* refers to a tongue of tissue, whereas the word *pedicle* refers only to the base or stem of the flap. The term *pedicle flap* is redundant (1). *Rotation* and *transposition* refer to specific types of flap and should not be used as general adjectives.

CLASSIFICATION

Classification of flaps is useful because it helps the surgeon to understand the properties of a particular procedure. The two most common classification systems are based on either the movement of the flap or the vascular anatomy of the flap. Classification based on the vascular anatomy is most important, particularly in the lower extremity where the blood supply to flaps is less reliable than other in areas of the body. With this in mind, there are two general types of flaps: random and axial pattern.

Random-pattern flaps (cutaneous flaps) derive their blood supply from the cutaneous dermal-subdermal plexus. Most skin flaps are of this type (1). They lack any axial arteries and depend on the perfusion pressure of the cutaneous vessels for survival. These flaps are subject to limitations based on their dimensions, particularly in terms of the length/breadth ratio. Because they do not have a large-caliber axial artery, they are dependent on the size of the dermal-subdermal plexus at the base of the flap (45). Consequently, the base of these flaps must be wide enough to support the length of the flap. This is particularly true in the lower extremity, where the breadth of the flap should be at least as great as its length. Use of a delay procedure (to be discussed later) can increase the rate of survival of these flaps by 50% to 100% (1).

Axial-pattern (arterial) flaps contain a direct cutaneous artery that arises from a larger direct vessel. The surviving length of the flap is dependent on the axial artery's dimensions, not on the width of the pedicle (base). This makes it possible to construct a flap at least as long as the territory of the axial artery (46). The portion of the flap that is distal to the axial artery is supplied by the dermal-subdermal plexus and is, in effect, a random flap. With delay procedures they can be made even longer. These arterialized flaps are safer, more robust, and more free from dimensional restrictions than are random flaps. An example of this approach in the lower extremity is the dorsalis pedis flap.

Axial-pattern flaps have certain variations, including the island and free flaps. An island flap is an arterial flap because it has a cutaneous artery, but there is no skin bridge. The advantage of this flap is that there is greater flexibility in rotation of the tissue. A free flap is transferred from a distant site with its vascular supply reattached by microvascular surgery. With recent advances and experience in microsurgical techniques, the free flap is being used more frequently in lower extremity reconstructive surgery (Fig. 49.44). An example of a free flap's use is a latissimus dorsi transfer for reconstruction of a defect over the tibia.

Skin flaps may also be classified as to transposition site. This classification includes local flaps (those lying adjacent

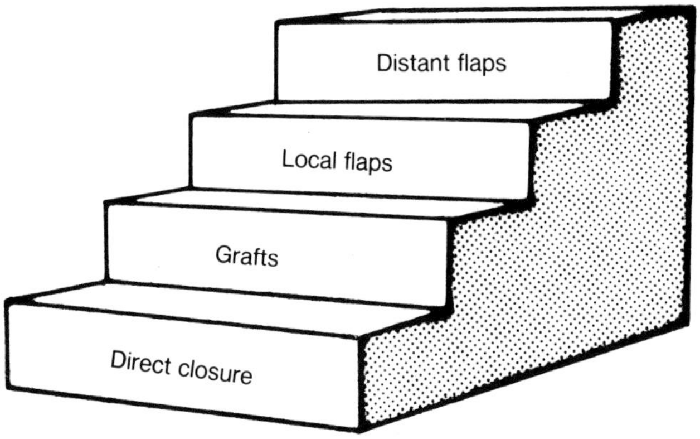

Figure 49.43. Illustration of "ascending" approach to wound coverage. The simplest technique should be considered first.

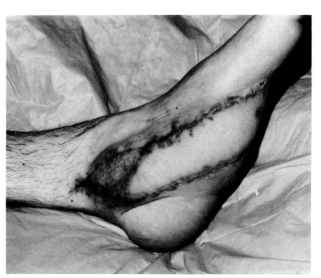

Figure 49.44. Latissimus dorsi free flap used for coverage of the medial and plantar sides of the foot.

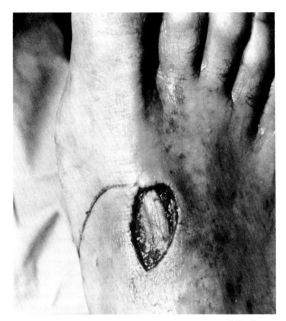

Figure 49.45. Rotation flap over the dorsum of the foot.

to the defect) and distant flaps (those transferred from a distance, either directly or by means of a carrier). Indirect distant flaps are most commonly transposed by using the wrist as the carrier. Using the wrist as a carrier allows a flap to be raised from a quite remote site and still be used at the defect site.

LOCAL FLAPS

Local flaps are of two basic types: those that rotate about a pivot point (rotation, transposition, and interpolation flaps) and advancement flaps (V-Y, Y-V, single, and bipedicle advancement).

Rotation flaps pivot about a fixed point to resurface an adjacent defect (Fig. 49.45). The donor site can be closed directly with sutures or with a skin graft (partial or full-thickness). The ideal shape of the rotation flap is a half-circle. The larger the circle, the less tension there is at any particular point on the flap. When excessive tension is present, it usually occurs at the pivot point. This can be alleviated by use of a back cut or excision of a Burow's triangle. A back cut is an incision placed on the diameter line of the half-circle adjacent to the pivot point. This back cut releases tension for closure of the flap over the primary defect but creates a secondary defect that must be closed either by direct suture or by skin grafting. Tension may also be released by excision of a triangle of skin adjacent to the pivot point (Burow's triangle). A dog-ear is often created at the apex of the triangulated defect. Excision of the dog-ear is usually done at a later date so that the blood supply of the flap is not jeopardized.

A transposition flap is usually rectangular or square and rotates about a pivot point to cover an adjacent defect (Fig. 49.46). The major difference between the rotation flap and

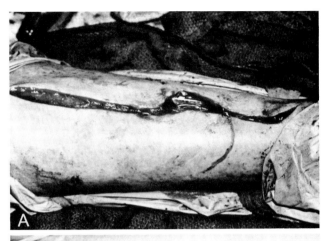

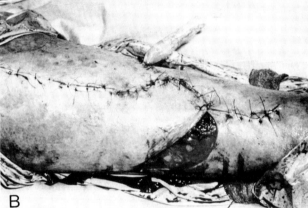

Figure 49.46. Transposition flap for coverage over the tibial plate. **A.** Defect and flap outline. **B.** Flap sutured in place. Note the donor defect that was subsequently covered with a split-thickness skin graft.

the transposition flap is that the transposition flap movement occurs mainly in a lateral direction as opposed to the movement about an arc that occurs with the rotation flap. It is quite common for a particular flap to possess elements of both rotation and transposition, in which case the flap is named according to the predominant motion (47). The ideal length/breadth ratio is variable, depending on the location, but in the lower extremity the ratio should probably not exceed 1:1. This aids the vascular supply to the flap by providing adequate pedicle width for the entrance of sufficient vessels from the dermal-subdermal plexus. As in some other local flaps, the defect must be triangulated first to allow for proper rotation of the tissue. The flap is designed to be longer than the adjacent defect to prevent excessive tension. Tension can be released by means of the back cut or Burow's triangle. The donor site (or secondary defect) may be closed by direct closure, skin grafting, or a secondary flap from adjacent lax skin (47). An example of this type of flap is the bilobed flap. Another example of the transposition flap is the Limberg flap for closure of a rhomboid defect.

Advancement flaps are moved directly forward to cover a defect without any rotation or lateral movement (Fig.

49.47). The single-pedicle advancement flap is square or rectangular and is stretched forward. The tissue is advanced by making use of the skin's elasticity. Tension occurs at the base of the flap and can be relieved by excision of Burow's triangle or by using back cuts. The tension created at the base limits this technique to coverage of small areas. Elongation may also be aided by a Z-plasty on each side of the base of the flap. Each of these techniques acts to relieve tension in a longitudinal direction while exaggerating transverse tension across the base. A bipedicle advancement flap can also be used. This is created by making a longitudinal incision parallel to the longitudinal axis of the defect. The interposed skin is then undermined and advanced laterally over the primary defect. The secondary defect may be covered with a skin graft. Other types of advancement flap include the V-Y and Y-V techniques.

DISTANT FLAPS

In addition to local flaps, skin coverage may be obtained from a site distant from the defect. In the lower extremity, indirect distant flaps by means of a carrier are seldom used. Direct flaps in the lower extremity are primarily transferred from the opposite extremity. The first step in the technique for this cross-leg flap consists of raising the flap on the donor leg (Fig. 49.48). This creates a donor defect that can be covered with a split-thickness skin graft at the time of the

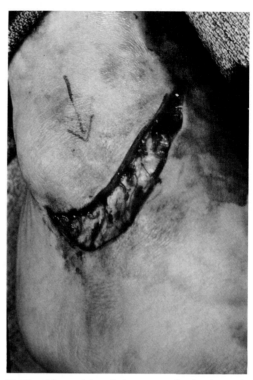

Figure 49.47.   After excision of a burn scar, a flap is advanced to cover the defect.

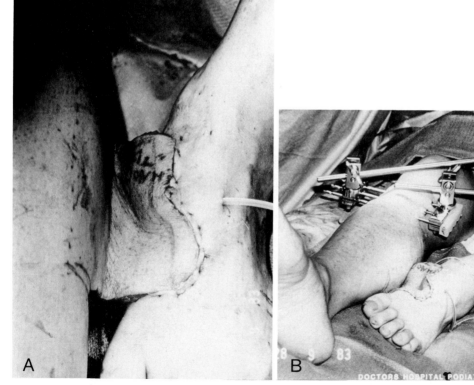

Figure 49.48.   Cross-leg flap from the contralateral calf. **A.** A flap is raised and sutured into the recipient site. **B.** An external fixator is used to stabilize both limbs until the flap can be divided from the donor site.

initial surgery. The raised flap is then applied to the recipient site and sutured in place with a hinged edge still attached to the donor leg for its blood supply. The two limbs must be immobilized (casting, pins in plaster, or external fixation) until the flap is ready for division and insetting into the recipient site (47, 48). In older patients this may result in serious joint stiffness. At 14 to 21 days the flap may be separated from the donor leg and the hinged edge sutured into place at the recipient site. Taylor and Hopson (49) have described a cross-foot flap that can be used to cover a heel defect with a flap from the contralateral medial arch. Disadvantages of cross-leg flaps include the prolonged hospitalization and immobilization, which results in significant morbidity, and the insensitive and relatively avascular nature of the flaps. Cross-extremity flaps are used less frequently now because of advances in the techniques of muscle flaps, myocutaneous flaps, and free flaps.

The free flap is a combination of skin and subcutaneous tissue transferred in one stage to a distant site with a blood supply that is restored by microvascular anastomosis (50). Other tissues such as bone and muscle may be transferred at the same time. The transfer of muscle has been suggested as a treatment for chronic osteomyelitis of the lower extremity (51). The concept behind this is to provide greater vascularity and antibiotic perfusion to the infected area than would be possible with local flaps. The technique is a valuable adjunct to therapy of this very difficult problem and must be combined with standard principles such as debridement of infected tissue and perioperative administration of antibiotics (51). It may also be used for the management of acute bone exposure wounds to reduce the incidence of bone infections (52, 53).

Common donor sites for free flap transfers include the groin (54), the dorsalis pedis territory of the first web space (55), the latissimus dorsi myocutaneous flap (56), and the tensor fascia lata (57).

The advantages of free flaps include the one-stage nature of the procedure, excellent vascularity to the recipient area, full-thickness coverage provided to the area (including muscle and bone if needed), and less hospitalization time than with other techniques for similar indications. The disadvantages include the technical difficulty of the procedure, the prolonged anesthesia time, the excessive bulk of certain flaps, and the risk of loss of the flap. Venous or arterial thrombosis is a major risk (58).

Specific indications in the foot include trauma subsequent to motor vehicle accident and high-velocity gunshot wounds with significant soft tissue loss (59, 60). Often the only alternative for these patients is amputation. The free groin flap is valuable in areas where coverage is needed without excessive bulk.

MUSCLE AND MYOCUTANEOUS FLAPS

Muscle and myocutaneous flaps can provide bulk, padding, skin coverage, and vascularity to an area. The decision to use muscle flaps should be based on knowledge of the anatomy, function, and reliability of the muscle. The preoperative evaluation must include the viable length of the muscle on the dominant vascular pedicle, the point and arc of rotation of the flap, the effect of loss of function of the muscle, and the possible size of the cutaneous segment to be transferred with the muscle (61). In general, muscle may support a cutaneous segment 50% larger than the size of the muscle, although this must be individualized.

Muscle flaps can be used in both the leg and the foot. The leg can be conveniently divided into three regions, where muscle flap use will vary according to the accessible muscles. In the upper third of the leg, muscle coverage can be obtained with the gastrocnemius or soleus muscles. The middle third of the leg can best be covered with the soleus, although the gastrocnemius, flexor digitorum longus, and tibialis anterior muscle flaps may also be used. In the lower third of the leg, local muscle flaps include the soleus muscle with skin graft and the peroneus brevis (Fig. 49.49). Distally based flaps of soleus, extensor digitorum longus, and extensor hallucis longus muscles may be used when minor vascular pedicles are intact (62-66).

In the foot, coverage of the heel may be obtained with the flexor digitorum brevis muscle and a skin graft (67, 68). (Heel coverage can be quite problematical and is discussed in greater detail later in the chapter.) The flexor digitorum brevis is supplied by both the medial and lateral plantar arteries, with the dominant supply from the lateral plantar artery. The flap is approached through a midline plantar incision, with superficial fascia reflected off the plantar fascia and retracted medially and laterally. The four tendons of the muscle are divided distally, and the muscle is reflected back on itself (Fig. 49.50). When the defect is more proximal, the origin of the muscle may be detached from the calcaneus to allow for more mobility of the flap (69) (Fig. 49.51).

The extensor digitorum brevis (EDB) has also been described for use as a muscle flap. The EDB has three slips originating from the distal and lateral surfaces of the calcaneus and is pedicled on the lateral tarsal artery. It has

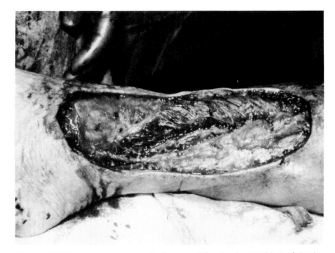

Figure 49.49. A soleus muscle flap used for the lower third of the leg with subsequent split-thickness skin graft coverage.

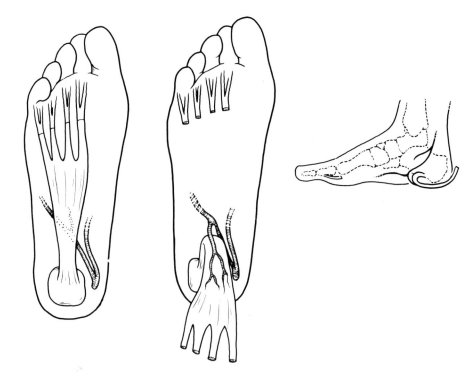

Figure 49.50. Diagram of a conventional flexor digitorum brevis muscle flap for inferior heel defects.

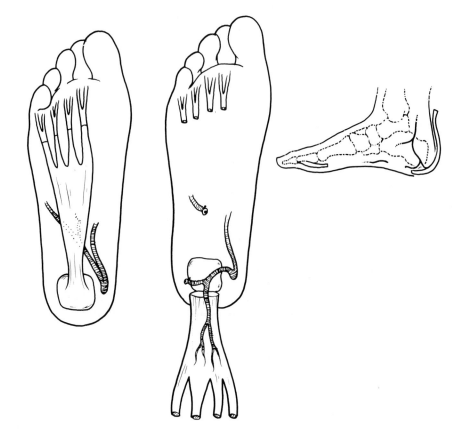

Figure 49.51. Division of the origin of the flexor digitorum brevis allows coverage of more proximal defects.

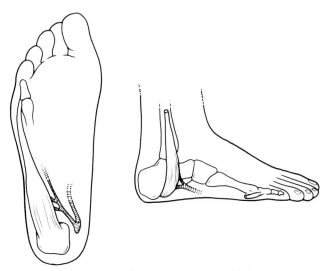

Figure 49.52. Diagram of the abductor digiti minimi muscle flap for coverage of lateral defects.

good mobility and provides effective, well-vascularized soft tissue coverage for the lateral malleolus. The muscle can also be detached and transferred by a microvascular technique. In either instance, the flap may be covered primarily or secondarily skin grafted.

The abductor hallucis can be used for coverage below the medial malleolus. The muscle is supplied by proximal and distal branches of the medial plantar artery. The tendon may be detached distally and reflected over itself to cover the defect along the medial arch below the medial malleolus. Division of the distal branches of the medial plantar artery that supply the muscle will allow greater proximal coverage (69).

The abductor digiti minimi may be used for the coverage of defects below the lateral malleolus (Fig. 49.52). This small muscle is supplied by the lateral neurovascular bundle. Division of the distal vascular pedicles allows for greater proximal mobility (69).

Ger (70), who pioneered the development of muscle flaps, has also described the use of the flexor hallucis brevis muscle flap in the management of neuropathic ulcerations of the forefoot.

Complications with muscle flaps may include surgical errors resulting from improper knowledge of vascular anatomy or poor dissection technique (71). Traction, twisting, and transection of the vascular pedicle are the most feared complications. The consequences of failure can be devastating because a defect larger than the original may be created.

SPECIFIC LOCAL FLAPS

Two examples of specific local pedal arterial flaps are the lateral calcaneal arterial flap and the dorsalis pedis flap. Both take advantage of specific arterial vessels to provide a flap that is more reliable and robust than a random-pattern flap. The lateral calcaneal artery skin flap was described by Grabb

and Argenta (72). According to cadaver and Doppler studies, the lateral calcaneal artery is a consistent vessel that usually arises from the peroneal artery as a terminal branch but may originate from the posterior tibial artery. The artery can be found 5 to 8 mm lateral to the Achilles tendon, posterior to the lateral malleolus. The artery then curves inferiorly along the peroneal tendons and courses distally to the base of the fifth metatarsal. Candidates for this flap should be evaluated with Doppler studies. If the presence of the dorsalis pedis or posterior tibial arteries is in question, an arteriogram should be performed. The flap has two versions, long and short. In both versions the base of the flap is approximately 4.5 cm wide, beginning at the level just above the lateral malleolus. The short version is approximately 8 cm long and courses along the lateral aspect of the calcaneus. This version is used for posterior heel defects. The long version is approximately 14 cm long and ends proximal to the base of the fifth metatarsal. Either flap may contain the sural nerve to provide a sensate flap, a particularly important consideration in contact areas such as the inferior and posterior aspects of the heel. The small saphenous vein may be transferred with the flap to assure adequate venous drainage.

The technique begins with an initial incision lateral to the Achilles tendon (Fig. 49.53). Dissection is carried distally and down to the level of the periosteum over the lateral side of the calcaneus. The anterior incision is then made close to the lateral malleolus, and the dissection is directed from distal to proximal, with gentle elevation of the flap and visualization of the neurovascular structures. After rotation of the flap, the donor site defect that has been created may be covered with a partial-thickness skin graft, either immediately or after a few days, to allow granulation tissue to grow over the periosteum. This provides a finer cosmetic result.

Before the distal end of the long version of the flap is divided, a fluorescein test should be performed. The flap is undermined and the distal end of the flap is gently clamped while the fluorescein test is performed. If the fluorescence continues to the distal extent of the flap, then the end may be divided. If the fluorescence does not extend to the tip of the flap, then the distal end must be divided in delayed stages, beginning 5 to 7 days after the initial surgery (72). Grabb and Argenta (72) report that this flap is useful in persons with diabetes.

Holmes and Rayner have described an island version of the flap, which can be moved to cover areas on the medial side of the ankle (73). Gang (74) described results of 11 island flaps averaging 4 cm in diameter, with the technique described by Holmes and Rayner. There were no failures due to necrosis. Two patients had abnormal sensations in the donor area, which improved after 4 to 6 months.

Argenta recommends splinting the foot in plantarflexion for some time in order to prevent pressure on the vascular pedicle during dorsiflexion (75). Yanai and associates noted that the disadvantages of the flap are skin depression at the donor site and disruption of the sural nerve (76). Horris and co-workers (77) also noted donor site complications in

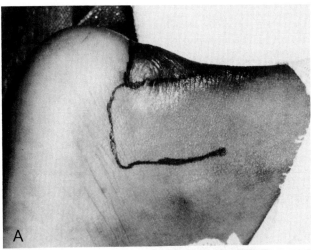

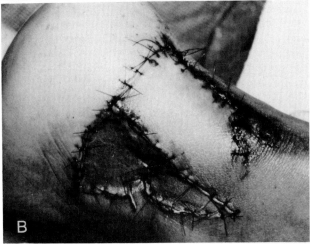

Figure 49.53. Lateral calcaneal artery flap used after the excision of a painful hypertrophic scar on the posterior heel. **A.** Outline of the flap and scar area to be excised. **B.** Flap rotated and sutured in place with split-thickness skin graft coverage of the donor site.

their series of seven patients with short versions of the lateral calcaneal artery flap (78). Each of their patients was able to return to closed shoes, which they previously had been unable to wear. The author's experience has been with young, healthy persons who had posterior heel defects (77).

Masquelet and associates have described a different laterally based flap, the lateral supramalleolar flap (79). The tissue is supplied by the perforating branch of the posterior peroneal artery. There are two versions of this flap. A rotation flap based on flow from the perforating branch of the peroneal artery may be used for coverage of wounds in the distal one-third of the leg. A second version of the flap is based on the retrograde flow from the anastomotic vascular circle at the sinus tarsi. This second version may be rotated for more distal coverage. In both versions the donor site is covered with a skin graft.

The arterialized dorsalis pedis flap may be used as either a local or a distant flap (80). The advantages include the thin and hairless skin, the large-caliber vessels, an available nerve supply, and the relatively low morbidity of the donor site. The flap is useful in the coverage of defects of the lower third of the leg, as well as the dorsum of the foot and the heel (81).

A 12 × 9 cm flap can be provided in an adult. The flap is outlined to be symmetrical with the dorsalis pedis. The dorsal venous arcade is included in the tissue (45). The flap is approached through the medial side, and the dorsalis pedis, dorsal first metatarsal, and plantar perforating arteries are isolated. The plantar perforating artery is ligated, and the flap is elevated. Sufficient vascular tissue is left over the dorsum of the foot to accept a split-thickness skin graft after the procedure.

Careful use of the dorsal vessels for an arterialized flap is based on precise knowledge of the anatomy of the area and potential anatomical variations (55, 82). Arteriography is often necessary for preoperative evaluation.

PERIOPERATIVE MANAGEMENT OF FLAPS

The two most important considerations for success are careful planning of the procedure, based on the blood supply of the flap, and use of a flap large enough for its intended function. A flap that is too small is subject to excessive tension and kinking that will result in failure. The surgeon who is unfamiliar with these techniques often designs the flap to be as small as possible, hoping that in case of failure, he or she will have minimized the disaster. Unfortunately, this defensive thinking results in a flap that must be stretched excessively to cover the defect. This tension creates vasospasm and ends with necrosis of the tissue.

The vascular status of the flap is of prime concern in the planning and execution of the surgery and during the postoperative care. Vascular status implies both arterial perfusion and venous drainage. Complications with the use of flaps usually stem from some form of circulatory embarrassment.

One of the most useful techniques is employment of a delay procedure whenever the vascular status of a flap is in question. A delay procedure involves sequentially dividing the blood supply to the tissue with incisions and undermining over several days. This reduces the area for vascular inflow in a gradual fashion, allowing the flap to adjust to the decrease in circulation. The adjustment occurs by means of an increase in the size and number of blood vessels in the flap, as well as reorientation of the vessels in the direction of the long axis of the flap. The mechanism for this effect is still unknown, although there is evidence that the main effect is vasodilation produced by a local sympathectomy and ischemic stimulation (47). The local sympathectomy in a delayed flap gradually produces a hypersensitivity to catecholamines, which contraindicates the use of epinephrine for this technique (83). The delay procedure may result in an increase in the surviving length of the random flap by 60% to 100% (47). Because local flaps in the foot and leg are often random (cutaneous) in their blood supply, the delay procedure may be particularly helpful.

The technical execution of the delay procedure for a rectangular transposition flap might involve creation of a bipedicle flap by making two parallel incisions and undermining between them. One week later the third incision is made, creating a single pedicle flap (one base) over a period of 2 or 3 days, or the flap is transferred after another few days (total time, 10 to 14 days). The benefits of the delay procedure are considerable in terms of increased circulation to the flap. These benefits must be weighed against the increased tissue reaction caused by elevation of a flap through undermining. Tissue reaction causes increased fibrosis, which can make transfer of the flap more difficult. Existing tissue planes should be used during the transfer to minimize tissue reaction.

There have been experimental attempts to duplicate the surgical delay phenomenon with pharmacological agents. The mechanism behind the technique is still controversial, but pharmacological delay has the potential to be useful as a means of achieving the delay phenomenon without the risks of infection, fibrosis, and hematoma associated with surgical delay.

PLANNING AND EXECUTION OF THE FLAP

Before planning the type of flap to be used, one must assess the defect. Size, shape, and location are important in determining the type of coverage. The condition of the surrounding skin is also important. Both the type of flap to be used and the actual execution of the flap need to be well planned in advance. Initially, one should determine whether the coverage will come from surrounding local tissue or from distant tissue. Because a local flap has to be greater in size than the defect it is designed to cover, the amount of surrounding healthy, pliable tissue will determine whether a local flap might be used. Once it has been decided that a local flap should be used, a rotation or transposition flap can be selected, depending on the given situation. There are numerous specific flaps that are designed for coverage of various geometrical shapes. The Limberg flap, for example, is designed to provide coverage of rhomboid defects without creating a secondary defect (84).

The planning of the actual transfer of the flap begins with the technique called "planning in reverse." A sterilizable, flexible material is cut to the shape of the flap. The pattern is then placed over the defect, and the steps are reversed from the actual transfer. This gives a more accurate picture of the amount of tissue required and indicates how best to design the flap. Eyeballing the flap saves time in the short run and risks disaster in the long run. It is better to err on the side of an excessively large flap rather than a small flap that would be placed under excessive tension. Frequently a small amount of tissue must be sacrificed to triangulate the recipient site defect for proper fit of the flap. The flap itself is usually divided at the natural tissue separation. In the lower extremity a natural tissue separation means separation at the junction between the superficial and deep fascia.

POSTOPERATIVE EVALUATION AND MANAGEMENT

There are a number of techniques available for monitoring the circulation in a flap (46). If a flap is failing, early recognition can permit appropriate surgical or medical management. A flap may also be assessed during its transfer. This may indicate to the surgeon that the flap would do better if delayed than if transferred immediately.

Many of the techniques that are available for monitoring the circulation in a flap have serious limitations. Clearance studies with radioactive isotopes are limited by the small area that they measure and because they may only be repeated, at the most, daily. Doppler studies can measure pulse flow, but not dermal circulation. Percutaneous pO_2 measurements have the advantage of being a noninvasive system for assessment. However, nitrous oxide and halothane appear to interfere with the instrumentation (85). Skin flap temperature may also be useful because it is noninvasive, inexpensive, and repeatable. Consistent results require temperature equilibrium for approximately 45 minutes, and this can be a serious limitation. Other tests of flap circulation include angiography, plethysmography, and intravenous fluorescein (86). The fluorescein test appears to be the most useful in terms of assessing the viability of the flap and is widely used for intraoperative assessment.

Fluorescein is a nontoxic dye that diffuses rapidly into the extracellular space after intravenous administration (87). Vascularized tissue will fluoresce yellow-green under ultraviolet light. Nonvascularized tissue will appear dark blue. Mottled areas are of questionable circulation and will usually have a superficial slough. The flap may have to be stroked for visualization of the fluorescence.

The drug fluorescein is excreted virtually unchanged through the kidneys within 24 hours (88). A dose of 15 mg/kg is usually sufficient (1 to 2 g), with darker-skinned individuals requiring a higher dosage range (89). Equilibration is allowed to occur for 10 to 20 minutes, and the flap is inspected under ultraviolet light. Quantification of the amount of fluorescence is possible for a more objective assessment (90, 91). Fluorescein is a relatively safe drug. One study found a 0.41% incidence of major reactions, consisting principally of hypotension (88).

COMPLICATIONS AND SALVAGE

Failure of a flap often creates a deficit that is larger than the original defect. The most frequent cause of flap failure or necrosis is vascular embarrassment. There are numerous potential reasons for this, including mechanical tension, kinking of the flap causing obstruction of flow, excessive edema or pressure, inflammation, infection, hematoma, or seroma.

Many times disaster can be avoided if the underlying cause of the necrosis is treated. Tension may be released by means of a back cut or Burow's triangle. This should be carried out within 4 hours of the onset of the tension to prevent necrosis. Skin grafting the flap donor site, rather than primarily repairing it, can also reduce tension.

Edema and excessive pressure from the dressing are detrimental factors that can be corrected by quick action. Hematoma must be evacuated promptly, although absolute intraoperative hemostasis is the best prevention. Infection may lead to disaster in a flap because of the flap's tenuous circulatory status. Kinking of the flap may be the result of a shearing force on the base of the flap. Proper positioning of the flap, combined with immobilization, can help prevent kinking.

Flap necrosis in a random-pattern flap is manifested by congested skin, cyanosis, and blistering. This is an acute process resulting in demarcation at a level where the vascular capacity is insufficient for both the ordinary metabolic load of the tissue and the adjoining necrosis of the failing portion of the flap. Necrosis in an axial-pattern flap may take several days to develop, and because of this it may result in a necrotic island in the middle of the flap as opposed to loss of the whole flap.

No treatment for flap necrosis is as effective as proper initial planning. Once necrosis has occurred, intervention must be rapid. Although the literature is replete with studies of various techniques to treat flap necrosis, most have not been clinically proven. Some suggested methods include cooling of the tissue to reduce metabolic demand, hyperbaric oxygen, closed suction drainage, leeches for the removal of venous congestion, postural assistance to venous return, and low-molecular-weight dextran. Infected necrotic tissue should be excised as it becomes apparent. The desperation measures just enumerated probably will do little to treat a progressing necrosis. Pharmacological manipulation has been reported with nitroglycerine (92), isoxuprine (93, 94), phenoxybenzamine (95), reserpine (95), propranolol (96), and heparin (96). Vasodilator drugs, such as isoxuprine, have generated the most interest because of their pharmacological delay effect.However, prostaglandin synthesis inhibitors have also been reported to be effective in increasing skin viability in animal studies (97). Mechanical barriers to desiccation, such as certain topical dressings, have been demonstrated to be effective for reducing the depth of skin loss in a failing flap (98).

More important (and effective) than treating flap necrosis is the prevention of necrosis. When designing the flap, one should allow for the increased tension that will be caused by normal edema. One should know the anatomy of the blood supply of the flap and not exceed its capacity. A delay procedure should be used whenever there is any question as to the blood supply. Prevention of hematoma with proper hemostasis and use of a closed suction drain and/or pressure dressing is of critical importance

WOUND COVERAGE IN PROBLEM AREAS

Certain areas of the foot and ankle are particularly troublesome when wound coverage is necessary. The heel, sole, and Achilles tendon are difficult areas for wound coverage because of the type of tissue required as well as the tissue that is available.

The heel is probably the most difficult area for wound coverage because of the weight-bearing forces that are directed through it. Heel defects may result from trauma, resection of tumors, neurotrophic ulcerations, ischemic ulcerations, and infection. The calcaneal heel pad is a highly specialized soft tissue structure that is essentially irreplaceable as a shock-absorbing structure. When defects of the heel pad are small (less than 50% of the heel pad), adjoining tissue may be mobilized or transferred for coverage with the identical tissue type (99). When defects are larger, other types of coverage must be considered, including skin grafts, local flaps, muscle flaps, and free neurovascular flaps. The type of coverage chosen will depend on the size and location of the defect, the cause of the defect, and the functional requirements of the patient.

Skin grafts are not the ideal coverage for deep defects of the heel pad. The graft does not provide significant padding and is usually not innervated. An exception to this is the technique described by Lister (100) for an innervated skin graft from the adjacent sural nerve dermatome. The technique involves microsurgical dissection to preserve the fine branches of the sural nerve. If a skin graft is to be used for coverage of a deep heel pad defect, a thick split-thickness skin graft or a full-thickness skin graft must be used.

Local flaps can be rotated from adjacent calcaneal heel padding if the defect is small. For larger defects, local flaps based on the calcaneal, medial plantar, or lateral plantar arteries can be rotated (101, 102). The long version of the lateral calcaneal artery flap can be used for coverage of plantar heel defects (72). An island flap created from the instep and based on vessels from the medial plantar artery has been suggested as a useful means of covering the heel with a durable tissue (103). This flap is raised between the plantar fascia and the first layer of plantar muscles. The skin overlying the lateral border of the foot should not be harvested because of its propensity to ulcerate when covered with a skin graft (104).

Muscle flaps can be quite useful for the coverage of heel defects because of their durability. Flexor digitorum brevis and abductor hallucis muscle flaps have been suggested (67, 68, 99, 105). These muscle flaps must be covered with a split-thickness skin graft. A musculocutaneous version of the flap has also been described (106, 107).

Larger, more complex defects of the heel may be treated with free composite tissue transfers. These have largely replaced cross-limb and thigh flaps, although these still have a place in the armamentarium of procedures used in this difficult area (108, 109).

The sole of the foot is an equally troublesome area for wound coverage. It is most important to determine whether the area to be covered is a weight-bearing area in this individual, a stressed area, or a recessed area. This will depend on the foot type, individual anatomical variations, and gait function. In weight-bearing or stressed areas, full-thickness skin grafts or flaps are most successful because of their mobility, sensation, and thickness (110).

Split-thickness skin grafts are most useful in recessed areas that are not subject to weight bearing or shearing stress. In some situations it is possible to take neurovascular flaps from recessed areas and use them to cover a weight-bearing defect (111, 112). Split-thickness grafts can then be used to cover the donor defect.

The Achilles tendon region also presents special problems for wound coverage. Skin loss in this area may result from trauma, postoperative slough, neurotrophic ulceration, burns, and pressure ulcerations from dressing or casts. The major difficulty with coverage in this region is encountered when the Achilles tendon is exposed. Allowing the area to granulate is a slow process that usually results in a painful hyperkeratotic scar. If the area is infected, the tendon may undergo necrosis because of exposure and the infective process.

If the tendon is covered with paratenon, a split-thickness skin graft may be used. More commonly bare tendon is exposed, and this requires flap coverage. In very severe injuries, composite free flaps may be used to cover the area. These have the disadvantages of excessive bulk, prolonged operating time, and technical difficulty. Cross-limb flaps or ipsilateral buttock flaps may also be used, although they require prolonged hospitalization and uncomfortable immobilization. Local flaps may be rotated for coverage either medially or laterally. Medially based flaps should be rotated after a double-delay procedure (113). The lateral calcaneal artery flap can be rotated without delay for posterior heel coverage and coverage of the lower 3 to 5 cm of the Achilles tendon (72). Regardless of the type of procedure that will be used, early coverage of this area is recommended to prevent further tissue loss, particularly with regard to tendon.

SKIN PLASTIES

Skin plasties consist of rearrangement or removal of skin to change the position of a part. Skin plasties in the digits and forefoot are valuable adjuncts to osseous surgical procedures. Some of the general purposes for skin plasties include: (a) skin lengthening (V-Y plasty, Z-plasty), (b) reduction of redundant skin after bone removal, (c) redirecting of old scars (Z-plasty), and (d) derotational skin plasties (e.g., repair of curly fourth toes).

Derotational Skin Plasties

Skin plasties can be particularly useful in digits where the deformity includes a rotational component. The two best examples of this situation are repair of congenital clinodactyly of the fourth toe (curly toe) and arthroplasty of the fifth toe when the toe is rotated in adducto varus. In rotated fifth toes one often sees lateral nail pathosis caused by weight-bearing pressure on the side of the toe (Fig. 49.54).

The primary guiding principle in derotation skin plasties is that the skin wedge must be placed perpendicular to the axis of rotation of the toe. Therefore the direction of the two semi-elliptical incisions must be carefully planned for each individual deformity. A skin scribe is helpful in designing the incisions. The skin wedge for a toe in which the

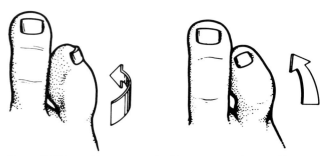

Figure 49.54. Adductovarus and adductus types of rotated fifth toes.

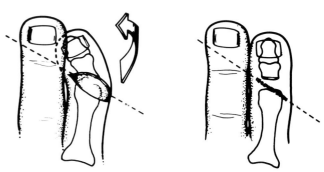

Figure 49.55. Placement of a skin wedge for clinodactyly repair in conjunction with hemi middle phalangectomy.

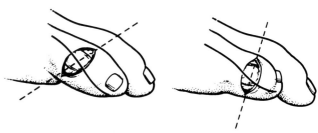

Figure 49.56. Two types of skin wedges that would be used in correction of adductovarus and adductus fifth toes. Note that after removal of the skin wedge, the neurovascular structures are still intact.

primary deformity is adductus will be quite different from a toe in which the deformity is adducto varus.

The second principle in using derotation skin plasties is that removal of the skin wedge is accomplished initially by dissection through the epidermis and dermis only. The superficial fascia is left intact. The incision is deepened through superficial fascia only when this is critical for exposure. This enhances preservation of neurovascular structures, a critical requirement in digital surgery. An example of this is clinodactyly repair. Two semi-elliptical incisions are made dorsally in a distal-medial to proximal-lateral direction. The wedge is placed over the portion of bone that is to be resected (Fig. 49.55).

For the fifth toe in adducto varus rotation, a skin plasty may be performed to derotate the toe. This incision is a modification of the "lazy S" approach. It provides exposure to the proximal, middle, and distal phalanges, as well as derotating the toe via a skin wedge (Fig. 49.56).

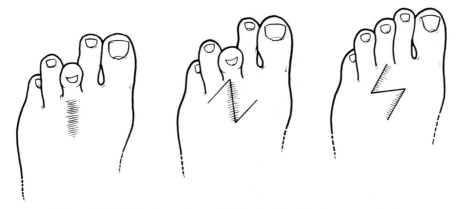

Figure 49.57.   Z-plasty may be used to "break up" and lengthen scar contracture.

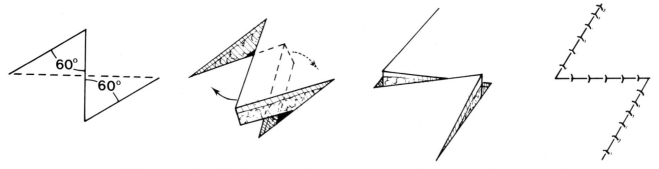

Figure 49.58.   Construction of the Z-plasty should be drawn on the skin before execution of the procedure. The procedure is based on the transposition of two flaps.

Figure 49.59.   Proper dissection at the flap tip prevents necrosis of the tip after Z-plasty. **A.** Proper technique. **B.** Sciving of the flap tip strips the skin of its blood supply.

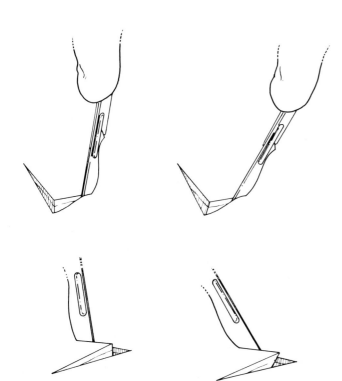

A   B

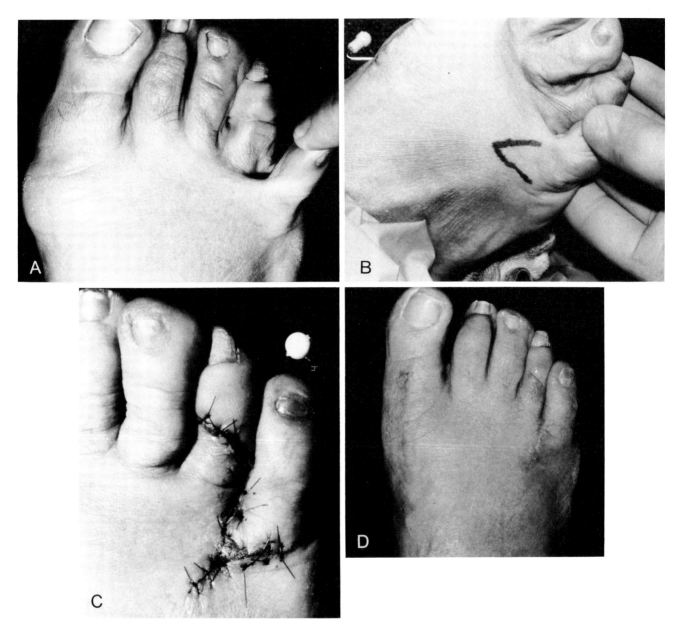

Figure 49.60. V-Y plasty technique used as part of overlapping fifth toe repair. **A.** Note the band of tight skin. **B.** V-incision diagram. **C.** Four days postoperatively (note skin wedge repair of fourth toe). **D.** Eight weeks postoperatively with excellent healing (hallux valgus repair has also been performed).

Z-Plasty

The Z-plasty is a very useful technique that consists of the transposition of two triangular flaps. This creates a lengthening effect in one axis and a shortening effect in a perpendicular axis (Fig. 49.57). The Z-plasty also creates a change in direction of the common limb of the Z. These two properties make the Z-plasty particularly useful in treating linear scar contractures.

Two factors are particularly important to consider when one is planning a Z-plasty (114-117). One is that the desired gain in length is created at the expense of transverse short-ening. In most areas of the body this does not present a problem. In the hand and foot, the skin is less mobile. The digits in particular have less room for transverse shortening than other areas of the body. One modification that helps circumvent these problems is the multiple Z-plasty. Instead of one large Z-plasty, multiple smaller Z-plasties are created. These may be continuous or separate. The multiple smaller Z-plasties summate to create a length increase equal to the large Z-plasty, with less total transverse shortening.

In addition to the problem of skin mobility, the foot is marked by transverse skin creases caused by the motion of underlying joints. If a Z-plasty is contemplated in such an area, it should be planned so that the transverse scar lies in the skin fold line.

The Z-plasty should be drawn on the skin before the procedure is performed. The arms of the Z should be equal, and the angle of the flap tips is usually 60° (Fig. 49.58). The flap tip angle must be at least 35° and preferably 60° to ensure a sufficient vascular base. The angle of the flap is important because it determines the ratio of the increase in length. An angle of 30° results in a 25% increase in length, whereas an angle of 60° results in a 75% increase in length. Increasing the angle beyond 60° results in increased length, but at the expense of increased transverse shortening. For this reason, 60° is generally considered to be the most efficient angle. In addition to angle size, limb length is another critical factor. The length of the limbs in the Z-plasty controls the actual increase in length; a larger Z increases the real length gain.

Proper preoperative planning can prevent most complications with the Z-plasty. However, necrosis of the tip can occur, particularly in thick scar tissue. Increasing the vascular supply and decreasing tension on the flaps can prevent tip necrosis (Fig. 49.59). Vascular supply can be maximized by keeping the flaps broad at the tip, maintaining thickness, and avoiding scar tissue across the base. Tension can be decreased with the use of multiple Z-plasties and with the part bandaged in midposition, not in maximal tension. Meticulous hemostasis is critical.

The Z-plasty is not a difficult procedure, but it does require meticulous planning. It is most useful where there is a thin linear scar contracture. It is also useful in other areas that require lengthening because it redistributes tension in the scar into different planes. This produces less chance of contracture or thick scarring.

V-Y And Y-V Plasties

The V-Y plasty is a popular technique for skin lengthening (Fig. 49.60). Its most desirable feature is that it allows some variability in the amount of length achieved. It is most appropriate in situations in which previous scar contracture is not a factor. The procedure begins with a V-shaped incision. The wider the angle of the V, the better the blood supply to the flat tip. In the foot the apex of the V should be proximal so that the V flap can be advanced distally. The skin is then advanced to the desired position, creating a Y-shaped incision. The entire V flap may be undermined beneath the superficial fascia for exposure purposes. When using the V-Y plasty in conjunction with digital surgery, one creates an initial Y-shaped incision. The V portion is located over the metatarsophalangeal joint with the stem of the Y over the toe itself. This provides excellent exposure for the surgery and allows for the desired lengthening.

An alternative lengthening procedure is the Y-V plasty (118) (Fig. 49.61). In this procedure a Y-shaped incision is made initially. Skin is advanced toward the stem of the Y, creating a V-shaped incision. Lengthening occurs perpendicular to the Y-V incisions, and shortening occurs in the

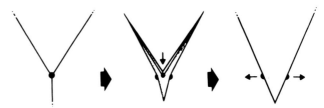

Figure 49.61. Diagram illustrating steps in Y-V plasty.

direction of the stem of the Y. As in other situations, the amount of lengthening that can be achieved depends on the mobility of the skin and the amount of shortening that can be tolerated by adjacent tissues.

Redundant Skin Plasties

Any time that bone is removed, redundant skin is created. This redundant skin is cosmetically unappealing and is sometimes a functional disadvantage. Hallux and lesser digit fusions often result in excessive soft tissue, particularly when the fusion is performed intentionally to shorten the digit.

In the hallux two semi-elliptical incisions are placed over the joint. The width of the skin wedge is designed to accommodate for the shortening that will occur after resection of the joint surfaces.

In the lesser digits this approach alone is often not possible because access is required to the extensor tendon, hood, and metatarsophalangeal joint capsule. In this case, a linear incision is placed over the dorsum of the toe, extending from the metatarsophalangeal joint to the proximal interphalangeal joint. Two transverse semi-elliptical incisions are then placed over the proximal-interphalangeal joint and a skin wedge is removed down to the superficial fascia. The dorsal neurovascular structures are reflected medially and laterally. This eliminates skin redundancy, and a superior cosmetic result is achieved.

SUMMARY

The study of plastic techniques and their application in the foot and leg is fascinating and complex. Particular concerns for weight-bearing and pressure areas make the foot a most challenging area for wound coverage. The diversity of options open to the surgeon should be clearly understood. Because of the individual nature of each wound and each patient, each situation must be examined carefully for the best solution.

References

1. Grabb WC: Basic techniques of plastic surgery. In Grabb WC, Smith JS (eds): *Plastic Surgery*, ed 3. Boston, Little Brown, 1979, pp 3-74.
2. Borges AF: *Elective Incisions and Scar Revision*. Boston, Little Brown, 1973, p 18.
3. Charnley J: Compression arthrodesis of the ankle and shoulder. *J Bone Joint Surg* 33B:180-191, 1951.
4. Dupuytren G: Traite des blessures par arnes de guerre. Paris, 1:66, 1834. Cited by Kraissl CJ: The selection of appropriate lines for elective surgical incisions. *Plast Reconstr Surg* 8:1-28, 1951.

5. Langer K: Ueber die Spaltbarkeit der Cutis, Sitzunopb. d., K. Akad. d. Wissensch. *Math-naturw Cl* 43:23, 1861. Cited by Kraissl C: The selection of appropriate lines for elective surgical incisions. *Plast Reconstr Surg* 8:1-28, 1951.

6. Kocher T: *Chirurgische Operationslehre*. 1892. Cited by Cox HT: The cleavage lines of the skin. *Br J Surg* 29:234-240, 1941.

7. Cox HT: The cleavage lines of the skin. *Br J Surg* 29:234-240, 1941.

8. Borges AF, Alexander JE: Relaxed skin tension lines, z-plasties on scars, and fusiform excision of lesions. *Br J Plast Surg* 15:242-254, 1962.

9. Gardner JH, Raybuck HE: Development of cleavage line patterns in the human fetus. *Clin Plast Surg* 4:187-190, 1977. Reprinted from *Anat Rec* 118:745-754, 1954.

10. Borges AF: Relaxed skin tension lines (RSTL) versus other skin lines. *Plast Reconstr Surg* 73:144-150, 1984.

11. Courtiss EH, Longacre JJ, De Stefano GA, Brizio L, Holmstrand K: The placement of elective skin incisions. *Plast Reconstr Surg* 31:31-44, 1963.

12. Curtin JW: Fibromatosis of the planter fascia. *J Bone Joint Surg* 47A:1605, 1965.

13. Burns AE, Harvey CK: Plantar fibromatosis: surgical considerations and a case report. *J Am Podiatry Assoc* 73:141-146, 1983.

14. Miller SJ: Surgical technique for resection of Morton's neuroma. *J Am Podiatry Assoc* 71:181-188, 1981.

15. Burns AE, Stewart WP: Morton's neuroma. *J Am Podiatry Assoc* 72:135-141, 1982.

16. Evans D: Calcaneo-valgus deformity. *J Bone Joint Surg* 57B:270-278, 1975.

17. Mahan K: Evans calcaneal osteotomy for flexible flatfoot. In McGlamry ED, McGlamry RC (eds): *Comprehensive Conference in Foot Surgery, Thirteenth Annual Seminar*. Atlanta, Doctors Hospital Podiatric Education and Research Institute, 1984, pp 34-36.

18. Fairclough JA, Mackie IG, Mintowt-Czyz W, Phillips GE: The contaminated skin-knife: a surgical myth. *J Bone Joint Surg* 65B:210, 1983.

19. Crawford AH: The Cincinnati incision: a comprehensive approach for surgical procedures of the foot and ankle in childhood. *J Bone Joint Surg* 64A: 1982.

20. Borges AF: Dog-ear repair. *Plast Reconstr Surg* 69:707-713, 1982.

21. Krizek JJ, Robson MC: Biology of surgical infection. *Surg Clin North Am* 55:1261-1267, 1975.

22. Krizek TJ, Robson MC, Kho E: Bacterial growth and skin graft survival. *Surgery Forum* 18:518, 1967.

23. McGregor I: *Fundamental Techniques of Plastic Surgery and Their Surgical Applications*, ed 7. New York, Churchill-Livingstone, 1980, pp 55-99.

24. Snell GD: The terminology of tissue transplantation. *Transplantation* 2:655-657, 1964.

25. Vistnes LM: Grafting of skin. *Surg Clin North Am* 57:939-959, 1977.

26. Rothstein AS: Skin grafting techniques. *J Am Podiatry Assoc* 73:79-85, 1983.

27. Turek D: Skin grafts of the lower extremity. *J Am Podiatry Assoc* 67:28-32, 1977.

28. Peacock EE Jr: *Wound Repair*, ed 3. Philadelphia, WB Saunders, 1984, pp 218-234.

29. Birdsell DC, Hein KS, Lindsay RL: The theoretically ideal donor site dressing. *Ann Plast Surg* 2:535-537, 1979.

30. Dinner MI, Peters CR, Sherer J: Use of a semi permeable polyurethane membrane as a dressing for split-skin graft donor sites. *Plast Reconstr Surg* 64:112-114, 1979.

31. Rovee DT, Korowsky CA, Labun J: Effect of local wound environment in epidermal healing. In Maibach HI, Rovee ET (eds): *Epidermal Wound Healing*. Chicago, Year Book, 1972, pp 159-181.

32. Waris T: Reinnervation of free skin autografts in the rat. *Scand J Plast Reconstr Surg* 12:85-93, 1978.

33. Matev IB: Tactile gnosis in free skin grafts in the hand. *Br J Plast Surg* 33:434-439, 1980.

34. Teh BT: Why do skin grafts fail? *Plast Reconstr Surg* 63:323-332, 1979.

35. Berenak J, Faulk WP: Clinical and immunological studies of human extra embryonic membranes in wound healing. In *International Symposium on Tissue Repair*. Walnut Creek, CA, Symposia Medicus, 1983, p 30.

36. Burke HB, Confer HE, Kutlick DA, Reister G, Vidt L: The use of porcine xenografts in treatment of chronic ulcerations. *J Am Podiatry Assoc* 69:345-350, 1979.

37. Culliton P, Kwasnik RE, Novicki D, Corbin P, Patton G, Collins W, Terleckyj B, Axler DA: The efficacy of porcine skin grafts for treating non-healing cutaneous ulcers. Part I. Clinical studies. *J Am Podiatry Assoc* 68:1-10, 1978.

38. McCarthy DJ, Axler DA: The efficacy of porcine skin grafts for treating non-healing cutaneous ulcers. Part II. Microanatomical studies. *J Am Podiatry Assoc* 68:86-95, 1978.

39. Axler DA, Terleckyj B, McCarthy DJ, Kwasnik RE, Novicki D, Culliton P: The efficacy of porcine skin grafts for treating non-healing cutaneous ulcers. Part III. Microbiologic studies. *J Am Podiatry Assoc* 68:141-150, 1978.

40. Eaglstein WH: Effects of dressings and topical agents on wound healing. In *International Symposium on Tissue Repair*. Walnut Creek, CA, Symposia Medicus, 1983, pp 58-59.

41. Burke JF: Clinical experience with a physiologically acceptable skin replacement. In *International Symposium on Tissue Repair*. Walnut Creek, CA, Symposia Medicus, 1983, p 55.

42. Gallico GG III, O'Connor NE, Compton CC, Kehinde O, Green H: Permanent coverage of large burn wounds with autologous cultured human epithelium. *N Engl J Med* 311:448-451, 1984.

43. O'Connor NE, Gallico GG, Compton CC, Green H: Cultured epithelia in grafting of burn wounds. In *International Symposium on Tissue Repair*. Walnut Creek, CA, Symposia Medicus, 1983, p 49.

44. Eisinger M: Use of epidermal cells grown in tissue culture for wound coverage. In *International Symposium on Tissue Repair*. Walnut Creek, CA, Symposia Medicus, 1983, p 52.

45. Lombardo M, Aquino J: Local flaps for resurfacing foot defects: a vascular perspective. *J Foot Surg* 21:302-304, 1982.

46. Daniel RK, Kerrigan CL: Skin flaps: an anatomical and hemodynamic approach. *Clin Plast Surg* 6:181-200, 1979.

47. Converse JM, McCarthy JG, Brauer RO, Ballantyne DL Jr: Transplantation of skin: grafts and flaps. In Converse J (ed): *Reconstructive Plastic Surgery*, ed 2, vol 1. Philadelphia, WB Saunders, 1977, p 152.

48. Epstein LJ: Cross-leg flaps in reconstruction of lower extremity injuries. *J Am Podiatry Assoc* 67:33-37, 1977.

49. Taylor GA, Hopson WLG: The cross-foot flap. *Plast Reconstr Surg* 55:677-681, 1975.

50. Daniel RK, May JW Jr: Free flaps: an overview. *Clin Orthop* 133:122-131, 1978.

51. Weiland AJ, Moore JR, Daniel KK: The efficacy of free tissue transfer in the treatment of osteomyelitis. *J Bone Joint Surg* 66A:181-193, 1984.

52. May JW Jr, Gallico GG III, Lukash FN: Microvascular transfer of free tissue for closure of bone wounds of the distal lower extremity. *N Engl J Med* 306:253-257, 1982.

53. Mathes SJ: The muscle flap for management of osteomyelitis (editorial). *N Engl J Med* 306:294-295, 1982.

54. Garrett JC, Buncke HJ, Brownstein ML: Free groin-flap transfer for skin defects associated with orthopaedic problems of the lower extremity. *J Bone Joint Surg* 60A:1055-1058, 1978.

55. Hendel PM, Buncke HJ: Another use for the first web space of the foot: neurovascular island flap. *Plast Reconstr Surg* 66:468-470, 1980.

56. Chaikhouni A, Dyas CL Jr, Robinson JH, Kelleher JC: Latissimus dorsi free myocutaneous flap. *J Trauma* 21:398-402, 1981.

57. Nahai F, Hill HL, Hester TR: Experiences with the tensor fascia lata flap. *Plast Reconstr Surg* 63:788-799, 1979.

58. Morrison WA, O'Brien BMcC, MacLeod A: Clinical experiences in free flap transfer. *Clin Orthop* 133:132-139, 1978.

59. Guba AM: The use of free vascular tissue transfers in lower extremity injuries. *Adv Orthop Surg* 7:60-68, 1983.

60. Iwaya T, Harii K, Yamada A: Microvascular free flaps for the treatment of avulsion injuries of the feet in children. *J Trauma* 22:15-19, 1982.

61. McCraw JB, Vasconez LO: Musculocutaneous flaps: principles. *Clin Plast Surg* 7:9-14, 1980.

62. Mathes SJ, Nahai F: Lower extremity: a systematic approach to flap selection. In Mathes SJ, Nahai F (eds): *Clinical Applications for Muscle and Musculocutaneous Flaps*. St Louis, CV Mosby, 1982, p 510.

63. Janecka IP: Lower extremity reconstruction using myocutaneous flaps. *Orthopaedics* 3:1097-1101, 1980.

64. Jackson IT, Scheker L: Muscle and myocutaneous flaps on the lower limb. *Injury* 13:324-330, 1982.

65. Solimbeni-Ughi G, Santoni-Rugiu P, de Vizia GP: The gastrocnemius myocutaneous flap (GMF): an alternative method to repair severe lesions of the leg. *Arch Orthop Trauma Surg* 98:195-200, 1981.

66. Arnold PG, Hodgkinson DJ: Extensor digitorum turn-down muscle flap. *Plast Reconstr Surg* 66:599-604, 1980.

67. Mathes SJ, Nahai F: Foot: a systematic approach to flap selection. In Mathes SJ, Nahai F (eds): *Clinical Applications for Muscle and Musculocutaneous Flaps.* St Louis, CV Mosby, 1982, p 585.

68. Nelson E, Scurran B, Tuerk D, Sihani S, Karlin J: Reconstruction of plantar heel defects: a review with case report. *J Am Podiatry Assoc* 73:235-239, 1983.

69. Scheflan M, Hanai F: Foot: reconstruction. In Mathes SJ, Nahai F (eds): *Clinical Applications for Muscle and Musculocutaneous Flaps.* St Louis, CV Mosby, 1982, p 594.

70. Ger R: Muscle transposition in the management of perforating ulcers of the forefoot. *Clin Orthop* 175:186-189, 1983.

71. Vasconez LO, McCraw JB, Hall EJ: Complications of musculocutaneous flaps. *Clin Plast Surg* 7:123-132, 1980.

72. Grabb WC, Argenta LC: The lateral calcaneal artery skin flap (the lateral calcaneal artery, lesser saphenous vein, and sural nerve skin flap). *Plast Reconstr Surg* 68:723-730, 1981.

73. Holmes J, Rayner CRW: Lateral calcaneal artery island flaps. *Br J Plast Surg* 37:402, 1984.

74. Gang R: Reconstruction of soft-tissue defect of the posterior heel with a lateral calcaneal artery island flap. *Plast Reconstr Surg* 79:415-421, 1987.

75. Argenta LC: Discussion: Reconstruction of soft-tissue defect of the posterior heel with a lateral calcaneal artery island flap. *Plast Reconstr Surg* 79:420-421, 1987.

76. Yanai A, Park S, Iwao T, Nakamura N: Reconstruction of a skin defect of the posterior heel by a lateral calcaneal flap. *Plast Reconstr Surg* 75:642-646, 1985.

77. Horris S, Hofman A, Van der Meulen J: Experiences with the lateral calcaneal artery flap. *Ann Plast Surg* 21:532-535, 1988.

78. Mahan KT: Lateral calcaneal artery skin flap for posterior heel coverage. *Clin Podiatr Med Surg* 3:277-287, 1986.

79. Masquelet A, Beveridge J, Romana C, Gerber C: The lateral supramalleolar flap. *Plast Reconstr Surg* 81:74-81, 1988.

80. Ohtsuka H, Shioya N, Hoshi E, Ogino Y: A free dorsalis pedis flap from the other foot combined with a dorsalis pedis pedicle flap from the same foot to close foot ulcers. *Br J Plast Surg* 32:3-8, 1979.

81. Krag C, Riegels-Nielsen P: The dorsalis pedis flap for lower leg reconstruction. *Acta Orthop Scand* 53:487-493, 1982.

82. Man D, Acland RD: The microarterial anatomy of the dorsalis pedis flap and its clinical applications. *Plast Reconstr Surg* 65:419-423, 1980.

83. Wu G, Calamel PM, Shedd DP: The hazards of injecting local anesthetic solutions with epinephrine into flaps. *Plast Reconstr Surg* 62:396-403, 1978.

84. Borges AF: Choosing the correct Limberg flap. *Plast Reconstr Surg* 62:542-545, 1978.

85. Harrison DH, Girling M, Mott G: Experience in monitoring the circulation in free-flap transfers. *Plast Reconstr Surg* 68:543-553, 1981.

86. Prather A, Blackburn JP, Williams TR, Lynn JA: Evaluation of tests for predicting the viability of axial pattern skin flaps in the pig. *Plast Reconstr Surg* 63:250-257, 1979.

87. Thorvaldsson SE, Grabb WC: The intravenous fluorescein test as a measure of skin flap viability. *Plast Reconstr Surg* 53:576-578, 1974.

88. Zahr KA, Sherman JE, Chaglassian T, Lane JM: Prediction of skin viability following en bloc resection for osteogenic sarcoma with fluorescein. *Clin Orthop* 180:287-290, 1983.

89. Singer R, Lewis CM, Franklin JD, Lynch JB: Fluorescein test for prediction of flap viability during breast reconstructions. *Plast Reconstr Surg* 61:371-375, 1978.

90. Graham BH, Walton RL, Elings VB, Lewis FR: Surface quantification of injected fluorescein as a predictor of flap viability. *Plast Reconstr Surg* 71:826-831, 1983.

91. Sasaki GH: Discussion: surface quantification of injected fluorescein as a predictor of flap viability. *Plast Reconstr Surg* 71:832-833, 1983.

92. Rohrich RJ, Cherry GW, Spira M: Enhancement of skin-flap survival using nitroglycerine ointment. *Plast Reconstr Surg* 73:943-948, 1984.

93. Finseth F, Adelberg MG: Experimental work with isoxuprine for prevention of skin flap necrosis and for treatment of the failing flap. *Plast Reconstr Surg* 63:94-100, 1979.

94. Finseth F: Clinical salvage of three failing skin flaps by treatment with a vasodilator drug. *Plast Reconstr Surg* 63:304-308, 1979.

95. Kerrigan CL, Daniel RK: Pharmacologic treatment of the failing skin flap. *Plast Reconstr Surg* 70:541-548, 1982.

96. Wray RC, Young VL: Drug treatment and flap survival. *Plast Reconstr Surg* 73:939-942, 1984.

97. Sasaki GH, Pang CY: Experimental evidence for involvement of prostaglandins in viability of acute skin flaps: effects on viability of mode of action. *Plast Reconstr Surg* 67:335-340, 1981.

98. McGrath MH: How topical dressings salvage "questionable" flaps: experimental study. *Plast Reconstr Surg* 67:653-659, 1981.

99. Scherlan M, Nahai F, Hartrampf CR: Surgical management of heel ulcers—a comprehensive approach. *Ann Plast Surg* 7:385-406, 1981.

100. Lister GD: Use of an innervated skin graft to provide sensation to the reconstructed heel. *Plast Reconstr Surg* 62:157-161, 1978.

101. Reiffel RS, McCarthy JG: Coverage of heel and sole defects: a new subfascial arterialized flap. *Plast Reconstr Surg* 66:250-260, 1980.

102. Jurkiewicz MJ: Discussion: coverage of heel and sole defects: a new subfascial arterilized flap. *Plast Reconstr Surg* 66:261-263, 1980.

103. Morrison WA, Crabb D McK, O'Brien B McC, Jenkins A: The instep of the foot as a fasciocutaneous island and as a free flap for heel defects. *Plast Reconstr Surg* 72:56-63, 1983.

104. Harrison DH, Morgan BDG: The instep island flap to resurface plantar defects. *Br J Plast Surg* 34:315-318, 1981.

105. Hartrampf CR, Schflan M, Bostwick J III: The flexor digitorum brevis muscle island pedicle flap: a new dimension in heel reconstruction. *Plast Reconstr Surg* 66:264-270, 1980.

106. Ikuta Y, Murakami T, Yoshioka K, Tsuge K: Reconstruction of the heel pad by flexor digitorum brevis musculocutaneous flap transfer. *Plast Reconstr Surg* 74:86-94, 1984.

107. Hartrampf CR Jr: Discussion: reconstruction of the heel pad by flexor digitorum brevis musculocutaneous flap transfer. *Plast Reconstr Surg* 74:95-96, 1984.

108. Irons G, Verheyden C, Peterson H: Experience with the ipsilateral thigh flap for closure of heel defects in children. *Plast Reconstr Surg* 70:562-567, 1982.

109. Shubailat M, Ajluni N, Kuresh B: Reconstruction of heel with ipsilateral tensor fascia lata myocutaneous flap. *Ann Plast Surg* 4:323-325, 1980.

110. Sommerlad BC, McGrouther DA: Resurfacing the sole: long-term follow-up and comparison of techniques. *Br J Plast Surg* 31:107-116, 1978.

111. Colen LB, Buncke HJ: Neurovascular island flaps from the plantar vessels and nerves for foot reconstruction. *Ann Plast Surg* 4:327-332, 1980.

112. Riegels-Nielsen P, Krag C: A neurovascular flap for coverage of distal plantar defects. *Acta Orthop Scand* 53:495-498, 1982.

113. DeMars RV, Graham WP III, Davis TS, Blomain EW: Wound coverage in the Achilles region. *Am J Surg* 144:376-378, 1982.

114. McGregor IA: The z-plasty. *Br J Plast Surg* 19:82-87, 1966.

115. McGregor IA: The z-plasty in hand surgery. *J Bone Joint Surg* 49B:448-457, 1967.

116. Cangialosi CP: Z-plasty skin lengthening: an adjunct to hammer toe correction. *Curr Podiatry* 30:13-15, 1981.

117. Longacre JJ, Berry HK, Basom CR, Townsend SF: The effects of Z plasty on hypertrophic scars. *Scand J Plast Reconstr Surg* 10:113-128, 1976.

118. Shaw DT, Li CS: Multiple Y-V plasty. *Ann Plast Surg* 2:436-440, 1979.

Additional References

Arnold PG, Irons GB: Lower extremity muscle flaps. *Orthop Clin North Am* 15:441-449, 1984.

Baker G, Newton E, Franklin J: Fasciocutaneous island flap based on the medial plantar artery: Clinical applications for leg ankle and foot. *Plast Reconstr Surg* 85:47-58, 1990.

Branch JD, Brownstein ML, Szabo Z: Microscopic surgery of the foot and lower leg: an introduction. *J Foot Surg* 20:3-13, 1981.

Byrd HS, Cierny G III, Tebbetts JB: The management of open tibial fractures with associated soft-tissue loss: external pin fixation with early flap coverage. *Plast Reconstr Surg* 68:73-79, 1981.

Cannon B, Constable JD, Furlow LT, Hayhurst JW, McCarthy JG, McCraw JB. Reconstructive surgery of the lower extremity. In Converse J (ed): *Reconstructive Plastic Surgery*, ed 2, vol 7. Philadelphia, WB Saunders, 1977, p 3521.

Cohen L, Replogle S, Mathes S: The V-Y plantar flap for reconstruction of the forefoot. *Plast Reconstr Surg* 81:220-227, 1988.

Crocker A, Moss A: The extensor hallucis brevis muscle flap. *J Bone Joint Surg* 71B:532, 1989.

Gibson T, Kenedi RM: Biomechanical properties of skin. *Surg Clin North Am* 47:279-294, 1967.

Davenport M, Daly J, Harvey I, Griffiths R: The bolus tie-over "pressure" dressing in the management of full thickness skin grafts. Is it necessary. *Br J Plast Surg* 41:28-32, 1988.

Fleetwood J, Barrett S, Day S: Skin flaps: the Burow advancement flap for closure of plantar defects. *J Am Podiatr Med Assoc* 77:246-249, 1987.

Giordano P, Argensen C, Pequignot, JP. Extensor digitorum brevis as an island flap in the reconstruction of soft-tissue defects in the lower limb. *Plast Reconstr Surg* 83:100-109, 1989.

Hallock G: Free-flap coverage of the exposed Achilles tendon. *Plast Reconstr Surg* 83:710-716, 1989.

Harashina T: Analysis of 200 free flaps. *Br J Plast Surg* 41:33-36. 1988.

Harii K: Microvascular surgery and its clinical applications. *Clin Orthop* 133:95-105, 1978.

Harrison DH: Discussion: the instep of the foot as a fasciocutaneous island and as a free flap for heel defects. *Plast Reconstr Surg* 72:64-65, 1983.

Hedley AK: Discussion: the management of open tibial fractures with associated soft-tissue loss: external pin fixation with early flap coverage. *Plast Reconstr Surg* 68:80-82, 1981.

Hinderer UT: Prevention of unsatisfactory scarring. *Clin Plast Surg* 4:199-206, 1977.

Ishikawa K, Isshiki N, Suzuki S, Shimamura S: Distally based dorsalis pedis island flap for coverage of the distal portion of the foot. *Br J Plast Surg* 40:521-525, 1987.

Jacobs HB: Skin knife-deep knife: the ritual and practice of skin incisions. *Am Surg* 179:102-104, 1974.

Kischer CW, Shetlar MR, Shetlar CL, Chvapil M: Immunoglobulins in hypertrophic scars and keloids. *Plast Reconstr Surg* 71:821-825, 1983.

Kumagai N, Nishina H, Tanabe H, Hosaka T, Ishida H, Ogino Y: Clinical application of autoLogous cultured epithelia for the treatment of burn wounds and burn scars. *Plast Reconstr Surg* 82:99-110, 1988.

Landi A, Soragni O, Monteleone M: The extensor digitorum brevis muscle island flap for soft-tissue loss around the ankle. *Plast Reconstr Surg* 75:892-897, 1985.

Leitner D, Gordon L, Buncke H: The extensor digitorum brevis as a muscle island flap. *Plast Reconstr Surg* 76:777-780, 1985.

Linares HA: Measurement of collagen-proteoglycan interaction in hypertrophic scars. *Plast Reconstr Surg* 71:818-820, 1983.

Locke RK, Frykberg RG: An effective surgical technique in the treatment and prevention of intractable plantar scars. *J Am Podiatry Assoc* 67:70-78, 1977.

Macht SD, Frazier WH: The role of endogenous bacterial flora in skin flap survival. *Plast Reconstr Surg* 65:50-55, 1980.

Marcinko D, Tursi F: Pedal burn contractures. *J Am Podiatr Med Assoc* 78:396-398, 1988.

Maxwell GP, Hoopes JE: Management of compound injuries of the lower extremity. *Plast Reconstr Surg* 63:176-185, 1979.

Massin P, Romana O, Masquelet, A: Anatomic basis of a pedicled extensor digitorum brevis muscle flap. *Surg Radiol Anat* 10:267-272, 1988.

Maruyama Y, Iwahira Y, Ebihara H: V-Y advancement flaps in the reconstruction of skin defects of the posterior heel and ankle. *Plast Reconstr Surg* 85:759-763, 1990.

Masquelet A, Romana M: The medialis pedis flap: a new fasciocutaneous flap. *Plast Reconstr Surg* 85:765-771, 1990.

McGraw JB: Selection of alternative local flaps in the leg and foot. *Clin Plast Surg* 6:227-246, 1979.

McLean N, Ellis H: Does remote sepsis influence the patency of microvascular anastomoses *Br J Plast Surg* 41:395-398, 1988.

Miller WE: Operative incisions involving the foot. *Orthop Clin North Am* 7:785-793, 1976.

Millikan LE: Skin anatomy in wound healing. *Osteopathic Annals* 10:148-155, 1982.

Morian WD: Soft-tissue reconstruction of below-knee defects. *Am J Surg* 139:495-501, 1980.

Mouzas GL: Conservative treatment of traumatic avulsion of tissue of fingers and toes. *Br J Clin Pract* 36:276-279, 1982.

Nanchahal J: Stretching skin to the limit: a novel technique for split skin graft expansion. *Br J Plast Surg* 42:88-91, 1989.

Pensler J, Steward R, Lewis S, Herndon D: Reconstruction of the burned palm: full-thickness versus split-thickness skin grafts —long term follow-up. *Plast Reconstr Surg* 81:16 19, 1988.

Riegels-Nielsen P, Krag C, Medgyesi S, Pers M: The repair of soft tissue defects in the lower leg. *Acta Orthop Scand* 54:772-776, 1983.

Robinson DW: Simple revision of scars. *Clin Plast Surg* 4:217-222, 1977.

Roggendorf E: The oblong parallelogram-shaped "schwenklappen"-plasty. *Plast Reconstr Surg* 65:635-655, 1980.

Scurran BL: Plantar approaches to foot surgery. *J Am Podiatry Assoc* 67:66-69, 1977.

Serafin D, Sabatier RE, Morris RL, Georgiade NG: Reconstruction of the lower extremity with vascularized composite tissue: improved tissue survival and specific indications. *Plast Reconstr Surg* 66:230-241, 1980.

Shah A, Pandit S: Reconstruction of the heel with chronic ulceration with flexor digitorum brevis myocutaneous flap. *Lepr Rev* 56:41-48, 1985.

Shapiro GD, Brownstein M, Coulter KR, Woodcox LH: A nondiabetic neurotrophic ulcer of the heel. *J Foot Surg* 21:285-291, 1982.

Smith DJ Jr, Loewenstein PW, Bennett JE: Surgical options in the repair of lower-extremity soft-tissue wounds. *J Trauma* 22:374-381, 1982.

Topol BM, Lewis VL Jr, Benveniste K: The use of antihistamine to retard the growth of fibroblasts derived from human skin, scar, and keloid. *Plast Reconstr Surg* 68:227-230, 1981.

Tring FC: Microtopography of the skin and scar formation. *J Dermatol Surg Oncol* 2:403-405, 1976.

Tsur H, Daniller A, Stravch B: Neovascularization of skin flaps: route and timing. *Plast Reconstr Surg* 66:85-93, 1980.

Vasconez LO, Bostwick J III, McCraw J: Coverage of exposed bone by muscle transposition and skin grafting. *Plast Reconstr Surg* 53:526-530, 1974.

Vidas MC, Weisman RA, Silverman OG: Serial fluorometric assessment of experimental neurovascular island flaps. *Arch Otolaryngol* 109:457-462, 1983.

Wiseman GG: Multiple recurring plantar fibromatosis and its surgical excision. *J Foot Surg* 22:121-125, 1983.

Wei F-C, Chen H-C, Chuang C-C, Noordhoff M: Reconstruction of Achilles tendon and calcaneus defects with skin-aponeurosis-bone composite free tissue from the groin region. *Plast Reconstr Surg* 81:579-587, 1988.

Welch JD: The photography of fluorescein. *Plast Reconstr Surg* 69:990-994, 1982.

Yoshimura M, Shimada T, Matsuda M, Itosokawa M, Imura S: Treatment of chronic osteomyelitis of the leg by peroneal myocutaneous island flap transfer. *J Bone Joint Surg* 71B:593-596, 1989.

Yoshimura Y, Nakajima T, Kami T: Distally based abductor digiti minimi muscle flap. *Ann Plast Surg* 14:375-377, 1985.

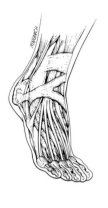

CHAPTER **50**

Principles of Muscle-Tendon Surgery and Tendon Transfers

Stephen J. Miller, D.P.M.

> One of man's greatest attributes is his ability to move. Purposeful active movement is dependent on many factors, but primarily on the ability of a myocyte to contract and thereby reduce its length. This motion is transmitted to the skeleton through a collection of longitudinally oriented collagen fibers: a tendon.
>
> —*Lawrence N. Hurst* (1)

Enhanced understanding of the biomechanics of foot function and the pathomechanics of abnormal foot structure have led to the effective use of muscle tendon transfers by the foot and leg surgeon. The goal of these procedures is to improve foot function through selective motor redistribution, with or without associated tarsal stabilization. As stated by Hackenbroch, "Tendon transplantation produces some benefits, redirects the powers, and is conservative in maintaining function as well as form. It does not create a new source of movement, but it utilizes efficiently the available power by eliminating less important motions and directing it to better advantage" (2). Tendon transfer is best applied in flexible deformities in which there is a dynamic muscular imbalance, such as in the conditions listed in Table 50.1.

The clinical foundations for various types of tendon transfers were developed largely in Germany and then further evolved in America (2-4) (Table 50.2). The first recorded tendon transfer was that of a peroneus longus muscle by Nicoladoni in Vienna on April 15, 1881. Ten years later intense interest developed in this area, pioneered by the German authors Lange, Biesalski, Vulpius, and Stoffel. However, Mayer stands out as the anatomical, literary, and clinical father of the modern concepts of tendon transfer (3, 5-10). Bernstein (11, 12), Steindler (13, 14), Ober (15), and Bunnell (16-19) in the United States added much to Mayer's work.

Development of major tendon transfer work in the podiatric community was first published by McGlamry and associates (20) in 1973. They reported modifying the split

Table 50.1.
Some Applications for Tendon Transfer

Postpoliomyelitis
Leprosy
Duchenne muscular dystrophy
Charcot-Marie-Tooth disease
Cerebral palsy
Discogenic disease
Sciatic nerve palsy
Common peroneal nerve palsy
Drop foot
Dorsal bunions
Recurrent clubfoot
Flexible flatfoot
Forefoot equinus
Hallus valgus
Hallus varus
Flexible hammer toes
Ankle stabilizations

Table 50.2.
Early Pioneers of Tendon Transfers

Nicoladoni	1882	Vienna
Drobnik	1892	Germany
Parrish	1892	New York
Milliken	1895	New York
Goldthwait	1895	Boston
Bradford	1897	Boston
Vulpius	1898	Heidelberg
Codavilla	1899	Italy
Lange	1902	Germany
Hoffa	1904	Germany
Jones	1908	England
Biesalski	1910	Germany
Mayer and Biesalski	1913	Germany
Vulpius and Stoffel	1913	Heidelberg/Mannheim
Mayer	1916	New York
Steindler	1918	Iowa
Bernstein	1919	Chicago
Bunnell	1921	Baltimore
Ober	1933	Boston

tibialis anterior tendon transfer (21), Young's tendosuspension (22, 23) for weak foot, and Jones's metatarsal suspension (24). Principles of tendon surgery were then incorporated into the treatment of the equinus foot by McGlamry and associates (25, 26). Sgarlato (27) presented the flexor tendon transfer for hammer toes in 1970.

The redistribution of the torque forces about the foot and ankle requires the application of specific principles based on an accurate knowledge and understanding of the anatomy, physiology, and mechanics of the musculotendinous structures involved. The foundation includes a knowledge of tissue histology, support structures, circulation, healing processes, and biomechanics that affect tendon function.

DEFINITIONS

Tendon Transfer

The detachment of a tendon of a functioning muscle at its insertion and then its relocation to a new insertion or attachment constitute a tendon transfer (28).

Tendon Transposition

The rerouting of the course of a normal muscle tendon without detachment to assist other functions is a tendon transposition (29). It is sometimes known as a *tendon translocation* (28). However, translocation refers more to the rerouting of a tendon, whether detached or not detached.

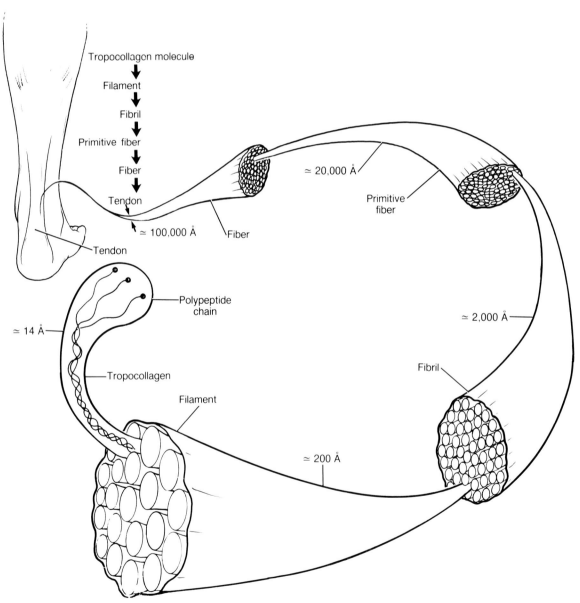

Figure 50.1. Schematic diagram: organization of components of collagen fiber, many of which make up tendon. (From Bryant WM, Greenwell JE, Weeks PM: Collagen organization during dilatation of cervix uteri. *Surg Gynecol Obstet* 126:27, 1968.)

Muscle-Tendon Transplantation

The detachment of a muscle tendon at both its origin and its insertion and moving it to a new location along with its neurovascular support structures constitute a muscle-tendon transplantation (28).

Tendon Suspension

Also known as tenosuspension, tendon suspension refers to those tendon procedures designed to support a structure (e.g., Young tenosuspension, Jones tenosuspension).

ANATOMY AND PHYSIOLOGY

Anatomical Considerations

DEFINITION AND DESCRIPTION

Tendons are integral parts of muscles, providing their connections to bone and transmitting their forces to provide movement. In essence they are smooth, cordlike, flat or round structures composed of parallel fibers that allow flexibility yet maintain great tensile strength (anisotropism). Their flexibility enables them to be angulated around bone surfaces or deflected beneath retinacula. Their inelasticity helps resist or transmit linear forces to develop torque about joint axes.

A tendon is composed largely of collagenous bundles lying parallel to each other and along the course of the tendon interposed with a few specialized fibroblasts (tenocytes) lying between the fibers. Construction begins with the basic *tropocollagen* molecules that are also oriented parallel to each other and are laid down in such a manner that each molecule overlaps the adjacent ones by 10% to 25% of its length. The tropocollagen subunits then polymerize to form collagen *filaments* that have a characteristic banding seen in the light microscope at 640 angstroms (Å). These filaments aggregate into *fibrils* of about 2000 Å in diameter, which in turn accumulate to make up the basic collagen *fiber* found in skin and connective tissue (Fig. 50.1).

Collagen fibers are condensed into *fasciculi* and surrounded by *endotenon,* a loose and relatively acellular tissue carrying blood vessels. The fascicule then combine to form the tendon that is surrounded by the *epitenon,* a one to two cell fibroblastic and synovial layer found on the surface of most tendons and closely related to the endotenon septa. The epitenon covering the tendon is sometimes referred to as the visceral layer, and it moves with the tendon (Fig. 50.2).

STRAIGHT COURSE

The supporting or surrounding tissue of a tendon varies, depending on whether the tendon has a straight pull or must travel around a corner. Along its straight course a tendon is surrounded by a loose elastic areolar tissue known as the *paratenon.* This areolar tissue is continuous with the epitenon and perimysium, as well as the coverings of the nerves and blood vessels that it carries to the tendon. The

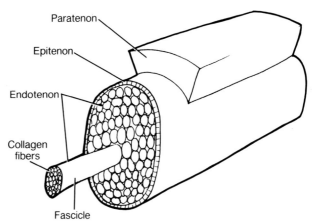

Figure 50.2.   Tendon anatomy showing various bundles and their coverings. (From Hurst LN: The healing of tendon. In Kernahan DA, Vistnes LM [eds]: *Biological Aspects of Reconstructive Surgery.* New York, Little, Brown & Co, 1977, p 384.)

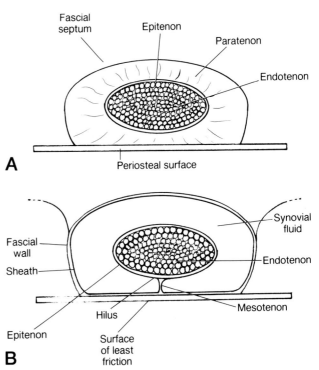

Figure 50.3.   **A.** Tendon with paratenon shown in cross-section. **B.** Tendon with sheath shown in cross-section.

supporting tissue fills the fascial space in which the tendon passes, and its elasticity enables the paratenon safely to stretch several centimeters with tendon movement. Together the epitenon and paratenon are called the *mesotenon* (Fig. 50.3).

ANGLED COURSE

Where a tendon rounds past a corner, changes direction, or passes under ligamentous structures, it is surrounded by a *tendon sheath*, through which the tendon is prevented from bowstringing across a joint. The tendon sheath is a tubular structure lined for the most part with synovial cells and within which the tendon glides back and forth much like a piston within a cylinder. Similar to the peritoneum it consists of two layers: the epitenon corresponding to the visceral layer and the inner side of the sheath corresponding to the parietal layer. Just as the intestinal mesentery is formed, these two layers reflect on themselves to form the *mesotenon*, a thin, delicate elastic membrane that will stretch several centimeters and that carries the tortuous blood and lymphatic vessels to the tendon. The point at which it is attached to the epitenon of the tendon is termed the *hilus*. The mesotenon is always located on the longitudinally convex side of the tendon where there is the least friction, and it is continuous with the areolar tissue surrounding the tendon proximal and distal to the sheath (Fig. 50.4). At those locations on either end of the sheath the connective tissue covering is doubled on itself to form invaginating folds known as *plicae*. These plicae provide for free pistoning motion of the tendon, stretching or folding in accordance with the tendon pull, thus protecting the vital mesotenon from excessive tension.

GLIDING MECHANISM

The gliding mechanism of the tendon is therefore dependent on these delicate tissues that contain the life support structures. In a straight course the paratenon assumes such responsibility, whereas around corners the mesotenon assisted by the plicae will allow liberal to-and-fro motion. The width of the mesotenon determines the degree of motion allowable between tendon and bone. These fine stretchable tissue coverings must be carefully preserved and repaired as necessary during surgery if one is to avoid tendon adhesions.

When the tendon sheath is absent, the tendon and overlying paratenon are enveloped in fatty areolar tissue. On the other hand, in some situations there is no mesotenon accompanying the tendon within the tendon sheath. Mayer (4) found this to be the case with the tendon of the tibialis posterior 100% of the time, the flexor hallucis longus 70% of the time, and the flexor digitorum longus in 50% of the specimens. To avoid confusion the term *peritenon* refers to all the connective tissue structures associated with the tendon, including the paratenon, mesotenon, epitenon, and endotenon (Fig. 50.5).

TENDON CIRCULATION

A tendon receives its blood supply via three sources: *(a)* a small part comes from the central blood vessels originating in the muscle belly; *(b)* some is derived from vessels of the bone and periosteum near the point of insertion of the tendon; *(c)* but the majority of the blood supply comes from the small vessels running in the paratenon or through the mesotenon, entering by the way of the hilus. These vessels then travel longitudinally in the epitenon and branch out,

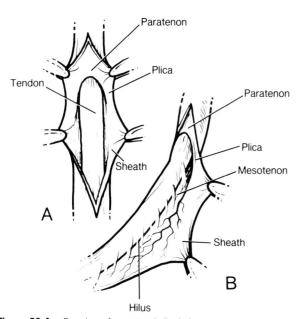

Figure 50.4. Drawing of extensor hallucis longus tendon to show relationship of paratenon, mesotenon, and sheath to tendon itself. **A.** Anteroposterior view. **B.** Lateral view. (From Bernstein MA: The surgery of tendon transposition with special reference to the importance of the tendon sheath. *Surg Gynecol Obstet* 29:55, 1919.)

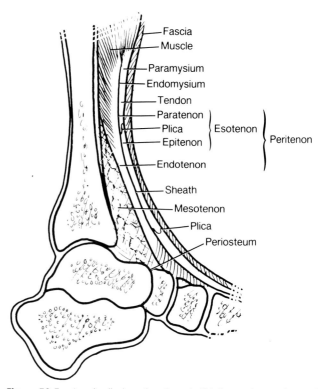

Figure 50.5. Longitudinal section through tibialis anterior tendon and surrounding structures. (From Mayer L: The physiologic method of tendon transplantation. I. Historical; anatomy and physiology of tendons. *Surg Gynecol Obstet* 22:182-197, 1916.)

anastomosing freely, also to penetrate the endotenon where they supply the fasciculi of tendon (Fig. 50.6). Where the mesotenon is absent within a tendon sheath, the blood is carried to the tendon through the elastic membranous tissue called *vincula,* another term for plicae, at each pole of the sheath (4, 12). Tendons also receive nutrition from local lymphatic and synovial fluid because between these major sources of blood supply are zones of apparent avascularity (1). Studies suggest that the synovial fluid diffusion can provide nutrition at least equal to that of the vincula vessels (30, 31).

ATTACHMENT TO BONE

Tendon insertion to bone must both transmit and disperse enormous stresses that are applied through the corresponding muscle. Force is dispersed first by the relatively expansive nature of the tendon at its insertion. The actual attachment to bone then transmits stress by means of a gradual tissue transition from tendon collagen fibers to fibrocartilage, which becomes calcified and organized into bone (32-34). The term *Sharpey's fibers* is not exactly correct because this is not the structure of attachment that Sharpey first observed (33, 35).

Tendon Healing

PROCESS

The goal of tendon healing is to produce an anastomosis of great tensile strength while providing unrestricted gliding function (36).

Research has shown that the epitenon is the most proliferative structure in the tendon repair process. After a short delay period it is augmented by the endotenon and interfascicular vessels. The tendon sheath, however, contributes little if anything to tendon repair. Even with complete sheath excision intact tendon function remains excellent as a new sheath develops and adhesion formation is minimal (37).

The origin of the fibroblast necessary for repair remains controversial. Lindsay and Thomson (37) and Lindsay and Birch (38) refined the peripheral healing theory of extrinsic processes. They believed that all connective tissue cells supporting a tendon are capable of producing the fibroblasts that will migrate into the tendon callus. Those in the less specialized tissues, the epitenon and endotenon, tend to react earlier. This theory was also advocated by Potenza (39) and Matthews and Richards (40) who concluded that tendon healing also requires the development of scars as a source of vascularity and fibroblasts necessary for collagen synthesis.

Using radioactive labeling and other techniques, researchers have been able to show that the tendon cells, or tenocytes, have the capability of producing cells for intrinsic tendon repair (31, 40-42). These more specialized cells tend to react later, usually after 2 weeks. Intrinsic repair appears to occur only under ideal experimental and clinical situations (40).

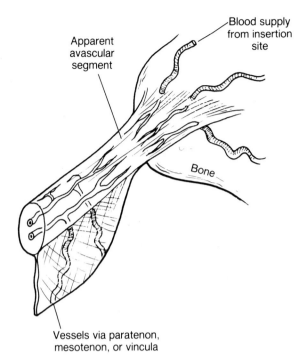

Figure 50.6. Blood supply as depicted to tendon in digital sheath. (From Hurst LN: The healing of tendon. In Kernahan DA, Vistnes LM [eds]: *Biological Aspects of Reconstructive Surgery.* New York, Little, Brown & Co, 1977, p 385.)

It is evident that both intrinsic and extrinsic processes have important roles in tendon healing. The degree of contribution from each is dependent upon the extent of local damage and the quality of the repair (30).

In summary, the integrity of the peritendinous structures is of paramount importance in the healing process. Proliferative reparative processes are much more efficient when healing occurs within paratenon as opposed to synovial tendon sheath. Whenever possible, tendon procedures should be performed in areas where paratenon is present, because the resultant scar will be able to glide with the areolar tissue of the paratenon, as well as the tendon itself.

When a tendon is separated from its normal surrounding structures, disturbances in nutrition and adhesion formation will lead to surgical failure. A tendon should not be stripped of paratenon in the process of transposition. For optimal healing all its necessary peritendinous tissues should accompany the tendon with a minimal amount of trauma during the transfer procedure for optimal healing (12).

CHRONOLOGY

When severed tendons are reapproximated end-to-end and maintained with suture, the healing process is one of progressive fibrosis and reconstitution of the tendon (cicatrization and tendonization) (43). The changes in tensile strength conform to the histological phases during the process of repair.

The stages of tendon healing are *(a)* the initial inflammatory (exudative) phase, *(b)* the fibroblastic (formative) phase, and *(c)* the remodeling (organizational) phase of maturation and differentiation. The first phase takes about 48 to 72 hours, whereas the second phase begins at approximately 5 days inasmuch as collagen fibers are formed in a random disorganized pattern. Fibroplasia predominates by the tenth day as the increased collagen and fibroblasts are oriented perpendicular to the long axis of the tendon. The third phase begins gradually from 15 to 28 days as the new collagen begins to align itself with the tendon (30, 40, 44, 45).

It takes about 4 weeks before healing is sufficient after tendon repair to allow a gradual return to activity, although passive motion should be started after the third week. The histological stages tend to overlap and vary with the individual's physiological response and ability to generate collagen, but generally patients progress through the following chronology (1, 3, 37, 40, 44, 46).

WEEK ONE. During the first week there is a reactive process whereby the tendon ends retract and become red and swollen with increased vascularity. An inflammatory cell exudate accumulates in the perisheath tissue and gap zone to form a jellylike bridge of serous and granulation tissue called a *fibroblastic splint* or *tendon callus.* Indeed, in 48 hours there is a vigorous fibroblastic proliferation and migration from the epitenon, mesotenon, and paratenon. Two days later the cells of the endotenon, followed by the tenocytes themselves, contribute to this proliferative cellular response. Initially the cells have a phagocytic function to clean up debris. At this stage sutures have reduced holding power in the softened tendon and may easily pull out.

WEEK TWO. During this week the vascularity of the paratenon increases as does the redness and edema of the tendon ends. Fibroblastic cells continue to proliferate into the amorphous mass to bridge the gap zone within 10 to 14 days. Still, there is no tensile strength and rupture may occur easily, although muscle tone is probably helping to stimulate repair. Active function of the tendon during the first 15 days will cause further irritation and swelling of the tendon, resulting in more adhesions, not a stronger union.

WEEK THREE. Now there is a vigorous production of collagen fibers that coalesce and begin to align themselves longitudinally to form new tendon fibers across the gap. The juncture is firmer and a cleavage begins between the tendon and surrounding tissue in preparation for movement. A moderate degree of bond strength is now present. Gentle mobilization after the third week will increase the strength of the union and discourage adhesion formation.

WEEK FOUR. Resolution reduces the swelling and vascularity during the fourth week. The tendon continues to be loosened from surrounding tissues to increase gliding function. Applied force through passive motion and muscle contraction will stimulate the collagen fibers into parallel formation so as to give optimum strength to the union. There should be only a progressive or gradual return to maximum contracture at this stage because complete strength has not yet been fully restored.

Gradually, the amount of collagen in the healing area diminishes as the remaining fibers establish a longitudinal orientation, maturing by about 8 weeks. Tissue strength increases with the development of multiple cross-linkages. However, there is minimal tensile strength until the tendon is stressed (47, 48).

Adhesions are either weakened or lysed as the gliding mechanism is restored or, if fixed, they contract and restrict motion.

PROGRESSIVE STRENGTH OF THE HEALING TENDON

This chronology will help in judging how long to immobilize a tendon after repair. Immediately after the surgery the strength of the union is no greater than that of the suture material. After 2 weeks the suture can withstand little strain. Limited isometric or passive range of motion exercises can be initiated after the third week as the union increases in strength. When 4 weeks have passed, there is no need for further immobilization because the danger of rupture is over. A gradual return to full function is advised (49) (Table 50.3).

FACTORS AFFECTING ADHESION FORMATION

It would greatly simplify clinical practice if tendons could heal in isolation, but they do not. The healing process was placed in perspective by the one wound—one scar concept advocated by Peacock who, with Van Winkle (50, 51), showed that each structure in the wound is connected with all others during healing, permeated by a single viscous gel. Thus the surrounding tissue heals in conjunction with tendon healing, and connections are necessary to revascularize the tendon repair. Initially, by the sixth to eighth day, the normal vascular anatomy is replaced by a haphazard arrangement of multiple small vessels with frequent anastomoses (12). During the resolution stage of healing the vascular pattern resumes a more normal configuration, and by 8 weeks the longitudinal supply has been reestablished (52).

Thus adhesions are not necessarily a complication of sur-

Table 50.3.
Summary of Chronology of Tendon Healing

Time	Histological Process	Strength	Treatment
Week one	Softening. Production of jelly-like "fibroblastic splint"	Suture	Immobilize
Week two	Increased vascularity and proliferation of fibroblasts	Suture	Immobilize
Week three	Vigorous production of collagen fibers	Moderate bond strength	Gentle motion or isometric exercises
Week four	Collagen fiber alignment; cleavage from local tissues	Gradual return to not quite full strength	Progressive muscular force

gery in themselves. They are indeed an integral part of the healing process (53). However, additional factors have been shown to influence proliferation of excess adhesions that impede tendon function.

Matthews and Richards (54) studied the effects of immobilization, suture, and sheath excision during tendon healing and monitored for adhesion formation. The results indicated that all three factors work in concert to contribute to adhesion formation rather than just one factor being solely responsible. Sutures produced the most adhesions, although at times none formed. Their constriction and trauma tend to devitalize the enclosed tendon, with fibrous proliferation occurring throughout the sutured area and not just the stump region. Immobilization alone does not evoke the development of adhesions. Excision of the sheath results in repair through the formation of granulation tissue, but this tissue does not contribute to, nor interfere with, the healing of tendon. The synovial layers are subsequently regenerated.

Other authors have shown that adhesions will form at every point of trauma to the tendon (12, 55, 56). Scar tissue will also form wherever blood is left to clot and organize (57).

As described previously, healing is most satisfactory when it occurs within the paratenon. Here the possibility of adhesion formation is diminished. When transferred, the paratenon should accompany the tendon only in small amounts. A thin film will allow the scar tissue to remodel so that it has the same characteristics as normal paratenon (36). If large amounts of paratenon are transferred, dense restrictive scar tissue is produced. When scar conditions are already present, autogenous paratenon or thin Silastic sheets (0.13 mm) can be interposed between the tendon and skin to prevent adhesion formation (58, 59).

Finally, the epitenon should never be stripped from the tendon unless scar tissue formation is desired as in side-to-side anastomosis. Ober (15) showed that the best way to restore and maintain gliding function is to pass the transferred tendon down the compartment of the paralyzed tendon. If necessary the paralyzed tendon can be withdrawn. Early, protected motion will help diminish the formation of restrictive adhesions during tendon healing (30).

Muscle-Tendon Physiology

TENDON FUNCTION

Definition and Function

A tendon is a nonelastic structure suitable for transferring large tensile forces produced by the contraction of muscle so that distant movement can occur about joint axes. It requires smooth gliding along its course and flexibility of associated joints to function properly.

Duchenne made the cogent observation early in his studies that the isolated action of any muscle is not physiological. Instead each muscle works in concert with and is affected

by other muscles or groups of muscles either synergistically or antagonistically. For example, muscle tone is required to maintain an extremity in its normal position at rest using these same subtle forces. Therefore, just as paralysis or loss of any single muscle must adversely affect others, similarly the selection of a muscle for transfer must be weighed for benefits with an understanding of the potential effects of the loss.

Concept of Tension

Blix (60) established that there exists a muscular length at which its contractile force is the strongest and most efficient. Thus the degree of tension developed by the muscle is directly related to the length of the muscle at the time of contraction (4, 60-62) (Fig. 50.7).

Muscles tend to produce their greatest force at about 120% of their resting length (see section on tension curve). Therefore it is important to reestablish normal muscle tension in the transfer of a musculotendinous unit, which is accomplished by maintaining the physiological length, a term coined by Stoffel (60-62). As Mayer (4) points out, based on his findings, this is done surgically by approximating the origin and insertion of a muscle—placing the foot in the position produced by maximal contraction of the transfer—and then removing all the slack from the tendon. By definition, zero tension is achieved when the patient is relaxed through general anesthesia. In other words, if the tendon were severed while in this position, the two ends would not separate. Using the tibialis anterior as an example, when the foot is placed in maximum dorsiflexion and moderate inversion, the tension on the tendon would be zero (Fig. 50.8).

Tension decreases as muscle fibers shorten. When they

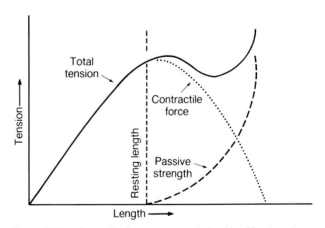

Figure 50.7. Contractile force curve as devised by Blix. Actual contractile force of muscle is greatest at about 120% of its resting length. Tension falls off markedly in both directions, indicating that muscle must have optimum length for function, and deviations from this length in either direction will reduce contractile force of muscle. (From Bechtol CO: Muscle physiology. *American Association of Orthopaedic Surgeons Instructional Course Lectures* 5:181, 1948.)

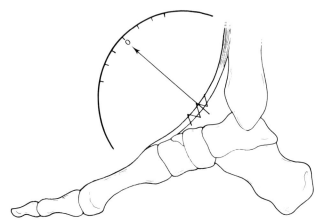

Figure 50.8. Determining zero tension for transferred tendons. Essentially foot is placed in desired position for correction (usually by dorsiflexing foot to right angle on leg). Then all slack is removed from tendon, and it is fixated in place with 0 pounds of tension. (From McGlamry ED, Butlin WE, Ruch JA: Treatment of forefoot equinus by tendon transpositions. *J Am Podiatry Assoc* 65:872-888, 1975.)

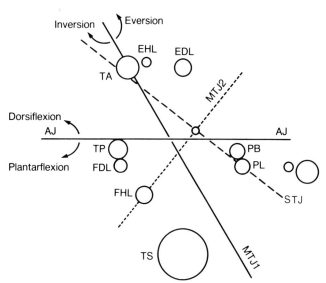

Figure 50.9. Cross-section in transverse plane through ankle joint showing relationship of various tendons with axes of ankle (AJ), subtalar (STJ), and midtarsal (MTJ) joints. Tendons are identified by letters representing their corresponding muscles. TA, tibialis anterior; EHL, extensor hallucis longus; EDL, extensor digitorum longus; MTJ, midtarsal joint; AJ, ankle joint; PB, peroneus brevis; PL, peroneus longus; STJ, subtalar joint; TS, triceps surae; FHL, flexor hallucis longus; TP, tibialis posterior. (From Elftman H: Dynamic structure of the human foot. *Artif Limbs* 13:49-58, 1969.)

reach approximately 60% of their resting length, zero tension is present.

Levers, Fulcrums, and Axes. Fulcrums are available to increase the angle of application and to improve the efficiency of tendon function. The sesamoids are fulcrums for the flexor hallucis brevis whereas the cuboid has the same function for the peroneus longus tendon.

The ratio of torque produced by the anterior and posterior leg muscles in controlling foot function is roughly 1:4, respectively. This discrepancy is offset by the long lever arm of the forefoot, which increases the force of the anterior leg muscles. Comparatively, the powerful triceps possesses a short lever arm through the posterior calcaneus.

The proximity of a tendon to a joint axis will determine whether its force is primarily stabilizing or rotatory (Fig. 50.9). The cross-sectional mass will determine the strength of the force (63-65).

PHASE FUNCTION/CONVERSION

Muscles with insertions in the foot can be generally divided into swing phase or stance phase muscles, depending on their function. For the most part the tibialis anterior, extensor hallucis longus, extensor digitorum longus, and peroneus tertius are swing phase muscles. The remainder are active during stance (Fig. 50.10).

Close and Todd in 1959 (66) evaluated the ability of transferred muscles to maintain or change phase, using electromyography (EMG) and cinematographic techniques. They found that muscles transferred to function in the same phase would rapidly regain their activity in as little as 7 or 8 weeks. Muscles transferred to function out of phase were generally unable to fire in their new position. However, such change in function was not entirely impossible. When transferred posteriorly into the calcaneus, the tibialis anterior showed activity in four of thirteen patients. When the per-

oneus longus and brevis were studied after transfer to the dorsum of the foot, the brevis was shown to readily convert its function as early as 3 months after surgery, whereas the longus only rarely demonstrated complete functional conversion. When transferred to the dorsum of the foot, the tibialis posterior tendon for the most part retained its stance phase activity (66). Other authors have also reported difficulty in getting the posterior tibial muscle to change phase (67). These authors also noted that muscles transferred alone to another phase were more likely to adapt than if they were transferred with additional muscles of the phase to be corrected.

Clinical experience has shown that it is more important to obtain a functional conversion than a phase conversion of a muscle, particularly when treating drop foot. For example, even though the transferred tibialis posterior muscle might not fully transfer phase in gait, it can still be trained to fire voluntarily at its new location in all but the most resistant patients. Even without functional conversion, such a tendon transfer can eliminate the need for a drop foot brace because of the resting tone stabilizing effect of the muscle. Active tenodesis can work as a rein or sling to hold the foot and ankle in a neutral position.

With the development and refining of techniques in biofeedback and electromyography, the retraining of muscles has improved dramatically (61, 62). Even changing phases can be more readily accomplished. However, it requires close cooperation with rehabilitation specialists for intensive conversion training. By teaching the patient how to isolate the desired motor activity before surgery, less difficulty will

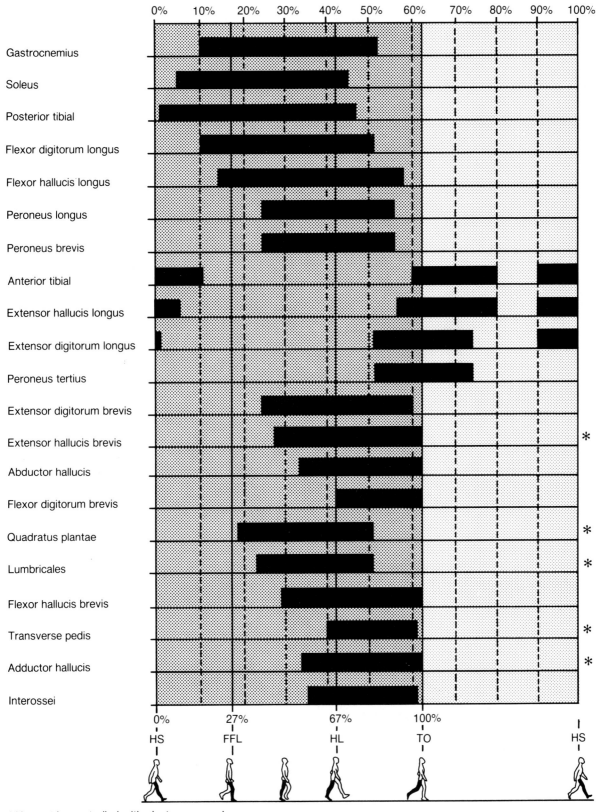

* Has not been studied with electromyography

Figure 50.10. Phasic activity of muscles controlling foot during normal gait. HS, heel strike; FFL, forefoot loading; HL, heel lift; TO, toe off. (From Root ML, Orien WP, Weed JH: *Normal and Abnormal Function of the Foot.* *Clinical Biomechanics,* vol II. Los Angeles, Clinical Biomechanics Corp, 1977.)

be encountered in learning how to voluntarily control and use the motor unit postoperatively.

PRINCIPLES OF TENDON TRANSFER SURGERY

Objectives

The goals of motor redistribution about the foot and ankle are primarily to provide active motor power where it is lost and thereby restore function and/or balance. To provide such motion surgery must be performed in an environment of flexible joints, unimpeded by contractures or bony deformities. The goals are as follows:

1. To improve motor function where weakness and imbalance exist and thereby prevent contractures and further deformity
2. To eliminate deforming forces
3. To provide active motor power for restoration of a lost essential motor function
4. To produce better stability by establishing better muscle balance
5. To eliminate the need for bracing
6. To improve cosmetic appearance

Muscle-Tendon Transfers

As tendon surgery has been refined over the last century, specific principles have evolved, the goal of which are to obtain optimum function. Several authors have clarified these principles so they may be applied universally, whatever the nature of the particular tendon surgery proposed (3, 6, 8, 13, 15, 68-70) (Fig. 50.11).

Selecting Suitable Cases

A necessary consideration in selecting a patient for a tendon transfer is the potential for rehabilitation. The nature of the disease, the patient's mental capacity, and the attitude toward the proposed operation all enter into the decision-making process, even for children and parents. The cause of the patient's disability must be analyzed in terms of its progressive nature, spasticity, flaccidity, and flexibility, as well as the remaining strength of the muscle. The transfer must be considered in relation to the total plan for rehabilitation of the patient.

In reviewing these factors it is also important for the surgeon and the patient to be realistic in determining and understanding the goal of the proposed muscle tendon transfer. A loss of one grade of muscle strength may be associated with many tendon transfers, and the patient or parents should be made aware of this factor in advance. However, most often, it is impossible to detect any loss, and often there appears to be a gain in strength. This occurs because of the change in leverage made possible with many transfers.

UNDERSTANDING ANATOMY AND PHYSIOLOGY INVOLVED

Paramount to preoperative planning is a thorough knowledge of the anatomy, pathology, and altered function of the involved area. The anatomy should be reviewed, and the examination should be comprehensive, including manual muscle testing and neurological evaluation. Gait analysis is mandatory to appreciate the pathomechanics involved. The examiner should be humble enough to reevaluate on several different occasions if at all unsure of the accuracy of findings. Cinematographical studies are an asset, particularly when slow motion is used for visual analysis. This is becom-

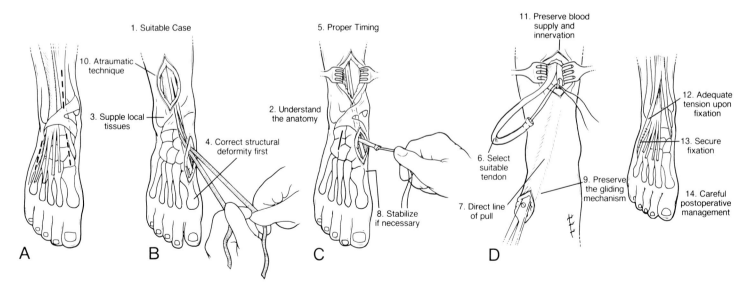

Figure 50.11. STATT technique. **A.** Placement of incisions. **B.** Splitting of tibialis anterior tendon. Must always be performed from proximal to distal. **C.** Split portion of tendon ready for transfer. Passing split portion of tendon laterally using retrograde tendon retriever. Curved Kelly or Boze-man forceps may be used. **D.** Attachment of split portion of tendon to peroneus tertius tendon. (As described in McGlamry ED, Ruch JA, Green DR: Simplified technique for split tibialis anterior tendon transposition [STATT] procedure. *J Am Podiatry Assoc* 65:927-937, 1975.)

Table 50.4.
Timing of Tendon Transfers in Certain Diseases

Disease	Suggested Timing	Reference
Cerebrovascular accident	6 mo	Edmonson and Crenshaw, 1980
Cerebral palsy	1 yr old—tendon lengthenings	Goldner, 1971
	4 yr old—tendon transfers	
Brain injury (children)	1 yr old	Samilson, 1976
	2 yr old	Hoffer, Reiswig, Garrett, and Perry, 1974
Lower level	6 mo to 8 yr old	Janda, Skinner, and Barto, 1984
Spinal dysplasia (e.g., myelomeningo-coele)	After 9 mo	Edmonson and Crenshaw, 1980
Poliomyelitis	2–3 yr after acute onset (during the early residual stage)	Peabody, 1949
		Edmonson and Crenshaw, 1980
	Better over 10 yr old	
Charcot-Marie-Tooth disease	Variable because of different ages of onset	
Leprosy	6 mo after onset of palsy (arm)	Brandsma and Lijftogt, 1983
	1 yr after onset of palsy (drop foot)	
Muscular dystrophy	Variable because different ages of onset	

ing more universally available with the affordability of more sophisticated modern video systems.

EVALUATING THE LOCAL TISSUES FOR SUPPLENESS

The tissues in the area of the transfer must be healthy. Severe scarring or scarring with concomitant tissue loss from previous trauma will not allow free tendon movement and may even result in further scar formation if surgery is attempted. Partial- and full-thickness burns tend to damage tendons in the area, leaving them indurated and often bound to the surrounding tissues.

CORRECTING FIXED OR STRUCTURAL DEFORMITIES FIRST

Tendon transfer cannot be expected to overcome a fixed deformity. For a transferred tendon to be effective, the functional defect or deformity must be entirely flexible. In other words, the associated joint should demonstrate a reasonable range of passive motion.

If a concurrent deformity is fixed, whether structural or as a contracture, it must be corrected at a prior surgery or at the same operation, provided it is done before the tendon is transplanted. Such fixed deformities can be altered by joint releases, tendon lengthenings, osteotomies, and arthrodeses.

SELECTING PROPER TIME FOR TRANSFER

Timing refers to the age of the patient and the course of the disease. Age is important if osseous stabilizing operations, which require adequate mature bone stock, are considered. However, it is not necessarily wise to delay tendon transfers several years if there exists a dynamic muscular imbalance, especially in younger patients who require or who resist brace protection. Early tendon surgery will prevent further deformity, thus facilitating the performance of future operations.

Although a child patient should be old enough to coop-

Table 50.5.
Grading System for Manual Muscle Testing

Grade	Description
5, Normal	Full resistance at end range of motion
4, Good	Some resistance at end range of motion
4+	Moderate resistance at end range of motion
4−	Mild resistance at end range of motion
3, Fair	Able to move against gravity alone
2, Poor	Able to move with gravity eliminated
1, Trace	Can palpate or visualize muscle contraction
0, Zero	No evidence of muscle contraction

erate in the retraining process, this is not always necessary. For example, in the dynamic and progressive talipes calcaneus deformity, early transfer can often arrest the progress of the deformity even though the patient may not fully understand the new function of the muscle (71-73).

Timing during the disease process is most important when the disease is of a progressive nature. When there is brain damage, surgery should be delayed until the most intense stage of spasm has passed. Other disorders have individual times suitable for tendon transfer that vary according to their nature (Table 50.4).

SELECTING SUITABLE TENDON OR TENDONS

An initial consideration is whether there is sufficient power in the remaining muscles to provide adequate function once the desired tendon is harvested. In other words, is the muscle to be transferred truly expendable?

It is also important to be realistic about the muscle's capability—its *strength* and *adaptability*—to perform its new function. Strength can be approximately assessed by estimating the cross-sectional mass of the muscle itself. Table 50.5 supplies helpful information for the selection of tendons of sufficient capability.

Choosing muscles that are functionally similar (i.e., stabilizers vs. accelerators) or within the same phase (i.e., stance or swing) is ideal but not absolute. In electing to use a muscle of the opposite phase, it is better to select one that has a high potential for conversion (e.g., the peroneus brevis).

In regressive neuromuscular conditions such as Charcot-Marie-Tooth disease, the potential for future deterioration of the muscle to be transferred must be as accurately ascertained as possible. Even if only several years of function remain, it can still serve to delay disability.

PROVIDING DIRECT OR MECHANICALLY EFFICIENT LINE OF PULL

The individual fibers of a muscle are set and arranged according to the optimal line of function. When this line of application is altered, the muscle must undergo a certain amount of readjustment. The more the line of pull is changed, the greater the demand on the muscle for adaptability, of which there is a definite limit (74).

Maximum physiological efficiency is obtained when a tendon pulls in a straight line. Therefore, changes in the direction of tendon contraction, that is, retinacula, reduce the maximal effectiveness of the muscle. When tendons are transferred, angulations should be avoided as much as possible because any degree of angulation will cause a loss of amplitude. Despite these considerations it is usually preferable to transfer the tendon along an anatomical course. Transferring the tendon subcutaneously will enhance its power but will result in bowstringing against the skin and also introduces an unpredictable degree of torsion against the involved joints.

In addition, as the lever arm increases, the force vectors change in amplitude. Generally the longer the lever arm, the more effective the muscular force. However, if the line of contracture is parallel to the lever, then additional length will have little effect. A good example is a tendon transfer to the dorsum of the foot beneath the extensor retinaculum (Fig. 50.12). Extensor tendons that are transferred to a more proximal location on the foot have a more effective force of ankle dorsiflexion compared with the distal metatarsophalangeal location.

PERFORMING STABILIZATION PROCEDURES IF NECESSARY

Tendon transfers require rigid lever arms on which to function, regardless of their distance from the joint axes. When such stability is not present, then it must be constructed by way of arthrodeses, regardless of whether in the toes or the tarsus.

Stabilization procedures must be performed before the tendon transfer, either at a prior surgery or during the same operation.

PRESERVING THE GLIDING MECHANISM

The most perplexing problem in tendon transfer surgery has been that of adhesions restricting function. All major tendon surgeons agree that the only satisfactory way to prevent adhesions is to preserve or reconstruct the physiological

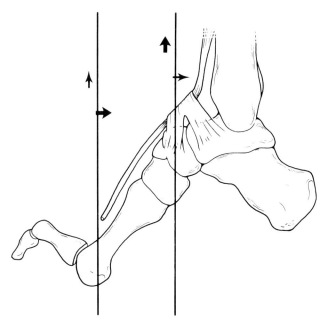

Figure 50.12. Vector force of effective lever arm of tendon. Arrows indicate relative direction and amount of force of tendons transposed at different levels. More proximal transfer insertion makes available greater dorsiflexory power. More distal insertion line of pull tends to parallel lever arm, and mechanical advantage of dorsiflexion is lost. (From McGlamry ED, Butlin WE, Ruch JA: Treatment of forefoot equinus by tendon transpositions. *J Am Podiatry Assoc* 65:872-888, 1975.)

gliding mechanism of the tendon. This is best accomplished through absolute atraumatic surgery, restoration of the tendon-sheath relationship, and use of existing sheaths or establishment of a subcutaneous tunnel. If possible, the peritendinous structures, including the paratenon and especially the epitenon, should be transplanted with the tendon.

Retention of the physiological relationship between the tendon and sheath can be obtained by passing the transferred tendon within the sheath of the paralyzed tendon. When this is not possible, a gliding channel can be fashioned within subcutaneous adipose tissue by establishing a channel with forceps or other blunt instruments. The channel will eventually be lined with smooth cells to permit gliding of the tendon.

Early protective mobilization exercises will help restore the gliding mechanism (75). Ultimately, the transferred tendon should have similar excursion to the one it replaces.

UTILIZING ATRAUMATIC TECHNIQUE AT ALL TIMES

The principle of atraumatic technique was first proposed and the term coined by the master tendon surgeon, Bunnell (76), in 1921. It is the central factor that contributes to preservation of the gliding function of the transferred tendon, reiterated time and again by many authors. Although it is a term heard often by the reconstructive surgeon, several aspects apply especially to tendon surgery.

Atraumatic technique begins with the incision. It should

not be placed directly over the tendon itself and, when practical, should parallel local skin creases to minimize the development of thick, nonpliable cicatrix.

Careful planning will allow the operation to be performed precisely, yet as quickly as possible, exposing tissues to air for the briefest time only. Absolute hemostasis is essential. An adhesion can be expected to form at every place a small clot of blood is allowed to remain. Thus the wound should be irrigated frequently and liberally, preferably with Ringer's solution, not only to keep the tissues moist but also to remove blood clots and other tissue debris that might adversely affect the healing process. Tissues must not be torn or crushed, except for the tendon end that is to be fixated and where fibrous production is desired.

Any damage to the gliding surface of the tendon, covered with smooth delicate cells, will readily cause adhesions to form. The tendon to be moved should be left in place until its new course and insertion are made ready to receive it. It should be manipulated very gently, using toothless forceps, Penrose drains or a wet gloved hand. Even a moistened sponge can be too rough. The paratenon and epitenon should be left intact and transferred with the tendon, which should be kept moist at all times. The tendon should never be allowed to lie on the local drapes. Mesotenon, when present, should be sharply and gently extricated.

PRESERVING BLOOD SUPPLY AND INNERVATION

Sometimes considerable traction is required to harvest a tendon for transfer. If this is excessive, the nerve supply to the tendon can pull free. Similarly, rough handling or indiscriminate dissection may lacerate the main blood vessel of the tendon, usually found running in the lower muscle fibers. Smaller vessels running in the mesotenon can be divided with impunity.

PROVIDING ADEQUATE MUSCLE-TENDON TENSION ON FIXATION

The concept of zero tension has already been described. Where too little tension will cause the muscle to shorten, leaving a loss of power, the strain of excess tension will cause rapid degeneration of the muscle tissue over a period of only weeks (5, 9). The goal is to establish tension that corresponds to the normal physiological conditions under which the muscle and tendon work. In other words, the physiological length of the muscle must be maintained. Yet, no matter how well the technique is described, fastening a tendon under zero tension is a skill that each surgeon develops with experience because it varies from one muscle to another.

USING SECURE FIXATION TECHNIQUES

A tendon transfer is only as good as the security of its point of fixation. The first recorded effort by Nicoladoni (3, 5-10) failed because the tendon pulled free, leaving other surgeons skeptical of the procedure.

Ideally the tendon should be secured as close as possible to the insertion of the paralyzed tendon. If this is not feasible, then consideration must be given to a location in which leverage will provide sufficient power and balance. When a tendon is split to balance its pulling force, care must be taken to fixate each branch under equal tension. If unbalanced, the resulting motion will go to the tightest branch.

Tendon may be attached in one of three ways: tendon to tendon, tendon to periosteum, or tendon to bone. The last provides the most secure fixation. Specific techniques will be described for each of these methods.

PROVIDING DETAILED POSTOPERATIVE MANAGEMENT

Postoperative care is crucial to a successful outcome. It is vital that the patient and, when necessary, the parents understand the requirements of immobilization, convalescence, and rehabilitation following tendon transfer surgery.

The cast should be applied at the time of surgery if possible. Manipulation during dressing changes or cast applications early in the healing period may cause the tendon to pull free.

Motion should be started early, as soon as the surgeon is reasonably certain that healing has provided firm anchorage of the tendon. Gentle isometric exercises within the cast can be started as early as 3 weeks.

Strengthening exercises begin the rehabilitation program immediately after removal of the cast. Then retraining the muscle to contract appropriately in its new location becomes the goal of therapy. If phasic conversion is required, intense training must be ~~intense~~ accompanied by rehabilitation techniques. These methods will be detailed later.

FIXATION OF TRANSFERRED TENDONS

Tendon to Tendon

Side-to-side anastomosis of a transferred tendon provides the most physiological pull; the greatest danger in such attachment is that of slippage. The adjoining surfaces should be roughened and the epitenon scraped free. Scarring the tendons with light cross-hatching will also encourage fibrous union (Fig. 50.13).

Polygalactic or polyglycolic acid sutures provide sufficient strength for sewing tendons, but they may be reinforced with a nonabsorbable polyester suture to increase strength over time as the former are absorbed.

Tendon to Bone

Four main techniques are used to anchor tendon into bone. All heal the same way physiologically in that the tendon is actually incorporated into the bone by ossification (77, 78). Ossification is most marked in the cortical area and only minimal in the medullary bone. The limb must be immobilized during the early phase but for not longer than 21 days. Prolonged immobilization will retard the tensile strength of the union. The relative size of the tendon to

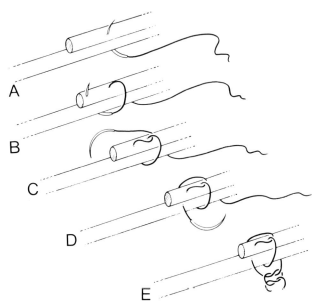

Figure 50.13. **A** to **E.** Suture technique for side-to-side anastomosis.

drill hole has little effect on the rate of union of tendon to bone.

TREPHINE PLUG. Michele vertebral trephines are ideal hand instruments for creating a drill hole and preserving the plug of bone for future replacement (79) (Fig. 50.14). Power trephines can also be used. The tendon end is inserted into the hole, and the plug is tapped into place. Anchor sutures are then placed in the surrounding fascia and periosteum. In the absence of a trephine, a cortical window may be fashioned with use of osteotomes or a drill.

CHINESE FINGER-TRAP SUTURE. This technique facilitates the drawing of a tendon through a drill hole (80). A polyester suture (1-0 or 2-0) is wrapped around the tendon in a criss-cross fashion proceeding from about 3 or 4 cm to the end. A knot is tied and the suture tails left long. A second suture is then wrapped criss-cross around the tendon, out of phase with the first suture and tied in a knot at the end. The ends of the suture are then passed through the drill hole to draw the tendon through. Finally, the sutures are cut to relieve tension around the tendon (Fig. 50.15).

THREE-HOLE SUTURE. This technique consists of anchoring the transposed tendon end with a double-armed suture, then placing it into one large drill hole. It is secured by drawing the suture ends out through two small adjacent

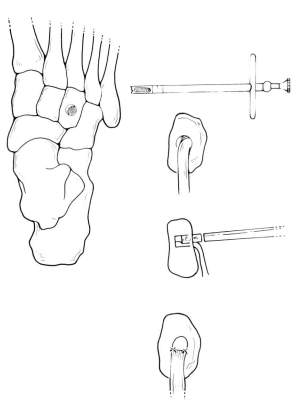

Figure 50.14. Insertion of tendon in trephined hole in bone. Michele vertebral trephine or power trephine may be used. (From Gould N: Trephining your way. *Orthop Clin North Am* 4:157-164, 1973.)

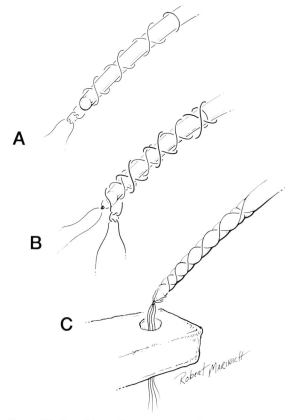

Figure 50.15. Chinese finger-trap suture. **A.** First criss-cross suture. **B.** Second criss-cross suture. **C.** Tendon compressed as it is drawn through the drill-hole in bone.

drill holes and tying them firmly. A nonabsorbable polyester suture is recommended (26) (Fig. 50.16).

BUTTRESS AND BUTTON ANCHOR. By this method a bone hole is drilled for tenodesis at the desired site. The suture is anchored in the tendon, and one or two straight Keith needles are then passed through the drill hole and out the other side of the foot. A button provides the anchor on which to tie the suture ends, but a sterile buttress material, such as foam or gauze, must be interposed between the button and the skin to disperse the pressure and to avoid ischemic necrosis (Fig. 50.17).

TUNNEL WITH SLING. Only when there is sufficient length of tendon available can this technique be used. It consists of drilling a hole completely through a bone and then passing the tendon all the way through so it can be sutured back on itself. In this manner the tendon becomes something of a sling. It has its greatest application in the Jones first meta-tarsal tendon suspension (26, 79) and in ankle stabilization procedures such as the one described by Watson-Jones (79) (Fig. 50.18).

TENDON WITH BONY INSERTION. Instead of severing the tendon at its insertion, the portion of bone to which it is attached is carefully removed with an osteotome or power saw. The plug of bone is then inserted into the new site where a similarly sized piece of cortical bone has been removed. The main disadvantage is that adjustment of the tendon length for proper tension is extremely limited.

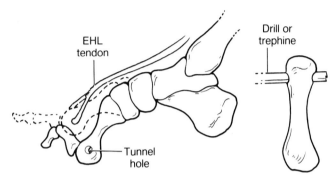

Figure 50.18. Securing tendon using tunnel and sling technique. Hole can be trephined or drilled. It is not necessary to replace plug of bone.

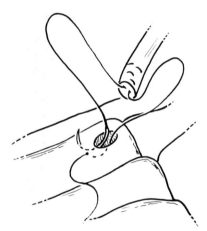

Figure 50.16. Three-hole suture technique for anchoring tendon to bone. (From McGlamry ED, Butlin WE, Ruch JA: Treatment of forefoot equinus by tendon transpositions. *J Am Podiatry Assoc* 65:872-888, 1975.)

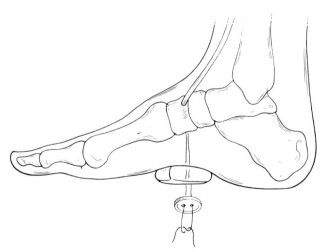

Figure 50.17. Tendon anchor into bone using external button with buttress to secure suture. (From McGlamry ED, Butlin WE, Ruch JA: Treatment of forefoot equinus by tendon transpositions. *J Am Podiatry Assoc* 65:872-888, 1975.)

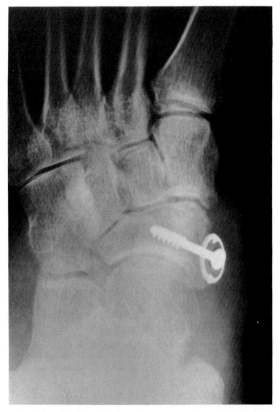

Figure 50.19. Radiograph showing screw and polyacetyl washer in place to attach posterior tibial tendon to navicular bone in modified Kidner procedure.

Screw and Washer. The use of a cleated polyacetyl washer and cancellous bone screw is a helpful method for securing a tendon at its new location. It is especially suited where there is little soft tissue to which the transferred tendon can be sutured or where other bone attachments are difficult. A good example is the anterior advancement of the posterior tibial tendon (Fig. 50.19).

OTHER CONSIDERATIONS IN TENDON SURGERY

Tendon Repair

Whether a tendon disruption is traumatically or iatrogenically induced, there are several methods of repair that will provide effective apposition for healing. Several principles should be observed.

The primary function of the suture is to reduce tension at the tendon ends so that gaping is minimized and healing can take place. It is vital that the microcirculation be preserved. For this reason, care must be taken not to encircle and strangulate large amounts of tendon tissue with suture.

Although close apposition is important, the tendon ends must not bunch or overlap excessively. Further, the tendon-to-tendon approximation must be equal. Excess on either side will allow outgrowths of fibrous tissue (pseudopodium) from the epitenon that will bind to surrounding structures and restrict motion.

The principles of immobilization for tendon healing remain the same, as already discussed. Critical to tendon repair then is utilization of the appropriate suture technique. Several are listed here and illustrated.

Bunnell End-To-End Suture. This has become a standard for years, although it does cause considerable tissue constriction (81) (Fig. 50.20).

Double Right-Angle Suture. This is good for quick repair of small tendons where there is little tension (Fig. 50.21).

Lateral Trap Suture. Designed after the oriental finger trap, this technique firmly grips the outside tendon fibers and thereby avoids constricting the microcirculation in the central area of the tendon (44) (Fig. 50.22).

Bunnell Pull-Out Suture. A pull-out stitch is simply a nonabsorbable suture, preferably stainless steel, that anchors a deep stitch to the outside of the skin so it can be extracted once healing is complete. Excellent for tenodesis, it may be applied anywhere (Fig. 50.23).

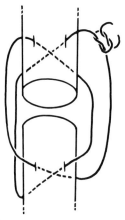

Figure 50.21. Double right-angle suture technique. (From Pulvertaft RG: Suture material and tendon junctures. *Am J Surg* 109:346-380, 1965.)

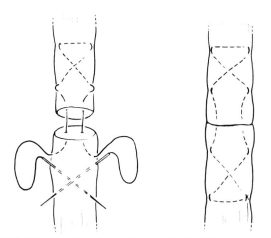

Figure 50.20. Bunnell end-to-end suture. Gentle tightening at gap site will produce accordion effect. (From Lawton JH: Repair of tendons and soft tissues. In Marcus SA, Block BH [eds]: *American College of Foot Surgeons—Complications in Foot Surgery, Prevention and Management,* ed 2. Baltimore, Williams & Wilkins, 1984, pp 129-162.)

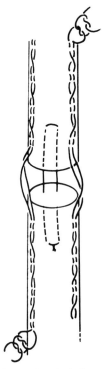

Figure 50.22. Lateral trap suture technique. Central mattress suture serves as temporary anchor to avoid multiple forceps manipulation of tendons. It can be removed once trap suture is in place. (From Ketchum LD, Martin NL, Kappel DA: Experimental evaluation of factors affecting the strength of tendon repairs. *Plast Reconstr Surg* 59:708-719, 1977.)

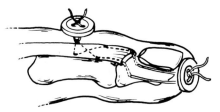

Figure 50.23. Bunnell pull-out suture. Buttons can be used to anchor suture externally. With this technique suture material must exit skin at two locations, one to cut stitch and one for extraction. (From Lawton JH: Repair of tendons and soft tissues. In Marcus SA, Block BH [eds]: *American College of Foot Surgeons—Complications in Foot Surgery, Prevention and Management,* ed 2. Baltimore, Williams & Wilkins, 1984, pp 129-162.)

Tendon Lengthening and Tenotomy

Tendon lengthening and tenotomy have limited indications when abnormal contracture of a musculotendinous unit compromises the normal function or position of a part. In fact, absolute tenotomy has few applications in reconstructive foot and ankle surgery.

The purpose of a tenotomy is to release a contracture and gain length, with the intention that the severed ends will allow for callous formation and eventual healing within their peritendinous structures. Research has shown that ruptured tendons heal within paratenon but not within sheath. Often, however, the gap is too great to allow for effective healing.

Unfortunately tenotomies can lead to an imbalance of forces so that even the slightest remaining antagonistic muscle is totally unopposed. Without sound judgment the result may be further deformity. Therefore tendon lengthening is often more desirable. Tendon lengthenings will often result in a loss of muscle strength roughly equal to one grade of manual examination once healed.

INDICATIONS AND TECHNIQUES

One of the digital tenotomies used in the foot is that of the flexor digitorum longus tendon slip to relieve mallet toe especially where there is a painful distal hyperkeratotic lesion. Splinting is advised for about 1 month to achieve proper alignment (28). Digital tenotomies are best performed through medial or lateral stab incisions with small blades, care being taken to avoid damage to the nearby neurovascular bundles (Fig. 50.24).

The Strayer (82, 83) technique for lengthening the gastrocnemius muscle requires complete severance of the aponeurosis and casting the foot in neutral position to allow healing at the new length. Another indication for tenotomy is to release the adductor hallucis tendon during hallux valgus repair, but it should be reattached to the neck of the first metatarsal to maintain intrinsic tone.

Flexible or functional hammer toes may be treated by lengthening the digital extensor tendons with or without capsulotomies (Fig. 50.25). The sliding Z-plasty is often the preferred technique for such a lengthening (Fig. 50.26). The same method can be applied to any other tendon in the foot.

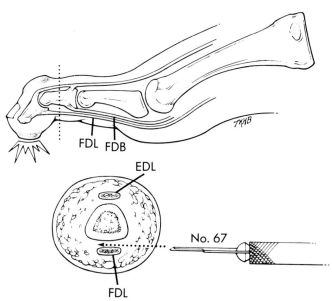

Figure 50.24. Long digital flexor tenotomy. Enter midway on lateral surface of digit just proximal to distal interphalangeal joint and keep blade horizontal passing between phalanx and FDL tendon. Rotate No. 67 blade plantarly and hyperextend distal toe until release is felt. FDL, flexor digitorum longus; FDB, flexor digitorum brevis; EDL, extensor digitorum longus.

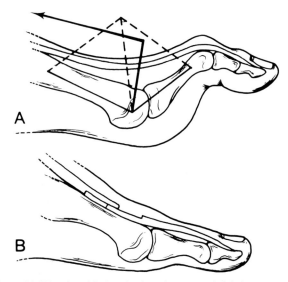

Figure 50.25. **A** and **B.** Lengthening of contracted digital extensor tendon releases vector forces that were causing retrograde buckling of toe. (From: Lawton JH: Repair of tendons and soft tissues. In Marcus SA, Block BH [eds]: *American College of Foot Surgeons—Complications in Foot Surgery, Prevention and Management,* ed 2. Baltimore, Williams & Wilkins, 1984, pp 129-162.)

It requires gentle stabilization of the tendon with atraumatic forceps for the duration of the procedure (Fig. 50.27). Otherwise the tendon will roll, and the fibers to be severed will cross planes. Approximately two thirds of the fibers should be cut on one side of the stabilizing instrument followed by two thirds of the fibers on the opposite side, 1 to

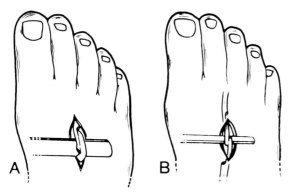

Figure 50.26. **A** and **B.** Technique for Z-plasty lengthening of contracted tendon. (From Lawton JH: Repair of tendons and soft tissues. In Marcus SA, Block BH [eds]: *American College of Foot Surgeons—Complications in Foot Surgery, Prevention and Management,* ed 2. Baltimore, Williams & Wilkins, 1984, pp 129-162.)

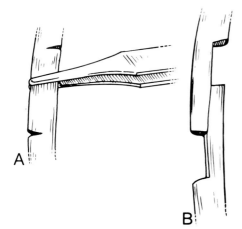

Figure 50.27. **A** and **B.** Stabilizing tendon for Z-plasty lengthening procedure.

3 cm more, from the first cut. The toe or foot should be gently forced away from the tendon to cause it to slide. Pulling at the slide site will usually cause it to rupture. It is not always necessary to strip the paratenon from the tendon. The blade can simply be stabbed through the paratenon parallel to the tendon fibers and rotated to the edge to sever the appropriate width of tendon.

Another indication is to lengthen the peroneus longus tendon for treatment of a functionally plantarflexed first metatarsal that is causing painful symptoms. Finally, dramatic results can often be seen by lengthening the Achilles tendon or triceps surae aponeurosis, the contracture of which is a major contributor to painful foot conditions.

An alternative lengthening method is known as the tongue-in-groove recession. If the outer third of the fibers proximally or distally and the central third a few centimeters away are cut, the tendon will then recess or slide in a tongue-and-groove fashion. Minimal suture repair is necessary. The most common application is for lengthening the triceps surae complex (84).

TENDON GRAFTS

Incorporation and Healing

Two schools of thought have existed over the years regarding the fate of an autogenous tendon graft in its new environment. One school believes that the transplanted tendon remains alive for the most part, whereas the other group holds that the graft undergoes necrosis, acting solely as a strut for ingrowing tendon cells from the stumps. Flynn and Graham (85) performed detailed histological studies and found that, although the healing process is slower yet similar to that for sutured tendons, the grafts completely necrosed and were replaced by tenoblasts from the stumps. However, the autograft does provide more than just a framework for collagen synthesis.

By 3 days the suture union is secured with a proliferation of sheath and peritendinous tissue between the stump and the graft. Young tenoblasts are seen in the stump, whereas the graft undergoes ischemic necrosis, and new capillaries abound.

After 1 week the tenoblasts invade the gap, and by the end of 3 weeks there is sufficient tensile strength and sheath healing to permit full gliding of the newly formed tendon so that guarded exercise can be initiated. Finally, by the seventh week adult tendon cells have developed across the gap and the fibers mature over the next several weeks so that the stumps and the graft appear homogenous (85).

Donor Tendons

Not only must the harvested tendon graft be long, thin, and resilient but it also must be handled absolutely atraumatically in a moist environment (86). Traction sutures prevent excessive handling and crushing. Donor grafts for foot surgery are the tendons of the plantaris, peroneus tertius, and slips of the extensor digitorum longus or brevis. If necessary small strips of fascia lata or Achilles tendon can be used.

Staged Tendon/Sheath Reconstruction

Reestablishing the gliding function of damaged tendon sheaths with synthetic material has been an elusive goal of tendon surgeons since the 1930s (87). The two-stage technique was developed about this time by Mayer and Ransohoff (88, 89), but it was not widely practiced until 1951, when a suitable inert material was incorporated, namely silicone rod implants (90, 91).

The primary indication for a staged gliding tendon graft is in patients in whom the gliding bed has been damaged, whether the injury is seen immediately or secondarily (92). The first stage consists of placing the silicone rod implant (93) in the desired tendon route while at the same time excising damaged tendon and scar tissue. The implant is sutured to existing muscle/tendon structures so it can glide during functional exercises. Over the next 6 weeks to 6 months the prosthesis acts as a template around which a pseudosynovial sheath forms. The second stage, usually performed 3 months after the first stage, requires removal of the silicone rod and inserting in its place an autogenous free tendon graft (92, 94, 95).

The remarkable result of this procedure is to restore function by way of a smooth gliding tendon within the newly formed pseudosheath (96, 97).

The most frequent complication of staged tendon reconstruction is synovitis. The technique was developed mainly within the subspecialty of hand surgery; to date there has been only occasional application to foot and leg reconstruction.

Tendon Xenografts

Considerable interest in tendon xenografts has been expressed in the European literature as long ago as 1881 (98). The key to preventing immunogenic host reactions to the foreign tendon tissue appears to be destruction of the cellular components of the xenograft. This is done by preserving the tendon graft in an organic solution such as glutaraldehyde. Lack of an overt foreign body reaction avoids adhesion formation when the graft is placed in a moving or dynamic environment. The same principles apply to allografts.

It is agreed by most investigators that tendon xenografts simply provide a bridge or scaffold for the ingrowing of host collagen. A typical healing response includes encapsulation and an opportunistic invasion by host fibrotic material migrating inward from each anastomosis (98).

The Tendon Xenografts Bioprosthesis Model GR6 mm has been used for lateral ankle stabilization procedures in cases in which suitable autogenous tendon is inadequate or best left undisturbed (99). A longer time of immobilization and non-weight-bearing is required for the xenograft to attach into bone, usually 8 weeks.

Surgical procedures for handling and implanting xenografts are essentially the same as those used for autologous grafting or primary repair procedures. Care must be taken to maintain sterile technique and to rinse the tendon xenograft thoroughly before implantation.

MUSCULAR DYNAMICS OF THE FOOT

To appreciate deformity and tendon imbalance it is necessary to understand muscle function as it affects the foot, whether intrinsic or extrinsic in its origin. The biomechanics of each individual muscle must of course be a part of that basic knowledge. However, as shown with such vivid insight by Duchenne in his 1867 monumental study entitled *Physiology of Motion,* the isolated action of muscles is not physiological. Using faradic stimulation, coupled with his own astute clinical observations, Duchenne accurately demonstrated the concept of synergistic function of muscle groups. In addition, he described the concept of multiple muscle tone maintaining an extremity in a normal position at rest "as so many springs which act to maintain the position of an extremity." When one spring is weakened or paralyzed, the stage is set for imbalance and abnormal position because of the pull or the tone of those remaining (100).

It is not the purpose of this chapter to describe in detail the function of each muscle. That should be fundamental knowledge of the reader. In addition, there should be a general appreciation of the muscles involved in the gross motions of the foot and specific knowledge of the major agonists or antagonists of each group. From this perspective deformities may be understood and appropriate muscle/tendon units selected for transfer.

A thorough biomechanical and neurological examination must be performed on patients for whom muscle tendon transfers may be considered. A highly useful tool is the standardized manual muscle testing described by Daniels and Worthingham (101), which uses a grading system for strength. Each muscle, placed at its end range of motion, is tested by applying manual force against it. The patient will best comprehend the test if the foot is placed with the desired muscle under maximum contraction and the patient is asked to hold it against the examiner's resistance. If considerable force is required to break the muscle, it is graded at five or normal. Grades then descend with appropriate reductions in strength (Table 50.5). On the basis of the examiner's experience, plus or minus may be used when the muscle test falls slightly above or below any one grade.

Cinematographical gait studies, particularly when obtained with a high-speed camera that will demonstrate detailed slow motion, may be invaluable in appreciating muscle imbalance and functional deficits or compensation. Instant videotape systems may also be used with some sacrifice of detail.

Finally, electromyographic studies can provide detailed information about a muscle. An experienced examiner can determine roughly what percentage of the motor units are still functional. Also the nature and often the stage of degeneration through which a muscle is passing may be assessed by analyzing the electrical activity within its fibers (101-106). Kinetic or dynamic electromyography may be used to determine phase function activity (107, 108).

TENDON TRANSFERS ABOUT THE FOOT AND ANKLE

A review of the literature reveals that almost every imaginable type of tendon transfer, or combination of transfers, has been attempted. Detailing every possible procedure would be impractical. However, for each deformity there exists an insufficiency, or muscle imbalance, to be corrected. The main procedures that are favored are herein described. This does not imply that other tendon transfers are not indicated under specific circumstances.

Conditions Amenable to Treatment by Tendon Transfer

WEAKNESS OR INSUFFICIENCY

Muscular weakness may be augmented and function enhanced by appropriate tendon transfers. Extensor insufficiency involving any of the three primary extensor muscles is amenable to tendon transfer correction. Total or partial loss of the tibialis anterior, long extensors, or either peroneal muscle is an indication for transfer. The replacement tendon selected will depend on the length of time of the deformity and the available tendons remaining.

Tibialis posterior weakness or dysfunction resulting in a collapsing flatfoot may be treated by transferring local tendons into the navicular or existing posterior tibial tendon.

TRICEPS SURAE INSUFFICIENCY

Weakness or paralysis of the triceps surae will cause a calcaneus deformity because of unopposed extensor activity. Also, loss of resistance against contraction of the intrinsic muscles during stance phase may result in forefoot equinus and, therefore, a calcaneocavus deformity. If there is concurrent loss of the peroneals a calcaneovarus deformity will develop, and loss of the tibialis posterior will produce calcaneovalgus deformity. Paralysis of the triceps surae in childhood will retard the growth of the calcaneal apophysis (109), resulting in a hypoplastic heel.

The triceps surae is the strongest muscle controlling the foot by a ratio of about 4:1. Therefore any transfer designed to offset the progression of the calcaneus deformity and restore propulsion must use two or more muscles. Selection may be made from the tibialis posterior, long flexors, and peroneals for posterior transfer into the calcaneus inasmuch as these are already stance phase muscles. In cases of complete paralysis all might be used. For isolated instances of triceps surae weakness a suggested transfer might include both long flexors and the peroneus longus, thus leaving the medial and lateral stabilizing muscles intact (tibialis posterior and peroneus brevis).

If all plantarflexory muscles are paralyzed, or are of insufficient strength, then phasic conversion transfer of the tibialis anterior is indicated. The tibialis anterior is a strong muscle, and if phasic conversion succeeds, its transfer will result in reasonably effective propulsion. Close and Todd (66) found that four of thirteen transfers underwent conversion and advised that such a change is much more likely if the tibialis anterior is transferred by itself. This information points to the necessity for a vigorous phase-conversion rehabilitation program for these patients.

SPASTICITY

In most cases muscle spasticity is the result of upper motoneuron lesions caused by cerebral palsy, direct trauma, or cerebrovascular accident. Loss of inhibitory impulses allows for greatly increased muscle tone, exaggerated stretch reflex, and frank spasticity. In these patients there are several special considerations to be observed regarding tendon transfers. If an associated disorder such as rigidity, dystonia, ataxia, or athetosis is present, tendon transfers are quite unpredictable. In general clonus is a poor prognostic sign for the successful outcome of these procedures (110). Any tension at all will maintain muscle spasm.

The most common foot deformity seen in cerebral palsy is that of equinus (84, 110-114). The gastrocnemius is affected more frequently than is the soleus by spasticity (84, 115), but the deformity may be the result of involvement of both muscles. Examination is important because the equinus deformity may be the result of relative central weakness of the dorsiflexors rather than spasticity of the triceps itself (109). Lengthening of either the gastrocnemius muscle or Achilles tendon when spasticity is present requires special considerations and involves selection from several different procedures. These are presented in the chapter on equinus surgery. A highly valuable tendon transfer for relief of spastic triceps equinus is the anterior advancement of the Achilles tendon insertion as described by Murphy in 1972 (111, 116-118).

Spastic equinovalgus is another deformity associated with cerebral palsy, seen in up to 90% of spastic equinus deformities (119). Tendon transfer alone will not correct the valgus component. Stabilizing procedures such as subtalar joint arthrodesis in adults, extra-articular subtalar arthrodesis, or calcaneal osteotomies are necessary adjuncts to maintain foot alignment (119-121).

Equinovarus is also frequently associated with spastic disease, caused principally by the tibialis posterior muscle. In these cases lengthening, transferring, or tenodesis of the tibialis posterior tendon has been successful (107, 122).

Perry and Hoffer stated that "the difficulty in achieving predictable results after tendon transfers in children with cerebral palsy is due to lack of understanding of the behavior of the muscle to be transferred" (108). They believed the key was dynamic electromyographic information obtained during active gait.

In terms of the tibialis posterior tendon transfer, best results were obtained when the tendon was shown preoperatively to be active only in the stance phase. If it was active throughout the gait cycle, then tendon lengthening or the split tendon transfer will be more successful (107, 109, 110, 123, 124).

Other authors believe that for cerebral palsy, careful preoperative clinical evaluation alone is sufficient to determine the appropriateness of a tibialis posterior tendon transfer (122, 125). For example, a positive tiptoe test result indicates that the posterior tibial tendon is most likely the active deforming force (126).

Whether the patient has paraplegia or hemiplegia does not seem to make any difference (107). However, tendon transfer is not recommended for the quadriplegic individual (122).

Because of the large incidence of reverse deformity, tendon transfer for the spastic patient must be selected judiciously on the basis of these principles. Attention must first be paid to the equinus. In fact, when equinovalgus or equinovarus is evident, the frontal plane component of the deformity may reduce with correction of the equinus (127).

Finally, in dealing with spastic muscles, it is usually desirable that the muscle be weakened to reduce the effects of the spasticity. The fact that muscles lose about one grade of strength when they are transferred helps fulfill this objective.

CONDITIONS INVOLVING THE FIRST METATARSOPHALANGEAL JOINT

A useful tendon transfer for maintenance of hallux abductovalgus correction is that of the adductor hallucis. On its release the tendon may be reattached to the medial intracapsular tissue or to the lateral extracapsular structures. The principle involved is to release the deforming force from the hallux and apply it as a dynamic method to assist in maintaining first metatarsal alignment. Details of the technique are discussed in the chapter on hallux abductovalgus surgery.

Transfer of the tendon of the abductor hallucis from the medial to the lateral side of the hallux is effective in tendon-capsule balance correction of hallux varus deformity (128). The tendon is routed through a channel created between the plantar first metatarsal and the flexor hallucis brevis.

The Jones tendon transfer in conjunction with interphalangeal joint fusion of the hallux will correct a reducible hammered great toe deformity (129). The transfer is useful to prevent extension contracture or hammering of the great toe, when both hallucal sesamoid bones must be removed.

Transfer tenodesis of the flexor hallucis longus tendon into the plantar proximal phalanx has been effective for correction of paralytic clawing of the hallux in children (130). This approach has the advantage of avoiding arthrodesis of the interphalangeal joint, a difficult procedure in young children and one that may retard the growth of the hallux. It is also a useful adjunctive procedure to prevent hammering of the hallux when both sesamoids are removed.

CONDITIONS INVOLVING THE LESSER TOES

Flexible hammer toes can achieve a dynamic correction by means of transfer of the flexor digitorum longus tendon slip dorsally around the shaft of the proximal phalanx (131-133). The tendon may either be wrapped around the bone and sutured on itself (134), split and sutured together dorsally (131), or passed through a drill hole in the neck of the proximal phalanx and sutured into the extensor tendons dorsally (135, 136). If the hammer toe is less reducible, the head of the proximal phalanx may be resected and the tendon anchored about the remaining shaft (131). This tendon transfer is quite effective when a noncorrectable triceps equinus deformity is the source of the muscle imbalance causing the hammer toes.

The Hibbs procedure releases the extensor tendon contractures that produce hammer toes and then increases dorsiflexory power of the foot by bunching the tendon slips together and transferring them into the midfoot. If necessary the extensor hallucis longus can be included and the hallux interphalangeal joint fused. The distal stumps of the longus tendons are sutured into their corresponding brevis tendons to allow for active dorsiflexion of the toes. The proximal interphalangeal joints require arthrodesis only if they are nonreducible in the face of a flexible forefoot equinus deformity.

Tendon transfer procedures for correction of fifth toe deformities are discussed in detail elsewhere in the text. It

should be remembered that for tendon transfers to be successful for digital realignment the deformities must be reducible.

EQUINUS FOOT

Of the various types of equinus deformities of the foot, forefoot and metatarsal equinus responds best to treatment with tendon transpositions about the dorsum of the foot. Each deformity, defined by the level of the foot at which plantarflexion of the distal structures takes place, is best seen with the foot hanging at rest (Fig. 50.28). Any existent triceps contractures or osseous ankle equinus must be first corrected if tendon transfers are to be effective in treating forefoot or metatarsal equinus (25, 26).

The goal of these tendon transpositions is to eliminate the retrograde force of the hyperextended or contracted digits on the metatarsal heads that, when present, results in an increased angle of declination of the metatarsal bones, plantar keratoses, and clawtoes (Fig. 50.29). Specifically the idea is to eliminate the swing phase substitution and resting forefoot equinus caused by loading of the long extensors to the toes (25). Such retrograde forces serve only to perpetuate the metatarsal equinus and produce clawtoes that will become less flexible the longer they are left untreated. The resulting deformities seen with forefoot equinus have been variously described as claw foot, clawtoes, Shaffer's foot, and cavovarus foot (67).

Tendon transfers to manage forefoot equinus have been reviewed (26) and include the Hibbs tendosuspension (134), the split tibialis anterior tendon transposition (STATT) (21,

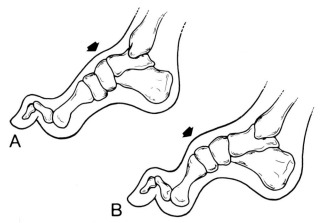

Figure 50.28. **A.** Forefoot equinus. This deformity consists of plantarflexion of forefoot on rearfoot at level of midtarsal joint. Note pathognomonic bulge overlying head of talus on dorsum of foot. Also, dorsally contracted digits apply retrograde plantarflexion at metatarsal heads, further accentuating deformity. **B.** Metatarsal equinus. This deformity consists of plantarflexion of forefoot on lesser tarsus occurring at tarsometatarsal joint level. Note pathognomonic bulge dorsally at metatarsal cuneiform joint level. Again, dorsally contracted digits apply retrograde plantarflexion at metatarsal heads, further accentuating deformity. (From McGlamry ED, Butlin WE, Ruch JA: Treatment of forefoot equinus by tendon transpositions. *J Am Podiatry Assoc* 65:872-888, 1975.)

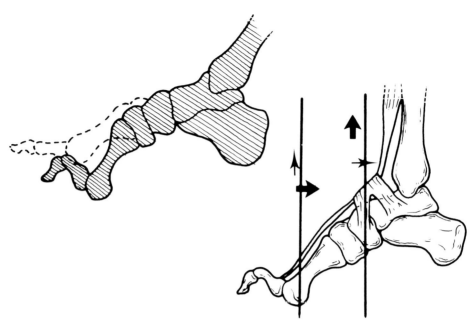

Figure 50.29. Realigning forefoot into more dorsiflexed position requires insertion of transferred tendon into dorsum of foot. Most effective lever arm for dorsiflexion is provided by proximal insertion of tendon where there is sharp angle of approach. More distal insertion less dorsi-flexory power. (From McGlamry ED, Butlin WE, Ruch JA: Treatment of forefoot equinus by tendon transpositions. *J Am Podiatry Assoc* 65:872-888, 1975.)

137), the tibialis anterior tendon transposition (20, 67), the Jones or Heyman pan metatarsal suspension (24, 138, 139), the peroneus longus tendon transposition (15, 67), and the tibialis posterior transposition (106, 140).

FLATFOOT

It is fairly well accepted that tendons by themselves will not provide architectural support for the medial longitudinal arch of the foot. However, they do provide a considerable amount of stability, the loss of which is readily seen when an important muscle such as the tibialis posterior loses its integrity or power. A progressive pes planovalgus deformity ensues, usually with a significant amount of forefoot abduction. Thus the use of tendons in treating flatfoot is intended to take advantage of their stabilizing influence.

The Young procedure is really a tendon transposition because it is rerouted through a key slot in the navicular (22, 23, 141). The Kidner procedure actually requires advancement of the tibialis posterior tendon, classically inferior to the navicular bone (142) or modified to the medial cuneiform to increase its adductory influence on the forefoot. Both procedures are reviewed in the chapter on pes valgus deformity.

ANKLE INSTABILITY

Tendons or portions of tendons are used in a variety of procedures to stabilize the ankle joint laterally. In these surgeries the transferred or translocated tendon is actually converted into a ligament as far as func-tion goes. Nevertheless tendon transfer principles must be carefully observed, especially in harvesting the tendon. This subject is covered in detail in chapter on ankle surgery.

Descriptions of Common Tendon Transvers

Several tendon surgeries have passed the test of time and experience and are very useful tools in foot and leg surgery. These have been reviewed and this section follows much of that format (29). It may be necessary to transfer various combinations of tendons to achieve optimal results. This should pose no problem as long as the principles described are followed in detail.

JONES SUSPENSION PROCEDURES

TECHNIQUE. The extensor hallucis longus tendon is first transected at the interphalangeal joint of the hallux. It is then rerouted through a medial-to-lateral drill hole in the head of the first metatarsal and sutured back to itself dorsally. The stump of the longus is then attached to the extensor hallucis brevis tendon to maintain some extensor function to the great toe. To prevent hammering of the hallux the interphalangeal joint requires arthrodesis (Fig. 50.30).

GOALS. The Jones suspension procedure is used to correct or prevent cockup of the hallux by eliminating the deforming force on the digit. Thus the retrograde buckling at the first metatarsophalangeal joint is released, and the extensor hallucis longus tendon changes function to dorsiflex the first

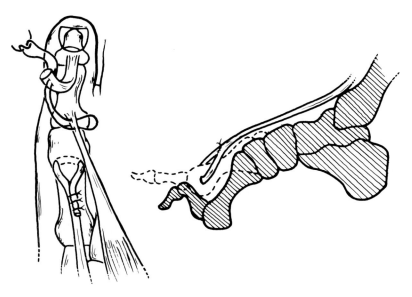

Figure 50.30. Jones suspension procedure. Extensor hallucis longus tendon is released and rerouted through first metatarsal neck, with distal stump attached to extensor hallucis brevis tendon.

metatarsal. This procedure is recommended for the following circumstances:

1. Flexible cavus foot (143)
2. Flexible plantarflexed first ray, with or without hammered hallux (26, 143)
3. Prophylaxis when both hallucal sesamoid bones are removed

RESULTS AND COMPLICATIONS. The panmetatarsal Jones suspension (25, 139, 144) for lesser metatarsals was found to be inadequate over longer periods (24). In young children the procedure is unsatisfactory because of the tendency of the long extensor to regenerate and return to its normal insertion at the distal phalanx and because of difficulty in fusing the interphalangeal joint near a growth center (130).

HIBBS TENDOSUSPENSION

TECHNIQUE. Through two separate incisions or one curvilinear incision the extensor digitorum longus tendons are detached far enough distally so they may be combined and undergo tenodesis into the midfoot (134). The ideal location is the base of the third metatarsal or the third cuneiform bone. The distal stumps of the longus tendons are sutured to the corresponding brevis tendon. The fourth and fifth longus slips must be attached to the fourth brevis slip (Fig. 50.31).

In addition, the tendon of the extensor hallucis longus can be similarly released and transferred with those of the extensor digitorum longus. Another modification is to combine a Jones tendon suspension with the basic Hibbs procedure if the medial segment of the foot needs adjustment (25, 26, 67) (Fig. 50.32).

GOALS. The Hibbs procedure is performed primarily to release the retrograde buckling at the metatarsophalangeal

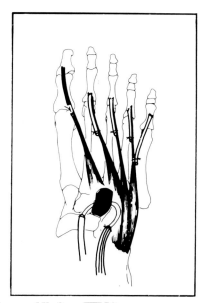

Figure 50.31. Modified Hibbs tendosuspension technique. Extensor hallucis longus tendon can be included in transfer if deemed necessary. (From McGlamry ED, Kitting, RW: Surgery of the equinus foot. In McGlamry ED [ed]: *Reconstructive Surgery of the Foot and Leg.* Miami, Symposia Specialists, 1974, p 347.)

joints. The plantarflexory forces causing the flexible forefoot equinus are released, and the dorsiflexory power of the foot is enhanced. This procedure or its modification is recommended for the following conditions:

1. Flexible forefoot or metatarsal equinus with or without clawtoes (26)
2. Flexible cavus deformity with clawtoes secondary to extensor substitution phenomenon (25, 67, 134)

RESULTS AND COMPLICATIONS. Skin sloughs from the dorsal foot may occur if there is sufficient disruption of vascular

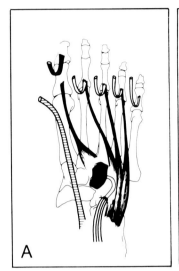
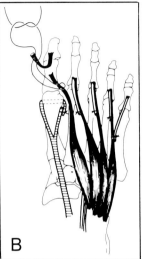

Figure 50.32. **A** and **B.** Combination Hibbs tendosuspension and Jones tendosuspension procedures. (From McGlamry ED, Kitting, RW: Surgery of the equinus foot. In McGlamry ED [ed]: *Reconstructive Surgery of the Foot and Leg.* Miami, Symposia Specialists, 1974, p 347.)

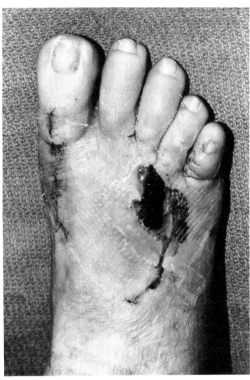

Figure 50.33. Ulcer from dorsal skin slough following Hibbs procedure. Patient developed hematoma in cast after fall.

vascular supply (Fig. 50.33). Dorsal anesthesia may be avoided by observing for and protecting the branches of the superficial peroneal nerve during dissection. Excessive tension may produce a tendonitis of the long extensor tendons beneath the cruciate ligaments, best treated with compression bandages and moist heat.

The major question is whether to fuse the proximal interphalangeal joints of the lesser toes. A simple rule to follow is that if the toes are completely flexible at the metatarsophalangeal and interphalangeal joints as evidenced by the Kelikian push-up test, then arthrodesis is not necessary. If the toes do not lie down after release of the long extensors, metatarsophalangeal joint releases must be done.

SPLIT TIBIALIS ANTERIOR TENDON TRANSFER

TECHNIQUE. The STATT procedure requires three incisions to move approximately one half of the tibialis anterior tendon laterally. The first incision is near the tendon's insertion, and the second is over the tibialis anterior at the anterior surface of the leg just above the transverse cruciate ligament. The tendon is split to its insertion, and the lateral fibers are drawn up through the second wound. A third incision is made over the peroneus tertius tendon about 1 inch proximal to its insertion, and the foot is placed in a position of slight eversion while dorsiflexed to neutral. The split tendon is then passed down through the peroneus tertius sheath (same as the extensor longus) and sutured to its tendon. If it is absent (and this should be known before surgery), then the transposed fibers must undergo tenodesis into the cuboid bone or attached to all or part of the peroneus brevis tendon (21, 145) (Figs. 50.11 and 50.34).

GOALS. The goal of the STATT procedure is to increase the true dorsiflexion of the foot by balancing its power laterally, somewhat like a yoke (145). Swing-phase loading of the long extensors on the toes is relieved, and the foot no longer assumes a varus or cavovarus position that would otherwise lose its flexibility over time (26).

Other adjunctive procedures may have to be performed. These include dorsiflexory osteotomy of the first metatarsal, claw-toe correction, calcaneal osteotomy, or triceps lengthening. The STATT procedure is recommended for the following conditions:

1. Spastic rearfoot varus (145)
2. Fixed equinovarus (145)
3. Excessive invertor power relative to evertor power (29)
4. Forefoot equinus with swing-phase extensor substitution and claw toes (21)
5. Flexible cavovarus deformity (137)
6. Excessive supination in gait (29)
7. Dorsiflexory weakness (29)

RESULTS AND COMPLICATIONS. Transient tenosynovitis is the most common complication, with the same mechanism and treatment previously described. Nerve damage may also occur but with attention to detail should be rarely encountered.

The STATT procedure has been successful in converting spastic varus dorsiflexion by the tibialis anterior muscle into pure dorsiflexion (145). It is a relatively simple procedure with little danger of overcorrection (137).

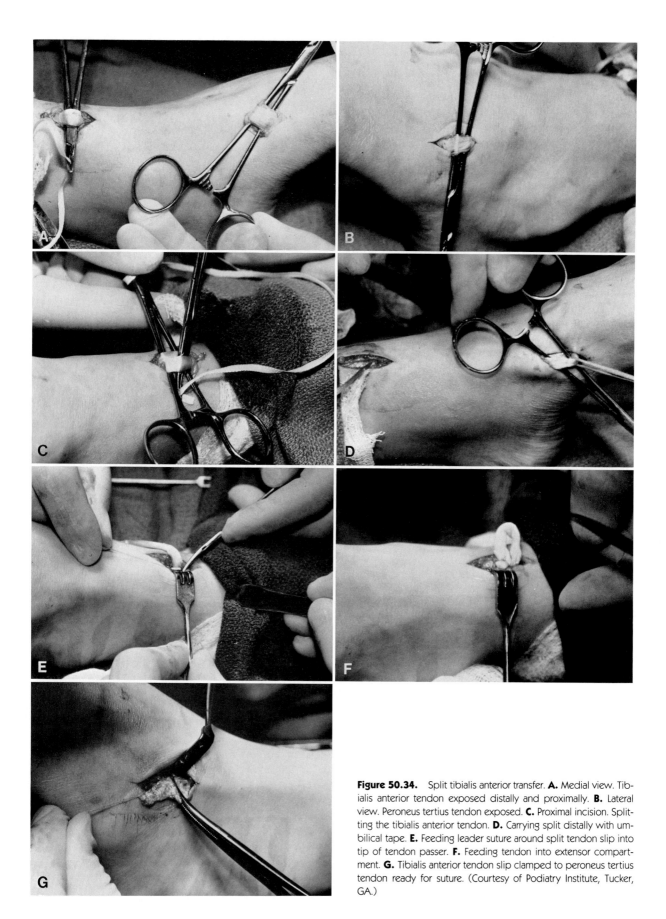

Figure 50.34. Split tibialis anterior transfer. **A.** Medial view. Tibialis anterior tendon exposed distally and proximally. **B.** Lateral view. Peroneus tertius tendon exposed. **C.** Proximal incision. Splitting the tibialis anterior tendon. **D.** Carrying split distally with umbilical tape. **E.** Feeding leader suture around split tendon slip into tip of tendon passer. **F.** Feeding tendon into extensor compartment. **G.** Tibialis anterior tendon slip clamped to peroneus tertius tendon ready for suture. (Courtesy of Podiatry Institute, Tucker, GA.)

TIBIALIS ANTERIOR TENDON TRANSFER

TECHNIQUE. Transfer of the tibialis anterior tendon involves releasing it from its insertion (first incision), drawing it proximally through its sheath to the anterior lower leg (second incision), and moving it laterally. Usually it is transferred into the third cuneiform bone (third incision) once it has been transposed through the long extensor sheath within the same muscle compartment (25, 26, 67). The foot must be positioned in neutral or slight plantarflexion for fixation (Fig. 50.35).

GOALS. The principal goal of the tibialis anterior tendon transfer is to reduce supinatory forces in the foot. It will also increase dorsiflexion strength if other dorsiflexors are weak or absent as in drop foot of most etiologies. The procedure is recommended for the following conditions:

1. Recurrent clubfoot (20, 146, 147)
2. Flexible forefoot equinus (20, 26)
3. Drop foot (20)
4. Tarsometatarsal amputation (148)
5. Charcot-Marie-Tooth deformity (147, 149, 150)

Other procedures may be required to provide stabilization through which the transferred tendon can function effectively. Triceps or gastrocnemius lengthening may be necessary.

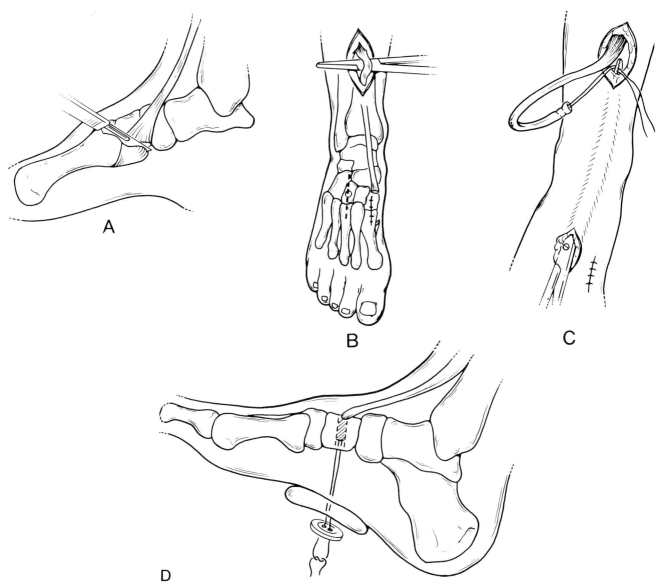

Figure 50.35. Tibialis anterior tendon transfer technique. **A.** Detachment of tibialis anterial tendon. **B.** Retrieval of tendon through proximal incision. **C.** Passing of tendon through extensor compartment using retrograde tendon passer. **D.** Attachment of transferred tendon into third cuneiform. This site can be selected anywhere on dorsal structures to balance foot. (From McGlamry ED, Kitting, RW: Surgery of the equinus foot. In McGlamry ED [ed]: *Reconstructive Surgery of the Foot and Leg*. Miami, Symposia Specialists, 1974, p 347.)

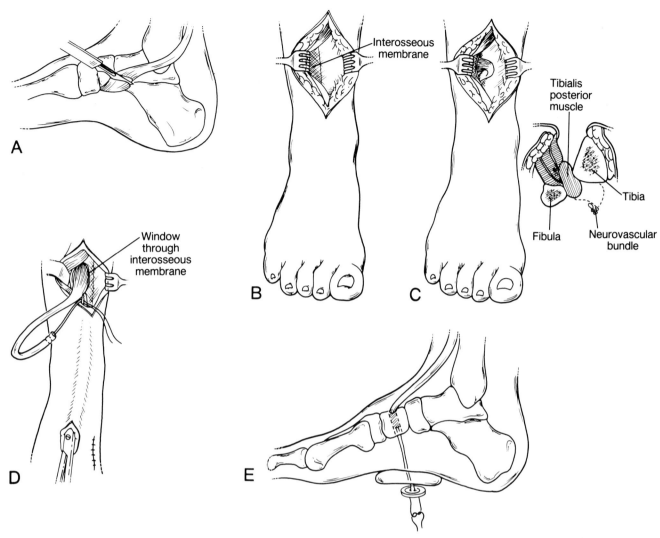

Figure 50.36. Tibialis posterior tendon transfer through interosseous membrane (technique 1). **A.** Detachment of tibialis posterior tendon at medial navicular bone. **B.** Exposing interosseous membrane and locating surrounding structures. **C.** Retrieving posterior tibial muscle and tendon. Tibialis posterior muscle belly lies immediately beneath interosseous mem-brane. Note location of neurovascular structures. Care must be taken not to detach muscle from its nerve and blood supply. **D.** Passing posterior tibial tendon distally through extensor compartment beneath retinacula. **E.** Attachment of tendon into dorsal bony structures.

RESULTS AND COMPLICATIONS. Great controversy exists over the use of tibialis anterior tendon transfer for correction of clubfoot deformities, especially those that are congenital or recurrent (109, 146, 147, 150-152). This is best discussed in the chapter dealing with clubfoot. Lehman also gives a clear and concise review of its application (152).

Tenosynovitis at the cruciate ligaments and nerve damage may be complications. If the tendon is transferred too far laterally, a severe pes planovalgus deformity may result. Excessive tension may similarly lead to disaster (67). If the muscle goes into tension-induced spasm, muscle relaxants may be required until the tissue accommodates itself. Generally, the STATT modification has proved more reliable without sacrificing any of the benefits of complete tendon transfer.

TIBIALIS POSTERIOR TENDON TRANSFER

TECHNIQUE. Two main techniques have been described for transferring the tibialis posterior tendon to the dorsum of the foot. The first uses three incisions: one to release the tendon, one to fixate the transferred tendon, and one on the anterior leg by which to draw the tendon through the interosseous membrane. Initially the tendon is released from its attachments at the navicular bone. Then the incision is made on the anterior leg just at the level of the middle and distal third and about 1 cm lateral to the tibial crest. The tibialis anterior muscle belly is separated from the lateral surface of the tibia and the interosseous membrane exposed. The latter structure is gently windowed. Usually visible when the posterior muscle mass is compressed, the tibialis posterior tendon is maneuvered through the window with blunt curved Kelly forceps and moist sponges. Care must be taken not to damage the neurovascular bundle lying just under the tibialis posterior muscle belly (Fig. 50.36). Now the muscle and tendon are drawn up through the opening. Often there are small segments of muscle attached distal to the window. These must be gently pulled free. Finally, an instrument (Bozeman forceps, Ober tendon passer, uterine packing forceps) is retrograded through the third incision up the extensor sheath to accept the tibialis posterior tendon and to draw it distally. It is fixated to the third cuneiform with the foot in a neutral position relative to the leg (15, 71, 106, 109, 140).

The second technique, with four incisions, consists of the same two approaches for release and attachment of the tendon but uses a posteromedial incision on the leg to pass the tendon anteriorly through the interosseous membrane. This approach helps free the tibialis posterior from its attachments to the tibia. The anterior leg incision is still necessary to draw the tendon distally through the extensor compartment (152-155) (Figs. 50.37 and 50.38).

As an alternative to bony insertion on the dorsum of the foot, the posterior tibial tendon may be split, with one half passed laterally to attach to the peroneus tertius tendon and one half passed medially through the sheath of the tibialis anterior to attach to the tendon near its insertion (29). The tendon must be split from proximal to distal, preferably with umbilical tape. The appropriate sheath must be used through which to pass the split tendons.

GOALS. The tibialis posterior is a very strong muscle and has the potential to provide good dorsiflexory power when replacement is needed. Transfer to the dorsum of the foot involves switching it from a stance-phase muscle to a swing-

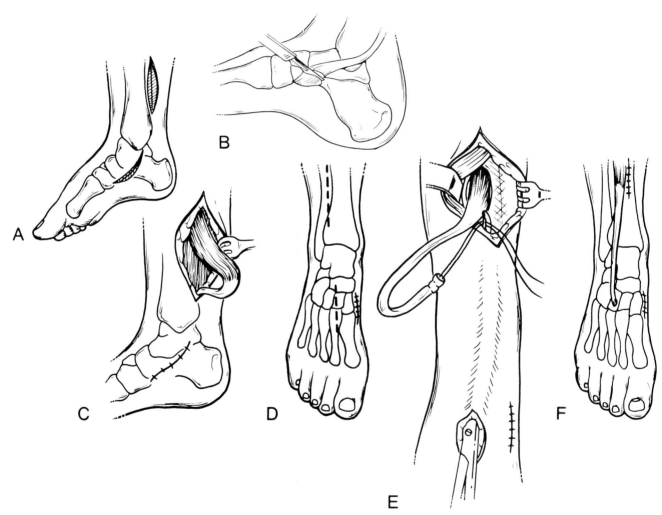

Figure 50.37. Tibialis posterior tendon transfer through interosseous membrane (technique 2). **A.** Location of medial foot and leg incisions. **B.** Detachment of posterior tibial tendon at its insertion. Preservation of maximum length is important. **C.** Retrieval of posterior tibial muscle and tendon into proximal wound using two-hand sponge technique. **D.** Location of incisions on the anterior leg and dorsal foot. **E.** Tendon is delivered through interosseous membrane and passed down extensor compartment beneath retinacula. **F.** Attachment of tendon into dorsal osseous structures. Posterior tibial tendon can be split and attached to tibialis anterior and peroneus tertius tendons, respectively, for more balanced suspension.

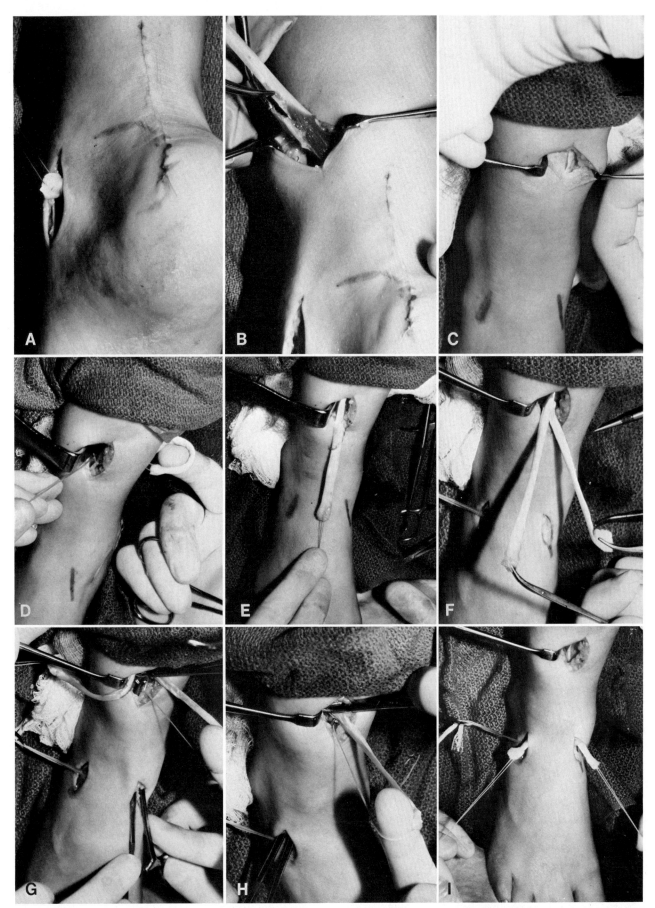

Figure 50.38. Tibialis posterior tendon transfer (technique 2). **A.** Posteromedial view of heel and ankle (tendon of Achilles lengthening has been performed). Tibialis posterior tendon released from insertion. **B.** Tendon drawn up through posteromedial incision. **C.** Anterior lower leg. Exposing interosseous membrane. Note transfer incisions marked distally. **D.** Passing tendon from posteromedial through interosseous membrane anteriorly. **E.** Tendon delivered anteriorly. **F.** Tendon split. **G.** Tendon forceps in tibialis anterior tendon compartment for medial slip of tibialis posterior tendon. **H.** Tendon forceps in extensor compartment preparing to pass lateral slip of tibialis posterior tendon to peroneus tertius. **I.** Split posterior tibial tendons in position to anchor.

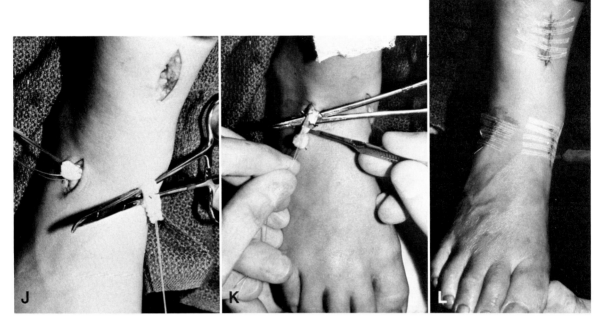

Figure 50.38. **J-L.** **J.** Suturing medial slip to tibialis anterior. **K.** Suturing lateral slip to peroneus tertius. **L.** Final closure with foot in neutral position. (Courtesy of Podiatry Institute, Tucker, GA.)

phase muscle. This will require well-planned physical therapy and retraining that ideally should begin even before surgery. The fact is that preoperative muscle education is helpful in postsurgical rehabilitation. Because the procedure is technically difficult, case selection is important. Tibialis posterior tendon transfer is recommended for the following conditions:

1. Weak or paralyzed anterior muscle group (106, 156)
2. Equinovarus deformity (106, 140, 157, 158)
3. Spastic equinovarus deformity (107, 122, 159-161)
4. Recurrent clubfoot deformity (106, 152, 162-165)
5. Drop foot (154, 166)
6. Charcot-Marie-Tooth disease foot deformities (147, 150, 167)
7. Permanent peroneal nerve palsy (168, 169)
8. Leprosy (170, 171)

RESULTS AND COMPLICATIONS. Controversy exists regarding the effectiveness of this transfer in spastic conditions. In many instances it may lead to worse deformities than those present before surgery (67, 106, 172-174). Because the tibialis posterior stabilizes the subtalar and midtarsal joints against pronation, loss of its insertion can lead to the rapid development of severe pes planovalgus deformity with a prominent abductory component (29, 175). The tendency for subsequent deformity may be largely circumvented by concomitant triple arthrodesis. A procedure of this nature is required in many instances because of the nature of the coexistent disease process.

Considerable success has been reported by others in correcting spastic equinovarus deformity with this tendon transfer in patients with cerebral palsy (120, 122, 160, 161). Active dorsiflexion may be accomplished in the majority of cases, especially when swing phase firing is present on the preoperative electromyography study (107, 108, 159). Phasic conversion is not to be expected with spastic disease.

Tibialis posterior tendon transfer may be used in recurrent clubfoot if there is lateral weakness in the foot. Here it can correct residual or recurrent equinovarus deformity. It will not be effective in the face of fixed deformities (152).

In general, tibialis posterior tendons transferred to the dorsum of the foot tend to regain their function (67, 109, 140, 168). However, as accurately depicted by Close and Todd (66) in their study using electromyographic oscillograms, the tibialis posterior muscle, for the most part, retains its stance-phase activity. In most cases the patient can achieve a level of voluntary and active dorsiflexion with the transferred muscle but without conversion to automatic swing phase function.

Even though the tibialis posterior tendon is a relatively strong muscle, it has a short excursion compared with the full range of motion available at the ankle. Therefore ankle dorsiflexion will be limited for this tendon transfer (159).

McGlamry has pointed out that tendons transferred for correction of equinus or drop foot serve a useful function by providing a check-rein effect on the foot, preventing it from dropping into equinus—even when there is no phase conversion. It does so by means of the stretch reflex. When a resting muscle is stretched, it responds by contracting. Thus, as the forward transferred tibialis posterior tendon and muscle are fixed under physiological tension, a constant tone of contraction can be elicited through the stretch reflex. Such tone will provide a constant monitoring or check-rein against the foot dropping into unopposed equinus (67). This same physiological principle, sometimes called *tenodesis effect* (107), may be applied to any other tendon transferred to the dorsum of the foot.

PERONEUS LONGUS TENDON TRANSFER

TECHNIQUE. The initial incision for this procedure is made at the junction of the middle and lower third of the lateral leg. The peroneus longus tendon lies superficial to the brevis; thus it is quickly isolated. The second incision is made along the lateral cuboid where the peroneus longus courses inferiorly into the plantar peroneal tunnel. The tendon is identified by tugging gently on it at the proximal incision; then it is sutured to the peroneus brevis before its release, so that the first metatarsal has some resistance against the tibialis anterior. The tendon is then withdrawn proximally and transferred into the anterior compartment through the anterolateral intermuscular septum. The tendon is delivered down the extensor pathway beneath the cruciate retinaculum and attached into the base of the third metatarsal, third cuneiform, or split and sutured by means of the technique already described (15, 26, 29, 67) (Fig. 50.39).

GOALS. The peroneus longus tendon transfer is an effective treatment for loss of dorsiflexory muscle power. It is surprisingly strong in its ability. Often it is combined with other tendon transfers to achieve the same purpose (67). Recommendations for its use include the following conditions:

1. Anterior muscle group weakness or paralysis
2. Drop foot deformity

Many other uses for this tendon have been described; however, the technique noted here is the one most commonly employed in foot surgery. The tendon has been translocated to replace a paralyzed tibialis posterior with consid-

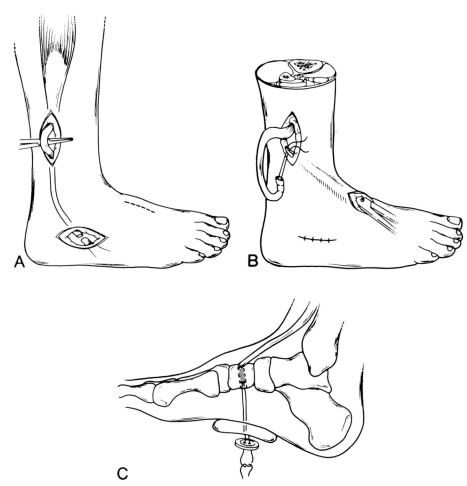

Figure 50.39. Peroneus longus tendon transfer technique. **A.** Locating peroneus longus tendon on lateral aspect of leg. It lies superficial to peroneus brevis. Detachment of peroneus longus tendon near cuboid bone. Stump of longus should be sutured to brevis tendon. **B.** Passing peroneus longus tendon through lateral intermuscular septum and down extensor compartment. **C.** Attachment of tendon into dorsum of foot. This tendon can also be split and attached to tibialis anterior and peroneus tertius tendons to balance suspension.

erable success (175). Further, the peroneus longus is a popular muscle for transfer into the posterior calcaneus to function effectively as a plantarflexor in paralytic calcaneus deformities (72, 121, 176-178).

RESULTS AND COMPLICATIONS. In a high percentage of cases the peroneus longus can switch gait phases (66). It is a fairly strong muscle, lending to its versatility. The complications are generally the same as for other transfers, but few have been reported.

PERONEUS BREVIS TENDON TRANSFER

TECHNIQUE. The peroneus brevis tendon transfer is approached and performed in a manner similar to that for the peroneus longus. It is a relatively simple task that is modified by the purpose for which the tendon is transferred (179).

GOALS. The goals of this transfer are very similar to those for the peroneus longus. It is an easy tendon to access and move.

RESULTS AND COMPLICATIONS. The peroneus brevis will change phases almost spontaneously when required to do so (66, 104). It is the tendon of choice for most ankle stabilizations. Complications are similar to those found in previous discussions (179).

Postsurgical Treatment

IMMOBILIZATION

Tendon must remain quiescent to heal and reestablish local vasculature. It is best to immobilize the limb in a cast at the time of the surgery, making the necessary allowances for swelling. Redressings and cast changes will only increase the possibility of rupturing the tendon from its new insertion. The cast may be removed at 4 weeks following a tendon repair or tendon-to-tendon anastomosis. If additional surgery is performed, such as arthrodesis, then immobilization must be for the full 6 weeks or more, although the cast may be changed after the third week. With a bivalved cast, gentle active exercise against no resistance can be instituted after 3 weeks. The latter approach assumes solid internal fixation of any arthrodeses that may have been performed. The foot should always be immobilized in a neutral position and at a right angle to the leg.

MOVEMENT

Early movement is essential to prevent long-lasting adhesion formation. By about 3 weeks after the surgery the callus of granulation tissue about the tendon will begin to release itself. At this stage early passive range of motion exercises will help mobilize the tendon and prevent restriction. The recovery of strength is not necessary to achieve this purpose. Converting immobilization by bivalving a cast will allow the patient the freedom to perform these exercises and then reapply the cast for other activities.

ESTABLISHING FUNCTION

Obtaining adequate strength and initiating function are dual goals for rehabilitation of tendon transfers. Often about the third week in a cast, gentle isometric efforts against the cast will help stimulate and strengthen the muscle. With such stimulation the randomly placed collagen fibers will realign themselves parallel for strength (41, 42). Once active range of motion has been achieved after appropriate immobilization, strength may be built at first simply with progressive weight-bearing exercise.

Sometimes passive range of motion movements are necessary to stretch the muscle-tendon unit and familiarize it with its desired function. Early passive motion also helps prevent adhesions.

Electrical stimulation, if used, should be applied only during the very early stages of rehabilitation. Because the transferred muscle is already innervated, voluntary stimulation and activity are the ultimate goals.

Isometric exercises are the mainstay for increasing strength through voluntary contraction. Any contraction will produce tension within a muscle. Duration or even force of the contraction is not nearly as important as is repetition. Once the desired movement can be made with sufficient strength, isokinetic exercise may be prescribed to develop smooth, coordinated contraction through the muscle's range of motion.

ESTABLISHING PHASE

If a muscle is transferred to function within its own phase, then simply establishing its contractile ability and strength is often sufficient. Sometimes reeducation at its new function requires a little more concentration. At first the patient is carefully instructed as to the desired function of the muscle at its new position. Then the patient is told to perform the function the muscle did before the transfer. This is repeated until the patient begins to see the new function and performs it well. When it can be performed automatically and with little effort, then the patient is ready for gait training to incorporate the newly functioning tendon.

Whether a muscle is transferred within its phase, but especially when transferred out of its phase, postoperative reeducation is greatly facilitated by teaching the patient to localize and contract the involved muscle before surgery. Once the cast has been removed, the patient is asked to carry out the same motion that produced a good contraction before the operation. As this is done, the foot will perform its new function (e.g., dorsiflexion) by way of the newly transferred tendon. This activity is repeated until the movement is performed without premeditation.

Now the involved muscle must be incorporated into the normal gait pattern using its new function. This is accomplished by first having the patient practice taking a single step. This is methodically repeated, slowly at first, making sure the muscle contracts through the appropriate phase of gait, until it becomes a conditioned reflex. Finally, the patient is permitted to accelerate the gait cycle as the function becomes automatic.

Visual and electromyographic biofeedback techniques may be used as adjunctive therapy, useful for reeducating transferred muscles. Mirrors can provide visual reinforcement for the patient who can see movement produced at his or her own volition. However, audiovisual facilitation may be produced by means of electromyographic biofeedback. Small portable myotrains can be taken home with the patient for continued therapy. By observing the meter on the myotrainer, with electrodes in place, the patient and the therapist actually see the muscle functioning, and this reinforcement helps achieve better control. Most myotrainers have threshold levels of sensitivity that can be preset by the operator. When muscle activity exceeds this threshold, as the instrument picks up the local electrical activity, a tone or meter needle will register a response. This allows the patient or therapist to set specific goals during muscle reeducation (160-162, 180-183).

INTRATENDINOUS LESIONS

Lesions occurring within the substance of a tendon must be clearly differentiated from peritendinous or synovial lesions.For example, tuberculosis will affect only tendon sheath and will not become intratendinous (184). However, ganglion cysts may arise from the peritendinous tissue and then localize and enlarge among the tendon fibers (185, 186)(Table 50.6).

Tumors

GIANT CELL TUMOR OF TENDON SHEATH

Giant cell tumor of tendon sheath is a peritendinous lesion made up of cells derived from the synovial tissue. It is a slow-growing mass, generally benign and reactive in nature. It is thought to form in response to trauma bordering in the category of a true neoplasm. Histologically, the lesion has been described as a variant of pigmented villonodular synovitis (187). Hemosiderian deposits and fatty infiltration account for the brownish yellow to rusty color of this tumorous mass. Treatment of choice is surgical extirpation

Table 50.6.
Intradendinous Lesions

Tumors
    Giant cell tumor of tendon sheath
    Fibroma of tendon sheath
    Synovial sarcoma
    Clear cell sarcoma of tendons and aponeuroses
Non-Tumors
    Xanthoma
    Ossifications
    Rheumatoid nodule
    Necrosis

with definitive removal inasmuch as recurrence rates are high (188).

FIBROMA OF TENDON SHEATH

Although related to the giant cell tumor, fibroma of tendon sheath differs in that it is composed of fibroblastic cells and also grows in the peritendinous tissue (189, 190). Trauma is also thought to be an inciting factor. As with the other benign lesions, when found within tendon, the mass must be excised and the tendon reconstructed, either locally or with a free tendon graft.

SYNOVIAL SARCOMA

Synovial sarcoma is a primary malignant tumor of mesenchymal origin that arises usually from joints but can also arise from tendons or bursae. The affected patient is typically young, generally 20 to 40 years, with males more commonly afflicted.The lesions occur mostly about the feet and ankles, growing slowly with distant metastases being spread via blood and lymph transport. Synovial sarcoma is not radiosensitive. Treatment consists of wide resection or amputation with or without follow-up chemotherapy. Even with treatment, the 5-year survival rate ranges from 35% to 50%.

CLEAR CELL SARCOMA OF TENDONS AND APONEUROSES

Clear cell sarcoma is a rare, malignant, slow-growing, and usually painless tumor found mostly in the foot and ankle region (191). It may be melanocytic or mesenchymal in origin, the latter similar to synovial sarcoma. Arising from tendon and aponeuroses, this neoplasm lacks aggressiveness although metastases are common. Wide excision with regional lymph node dissection or amputation if around articulations are treatments of choice. Recurrence is common with a mortality rate of about 50% (192).

NON-TUMORS

XANTHOMA. There have been several case reports of intratendinous xanthomas throughout the literature, usually involving the Achilles tendon (193-197). The tumor-like nodules result from accumulated endocytosis of circulating lipids by mesenchymal cells (typically histiocytes). Foam cells with multinucleated giant cells are characteristic histological features. The lesions are associated with familial types II and III hyperbetalipoproteinemia. Biopsy specimens may show birefringent crystals, which must be differentiated from calcium pyrophosphate dihydrate crystals. When the condition is painful and unresponsive to conservative measures, surgical excision is recommended. When there is extensive involvement, total or subtotal tendon resection is necessary, requiring tendon reconstruction with autografts or fascia.

OSSIFICATIONS. Extra-articular ossification commonly occurs in the Achilles tendon, usually just proximal to its insertion (193, 198-200). Trauma or irritation are thought to be instigating factors. Pain may be a consequence of fracture or chronic inflammation, and the calcific deposits should be extirpated in these instances. If extensive, they should be totally resected and the tendon reconstructed.

RHEUMATOID NODULE. Usually seen in patients with well-established rheumatoid arthritis, rheumatoid nodules can occur adjacent to or extend within tendons. They are often symmetrical and bilateral and have a multilobulated appearance when excised. When painful, they should be removed surgically, although there is a very high recurrence rate.

NECROSIS. Chronic inflammation and repetitive trauma may lead to areas of intratendinous necrosis. Sometimes these areas are palpably enlarged. Untreated, they may lead to rupture of the tendon. The Achilles tendon is most commonly involved, especially the relatively avascular area 2 to 6 cm proximal to the Achilles insertion (201, 202). Surgical intervention is aimed at excising the degenerated portion of the tendon and reconstructing it with grafting if necessary.

References

1. Hurst LN: The healing of tendon. In Kerahan DS, Vistnes LM (eds): *Biological Aspects of Reconstructive Surgery.* New York, Little Brown & Co, 1977, pp 383-389.
2. Erlacher PJ: The development of tendon surgery in Germany. A review of the history and an evaluation of the treatment. *American Academy of Orthopaedic Surgeons Instructional Course Lectures* 13:110-115, 1956.
3. Herndon CH: Tendon transplantation at the knee and foot. *American Academy of Orthopaedic Surgeons Instructional Course Lectures* 18:145-167, 1961.
4. Mayer L: The physiologic method of tendon transplantation. I. Historical, anatomy and physiology of tendons. *Surg Gynecol Obstet* 22:182-197, 1916.
5. Biesalski K, Mayer L: Die physiologische Sehnenver planzung, vol 14. Berlin, Julius Springer, 1916. Quoted in Mayer L: The physiological method of tendon transplantation. I. Historical anatomy and physiology of tendons. *Surg Gynecol Obstet* 22:182-197, 1916.
6. Mayer L: The physiologic method of tendon transplantation. II. Operative technique. *Surg Gynecol Obstet* 22:298-306, 1916.
7. Mayer L: The physiologic method of tendon transplantation. III. Experimental and clinical experiences. *Surg Gynecol Obstet* 22:472-481, 1916.
8. Mayer L: Tendon transplantations on the lower extremity. *American Academy of Orthopaedic Surgeons Instructional Course Lectures* 6:189-200, 1949.
9. Mayer L: The physiologic method of tendon transplants. Reviewed after forty years. *American Academy of Orthopaedic Surgeons Instructional Course Lectures* 13:116-120, 1956.
10. Mayer L: The physiological method of tendon transplantation in the treatment of paralytic dropfoot. *J Bone Joint Surg* 19:389, 1937.
11. Bernstein MA: The clinical aspect of tendon transplantation. *Surg Gynecol Obstet* 34:84, 1922.
12. Bernstein MA: The surgery of tendon transposition with special reference to the importance of the tendon sheath. *Surg Gynecol Obstet* 29:55, 1919.
13. Steindler A: Nutrition and vitality of the tendon in tendon transplantation. *Am J Orthop Surg* 16:63, 1918.
14. Steindler A: *Orthopedic Operations.* Springfield IL, Charles C Thomas, 1940, pp 125-154.
15. Ober FR: Tendon transplantation in the lower extremity. *N Engl J Med* 209:52-59, 1933.
16. Bunnell S: An essential in reconstructive surgery—"atraumatic" technique. *Calif State J Med* 19:204, 1921.
17. Bunnell S: *Surgery of the Hand.* Philadelphia, JB Lippincott, 1956.
18. Bunnell S: Repair of the nerves and tendons of the hand. *J Bone Joint Surg* 10:1, 1928.
19. Bunnell S: Primary repair of severed tendons. The use of stainless steel wire. *Am J Surg* 47:502, 1940.
20. McGlamry ED: Transfer of the tibialis anterior tendon. *J Am Podiatry Assoc* 63:609-617, 1973.
21. McGlamry ED, Ruch JA, Green DR: Simplified technique for split tibialis anterior tendon transposition (STATT procedure). *J Am Podiatry Assoc* 65:927-937, 1975.
22. Beck EL, McGlamry ED, Kitting RW: The Young weakfoot suspension. *J Am Podiatry Assoc* 63:528-529, 1973.
23. Beck EL, McGlamry ED: Modified Young tendosuspension technique for flexible flatfoot analysis of rationale and results: a preliminary report on 20 operations. *J Am Podiatry Assoc* 63:582-604, 1973.
24. McGlamry ED: Unfavorable long-term results in the Jones metatarsal suspension. *J Am Podiatry Assoc* 65:479-480, 1975.
25. McGlamry ED, Kitting RW: Equinus foot: an analysis of the etiology, pathology, and treatment techniques. *J Am Podiatry Assoc* 63:165-184, 1973.
26. McGlamry ED, Butlin WE, Ruch JA: Treatment of forefoot equinus by tendon transpositions. *J Am Podiatry Assoc* 65:872-888, 1975.
27. Sgarlato TE: Transplantation of flexor digitorum longus in hammertoe. *J Am Podiatry Assoc* 60:383-388, 1970.
28. Lawton JH: Repair of tendons and soft tissues. In Marcus SA, Block BH (eds): *American College of Foot Surgeons—Complications in Foot Surgery, Prevention and Management,* ed 2. Baltimore, Williams & Wilkins, 1984, pp 129-162.
29. Fenton CF, Gilman RD, Jassen M, Dollard M, Smith GA: Criteria for selected major tendon transfers in podiatric surgery. *J Am Podiatry Assoc* 73:561-568, 1983.
30. Strickland JW: Flexor tendon injuries. I. Anatomy, physiology, biomechanics, healing, adhesion formation around a repaired tendon. *Orthop Rev* 15:632-645, 1986.
31. Lundborg G, Rank F: Experimental intrinsic healing of flexor tendons based upon synovial fluid nutrition. *J Hand Surg* 3:21-31, 1978.
32. Strates BS: Calcification implants of tendon. *Experientia* 25:924, 1969.
33. Cooper RR, Misol S: Tendon and ligament insertion. *J Bone Joint Surg* 52A:1-20, 1970.
34. Myskiw PM, Pattinian HR, Ricken JA, Solinene A: The attachment of tendon to bone. *J Am Podiatry Assoc* 68:308-312, 1978.
35. Sharpey W, Ellis GV: *Elements of Anatomy by Jones Quain,* vol 1, ed 6. London, Walton & Moberly, 1856.
36. Peacock EE Jr: *Wound Repair,* ed 3. Philadelphia, WB Saunders, 1984, pp 263-331.
37. Lindsay WK, Thomson HG: Digital flexor tendons: an experimental study. I. The significance of each component of the flexor mechanism in tendon healing. *Br J Plast Surg* 12:289-316, 1960.
38. Lindsay WK, Birch JR: The fibroblast in flexor tendon healing. *Plast Reconstr Surg* 34:223, 1964.
39. Potenza AD: Critical evaluation of flexor-tendon healing and adhesion formation within artificial digital sheaths. *J Bone Joint Surg* 45A:1217-1233, 1963.
40. Matthews P, Richards H: The repair potential of digital flexor tendons. *J Bone Joint Surg* 56B:618-624, 1974.
41. Manske PR, Gelberman RH, VandeBerg JS, Lesker PA: Flexor tendon intrinsic repair: a morphological study in vitro. *J Bone Joint Surg* 66A:385-396, 1984.
42. Gelberman RH, Manski PR, VandeBerg JS, Lesker PA: Tendon healing characteristics of the dog, chicken, rabbit and monkey in vitro. *J Orthop Res* 2:39-48, 1984.
43. Ketchum LD: Tendon healing. In Hunt TK, Dunphy JE (eds): *Fundamentals of Wound Management.* New York, Appleton-CenturyCrofts, 1979, pp 500-523.
44. Mason ML, Allen HS: The rate of healing of tendons—an experimental study of tensile strength. *Ann Surg* 113:424-459, 1941.
45. Ross R: The fibroblast and wound repair. *Biol Rev* 43:51-96, 1968.

46. Mason JL, Shearon CG: The process of tendon repair. An experimental study of tendon suture and tendon graft. *Arch Surg* 25:615, 1932.

47. Fukada E, Yasuda I: Piezoelectric effects in collagen. *Jpn J Physiol* 3:117, 1964.

48. Birdsell DC, Tustanoff ER, Lindsay WK: Collagen production in regenerating tendon. *Plast Reconstr Surg* 37:504, 1966.

49. Ketchum LD, Martin NL, Kappel DA: Experimental evaluation of factors affecting the strength of tendon repairs. *Plast Reconstr Surg* 59:708-719, 1977.

50. Peacock EE Jr, Van Winkle W Jr: *Wound Repair*, ed 2. Philadelphia, WB Saunders, 1976, pp 367-464.

51. Peacock EE Jr: Biological principles in the healing of long tendons. *Surg Clin North Am* 45:461-476, 1965.

52. Bergljung L: Vascular reactions after tendon suture and tendon transplantation; a stereomicroangiographic study on the calcaneal tendon of the rabbit. *Scand J Plast Reconstr Surg* [Supp] 4:7-63, 1968.

53. Potenza AD: Tendon healing within the flexor digital sheath in the dog. *J Bone Joint Surg* 44A:49-64, 1962.

54. Matthews P, Richards H: Factors in the adherence of flexor tendon after repair. *J Bone Joint Surg* 58B:230-236, 1976.

55. Potenza AD: Concepts of tendon healing and repair. In *American Academy of Orthopaedic Surgeons Instruction Course Lectures, Symposium of Tendon Surgery in the Hand*. St. Louis, CV Mosby Co, 1975, pp 18-47.

56. Potenza AD: Prevention of adhesions to healind digital flexor tendons *JAMA* 187:187-191, 1964.

57. Adams W: On the reparative process in human tendons after subcutaneous division for the cure of deformities. Transactions of London Pathology Society, 1854-5, vi, 358; also 1869-70 xxi, 417. Referenced in Bernstein MA: The surgery of tendon transposition with special reference to the importance of the tendon sheath. *Surg Gynecol Obstet* 29:55-69, 1919.

58. Stark HH, Boyes JH, Johnson L, Ashworth CR: The use of paratenon, polyethylene film, or Silastic sheeting to prevent restricting adhesions to tendons in the hand. *J Bone Joint Surg* 59A:908-913, 1977.

59. Holtz M, Midenberg ML, Kirsehenbaum SE: Utilization of a Silastic sheet in tendon repair of the foot. *J Foot Surg* 21:253-259, 1982.

60. Blix M: Die Lange und die spannung des Muskels. *Can Arch Physiol* 5:150-206, 1894.

61. Bechtol CO: Muscle physiology. *American Academy Orthopedic Surgeons Instructional Course Lectures* 5:181, 1948.

62. Elftman H: Biomechanics of muscle, with particular application to the studies of gait. *J Bone Joint Surg* 48A:363, 1966.

63. MacConaill MA: Some anatomical factors affecting the stabilizing functions of muscles. *Ir J Med Sci* 6:160, 1946.

64. MacConaill MA: The movements of bone and joints. *J Bone Joint Surg* 31B:100, 1949.

65. Steindler A: *Kinesiology of the Human Body*, ed 3. Springfield IL, Charles C Thomas, 1970.

66. Close JR, Todd FN: The phasic activity of the lower extremity and the effect of tendon transfer. *J Bone Joint Surg* 41A:189-208, 1959.

67. McGlamry ED, Kitting RW: Surgery of the equinus foot. In McGlamry ED (ed): *Reconstructive Surgery of the Foot and Leg*. Miami, Symposia Specialists, 1974, pp 347-376.

68. Basmajian JV: *Muscles Alive. Their Functions Revealed by Electromyography*, ed 4. Baltimore, Williams & Wilkins, 1979.

69. Basmajian JV (ed): *Biofeedback—Principles and Practice for Clinicians*. Baltimore, Williams & Wilkins, 1979.

70. Kuhlmann RF, Bell JF: A clinical evaluation of tendon transplantation for poliomyelitis affecting the lower extremities. *J Bone Joint Surg* 34A:915-926, 1952.

71. Green WT, Grice DS: The surgical correction of the paralytic foot. *American Academy of Orthopaedic Surgeons Instructional Course Lecture* 10:343-363, 1953.

72. Green WT, Grice DS: The management of calcaneus deformity. *American Academy of Orthopaedic Surgeons Instructional Course Lectures* 13:135-149, 1956.

73. Irwin CG: The calcaneus foot. *American Academy of Orthopaedic Surgeons Instructional Course Lectures* 15:135, 1958.

74. Bradford EH: Tenoplastic surgery. *Ann Surg* 26:153, 1897.

75. Gelberman RH, VandenBerg JS, Lundborg GN: Flexor tendon healing and the restoration of the gliding surface: an ultra-structural study in dogs. *J Bone Joint Surg* 65A:583-598, 1980.

76. Bunnell S: An essential in reconstructive surgery—atraumatic technique. *Calif State J Med* 19:204, 1921.

77. Kernwein G, Fahey J, Garrison M: The fate of tendon fascia and elastic connective tissue transplanted into bone. *Ann Surg* 108:285, 1938.

78. Kernwein G: A study of tendon transplantation into bone. *Surg Gynecol Obstet* 75:794, 1942.

79. Gould N: Trephining your way. *Orthop Clin North Am* 4:157-164, 1973.

80. Krackow KA, Cohn BT: A new technique for passing tendon through bone. *J Bone Joint Surg* 69A:922-924, 1987.

81. Boyes JH: *Bunnell's Surgery of the Hand*, ed 4. Philadelphia, JB Lippincott, 1964, pp 404-481.

82. Strayer LM Jr: Recession of the gastrocnemius. An operation to relieve spastic contracture of the calf muscles. *J Bone Joint Surg* 32A:671-676, 1950.

83. Strayer LM Jr: Gastrocnemius recession. Five year report of cases. *J Bone Joint Surg* 40A:1019, 1958.

84. Silver CM, Simon DD: Gastrocnemius muscle recession (Silverskiöld operation) for spastic equinus deformity in cerebral palsy. *J Bone Joint Surg* 41A:1021, 1959.

85. Flynn JE, Graham JH: Healing of tendon wounds. *Am J Surg* 109:315-345, 1965.

86. Tubiana R: Incisions and techniques in tendon grafting. *Am J Surg* 109:339-345, 1965.

87. Hanisch CM, Kleiger B: Experimental production of tendon sheaths. *Bull Hosp Joint Dis* 11:22-31, 1950.

88. Mayer L, Ransohoff NS: Contribution to the physiological method of repair of damaged finger tendons. Preliminary report on reconstruction of the destroyed tendon sheath. *Am J Surg* 31:56, 1936.

89. Mayer L, Ransohoff NS: Reconstruction of the digital tendon sheath. A contribution to the physiological method of repair of damaged finger tendons. *J Bone Joint Surg* 18:607, 1936.

90. Carroll RE, Bassett AL: Formation of tendon sheath by silicone rod implants. Proceedings of the American Society for Surgery in the Hand. *J Bone Joint Surg* 45A:884, 1963.

91. Hunter J: Artificial tendons. Early development and application. *Am J Surg* 109:325-338, 1965.

92. Hunter JM, Jaeger SH: Tendon implants: primary and secondary usage. *Orthop Clin North Am* 8:473-489, 1977.

93. Salisbury RE, Mason AD Jr, Levine NS, Pruit BA, Wade CWR: Artificial tendons: design, application and results. *J Trauma* 14:580-586, 1974.

94. Unter JM, Schneider LH: Staged tendon reconstruction. In *American Academy of Orthopaedic Surgeons, Instructional Course Lectures*, vol 26. St Louis, CV Mosby Co, 1977, pp 134-144.

95. Sakellarides HT: Severe injuries of the flexor tendons in no man's land with excess scarring and flexion contracture treated with silicone rod and tendon grafting. *Orthop Rev* 6:51-54, 1977.

96. Mahoney J, Farkas LG, Lindsay WK: Silastic rod pseudosheaths and tendon graft healing. *Plast Reconstr Surg* 66:746-750, 1980.

97. Farkas LG, Lindsay WK: Functional return of tendon graft protected entirely by pseudosheath: experimental study. *Plast Reconstr Surg* 65:188-194, 1980.

98. Van Der Meulen JC, Leistikow PA: Tendon healing. *Clin Plast Surg* 4:439-458, 1977.

99. Dockery GL: Bovine tendon lateral ankle stabilization procedure: xenograft bioprosthesis model GR 6 mm. *J Foot Surg* 25:469-471, 1986.

100. Chase R: Muscle tendon kinetics. *Am J Surg* 109:277-282, 1965.

101. Daniels L, Worthingham C: *Muscle Testing*, ed 3. Philadelphia, WB Saunders, 1972.

102. Basmajian JV: Functional and anatomical considerations in major muscle tendon imbalance. *J Am Podiatry Assoc* 65:723-731, 1975.

103. Basmajian JV: *Muscles Alive*, ed 3. Baltimore, Williams & Wilkins, 1974.

104. Mann RA: Tendon transfers and electromyography. AOFS surgery of the foot. *Clin Orthop* 85:64-66, 1972.

105. Caldwell GD: Correction of paralytic footdrop by hemigastrosoleus transplant. *Clin Orthop* 11:81-84, 1958.

106. Turner JW, Cooper RR: Anterior transfer of the tibialis posterior through the interosseous membrane. *Clin Orthop* 83:241, 1972.

107. Lagast J, Mylle J, Fabry G: Posterior tibial tendon transfer in spastic equinovarus. *Arch Orthop Trauma Surg* 108:100-103, 1989.

108. Perry J, Hoffer, MM: Preoperative and postoperative dynamic electromyography as an aid in planning tendon transfers in children with cerebral palsy. *J Bone Joint Surg* 59A:531-537, 1977.

109. Tachdjian MD: *Pediatric Orthopedics*. Philadelphia, WB Saunders, 1972.

110. Samilson RL: Tendon transfers in cerebral palsy. *J Bone Joint Surg* 53B:153-155, 1976.

111. Pierrot AH, Murphy OB: Heel cord advancement. A new approach to the spastic equinus deformity. *Orthop Clin North Am* 5:117-126, 1974.

112. Giannestras NJ: *Foot Disorders: Medical and Surgical Management*, ed 2. Philadelphia, Lea & Febiger, 1973.

113. McCarroll HR: Surgical treatment of spastic paralysis. In *American Association of Orthopaedic Surgeons Instructional Course Lectures* 6:134-151, 1949.

114. Pollock GA: Surgical treatment of cerebral palsy. *J Bone Joint Surg* 44B:68-81, 1962.

115. Craig JJ, Van Vuren J: The importance of gastrocnemius recession in the correction of equinus deformity in cerebral palsy. *J Bone Joint Surg* 58B:84-87, 1976.

116. Smith SB, Weil LS: Anterior advancement of the tendo Achillis for spastic equinus deformity. *J Am Podiatry Assoc* 64:1016-1023, 1974.

117. Jay RM, Schoenhaus HD: Further insights in the anterior advancement of the tendo Achillis. *J Am Podiatry Assoc* 71:73-76, 1981.

118. Sharrard WJW, Bernstein S: Equinus deformity in cerebral palsy. A comparison between elongation of the tendo calcaneus and gastrocnemius recession. *J Bone Joint Surg* 54B:272-276, 1972.

119. Banks HH: The management of spastic deformities of the foot and ankle. *Clin Orthop* 122:70-76, 1977.

120. Baker LD, Hill LM: Foot alignment in the cerebral palsy patient. *J Bone Joint Surg* 46A:1-15, 1964.

121. Baker LD, Basset FH, Dyas EC: Surgery in the rehabilitation of cerebral palsied patients. *Dev Med Child Neurol* 12:330-342, 1970.

122. Root L, Miller SR, Kirz P: Posterior tibial—tendon transfer in patients with cerebral palsy. *J Bone Joint Surg* 69A:1133-1139, 1987.

123. Samilson RL (ed): *Orthopaedic Aspects of Cerebral Palsy*. Clinics in Developmental Medicine, vol 52 and 53. London, Heinemann, 1975, pp 35-70, 282-291.

124. Medina PA, Karpman RR, Young AT: Split posterior tibial tendon transfer for spastic equinovarus foot deformity. *Foot Ankle* 10:65-67, 1989.

125. Kling TF, Kaufer H, Hensinger RN: Split posterior tibial-tendon transfers in children with cerebral spastic paralysis and equinovarus deformity. *J Bone Joint Surg* 67A:186-194, 1985.

126. Root L: Functional testing of the posterior tibial muscle in spastic paralysis. *Dev Med Child Neurol* 12:592-595, 1970.

127. Banks H: The correction of equinus deformity in cerebral palsy. *J Bone Joint Surg* 40A:1359-1379, 1958.

128. Clark WD: Abductor hallucis tendon transfer for hallux varus. *J Foot Surg* 23:146-148, 1984.

129. Woodhams LE: A three-year follow-up study of hammer digit syndrome of the hallux. *J Am Podiatry Assoc* 64:955-966, 1974.

130. Sharrard WJW: Tenodesis of flexor hallucis longus for paralytic clawing in the hallux in childhood. *J Bone Joint Surg* 58B:224, 1976.

131. Sgarlato TE: Transplantation of the flexor digitorum longus muscle tendon in hammertoes. *J Am Podiatry Assoc* 60:383-388, 1970.

132. Parrish TF: Dynamic correction of clawtoes. *Orthop Clin North Am* 4:97-102, 1973.

133. Taylor RG: The treatment of claw toes by multiple transfers of flexors into extensor tendons. *J Bone Joint Surg* 33B:539, 1951.

134. Hibbs RA: An operation for "clawfoot." *JAMA* 73:1583, 1919.

135. Kuwada GT, Dockery GL: Modification of the flexor tendon transfer procedure for the correction of flexible hammertoes. *J Foot Surg* 19:38-40, 1980.

136. Kuwada GT: A retrospective analysis of modification of the flexor tendon transfer for correction of hammertoe. *J Foot Surg* 27:57-59, 1988.

137. McGlamry ED, Bouchard JL: Split tibialis anterior tendon transfer (STATT)—a review of the procedure and an analysis of its effectiveness. *J Am Podiatry Assoc* 67:883-890, 1977.

138. Jones R: Arthrodesis and tendon transplantation. *Br Med J* 1:728, 1908.

139. Heyman CH: The operative treatment of clawfoot. *J Bone Joint Surg* 14:335, 1932.

140. Watkins M, Jones JB, Ryder CT, Brown TH: Transplantation of the posterior tibial tendon. *J Bone Joint Surg* 36A:1181, 1964.

141. Young CS: Operative treatment of pes planus. *Surg Gynecol Obstet* 68:1099, 1939.

142. Kidner FC: The pre-hallux in relation to flatfoot. *JAMA* 101:1539, 1933.

143. Jones R: The soldier's foot and the treatment of common deformities of the foot. *Br Med J* 1:749, 1916.

144. Chuinard EG, Baskin M: Claw-foot deformity. *J Bone Joint Surg* 55A:351, 1973.

145. Hoffer MD, Reiswig JA, Garrett AM, Perry J: The split anterior tibial tendon transfer in the treatment of spastic hindfoot varus of childhood. *Orthop Clin North Am* 5:31-38, 1974.

146. Garceau GJ, Palmer RM: Transfer of the anterior tibial tendon for recurrent clubfoot. *J Bone Joint Surg* 49A:207-332, 1967.

147. Levitt RL, Canale ST, Cooke AJ Jr, Gartland JJ: The role of foot surgery in progressive neuromuscular disorders in children. *J Bone Joint Surg* 55A:1396-1410, 1973.

148. Turan I: Tarsometatarsal amputation and tibialis anterior tendon transposition to first cuneiform. *J Foot Surg* 24:113-115, 1985.

149. Roper BA, Tibrewal SB: Soft tissue surgery in Charcot-Marie-Tooth disease. *J Bone Joint Surg* 71B:17-20, 1989.

150. Jacobs JE, Carr CR: Progressive muscular atrophy of the peroneal type (Charcot-Marie-Tooth disease). *J Bone Joint Surg* 32A:27-30, 1950.

151. Kite JH: *The Clubfoot*. New York, Grune & Stratton, 1964, pp 36-39.

152. Lehman WB: *The Clubfoot*. Philadelphia, JB Lippincott, 1980, pp 79-86.

153. Hsu JD, Hoffer MM: Posterior tibial tendon transfer anteriorly through the interosseous membrane. A modification of the technique. *Clin Orthop* 131:202-204, 1978.

154. Gunn DR, Molesworth BD: The use of the tibialis posterior as a dorsiflexor. *J Bone Joint Surg* 39B:674, 1957.

155. Williams PF: Restoration of muscle balance of the foot by transfer of the tibialis posterior. *J Bone Joint Surg* 56B:217, 1976.

156. Eyring EJ, Earl WC, Brockmeyer JR: Posterior tibial tendon transfer in neuromuscular conditions other than anterior poliomyelitis. *Arch Phys Med Rehabil* 55:279, 1973.

157. Spector EF, Todd WF, Wilson F: A review of selected posterior tibial tendon transfer procedures. A case report. *J Am Podiatry Assoc* 69:325-328, 1979.

158. Tuell JI: Anterior transposition of posterior tibial muscle in equinovarus. *Clin Orthop* 23:227, 1962.

159. Ranjit SB, Louis HG, Albano P: Transfer of tibialis posterior tendon in cerebral palsy. *J Bone Joint Surg* 58A:497-500, 1976.

160. Miller GM, Hsu JD, Hoffer MM, Rentfro R: Posterior tibial tendon transfer: a review of the literature and analysis of 74 procedures. *J Pediatr Orthop* 2:363-370, 1982.

161. Johnson WI, Lester EL: Transposition of the posterior tibial tendon. *Clin Orthop* 245:223-227, 1989.

162. Fried A: Recurrent congenital clubfoot. The role of the tibialis posterior in etiology and treatment. *J Bone Joint Surg* 41A:243, 1959.

163. Singer M: Tibialis posterior transfer in congenital clubfoot. *J Bone Joint Surg* 43B:717, 1961.

164. Gartland J: Posterior tibial transplant in the surgical treatment of recurrent clubfoot. A preliminary report. *J Bone Joint Surg* 46A:1217, 1964.

165. Gartland J, Surgent RE: Posterior tibial transplant in the surgical treatment of recurrent clubfoot. *Clin Orthop* 84:66-70, 1972.

166. Goldner JL, Irwin CE: Paralytic equinovarus deformities of the foot. *South Med J* 42:83-94, 1949.

167. Karlholm S, Nilsonne U: Operative treatment of the foot deformity in Charcot-Marie-Tooth disease. *Acta Orthop Scand* 39:101-106, 1968.

168. Lipscomb PR, Sanchez JJ: Anterior transplantation of the posterior tibial tendon for persistent palsy of the common peroneal nerve. *J Bone Joint Surg* 43A:60, 1961.

169. Cozer L: Management of the foot drop in adults after permanent peroneal nerve loss. *Clin Orthop* 67:151, 1969.

170. Richard BM: Interosseous transfer of tibialis posterior for common peroneal nerve palsy. *J Bone Joint Surg* 71B:834-837, 1989.

171. Sundararaj GD: Tibialis posterior transfer (circumtibial route) for drop-foot deformity. *Indian J Lepr* 56:555-562, 1984.

172. Gritzka TL, Stahlei LT, Duncan WR: Posterior tibial tendon transfer through the interosseous membrane to correct equinovarus deformity in cerebral palsy. An initial experience. *Clin Orthop* 89:201-206, 1972.

173. Scheider M, Balon K: Deformity of the foot following anterior transfer of the posterior tibial tendon and lengthening of the Achilles tendon for spastic equinovarus. *Clin Orthop* 125:113, 1977.

174. Goldner JL, Keats PK, Bassett FH, Chippinger FW: Progressive talipes equinovalgus due to trauma or degeneration of the posterior tibial tendon and medial plantar ligaments. *Orthop Clin North Am* 5:39-51, 1974.

175. Fried A, Hendel C: Paralytic valgus deformity of the ankle. Replacement of the paralyzed tibialis posterior by the peroneus longus. *J Bone Joint Surg* 39A:921-932, 1957.

176. Nicoladoni C: Nachtrag zum pes Calcaneus und zur Transplantation der Peronealsehnen. *Archiv Klin Chir* 27:660-666, 1881.

177. Bickel WH, Moe JH: Translocation of the peroneus longus tendon for paralytic calcaneus deformity of the foot. *Surg Gynecol Obstet* 78:627-630, 1944.

178. Makin M, Yossipovitch A: Translocation of the peroneus longus in the treatment of paralytic pes calcaneus. A follow-up study of thirty-three cases. *J Bone Joint Surg* 48A:1541-1547, 1966.

179. White RK, Kraynick BM: Surgical uses of the peroneus brevis tendon. *Surg Gynecol Obstet* 108:117, 1959.

180. Booker HE, Rubow RT, Coleman PJ: Simplified feedback in neuro-muscular re-training: an automated approach using electromyographic signals. *Arch Phys Med Rehabil* 50:621, 1969.

181. Baker M, Regenos E, Wolf SL, Basmajian JV: Developing strategies for biofeedback: applications in neurologically handicapped patients. *Phys Ther* 57:402-408, 1977.

182. Brown DM, Nahai F: Biofeedback strategies of the occupational therapist in total hand rehabilitation. In Basmajian JV (ed): *Biofeedback—Principles and Practice for Clinicians.* Baltimore, Williams & Wilkins, 1979, pp 43-56.

183. Takebe K, Hirohata K: EMG biofeedback in tendon transplantation for drop foot. *Arch Orthop Trauma Surg* 97:77-79, 1980.

184. Goldberg I, Avidor I: Isolated tuberculous tenosynovitis of the Achilles tendon. A case report. *Clin Orthop* 194:185-188, 1985.

185. Rayan GM: Intratendinous ganglion. A case report. *Orthop Rev* 18:449-451, 1989.

186. Rosenberg A: Dorsal tendosynovial cyst. *J Am Podiatr Med Assoc* 76:455-457, 1986.

187. Jaffe HD, Lichtenstein L, Sutro CJ: Pigmented vilonodular synovitis, bursitis and tenosynovitis. *Arch Pathol* 31:731, 1941.

188. Gold AG, Bronfman RA, Clark EA, Comerford JS: Giant cell tumor of the extensor tendon sheath of the foot. A case report. *J Am Podiatr Med Assoc* 77:561-563, 1987.

189. Sarma DP, Weilbaecher TG, Rodriguez FH Jr: Fibroma of tendon sheath. *J Surg Oncol* 32:230-232, 1986.

190. Gill PW, Rosenthal L, Wagreich CR: Tenosynovial fibroma. A case report. *J Am Podiatr Med Assoc* 78:368-369, 1988.

191. Enzinger FM: Clear cell sarcoma of tendons and aponeuroses: an analysis of 21 cases. *Cancer* 18:1163, 1965.

192. Langen RJ, Nyongo AJ, Huntralcoon M, Landry ME: Clear cell sarcoma of tendons and aponeurosis: histogenesis and mode of treatment. *J Foot Surg* 28:112-115, 1989.

193. Marcinko DE, Miller II, Read JM III: Achilles tendon hypercholesterolemic xanthoma. *J Foot Surg* 23:398-401, 1984.

194. Panman WF, Hamming JJ: Xanthoma of the Achilles tendon. *Neth J Surg* 38:155-157, 1986.

195. Karaharju E, Paavolainen P, Holmstrom T, Nikkari T: Xanthomas of the Achilles tendon. Case report. *Ital J Orthop Traumatol* 9:529-532, 1983.

196. Lee CK, Weiss AB: Xanthomas of the Achilles tendon. A case report. *Clin Orthop* 194:185-188, 1985.

197. Schumacher HR Jr, Michaels R: Recurrent tendonitis and Achilles tendon nodule with positively birefringent crystals in a patient with hyperproteinemia. *J Rheumatol* 16:1387-1389, 1989.

198. Kernohan J, Hallt AJ: Treatment of a fractured ossified Achilles tendon. *J R Coll Surg Edinb* 29:263, 1984.

199. Raynor KJ, McDonald RJ, Edelman RD, Parkinson DE: Ossification of the Achilles tendon. *J Am Podiatr Med Assoc* 76:688-690, 1986.

200. Postacchini F, DiCastro A: Subtotal ossification of the Achilles tendon. Case report. *Ital J Orthop Traumatol* 9:529-532, 1983.

201. Lagergren C, Lindholm A: Vascular distribution in the Achilles tendon: an angiographic and microangiographic study. *Acta Chir Scand* 116:491, 1958-1959.

202. Fox JR, Blazina ME, Jobe FW, Kerlan RK, Carter VS, Shields CL Jr, Carlson GJ: Degeneration and rupture of the Achilles tendon. *Clin Orthop* 107:221, 1975.

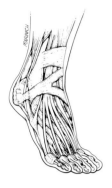

CHAPTER **51**

Ankle Arthroscopy

George Gumann, D.P.M.

HISTORY OF ARTHROSCOPY

Although it is a relatively new discipline, arthroscopy is proving to be a valuable modality to aid in the diagnosis and treatment of intra-articular conditions, especially in the knee (1, 2). The first endoscopic intra-articular observation occurred when Takagi examined a cadaveric knee in 1918 at the University of Tokyo. His original instrument was a cystoscope, but soon afterwards he developed a 7.3-mm instrument that he called an arthroscope (3). In Switzerland, Bircher (4) reported the first arthroscopic examination of a meniscus in 1921. Burman (5) in 1931 at the Hospital for Joint Diseases in New York City, using cadaveric specimens and a 4-mm arthroscope, described the arthroscopic appearance of most major joints. Of interest in this classical paper is Burman's view that the ankle was not suitable for arthroscopic evaluation because of its narrow joint space. The first person to successfully perform an ankle arthroscopy was Takagi (6) in 1939. His protege, Watanabe, developed a practical design in the No. 21 arthroscope for examining the knee in 1960. Watanabe and Takeda (7) also reportedly performed the first operative procedure with the arthroscope, a meniscectomy.

With the development of improved fiberoptics and self-focusing glass (Selfoc) in 1968, an incandescent bulb was no longer required at the end of the arthroscope, thereby allowing the use of smaller-diameter arthroscopes that facilitated entry into small joints (8). Selfoc was incorporated in the development of the Watanabe No. 24 arthroscope in 1970. Its outside diameter was 2.2 mm (9), and it was manufactured under the name Needlescope. Watanabe (10) subsequently reported on 28 patients undergoing ankle arthroscopy. Chen (11) in 1976 reviewed his experience with ankle arthroscopy on 67 patients and 17 cadavers. Both Plank (12) and Johnson (13) have discussed the indications and techniques of ankle arthroscopy. In 1981 Parisien and Shereff (14) reported on 30 cases and Drez and associates (15) on 56 cases of ankle arthroscopy. Heller and Vogler (16) reported in 1982 on 21 cases. The first seminar specifically for ankle arthroscopy was held in 1983 by Lundeen and associates in Indianapolis, Indiana (Lundeen RO, personal communication).

The views and opinions of the author are not to be construed as reflecting official policy of the Department of Defense or the U.S. Army Medical Department.

INSTRUMENTATION

To perform an arthroscopy one needs certain basic equipment and requisite skills. There are hollow cannulas into which both a sharp trocar and a blunt obturator are introduced. The trocar is used to pierce soft tissue and capsule, and the obturator is used to enter the joint. The cannula also serves to hold the arthroscope and to protect it. In addition, the cannula can serve to allow ingress or egress of the irrigating solution (Fig. 51.1).

Several companies manufacture arthroscopes. The arthroscope (Fig. 51.2) functions like a telescope and is available in sizes from 1.7 to 8.0 mm. It consists of a small-diameter metallic tube encompassing fiberoptic light bundles that transmit light into the joint and a Selfoc lens system that carries light from the joint to the eyepiece. Straight-on viewing is available, as well as various angled lenses that create an obliquity in the field of vision. The arthroscope also has a side arm for attachment of the light cable. The light cable is then attached to a light source, many of which consist of high intensity metal halide arc discharge lamps.

Although direct visualization is possible through the arthroscope, it is easier to use a camera and video display screen. This is easier on the eyes, frees both hands to manipulate the arthroscope and other instruments, and allows the entire surgical team to view the case, which alleviates boredom.

An irrigation system is necessary to distend the joint to allow better visualization of the joint structures. Irrigation also performs a therapeutic lavage of debris and hemarthrosis to maintain a clear field (14). Normal saline is used for this purpose. A gravity-assisted system with two 3000 ml bags of saline are preferably used and elevated above the operating table. Visualization is directly related to capsular distention and joint distraction created by both the volume and pressure of the saline.

With the basic instrumentation just described, diagnostic arthroscopy can be performed. However, for surgical arthroscopy, additional equipment is required, and there are a large number of instruments to aid in the operative treatment of joint problems. Biopsy forceps, scissors, grasping forceps, meniscal knives, and probes have been developed (Fig. 51.3). Power instrumentation is available as well. The intra-articular shaver system is a highly versatile and useful instrument employed for debridement of soft tissue and cartilage (Fig. 51.4). An arthroplasty system is also available

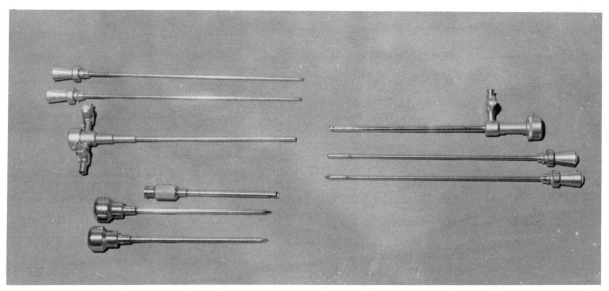

Figure 51.1. Various diameter cannulas with trocars (sharp point) and obturators (blunt point).

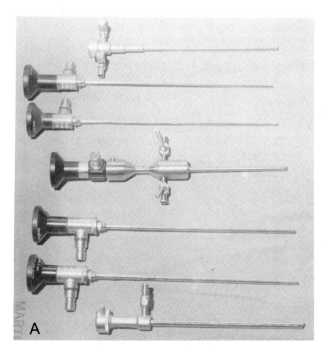

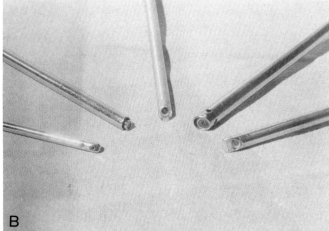

Figure 51.2. **A.** Arthroscopes. Top to bottom, 2.7-mm Wolf with 10° and 110° viewing; 4.0-mm Dyonics with 30° viewing; 4.5-mm Wolf with 25° and 70° viewing. **B.** Angled lenses on arthroscopes.

with burs to abrade articular defects to good bleeding bone for chondromalacia, osteochondral defects, and osteoarthritis (Fig. 51.5). However, one will find that some of these instruments are large and difficult to maneuver within the ankle joint. Therefore, small abraders have been manufactured. In addition, very small mosquito hemostats, sharpened nerve hooks, Kirschner wires (K-wires), modified pi-

tuitary forceps, and even small diameter needles are available.

ANATOMY

It is important to understand the extra-articular, as well as intra-articular, anatomy to successfully use arthroscopy with

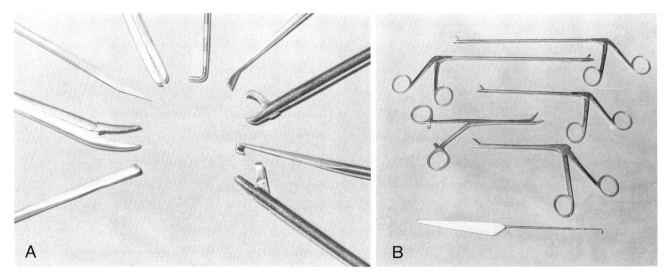

Figure 51.3. **A** and **B.** Accessory instruments.

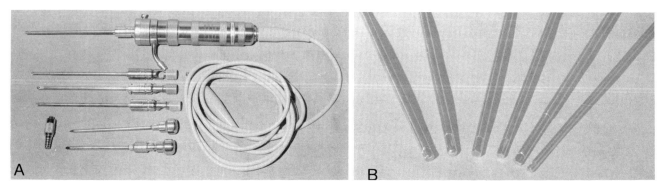

Figure 51.4. **A** and **B.** Dyonics' intra-articular cutter and shaver.

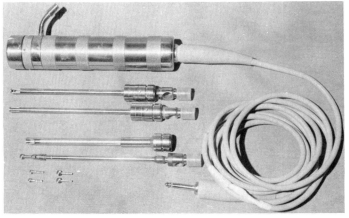

Figure 51.5. Dyonics' arthroplasty set.

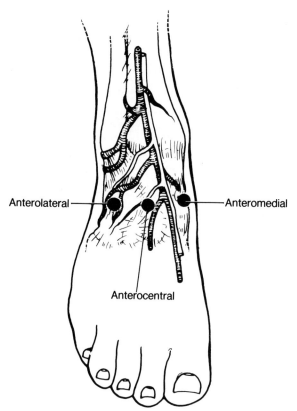

Figure 51.6. Anterior arthroscopic portals—anteromedial, anterocentral, anterolateral.

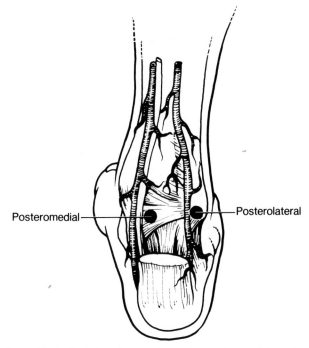

Figure 51.7. Posterior arthroscopic portals—posteromedial, posterolateral.

minimum morbidity. Drez and associates (15) have divided the ankle into an anterior and a posterior joint cavity that they further subdivide into a lateral, central, and medial compartment. There are five portals of entry to the ankle joint, three anteriorly and two posteriorly (Figs. 51.6 and 51.7). Consequently there is significant overlap of structures from adjacent portals.

ARTHROSCOPIC APPROACHES

Anterior Approaches

The anteromedial portal of the ankle is approached medial to the tibialis anterior tendon (1) (Fig. 51.8). The surgeon must be careful to avoid this tendon, the great saphenous vein, and the saphenous nerve. Through this portal one can see the tip of the medial malleolus, the deltoid ligament, the anteromedial synovial wall, the medial tibiotalar articulation, most of the articular facet on the medial aspect of the talus, the medial shoulder of the talus and tibia (medial bend), along the anterior aspect of the ankle, the anterior half of the talar dome, and the anterior synovial wall. Laterally one can view the fibula, tibiofibular synovial fringe, and the anterolateral aspect of the tibia (tubercle of Chaput) (Fig. 51.9). The lateral joint compartment inferiorly is very difficult to see without an angled scope.

The anterocentral portal is located lateral to the extensor hallucis longus tendon (2). The surgeon absolutely must locate and mark the anterior tibial artery and deep peroneal nerve to prevent injury via this approach. The extensor hallucis longus and extensor digitorum longus tendons are also subject to injury, as well as the terminal branches of the superficial peroneal nerve. From this portal the entire anterior aspect of the joint can be well viewed from medial to lateral, including the tibiofibular articulation. Structures seen include the anterior synovial wall, the anterior aspect of the distal tibia, and the trochlear surface of the talus.

Plantarflexion of the foot increases the visible portion of the talar dome. Laterally the tubercle of Chaput, the fibula, the tibiofibular synovial fringe (normal synovial outpouching), and inferior portion of the anteroinferior tibiofibular ligament are observed. However, the more inferior portions of the lateral and medial compartments are not well visualized. As one moves further along from the central portal, either medially or laterally, an angled scope will aid viewing.

The anterolateral portal is approached just lateral to the peroneus tertius or extensor digitorum longus (3). Care must be maintained to avoid injury to these tendons and the terminal branches of the superficial peroneal nerve. Through this portal one can observe the tip of the lateral malleolus, the anterior talofibular ligament, sometimes the posterior talofibular ligament, the talofibular joint, the anterolateral synovial wall, portions of the facet on the lateral aspect to the talus, the distal tibiofibular articulation, and the tibiofibular synovial fringe and recess.

The arthroscope can also be advanced medially along the anterior aspect of the ankle to the medial shoulder of the

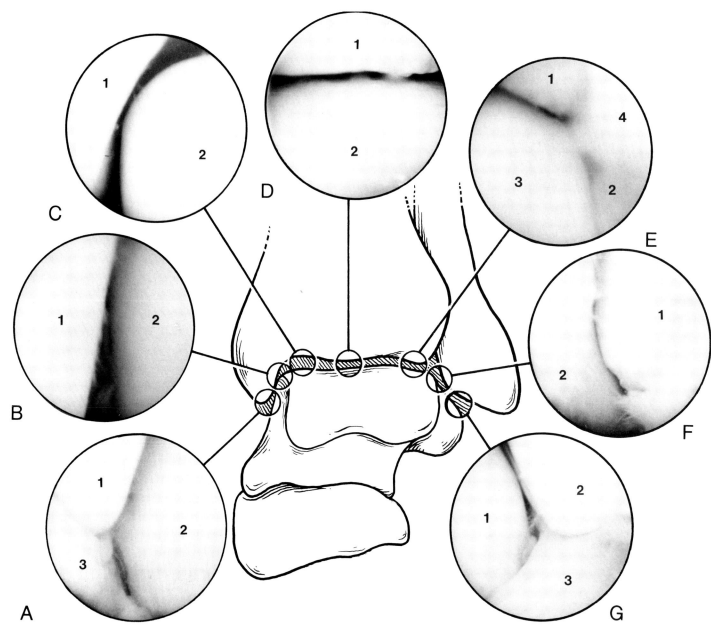

Figure 51.8. Normal arthroscopic intra-articular anatomy of the anterior aspect of the ankle. **A.** Deltoid ligament and inferior aspect medial malleolus, talus. (*1*, tip of medial malleolus; *2*, talus; *3*, deltoid ligament). **B.** Talar-medial malleolar joint (*1*, medial malleolus, *2*, talus). **C.** Medial shoulder to talotibial joint (*1*, tibia; *2*, medial shoulder of talus). **D.** Tibiotalar joint (*1*, tibia; *2*, talus). **E.** Tibiofibular-talar articulation (*1*, tibial; *2*, fibula; *3*, lateral shoulder of talus; *4*, tibiofibular synovial fringe). **F.** Talofibular joint (*1*, lateral malleolus; *2*, talus). **G.** Anterior talofibular ligament and inferior aspect of lateral malleolus, talus (*1*, talus; *2*, tip of lateral malleolus; *3*, anterior talofibular ligament).

talus and medial malleolus. However, the inferior portion of the medial compartment is not well seen without an angled scope. The distal tibiofibular joint is often partially obscured by the tibiofibular synovial fringe and the inferior aspect of the anterior inferior tibiofibular ligament (anterior syndesmosis). The tibiofibular synovial fringe thickens with chronic inflammation, which handicaps observation.

Posterior Approaches

The instrument enters the posterolateral portal lateral to the Achilles tendon (1) (Fig. 51.10). Care must be taken to avoid injury to this tendon, the peroneal tendons, the short saphenous vein, and the sural nerve. One can see most of the posterior joint cavity through this approach. Structures seen include the tip of the lateral malleolus, the posterior

Chapter 51: Ankle Arthroscopy   **1339**

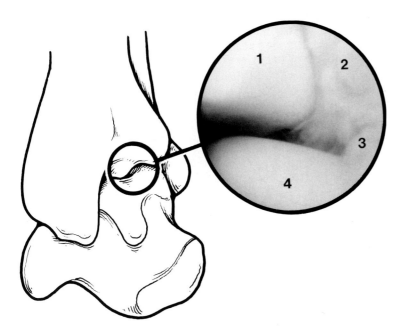

Figure 51.9. Distal tibiofibular articulation with the tibiofibular synovial fringe as seen from an anteromedial portal. (*1*, anterior lateral aspect of tibia; *2*, fibula; *3*, tibiofibular synovial fringe; *4*, lateral aspect of talar dome.)

talofibular ligament, the talofibular articulation, the postero-inferior tibiofibular ligament (posterior syndesmosis), the posterior aspect of the tibiofibular articulation, the posterior aspect of the distal tibia, the trochlear surface of the talus, the posterior synovial wall, the medial malleolus, and the posterior aspect of the deltoid ligament.

The posteromedial portal is medial to the Achilles tendon (2). Care must be exercised to avoid all the components of the tarsal tunnel region. This is a very dangerous approach, and the author has not used this portal because the posterolateral approach has allowed adequate visualization. Care must also be exercised so that with either posterior approach the arthroscope enters the ankle joint and not the subtalar joint.

It is most important to determine preoperatively which portal of entry one will use. The patient will be supine for an anterior approach and prone for a posterior approach. If both approaches need to be made, the patient will be in a lateral position or will have to be rotated, necessitating a change of gowns and drapes. Remember that distraction will enhance visualization, as will plantarflexion for anterior portals and dorsiflexion for posterior portals. Consequently, an assistant can greatly enhance the ease with which arthroscopy is performed by distracting and manipulating the joint.

The surgeon chooses a portal that will allow visualization of the compartment containing the abnormality. Also consider the use of a second portal to introduce surgical instruments or for an ingress/egress line. For example, if there is an osteochondral fragment laterally, the surgeon may want to place the arthroscope in the anterocentral portal and use the anterolateral portal for the necessary instrumentation. Also consider the placement of the arthroscope in regard to a possible surgical incision. If an arthrotomy is

required, an arthroscopic portal can be incorporated if necessary.

The author's approach to problems requiring arthroscopy usually emphasizes the anterior portals. One must also realize that arthroscopy has its limitations and there are some joint surfaces that will not be observed, such as along the interior surface of the facets on the lateral and medial malleolus, as well as the underside of the tibial plafond. Drez and associates (15) point out that the distal tibiofibular articulation is difficult to view. Visualization of the posterior aspect of the joint is also difficult.

PROCEDURE

It is important in the preoperative evaluation of the patient to include a history, physical examination, appropriate laboratory tests, including a screen for arthritis (if warranted) and conventional radiographs. The use of additional tests such as arthrocentesis, stress x-ray films, arthrogram, bone scan, tomograms, computed tomography (CT) scan, and a magnetic resonance imaging (MRI) can help to delineate pathological conditions.

Sterilization of the arthroscopes is done by ethylene oxide gas for the first case, followed by soaking in activated glutaraldehyde solution for 20 minutes if other cases are to follow. Arthroscopes cannot be autoclaved because the process will eventually cause deterioration of the adhesive seals between the lenses. Using this type of sterilization, Johnson (17) reported only four infections in 7240 cases from October 30, 1972, through June 30, 1979.

The patient can be positioned supine on an operating table with the surgeon standing, or if the thigh is placed in a knee holder, the end of the table may be dropped 90° and the surgeon may sit. Both methods have been employed by

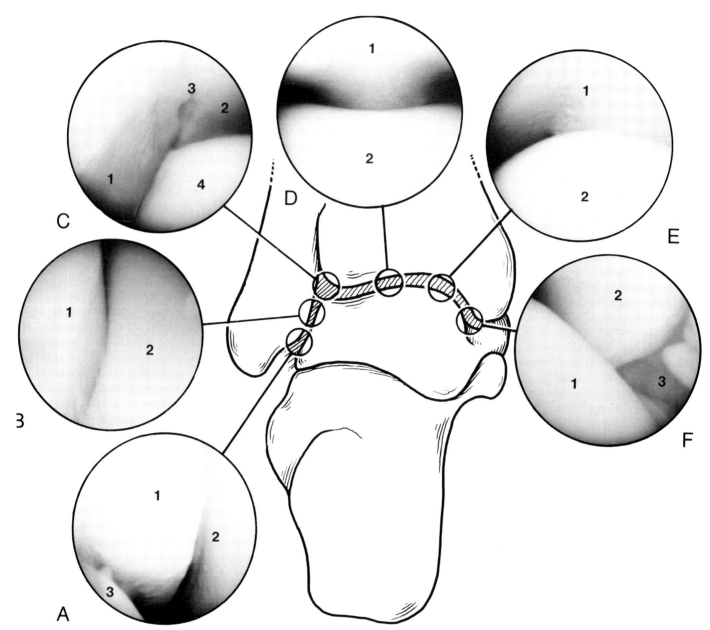

Figure 51.10. Normal arthroscopic intra-articular anatomy of posterior aspect of ankle as seen through posterolateral portal. **A.** Posterior talofibular ligament, inferior aspect of lateral malleolus, talus. (*1*, tip of lateral malleolus; *2*, talus; *3*, posterior talofibular ligament.) **B.** Talofibular joint (*1*, lateral malleolus; *2*, talus). **C.** Tibiofibular joint (*1*, fibula; *2*, tibia; *3*, tibiofibular joint; *4*, talus). **D.** Tibiotalar joint (*1*, tibia; *2*, talus). **E.** Medial shoulder of talus (*1*, tibia; *2*, talus). **F.** Inferior aspect of medial malleolus, deltoid ligament, talus (*1*, talus; *2*, medial malleolus; *3*, deltoid ligament).

the author, and both have been found to be useful. The author's preference is to stand because distraction and manipulation of the foot are easier to perform in this position.

Anesthesia can be local, regional, or general. The author has not used local anesthesia because regional or general anesthesia allows muscle relaxation for better manipulation and distraction. However, Lundeen (personal communication and unpublished observations) reports using local anesthesia to perform ankle arthroscopy. The skin, subcutaneous tissue, and capsule are anesthetized intra-articularly

with 2% lidocaine with or without epinephrine. An ankle tourniquet is used, and patient tolerance has been reported to be excellent. The ankle is prepared and draped in the usual sterile manner. The use of a thigh tourniquet is optional with regional or general anesthesia. The author recommends a tourniquet because intra-articular hemorrhage can obscure the field of view and is not always controlled by continuous irrigation.

The first step is to outline the joint and identify extra-articular structures such as the anterior tibial artery, especially if an anterocentral portal is to be used (Fig. 51.11). To prevent loss of landmarks the arthroscopic portals to be used should be marked prior to joint distention. Next a 50-ml syringe filled with normal saline and attached to an 18-gauge 1½-inch needle is inserted into the ankle joint. Successful insertion will be confirmed by the ease with which saline may be injected, the ability to aspirate the saline, and the obvious distention of the capsule. Distention usually requires about 20 to 25 ml. If one can inject only 10 to 12 ml, then this is probably due to capsular adhesions and fibrosis. With the capsule distended, a stab incision is made over the portal of entry, usually in a vertical manner.

Parisien and Shereff (14) recommend the anteromedial portal, but the author selects the entry site based upon the specific needs of the individual patient. The surgeon can use a hemostat to bluntly dissect a channel to the capsule or just insert the arthroscopic cannula with trocar to pierce the soft tissue and capsule (Fig. 51.12). The trochar is replaced with an obturator to penetrate the synovium and prevent iatrogenic cartilaginous damage. If done properly, when the obturator is removed, saline will leach out of the cannula. Then the arthroscope, to which the light source cable and the camera are attached, can be inserted (Fig. 51.13). The intra-articular picture will appear on the monitor screen.

While viewing the joint, the surgeon introduces a second cannula under direct vision for the outflow (Fig. 51.14). The outflow can be connected to the arthroscope cannula, or it can be placed through the second cannula. The author has

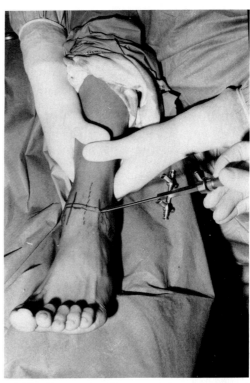

Figure 51.12. The cannula with a trocar is introduced through a stab incision over the anterolateral portal to pierce soft tissue and capsule. The trocar is replaced by an obturator to pierce synovium and enter the joint.

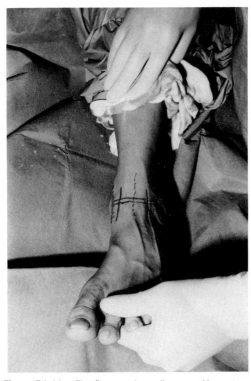

Figure 51.11. The first step is to diagram ankle anatomy.

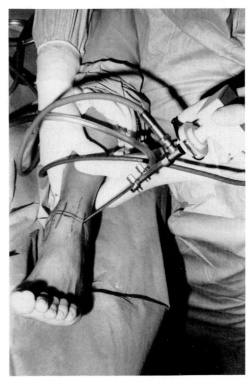

Figure 51.13. Arthroscope with the camera in the anterolateral portal.

discarded the technique of maintaining joint distention by using a saline-loaded syringe connected by intravenous (IV) tubing to the inflow cannula. Instead, two 3000-ml bags of saline are suspended on an IV pole about 7 feet above the floor and connected to the arthroscope cannula. The author generally uses the arthroscope cannula for the inflow because it tends to push the synovium and debris away from the end of the instrument. The second cannula is used for the outflow, as well as to allow the insertion of other instruments such as biopsy forceps, probes, or a power cutter.

Once these steps have been accomplished, one can visually inspect the joint in a systematic manner (Fig. 51.15). Again visualization is a matter of distention of the joint capsule and distraction of the joint. To enhance visualization it is necessary not only to dorsiflex and plantarflex the ankle but also to invert and evert the foot. On penetrating the ankle joint, the surgeon must make every effort to identify a familiar structure to become oriented. This can be difficult

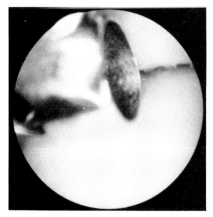

Figure 51.14. Arthroscopic view of the egress cannula.

because synovial thickening, chondromalacia, or capsular adhesions may prevent visualization by obscuring the end of the arthroscope or joint surfaces. Also, only a small portion of the joint can be seen through the scope and this is magnified. Consequently, the surgeon must use three principles in performing arthroscopy: scanning, pistoning, and rotation.

Scanning is the sweeping across the joint from side to side or up and down. The goal is to go from known areas to unknown areas in an attempt to delineate normal versus pathological anatomy. Pistoning is the moving of the arthroscope toward and away from some portion of the joint. As one moves toward an object in the joint, it becomes larger and the field of vision narrows. The farther the arthroscope moves away, the smaller the appearance of the object but the greater the field of vision. Rotation involves turning the arthroscope about its axis, taking advantage of the angled tip to increase the field of vision.

With the completion of either the diagnostic or operative arthroscopy, the joint is compressed to extrude the remaining irrigation solution, and the stab incision may be either closed with Steri-Strips or, preferably, sutured. A bulky dressing is applied followed by an elastic bandage. Sometimes a plaster splint is applied with the foot positioned at 90°. From the recovery area, the patient is returned to the room with routine orders for ice, elevation, evaluation of neurovascular status, and analgesics. With diagnostic arthroscopy, or synovectomy, range of motion exercises are encouraged with partial weight bearing with crutches beginning that evening or the next day under physical therapy guidance. The patient progresses to full weight bearing as tolerated and is usually discharged the next day. In the civilian sector, arthroscopy can be done on an outpatient basis.

If abrasion arthroplasty is performed for chondromalacia,

Figure 51.15. Intraoperative photograph of an ankle arthroscopy. The arthroscope is in the anteromedial portal, and an assistant is manipulating the ankle. Progress is followed on a video screen.

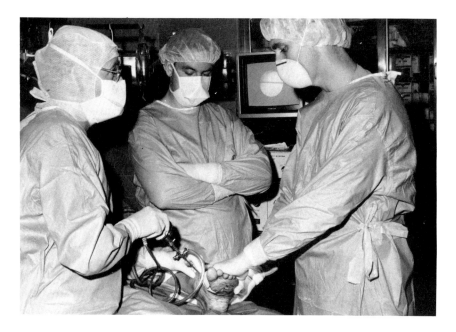

Table 51.1.
Indications for Arthroscopy

1. Persistent ankle joint pain
2. Osteochondral and chondral fractures/defects
3. Synovitis—diagnostic/debridement
4. Arthritis—rheumatoid, osteoarthritis
5. Anterior impingement exostosis
6. Chronic ankle instability
7. Preoperative planning—evaluation of articular surfaces
8. Chondromalacia
9. Adhesive capsulitis
10. Meniscoid body
11. Ankle fusion
12. Fracture

or after excision of a transchondral fracture, the patient abstains from weight bearing for 6 weeks while undergoing range of motion exercises. Continuous passive motion for the first 7 to 10 postoperative days would be an excellent adjunct. Edema may remain for several months, but patients many times can return to full activity in 1 to 3 months, depending upon the specific procedure performed.

INDICATIONS (Table 51.1)

Persistent Ankle Joint Pain

After injury there may be continuing clinical evidence or supportive tests that indicate a pathological condition within the ankle. This is one of the primary indications for ankle arthroscopy and is the most common indication for the author. The typical patient has a history of ankle injury, usually 6 to 8 months prior to seeking attention but at times many years previous. Complaints usually elicited are those of diffuse pain, swelling, and a decrease in activity. The patient may report any (or none) of the following symptoms: limitation of motion, instability, recurrent sprains, locking, popping, or grinding. Clinically, there is usually no discoloration or increased warmth about the ankle. Mild edema or joint effusion may be present. Tenderness is diffuse and may involve the entire ankle joint. The range of motion may be limited. Many times there are no indications of ankle instability. Routine radiographs show normal findings. Results of special studies, including stress radiography, CT scan, MRI, and laboratory work-up for arthritis, are all normal. The only positive finding may be a bone scan, with diffuse uptake at the ankle.

Upon arthroscopic examination, many intra-articular soft tissue conditions may be identified. One may find fibrous bands (Fig. 51.16) as described by Johnson (13). After injury an initial hyperemia of the synovium can lead to hypertrophy of the synovial villi. With chronic irritation the longer, broader portions form fibrous bands. Wolin and associates (18) reported on the hyalinization of unresorbed hemorrhage and fibrin exudate which produced a symptomatic meniscoid body along the anterior talofibular ligament (Fig. 51.17) Loose chondral bodies (Fig. 51.18), adhesive capsu-

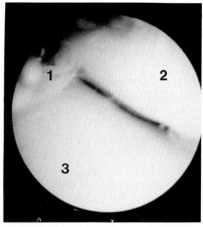

Figure 51.16.   Fibrous bands *(1)* along anterior aspect of ankle *(2)* tibia, *(3)* talus.

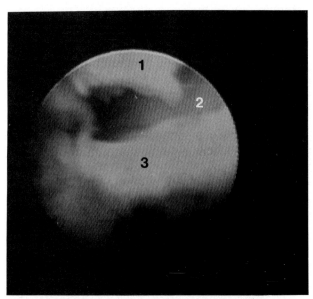

Figure 51.17.   Meniscoid body *(3)* *(1,* tibia; *2,* talus).

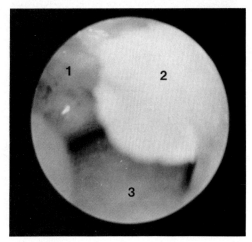

Figure 51.18.   Chondral loose body *(2)* *(1,* tibia; *3,* talus).

litis, traumatic arthritis, or hypertrophic synovitis, may also be found.

Watanabe and Takeda (19) have noted the therapeutic value of arthroscopic lavage of a joint, using large quantities of saline, that they termed *joint perfusion*. Experience has demonstrated this to be true. However, the author's patients who have had definite arthritic changes have not done as well as those reported by others. In these cases the effects have been temporary and unpredictable. Another benefit of the procedure has been an increased range of motion from lysis of capsular adhesions by joint distention, manipulation during the procedure, synovectomy, or with release by a meniscal knife under arthroscopic control. Jackson (20), in reviewing his own work, reports that approximately 21% of the symptomatic relief achieved with diagnostic arthroscopy can be attributed to joint lavage and 4% to the lysis of adhesions.

Synovitis

Patients with persistent synovitis may be evaluated and a synovial biopsy specimen obtained. This can help diagnose problems such as rheumatoid arthritis or pigmented villonodular synovitis. Cultures can help determine the presence of infectious synovitis, and specimens should be cultured for bacteria, fungus, and acid-fast organisms. However, these tests have never helped the author. Synovial biopsy specimens have always returned with a diagnosis of chronic synovitis. Experience has shown that chronic ankle conditions produce a significant amount of synovitis. This tends to obscure the visualization of joint surfaces and will require

debridement,which is a time-consuming procedure. A full-radius synovial resector is used to debride the hypertrophic synovitis. In addition, capsular adhesions will limit distention of the joint, further hindering joint inspection.

Osteochondral and Chondral Fractures

One can evaluate an osteochondral fracture (Fig. 51.19) in regard to size, depth, and amount of displacement. Berndt and Harty (21) described and classified these lesions as trans-

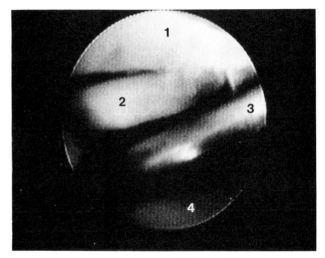

Figure 51.19. Osteochondral fracture *(2)* (stage IV), anterolateral aspect of talar dome *(1,* tibia; *3,* probe; *4,* talus).

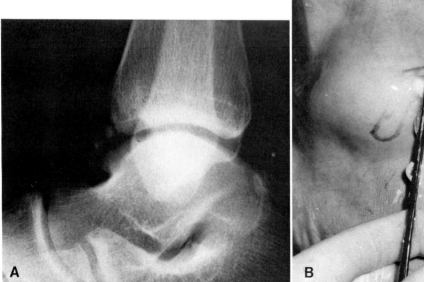
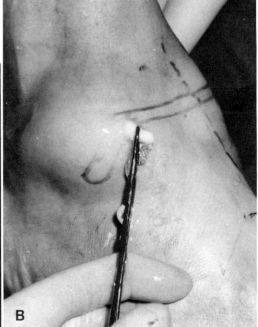

Figure 51.20. **A.** Lateral radiograph demonstrating multiple old lateral transchondral fractures of the talar dome. **B.** Intraoperative photograph showing excision of fracture fragments through an anterolateral portal.

chondral fractures. Stage I is a compression of the articular cartilage. Stage II is an incomplete fracture. Stage III is a complete fracture that is nondisplaced. Stage IV is a displaced fracture. Transchondral fractures are the second most common reason for the author to perform ankle arthroscopy.

Transchondral fractures are classically described as occurring on either the lateral or the medial talar dome. The lateral lesions are described as shallow, wafer-shaped, and occurring on the anterior half of the talar dome. This anterior location has traditionally allowed easy excision by means of an anterolateral arthrotomy. This position also facilitates arthroscopic excision through the anterior portals. Because most acute stage IV lateral talar dome fractures have a concomitant grade III rupture of the fibular collateral ligaments, the author excises or occasionally performs open reduction with internal fixation of the fragment by arthrotomy. The ruptured anterior talofibular and calcaneofibular ligaments can then be primarily repaired.

Arthroscopy is reserved for those cases having old lateral talar dome fractures, with or without associated chronic instability (Fig. 51.20). The arthroscope is placed in the anteromedial portal, and the anterolateral portal is used for instrumentation to excise the fragment. A full-radius synovial resector is used first to debride the hypertrophic synovitis, which always obscures the anterolateral aspect of the joint. Then the fragment is freed with a probe and/or a banana-blade knife. The fragment is grasped with a small Kocher hemostat and removed through the anterolateral portal. The portal may have to be extended to excise a large fragment. Finally, the remaining defect is abraded down to bleeding bone, and the irregular cartilaginous ends are smoothed with a synovial shaver. Sometimes the defect is percutaneously drilled with a K-wire under arthroscopic control. If chronic ankle instability is present with only anterior talofibular ligament insufficiency, this can be addressed at the same time with an arthroscopic stapling.

Medial talar dome lesions are described as being deeper, cup-shaped, and located on the posterior third of the talar dome. It is the posterior location that has made the approach to this lesion difficult. The most commonly reported approach has been with a medial malleolar osteotomy. However, the author has successfully removed the majority of medial talar dome transchondral fractures with the arthroscope. Some of the fractures are large or located more anteriorly than normal and, therefore, can be approached through the anterior portals. The arthroscope is placed in the anterolateral portal for visualization. The anteromedial portal is used for surgical instrumentation to remove the fragment. If there is a degree of joint laxity or some instability, then access to the posterior aspect of the medial talar dome is even easier. Usually an assistant will plantarflex and distract the ankle for visualization.

An additional technique, introduced by Guhl (22), which has been useful, is to apply a mechanical distraction device (Fig. 51.21). One pin is placed in the tibia and another in the calcaneus. The device is attached and the joint is dis-

tracted, allowing better access to the lesion. The fragment is freed, grasped, and removed. Guhl also reported on the drilling of the defect by passing a K-wire through the medial malleolus under arthroscopic and fluoroscopic control. The ankle is then dorsiflexed and plantarflexed to allow drilling of different areas of the defect. Obviously, the pins used for the distractor adds morbidity to the case and increases the possibility of complications such as fracture. To date, no neurovascular or ligamentous damage has been noted. The distractor does not need to be used routinely for ankle arthroscopy. If the arthroscopic approach is unsuccessful, a posteromedial arthrotomy is used to remove the fragment. Lundeen uses arthroscopy to approach the medial lesion but abrades a groove posteriorly along the medial bend of the tibia until the fracture can be reached (Lundeen RO, personal communication).

After arthroscopic removal, the patient abstains from weight bearing for 6 weeks, and if it is available, continuous passive motion is used for the first 7 to 10 days (23). This is followed by active and passive range of motion exercises. The patient is placed in a removable plaster splint or fracture brace. If an arthroscopic stapling was performed at the same time, a non-weight-bearing short-leg cast is employed for 6 weeks.

Anterior Impingement Exostosis

An osteophyte located on the anterior aspect of the tibia is another problem easily addressed by arthroscopy (Fig. 51.22). From either the anteromedial or anterolateral portal, a small osteotome can be used to resect the osteophyte. The progress of the resection can be followed with the arthroscope. The bony fragment is then grasped and removed through one of the portals. The resected area of the anterior tibia can be further remodeled with an abrader. The adequacy of the resection may be confirmed with intra-operative radiographs. If the exostosis is small, it can be remodeled with the abrader alone. However, if there is a corresponding exostosis located on the neck of the talus, it may not be visible if it is extracapsular.

Arthritis

Arthroscopy can help establish a diagnosis of rheumatoid arthritis by the appearance of the synovium and synovial biopsy (Fig. 51.23). When indicated, synovectomy can be performed with the arthroscope and synovial resection. Again Watanabe and Takeda (19) have reported on the clinical benefits of arthroscopic debridement and joint lavage. Johnson (24) notes that in the knee, rheumatoid synovitis is characterized by fingerlike projecting villi (dumbbell-shaped) with rounded ends. This differs from degenerative arthritis in which the villi are finer and fimbriated. Lundeen has observed gouty arthritis with tophaceous deposits at synovial reflections invariably imbedded in fibrous tissue (personal communication and unpublished observations). Areas of chondromalacia can be abraded to allow a resurfacing phenomenon with fibrocartilage.

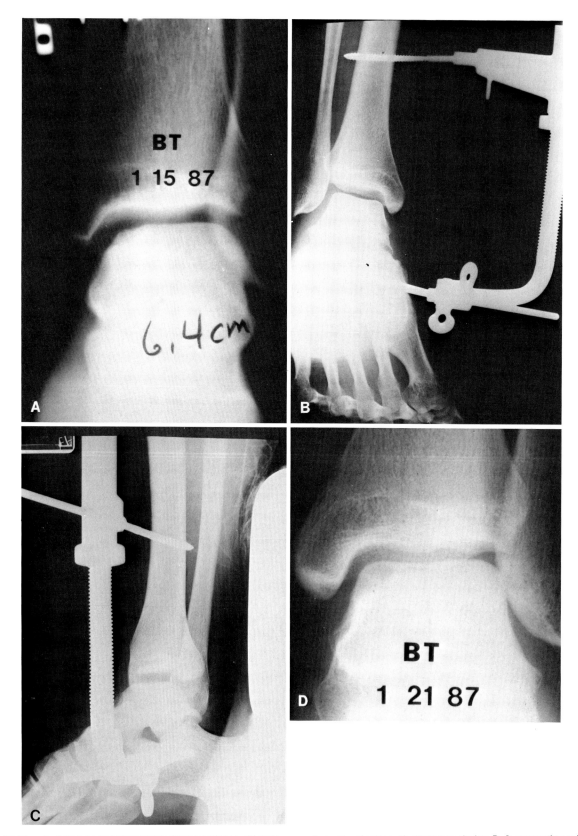

Figure 51.21. **A.** Anteroposterior tomogram demonstrating an old stage III medial talar dome transchondral fracture. **B** and **C.** Mortise and lateral radiographs of ankle with distraction device. **D.** Postoperative radiograph after excision of the medial transchondral fracture.

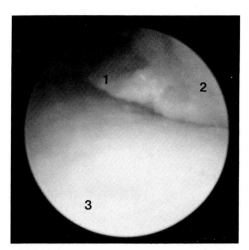

Figure 51.22.   Anterior tibial osteophyte *(1)* (*2,* tibia; *3,* talus).

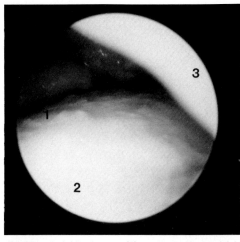

Figure 51.23.   Arthritic changes *(1)* on dome of talus *(2)* (*3,* tibia).

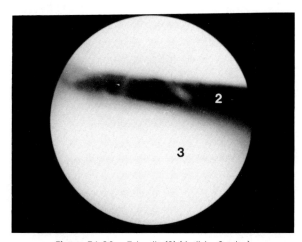

Figure 51.24.   Talar tilt *(2)* (*1,* tibia; *3,* talus).

Ligament Injuries

Because portions of the collateral ligaments are intracapsular, ligamentous injuries can be evaluated and tested for stability (Fig. 51.24). The author has used arthroscopy in four patients with acute lateral ankle ligament disruptions (grade III). The ruptured ends of the anterior talofibular ligament were observed, and in one case the site where the ligament avulsed off the lateral malleolus was visible. In two of these cases, transchondral fractures on the lateral aspect of the talar dome were visible on radiograph. In three of the cases both anterior displacement of the talus out of the mortise and talar tilt could be observed on stress testing. Care must be exercised in acute trauma so that the irrigation solution does not escape through the capsular tears and infiltrate into the surrounding fascial planes, which could result in a compartment syndrome. In one case arthroscopy was discontinued because of this problem prior to the development of a compartment syndrome. All required arthrotomy for primary repair of the ligaments and excision of transchondral fracture. The role for ankle arthroscopy in the acutely injured patient is limited.

To date there are no percutaneous techniques for primarily repairing ankle ligaments with arthroscopy. However, chronic lateral ankle instability may be amenable to arthroscopic surgery in selected cases of anterior talofibular ligament instability. Lundeen and Hawkins (25) have performed arthroscopic stapling and reported promising early results. They describe a ballooning of the lateral capsule and anterior talofibular ligament, which is visible at the time of surgery.

The author has performed arthroscopic staplings, all on active-duty soldiers with isolated anterior talofibular ligament insufficiency (Fig. 51.25). A 25° 4.0-mm arthroscope is placed in the anteromedial portal for visualization. A 4.2/5.5-mm full-radius synovial resector is employed to debride the hypertrophic synovitis in the lateral compartment through an anterolateral portal. The 25° arthroscope is exchanged for a 70° arthroscope to enable the surgeon to look inferiorly into the lateral joint compartment. With the 70° arthroscope, one can easily see the tip of the lateral malleolus, anterior talofibular ligament, anterolateral capsule, and the lateral surface of the talar body.

A 4.5-mm abrader is introduced through the anterolateral portal and used to create a trough on the anterior aspect of the lateral talar body. Then an accessory portal is made along the anterior and inferior aspects of the lateral malleolus over the anterior talofibular ligament. The soft tissues are spread with a hemostat to make sure no nerve is in the way. An arthroscopic staple is placed through this accessory portal, and the attenuated anterior talofibular ligament/capsular tissue is grasped between the prongs of the staple. With the arthroscope, one will see the tip of the staple protrude through the ligamentous/capsular tissue. The tips of the staple are positioned into the abraded area on the lateral aspect of the talus with the ankle dorsiflexed. The staple is impacted into the talus with a mallet, and radiographs are obtained to confirm its position. This is basically a tightening of the anterior talofibular ligament and anterolateral cap-

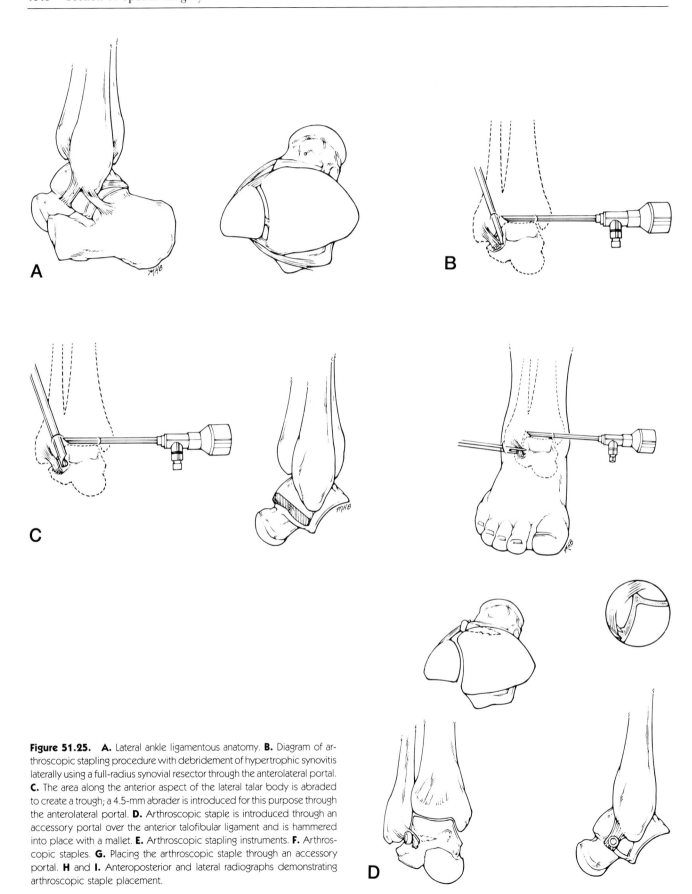

Figure 51.25. **A.** Lateral ankle ligamentous anatomy. **B.** Diagram of arthroscopic stapling procedure with debridement of hypertrophic synovitis laterally using a full-radius synovial resector through the anterolateral portal. **C.** The area along the anterior aspect of the lateral talar body is abraded to create a trough; a 4.5-mm abrader is introduced for this purpose through the anterolateral portal. **D.** Arthroscopic staple is introduced through an accessory portal over the anterior talofibular ligament and is hammered into place with a mallet. **E.** Arthroscopic stapling instruments. **F.** Arthroscopic staples. **G.** Placing the arthroscopic staple through an accessory portal. **H** and **I.** Anteroposterior and lateral radiographs demonstrating arthroscopic staple placement.

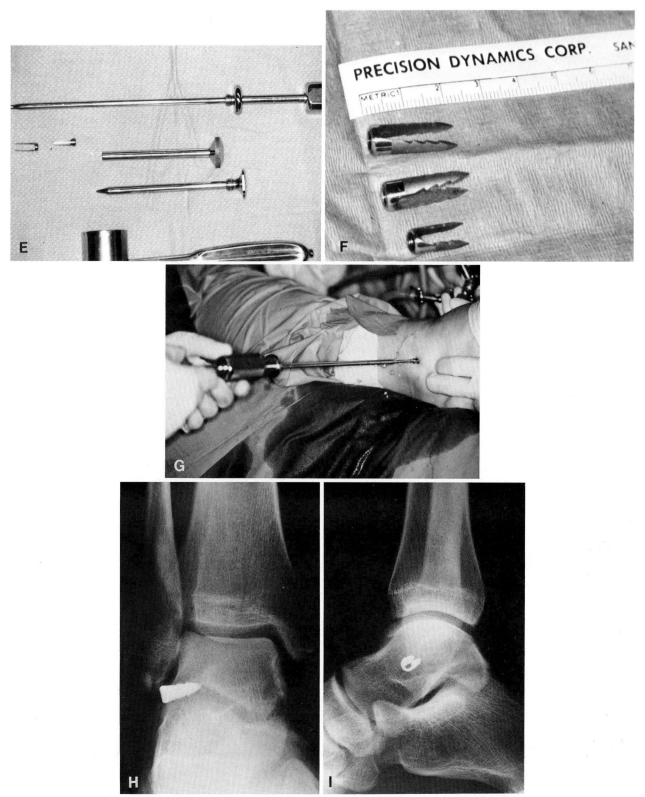

Figure 51.25. E-I.

sule. The arthroscopic portals are sutured, and a short-leg cast is applied.

To date, instability has persisted in one of ten patients and has required ankle reconstruction. One patient continued to demonstrate a slight anterior drawer sign, but less than before surgery. The other patients have remained stable.

Evaluation of Articular Surfaces and Preoperative Planning

In contemplating reconstructive procedures such as lateral ligament reconstruction or fibular osteotomy, arthroscopic evaluation can determine whether articular degeneration has occurred.

Chondromalacia

The effects of chondromalacia on the articular cartilage can be evaluated and staged: stage I is softening or swelling of the cartilage, stage II represents articular fissuring, stage III demonstrates fibrillation of cartilage with a crab-meat, sawtooth appearance. Exposure of subchondral bone represents stage IV (26) (Fig. 51.26). In 1979 Johnson (27) introduced the technique of abrasion arthroplasty of chondromalacial defects of the patella. By debriding full-thickness cartilaginous defects with a high-speed bur to a depth of 1 mm, underlying capillaries were exposed. If the joint underwent rehabilitation with range of motion exercises and non-weight-bearing, a layer of fibrocartilage was produced. Histologically, this is not normal cartilage, but pain is alleviated by a resurfacing phenomenon. However, Salter et al. (23) reported that the addition of a continuous passive mo-

tion machine to the postoperative regimen significantly increased the amount of replacement by normal hyaline cartilage.

CONTRAINDICATIONS

Soft tissue infection over a joint is a contraindication to arthroscopy. Also, in acute trauma moderate to severe edema would increase the morbidity in any surgical procedure.

COMPLICATIONS

Small (28) reported in a prospective study that 21 experienced arthroscopists performing 146 ankle arthroscopies encountered only one complication: an infection. However, Guhl (29) reported 13 complications in 131 cases, for a complication rate of 7.6%. These included three painful scars, one scarring of the peroneal tendons from a distraction device, four nerve injuries, two infections, two misdiagnoses, and one broken pin. Martin and associates (30), in 58 cases, reported a 15% complication rate, with a higher rate of nerve injury. Barber and associates (31) reported a 17% complication rate in 53 consecutive ankle arthroscopies. There were three wound infections, three nerve injuries, one reflex sympathetic dystrophy, and two synovial fistulas. Nevertheless, Guhl reported that his complication rate decreased with experience.

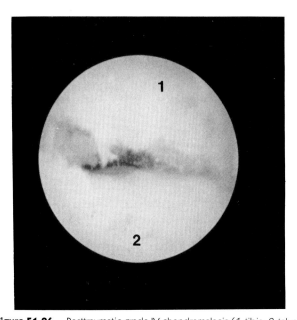

Figure 51.26. Posttraumatic grade IV chondromalacia (1, tibia; 2, talus). (Courtesy of R. Lundeen.)

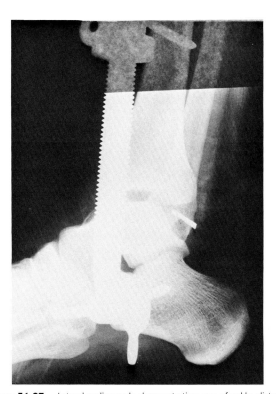

Figure 51.27. Lateral radiograph demonstrating use of ankle distractor with a broken knife blade in the posterior aspect of the ankle joint.

The author's most common postoperative complication has been the recurrence of symptoms. This has occurred in patients with findings of traumatic arthritis. There have also been one infection, two nerve injuries, one broken knife blade (Fig. 51.27), which was successfully retrieved, and one misplacement of an arthroscopic staple.

CONCLUSION

Arthroscopy of the ankle is no longer in its infancy. Today there are many practitioners employing this modality. Like any procedure, it is not a panacea for all ankle problems. However, direct visualization of intra-articular abnormalities and the low morbidity associated with the procedure make this an exciting and challenging area. Its indications and limits are established. With increased clinical consciousness, smaller surgical instrumentation, and longer-term follow-up, diagnostic and surgical arthroscopy of the ankle will become a more important surgical technique.

References

1. Cassell SW: Arthroscopy of the knee joint, a review of 150 cases. *J Bone Joint Surg* 53A:287, 1971.
2. Jackson RW, Abe I: The role of arthroscopy in the management of disorders of the knee: an analysis of 200 consecutive examinations. *J Bone Joint Surg* 54B:310, 1972.
3. Watanabe M: *Atlas of Arthroscopy*, ed 2. Tokyo, Igaku Shoin, LTD, 1969.
4. Bircher E: Die Arthroendoskopie. *Zentralbl Chir* 48:1460-1461, 1921.
5. Burman MS: Arthroscopy or direct visualization of joints—an experimental cadaver study. *J Bone Joint Surg* 13:669-695, 1931.
6. Takagi K: The arthroscope. *J Jpn Orthop Assoc* 14:359-411, 1939.
7. Watanabe M, Takeda S: The number 21 arthroscope. *J Jpn Orthop Assoc* 34:1041, 1960.
8. O'Connor RL: *Arthroscopy*. Philadelphia, JB Lippincott, 1972.
9. Watanabe M: *Selfoc-Arthroscope (Watanabe No. 24 Arthroscope)* (monograph). Tokyo Teishin Hospital, Tokyo Department of Orthopaedic Surgery, 1972.
10. Watanabe M: Arthroscopy of small joints. *J Jpn Orthop Assoc* 45:908, 1971.
11. Chen YC: Clinical and cadaver studies on ankle joint arthroscopy. *J Jpn Orthop Assoc* 50:631, 1976.
12. Plank E: Die Arthroskopie des oberen Sprunggelenkes. *Helfe Unfallheinkunde* 131:245-251, 1978.
13. Johnson LL: *Diagnostic and Surgical Arthroscopy: The Knee and Other Joints*, ed 2. St Louis, CV Mosby, 1981, pp 412-419.
14. Parisien JS, Shereff MJ: The role of arthroscopy in the diagnosis and treatment of disorders of the ankle. *Foot Ankle* 2:144-149, 1981.
15. Drez D, Guhl JF, Gollehon DL: Arthroscopy: techniques and indications. *Foot Ankle* 2:138-143, 1981.
16. Heller AJ, Vogler HW: Ankle joint arthroscopy. *J Foot Surg* 21:23-29, 1982.
17. Johnson LL: *Diagnostic and Surgical Arthroscopy: The Knee and Other Joints*, ed 2. St Louis, CV Mosby, 1981, p 23.
18. Wolin I, Glassman F, Siderman S, Levinthal DH: Internal derangement of the talofibular component of the ankle. *Surg Gynecol Obstet* 91:193-200, 1950.
19. Watanabe M, Takeda S: *Atlas of Arthroscopy*. Tokyo, Igaku Shoin, 1957, p 6.
20. Jackson RW: The current role of arthroscopy in the management of knee problems. Proceedings of the combined meeting of the orthopedic associations of the English-speaking world. *Orthop Trans* 6:469, 1982.
21. Berndt AL, Harty M: Transchondral fractures (osteochondritis dessicans) of the talus. *J Bone Joint Surg* 41A:988-1018, 1959.
22. Guhl JK: New techniques for arthroscopic surgery of the ankle: preliminary report. *Orthopedics* 9:261-269, 1986.
23. Salter RB, Simmonds DF, Malcolm BW, Rumble EJ, MacMichael D, Clemons N: The biological effect of continuous passive motion on the healing of full thickness defects in articular cartilage. *J Bone Joint Surg* 62A:1232-1251, 1980.
24. Johnson LL: *Diagnostic and Surgical Arthroscopy: The Knee and Other Joints*, ed 2. St Louis, CV Mosby, 1981, pp 203-204.
25. Lundeen RO, Hawkins R: Arthroscopic lateral ankle stabilization *J Am Podiatry Assoc* 75:372-376, 1985.
26. Wiles P, Andrews P, Devas M: Chondromalacia of the patella. *J Bone Joint Surg* 38B:95, 1956.
27. Johnson LL: Healing of human articular cartilage: an arthroscopic review (Presented at the American Academy of Orthopaedic Surgeons). *Orthop Trans* 5:400, 1981.
28. Small NC: Complications in arthroscopic surgery performed by experienced arthroscopists. *Arthroscopy* 4:215-221, 1988.
29. Guhl JF: New concepts (distraction) in ankle arthroscopy. *Arthroscopy* 4:160-167, 1988.
30. Martin DF, Baker CL, Curl WW, Andrews JR, Robie DB, Haas AF: Operative ankle arthroscopy, long term follow-up. *Am J Sports Med* 17:16-23, 1989.
31. Barber FA, Click J, Britt DT: Complications of ankle arthroscopy. *Foot Ankle* 10:263-266, 1990.

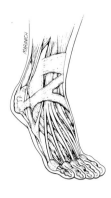

CHAPTER **52**

The Neuropathic Foot

Vincent J. Hetherington, D.P.M.

The neuropathic foot is defined as the foot affected by one of several disease states that are manifested by an altered neural function. This affects sensory, motor, and vascular elements to varying degrees. Pathology results through a combination of external and internal factors. The external environment includes the home or workplace, occupation, floor surfaces, and shoes. The internal environment encompasses altered musculoskeletal function, deformity, vascular modifications, and skin dysfunction.

The purpose of this chapter is to discuss the role of internal changes, their relationship to external factors, the development of pathological conditions, and their management with regard to the neuropathic foot. The exact pathology of each individual disease process is beyond the scope of this chapter. The points discussed here represent the pedal manifestations of these diseases. The conditions most commonly seen by the average clinician are those associated with diabetes mellitus, and thus the primary emphasis of discussion is premised on this disease entity.

NEUROPATHY

In many patients nerve damage does not involve a few select fibers but, rather, is manifested as a peripheral polyneuropathy. This is particularly true in patients with diabetes. The clinician should be aware of all the forms of this process as they appear in the foot and leg. Table 52.1 lists the prevalence of the various subtypes of symmetrical diabetic polyneuropathy. Most clinicians are acutely aware of the sensory deficit so commonly associated with diabetes. However, other components of the neuropathic process are of equal importance in the development of complications. Approximately 70% of diabetic patients will have involvement of all three nerve fiber types, as opposed to sensory neuropathy alone (1). Motor and autonomic dysfunction are components of the process that are largely not included in the

Table 52.1.
Fiber Involvement in Distal Symmetrical Diabetic Polyneuropathy

Subtype	% of cases
Mixed sensory-motor-autonomic	70
Predominantly sensory	30
Predominantly motor	<1
Predominantly autonomic	<1

Adapted from Brown MJ, Asbury AK: Diabetic neuropathy. *Ann Neurol* 15: 2-12, 1984.

assessment of the neuropathic patient and yet are of great importance.

Sensory Neuropathy

Diseases that result in diminished sensation of the foot vary in their presentation and etiology. Table 52.2 presents a compilation of some of these conditions. Although sensory dysfunction may be the most obvious neurologic deficiency, the clinician should be aware that there may be other aspects of neuropathy involving the extremity.

Motor Neuropathy

The motor neuropathy that accompanies diabetic polyneuropathy most often affects the intrinsic muscles of the foot. Some authors have even referred to this condition as the intrinsic minus foot (2, 3), or one lacking intrinsic muscle function. Once these small muscles lose the ability to function effectively, digital contractures will begin to develop. Many patients will have a biomechanical imbalance that predisposes them to the development of hammer toes, which is, in turn, exacerbated by the intrinsic atrophy.

Digital contractures place the patient at risk of the development of clavi, which, when combined with sensory deficits, may lead to ulceration. An often unrecognized consequence is thickening of the distal nail. Nails will respond to chronic pressures, and, with fixed contractures of the digit, weight is primarily shifted to the tip of the toe as opposed to the plantar pulp. This increases the pressures at the hyponychium and leads to onychauxis. Many times this is misinterpreted as being a consequence of onychomycosis.

Hammer toe deformities are usually associated with dorsal contractures of the metatarsophalangeal joint. This buckling effect increases the pressures in the ball of the foot, potentially leading to hyperkeratotic lesions and/or ulceration.

Although intrinsic atrophy is the most common form of motor dysfunction in the diabetic limb, a number of patients will also have weakness in the leg. The anterior or extensor compartment appears to be the muscle group most commonly involved. Although weakness may also be evident in other muscle groups, the extensors appear to suffer to a greater extent. In a few patients this may be profound enough to cause a drop foot. In most individuals the involvement is more subtle. However, the net effect is that the normal antagonism between muscle groups is lost. Therefore, the triceps achieve a mechanical advantage that,

Table 52.2.
Outline of Diseases and Processes Resulting in a Neuropathic Foot

I. Neuropathy Associated With Systemic Disease
   Diabetes mellitus
   Uremia
   Amyloidosis
II. Neuropathy Associated With Nutritional Disturbances
   Alcoholism
   Pernicious anemia
III. Neuropathy Associated With Infectious Diseases
   Leprosy
   Syphilis
   Poliomyelitis
IV. Neuropathy on a Vascular Basis
   Cerebral vascular accident
   Spinal cord infarction
   Diabetic mononeuropathy
   Arteritis
   Peripheral vascular disease
V. Hereditary Motor and Sensory Neuropathy (HMSN)
   Roussy-Lévy syndrome
   Charcot-Marie-Tooth disease
VI. Hereditary Sensory and Autonomic Neuropathy (HSAN)
   Hereditary sensory neuropathy
   Congenital sensory neuropathy
   Dysautonomia (Riley-Day syndrome)
VII. Cerebellar Degeneration
   Friedreich's ataxia
VIII. Motor Neuron Disease
   Amyotrophic lateral sclerosis
IX. Diseases of the Spinal Cord
   Spina bifida
   Syringomyelia
X. Trauma
   Spinal cord injury
   Peripheral nerve injury
   Spinal root trauma
XI. Compressive Neuropathy
   Spinal cord tumor
   Peripheral nerve compression
XII. Toxic Neuropathy
   Lead poisoning
XIII. Other
   Cerebral palsy

in turn, favors the development of an ankle equinus.

Once equinus develops, the long extensor muscles will fire prematurely in gait as the patient attempts to overcome the anterior leg weakness and to achieve adequate dorsiflexion. Even with normal intrinsic function, digital instability is created by the extensor substitution. Therefore, digital contractures are once again favored. Equinus also increases the pressures plantar to the metatarsal heads, compounding plantar keratoses. Compensation for the loss of ankle dorsiflexion usually takes place in the midfoot and rearfoot areas. Typically this is a symptomatic process, but sensory neuropathy eliminates the protective mechanism of pain.

Autonomic Neuropathy

Within the lower extremity the sympathetic nerves primarily control the vascular tone of the arterioles and regulate sweat gland function. Once autonomic neuropathy develops, the arterioles lose the ability to constrict. When this is combined with altered sweat gland function, the patient with autonomic neuropathy has a warm, dry, anhidrotic foot.

Throughout the last decade a greater understanding of the role of autonomic neuropathy has been achieved. Boulton and associates (4) demonstrated that the pO_2 of venous blood in patients with neuropathic feet was significantly higher than that in control subjects. Autonomic neuropathy was thought to increase arteriovenous shunting and result in a rapid shift of blood from the arterial to the venous capillary bed (5). Venous occlusion plethysmography demonstrated that, on average, blood flow to the diabetic neuropathic foot was five times greater than to the control foot (6). In fact, the mean skin temperature was noted to be approximately 7° C greater in the neuropathic limbs.

Edmonds and associates (7) demonstrated that the uptake of technetium was greater in all three phases in patients with diabetic neuropathy than in control patients. The authors attributed this phenomena to an increased blood flow secondary to sympathetic denervation.

Another consequence of autonomic neuropathy is vascular calcification. After sympathetic dysfunction the muscles within the media of the arterioles will atrophy and secondarily calcify (8). Calcification of arterioles was reported by Goebel and Fuessel (9) in both diabetic and nondiabetic patients after surgical sympathectomy. Edmonds and associates (10) found that vascular calcification was most closely related to the degree of neuropathy, not to age or duration of diabetes. Fifteen of 20 patients with neuropathy were noted to have vascular calcification in the feet, compared with only 4 of 20 diabetic patients without neuropathy. Furthermore, two large studies of Charcot foot deformity found that 78% and 90%, respectively, demonstrated radiographic evidence of vascular calcification (11, 12).

This finding, in and of itself, should not be interpreted as evidence of peripheral vascular disease. The tissue that undergoes this process is within the tunica media of the vessel. Therefore, the internal diameter of the arteriole is unchanged and blood flow to the limb is not diminished (13). However, calcification may alter vessel elasticity, making it difficult to palpate the pulses in some individuals. Studies have shown that ankle/arm indices are consistently higher in patients with neuropathic feet than in control subjects (5, 14). At times one may find it impossible to occlude the arteries with a sphygmomanometer. However, more sophisticated vascular studies will confirm the circulatory status of the limb.

Gilbey and associates (15) in examining patients with diabetic nephropathy and autonomic neuropathy found that vascular calcification was common and extensive and yet did not indicate tissue ischemia. They concluded, despite this finding, that there was a high peripheral blood flow and normal transcutaneous pO_2 at rest. Chantelau and associates (16) examined diabetic patients who had medial arterial calcification and found no evidence of peripheral vascular disease. They noted that transcutaneous pO_2 increased significantly after exercise. It was suggested that this was due to the increased blow flow found in the neuropathic limb.

The hyperemia that occurs as a consequence of autonomic neuropathy does not selectively involve the soft tissues. Numerous authors have shown that the bone is highly innervated with sympathetic fibers and that sympathectomy results in an increase of between 10% and 115% in blood flow to the bone (17-20). Edmonds and associates (7) indicated that the increased uptake of technetium in the third phase of bone scans in the neuropathic limb was due to this denervation. This effect was isolated to the feet; therefore other metabolic causes of hyperemia were excluded.

VASCULAR OCCLUSIVE DISEASE

The patient with diabetes appears to have a greater and more significant degree of peripheral macrovascular disease than the normal patient. Conrad (21) performed an extensive comparison of large- and small-vessel disease in diabetic and nondiabetic individuals. One of his major conclusions was that the variation and pattern of obstruction differ in diabetics and nondiabetics. In diabetics there appears to be an increase in disease in the vasculature of the calf. Arterial sclerosis in the diabetic appears to occur distally, and it progresses in a distal-to-proximal fashion. As a result of this more distal origin of the arterial sclerosis and the manner of progression, a less effective collateral circulation appears to develop.

However, Conrad believed that the existence of a diabetic small artery disease could not be supported by conclusive evidence. Any decrease in blood flow to the digits could be explained by an increase in resistance of the more proximal calf arteries and would not be evidence of distal arterial disease. Poor collateralization often occurs because of involvement of the genicular circulation that is affected by diabetes.

Numerous other authors (22-24) have subscribed to the theory that microvascular insufficiency develops in the diabetic via a variety of means. Various aspects of these factors have been investigated. These include (a) functional changes in the endothelium, (b) endothelial injury (25), (c) platelet adhesion and aggregation (26, 27), (d) basement membrane thickening (28-32), (e) increased plasma viscosity, (f) red blood cell aggregation and microthrombosis (33), (g) microaneurysm (23, 34), and (h) altered fibrinolysis (33).

A dermal microangiopathy has been identified in the toes of diabetics, by both light and electron microscopy, as a thickening of the capillary basement membrane (31, 32). Histologic changes seen in skeletal muscle, capillary basement thickening, pericyte degeneration, and acellular capillaries occurred with increasing frequency from neck to foot in diabetics. Tilton and his coauthors (35) believed this to be due to increased venous pressure. They surmised that these capillary degenerative changes are more prevalent in the foot and may be consistent with accelerated vascular disease.

Hyperglycemia in the diabetic appears to lead directly to increased enzymatic incorporation of carbohydrate into the basement membrane. There is an increased ability of the red blood cells to aggregate, and there is a hyperviscosity of the plasma. In diabetics, there also appears to be a decreased fibrolytic activity of the blood, as well as an increased ability of the platelets to aggregate.

Despite these findings, however, there is evidence that the changes that occur within the small vessels of the lower extremity do not result in a functional loss of perfusion to the tissues. LoGerfo and Coffman (36) noted that ". . . the idea that diabetic patients have occlusive microvascular disease has not been confirmed by light microscopy, vascular casting, or physiologic studies. It has, however, been a tenacious misconception . . . which can lead to inappropriate care of the foot in the diabetic patient. . . ." These authors note that, although there is a capillary basement membrane thickening in vessels of diabetics, there is ". . . no evidence of capillary narrowing or occlusion."

Flynn and associates (37) used both television microscopy and laser Doppler flowmetry to study the microcirculation in diabetic neuropathic feet. They concluded that the skin capillary blood flow was increased in diabetics with neuropathy. Furthermore, there was no evidence to support the premise of capillary ischemia under resting conditions.

These findings are confirmed every day by those who treat the neuropathic foot. Provided there is no proximal occlusion and no infection, stress is alleviated, and wound care is provided, diabetic patients have the capacity to heal. The clinical appearance of many feet at the time of presentation also argues against a functional microangiopathy. In many individuals the degree of inflammation associated with some of the neuropathic complications (i.e., infection, pathologic fracture) is severe. The capacity to mount an acute inflammatory response is dependent on good circulation.

The key factor is that one should not immediately assume that, simply because the patient may have diabetes peripheral vascular disease is also present. Today there are a number of noninvasive modalities that may be used to aid the clinician in determining the peripheral perfusion, thereby providing the patient with a better evaluation, treatment, and prognosis. Although the concepts with regard to microvascular disease in the diabetic appear to be changing, there is still universal agreement that these individuals are more susceptible to the development of occlusive disease in the larger vessels.

SOFT TISSUE BIOMECHANICS

The pathogenesis of soft tissue lesions in the neuropathic foot is closely related to the biomechanical properties of the skin. Because of its complex constituents, the skin serves various functions. Among these is the ability to adapt to the absorption and dissipation of energy. To function properly, the skin must have adequate sensibility, pliability, and vascularity.

The skin may be regarded as a series of networks as described by Gibson and Kenedi (38). The collagen fiber network of the integument functions so that if stretched in any direction most of the fibers will be oriented parallel to the lines of stretch. At low loads few fibers may be involved. As the load increases, the number of fibers will also increase to resist further tissue extension. The elastic fiber network is intimately related to the collagen fibers and acts as an energy-storage device or spring to return the collagen to its relaxed position.

The interstitial fluid that surrounds the network acts to lubricate the mechanism and serves as a buffer against sudden changes. The interstitial fluid is also important in the dissipation of heat. An increase in the amount of interstitial fluid increases the resistance of the skin to deformity. The skin, therefore, has viscoelastic properties. Fluid is forced

out of the tissue during deformation and returns during a recovery period (39). The function of the interstitial fluid has been compared to that of a shock absorber.

In diabetes, glycosylation of structural proteins such as collagen and keratin may result in the loss of flexibility of the dermis and superficial layers of the skin (40). This may also affect tendons and joint structures, resulting in limited joint mobility. It has been noted that limited joint mobility in the foot predisposes the patient to a greater risk of ulceration (41). It also compounds the muscular imbalances created by motor neuropathy, making contracture more rigid.

Dryness due to autonomic dysfunction will further reduce the capacity of the skin to resist stress. Therefore, supple-

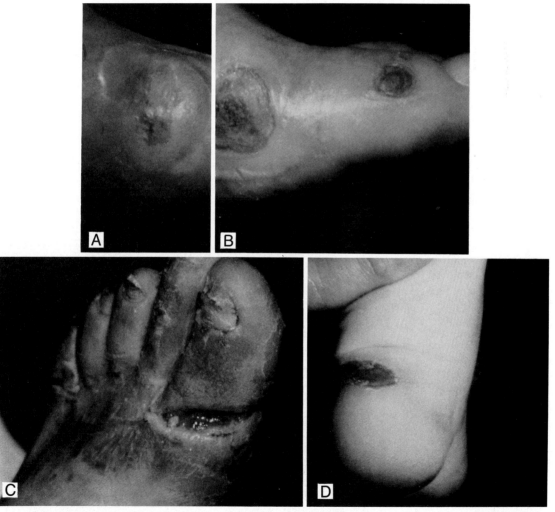

Figure 52.1. **A.** A small skin irritation that developed in a diabetic patient with advanced peripheral vascular disease. **B.** Ischemic ulceration with penetration through the subcutaneous tissues. The capsular structures are exposed on the lateral aspect; medially an eschar of necrotic tissue covers the lesion. The lesions were progressive, and the patient's vascular disease was not amenable to reconstruction. Infection ensued and amputation was required. **C.** Neurotrophic ulceration caused by continuous pressure developed as a result of a home shoe modification. The patient has peripheral neuropathy secondary to chronic ethanol abuse. The ulcer was caused by a shoelace. **D.** Painless ulcer developed on posterior portion of heel in 2½-year-old child with spina bifida because of improperly fitting shoe. A seam in the shoe rested directly over the ulcer site.

mentary agents are important for many patients to help enhance hydration of the tissues.

MECHANISM OF THE DEVELOPMENT OF NEUROPATHIC ULCERATION

The mechanisms or pathogenesis of the development of plantar ulcers have been discussed by Brand (42) and Hall and Brand (43) and are listed as follows: *(a)* continuous pressure, *(b)* concentrated high pressure, *(c)* repetitive mechanical stress, and *(d)* thermal injury. Skin defects that result from continuous pressure are caused by a relative lack of blood supply. Kosiak (44) points out that intense pressures of short duration are as detrimental as low pressures applied for extended periods. Regardless of the specific mechanism, localized ischemia leads to irreversible tissue damage and necrosis. The normal capillary blood pressure ranges from 13 to 33 mm Hg. Pressures above this level result in blockage of capillary flow. Therefore the extent of tissue involvement secondary to continuous pressure is dependent on time and pressure and can extend from skin to bone.

Ulcerations that arise from continuous pressure are those in the decubitus type. In the foot this occurs commonly on the heel. This type of lesion will also develop over a bony prominence, such as the first metatarsophalangeal joint in a shoe that is excessively tight. The constant pressure exerted by the shoe over the bony prominence causes compression of the capillary blood flow, leading to necrosis. The eventual outcome for this type of lesion need not be related to the patient's underlying blood supply. Should a pressure ulcer develop over the first metatarsophalangeal joint in a diabetic who has peripheral neuropathy but adequate circulation, healing will follow quite unremarkably, provided there is no infection. However, if this type of ulceration occurs in a patient with compromised circulation it may initiate a progressive ischemic lesion (Fig. 52.1 A and B.). Defects caused by concentrated high pressure are usually the result of a sudden trauma, such as stepping on a piece of glass or a nail. The force supplied exceeds the sheer stress of the skin, resulting in tissue tearing. The force required to cause such a break is approximately 600 to 700 pounds per square inch (42).

Figure 52.2. **A.** Typical plantar ulcers in a diabetic patient as a result of repetitive mechanical stress. **B.** A diabetic patient with hallux rigidus in whom neurotrophic ulceration developed on the plantar aspect of the great toe.

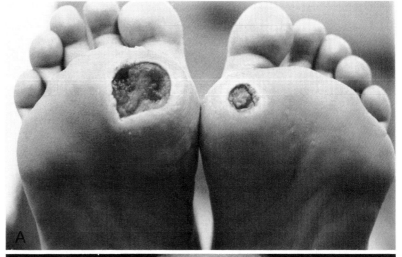

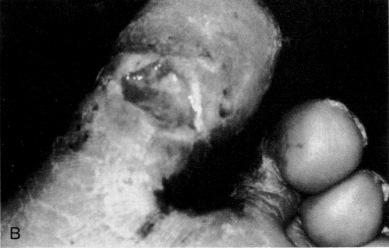

Table 52.3.

Factors Contributing to the Formation of Neurotrophic Ulceration as a Result of Repetitive Cyclical Biomechanical Trauma (Moderate Repetitive Mechanical Stress)

Insensitivity
Hyperkeratosis
Muscle weakness
Fat pad and soft tissue atrophy
Deformity
Stress exceeds mechanical limits of skin
Autolysis
Soft tissue dissection by fluid, blood, or pus
Microvascular insufficiency

Tissue necrosis may develop in active patients as a result of repetitive mechanical stress (Fig. 52.2). The events that lead to ulceration are inflammation and autolysis. Brand (42) relates that the part of the foot that ulcerates most commonly is exposed to pressures between 1 and 5 kg/cm² at every step. Traumatic inflammation occurs and, with repeated trauma, inflammation gives way to necrosis when the mechanical limits of the skin and subcutaneous tissue are exceeded.

Part of the necrosis is caused by the enzymes of inflammatory cells from the initial trauma, which in turn are stimulated to release enzymes during a subsequent episode. A seroma or hematoma develops within the deeper layers of the subcutaneous tissue and the dermis. Dissection of the subcutaneous tissues evolves with pressures and shear from walking. Continued pressure and injury eventually leads to breakdown of the skin and rupture through the plantar surface of the foot. Continued aggravation of the lesion enlarges and deepens the lesion so that subsequent infection readily occurs. Factors contributing to the development of these types of ulcers are listed in Table 52.3.

Repetitive mechanical stress is multifactorial in the development of ulcerations. Ulceration may develop as a result of cyclical biomechanical trauma under areas of weight bearing or under areas of bony prominence. Resulting ulcers are usually located on the plantar surface of the foot and are frequently referred to as mal perforans lesions. This type of ulceration may occur on dorsal digital surfaces in association with hammer toe deformity (Fig. 52.2).

Manley and Darby (45), in their research of mechanical stress and the development of foot ulcerations in rats, reached the following conclusions:

1. Repetitive mechanical stress of a magnitude and repetition rate within physiological limits can stimulate the formation of foot ulcers if the foot is subjected to a significant number of stress repetitions.
2. With the increase in the daily number of repetitions a shorter time period is required for ulcer formation.
3. Denervation predisposes the foot to the formation of plantar ulcers.

A healed ulcer may contribute to the formation of further lesions because the scar tissue binds the skin to the fascia

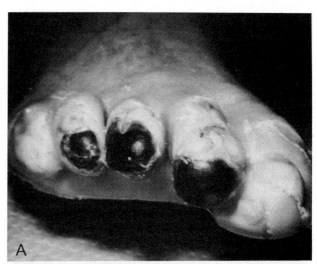
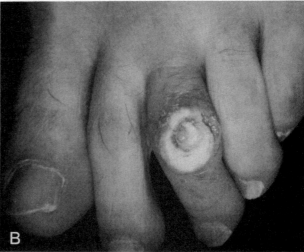

Figure 52.3. **A.** Full-thickness chemical burns in a diabetic patient with peripheral neuropathy caused by a home remedy. **B.** Full-thickness skin loss with exposure of the underlying bone in this diabetic patient caused by a commercially available corn remover.

and ultimately to the bone. The skin is placed at a mechanical disadvantage because the collagen network is replaced with fibrous scar tissue. This tissue does not have the same capacity to adapt and dissipate energy.

Thermal injuries, such as burns or frostbite, are common in insensitive feet. Patients who sustain such injury and who are unaware of the problem can often, because of unintentional neglect, convert a partial-thickness tissue loss to full-thickness loss by continued ambulation on the foot with subsequent development of infection (Fig. 52.3).

In addition to these ulcerative problems, other means of skin compromise may develop. Ischemic ulceration may occur in some diabetics. The clinical presentation is often accompanied by gangrene of the digits or the appearance of small ischemic punched-out ulcers.

An insidious type of lesion causing ulceration and infection in the neuropathic foot is that of sinus formation. This commonly originates between the fourth and fifth digits under a heloma molle. Fissuring may occur, especially about the heel, in these patients because of dyshidrosis (Fig. 52.4).

The last clinical entity is a traumatic vascular type of injury that results in an inflammatory thrombosis. This may be seen in diabetics with advanced vascular insufficiency. Some minor traumatic episode, such as stubbing the toe, may set up inflammation that will lead to thrombosis of the small vessels and ultimately gangrene.

Neurotrophic ulcers have been classified by various methods. The most widely used is the six-grade classification of Wagner (46):

Grade 0. The skin is intact, but there may be some osseous deformity placing the foot at risk
Grade 1. Localized superficial ulcer
Grade 2. Deep ulcer with extension to tendon, bone, ligament, or joint
Grade 3. Deep abscess with osteomyelitis
Grade 4. Gangrene of the toes or forefoot
Grade 5. Gangrene of the whole foot

ALTERATIONS IN FOOT BIOMECHANICS

Weight-bearing studies have been performed by various authors on the neurotrophic foot. Stokes and associates (47, 48) found that in diabetics peak loads were shifted laterally on the foot and that greater abnormalities in loading were consistent with an increase in peripheral neuropathy. Their most striking finding was the reduction of loading of the toes, which is significant in the diabetic, even without evidence of ulceration. The position of maximum load was found in each case to correspond to the position of the ulcer in patients in whom cutaneous compromise did develop. Callosities were evident at sites of heavy loading.

Barrett and Mooney (49) found that the plantar aspect of the forefoot demonstrated high pressure in areas of ulcer formation. This was also confirmed by Sabato and associates (50) in patients with Hansen's disease. In the analysis of vertical forces acting on the diabetic patient with neurotrophic ulcerations, Ctercteko and associates (51) found that toe loading was significantly reduced in diabetics, both with and without ulceration. Their findings differed from those of the Stokes group, and they found a medial shift in loading

Figure 52.4. **A.** Massive soft tissue and plantar space infections of the left foot that originated as a sinus tract forming between fourth and fifth digits. **B.** The result of an untreated heel fissure.

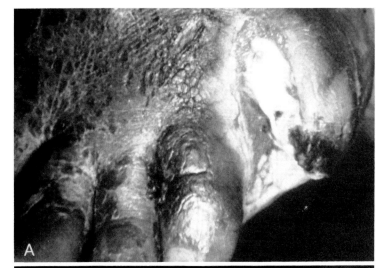
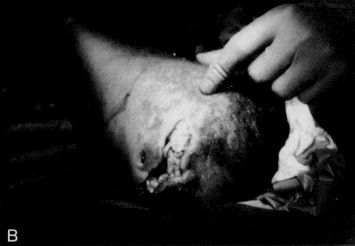

in the metatarsal region. They also found significantly greater forces acting on the first ray area in diabetics, both with and without ulceration. All ulcers in the metatarsal region occurred at the sites of maximum force, and the peak force was also significantly greater in the ulcerated feet. No significant correlation between contact time and severity of the neuropathy was demonstrated.

Anterior displacement of body weight was also not noted by Burman and Perls (52) in 1958. Ellenberg, in 1968 (53), attributed the hammering and contracture of the digits in the diabetic with neuropathy to imbalances and weakness of the intrinsic muscles of the foot. Pati and Behera (54) found clawing of the toes in 50 of 57 cases of ulceration beneath the metatarsal head in patients with leprosy. Amputation of the toe was an associated finding in the remaining seven.

OSSEOUS AND RADIOGRAPHIC CHANGES ASSOCIATED WITH THE NEUROPATHIC FOOT

The patient with a neuropathic foot not only is susceptible to cutaneous compromise but may suffer a loss of osseous integrity as well. These pathologic fractures and dislocations have been termed Charcot joints or neuroarthropathy. Classically, Charcot joints have been described as being due to constant repetitive stress in an insensitive foot. Joint fatigue develops, leading to subluxation, microfracture, and further compromise. This process has been termed the neurotraumatic etiology.

However, newer evidence, reinterpretation of basic research, and a more complete understanding of the components of polyneuropathy have led to a resurgence of the hypervascular theory to explain the evolution of Charcot joints. Autonomic neuropathy results in an increase in the peripheral perfusion to the lower extremity as previously described. This, in turn, weakens the osseous structures through the washout of bone mineral, thus rendering the bones much more susceptible to fracture.

However, attempts to attribute the Charcot foot deformity to a single component of neuropathy fail to take into account all aspects of this involved process. A more logical approach or unified theory has been proposed to account for all factors involved (55, 56)(Table 52.4). In most instances all three forms of peripheral neuropathy—autonomic, motor, and sensory dysfunction—will be implicated in the development of a Charcot foot.

Autonomic neuropathy appears to be essential for the development of these pathologic injuries. Although it does not have to be the initial manifestation of nerve pathosis, there is evidence to support the fact that autonomic fibers may be damaged first in the periphery in diabetics (57-60). Reinhardt (61) has described several prediabetic radiographic findings of injury as being present prior to the onset of clinical sensory deficit or diabetes. A logical explanation of these findings is that the subclinical or prediabetic state provides the initial osteopenia which renders the patient susceptible to injury (56).

Motor neuropathy is important in establishing mechanical

Table 52.4.
Evolution of Charcot Joints

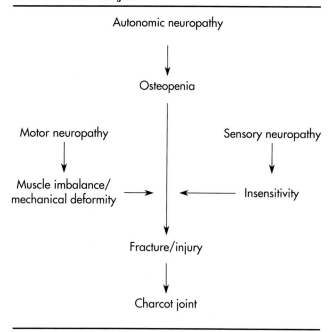

deformity and imbalance, which may apply additional stress to the foot. Furthermore, limited joint mobility may ensure that these deformities are more rigid and problematic. Sensory neuropathy ensures that the patient will not be aware of the stresses, that are occurring. Therefore, the joints are not placed at rest but are subjected to further trauma. As pointed out by Brower and Allman (55), there must first be some underlying osseous problem to permit the development of fractures.

Osseous changes associated with the neuropathic foot may be of two types: atrophic and hypertrophic. The atrophic arthropathy exhibits radiographic osteoporosis, atrophy, destruction, and the disappearance of bone substance (27, 62-70). Dislocation of the joints has also been noted to occur. The joints are usually free of osteophytes, sclerosis, or eburnation and fragmentation.

Pogonowska and associates (66) discuss the bone absorption patterns of diabetes. The pattern is described as initially affecting the forefoot. The metatarsals and phalanges are usually affected first. They summarize the changes as follows: *(a)* osteoporosis, *(b)* juxta-articular cortical bone defects, *(c)* osteolysis, *(d)* apparent destruction of the entire bone, *(e)* occurrence of reconstruction, *(f)* slight periosteal reaction, and *(g)* sclerosis of the shaft of the bone.

Many of these changes, that were related to diabetic osteopathy also occur in other types of neuropathic osteopathy. Examples are seen in alcoholic neuropathy (69, 71) and in the distal absorption seen in the bones of the foot in leprosy (68, 70).

Kraft (72), in discussing the diabetic foot, stated that in the absorptive type of arthropathy, the bone becomes sclerotic, simulating the appearance of osteomyelitis. Schwarz and associates (65) postulated that the absorptive type is caused by autosympathectomy in addition to impaired sensation. Friedman and Rakow (67) believed that both types were etiologically related to increased blood flow.

Radiographically, the bones may appear to exhibit penciling or a sucked-candy deformity. The pathological process usually involves gradual resorption of the metatarsals and phalanges of the foot, beginning distally, progressing gradually toward the base, and terminating with a distal pointed deformity. The epiphyseal ends are lost, and the remaining points may tend to become sclerotic. The joints may take the appearance of the described mortar-and-pestle deformity (Fig. 52.5). Absorption of the small long bones in the foot is manifest in one of three ways (73) (Fig. 52.6): distal absorption, concentric absorption, or a combination of the two (61).

The radiographic presentation of the hypertrophic arthropathy has been discussed by numerous authors (74-79). General findings include moderate to marked osseous overgrowth and osteophytes, sclerosis of the affected joints, eburnation, and fragmentation of bone (Fig. 52.7). This is most commonly noted in the midtarsus and tarsus of the foot. A pes valgus deformity is the classic presentation, and plantar ulceration due to osseous prominence is common.

Specific patterns of tarsal destruction have been described

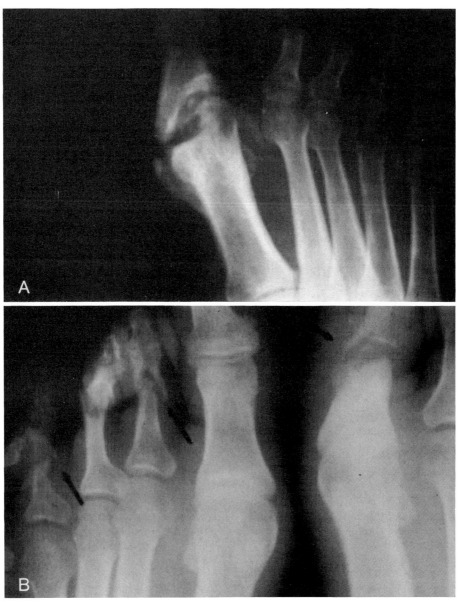

Figure 52.5.   Joint deformities observed in the forefoot of patients with peripheral neuropathy. **A.** Destruction of the first metatarsophalangeal joint in a diabetic. **B.** Mortar-and-pestle appearance of the lesser digits of the left foot caused by chronic alcohol abuse. Osteomyelitis was confirmed by biopsy of the right hallux.

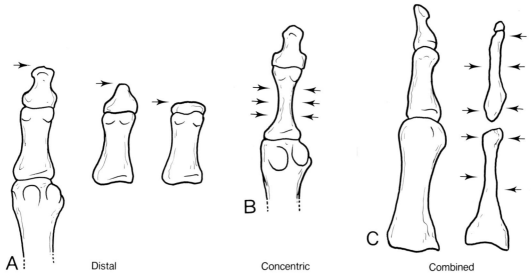

Figure 52.6. Methods of absorption of small bones. (Modified from Enna CD: The foot in leprosy. In McDowell F, Enna CD (eds): *Surgical Rehabilitation in Leprosy.* Baltimore, Williams & Wilkins, 1974, p 299.)

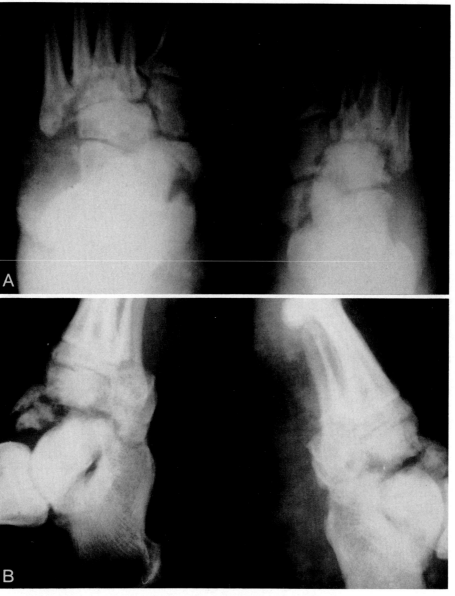

Figure 52.7. Dorsoplantar **(A)** and lateral **(B)** projections of hypertrophic neuroarthropathy.

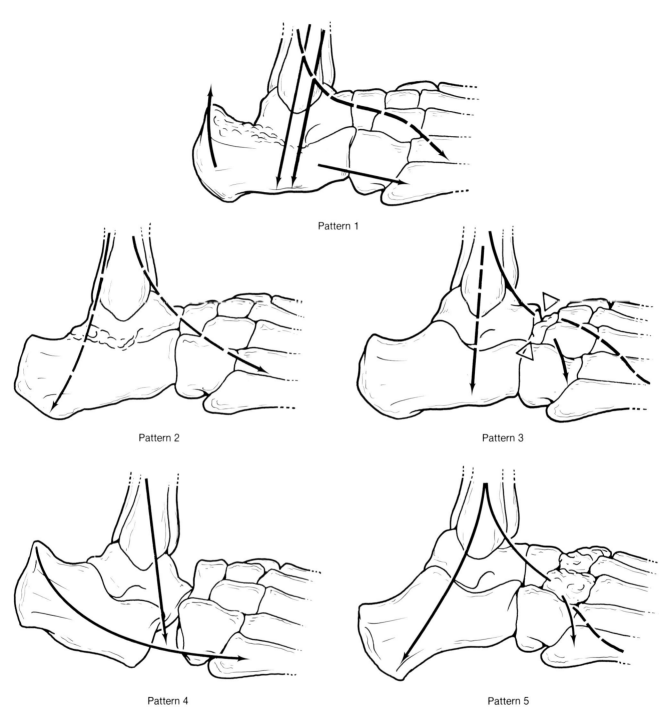

Pattern 1

Pattern 2

Pattern 3

Pattern 4

Pattern 5

Figure 52.8.   Patterns of tarsal degeneration. (Modified from Harris JR, Brand PW: Patterns of disintegration of the tarsus in the anesthetic foot. *J Bone Joint Surg* 48A:14-16, 1966.)

by Harris and Brand (80). This was divided into five patterns of degeneration (Fig. 52.8).

Pattern 1 involves the posterior pillar in which the calcaneus is injured most frequently. The resulting fracture may not be clear but is the consequence of internal trabecular breakdown with flattening of the bone. An incongruity of the subtalar joint may be associated with an ulcer of the

heel. The patient also may have a swollen heel and vague pain and local warmth. Once the damage has occurred, there is a tendency toward progressive change of shape. With increased destruction, the body weight is transmitted directly through the center of the foot.

Pattern 2 shows destruction of the body of the talus. It is common for the talus to be the primary focus of disinte-

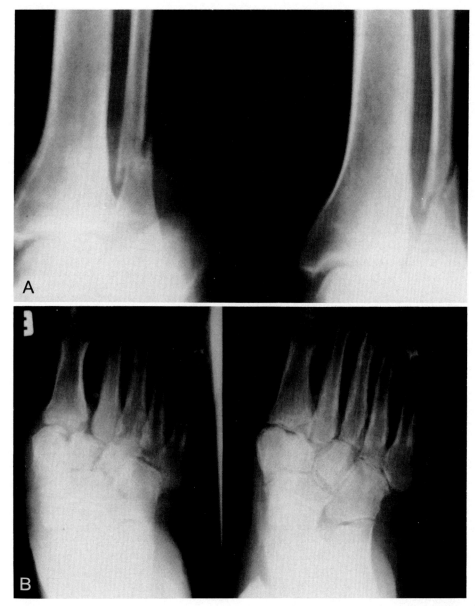

Figure 52.9.   Fractures in two diabetic patients caused by insensitivity. **A.** Fracture of the fibula. **B.** Dislocation of the tarsometatarsal articulation and metatarsal fractures.

gration. When the body of the talus is lost, stability of the foot is also sacrificed and the tibia may rest directly on the ground.

Pattern 3 demonstrates destruction of the anterior pillar of the medial arch. This is a common and consistent pattern, which may progress to complete collapse of the medial arch, disintegration of the navicular, and involvement of the head of the talus. Once the fracture of the navicular occurs, continued weight bearing forces the head of the talus into the navicular, resulting in ultimate destruction. The medial arch loses its continuity and tends to flatten with a plantar declination of the head of the talus.

Pattern 4 is characterized by destruction of the anterior pillar and lateral arch and is described by Brand as dominated by sepsis. Perforating ulcers may occur under the base of the fifth metatarsal and cuboid. The destruction of part of the midtarsal joint interferes with the stability of the foot. The pull of the Achilles tendon eventually leads to the collapse of the bony architecture of the foot. The calcaneus will tend to be drawn posteriorly and dorsally, thrusting the head of the talus plantarly to complete subluxation of the talonavicular joint (Fig. 52.9).

Pattern 5 shows disruption of the cuneometatarsal joints and appears to be related to trauma.

Table 52.5.

Comparative Radiographic Appearances in Osteomyelitis Seen in or Mimicked by Neuropathic Bone Disease

Osteomyelitis	Neuropathic
Bone destruction present	Bone destruction and fragmentation
Increased soft tissue density	Increased soft tissue density
Changes in bone density with early sclerosis and osteoporosis in later progression	Sclerosis may be present and osteoporosis may present as diabetic osteolysis
Progressive reabsorption of bone occurs	Progressive reabsorption usually is not present
Sequestrum formation occurs	Sequestum formation may be mimicked by fragmentation
Subperiosteal new bone formation occurs	Subperiosteal new bone formation occurs

COMPLICATIONS

The diagnosis of osteomyelitis in previously diseased bone may be difficult, as radiologic changes due to osteomyelitis and to Charcot degeneration may be similar (76) (Table 52.5). Radioisotope evaluation of the neurotrophic foot may also be somewhat misleading (73-81). There is some difficulty with interpretation of the technetium scan of the neurotrophic foot, in that the bone has been previously diseased. A positive technetium scan results from basic physiological changes seen in various disease and infectious processes, such as a hyperemia or an increase in blood supply to the affected bone. Regardless of the initiating factor, osseous injury will lead to increased blood supply to the site. This is true in fractures, in infection, and in neurotrophic disease as the body attempts to initiate repair. Therefore, focal uptake is not necessarily a reflection of osteomyelitis but may represent the repair process for the earlier destruction.

Prolonged increases in technetium uptake are the consequences of new vessel formation. Increased uptake has also been attributed to the autonomic neuropathy that increases the blood flow to the extremity (7). This would affect both the technetium and the initial gallium scans.

Hoffer (82) describes four methods of gallium localization: increased permeability of blood vessels, leukocyte localization, lactoferrin binding at the infected site, and direct bacterial uptake. With neurotrophic changes, however, reparative processes require the presence of white blood cells and lysosomal activity in the repair area. The increased permeability of the blood vessels surrounding the Charcot joint would be expected to contribute to an increased uptake of gallium in the area. Glynn (83) noted a marked accumulation of gallium in neuroarthropathy.

Although radioisotopic studies may be helpful in evaluating the neurotrophic foot, care must be given to their interpretation. Future methods of radioisotopic detection of infection such as the white blood cell scan, may prove valuable.

Because of the limitations of standard radiographs and the scanning techniques, bone biopsy is recommended as a means of providing a definitive diagnosis when osteomyelitis is suspected in the neuropathic foot (56, 77, 84).

EVALUATION OF A PATIENT WITH NEUROPATHY

Practitioners sometimes see patients who have no idea that they have a foot that is affected by neuropathy. In fact, some

Table 52.6.

Signs and Symptoms Associated With the Neuropathic Foot

1. Paresthesias
2. Hypoesthesia
3. Anesthesia
4. Nocturnal cramping
5. Diminished or absent deep tendon reflexes
6. Diminished or absent vibratory sensation
7. Diminished or absent temperature or pain sensation
8. Anhydrosis
9. Callous formation
10. Ulceration
11. Intrinsic muscle atrophy
12. Digital deformity
13. Cavus foot deformity or pes valgus deformity
14. Increased skin temperature
15. Edema
16. Change in function (drop foot)

From Schuster S, Jacobs AM: Diabetic autonomic neuropathy in the surgical management of the diabetic foot. *J Foot Surg* 21: 16-22, 1982.

of these patients will not be aware of their underlying disease process. Therefore such symptoms as paresthesia, anesthesia, hyperesthesia, or change in function may be of importance (84). Patients who complain of paresthesias or "pins and needles" and a sensation of swollen or burning feet are in this category. Paresthesia may precede the diagnosis of neurologic disease. This is frequently the cause of foot discomfort in patients with undiagnosed diabetes mellitus. Burning feet may be the primary indication of an inherited peripheral neuropathy (85). Patients who complain of difficulty climbing stairs, dragging of the toes, or frequent tripping may also be candidates for an evaluation of neurological dysfunction (Table 52.6).

In the patient with a suspected peripheral neuropathy, a thorough medical history should be obtained, especially with regard to the onset, duration, and progression of the symptoms. One should inquire as to the presence of diabetes, peripheral vascular disease, collagen disorders, vitamin deficiencies, anemia, uremia, prolonged illness, infection, trauma to the nervous system, exposure to toxins such as ethanol, and a history of any congenital defect. Family history is extremely important in determining inherited forms of peripheral neuropathy. A thorough history of current medications and allergies should also be elicited.

The physical examination presented here is directed toward the evaluation of the lower extremity. In general, the examination should include inspection, palpation of the muscle mass, and observation of atrophy of the intrinsic muscles. The hand may also be extremely useful in detecting atrophy caused by peripheral neuropathy. In such instances the hand may demonstrate weakness, loss of intrinsic muscle tone and mass, and an increase in noticeable bony prominences.

Vibratory sensation (86, 87) and light-touch evaluation (88) are important clinical means of determining changes in the patient's sensorium as related to peripheral neuropathy. Recently more sophisticated types of electronic equipment have become available. However, there still remains a limitation to the ability of multiple observers to generate reliable, reproducible data regarding sensory neuropathy among different sets of patients.

The joints of the lower extremity should be evaluated for gross deformity. The range of motion should be evaluated for the presence of crepitation or limited motion. Equinus, if noted, will have to be accommodated. From a conservative standpoint, this may be managed by increasing the heel height to offset the tension in the Achilles tendon. Manual muscle testing may also be included as part of the neurological evaluation.

One should also be alert for the presence of swelling and heat, which would accompany the development of neuropathic joints. Bergtholdt (89) recommends a temperature-assessment program to monitor risk patterns. Increased physical activity or ill-fitting footwear may be indicated by increased temperature at local areas of stress. Bergtholdt terms this method a "pain substitute" that can detect areas sensitive to ulceration. Thermography is also useful in the early diagnosis of Charcot joints because of increased heat in the area of the involved joints (90-92). The earliest indicator of a Charcot joint collapse is the localized increase in temperature of the part. However, thermography is not practical in the average clinical setting. Manual palpation of the part remains a fairly reliable means of gauging temperature differentials and assessing risks.

The skin should be evaluated for evidence of ulceration, healed scars, or skin lesions that show no response to pin prick. Dry skin should be moisturized to maintain the maximal degree of hydration.

Electrophysiological findings may be used in limited circumstances to aid in the diagnosis and determination of the extent of involvement of the patient with peripheral neuropathy. Diagnosis may also require the use of sural nerve biopsy.

Diabetic patients who complain of symptoms in the legs must be carefully evaluated, because the symptoms may also be caused by such factors as lumbosacral strain, sciatic neuropathy, arthritis, peripheral vascular disease, and obesity.

The initial vascular examination consists of simple clinical tests such as assessment of peripheral pulses, capillary filling time, and skin temperature. One should keep in mind that autonomic neuropathy may result in vessel calcification, which may render pulses nonpalpable. More involved evaluation, including sophisticated noninvasive testing, may be required. From the evaluation, one basically wants to determine (a) how much circulation exists in the extremity; (b) whether the circulation is adequate to treat the prob-

lem; and (c) whether invasive vascular procedures are indicated.

In the past a great deal of emphasis regarding the circulation has been placed in the ankle/arm ischemic index. Wagner (93) found that in nondiabetics a surgically treated ulcer may heal with an index as low as 3.5. In the diabetic patient surgery on an ulcer was not recommended if there was a reading lower than 4.5. However, vascular calcification may influence the ankle/arm ratio if the vessels are difficult to occlude.

A LOGICAL APPROACH TO MANAGEMENT OF NEUROPATHIC FEET

For purposes of management, the neuropathic foot may be classified into three categories (Table 52.7). The first is the foot with no ulcerations, with or without osseous deformity, and no evidence of active bony destruction.

Enna (94), in 1982, classified the insensitive foot into four groups as they related to the need for orthotic care. Group 1 has only one deficit, loss of plantar sensation. A soft insole of microcellular rubber, such as Spenco, is provided as a means of prophylaxis.

Group 2 has two defects—loss of plantar sensation and deficiency of the subcutaneous soft tissue, with or without scarring of the plantar skin. In this foot type a molded material, such as plastizote, with or without a layer of microcellular rubber, is advantageous. Any increase in the mass of the material is accompanied by the use of an extra-depth shoe to accommodate the thickness of the insole.

Group 3 includes three deficits. In addition to loss of sensation and the presence of plantar scarring, gross deformity is present and may require surgical intervention. The surgical intervention may include both resection of prominent osseous structures and, in some cases, judicious arthrodesis of the involved joints. Molded shoes with the appropriate insole materials would be required to manage this type of deformity.

Group 4 patients have short, deformed, rigid feet. A molded shoe is fabricated to the dimensions of the foot. In this type of deformity the sole of the shoe requires a rocker bottom to allow a more normal gait and reduce the forces interacting with the insensitive foot.

The use of insoles and shoes as outlined here is also applicable to the follow-up care of patients after they have been successfully treated for superficial or deep ulcerations (95-98). Modifications of shoes may require application of a rocker-bottom sole, an anterior heel, a metatarsal bar, or a platform. Bracing may also be of benefit in reducing weight-bearing stress to the foot.

The second category of the neuropathic foot includes patients who have active neuroarthropathy (99). Rest is required until clinical and radiological evidence of healing is seen. Lennox (100) advises bed rest followed by the use of curtches with no weight bearing, partial weight bearing, and then the use of gait-assisted devices over a period of some weeks until union is achieved. "This sequence is ideal, as it insures an initial period of absolute rest, and then a gradual return to function" (100). However, weight bearing prior

Table 52.7.
Logical Approach to Management of the Neuropathic Foot

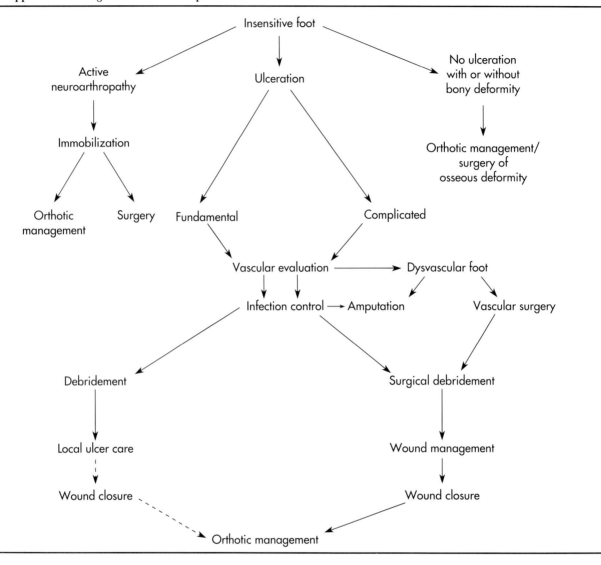

to complete consolidation, even when supported by braces or other devices, risks further complications and delays healing. If a patient is unable to use crutches, then a wheelchair is employed.

Compression dressings may be applied initially until the edema has stabilized, after which traditional casts may be used. If the foot is moldable, then one may position the part so as to encourage consolidation in a more suitable alignment. The period of immobilization required before consolidation may last from 3 to 4 months or more.

Return to activity should be gradual, and the patient should be followed up after the resumption of weight bearing to monitor the limb for the development of heat or swelling. These factors could be indicative of incomplete healing, and further abstinence from weight bearing and immobilization are in order. Ambulation may begin in either

a weight-bearing cast or a removable brace. With time, the length of ambulation is increased while the use of external support is reduced. However, in patients with severe deformity or in whom there remains some degree of instability, bracing may be required on a more permanent basis. These measures, along with appropriate shoes and orthotic support, reduce the stress to the susceptible areas of the foot.

Arthrodesis of major foot joints may be indicated in selected cases. The aims of surgery are (a) to simplify and stabilize the remaining skeleton, (b) to restore the foot to a plantigrade position without deviation, (c) to restore a functional foot for ambulation, and (d) to prevent further deformity (56, 100). The use of bone grafts and internal fixation may also be indicated.

The third category of neuropathic foot includes those with ulceration and may be divided into fundamental and complicated conditions. The fundamental type includes the foot with simple neurotrophic ulcers where soft tissue infection may be present. The complicated type includes the ulcer that extends past the subcutaneous tissue into the deeper layers of the foot. Such ulcers may be associated with deep plantar space infection that involves underlying bone and muscle. At times these ulcers are complicated by osteomyelitis, systemic infection, or active neuroarthropathy.

In the fundamental uncomplicated ulcer the goal of local care is to remove necrotic tissue, reduce the existing bacterial level, and promote healing. In managing this type of ulcer one should first treat the soft tissue skin infection, if one is present. The simple presence of bacteria does not necessarily imply the presence of an infectious process. The possibility of colonization of the ulcer must be considered. Systemic antibiotics are not indicated for bacterial colonization. One should also look for evidence of systemic infection and deep local infection, such as abscess formation.

The literature has shown that the majority of diabetic infections are polymicrobial in nature (101-104). The most common are caused by gram-positive aerobic cocci. It is recommended that proper anaerobic cultures also be taken. Of interest is the poor correlation of culture findings between swabs of an ulcer and those obtained from uncontaminated deep-tissue specimens (102, 105). Much better results are obtained with needle aspirates and direct biopsy of these specimens rather than swabs of the ulcers.

Although treatment may include the use of intravenous antibiotics, antibiotics do not always appear to eradicate organisms in the deep tissues. A surgical debridement is often required for drainage and definitive treatment.

Various supportive measures have been recommended for use in the ulcerated patient. These include overall nutritional support and the use of various vitamin and zinc supplements (106).

One modality that has been advocated for a number of neuropathic foot complications, including ulcers, is total contact casting (107-112). Total contact weight bearing allows the weight of the foot to be more evenly distributed and can prevent localized areas of focal pressure that may lead to ulceration. Weight-bearing pressure is also distributed into the leg area. The cast precludes ankle motion, obviating the bending force within the foot, which may perpetuate ulcerations. Although the contact cast is probably most effective in providing these benefits, a standard cast may also be employed with success.

However, there is a risk that potential infection may be concealed by a plaster cast. One should also note that these patients are prone to cast-related problems. Specifically, in the neuropathic patient a cast may conceal a potential infection and, more specifically, an ill-fitting cast may lead to the development of pressure-type ulcerations, further complicating their management. Frequent cast checks are mandatory. Changing the cast on a frequent basis is preferred to windowing the cast for the management of pedal ulcerations.

Fundamental ulcerations may be managed by a variety of methods provided the pressure to the area is alleviated.

Management of the complicated ulceration requires precise and accurate surgical treatment (113-116). Debridement and resection of necrotic tissue, including tendon and bone, are required. This usually involves a radical debridement, which is exactly what the term implies—aggressive excision of all necrotic and infected tissue. It may include bone, tendon, and muscle. All necrotic tissue must be removed to allow healing. A large area may have to be resected and the wound deepened. Guidelines have been established for radical debridement and include (a) never sacrifice blood supply, (b) allow adequate incisions for drainage, and (c) avoid weight-bearing areas if at all possible.

After radical debridement, depending on the amount of exposure that is required, treatment usually consists of local wound management until a healthy granulating base is obtained. Debridement may be required on more than one occasion. Exposed bone will cover spontaneously with granulation tissue followed by epithelium or will sequestrate and then cover, provided there is adequate circulation at the wound site (117). A variety of closure methods, including delayed primary closure, skin grafts, flaps, or muscle transfers, may be employed to enhance the end result and function.

References

1. Brown MJ, Asbury AK: Diabetic neuropathy. *Ann Neurol* 15:2-12, 1984.
2. Lippmann HI: Must loss of limb be a consequence of diabetes mellitus? *Diabetes Care* 2:432, 1979.
3. Lippmann HI, Farrar R: Prevention of amputation in diabetes. *Angiology* 30:649, 1979.
4. Boulton AJM, Scarpello JHB, Ward JD: Venous oxygenation in the diabetic neuropathic foot: evidence of arteriovenous shunting? *Diabetologia* 22:6-8, 1982.
5. Edmonds ME, Roberts VC, Watkins PJ: Blood flow in the diabetic neuropathic foot. *Diabetologia* 22:9-15, 1982.
6. Archer AG, Roberts VC, Watkins PJ: Blood flow patterns in painful diabetic neuropathy. *Diabetologia* 27:563-567, 1984.
7. Edmonds ME, Clarke MB, Newton JB, Barrett J, Watkins PJ: Increased uptake of bone radiopharmaceutical in diabetic neuropathy. *Quarterly J Med* 57:843-855, 1985.
8. Kerper AH, Collier WD: Pathological changes in arteries following partial denervation. *Proc Soc Exp Biol Med* 24:493-494, 1926.
9. Goebel FD, Fuessel HS: Monckeberg's sclerosis after sympathetic denervation in diabetic and nondiabetic subjects. *Diabetologia* 24: 347-350, 1983.
10. Edmonds ME, Morrison N, Laws JW, Watkins PJ: Medial arterial calcification and diabetic neuropathy. *Br Med J* 284:928-930, 1982.
11. Sinha S, Munichoodappa CS, Kozak GP: Neuro-arthropathy (Charcot joints) in diabetes mellitus. *Medicine* 51:191-210, 1972.
12. Clouse ME, Gramm HF, Flood T: Diabetic osteoarthropathy. Clinical and roentgenographic observations in 90 cases. *AJR* 121:22-34, 1974.
13. Bevan RD, Tsuru H: Long term denervation of vascular smooth muscle causes not only functional but structural change. *Blood Vessels* 16:109-112, 1979.
14. Scarpello JH, Martin TR, Ward JD: Ultrasound measurements of pulse wave velocity in the peripheral arteries of diabetes subjects. *Clin Sci* 58:53-57, 1980.
15. Gilbey SG, Walters H, Edmonds ME, Archer AG, Watkins PJ, Parsons V, Grenfell A: Vascular calcification, autonomic neuropathy, and peripheral blood flow in patients with diabetic nephropathy. *Diabetic Med* 6:37-42, 1988.
16. Chantelau E, Ma XY, Hernberger S, Dohmen C, Trappe P, Baba T: Effect of medial arterial calcification on O_2 supply to exercising diabetic feet. *Diabetes* 39:938-941, 1990.

17. Duncan CP, Shim SS: The autonomic nerve supply of bone. *J Bone Joint Surg* 59B:323-330, 1977.
18. Trotman NM, Kelly WD: The effect of sympathectomy on blood flow to bone. *JAMA* 183:121-122, 1963.
19. Yu W, Shim SS, Hawk HE: Bone circulation in hemorrhagic shock. *J Bone Joint Surg* 54A:1157-1166, 1972.
20. Shim SS, Copp DH, Patterson FP: Bone blood flow in the limb following complete sciatic nerve section. *Surg Gynecol Obstet* 123:333-335, 1966.
21. Conrad MC: Contributions of large and small vessel disease to severe ischemia of the lower extremities in diabetics and nondiabetics. *Vasc Diag Ther* 2:17-28, 1981.
22. Colwell JA: Studies on the pathogenesis of diabetic vascular disease. *J S C Med Assoc* 77:267-272, 1981.
23. McMillan DE: Deterioration of the microcirculation in diabetes. *Diabetes* 24:944-957, 1975.
24. Arenson DJ, Sherwood CF, Wilson RC: Neuropathy, angiopathy, and sepsis in the diabetic foot (part two: angiopathy). *J Am Podiatry Assoc* 71:661-665, 1981.
25. Janka HU, Standl E, Schramm W, Mehnrt H: Platelet enzyme activities in diabetes mellitus in relation to endothelial damage. *Diabetes* 32:47-51, 1983.
26. Sinziner H, Silberbauer K, Kaliman J, Klein K: Vascular prostacyclin synthesis, platelet sensitivity, plasma factors and platelet function, arteriopathy with and without diabetes mellitus. In Noseda G, Lewis B, Paolett R (eds): *Diet and Drugs in Atherosclerosis.* New York, Raven Press, 1980, pp 93-95.
27. Bern MM: Platelet functions in diabetes mellitus. *Diabetes* 27:342-352, 1978.
28. Williamson JR, Kilo C: Small vessel disease: diabetic microangiopathy. *Angiology* 31:448-454, 1980.
29. Williamson JR, Vogler NJ, Kilo C: Microvascular disease in diabetes. *Med Clin North Am* 55:847-860, 1981.
30. Williamson JR, Kilo C: Capillary basement membranes. *Diabetes* 32:96-100, 1983.
31. Friedericki HHR, Tucker WR, Schwartz TB: Observations on small blood vessels of skin in the normal and in diabetic patients. *Diabetes* 15:233-250, 1966.
32. Banson BB, Lacy PE: Diabetic microangiopathy in human toes. *Am J Pathol* 45:41-50, 1964.
33. Almer L, Sundvist G, Lilja B: Fibrinolytic activity, autonomic neuropathy and circulation in diabetes mellitus. *Diabetes* 32:4-19, 1983.
34. Coster AA, Swedlow BL: Ultrastructural morphology of diabetic microangiopathy. *J Am Podiatry Assoc* 66:69-75, 1976.
35. Tilton RG, Faller AM, Burkhardt DL, Kilo C, Williamson JR: Pericyte degeneration and acellular capillaries are increased in the feet human diabetic patients. *Diabetologia* 28:895-900, 1985.
36. LoGerfo FW, Coffman JD: Vascular and microvascular disease of the foot in diabetes. *N Engl J Med* 311:1615-1618, 1984.
37. Flynn MD, Edmonds ME, Tooke JE, Watkins PJ: Direct measurement of capillary blood flow in the diabetic neuropathic foot. *Diabetologia* 31:652-656, 1988.
38. Gibson T, Kenedi RM: Biomechanical properties of skin. *Surg Clin North Am* 47:279-293, 1967.
39. Daly CH: Biomechanical properties of dermis. *J Invest Dermatol* 79:17-20, 1982.
40. Huntley AC: Cutaneous manifestations in diabetes: general considerations. In Jelinek JE (ed): *The Skin in Diabetes.* Philadelphia, Lea & Febiger, 1986, pp 23-30.
41. Delbridge L, Perry P, Marr S, Arnold N, Yue DK, Turtle JR, Reeve TS. Limited joint mobility in the diabetic foot: relationship to neuropathic ulceration. *Diabetic Med* 5:333-337, 1988.
42. Brand PW: Management of the insensitive limb. *Phys Ther* 59:8-12, 1979.
43. Hall OC, Brand PW: The etiology of the neuropathic plantar ulcer. *J Am Podiatry Assoc* 69:173-177, 1979.
44. Kosiak M: Etiology and pathology of ischemic ulcers. *Arch Phys Med Rehabil* 40:62-69, 1959.
45. Manley MT, Darby T: Repetitive mechanical stress and denervation in plantar ulcer pathogenesis in rats. *Arch Phys Med Rehabil* 61:171-177, 1980.
46. Wagner FW: The insensitive foot. In Kiene RH, Johnson KA (eds): *AAOS Symposium of the Foot and Ankle.* St Louis, CV Mosby, 1981, pp 135-158.
47. Stokes IAF, Faris IB, Hutton WC: The neuropathic ulcer and loads on the foot in diabetic patients. *Acta Orthop Scand* 46:839-847, 1975.
48. Stokes IAF, Hutton WC: The effect of the diabetic ulcer on the load bearing function of the foot. In Kenedi RM, Cowden JM (eds): *Bedsore Biomechanics.* Baltimore, University Park Press, 1976, pp 245-247.
49. Barrett JP, Mooney V: Neuropathy and diabetic pressure lesions. *Orthop Clin North Am* 4:43-47, 1973.
50. Sabato S, Yosipovitch Z, Simkin A, Sheskin J: Plantar trophic ulcers in patients with leprosy. *Int Orthop* 6:203-208, 1982.
51. Ctercteko GC, Chanendran M, Hutton WC, Lequesne LP: Vertical forces acting on the feet of diabetic patients with neuropathic ulceration. *Br J Surg* 68:608-614, 1981.
52. Burman M, Perls W: The weight stream in Charcot disease of joints. *Bull Hosp Joint Dis* 19:31-47, 1958.
53. Ellenberg M: Diabetic neuropathic ulcer. *J Mt Sinai Hosp* 35:585-594, 1968.
54. Pati L, Behera F: Metatarsal head pressure (MHP) sores in leprosy patients. *Lepr India* 53:588-593, 1981.
55. Brower AC, Allman RM: Pathogenesis of the neurotrophic joint: neurotraumatic vs. neurovascular. *Radiology* 39:349-354, 1981.
56. Banks AS, McGlamry ED: Charcot foot. *J Am Podiatr Med Assoc* 79:213-235, 1989.
57. Watkins PJ, Edmonds ME: Sympathetic nerve failure in diabetes. *Diabetologia* 25:73-77, 1983.
58. Fagius J: Microneurographic findings in diabetic polyneuropathy with special reference to sympathetic nerve activity. *Diabetologia* 23:415, 1982.
59. Guy RJC, Clark A, Malcolm PN, Watkins PJ: Evaluation of thermal and vibration sensation in diabetic neuropathy. *Diabetologia* 28:131-137, 1985.
60. Young RJ, Yue QZ, Rodriguez E, Prescott RJ, Ewing DJ, Clarke BF. Variable relationship between peripheral somatic and autonomic neuropathy in patients with different syndromes of diabetic polyneuropathy. *Diabetes* 35:192-197, 1986.
61. Reinhardt K: The radiologic residua of healed diabetic arthropathies. *Skeletal Radiol* 7:167-172, 1981.
62. Buchman NH: Bone and joint changes in the diabetic foot. *J Am Podiatry Assoc* 66:211-226, 1976.
63. Geoffroy J, Hoeffel JC, Pointel JP, Drouin P, Debry G, Martin R: The feet in diabetes. *Diagn Imaging* 48:286-293, 1979.
64. Enna CD: Skeletal deformities of the denervated hand in Hansen's disease. *J Hand Surg* 4:227-233, 1979.
65. Schwarz GS, Berenyi MR, Siegal MW: Atrophic arthropathy and diabetic neuritis. *Am J Roentgenol Rad Ther Nucl Med* 106:523-529, 1969.
66. Pogonowska MJ, Collins LC, Dobson HL: Diabetic osteopathy. *Radiology* 89:265-271, 1967.
67. Friedman SA, Rakow RB: Osseous lesions of the foot in diabetic neuropathy. *Diabetes* 20:302-307, 1971.
68. Riordan DC: The hand in leprosy: a seven year clinical study. *Diabetes* 42A:683-690, 1960.
69. Miller RM, Hunt JA: The radiological features of alcoholic ulceroosteolytic neuropathy in blacks. *S Afr Med J* 54:159-161, 1978.
70. Enna CD, Jacobson RR, Rausch RO: Bone changes in leprosy: a correlation of clinical and radiographic features. *Radiology* 10:295-306, 1971.
71. Thornhill HL, Richter RW, Shelton ML, Johnson CA: Neuropathic arthropathy (Charcot forefeet) in alcoholics. *Orthop Clin North Am* 4:7-20, 1973.
72. Kraft E, Spyropoulos E, Finby N: Neurogenic disorders of the foot in diabetes mellitus. *Am J Roentgenol* 124:17-24, 1975.
73. Enna CD: The foot in leprosy. In McDowell F, Enna CD (eds): *Surgical Rehabilitation in Leprosy and in Other Peripheral Nerve Disorders.* Baltimore, Williams & Wilkins, 1974.
74. Bruckner FE, Howell A: Neuropathic joints. *Semin Arthritis Rheum* 2:47-69, 1972.
75. Wolf DS, Raczka EK, Shevlin AM: Charcot's joint in a juvenile-onset diabetic. *J Am Podiatry Assoc* 67:200-203, 1977.

76. Sella AJ: Diabetic neurosteoarthropathy of the tarsus. *Conn Med* 43:70-74, 1979.
77. McNamara G, Shor RI: Diabetic neuropathic osteoarthropathy. *J Am Podiatry Assoc* 73:485-489, 1983.
78. Newman JH: Non-infective disease of the diabetic foot. *J Bone Joint Surg* 63B:593-596, 1981.
79. Weissman SD, Weiss A: Diabetic neurotrophic osteoarthropathy (Charcot joint). *J Am Podiatry Assoc* 70:196-200, 1980.
80. Harris JR, Brand PW: Patterns of disintegration of the tarsus in the anaesthetic foot. *J Bone Joint Surg* 48B:4-16, 1966.
81. Frykberg RG: The diabetic Charcot foot. *Arch Podiatr Med Foot Surg* 5:15-27, 1978.
82. Hoffer P: Gallium mechanisms. *J Nucl Med* 21:282, 1980.
83. Glynn TP: Marked gallium accumulation in neurogenic arthropathy. *J Nucl Med* 22:1016-1017, 1981.
84. Hetherington VJ: Technetium and combined gallium and technetium scan in the neurotrophic foot. *J Am Podiatry Assoc* 72:458-463, 1982.
85. Dyck PJ, Low PA, Stevens JC: "Burning feet" as the only manifestation of dominantly inherited sensory neuropathy. *Mayo Clin Proc* 58:426-429, 1983.
86. Nielsen NV, Lund FS: Diabetic polyneuropathy, corneal sensitivity, vibratory perception and Achilles tendon reflex in diabetes. *Acta Neurol Scand* 59:15-22, 1979.
87. Christensen NJ: Vibratory perception and blood flow in the feet of diabetics. *Acta Med Scand* 185:553-559, 1969.
88. Dyck PJ, Schultz PW, O'Brien PC: Quantitation of touch-pressure sensation. *Arch Neurol* 26:465-473, 1972.
89. Bergtholdt HT: Temperature assessment of the insensitive foot. *Phys Ther* 59:18-22, 1979.
90. Wilkinson JD: Section of dermatology: ulcerating and mutilating acropathy with thermographic findings. *Proc R Soc Lond* 69:513-515, 1976.
91. Dribbon BS: Application and value of liquid crystal thermography. *J Am Podiatry Assoc* 73:400-404, 1983.
92. Sandrow RE, Torg JS, Lapayowker MS, Resnick EJ: The use of thermography in the early diagnosis of neuropathic arthropathy in the feet of diabetics. *Clin Orthop* 88:31-33, 1972.
93. Wagner FW: Transcutaneous Doppler ultrasound in the prediction of healing and the selection of surgical level for dysvascular lesions of the toes and forefoot. *Clin Orthop* 142:110-114, 1979.
94. Enna CD: Rehabilitation of leprous deformity. *Ann Rev Med* 33:41-45, 1982.
95. Block P: The diabetic foot ulcer: A complex problem with a simple treatment approach. *Milit Med* 146:644-646, 1981.
96. Seder JI: Management of foot problems in diabetics. *J Dermatol Surg Oncol* 4:708-709, 1978.
97. Singleton EE, Cotton RS, Shelman HS: Another approach to the long term management of the diabetic neurotrophic foot ulcer. *J Am Podiatry Assoc* 68:242-244, 1978.
98. Brenner MA: An ambulatory approach to the neuropathic ulceration. *J Am Podiatry Assoc* 64:862-869, 1974.
99. Goldman F: Identification, treatment, and prognosis of Charcot joint in diabetes mellitus. *J Am Podiatry Assoc* 72:485-490, 1982.
100. Lennox WM: Surgical treatment of chronic deformities of the anesthetic foot. In McDowell F, Enna CD (eds): *Surgical Rehabilitation in Leprosy and in Other Peripheral Nerve Disorders.* Baltimore, Williams & Wilkins, 1974, p 350.
101. Louie TJ, Bartlett JG, Tally FD, Gorbach SL: Aerobic and anaerobic bacteria in diabetic foot ulcers. *Ann Intern Med* 85:461-463, 1976.
102. Sharp CS, Bessman AN, Wagner FW, Garland D, Reece E: Microbiology of superficial and deep tissues in infected diabetic gangrene. *Surg Obstet Gynecol* 149:217-219, 1979.
103. Sapico FL, Canawati HN, Witte JL, Montgomerie JZ, Wagner FW, Bessman AN: Quantitative aerobic and anaerobic bacteriology of infected diabetic feet. *J Clin Microbiol* 12:413-420, 1980.
104. Walsh CH, Campbell CK: The multiple flora of diabetic foot. *Ir J Med Sci* 149:366-369, 1980.
105. Mackowiak PA, Jones SR, Smith JW: Diagnostic value of sinus-tract cultures in chronic osteomyelitis. *JAMA* 239:2772-2775, 1978.
106. Engel ED, Erlick NE, Davis RH: Diabetes mellitus: impaired wound healing from zinc deficiency. *J Am Podiatry Assoc* 71:536-544, 1981.
107. Coleman WC, Brand PW, Birke JA: The total contact cast. *J Am Podiatry Assoc* 74:548-551, 1984.
108. Birke JA, Sims DS, Buford WL: Walking cast: effect on plantar foot pressures. *J Rehab Res Dev* 22:18-22, 1985.
109. Walker SC, Helm PA, Pullium G: Total contrast casting and chronic diabetic neuropathic foot ulcerations: healing rates by wound location. *Arch Phys Med Rehabil* 68:217-221, 1987.
110. Borssen B, Lithner F: Plaster casts in the management of advanced ischemic and neuropathic diabetic foot lesions. *Diabetic Med* 6:720-723, 1989.
111. Boulton AJM, Bowker JH, Gadia M, Lemerman R, Caswell K, Skyler JS, Sosenko JM: The use of plaster casts in the management of diabetic neuropathic foot ulcers. *Diabetes Care* 9:149-152, 1986.
112. Kaplan M, Gelber RH: Care of plantar ulcerations: comparing applications, materials and non-casting. *Lepr Rev* 59:59-66, 1988.
113. Robson MC, Edstrom LE: Conservative management of the ulcerated diabetic foot. *Plast Reconstr Surg* 59:551-554, 1977.
114. Kritter AE: A technique for salvage of the infected diabetic gangrenous foot. *Orthop Clin North Am* 4:21-30, 1973.
115. Rice JS: Diabetic infection, ulceration and gangrene. *J Am Podiatry Assoc* 64:774-781, 1974.
116. LaPorta GA, Richter KP, Marzzacco JC: Local radical amputation in the foot for arterial insufficiency. *J Am Podiatry Assoc* 67:192-197, 1977.
117. Brown PW: The fate of exposed bone. *Am J Surg* 137:464-468, 1979.

Additional References

Albert SF: Elective foot surgery and the alcoholic. *J AmPodiatry Assoc* 71:8-18, 1981.

Andersson R: Hereditary amyloidosis with polyneuropathy. *Acta Med Scand* 188:85-94, 1970.

Archer AG, Watkins PJ, Thomas PK, Sharma AK, Payan J: The natural history of acute painful neuropathy in diabetes mellitus. *J Neurol Neurosurg Psychiatry* 46:491-499, 1983.

Arenson D, Sherwood MS, Wilson RC: Neuropathy, angiopathy, and sepsis in the diabetic foot. *J Am Podiatry Assoc* 71:618-623, 1981.

Baker AB, Baker AH: *Clinical Neurology.* Philadelphia, Harper & Row, 1983, vol 4.

Child DL, Yates DAH: Radicular pain in diabetes. *Rheumatol Rehabil* 17:195, 1978.

Clements RS: Diabetic neuropathy—new concepts of its etiology. *Diabetes* 28:604-610, 1979.

Cofield RH, Morrison MJ, Beabout JW: Diabetic neuroarthropathy in the foot: patient characteristics and patterns of radiographic change. *Foot Ankle* 4:15-22, 1983.

Cooper CT: Hansen's disease: a podiatrist's experience. *J Am Podiatry Assoc* 65:300-309, 1975.

Cornblath DR, McArthur JC: Predominantly sensory neuropathy in patients with AIDS and AIDS-related complex. *Neurology* 38:794-796, 1988.

Dehen H, Willer JC, Prier S, Boureau F, Cambier J: Congenital insensitivity to pain and the "morphine-like" analgesic system. *Pain* 5:351-358, 1978.

Dyck PJ, Lambert EH, O'Brien PC: Pain in peripheral neuropathy related to rate and kind of fiber degeneration. *Neurology* 26:466-471, 1976.

Dyck PJ, Thomas PK, Lambert EH, Bunge R: *Peripheral Neuropathy,* ed 2. Philadelphia, WB Saunders, 1984, vol 1.

Dyck PJ, Thomas PK, Lambert EH, Bunge R: *Peripheral Neuropathy,* ed 2. Philadelphia, WB Saunders Co, 1984, vol 2.

Ellenberg M: Diabetic neuropathy: clinical aspects. *Metabolism* 25:1627-1655, 1976.

England AC, Brown DD: Severe sensory changes and trophic disorder in peroneal muscular atrophy (Charcot-Marie-Tooth type). *Arch Neurol* 67:1-22, 1952.

Ferrito JD, Biggs EW: Delayed primary closure in wound healing. *J Am Podiatry Assoc* 67:56-57, 1977.

Forgacs S: *Bones and Joints in Diabetes Mellitus.* The Hague, Netherlands, Hungary, Martinus Nijhoff Publishers, 1982.

Forgacs S: Clinical picture of diabetic osteoarthropathy. *Acta Diabetol Lat* 13:111-115, 1976.

Horibe S, Tada K, Nagano J: Neuroarthropathy of the foot in leprosy. *J Bone Joint Surg* 70B:481, 1988.

Julsrud ME: Diabetic neuropathy. *J Am Podiatry Assoc* 71:318-322, 1981.

Kaplan WE, Abourizk NN: Diabetic peripheral neuropathies affecting the lower extremity. *J Am Podiatry Assoc* 71:356-362, 1981.

McMillan DE: The effect of diabetes on blood flow properties. *Diabetes* 32:56-63, 1983.

Meyerson LB, Meier GC: Cutaneous lesions in acroosteolysis. *Arch Dermatol* 106:224-227, 1972.

Mishalanie MA, Dockery GL: Spina bifida and its effect on the lower extremities. *J Am Podiatry Assoc* 70:84-88, 1980.

Nelson PB, Nelson EW: Clinical applications of the Doppler ultrasound flow meter in lower extremity vascular disease. *J Foot Surg* 19:88-94, 1980.

Reynolds EH, Rothfeld P, Pincus JH: Neurological disease associated with folate deficiency. *Br Med J* 2:398-400, 1973.

Reynolds EH: The neurology of vitamin B2 deficiency metabolic mechanisms. *Lancet* 2:832-833, 1976.

Snider W, Simpson DM, Nielsen S, Gold JWM, Metroka CE, Posher JB: Neurological complications of acquired immune deficiency syndromes: analysis of 50 patients. *Ann Neurol* 14:403-418, 1983.

Snipley DE, Miner KM: The role of physical therapy in foot problems. In McDowell F, Enna CD (eds): *Surgical Rehabilitation in Leprosy.* Baltimore, Williams & Wilkins, 1974, p 301.

Spritz N: Nerve disease in diabetes mellitus. *Med Clin North Am* 62:787-798, 1978.

Wagner FW: Transcutaneous Doppler ultrasound in the prediction of healing and the selection of surgical level for dysvascular lesions of the toes and forefoot. *Clin Orthop* 142:110-114, 1979.

Winegrad AI, Greene DA: Diabetic polyneuropathy: the importance of insulin deficiency, hyperglycemia and alterations in myoinositol metabolism in its pathogenesis. *N Engl J Med* 295:1416-1420, 1976.

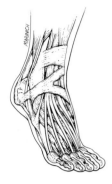

CHAPTER **53**

Elective Diabetic Foot Surgery

Alan S. Banks, D.P.M.

With respect to surgery in the diabetic limb, emphasis has centered on the treatment of acute problems, most often in the form of infection or ulceration. Little has been published regarding the surgical management of deformities prior to the development of these more advanced complications. Generally, surgical intervention for an acute problem is viewed as a terminal event, with little consideration given to the future consequences that may result or any thought toward rectifying the original deformities. It would seem that a more proactive form of treatment would be in order for this subset of patients who suffer a disproportionate share of foot maladies. The repair of those deformities that place the diabetic foot at risk would tend to reduce the likelihood of subsequent complications.

Surgeons in general have been fearful of the diabetic foot, certainly with some degree of justification. However, much of the irrational element of this anxiety should be tempered with some of the newer concepts of the way the disease process affects the lower extremity. The status of the peripheral vascular supply is perhaps the greatest fear regarding the diabetic patient. Although this is a source of concern, the autonomic neuropathy that is a feature of the disease process for some of these individuals actually enhances the blood supply to the lower extremity. Furthermore, today there are a number of reliable noninvasive modalities that can provide specific information on the circulatory status of the limb. Therefore it would not seem reasonable to withhold potentially valuable surgical treatment from a patient without further investigation of the vascular status.

INDICATIONS FOR SURGERY

Surgery on the diabetic foot may be considered for four distinct reasons (1), not all of which may be elective.

Incision and Drainage

Incision and drainage may be required for the adequate treatment of infection. This acute problem requires that all compromised tissues be thoroughly debrided. When possible, however, the surgeon should proceed with surgery in a manner that takes into consideration reconstruction that may be required in the future.

Biopsy

Biopsy is another form of surgery that is often indicated in the diabetic foot. Bone biopsy is the most reliable means of diagnosing osteomyelitis. The author prefers this technique to other modalities, such as radionuclide scans, in most instances in which bone infection is suspected. Bone cultures should be taken at the same time for a more definitive identification of the organisms involved, as sinus tract cultures are not considered a reliable indication of the true pathogens within the bone (2).

In some instances there may be radiographic changes that make it difficult to determine whether the patient has osteomyelitis or a Charcot joint. In such instances, a synovial biopsy specimen may be obtained with the bone specimen. Horwitz (3) described the characteristic microscopic appearance of the Charcot joint as consisting of multiple shards of bone and soft tissue embedded within the deep layers of the synovium. However, the clinician should be aware that both of these conditions may be present simultaneously.

When an open lesion is present, it is preferable to remove the bone biopsy specimen through an incision removed from the ulcer site. This will prevent contamination of the bone cultures with organisms from the sinus tract. The ulcer may be covered with an occlusive dressing to further assist in this goal. However, this approach may not always allow one to adequately visualize the bone in question, especially in the midfoot area. Biopsy material may have to be taken through the ulcer or the adjacent tissues.

Exostectomy

The factors that predispose the diabetic to foot ulceration have been discussed in the chapter on the neuropathic foot. Ulceration may become a significant source of disability as well as infection. When conservative measures have failed, or when the osseous structure is such that further ulceration is a distinct possibility, then removal of the offending bone may be considered.

Exostectomy has been typically performed in the midfoot area for plantar lesions associated with a Charcot foot. The severe collapse and dislocation that may accompany this process can render the patient susceptible to cutaneous compromise despite the best of conservative care. In the forefoot, resection of the metatarsal head may be performed to allow a chronic recalcitrant mal perforans ulceration to heal.

Harkless and Dennis advocate surgery for any ulcer that has been resistant to conservative care for more than 3 months (4).

There are three basic methods of performing an exostectomy in the presence of an open wound. Each may be applicable in certain situations. The first technique is to excise the bone from an incision site removed from the ulcer to minimize contamination of the underlying bone. An example would be resection of a metatarsal head through a dorsal incision for a plantar ulcer. The ulcer may be covered with an occlusive dressing. For a plantar midfoot ulcer, one may make an incision at either the medial or lateral aspect of the foot and work toward the prominent bone. Typically the ulcer is then allowed to granulate closed, although the surgical incision may be sutured.

The second approach is to excise the ulcer and then perform whatever osseous work is required through the same incision prior to primary wound closure. This technique was described by Leventen (5). Closed suction drainage can be employed, and if necessary the surgeon may culture the fluid to assess the wound for viable organisms. The advantage of excising the ulcer is that often the soft tissues are so fibrotic that it might be impossible for the wound to adequately granulate closed despite osseous resection. Excision ensures that healthy tissues are present for healing. It also reduces the time of further disability.

The final method of performing exostectomy consists of excising the ulcer to healthy wound margins and removing the problematic bone. However, the wound is then packed open and a delayed primary closure is performed at a later time. This gives one additional time to assess the wound and await the results of bone biopsies and cultures if osteomyelitis is suspected. If additional bone needs to be excised, then it can be readily resected. Daily packing and irrigations may reduce the bacterial count. The technique may also allow the tissues to stabilize and the wound to begin granulating, both of which may enhance the success of the closure.

Exostectomy may certainly be an effective means of alleviating or preventing ulcerative lesions in the diabetic foot. However, isolated metatarsal head resections are not without the potential for future problems. In time the associated digit will contract into the metatarsophalangeal joint space and assume a shortened, more dorsal location. The adjacent toes will deviate within the transverse plane to fill this digital void. Both of these processes place the foot at additional risk of digital ulceration. The uneven metatarsal parabola exacerbates the pressures imposed upon the adjacent metatarsal heads, again risking hyperkeratosis and ulceration. Furthermore, this may place enough additional stress upon the remaining metatarsals to lead to Charcot collapse.

The preferred approach is to envision metatarsal head resection as a stage of reconstruction. Once the ulcer has healed, the risk of future problems may be reduced by resection of the remaining metatarsal heads to even the weight-bearing parabola.

Exostectomy within the midfoot and rearfoot may be very successful in eliminating chronic lesions. If joint instability remains, however, further collapse may negate the benefits of the procedure. Furthermore, this will not alter the rocker-bottom alignment characteristic of so many of these feet. The procedure seems best suited to chronic Charcot feet that have achieved suitable autoarthrodesis of the joints. One also needs to ensure that the ankle equinus deformity, which accompanies most of the chronic Charcot feet, is addressed to provide a better chance of success.

Reconstructive Surgery

Reconstructive surgery may include any procedures, ranging from digital stabilization to major rearfoot arthrodesis. These measures have been discussed relatively infrequently. However, elective repair of foot deformities can be of benefit in certain persons.

Wagner (7) states that patients who develop ulcerative lesions or profound hyperkeratosis resistant to conservative measures are candidates for elective reconstruction of their deformities. O'Neal (6) says that serious consideration should be given to early correction of foot deformities. He noted that conditions that may be well tolerated initially should not be ignored until complications develop, at which time a reconstructive procedure may not be possible. Other authors have discussed positive experiences with elective intervention in diabetic patients (8-11).

It would be impossible to establish criteria for the selection of surgical candidates and the timing of surgical intervention. This should be based on the individual patients and their deformities, needs, and risks.

DIGITAL STABILIZATION

Contracture of the digits renders the patient susceptible to the formation of heloma. In addition, the associated buckling at the metatarsophalangeal joint shifts the fat pad anteriorly and increases the pressures within the plantar aspect of the foot. Both of these factors place the foot at risk of hyperkeratosis and subsequent ulceration.

The procedure preferred by the author for repair of digital contractures in the neuropathic foot is arthrodesis of the proximal interphalangeal joint. The fusion serves to create a rectus digit through which the long flexor tendon will direct plantarflexory force at the metatarsophalangeal joint level, eliminating retrograde buckling. Arthroplasty is usually performed in the fifth toe, as some flexibility is required for the digit to accommodate to the outer border of a shoe. If an arthroplasty is selected for digital reconstruction, then the toe is fixated with a Kirschner wire (K-wire) for 4 to 6 weeks. This allows for a more organized fibrosis of the joint space and tends to provide more postoperative stability. K-wire stabilization has also been recommended by Gudas (12).

Warren (13) noted that the problem of digital contracture could be partially corrected with a Girdlestone type of tendon transfer. However, the author has not attempted this approach.

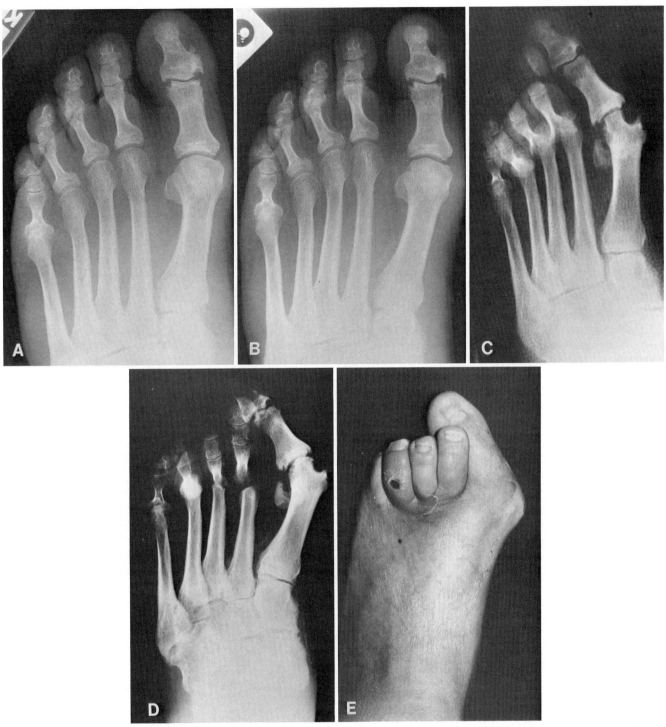

Figure 53.1. Sequential radiographs in an insulin-dependent diabetic. **A.** Initial radiograph in 1979. Note the Charcot involvement of the hallux interphalangeal joint, early hallux abducto valgus, and lesser digital contractures. **B.** Appearance in 1983 with progression of the hammer toe deformities. **C.** Appearance in 1985. Dislocation of the lesser metatarsophalangeal joints has allowed further progression of the hallux abducto valgus deformity. Severe plantar lesions are present, and the patient will subsequently undergo multiple hospitalizations for associated infections. **D** and **E.** Appearance in 1988. Although excision of the second and third metatarsal heads and bases of the proximal phalanges has alleviated the acute infectious processes, the foot is still grossly compromised and at risk. Certainly, panmetatarsal head resection is the best treatment option for this patient. Sometimes the most aggressive treatment is also the most conservative in light of this patient's deformity and subsequent prognosis.

METATARSALS/METATARSOPHALANGEAL JOINTS

Surgery on the metatarsals is usually performed for recalcitrant hyperkeratosis or ulceration. Classically, the approach has been to resect the offending metatarsal head. This is quite successful in alleviating isolated pressures, but it predisposes the patient to later deformity. As discussed previously, the ultimate plan should be to perform a panmetatarsal head resection at a later time, once the more acute problem has resolved. Such resections should be performed at precisely planned lengths so as to evenly distribute forefoot weight distribution (Fig. 53.1).

Panmetatarsal head resection has been reported as a successful procedure in the neuropathic foot. Jacobs (14) described this technique in 12 diabetic patients, some of whom were experiencing problems after metatarsal head resection or ray resection. There were no reported problems with wound healing. Two patients required vascular reconstruction prior to the resections. Jacobs believed the procedure should be considered as an alternative to transmetatarsal amputation.

Giurini and associates (15) reported good results with a total of 17 procedures in 15 patients. There were no problems with wound healing and no postoperative infections, despite the presence of open ulcers in some patients at the time of surgery. None of the patients required vascular reconstruction.

When performing panmetatarsal resections, the author

prefers to stabilize the metatarsophalangeal joint spaces with a K-wire for 6 weeks to enhance stability at this level. If there are open lesions contiguous with the bone or periosteum, however, this may be avoided. Concomitant digital stabilizations will further contribute to control and alignment at the metatarsophalangeal level (Fig. 53.2).

The use of implants within the first metatarsophalangeal joints of neuropathic patients is still an area in which there are no clear indications or contraindications. In the patient without neuropathy these devices generally provide better function. The author has seen first metatarsophalangeal implants used successfully in conjunction with panmetatarsal head resection for diabetic patients, albeit in a limited number of cases. At present there appears to be no advantage to lesser metatarsophalangeal joint implants over K-wire stabilization.

More recently metatarsal osteotomy has been advocated for plantar hyperkeratosis and preulcerative lesions. Daniels (16) reported that a tilt-up osteotomy that maintained the plantar cortex intact was successful in alleviating lesions in a number of patients. However, no specifics were provided. Tillo and associates (17) followed 49 diabetic patients for an average of 19 months after lesser metatarsal osteotomy for recalcitrant ulceration. Most of the procedures performed were osteoclasis. Transfer ulceration developed in 13 patients. Ten of these were managed conservatively. Three patients underwent additional surgery. Three patients had

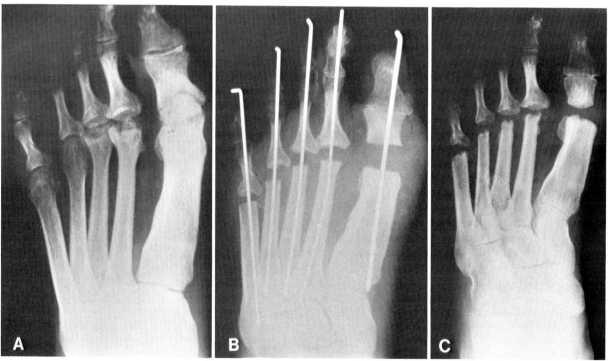

Figure 53.2. **A.** A 36-year-old insulin-dependent female patient with recurrent plantar first metatarsal ulceration due to Charcot degeneration with hallux limitus and hallux malleus. A previous tibial sesamoidectomy was only temporarily successful. Similar findings are also present at the second metatarsophalangeal joint. **B.** Following panmetatarsal head resection. **C.** Four months following surgery.

recurrent ulceration at the original site. Three patients required subsequent amputation consisting of ray resection. Despite the problems noted, overall, the authors were able to avoid amputation in 94% of those treated.

The author does not consider lesser metatarsal osteotomy as reliable as panmetatarsal head resection, especially considering the number of transfer and recurrent lesions experienced in nondiabetics (18). However, an osteotomy certainly involves less surgery and tissue disruption. In patients who have problems postoperatively, the procedure could easily be converted to a panmetatarsal head resection. Therefore this approach to plantar metatarsal problems may occasionally merit consideration.

Procedures that involve the first metatarsophalangeal joint alone are performed most commonly for isolated hallux abducto valgus or hallux limitus. Many of these patients will suffer from severe hallux abducto valgus, which encourages further deformity in the adjacent digits. The prominence created at both the dorsomedial and plantarmedial aspects of the first metatarsal head is a frequent area of ulceration. Although this site of pressure may be managed conservatively with a number of protective devices, there will come a time when this is inadequate.

The techniques employed for the repair of the hallux abducto valgus deformity may be the same as would be used for nondiabetics. However, arthroplasty procedures may be required more often in this patient group when motor neuropathy is significant. Concomitant medial column instability may be an indication for a first metatarsocuneiform arthrodesis. Retrospective studies on the repair of hallux abducto valgus in the neuropathic foot are lacking.

In the neuropathic patient with hallux limitus, an ulcer often develops on the hallux (19). This is logical, as the patient with insensitivity will continue to attempt a normal heel-toe gait since the hallux limitus will not be painful. Adequate motion is simply not available at the metatarsophalangeal joint to allow hallux dorsiflexion at heel-off. Major stress is placed on the great toe, exceeding the capacity of the soft tissue to adapt.

Daniels (19) successfully performed arthroplasties of the first metatarsophalangeal joints in 10 feet with recalcitrant hallux ulcers and hallux limitus. Bone was resected first from the phalangeal base in an angular manner to preserve the attachment of the short flexor tendons. In several patients it was necessary to remove additional bone from the metatarsal head. At 2½ years after surgery no patient had experienced any recurrence of lesions. The range of motion at the first metatarsophalangeal joint increased from 22° to 26° preoperatively to postoperative values ranging between 45° and 70°.

Downs and Jacobs (20) describe successful healing of lesions in six previously unresponsive patients after Keller arthroplasty. No recurrence of ulceration was noted after 2 to 5 years postoperatively. Interestingly, these authors indicate that there was no evidence of hallux rigidus, hallux valgus, or substantial pronation of the foot in any of these patients.

MIDFOOT, REARFOOT, AND ANKLE ARTHRODESIS

Major arthrodesis procedures for diabetics are performed primarily for the repair of Charcot foot deformities. Fusion of the affected joints affords stability and realignment of the deformity and reduces the risk of complications in these patients, many of whom are otherwise doomed to amputation. Reconstruction of the Charcot foot is not a new concept. Harris and Brand (21) stated that they would not hesitate to perform a fusion in a neuropathic foot where conservative measures had failed. Arthrodesis was successful, provided it was performed early in the disease process or later if the affected bone was resected.

One year later Johnson (22) published a thorough report on reconstructive measures for the neuropathic joint, including guidelines for the timing of the procedure and postoperative care. Johnson generally preferred to avoid ankle arthrodesis in favor of tibial osteotomies. Triple arthrodesis and exostectomy were deemed valuable in the foot. He proposed that, even if fusion did not occur, the new alignment that was created allowed the foot to better withstand weight-bearing stress.

Warren (13) stated that she and her colleagues had performed more than 4000 surgical procedures in neuropathic patients. Satisfactory results were noted in 39 of 48 patients (81%) who had undergone arthrodesis in either the foot or the ankle at least 2 years before follow-up. Failure to achieve arthrodesis was noted only in patients in whom external fixation had been employed or in those who had been immobilized for too short a time postoperatively.

However, the patients treated by Harris and Brand (21) and by Warren (13) were suffering from Hansen's disease. The patients under Johnson's care were primarily affected by tabes dorsalis (22). In fact, Johnson stated that surgery of this nature in the diabetic patient was not indicated "... because of potential circulatory problems." Over the ensuing years it became evident that the same process that led to development of the Charcot foot in other patient populations was also responsible for these deformities in the diabetic. In fact, good circulation is actually a prerequisite for the development of a Charcot foot, regardless of the underlying disease entity (1, 23).

Banks and McGlamry (1) discussed the concepts of Charcot joint reconstruction, particularly as they are applied in the diabetic patient. Reconstruction was considered in patients who had sufficient deformity or instability that future amputation was likely without intervention. Those who had lesser deformities but in whom further collapse or ulceration could be reasonably predicted were included as well. The authors noted the high rate of further ablative surgery in patients undergoing amputation as a primary rationale for elective intervention. In fact, arthrodesis in the Charcot foot was considered a form of limb salvage for many patients. The results were favorable and encouraging. Other experiences were similarly optimistic (8-11).

The principles of Charcot joint reconstruction today are very similar to the concepts proposed by Johnson in 1967. First, the foot must be in the quiescent state without active inflammation. The degree of edema, erythema, and warmth that accompany the acute Charcot collapse should dispel any notion of avascularity in this foot type. The immediate concern is to allow resolution of the acute stage before progressing with additional therapy. Initially, compression dressings are applied, followed by casts once the more active phase of swelling has passed.

The author strongly recommends that no weight be borne by the extremity until the quiescent phase has been achieved. Even with a cast, it is difficult to achieve this state if the patient continues weight bearing. Although crutches or a walker may suffice, the patient is encouraged to use a wheelchair. The additional stress borne by the contralateral extremity during the recovery process may lead to Charcot collapse in this limb as well.

Once the foot has entered the quiescent phase and equilibrated, one will note the dissipation of edema, the return of normal skin lines, and the restoration of a symmetrical temperature gradient with the contralateral limb. The latter is usually the final event in the recovery sequence.

Just as the patients must bear no weight while awaiting the quiescent state, they must also be willing to accept this aspect of care in the postoperative period. The preoperative requirement of no weight bearing is a good test of compliance. Premature stress to the foot prior to consolidation of the surgical areas risks complete dissolution of the arthrodesis.

Intraoperatively one will have to resect any bone of questionable quality. In some patients bone resection may be required, regardless of the quality of the bone. Once severe dislocation has occurred, it may be impossible to completely relocate the joints into an anatomical configuration because of soft tissue tension. Accordingly, the removal of bone is required to allow arthrodesis of the joints in a suitable position.

Fixation should be of the most rigid form available that will render stability. Sometimes screws fail to purchase the bone, and other forms of stabilization are required. In other instances there is simply not enough time to individually place a screw in every site, necessitating fixation. Therefore, staples, K-wires, and Steinmann pins are used for many areas. In particular, the pneumatic stapler enables one to fixate multiple joints in a minimum of time. Even when screws and staples appear to be adequate, one or two pins may be buried for additional support. This appears to be an effective way to minimize bending forces, which may disrupt the other forms of fixation.

Lisfranc's Joint

Lisfranc's joint is one of the areas most commonly affected by the Charcot process. In some patients the dislocation is primarily a transverse plane deformity, which lends itself to easier repair. In more severe cases the metatarsals may be dorsally dislocated over the cuneiforms and the cuboid. Restoration of full length to the foot is almost impossible because of the adaptive contracture of the soft tissues. Arthrodesis of the metatarsals directly to the navicular and cuboid or to the talus and calcaneus with graft interposition is often necessary.

In addition to resecting cartilage from the base of the metatarsals, care is taken to also resect the intermetatarsal articulations. This will encourage arthrodesis between the metatarsals, and it further contributes to stability.

The alignment at this joint level is important for an even distribution of weight across the ball of the foot postoperatively. Ideally, all the metatarsals should be on the same plane, with the forefoot in slight valgus position. When arthrodesis is limited to Lisfranc's joint, perhaps with additional involvement of the cuneiforms, one way to establish an appropriate parabola is to first temporarily pin the first and fifth metatarsal bases in position. This will create the weight-bearing plane for the forefoot. Next, while one is working from the second metatarsal laterally, the intermediate metatarsals are aligned and temporarily fixated in the same plane. Finally, the fifth metatarsal will usually require some adjustment for adequate juxtaposition to the fourth metatarsal. Permanent fixation may then be applied.

In other patients the relationship of the metatarsals to one another may be relatively consistent, and yet severe disruption of the tarsus and midfoot may be evident. Arthrodesis of the midfoot may require removal of the cuneiforms and cuboid, leaving one with poor proximal references and irregular surfaces for arthrodesis. The relationship of the metatarsals may actually be the most normal part of the anatomy. Therefore it may be advantageous to first fixate the metatarsals from side to side, creating an appropriate parabola, before reconstructing the midfoot. The metatarsals are then attached as a unit to the proximal portion of the foot.

When the intercuneiform and naviculocuneiform joints are affected without gross displacement, then the more proximal joints are stabilized before one proceeds distally (Figs. 53.3 and 53.4).

Triple and Pantalar Arthrodesis

More proximal stabilization will be required in many Charcot patients. Multiple joint involvement is often the rule unless one is able to intervene at an early stage. Often surgery will consist of fusing not only these joints but more distal segments as well. The relationship of the forefoot is predicated on the final position of the ankle and rearfoot. Again, the general principle is to perform proximal stabilization and alignment first and then to work distally.

It is preferable to avoid ankle arthrodesis if possible. Generally, previous authors have noted a high rate of nonunion when attempts have been made to perform ankle arthrodesis in neuropathic patients (24-26). This author has noted that talotibial and tibiocalcaneal fusion certainly do require a greater period of time for adequate consolidation in these patients. To date, however, there has not been a noticeable incidence of frank nonunion. This finding is similar to that of Warren (13), who noted nonunion only in cases in which external fixation was used in lieu of internal fixation and in which the period of immobilization was too short (Fig. 53.5).

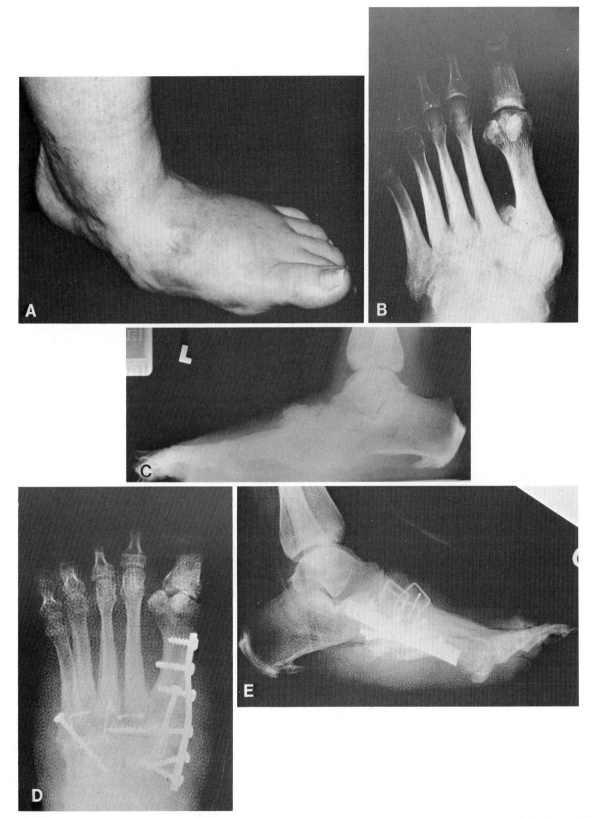

Figure 53.3. **A.** Diabetic female patient with Charcot deformity of the midfoot and equinus. Chronic pain is experienced despite molded shoes and other supportive measures. **B** and **C.** Radiographic appearance. **D** and **E.** Postoperative appearance following midfoot arthrodesis and tendo Achillis lengthening. **F.** Sixteen weeks postoperatively when weight bearing was resumed. All areas are well healed. **G.** Clinical appearance 9 months postoperatively. **H** and **I.** Radiographic appearance 9 months postoperatively.

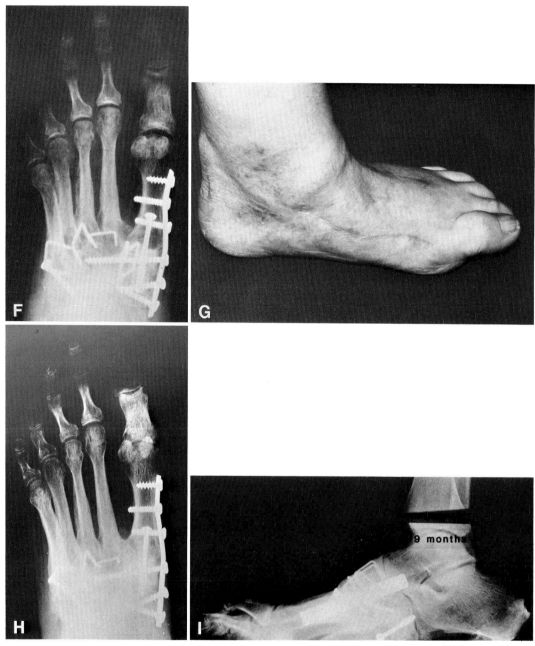

Figure 53.3. F-I.

TENDO ACHILLIS LENGTHENING

Equinus deformity will serve as the disruptive force that instigates Charcot collapse in many neuropathic patients. When there is no compensation for the equinus, the foot will usually fracture and/or dislocate at the weakest point. Typically this involves the tarsometatarsal articulation. Furthermore, equinus will continue to exacerbate the rocker-bottom foot, increasing the risk of ulceration or additional deformity. Neuromuscular imbalance exists in many diabetic patients, and if reconstruction is being performed then tendo Achillis lengthening is a logical means of eliminating this destructive force.

True ankle dorsiflexion may be difficult to assess preoperatively in the patient who has flexible dislocation within the foot. Therefore the decision as to whether or not to lengthen the Achilles tendon may be made intraoperatively after the foot has been stabilized and realigned. Even if a tendo Achillis lengthening is anticipated preoperatively, it is usually performed as the last procedure, once the final alignment of the foot is attained. This ensures that there

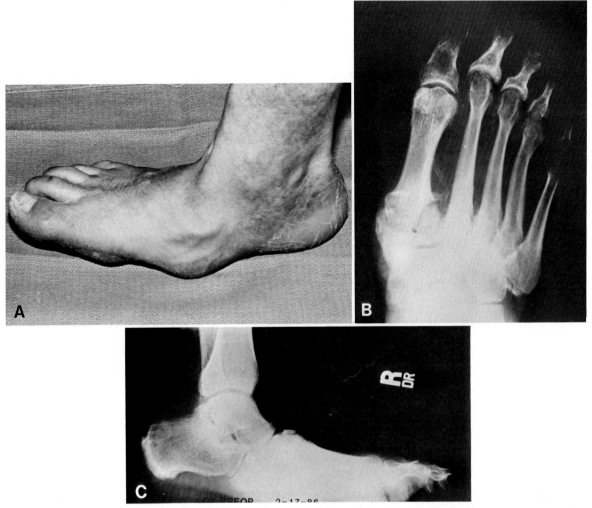

Figure 53.4.   **A.** Collapsed rocker-bottom Charcot foot deformity. **B** and **C.** Preoperative radiographic appearance. **D** to **F.** Appearance 1 year following midfoot arthrodesis and tendo Achillis lengthening. (From Banks AS, McGlamry ED. Charcot foot. *J Am Podiatr Med Assoc* 79:213-235, 1989.) **G** and **H.** Appearance 4 years following surgery.

will be adequate correction and that the equinus deformity will not persist.

The preferred lengthening is from an open frontal plane approach. This may be performed with the patient supine by external rotation of the limb and flexion of the knee. The specific degree of lengthening may be achieved and then maintained with sutures.

Many patients may never regain full strength of the triceps after surgery. However, leaving an ankle equinus uncorrected is an invitation to future joint collapse. The loss of a propulsive gait is more than offset by retention of the limb and return to meaningful weight-bearing function.

OTHER CONSIDERATIONS

One must remember that the diabetic patient has a systemic disease process and that facets of the neuropathy will be manifested not only in the lower extremity but in other 1areas as well. Cardiac dysfunction is the greatest concern, and often it is aggravated by loss of autonomic innervation. These patients are at risk of silent myocardial infarctions. In fact, during the preoperative evaluation several individuals have been found to have sustained recent infarction.

Autonomic neuropathy may also affect the urinary system. The medications provided both preoperatively and postoperatively may aggravate any pre-existing bladder dysfunction so that the patient is unable to void. Other complaints with regard to the gastrointestinal system, such as diarrhea, constipation, early satiety, and nausea, may be related to neuropathy.

Good control of the blood glucose and appropriate nutrition will maximize the potential for the patient to do well. In many of these individuals a true multidisciplinary team is required.

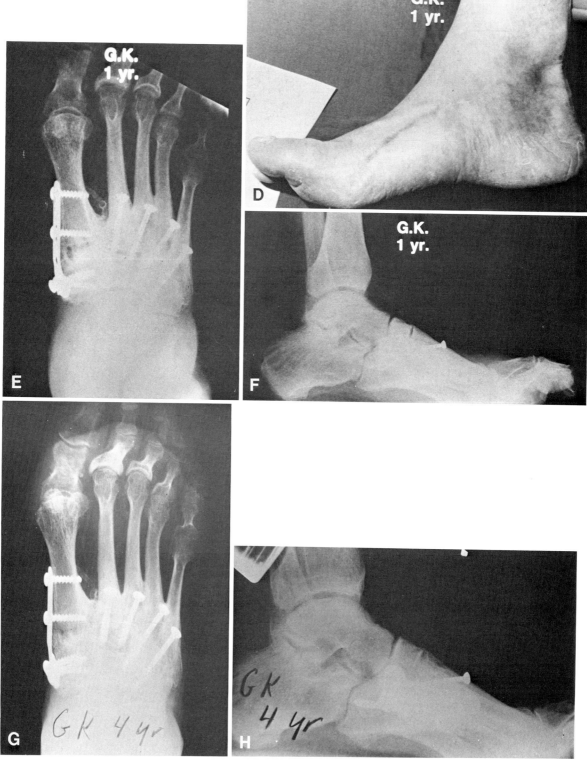

Figure 53.4.   D-H.

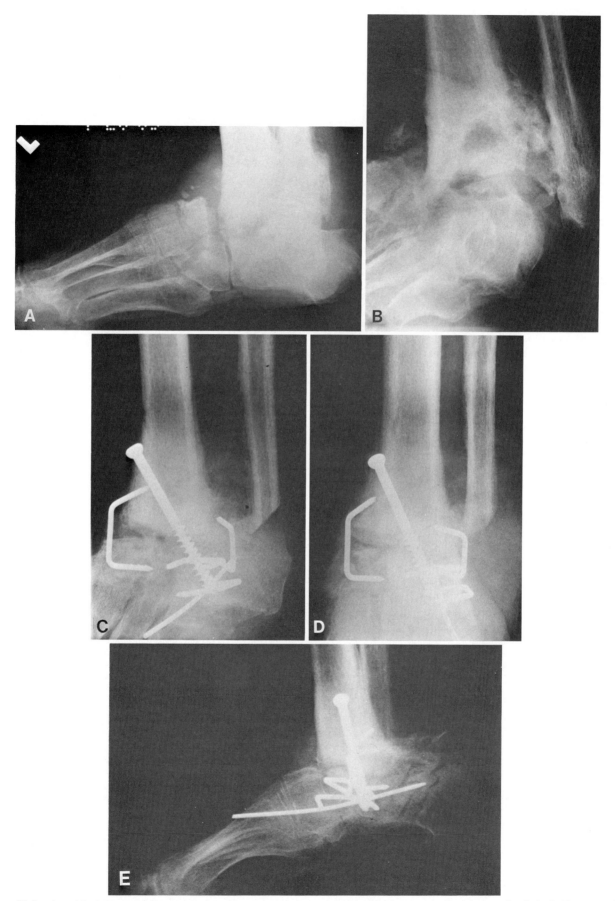

Figure 53.5. **A** and **B.** A 64-year-old non-insulin-dependent man with dissolution of the talus and gross instability. **C** and **D.** Following tibio- calcaneal and calcaneo-cuboid-navicular arthrodesis. **E.** Eleven months following surgery.

Postoperative Care

The postoperative care will vary for each patient, depending on which procedures are performed. Regardless of the surgery, a period of non-weight bearing may be instituted initially, even though this might not be required for similar procedures in nondiabetics. Patients with sensory neuropathy may tend to overextend their activities because of the lack of pain. This may encourage a greater degree of edema or hematoma formation.

For patients undergoing midfoot or rearfoot fusions the initial postoperative period consists of bed rest, elevation, compression dressings, and closed suction drainage. An initial dressing change is made 3 to 4 days after surgery, and compression dressings are reapplied until the edema and wound status have stabilized. Then a permanent cast may be applied. Generally speaking, there will be much less edema than would be anticipated if the same surgery were performed in a nondiabetic.

Casting and abstinence from weight bearing are maintained until there is radiographic evidence of suitable consolidation. The return to full weight-bearing status must be made in a progressive, graduated manner; otherwise there is risk of collapse. Bone is a living substance and will adapt to stress, provided the patient does not exceed the inherent strength of the osseous tissue in the interim period. Patients are initially allowed to bear weight in a standard cast or a removable walking brace. Either a walker or crutches are employed, and the duration of weight bearing is gradually increased over time. Appropriate shoes and orthotic support are also employed after a return to greater activity.

Complications

The complication rate after elective surgical intervention in the diabetic has not been inordinately high, provided the patient complies with the postoperative regimen. This is in direct contradiction of Gudas (12), who noted a fairly substantial incidence of postoperative infection. The risk of infection appeared to be directly related to the presence of previous ulceration as well as the duration of the lesion. Ulceration present for more than 1 year in a weight-bearing area appeared to have the greatest correlation with postoperative problems. This was attributed to possible residual bacteria within the scarred soft tissues. Interestingly, other papers fail to report infection as a complication, even when surgery was performed in the presence of open ulcerative wounds (5, 14, 15, 19, 20). However, several of these authors did maintain the patients on antibiotics for a number of days postoperatively (5, 14, 20).

Obviously, the more major arthrodesis procedures incur a greater risk of postoperative problems simply because of the degree of dissection and the number of joints affected. Very few patients have encountered complications with wound healing. In fact, most of the surgical wounds in these patients appear to heal as fast as, if not faster than, those in nondiabetics. For more isolated procedures (i.e., Lisfranc arthrodesis), osseous healing appears to be quite rapid.

However, the length of time for fusion generally increases somewhat proportionately with the number of additional areas that require concomitant surgery. Patients who require more extensive use of bone grafts similarly require a longer period for consolidation.

Infrequent complications in midfoot and rearfoot arthrodesis have included collapse at the fused joints after the resumption of weight bearing. Collapse of adjacent joints not fused has been seen in only one patient. In several other patients deformation has developed within the osseous structure at the site of surgery, but without collapse.

Although Charcot reconstruction in this patient population is still in the early stages of study, the results to date have generally been encouraging, especially when one considers that amputation is the alternative for many of these limbs.

References

1. Banks AS, McGlamry ED: Charcot foot. *J Am Podiatr Med Assoc* 79:213-235, 1989.
2. Mackowiak PA, Jones SR, Smith JW: Diagnostic value of sinus tract cultures in chronic osteomyelitis. *JAMA* 239:2772-2775, 1978.
3. Horwitz T: Bone and cartilage debris in the synovial membrane. Its significance in the early diagnosis of neuro-arthropathy. *J Bone Joint Surg* 30A:579-588, 1948.
4. Harkless LB, Dennis KJ: The role of the podiatrist. In Levin ME, O'Neal LW (eds): *The Diabetic Foot*, ed 4. St Louis, CV Mosby, 1988, pp.249-272.
5. Leventen EO: Charcot foot—a technique for treatment of chronic plantar ulcer by saucerization and primary closure. *Foot Ankle* 6:295-299, 1986.
6. O'Neal LW: Surgical pathology of the foot and clinicopathologic correlations. In Levin ME, O'Neal LW (eds): *The Diabetic Foot*, ed 4. St Louis, CV Mosby, 1988, pp 203-236.
7. Wagner FW: The dysvascular foot: a system for diagnosis and treatment. *Foot Ankle* 2:64-122, 1981.
8. Banks AS, McGlamry ED, Corey SV: Charcot joints. In McGlamry ED (ed): *Reconstructive Surgery of the Foot and Leg, Update '88*, Tucker, GA, Podiatry Institute Publishing Co, 1988, pp 68-79.
9. Corey SV: Elective surgery in the diabetic patient. In McGlamry ED (ed): *Reconstructive Surgery of the Foot and Leg, Update '89*. Tucker, GA, Podiatry Institute Publishing Co., 1989, pp 159-167.
10. Banks AS, McGlamry ED: Diabetic and diabetic Charcot foot reconstruction. In McGlamry ED (ed): *Reconstructive Surgery of the Foot and Leg, Update '89*. Tucker, GA, Podiatry Institute Publishing Co, 1989, pp 176-201.
11. McGlamry ED, Banks AS, Corey SV: Understanding diabetic and diabetic Charcot foot reconstruction. In DiNapoli DR (ed): *Reconstructive Surgery of the Foot and Leg, Update '90*. Tucker, GA, Podiatry Institute Publishing Co, 1990, pp 178-192.
12. Gudas CJ: Prophylactic surgery in the diabetic foot. *Clin Podiatr Med Surg* 4:445-458, 1987.
13. Warren AG: The surgical conservation of the neuropathic foot. *Ann R Coll Surg Engl* 71:236-242, 1989.
14. Jacobs RL: Hoffman procedure in the ulcerated diabetic neuropathic foot. *Foot Ankle* 3:142-149, 1982.
15. Giurini JM, Habershaw GM, Chrzan JS: Panmetatarsal head resection in chronic neuropathic ulceration. *J Foot Surg* 26:249-255, 1987.
16. Daniels EG: A preventative metatarsal osteotomy for healing pre-ulcers in American Indian diabetics. *J Am Podiatr Med Assoc* 76:33-37, 1986.
17. Tillo TH, Giurini JM, Habershaw GM, Chrzan JS, Rowbotham JL: Review of metatarsal osteotomies for the treatment of neuropathic ulcerations. *J Am Podiatr Med Assoc* 80:211-217, 1990.
18. Hatcher RM, Goller WL, Weil LS: Intractable plantar keratoses. A review of surgical corrections. *J Am Podiatr Assoc* 68:377-386, 1978.

19. Daniels E: Neuropathic foot ulcer prevention in diabetic American Indians with hallux limitus. *J Am Podiatr Med Assoc* 79:447-450, 1989.
20. Downs DM, Jacobs RL: Treatment of resistant ulcers on the plantar surface of the great toe in diabetics. *J Bone Joint Surg* 64A:930-933, 1982.
21. Harris JR, Brand PW: Patterns of disintegration of the tarsus in the anaesthetic foot. *J Bone Joint Surg* 48B:4-16, 1966.
22. Johnson JTH: Neuropathic fractures and joint injuries. *J Bone Joint Surg* 49A:1-30, 1967.
23. Frykberg RG, Kozak GP: The diabetic Charcot foot. In Kozak GP (ed): *Management of Diabetic Foot Problems*. Philadelphia, WB Saunders, 1984.
24. Brooks AL, Saunders EA: Fusion of the ankle in denervated extremities. *South Med J* 60:30-33, 1967.
25. Barrett G, Meyer L, Bray E, Taylor R, Kolb LF: Pantalar arthrodesis: a long-term follow-up. *Foot Ankle* 1:279-283, 1980.
26. Stuart MJ, Morrey BF: Arthrodesis of the diabetic neuropathic ankle joint. *Clin Orthop* 253:209-211, 1990.

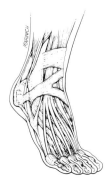

CHAPTER 54

Limb Salvage

Gary R. Bauer, D.P.M.

Compromise of the lower extremity may be encountered in situations of neurovascular insufficiency and massive infectious processes and after trauma to the cutaneous or musculoskeletal structures. Advances in medical technology have resulted in greater life expectancies, even in persons with morbid disease processes. As a result, there has been an increase in the number of individuals who are susceptible to loss of a limb.

The extent of vascular impairment is the ultimate factor that determines the potential for limb salvage. Traumatic disruption of major arterial supply may be associated with soft tissue laceration, transection of portions of the extremity, and blunt crushing or degloving injuries. Therefore the potential for surgical salvage is influenced by associated tissue injury and loss. Advances in microvascular reconstructive technology have greatly enhanced the ability to salvage limbs. Replantation is now technically possible, with an excellent expectation for survival. However, the indications for replantation of the lower extremity are limited because of the poor functional results (1-7). State-of-the-art external/internal fixator systems have enhanced the management of osseous and soft tissue injury by providing stability, which facilitates wound management.

Arteriosclerotic occlusive vascular disease is undoubtedly the major contributor to vascular impairment of the limb (8-10). This is essentially a developmental consequence of aging, influenced to a significant degree by the American life-style. The consumption of fatty foods, smoking, and stress factors all contribute to this process. Superimposed metabolic effects of diabetes mellitus may also tend to accelerate and alter the distribution of these arterial occlusive processes (11, 12). The involvement of vascular channels distal to the femoropopliteal trifurcation with a multisegmental distribution limits the feasibility and prognosis for vascular reconstruction. Recent advances in this realm have significantly improved the indications for and frequency of distal vascular reconstructions, which are now commonplace at most medical centers. Vascular impairment must be assessed and addressed prior to, or in combination with, any attempt at limb salvage.

The neuropathic extremity is predisposed to limb compromise. Diabetes mellitus and alcoholism account for the overwhelming majority of patients in this risk group. Sensory, motor, and autonomic involvement all contribute to this morbid process (11). Motor neuropathy leads to development of atrophy and imbalance of the extrinsic and intrinsic muscles of the foot. The resultant digital contractures

create a retrograde loading on the respective metatarsal segments, compounding plantar pressures. Gait aberrations may also augment this process.

Sensory neuropathy eliminates the protective mechanisms that would normally alert one to accommodate the pathological weight distribution.

Autonomic involvement results in trophic skin changes that diminish the ability of the integument to provide an effective protective barrier. Thinning with atrophy and distal migration of the intrametatarsal subcutaneous tissues further predisposes to mal perforans conditions. Interdigital fissuring is a common precipitator of tracking plantar space infection with resultant threat to life and limb (13).

Overwhelming infections that jeopardize the extremity include osteomyelitis and tracking closed-compartment processes. Osteomyelitis presents a locally invasive destruction of bone that is best addressed with en bloc resection of the affected segment. The large osseous void created presents a reconstructive dilemma. Historically, autogenous grafting procedures with staged attempts at bridging or bypassing the defect have produced unpredictable results (14-25).

Newer technologies to address this formidable problem are now on the horizon. Microvascular transplant of free osseous segments has met with some success. However, it poses many of the same risks as that of conventional procedures (26-30). Bone transport technology as pioneered by Ilizarov offers its greatest potential in these situations (31-37).

Controlled fracture callus distraction via segmental ring fixators has the capability of reconstructing large segmental defects without the need for donor tissues. The involved long bone is subjected to osteotomy near one or both metaphyseal regions, with care taken to preserve the periosteal blood supply. The ring fixator system is arranged about the osteotomy to allow distraction by regulated calipers. Once the desired length is achieved, fixation is maintained with the frame for a period approximately twice that required to achieve the lengthening. Distraction osteogenesis seems to offer the greatest potential for salvage in segmental osseous defects (Fig. 54.1).

Necrotizing fasciitis occurs as a fulminant, generally anaerobic invasion, with rapid proximal progression along the superficial fascial plane. Plantar space infections track between the deep spaces of the sole of the foot and may result in proximal extension along the deep fascial clefts of the leg (38-40). Limb salvage in these conditions is contingent on a high degree of suspicion, prompt recognition, and early

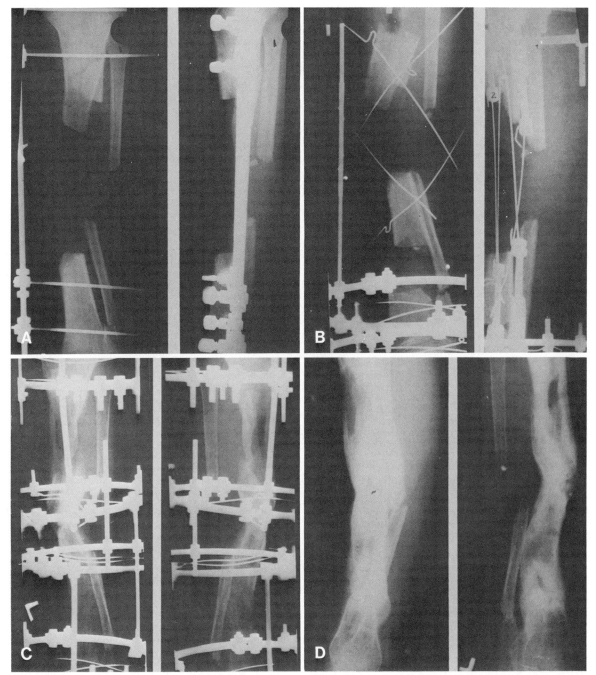

Figure 54.1. **A.** Anteroposterior and lateral roentgenograms following initial external fixator application for a 14 cm defect of the tibia and associated soft tissues. **B.** Anteroposterior and lateral roentgenograms after double corticotomy of the proximal and distal remainder of the tibia and application of Ilizarov type of ring fixator. **C.** Anteroposterior and lateral roentgenograms. Transported fragments are in contact, and frame has been revised for interfragmental compression. **D.** Final roentgenograms at 18 months. The patient was bearing full weight without an orthosis.

aggressive surgical decompression. These are true surgical emergencies. Delay of appropriate treatment by even several hours may significantly alter the potential for preserving a viable extremity.

Decompression is achieved through generous incisions centered over the affected compartment with care to pre-serve major neurovascular channels. Aggressive surgical debridement of all devitalized and necrotic tissue is followed by copious irrigation with a pressurized lavage system. Parenteral antibiotics should be instituted after procurement of deep aerobic and anaerobic cultures. The initial agent is determined empirically on the basis of the Gram stain and the character of the infection's presentation and is modified on the basis of serial sensitivity findings. Repeat debridement may be required, should the infectious process progress.

Surgical limb salvage after any ablative process must achieve not only skin and soft tissue coverage but a functional extremity as well. To this end, various principles of plastic surgery come into play, along with a sound biomechanical knowledge of load distribution in the compromised lower extremity.

Localized areas of soft tissue deficit are frequent after radical debridement for control of deep infection and in traumatic degloving injuries. Restoration of a stable, well-healed, and functional extremity may necessitate mobilization of local or distant soft tissues, including skin, subcutaneous tissue, and/or muscle. The simplest method that will achieve this state should be selected (41). Coverage with split thickness skin grafts may be sufficient in patients with good granular beds. Meshed grafts are useful when the recipient defect is large. Nonmeshed thick split-thickness skin is preferable in areas of weight bearing, since the greater dermal component provides additional resistance to loading. Full-thickness skin grafting is rarely feasible because of the donor defect created as well as the decreased probability of survival with marginal vascular status and potential instability. Stability of the recipient bed may be augmented by bolster-type horizontal mattress sutures, which secure the marginal wound tissues (Fig. 54.2). This minimizes the risk of postoperative sloughing of the graft.

Submetatarsal head mal perforans ulcers are best addressed with aggressive local wound care. If pressure is alleviated through accommodative padding or shoe modifications, healing should occur by local granulation and epithelialization. All hyperkeratosis marginal to the ulcer must be removed along with any devitalized or exuberant granulation tissue present in the ulcer bed. Residual marginal hyperkeratosis is a primary factor related to extension of the ulcerative process in the neuropathic foot. This encourages marginal undermining with extension of the skin defect and prevents epithelialization. After closure, accommodative insole fillers or prophylactic surgical procedures should be considered to prevent recurrence.

Larger defects that are not amenable to primary closure or skin grafting may require local flap transposition to mobilize adjacent vascularized soft tissue and skin into the area. Axial pattern flaps are preferable to random transfers because of the more predictable neurovascular profusion. Muscle transfer may be useful in conditions of chronic osteomyelitis where a relatively avascular segmental defect or exposed bone is present (42, 43). Muscle flaps are based on the extrinsic as well as the intrinsic vascular supply and may allow total or partial transfer, depending on the individual requirements and donor muscle being considered. The transposed muscle serves to fill the dead space as well as improve the local vascular environment. This provides an excellent bed that will readily accept a split-thickness skin graft. The limitations of local flap transfer are the availability of donor tissues and the vascular pedicle, which determines the arc of rotation.

Distant free vascularized tissue transfer (skin, subcutaneous, muscle, and/or bone) is a valuable procedure in selective limb salvage situations (44-47). Open fracture dislocations with exposed articular surfaces and the loss of overlying soft tissues are an indication for immediate free muscle or myocutaneous coverage. These procedures are technically demanding and time consuming. The potential benefits and risks must be weighed relative to alternate methods for limb salvage. The dysvascular and diabetic patient frequently manifests multisystem involvement. Cardiovascular and renal compromise, in addition to peripheral vascular concerns, make alternate methods of surgical limb salvage more desirable.

Local amputation may be useful to facilitate direct closure. Through selective osseous resection, the local vascular supply to the soft tissues may be preserved and the salvaged extremity may be more durable and functional than if more sophisticated methods of tissue mobilization are used (48-56). In addition, healing in these procedures is more predictable and is associated with less morbidity and risk. Free flap transfers may be bulky and mechanically unstable. The protective sensation achieved, even with neural anastomosis, is frequently less than desirable.

The goals of selective osseous resection are to restore a functional parabola that will evenly dissipate weight-bearing stresses over the structure and to make available viable soft tissues with retained protective sensation to achieve durable coverage/closure. Secondary objectives are to preserve a heel-to-toe gait pattern and provide a foot that may be accommodated in standard shoes with an innersole filler.

Accordingly, limitations are imposed on selective local foot amputation (41). Lateral column deficit must preserve the medial two rays and a portion of the third metatarsal. Medial column deficit must preserve the proximal third of the first metatarsal and a greater portion of the second and third rays. The oblique metatarsal break should be restored to a graded step-down pattern, if possible, to allow even weight distribution in propulsive gait. Central ray deficits require an accommodative spacer to prevent midline convergence of the marginal digits. There is significant risk of mal perforans ulcers developing under the retained first and fifth metatarsal heads. Immediate transmetatarsal amputation may be a more desirable form of salvage.

Figure 54.2. A. Large cutaneous defect following ablative debridement of severe diabetic necrotizing fasciitis. Note the undermined and unstable marginal skin. **B.** Plantar view demonstrates residual defect following resolution of severe plantar space infection. **C** and **D.** Reconstruction demonstrating stabilization of marginal skin with strategically positioned bolster sutures. A 3:1 meshed split-thickness graft has been applied dorsally and an unmeshed graft plantarly. **E** and **F.** One-year follow-up showing stable coverage. Patient wears a standard shoe with insole modification and demonstrates a propulsive gait pattern. **G.** Final radiograph demonstrates a symmetrical step-down pattern to the metatarsal parabola.

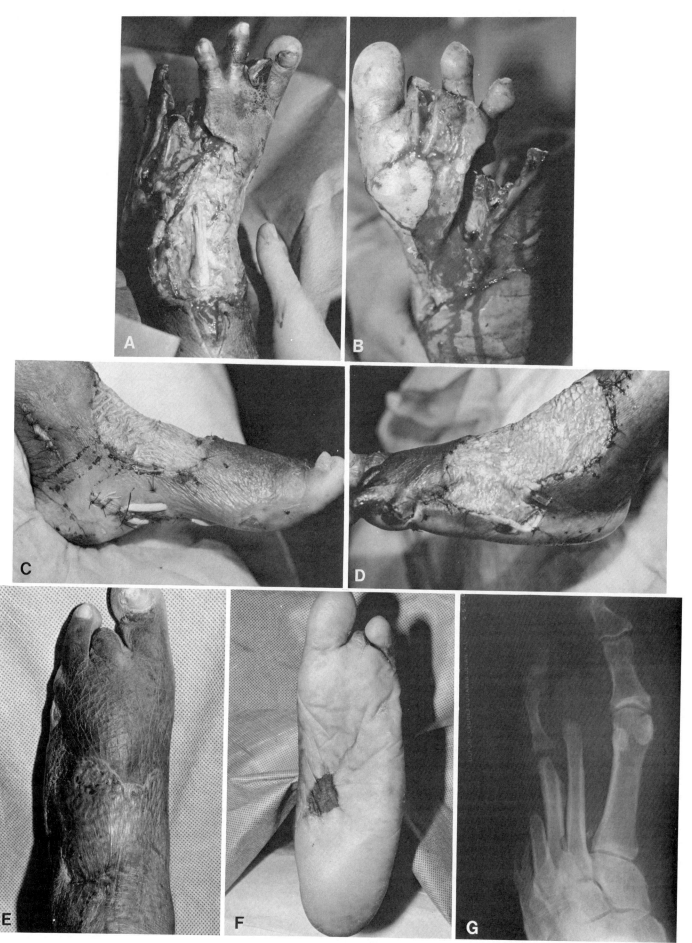

Figure 54.2. A-G.

Transmetatarsal amputation is a reliable salvage procedure for dysvascular conditions with resultant localized tissue loss distal to the digital sulcus (57-61). Classically, a symmetrical parabola of the metatarsal stumps is covered with a plantarly based flap to provide durable coverage in propulsion. Often the available tissues require creative modification and mobilization techniques to achieve closure.

Preservation of the first metatarsal base to maintain the tendon insertion of tibialis anterior is crucial to provide a durable and balanced functional extremity (62). The loss of tibialis anterior tendon function will result in progressive developmental equino varus because of the unopposed triceps surae action. Subsequently, increasing weight-bearing pressure will be concentrated on the distal lateral stump, with a risk of tissue breakdown.

Any partial foot amputation with osseous resection proximal to the Lisfranc level must provide dynamic muscle rebalancing (63-65). This may be addressed through attachment of the anterior musculature into the distal osseous stump while an attempt is made to preserve an effective lever arm. Transfer under physiological muscle tension will assure maximum functional efficiency. This may have to be augmented with such procedures as tenotomy or lengthening of the triceps to reduce the risk of equinus.

Skin closure may require a combination of plantarly or dorsally based flaps as well as grafting procedures, depending on the cutaneous tissues available after functional osseous contouring. Viable skin should never be sacrificed until stump coverage is assured. Toe fillet procedures may provide additional length to extend conventional flap coverage. Redundant cutaneous tissues may be incorporated in areas of more distant tissue deficit as either full- or split-thickness grafts.

Limb salvage poses a formidable challenge to the podiatric surgeon. Patient education and routine prophylactic care by means of palliation and accommodative devices are primary modalities in controlling the conditions that so frequently predispose the patient to loss of a limb. Recognition and prompt appropriate treatment of acute problems will limit the tissue deficit when a limb-threatening condition is present. A team approach may involve the services of internal medicine and infectious disease, as well as podiatric surgery. General health and nutritional status must be maximized to ensure the patient's ability to cope with and overcome the imposed traumatic and surgical insult (66).

The goals of surgical salvage are to produce a healed and functional extremity. To this end, a broad knowledge of the salvage options and the technical skill to implement them are mandatory. A well-informed and compliant patient is necessary to ensure the best potential for a favorable result. Realistic expectations must be observed to avoid subjecting the patient and physician to a prolonged course, the end result of which is failure. Appropriate protection of the salvaged extremity demands insole accommodation or bracing where indicated and a life-style modification consistent with the functional tolerance of the extremity. The reconstructed limb will forever be at increased risk of future compromise.

References

1. Fukui A, Inada Y, Sempuku T, Tamai S: Successful replantation of a foot with satisfactory recovery: a case report. *J Reconstr Microsurg* 4:387-390, 1988.
2. Cheng TH, Ping HL, Gung TK: Successful restoration of a traumatically amputated leg. *Chin Med J* 84:641, 1965.
3. Magee HR, Parker WR: Replantation of the foot: results after two years. *Med J Aust* 1:751, 1972.
4. Hoehn JB: Replantation of the foot. *Surg Round* 1:53, 1978.
5. Lesavoy MA: Successful replantation of the lower leg and foot, with good sensibility and function. *Plast Reconstr Surg* 64:760, 1979.
6. Van Beek AL, Wavak PW, Zook EG: Replantation of heel in a child. *Ann Plast Surg* 2:154, 1979.
7. Chen ZW, Zeng BF: Replantation of the lower extremity. *Clin Plast Surg* 10:103, 1983.
8. Towne J, Condon R: Lower extremity amputations for ischemic disease. *Adv Surg* 13:199-226, 1979.
9. Burgess E, Romano R, Zettl J, Schrock R: Amputations of the leg for peripheral vascular insufficiency. *J Bone Joint Surg* A: 874-890, 1971.
10. Wagner F: The dysvascular foot: a system for diagnosis and treatment. *Foot Ankle* 2:64-121, 1981.
11. Levin ME, O'Neal LW: *The Diabetic Foot*, ed 3. St Louis, CV Mosby Co, 1983.
12. Levin ME: The diabetic foot. *Angiology* 31:375-385, 1980.
13. Grodinsky M: Foot infection of peridigital origin. *Ann Surg* 94:274-279, 1931.
14. Cabanela ME: Open cancellous bone grafting of infected bone defects. *Orthop Clin North Am* 15:427-440, 1984.
15. Bickel WH, Bateman JG, Johnson WE: Treatment of chronic hematogenous osteomyelitis by means of saucerization and bone grafting. *Surg Gynecol Obstet* 96:265-274, 1953.
16. Coleman HM, Bateman JE, Dale GM: Cancellous bone grafts for infected bone defects. *Surg Gynecol Obstet* 83:392-398, 1946.
17. De Oliveira JC: Bone grafts and chronic osteomyelitis. *J Bone Joint Surg* 53B:672-683, 1971.
18. Hazlett W: The use of cancellous bone grafts in the treatment of subacute and chronic osteomyelitis. *J Bone Joint Surg* 36B:584-590, 1954.
19. Higgs SL: The use of cancellous chips in bone grafting. *J Bone Joint Surg* 28:15-18, 1946.
20. Hogeman KE: Treatment of infected bone defects with cancellus bone-chip grafts. *Acta Chir Scand* 98:576-590, 1949.
21. Knight MF, Wood GO: Surgical obliteration of bone cavities following traumatic osteomyelitis. *J Bone Joint Surg* 27:547-556, 1945.
22. Mowlem R: Cancellous chip bone-grafts. *Lancet* 2:746-748, 1944.
23. Robertson JM, Barron JN: A method of treatment of chronic infective osteitis. *J Bone Joint Surg* 28:19-28, 1946.
24. Sudmann E: Treatment of chronic osteomyelitis by free grafts of autologous bone tissue. *Acta Orthop Scand* 50:145-150, 1979.
25. Winter FE: The surgical treatment of pyogenic osteomyelitis. *Clin Orthop* 51:139-149, 1967.
26. Woad MB, Cooney WP: Vascularized bone segment transfers for management of chronic osteomyelitis. *Orthop Clin North Am* 15:461-472, 1984.
27. Chin-Tanc H, Chi-Wei C, Kuo-Li S: Free vascularized bone graft using microvascular technique. *Ann Acad Med Singapore* 8:459, 1979.
28. Weiland PJ, Daniel RK: Microvascular anastomoses for bone grafts in the treatment of massive defects in bone. *J Bone Joint Surg* 61A:98-104, 1979.
29. Weiland AJ, Moore JR, Daniel RK: The efficacy of free tissue transfer in the treatment of osteomyelitis. *J Bone Joint Surg* 66A:181-193, 1984.
30. Sowa DT, Weiland AJ: Clinical application of vascularized bone autografts. *Orthop Clin North Am* 18:257-273, 1987.
31. Ilizarov GA, Soybelman LM, Chirkova AM: Some roentgenologic and morphological data on regeneration of bone tissue in experimental distraction epiphysiolysis. *Ortop Travmatol Protez* 31:26, 1970.
32. Ring PA: Experimental bone lengthening by epiphyseal distraction. *Br J Surg* 46:69-73, 1958.
33. Eydelstein BM, Udalova F, Bochkarev GF: Dynamics of operative regeneration after lengthening by the method of distraction epiphysiolysis. *Acta Chir Plast* 15:149, 1973.
34. Monticelli G, Spinelli R, Bonucci E: Distraction epiphysiolysis as a

method of limb lengthening. I. Experimental study. *Clin Orthop* 154:284-291, 1981.

35. Monticelli G, Spinelli R, Bonucci E: Distraction epiphysiolysis as a method of limb lengthening. II. Morphological investigations. *Clin Orthop* 154:292-303, 1981.

36. Monticelli G, Spinelli R, Bonucci E: Distraction epiphysiolysis as a method of limb lengthening. III. Clinical application. *Clin Orthop* 154:304-315, 1981.

37. Monticelli G, Spinelli R: Limb lengthening by closed metaphyseal corticotomy. *Ital J Orthop Traumatol* 9:139-150, 1983.

38. Meade JW, Mueller CB: Major infection of the foot. *Med Times* 96:154-169, 1968.

39. Grodinsky M: A study of the tendon sheaths of the foot and their relation to infection. *Surg Gynecol Obstet* 51:460-472, 1930.

40. Grodinsky M: A study of the fascial spaces of the foot and their bearing on infection. *Surg Gynecol Obstet* 49:737-751, 1929.

41. Bauer G: Function reconstruction after ablative debridement for severe diabetic foot infection. *Clin Podiatr Med Surg* 7:509-521, 1990.

42. Fitzgerald RH Jr, Ruttle PE, Arnold PG: Local muscle flaps in the treatment of osteomyelitis. *J Bone Joint Surg* 67A:175-185, 1985.

43. Mathes SJ, Alpert BS, Chang N: Use of the muscle flap in chronic osteomyelitis: experimental and clinical correlation. *Plast Reconstr Surg* 69:815-828, 1982.

44. Irons GB, Fisher J, Schmitt EH: Vascularized muscular and musculocutaneous flaps for management of osteomyelitis. *Orthop Clin North Am* 15:473-480, 1984.

45. May JW Jr, Moore JR, Daniel RK: The efficacy of free tissue transfer in the treatment of osteomyelitis. *J Bone Joint Surg* 66A:181-193, 1984.

46. Weiland AJ, Moore JR, Daniel RK: The efficacy of free tissue transfer in the treatment of osteomyelitis. *J Bone Joint Surg* 66A:181-193, 1984.

47. Colen LB: Limb salvage in the patient with severe peripheral vascular disease: the role of free-tissue transfer. *Plast Reconstr Surg* 79:389-395, 1987.

48. Millsteir SG, McCowan SA, Hunter GA: Traumatic partial foot amputations in adults. *J Bone Joint Surg* 70B:251-254, 1988.

49. Pinzur MS, Sage R, Abraham M, Osterman H: Limb salvage in infected lower extremity gangrene. *Foot Ankle* 8:212-215, 1988.

50. Parziale JR, Hahn K: Functional considerations in partial foot amputations. *Orthop Rev* 17:262-266, 1988.

51. Braddeley RM, Fulford JC: A trial of conservative amputations for lesions of the feet in diabetes mellitus. *Br J Surg* 52:38-43, 1965.

52. Wagner FW: Amputations of the foot and ankle. *Clin Orthop* 122:62-69, 1977.

53. Kritter AE: A technique for salvage of the infected diabetic gangrenous foot. *Orthop Clin North Am* 4:21-30, 1973.

54. Larsson V, Andersson GB: Partial amputation of the foot for diabetic or arteriosclerotic gangrene. *J Bone Joint Surg* 60B:126-130, 1978.

55. Robson M, Edstrom LE: Conservative management of the ulcerated diabetic foot. *Plast Reconstr Surg* 59:551-554, 1977.

56. Robson M, Edstrom LE: The diabetic foot: an alternative approach to major amputation. *Surg Clin North Am* 57:1089-1102, 1977.

57. Bradham GB, Lee WH, Stallworth JM: Transmetatarsal amputation. *Angiology* 11:495-498, 1960.

58. McKittrick LS, McKittrick JB, Risley TS: Transmetatarsal amputation for infection or gangrene in patient with diabetes mellitus. *Ann Surg* 130:826-842, 1949.

59. Young AE: Transmetatarsal amputation in the management of peripheral ischemia. *Am J Surg* 134:604-607, 1977.

60. Wheelock FC: Transmetatarsal amputation and arterial surgery in diabetic patients. *N Engl J Med* 264:316-320, 1961.

61. Schwindt CD, Lulloff RS, Rogers SC: Transmetatarsal amputations. *Orthop Clin North Am* 4:31-42, 1973.

62. Spittler AW, Brennan J, Payne J: Syme amputation performed in two stages. *J Bone Joint Surg* 36A:37-41, 1954.

63. Roach J, Deutsch A, McFarlane D: Resurrection of the amputations of Lisfranc and Chopart for diabetic gangrene. *Arch Surg* 122:931-934, 1987.

64. Christie J, Clowes CB, Lamb DW: Amputation through the middle part of the foot. *J Bone Joint Surg* 62B:473-474, 1980.

65. MacDonald A: Chopart's amputation: the advantages of a modified prosthesis. *J Bone Joint Surg* 37B:468-470, 1955.

66. Dickhaut SC, DeLee JC, Page CP: Nutritional status: importance in predicting wound-healing after amputation. *J Bone Joint Surg* 66A:71-75, 1984.

Additional References

Pavot AP: Ankle disarticulation: a definitive type of amputation in adults. *Arch Phys Med Rehabil* 54:307-310, 1973.

Pinzur MS, Jordan C, Rana NA: Syme's two stage amputation in dysvascular disease. *Ill Med J* 160:23-27, 1981.

Turan I: Tarso metatarsal amputation and tibialis anterior tendon transposition to cuneiform. I. *J Foot Surg* 24:113-115, 1985.

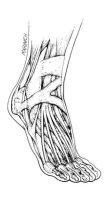

CHAPTER **55**

Amputations in the Foot

Jim L. Gregory, D.P.M.
Verdon Peters, D.P.M.
Lawrence B. Harkless, D.P.M.

HISTORY

Amputations have probably been performed since the beginning of mankind. Archaeological evidence dates to the Neolithic period when saws and knives made of stone were found with the skeletal remains of amputated limbs (1). The word *amputation* is derived from the Latin word *amputare*, which literally means cutting around (1). The term was originally used to describe the removal of limbs or portions of limbs by knife.

The history of amputations closely parallels the development of surgery itself. Since the ancient surgeon was primarily a military surgeon, most procedures were performed on battle casualties. The major contributions made by the amputation surgeon included the use of tourniquets and ligatures to control bleeding, tissue handling, secondary wound closure after infection, and recognition of the importance of cleanliness. Hippocrates (circa 500 BC) recommended amputation to remove diseased limbs (1). Celsus, in the first century AD, recommended amputation between healthy and gangrenous tissues (1, 2). During this time, ligatures were used to control bleeding. The medical indications for amputations were expanded to include tumors, ulcers, injuries, and deformities in addition to gangrene.

The Dark Ages (AD 200 to AD 1500) witnessed a decline in amputation technique, which eventually resulted in the abandonment of ligatures and the increasing use of cautery to control bleeding (1). Little refinement in surgical technique was noted during this period until the eleventh century AD when Albucasia, a Muslim surgeon, introduced the use of the constricting surgical bandage to control bleeding (1).

Ambrose Pare (1510 to 1590) made the most significant contributions to amputation surgery (1-3). He reintroduced the use of ligatures and discontinued the use of cautery to control hemorrhage. One of his innovations was the development of a spring-loaded artery forceps to hold blood vessels while ligatures were applied. Pare emphasized the importance of removing all dead tissue and advocated that amputation sites be selected with respect to future use of prosthesis.

The preanesthetic period, 1600 to 1846, witnessed improvements in surgical technique, site selection, soft tissue handling, stump coverage, prevention of infection, and postsurgical rehabilitation (1). The description of blood circulation by Harvey in 1616 led to the invention of more efficient tourniquets (1).

The primary problem encountered during this era was infection. Both the French surgeon Baron Dominique Carey (1766 to 1842) and the English surgeon George Guthrie (1785 to 1856) found that immediate amputation of traumatized limbs resulted in less incidence of infection and a lower mortality (2, 3). The hallmarks of modern surgery include the evolution of anesthesia and aseptic technique. With these developments, surgeons focused attention on improved technique and site selection. Attention in the latter half of the nineteenth century focused on the shape of amputation stumps and their weight-bearing possibilities. Thus far in the twentieth century, there have been many contributions regarding site selection, technique, rehabilitation, and the use of prosthetics.

RATIONALE FOR LIMB SALVAGE

The primary function of the lower extremity is locomotion; preservation of this function should be the surgeon's goal. McCollough (4) suggests thinking of amputation as a reconstructive procedure that eliminates a diseased, sometimes functionless extremity in order to restore ambulation. Amputation should not be considered in a completely negative sense but as an alternative method whereby the ability to walk may be regained.

The amount of energy expended in walking increases as the level of the amputation progresses proximally. There is a significant increase in energy expended when the knee joint is lost in above-knee amputation (4). The data from several studies indicate that energy expenditure is less for the below-knee amputee than for the above-knee amputee. Furthermore, the more distal the site of the below-knee stump, the less the energy is required in walking (4-6). Gonzales and associates (5) noted a 65% increase in oxygen consumption during ambulation in above-knee amputees.

In the same study the energy expenditure for the bilateral below-knee amputee was 25% less than for the unilateral above-knee amputee.

Waters and co-workers (6) compared gait parameters and the energy cost of walking with prostheses in 70 patients with unilateral traumatic and vascular amputations. They found that the rate of oxygen consumption, net oxygen cost, relative energy cost, and heart rate were less for the Syme's amputees than for below-knee and above-knee amputees. The authors stated that in both groups the performance was significantly better with more distal amputations. From this information, it is apparent that every effort should be made to perform amputations at the most distal site possible.

EPIDEMIOLOGY

Amputations are performed in the lower extremity for five major reasons: peripheral vascular disease, congenital deformities, trauma, infection, and tumors. Of these reasons, peripheral vascular disease is the leading cause of amputations in the western world (4). According to the National Center for Health Statistics national hospital discharge survey, 104,488 nontraumatic amputations were performed in private hospitals in 1985 (7). Published studies of patients who have undergone lower-extremity amputations consistently reveal that 70% to 90% are secondary to the complications of peripheral vascular disease (8-10).

Complications resulting from diabetes mellitus, which includes peripheral vascular disease, neuropathy, and infection, account for 45% to 70% of all lower-extremity amputations (11). The National Diabetes Advisory Board reports an estimated 5% to 15% of all diabetics will require an amputation at some time in their lives (11). It is expected that more than 1 million diabetics alive today will eventually require an amputation. The survival rate for diabetic amputees remains low. Survival rates are 50% for the first 3 years and 40% for the first 5 years after unilateral amputation (12). Sinnock and Most (11) studied the epidemiology of lower-extremity amputations in diabetic individuals and arrived at an age-adjusted lower-extremity amputation rate of 59.7/10,000 diabetics. They also found that amputation rates increased with age, that the rates were higher in males, and that the overwhelming majority of amputations either involved the toe or were above-the-knee. The authors concluded that diabetic patients were 15 times more likely to undergo a lower-extremity amputation than nondiabetic persons.

PATHOLOGICAL CONDITIONS

The most common underlying pathological conditions associated with amputations are peripheral vascular disease and neuropathy. These two factors are often complicated by the presence of infection. Infection, especially in diabetics, affords less predictable results because of an impaired immune status. Diminished circulation, loss of protective sensation, and a lowered host resistance to infection predispose the foot to breakdown.

The role of microvascular disease in the development of ischemic lesions is currently being challenged. Goldenberg and associates (13) suggested that microvascular occlusive disease and endothelial proliferation were the cause of ischemic lesions in diabetic limbs. Recently, LoGerfo and Coffman (14) reviewed the findings said to support the theory of microvascular disease. They concluded that a functional microangiopathy in diabetic patients had not been confirmed. They stated that the misconception of this process was responsible for many diabetic patients receiving inappropriate foot care (14).

Macrovascular disease is histologically similar in diabetic and nondiabetic patients (15). In diabetic patients, however, the distribution of atherosclerotic changes is more likely to occur farther distally in the tibial and peroneal vessels. The risk factors for peripheral vascular disease include smoking, hypertension, obesity, hyperlipidemia, and, of course, diabetes. The earliest symptom of peripheral vascular disease may be claudication. The degree of claudication is sometimes difficult to assess accurately from the history or even the physical examination. Pain is often neurogenic and musculoskeletal, rather than vascular in origin. Cardiopulmonary problems may limit the performance of elderly patients on exercise tests. Intermittent claudication often has a benign course. The patient may at first experience increasing disability because of rest pain and an inability to walk. Then collateral circulation may develop, with relief of the claudication and recovery of functional capacities. As the disease process progresses, rest pain, ischemic ulcers, and gangrene may develop as an end stage. These progressive changes often necessitate amputation.

Sensorimotor and autonomic neuropathy contribute to the pathosis of the diabetic foot through independent factors. The chronic effects of sensorimotor neuropathy lead to the characteristic abnormal posture of the neuropathic foot. An imbalance develops between flexors and extensors secondary to intrinsic muscle atrophy. This leads to clawing of toes and prominent metatarsal heads. The combination of insensitivity and high-pressure loads leads to callosities, and further pressure leads to plantar ulcers. Autonomic dysfunction frequently coexists with sensorimotor neuropathy. Autonomic neuropathy is characterized by reduced perspiration and increased blood flow. The dry skin is predisposed to callus and fissuring, whereas increased blood flow may place the patient at risk for the development of Charcot deformity.

DETERMINATION OF AMPUTATION LEVEL

The primary objective of amputation surgery is the maintenance of a functional stump at a level capable of healing. The surgeon must balance the concern for maintaining limb length against the need to obtain wound healing. The selection of the amputation level should be at the most distal point compatible with tissue viability and wound healing.

Clinical features that may provide some indication of wound healing potential include palpable pedal pulses, skin temperature, dependent rubor, degree of sensory loss, capillary return, and bleeding of the skin edges at the time of surgery. Palpable pulses have clinical significance only when present, and they provide a good indication of healing potential. Burgess and co-workers (16) concluded that palpable pulses reflect arterial inflow but not collateral circulation. In the ischemic limb the collateral circulation is the primary determinant of wound healing. They reported satisfactory healing after below-knee amputations in 66% of diabetics and 72% of non-diabetics with absent pedal pulses. In a series of 53 transmetatarsal amputations, Young (17) demonstrated that the presence of a popliteal pulse was unrelated to the outcome of the amputation. These results suggest that the status of peripheral pulses is a poor predictor of blood flow and should not be used in the selection of the amputation level (18). No correlation has been found between measurements of skin blood flow and the level of the most distal palpable pulse.

Skin temperature provides information about the collateral circulation and gives useful information for determination of an appropriate amputation level. Limb temperature should be compared with that of the opposite limb; a marked difference in temperature may provide useful input for assessment of healing potential. Dependent rubor is a clinical sign indicative of marginal viability of the skin. Moore (19) noted that an incision through dependent rubor will not heal.

Bleeding of the skin at the time of surgery has been found to be the most accurate clinical sign on which to base a prediction of wound healing. Little or no bleeding from the wound edge usually mandates a more proximal amputation when considered with other factors. McCollough (4) noted healing in 92% of 134 below-knee amputations when skin edges bled at the time of surgery (Fig. 55.1).

For more accurate assessment of the level of tissue viability, a number of noninvasive and invasive tests have been used (4). Burgess and Matsen (18) reviewed several of these tests. They stated that each of the techniques provided some useful information about the circulatory status of the limb and had a certain degree of predictive value. However, they concluded that no single modality could predict the outcome of an amputation in every circumstance. Techniques described in the literature include Doppler ultrasonography with segmental pressures (20-27), pulse volume recordings (25), digital photoplethysmography (26, 27), xenon 133 clearance (28), thermography or skin temperature (29, 30), transcutaneous oxygen tension (31-35), preoperative nutritional status (36), preoperative hemoglobin (37), fluorescein angiography (38), and laser Doppler (39).

Some of the most commonly used techniques include Doppler ultrasonography with segmental pressures, photoplethysmography, skin temperature measurement, and transcutaneous oxygen tension. Doppler-determined segmental pressure is perhaps the most widely used means of determining circulatory status. Early studies showed an association between ankle pressures and the success of healing

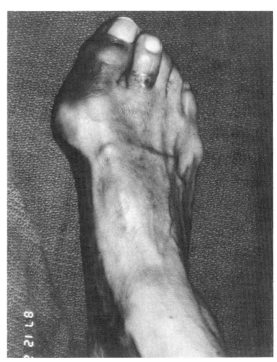

Figure 55.1. Prominent dorsal veins in a diabetic patient may be indicative of an arteriovenous shunting, consistent with autonomic neuropathy.

amputations. Pollack and Ernst (22) determined that a pressure of 55 mm Hg at the ankle or an ankle-brachial index of 0.3 would accurately predict healing. Wagner (20) obtained healing in more than 90% of amputations when the ankle-brachial index was over 0.45. More recent studies have been less favorable. Cederberg and associates (21) studied 67 below-knee amputations and found no correlation between ankle-brachial ratios and healing in diabetic and non-diabetic patients. Wagner and associates (32) also found Doppler segmental pressures and ratios unreliable for the prediction of healing. The authors stated that medial arterial calcinosis may spuriously raise the arterial pressure and mislead the surgeon. Single-toe amputation sites heal with ankle arterial pressures as low as 35 mm Hg, but forefoot amputations usually do not heal with ankle pressures of less than 55 to 60 mm Hg (40). In general, an ankle systolic pressure of more than 70 mm Hg is used to predict primary healing after toe, transmetatarsal, or Syme's amputations (40).

However, diabetic patients frequently have artificially elevated systolic pressures at all levels of the lower extremity, which may make Doppler assessment inaccurate. Segmental systolic pressure readings may be falsely elevated in more than half of the patients undergoing foot amputation and more than a third of those having below-knee amputations (40). Segmental pulse volume recordings (PVRs) provide correct predictions in only half of the total cases. Systolic pressures cannot be measured at all in 5% to 10% of diabetic patients because the vessels are stiff and noncompressible.

It is generally agreed that the absence of Doppler arterial signals in the popliteal space or more distally predicts wound failure in 85% of below-knee amputations.

Digital photoplethysmography (PPG) has been used to determine pulsatile circulation and pressure in the toes. Barnes and co-workers (24) compared digital PPG with Doppler segmental blood pressures to assess wound healing after 122 amputations. They found that healing was influenced by the presence of diabetes and correlated better with digit pulsation than with ankle pressure. Apelqvist and associates (26) also compared digital PPG with Doppler segmental pressures in 300 patients. The authors found that no patients healed with an ankle pressure less than 40 mm Hg and that 85% of the patients healed with a toe pressure greater than 45 mm Hg. They concluded that a combination of ankle and toe pressure was more useful for assessing healing potential than either pressure alone.

Transcutaneous oxygen tension ($TcpO_2$) has become a very popular noninvasive means of evaluating local cutaneous circulation in patients with peripheral vascular disease. The circulatory status of the extremity may be reflected by a transcutaneous pO_2 measurement. To measure the transcutaneous oxygen tension, the skin is locally warmed to 44° C. A Clark electrode applied to the extremity measures the oxygen emanating from the skin. Initial data indicated that below-knee amputations heal if the pO_2 level is greater then 40 mm Hg and fail to heal if below-knee transcutaneous pO_2 value is 26 mm Hg or less (40). Healing is variable if values are between 26 mm and 40 mm Hg. This measurement reflects a balance between oxygen delivery to skin and cutaneous oxygen consumption. Burgess and associates (34) measured $TcpO_2$ in 319 limbs in an approximately equal number of diabetics and nondiabetics. They found that limbs with $TcpO_2$ values below 20 mm Hg were more likely to have ulcers or rest pain or to require amputation. Wyss and co-workers (35) found that the preoperative value of $TcpO_2$ was a more consistent predictor of success or failure of healing after foot amputations than measurements of ankle systolic pressure. Oishi and associates (31) compared $TcpO_2$, Doppler segmental pressure, and skin temperature in 80 patients. The results of the vascular studies were correlated with the outcome of the amputation. Measurement of $TcpO_2$ was found to be the most accurate predictor of healing. They also found that, regardless of the initial $TcpO_2$ value, if the $TcpO_2$ increased by 10 mm Hg or more after inhalation of oxygen, healing of the amputation site could be predicted with a 98% sensitivity.

Amputations selected on the basis of clinical judgment at the time of surgery had a 90% sensitivity. Wound healing in patients with peripheral vascular disease is multifactorial. Factors other than blood flow may account for failure. Overall health status, nutritional status, operative technique, postoperative care including stump management, and the presence of infection may account for failure. It is probably unrealistic to think that a single modality may accurately predict success or failure of an amputation. Therefore, clinical judgment may also play a major role in selection of the amputation level. Noninvasive tests may improve clinical judgment, but should not replace it.

The degree of sensory loss is important in the patient who has ischemia associated with neuropathy. When amputations are performed in patients with a poor protective mechanism, there is a higher incidence of ulceration and eventual breakdown.

PREOPERATIVE EVALUATION

Patients who require amputation will invariably have other concomitant medical problems. A thorough evaluation by an internist or other appropriate specialists may be indicated before one proceeds with surgery. Diabetes is a predisposing factor for many amputations. Strict control of blood glucose and evaluation and management of any associated cardiovascular or renal disorders are mandatory. Patients with peripheral vascular disease also have a high incidence of ischemic heart disease (41-43). This is emphasized since the single most important factor in assessment of operative risk is a history of previous myocardial infarction (43).

In general, lower extremities that require amputation will fall into one of three categories: (a) the infected neuropathic foot, (b) the infected ischemic foot, and (c) the ischemic noninfected foot (41). Broad-spectrum antibiotics are initiated in all three groups, with adjustments made pending culture and sensitivity results if infection is present. The infected neuropathic foot usually has good circulation. Incision and drainage of the infection should be carried out as soon as the patient is stable. This will prevent the occurrence of excessive tissue necrosis secondary to the infectious process. A more definitive procedure may be performed at a later time. When the patient has an infected ischemic foot, the infection should be cleared, if at all possible, prior to the amputation. Incisions left open after drainage of abscesses do not heal well in the presence of ischemia. Before an ischemic foot is amputated, a vascular consultation should be obtained. If the patient is a candidate for arterial reconstruction, the amputation should be delayed until the revascularization procedure has been performed. The authors will generally allow the patient to recuperate a minimum of 3 to 4 days after the vascular surgery. Delaying the procedure will ensure an adequate blood supply at the time of the amputation, thereby enhancing the overall healing potential.

The type of anesthesia chosen depends on the patient's status and the amputation to be performed. Most anesthesiologists recommend spinal anesthesia and believe that this is the procedure of choice in diabetics undergoing lower extremity surgery (43). If the patient can withstand it, however, general anesthesia may be a safe alternative. In more proximal amputations the authors generally request a spinal or general anesthetic, as this allows the use of a thigh tourniquet. Use of a thigh tourniquet, provided the vessels are compressible, allows good hemostasis, facilitates surgical time, and, more important, improves technique. Most digital amputations may be performed with the patient under local anesthesia. On several occasions amputations have been performed without anesthesia in patients with neuropathy.

PRINCIPLES OF TECHNIQUE IN AMPUTATION SURGERY

Regardless of the specific amputation, certain basic principles must be followed to obtain an acceptable stump. It is of the utmost importance that tissues be handled gently and that stumps be fashioned in such a way as to prevent or minimize the potential for breakdown. Several authors have suggested that one consider each tissue encountered during an amputation and the role that each may have in later function (1, 44). Skin is the critical tissue that determines the healing capacity of an amputation stump. Care must be taken to minimize trauma to the skin by avoiding unnecessary instrumentation and excessive traction or pressure. Skin flaps should be designed with as broad a base as possible, and the length should be minimized. Dissection between tissue layers is avoided to preserve deep circulation. No dead space should remain prior to skin closure, or else the area should be drained and/or packed. Skin should be closed with fine, nonreactive material, usually a monofilament suture or fine wire. There should be no tension on the wound edges.

Retention of muscle function is essential to provide the limb with effective strength, shape, circulation, and the potential for ambulation. This aspect becomes extremely important when transmetatarsal or midfoot amputations are performed. Preservation of the tibialis anterior and peroneus brevis tendons is necessary to prevent equinus or equinovarus deformity. Muscle function depends on a fixed origin and insertion. Without fixed resistance against which muscle tissue may contract, progressive weakness and atrophy develops. The presence of ischemic muscle at the time of surgery is not an absolute indication for an above-knee amputation. Healing may occur if the skin is viable and the necrotic muscle is resected.

The free end of a severed nerve heals by neuroma formation. Attempts to prevent formation of stump neuroma have generally failed. Neuromas may become painful when subjected to pressure, traction, or shear (1). Nerves should be sectioned sharply while under traction and allowed to retract proximally away from the incision site. This allows the nerve stump to be protected from irritative forces of prostheses or shoes.

Blood vessels should be cauterized or ligated as needed. Larger blood vessels should be ligated. If a tourniquet is used, it is generally deflated before wound closure to allow for more adequate hemostasis and to prevent hematoma formation. This will also indicate the potential for wound healing as the time that elapses between release of the tourniquet and tissue hemorrhage is a reflection of the degree of circulation present.

Complications resulting from excessive bony prominences are the most common problems necessitating stump revision. Bone should be rounded before closure to provide a smooth contour (1). This principle has its most important application in transmetatarsal amputations. The formation

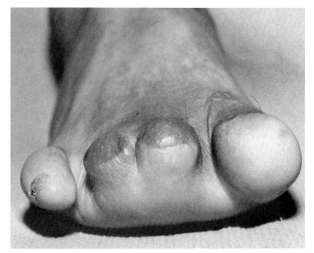

Figure 55.2. This amputation level usually results in poor function and the need for a secondary higher level of amputation.

of bone spurs may be minimized by careful resection of any retained periosteal elements flush with the cortical surface of the bone and by careful contouring of the metatarsals (Fig. 55.2).

No preoperative assessment method will ever predict the outcome of an amputation with total certainty because the healing process depends on the postoperative rather than the preoperative blood supply. The preoperative criteria used to select the amputation level may be entirely sound, and yet the amputation may fail because of intraoperative or postoperative factors.

Wound infection may ruin all efforts. When there is evidence of serious infection and ischemia, packing the wound open will probably result in a lower rate of wound complication without eventual reamputation at a higher level. Primary closure may be performed at a later time, once the tissues have stabilized. In the presence of local infection, antibiotics given preoperatively and postoperatively also enhance the results.

Further, successful wound healing depends on operative technique. In cases of peripheral vascular disease, surgery must be meticulous, with delicate handling of tissue and gentle retraction of the skin. Tension on tissue occludes small blood vessels and must be avoided. The length, shape, and source of the flap are other factors that affect the healing potential. Flaps should have adequate length so that closure may be accomplished without tension. Ligatures should be used with care to prevent incarceration of tissues adjacent to the vessel. The skin should be closed in a manner that will hold and yet not occlude the skin perfusion.

SURGICAL TECHNIQUE

Digital Amputations

Toe amputations are the most frequently performed peripheral amputations (45). The indications for digital resection include a localized gangrenous or infectious process distal to the proximal interphalangeal joint (Fig. 55.3). There should be no dependent rubor of the toes, and the venous filling time should be less than 25 seconds. Other signs consistent with good healing potential are a well nour-ished appearance of the skin and hair on the digits. If the gangrenous process is dry and not infected, the surgeon may choose to allow the toe to undergo autoamputation. If this approach is selected, then frequent observation is man-datory. The foot should be kept clean and well protected. If any sign of wet gangrene is noted, amputation should be expedited.

TECHNIQUE

The proper level of amputation should first be identified as previously discussed in this section. If a distal Syme's type of amputation is to be performed, then the following tech-nique is generally acceptable. A transverse incision is made in viable tissue over the distal phalanx. This incision, which should generally be straight, begins just above the midline of the toe medially and laterally. It is carried across the dorsum to an equidistant point on the opposite side. A sec-ond horizontal incision is then placed around the tip of the toe, joining both ends of the previous dorsal incision (Fig. 55.4). Both of these incisions should be carried directly from the skin to the bone with no attempt at additional soft tissue dissection. If the amputation is to be carried out through the distal tuft region of the bone, then the plantar skin flap is freed directly at the periosteal level and dissected to the most proximal margin of the incision (Fig. 55.5).

With the use of either power or manual bone-cutting in-struments, osteotomy of the tuft is performed, and the entire

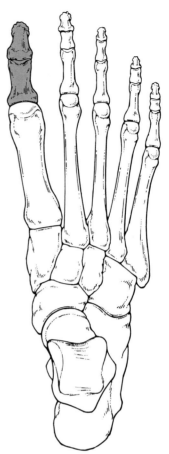

Figure 55.3. Digital amputation.

Figure 55.4. **A.** Dorsal approach to hallux am-putation. **B.** Plantar approach for amputation of the great toe or a lesser toe.

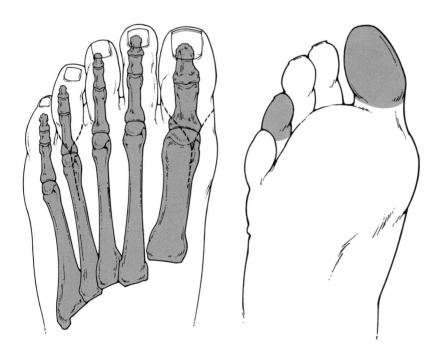

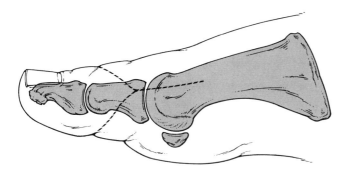

Figure 55.5. Dorsomedial approach for first metatarsophalangeal joint disarticulation or partial first-ray amputation.

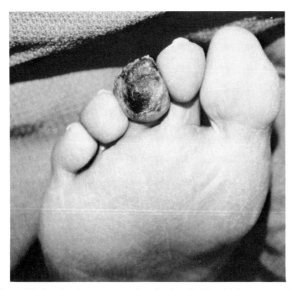

Figure 55.6. Focal gangrene at the distal end of the third toe, amenable to distal Syme's amputation.

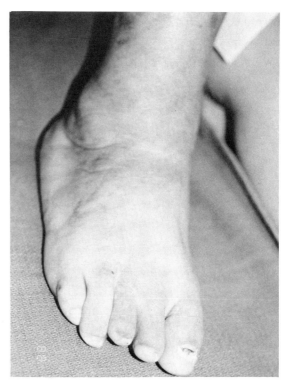

Figure 55.7. Well-healed foot after distal Syme's procedure of the second and third toes in the same patient as in Figure 55.6 some time later.

section of both bone and skin is removed in toto. The plantar skin flap is examined for any tendinous debris or other connective, fibrous, or periosteal tissue and debrided until only healthy adipose tissue remains. The skin flap should then be approximated to the dorsal incisional area and, if necessary, trimmed to allow accurate approximation. One must be cautious not to place the terminal flap under any tension. However, the flap should not have excessive bulk, which would create a dead space at the terminal area of the toe (Figs. 55.6 and 55.7).

If the surgeon selects an interphalangeal disarticulation instead of a distal tuft amputation, the technique is essentially the same except that it is usually easier to start the periosteal bone dissection at the joint level and to carry this dissection in a retrograde fashion distally, excising the entire phalanx and soft tissue. The wound should be copiously irrigated before closure. If a tourniquet is used, it should be released and the wound examined for any free bleeders. If these are found, they should either be clamped and co-agulated or ligated.

Closure after Syme's or terminal amputations of the toes is generally accomplished without deep sutures. The skin and subcutaneous tissues are approximated simultaneously under minimal tension with either interrupted monofilament sutures or, if necessary, vertical mattress sutures.

Digital amputations at the proximal interphalangeal joint level are accomplished in a manner similar to the Syme's procedure. Occasionally, however, a dorsal skin flap provides the most available viable tissue to use. Modification of the technique may be required, depending on the status of local tissues. The experience and judgment of the surgeon will be necessary for fashioning flaps of an unusual nature.

For amputation of the entire toe at the metatarsophalangeal joint, the dorsal incision is generally started 1 to 2 cm proximal to the metatarsophalangeal articulation. The incision extends distally to the joint level and, in a circumscribed fashion, up onto the proximal phalanx and around the plantar aspect of the toe, where it connects with the initial dorsal incision to form a teardrop shape. The incisions are carried directly from skin to bone. The metatarsophalangeal joint is identified, the capsule is incised, the base of the proximal phalanx is grasped with Kocher or towel forceps. Dissection is accomplished subperiosteally with the scalpel held close to the osseous structures as the toe is rotated and excised in toto. After removal of the toe the wound is copiously irrigated, and all tendon, capsule, and other dense fibrous connective tissue is debrided carefully. It is recommended that the articular cap of the metatarsal head be preserved to prevent the invasion of bacteria, particularly if the wound is of a septic nature. The skin and subcutaneous tissues are again approximated simultaneously with an interrupted nonabsorbable suture under light skin tension. If a dead space or pocket is fairly evident, a Penrose or other type of small drain should be placed in the wound for approximately 24 to 48 hours.

Disarticulations at the metatarsophalangeal joint of the hallux are accomplished in a similar manner. However, the incision is often located dorsomedially rather than directly dorsal. The sesamoids are usually excised, as well as any osteophytes, osseous projections, or spiculations in the plantar crista of the metatarsal head. Again, after copious irrigation and release of a tourniquet, the wound should be examined for any free bleeders before closure is attempted. Closure is usually accomplished by means of nonabsorbable sutures with minimal tension on the flaps. A small drain is usually placed before closure and is removed within 24 to 48 hours.

If any of these amputations are performed in association with sepsis, it is recommended that primary closure be delayed for a period of 3 to 5 days. Nonabsorbable sutures may be employed in a retention fashion without approximating the wound. This technique allows the wound to be closed at bedside, in many instances without anesthesia. After the larger digital amputations, however, such as amputation of the hallux, it may be best to take the patient back to the operating room to re-examine and explore the wound before closure. If there is any doubt as to whether closure should be accomplished initially, it is usually best to pack the wound open. Light tension may be applied to the skin flaps to prevent retraction if this is a concern.

RESULTS

Sizer and Wheelock (45) analyzed 552 diabetic patients who underwent 692 digital amputations during a 12-year period. A total of 206 operations were performed for removal of the hallux, and 436 lesser toes were amputated. An additional 50 patients underwent emergency operations for control of sepsis before either a transmetatarsal amputation or a leg amputation. The authors obtained a successful healing rate of 94% when the operations were performed for control of sepsis; the exceptions involved four patients who died postoperatively.

Amputation of a lesser digit generally results in little disturbance in gait. However, amputation of the great toe does result in an apropulsive gait. The attachments of the long and short extensors and flexors to the great toe are sacrificed. Long-term sequelae include hammering of the lesser digits and abnormal loading pressures under the lesser metatarsal heads, primarily the second (46)(Fig. 55.8). The authors have also observed patients with increased weight bearing under the first metatarsal head. This correlates with the findings of Sanders (47) as well as Brand (Paul W. Brand, FRCS, personal communication, 1986). It is extremely important that patients who have undergone hallux amputation be fitted with inlay depth shoes, orthotic devices, and

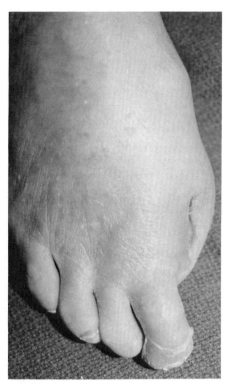

Figure 55.8. The second toe is often hammered and adducts after a hallux amputation.

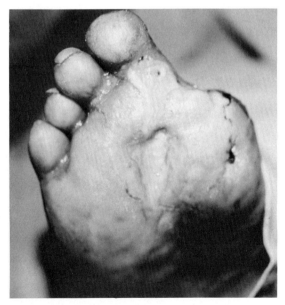

Figure 55.9. Grade III ulceration plantar to the second and third metatarsals 5 years after hallux amputation. This is often the result of inadequate follow-up with appropriate shoe modifications.

fillers to prevent further complications (Paul W. Brand, FRCS, personal communication, 1986) (Figs. 55.9 and 55.10).

Amputation of the second digit invariably results in hallux valgus (48). The second digit serves as a buttress, stabilizing the great toe against excessive abductory forces (Figs. 55.11 and 55.12). A prosthetic device or filler should be fabricated to slow the progression of the hallux valgus deformity. Plas-

tizote or a sponge rubber insert with appropriate shoe therapy is essential to prevent further morbidity.

Ray Resections

Ray resection is considered when infection extends to the web space or involves the metatarsophalangeal joint. The merits of performing a ray resection instead of a transmetatarsal amputation should be carefully scrutinized, especially when a central ray resection is contemplated. Resection of the first ray or removal of two or more lateral rays will lead to increased pressure under the remaining plantar surface.

TECHNIQUE

This procedure involves removal of the toe, as well as all or a portion of the involved metatarsal. Ray resections are usually reserved for the lesser metatarsals, since complete resection of the first metatarsal may lead to an afunctional foot. The technique generally involves a dorsal incision over the intended ray. The incision is carried directly from skin to bone in a distal direction to the metatarsophalangeal joint level, where a teardrop skin incision is carried through the sulcus and web space plantarly. If the entire ray is going to be resected, dissection is generally initiated at the metatarsophalangeal joint level in a subperiosteal fashion and continued in a proximal direction to the point of articulation of the base of the metatarsal.

Ray resections of the second through fourth metatarsals are usually partial ray resections, since removal of the entire metatarsal disrupts LisFranc's joint and the stability of the remaining metatarsals. Therefore, the metatarsal is generally transected at the flair of the metatarsal base. For ray resections of the fifth metatarsal, the ligamentous structures at the fifth metatarsal-cuboid articulation are severed and the entire bone is excised (Fig. 55.13). This is followed by copious irrigation. If a tourniquet is being used, it should be released.

The wound should be allowed to stabilize for approxi-

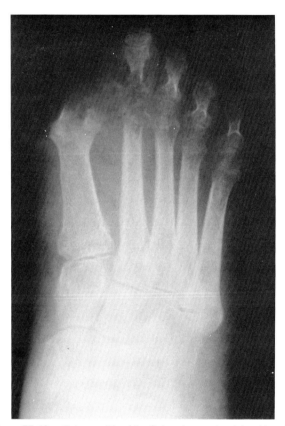

Figure 55.10. Osteomyelitis of the first and second metatarsal heads 5 years after hallux amputation.

Figure 55.11. Focal gangrene of the dorsal interphalangeal joint of the second toe 5 months after an ant bite.

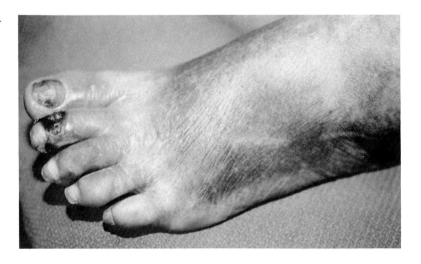

mately 1 to 2 minutes with gauze packing in place prior to examination. All tendons should be placed under tension and transected sharply at the proximal margin of the wound and allowed to retract. Nerve structures should be managed in a similar manner when identified. The skin flaps should then be lightly approximated. If redundant tissue is present, the flap may be remodeled when closure can be accomplished without tension or dead space. Again, closure should usually be accomplished without deep sutures with non-absorbable monofilament nylon or wire material. More recently, skin staples have been found to be adequate for closure (Figs. 55.14 to 55.16).

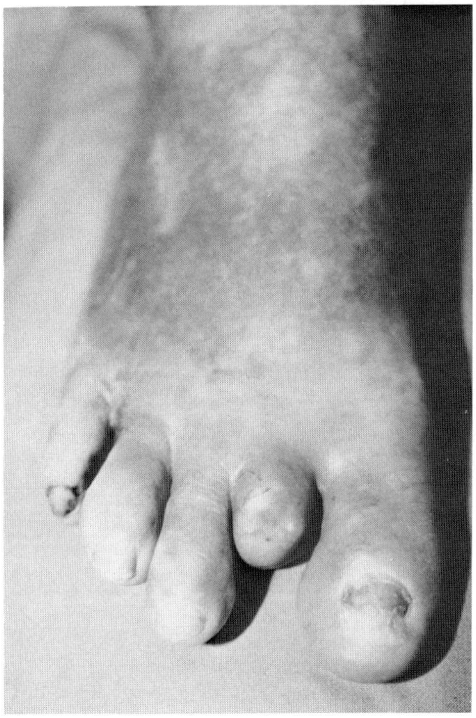

With ray resection of the second metatarsal, it is sometimes advisable to consider performing a closing base wedge osteotomy of the first metatarsal to assist in reducing the large space between the hallux and the third toe. This technique would be more suited to the patient who requires ray resection because of a neoplasm or trauma and probably would not be used in a dysvascular patient.

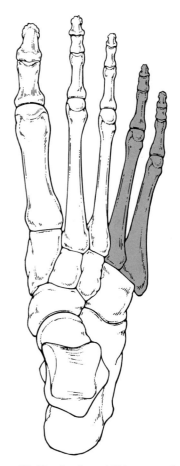

Figure 55.13. Fourth- and fifth-ray resections.

Figure 55.14. Grade III ulceration with cutaneous gangrene andosteomyelitis prior to partial first-ray resection.

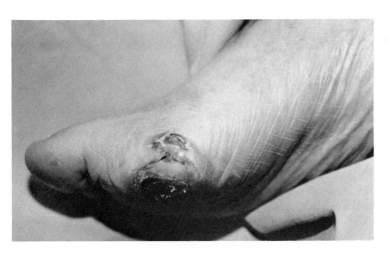

Figure 55.12. Three months following a partial second-toe amputation. Note that salvage at this point provides an adequate lateral buttress to resist hallux valgus deformity.

Figure 55.15. Two weeks after partial first-ray amputation. Note the Steri-Strip closure. Sutures are not always required for healing.

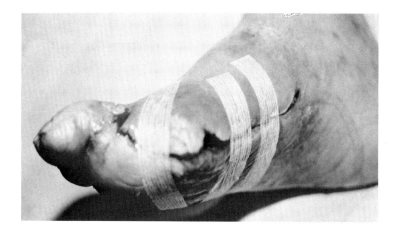

Figure 55.16. Eight weeks after partial first-ray resection with a well-healed wound demonstrating results of delayed primary closure.

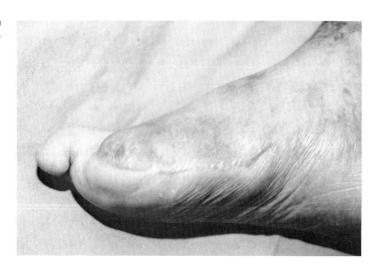

RESULTS

Gianfortune and associates (49) reviewed the results of ray resection in 28 patients who underwent 37 surgical procedures. They obtained a success rate of only 34%. The major reason for failure was transfer ulceration after resumption of ambulation. The highest success rate (50%) was obtained with ray resection involving the third metatarsal. Ray resection of the first, second, fourth, and fifth rays revealed lower success rates of 38%, 14%, 25%, and 23%, respectively. According to these authors, relative contraindications for the procedure included peripheral vascular disease, uncontrolled infection extending beyond a single metatarsophalangeal joint, peripheral neuropathy with significant sensory deficit, and static foot deformities that are ulcerative or potentially ulcerative.

Other authors have found the procedure successful when used for fourth or fifth ray resection. McCollough (4) recommends ray resection for infection or gangrene of the fourth or fifth toes. Similarly, Wagner (50) recommends the procedure for fourth or fifth rays where ray resection has an 80% success rate.

Transmetatarsal Amputations

McKittrick and associates (51) discussed the following indications for metatarsal amputation: (a) gangrene of one or more toes, provided the gangrene has stabilized and does not involve the dorsal or plantar aspect of the foot; (b) stabilized infection or open wound of the distal portion of the foot; and (c) an open infected lesion in a neuropathic foot.

Extension of an infectious process to the web space or plantar aspect of the foot is an indication for an open transmetatarsal amputation. This may be closed at a later time or allowed to heal by second intention. This amputation may be performed at any level of the metatarsals, provided the insertion of the tibialis anterior tendon is preserved (Fig. 55.17). Preservation of the tendon cannot be overemphasized as loss of function will result in an equinus deformity.

TECHNIQUE

The approach for transmetatarsal amputation is initially a dorsal transverse incision at the level of the intended bone resection (Figs. 55.18 and 55.19). The plantar incision is

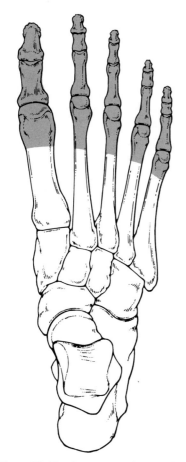

Figure 55.17. Transmetatarsal amputation.

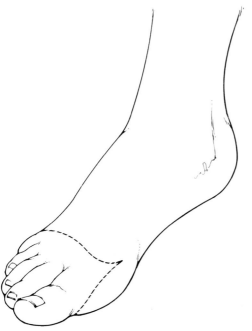

Figure 55.18. Standard dorsal approach for transmetatarsal amputation.

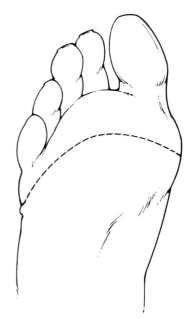

Figure 55.19. Continuation of dorsal incision plantarly.

then made distal to the metatarsal heads and is extended transversely at the level of the flexor crease of the toes. The incisions extend directly to bone as previously described. The plantar flap containing the subcutaneous fat and plantar muscles is reflected to the level of the intended bone resection. It is recommended that retraction and instrumentation on the skin edges be limited to the surgeon's and the assistant's gloved hands, rather than tissue forceps and/or other metallic retractors that are traumatic to the skin margins.

The metatarsals are then sectioned transversely in a slightly parabolic manner. All metatarsals are beveled on the plantar portion, with the first and fifth metatarsals being beveled on medial and lateral aspects, respectively. If any sesamoid bones are present in the plantar flap, they should be resected and excised in toto. Nerves and tendons are identified and divided so that they retract proximally. The plantar flap is then placed over the distal end of the bone and sutured to the shorter dorsal flap without tension (Fig. 55.20).

It is highly recommended that a small drain or Hemovac type of device be placed at the osseous level before closure of the flap. This is generally removed in 24 to 48 hours. Copious irrigation before closure is highly recommended. If tourniquets are used, the wound should be allowed to stabilize for 1 to 2 minutes and carefully inspected for active bleeders. Postoperative hematomas are more critical in the transverse metatarsal amputation than in single digital amputations or ray resection. An attempt should be made to minimize dog-ears on the corners of the closure.

Skin closure is accomplished with a nonabsorbable skin suture and/or skin staples. Deep closure is generally not recommended, since this may tend to create dysvascular compromise of the skin margins in portions of the wound.

The wound is dressed and a posterior plaster splint is applied until the drain is removed. It is generally acceptable to protect the foot in a short leg walking cast that is well padded for the initial 3 to 5 weeks postoperatively. Long-term follow-up of transmetatarsal amputations often indicates the need for a percutaneous Achilles tendon lengthening. As the fulcrum length of the foot is markedly shortened, the excessive pull generated by the Achilles tendon may cause irritation at the distal stump margin of the transmetatarsal amputation (Fig. 55.21).

RESULTS

McKittrick and associates (51) reviewed the results of 215 transmetatarsal amputations performed over a 5-year period. They were able to evaluate 202 of the amputations

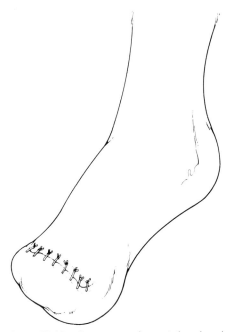

Figure 55.20.   Transmetatarsal amputation closed.

and reported a 67% success rate. The major reasons for failure were recurrent ulcerations at the stump site and inadequate healing of the wounds. Schwindt and co-workers (52) discussed the results of 92 amputations performed over an 8-year period. Overall, they obtained a 62% success rate. Results were better in diabetic neuropathic feet than in dysvascular extremities. Complications cited were ulceration at the stump, continued rest pain, and nonhealing of dysvascular stumps. Wagner (50) reported healing in 75% of his cases and attributed failures to spread of infection and gangrene. Postoperatively, he noted that 35% of his patients had pressure complications at the stump.

The two factors that usually account for failure of transmetatarsal amputations are abnormal pressure at the stump site and the development of equinus deformity. The risk of pressure ulceration may be minimized by rounding the stumps and beveling them plantarly. Equinus deformity should be evaluated at the time of amputation. If present, an Achilles tendon lengthening may be indicated. Also, if it is necessary to sacrifice the insertion of the tibialis anterior tendon, consideration should be given to transferring it laterally to the dorsum of the midfoot.

Prescription shoes are mandatory for patients who have undergone transmetatarsal amputation. We generally prescribe inlay depth shoes with a rocker sole and a rigid shank. The rigid shank and the rocker sole are necessary to help the foot clear the ground, for amputees lose the ability to push off adequately. A plastizote insert with a transmetatarsal filler is also employed.

Lisfranc and Chopart Amputations

Recently, there has been a resurgence of interest in midfoot amputations (Fig. 55.22). In the past these procedures were almost universally decried, as they invariably resulted in equinus or equinovarus deformity. Today, surgeons who perform these amputations recommend percutaneous Achilles tendon lengthening and/or extensor tendon transfer to resist any ensuing equinus forces. The indications for amputations at this level are conditions that are too ad-

Figure 55.21.   The left foot represents a proper and functional level of transmetatarsal amputation, whereas the patient's right foot required revision.

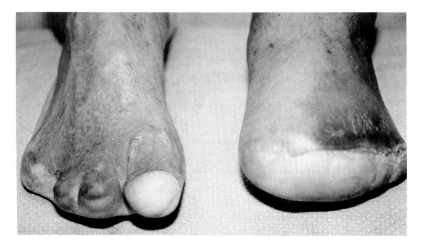

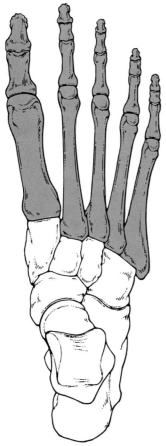

Figure 55.22. Lisfranc's amputation.

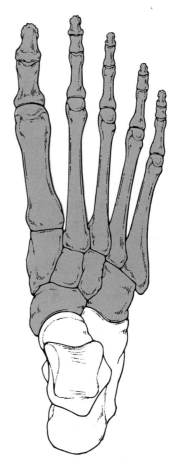

Figure 55.23. Chopart's amputation.

vanced for a transmetatarsal amputation and cases in which a Syme's or below-knee amputation may be avoided.

TECHNIQUE

Lisfranc Amputation

The incision begins at the base of the fifth metatarsal and extends distally along the lateral edge of the metatarsal shaft to the neck of the metatarsal. The incision is then carried down and across the plantar surface of the foot parallel and just proximal to the metatarsal heads. The medial arm of the incision extends proximal to the first metatarsocuneiform joint. The dorsal incision is curved with a distal convexity just distal and parallel to the line of the transverse metatarsal joints. The flaps are elevated at the periosteal level, exposing the tarsometatarsal articulations.

The lateral three metatarsals are disarticulated from their attachments to the cuboid and the lateral cuneiform. The first metatarsal is then separated from its attachment to the medial cuneiform. The second metatarsal is the last to be disarticulated and is often the most difficult to remove atraumatically. Modified techniques may have to be used. However, plantarflexion of the second metatarsal will

allow the surgeon to introduce a scalpel into the joint. Dissection proceeds along the articular surface, coursing around the base of the metatarsal with intermittent flexion being placed on the bone. This usually facilitates removal of the entire metatarsal from its keystone bed within the cuneiforms. The wound is copiously irrigated and the tourniquet is released. All vessels are ligated or bovied, and if the amputation is not close to septic areas, the flaps are approximated with nonabsorbable sutures. It is highly recommended that a rigid dressing be applied immediately and worn for approximately 6 to 8 weeks to resist equinus deformity.

Chopart Amputation

The initial skin incision is made just posterior to the navicular tuberosity and is carried distally along the medial border of the first metatarsal. Midway on the shaft of the metatarsal the incision is carried down across the plantar aspect of the foot and a plantar flap is fashioned. On the lateral side of the foot the incision is made proximally along the shaft of the fifth metatarsal to a point midway between the lateral malleolus and the base of the fifth metatarsal. The dorsal incision is curved, with a distal convexity parallel to the line of the metatarsal heads. The plantar flap is carefully elevated. The ligaments holding the talonavicular joint are divided, and the tibialis anterior tendon is firmly attached to the neck of the talus, usually via a drill hole. Division of the ligaments between the calcaneus and the cuboid completes the disarticulation (Fig. 55.23).

The wound is copiously irrigated during the entire procedure, all vessels are identified, bovied and/or clamped and tied, and ultimately the flaps are opposed without deep sutures. A rigid dressing is required to resist equinus deformity and is usually worn for 6 to 8 weeks (Figs. 55.24 and 55.25).

Technical problems encountered with Lisfranc and Chopart amputations include a fixed equinus deformity caused by loss of the distal attachments of the dorsiflexors. The consequences may include ulceration and ultimate infection. Therefore many surgeons state that Lisfranc's amputation should never be performed, and it has largely been discarded as an elective amputation in the English-speaking parts of the world. However, there are documented cases of amputees who have undergone both a tarsometatarsal amputation and a contralateral Syme's amputation and find that the midfoot amputation is superior. It is thought that if ankle equinus could be prevented it would make the tarsometatarsal amputation more desirable. For this reason, the following options should be considered as initial means of prevention and reconstruction when one is contemplating a Lisfranc or Chopart amputation: (*a*) tibialis anterior tenodesis, with or without extensor tendon augmentation; (*b*) the use of the peroneal or posterior tibial tendons as an anterior sling; (*c*) a subtalar wedge osteotomy with arthrodesis; (*d*) lengthening of the Achilles tendon; and (*e*) possible removal of the talus.

RESULTS

Pinzur and associates (53) reported the results of 64 amputations performed on 58 patients, each of whom had a diagnosis of gangrene or nonhealing ulcers. Amputations were performed at the transmetatarsal level when possible. If conditions required a more proximal level, a Lisfranc amputation was combined with a percutaneous lengthening of the Achilles tendon to prevent equinus deformity. Overall, they obtained an 81% success rate, and all of the patients who healed resumed ambulation. Roach and associates (54) obtained healing in 18 of 19 midfoot amputations. All wounds were left open to heal by secondary intention. The authors did not find it necessary to perform Achilles tendon lengthening or extensor tendon transfer to prevent equinus deformity. Postoperatively, the 18 patients who were able to resume ambulation were fitted with rocker-soled shoes and a plastic ankle/foot orthosis.

The authors recommend the following precautions for success: (*a*) the use of atraumatic technique without a tourniquet; (*b*) removal of all tendon, exposed cartilage, and joint surfaces to allow granulation tissue to form; (*c*) an ankle pressure of 60 mm Hg or an ankle/brachial index of 0.5 or greater, which indicates good healing potential; and (*d*) the

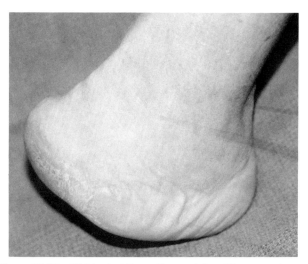

Figure 55.24. Well-healed Chopart's amputation, 10 years postoperatively.

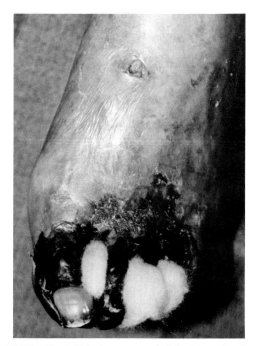

Figure 55.25. Grade V foot gangrene of all the toes, extending to the level of the metatarsophalangeal joint. This is not salvageable by Syme's amputation.

use of intravenous low-molecular-weight dextran to help poorly perfused flaps survive.

Syme's Amputations

Syme's amputation was described by Sir James Syme of Edinburgh in 1843 (Fig. 55.26) (55). The usefulness of the procedure in the diabetic or dysvascular foot has been somewhat controversial. Its major role in the past has been for

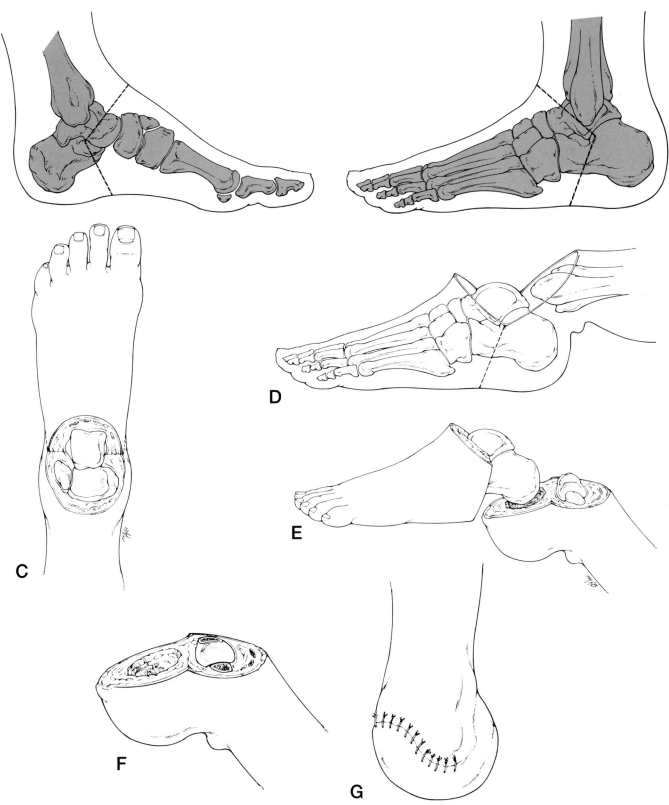

Figure 55.26. **A** to **G.** Incisional planning for Syme's amputation.

congenital defects and trauma. The advantages of performing a Syme's amputation rather than a below-knee amputation are as follows: (*a*) it provides a stump capable of transmitting the entire body weight; (*b*) because only the foot is removed, a stump with some leverage remains; and (*c*) it is less crippling than below-knee amputations and leaves the patient with less of a sense of mutilation (Fig. 55.27).

Harris (56) described the indications for the procedure and outlined technical points essential for obtaining a satisfactory end-bearing stump. Indications for the procedure are severe injuries of the foot, intractable infections of the bones of the foot, severe deformities, selected cases of vascular disease, frostbite, certain neurological conditions, and malignant lesions of the foot. Technical steps essential for success are (*a*) transection of the tibia and fibula just above the articular cartilage; (*b*) transection in a line parallel to the ground; (*c*) preservation of the weight-bearing adipose tissue in the heel by transection of the calcaneus subperiosteally; and (*d*) placement of the heel flap precisely beneath the tibia.

The two-stage Syme's amputation was described by Spittler and associates (57). The primary indications for the two-stage procedure are gross infection and sinuses. This offers an alternative to low circular below-knee amputations followed by higher revision. The first segment of the two-stage procedure is disarticulation of the foot with preservation of the anterior and posterior flaps. Once the infection has cleared the malleoli are transected and the wound is closed.

TECHNIQUE

The technique generally accepted today for a one-stage Syme's amputation is as follows. A plantar incision is used as initially described by Syme, and yet is advanced slightly more proximally to provide a larger heel flap. The foot is held at a right angle to the leg, and the plantar skin incision is made 2 cm proximal to the center of the malleolus. It is then carried directly across the plantar surface of the foot to a point two centimeters proximal to the other malleolus. The anterior incision over the dorsal aspect of the ankle is made from one malleolus to the other at a 45° angle to the sole of the foot and the long axis of the leg.

The ankle joint is entered through the anterior incision. The tibial and fibular collateral ligaments are divided from within the joint. Care must be taken to preserve the posterior tibial artery medially when the tibial collateral ligament is divided. The talus is then dislocated plantarly from the ankle mortise, and the Achilles tendon is carefully divided, with care being taken to avoid damage to the skin flap behind it. The talus, the calcaneus, and the foot are removed, avoiding damage to the posterior tibial artery. Great care must be taken to separate the heel flap from the calcaneus. If dissection is performed in the subcutaneous layers between the periosteum and the dermis, the septa will open and decompress the heel fat pad. If this is violated, the resistant properties of the elastic adipose tissue will be lost and unable to function as a hydraulic buffer. As Syme has stated, this amputation can be disastrous if performed incorrectly.

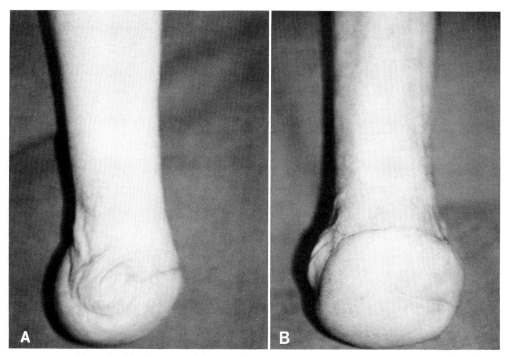

Figure 55.27. Long-term follow-up of Syme's amputation. **A.** Lateral. **B.** Anterior.

The malleoli and a subchondral portion of the distal tibia are then removed, preferably with power equipment, with maintenance of a broad weight-bearing surface. Care should be taken to place this osteotomy parallel to the ground when the patient is bearing weight. Therefore tibial varum or other lower extremity malalignment should be noted. It is rare that the osteotomy is placed in the same plane as the ankle joint. After copious irrigation, the wound should be packed with a laparotomy sponge and the tourniquet released. After the reactive hyperemia has stabilized, the subcutaneous tissue and the skin of the heel flap are sutured to the margin of the anterior incision across the front of the ankle. Skin staples are preferred for this amputation. If possible, the suture lines should be slightly above the anterior margin of the distal end of the tibia. If dog-ears are noted, these are generally not trimmed in a Syme's amputation but are merely allowed to shrink. It is paramount that a surgical drain be used in view of the dead space created by this amputation.

The preferred postoperative dressing is a tension type of amputation sock with a rigid plaster dressing and appropriate foam padding. It is paramount that the plantar fat pad of the heel be maintained directly beneath the tibial osteotomy. Displacement of the fat pad could result in poor positioning, thus preventing the shock-absorption quality that is afforded by this tissue. Sutures are generally removed in 2 to 3 weeks. In the dysvascular patient, weight bearing is usually deferred for a period of approximately 4 weeks and should be initiated only with the protection of a rigid postoperative dressing.

Two-stage Syme's Amputation

A two-stage Syme's amputation is advocated if there is an overt infection of the foot or if the plantar skin is compromised. The technique is basically as described for the one-stage procedure but does not include osteotomy of the malleoli or the distal tibia at the initial operative setting. The wound is copiously irrigated, a semibulky gauze drain is placed in the void produced by the calcaneus, and the flap is held in place by retention-type sutures without full closure. A rigid postoperative dressing is also recommended to protect the heel flap and pad. The wound is allowed to stabilize for approximately 3 to 5 days. The patient is then returned to the operating room and the flap is examined, the wound is copiously irrigated, osteotomies of the malleoli and distal tibia are then performed, and closure is accomplished as previously described. A success rate of nearly 95% has been claimed with this procedure (57). It is used on patients who have diabetes, arteriosclerosis, or other dysvascular conditions as long as the following indications are met:

1. Doppler systolic pressure at the ankle is 70 mm Hg or greater.
2. The heel pad is free of open lesions.
3. The patient has the potential to use a prosthesis.

4. There is no gross purulence at the amputation site or ascending lymphangitis.
5. The ratio of ankle to arm systolic pressure is over 0.45.
6. Bleeding occurs at the skin flaps within 3 minutes after release of the tourniquet.
7. There is no gas in the tissues proximal to the amputation site, as evaluated by palpation and radiographic examination.

RESULTS

The results of the two-stage Syme's amputation were discussed by Spittler and associates (57), who performed 36 of the procedures and obtained a healed stump in 30. Complications cited were three superficial peroneal nerve neuromas and one case of thrombophlebitis. Wagner (50) performed the two-stage procedure in more than 300 cases, with a total success rate of 70%. His criteria for success were satisfactory healing and the capacity to function with a prosthesis. Jany and Burkus (58) discussed their results in 10 patients over a 5-year period. Surgical wounds healed in 5 of the 10 patients. The patients who healed were fitted for a prosthesis, and no late complications were noted.

REFERENCES

1. Rang M, Thompson GH: History of amputation and prostheses. In Kostuik JP, Gillespie R (eds): *Amputation Surgery and Rehabilitation*. New York, Churchill Livingstone, 1981, pp 1-15, 43-46.
2. Wangensteen OH, Wangensteen SD: *The Rise of Surgery From Empiric Craft to Scientific Principle*. Minneapolis, University of Minnesota Press, 1978, 18-52, 279, 378.
3. Malone JW, McIntyre KE, Rubin JR, Ballard J: Amputation for trauma. In Moore WS, Malone JW(eds): *Lower Extremity Amputations*. Philadelphia, WB Saunders, 1989, pp 320-329.
4. McCollough NC: Principles of amputation surgery in vascular disease. In Evarts CM (ed): *Surgery of the Musculoskeletal System*. New York, Churchill Livingstone, 1983, vol 4, pp 25-42.
5. Gonzalez EG, Corcoran PJ, Reyes RL: Energy expenditure in below-knee amputees: correlation with stump length. *Arch Phys Med Rehabil* 55:111-119, 1974.
6. Waters RL, Perry J, Antonelli EE, Hilsop H: Energy cost of walking of amputees: the influence of level of amputation. *J Bone Joint Surg* 58A:42-46, 1976.
7. Bild DE, Selby JV, Sinnock P, Browner WS: Lower-extremity amputation in people with diabetes: epidemiology and prevention. *Diabetes Care* 12:24-29, 1989.
8. Condon RE, Jordon PM: Below-knee amputation for arterial insufficiency. *Surg Gynecol Obstet* 130:641-648, 1970.
9. Potts JR, Wendelken JR, Elkins RC: Lower extremity amputation: review of 110 cases. *Am J Surg* 133:924-928, 1979.
10. Murdoch G: Amputation surgery in the lower extremity. Part II. *Prosthet Orthop Int* 1:183-192, 1977.
11. Sinnock P, Most RS: The epidemiology of lower extremity amputations in diabetic individuals. *Diabetes Care* 6:87-91, 1983.
12. Knighton DR, Fiegel VD, Doucette M: Treating diabetic foot ulcers. *Diabetes Spectrum* 3:51-56, 1990.
13. Goldenberg SG, Josh RA, Alex M: Nonatheromatous peripheral vascular disease of the lower extremity in diabetes. *Diabetes* 8:261-73, 1959.
14. LoGerfo FW, Coffman JD: Vascular and microvascular disease of the foot in diabetes. *N Engl J Med* 311:1615-1618, 1984.
15. Boulton AJ: The diabetic foot. *Med Clin North Am* 72:1517-1530, 1988.
16. Burgess EM, Romano RL, Zettle JH: Amputations of the leg for peripheral vascular disease. *J Bone Joint Surg* 53A:874-890, 1971.

17. Young AE: Transmetatarsal amputation in the management of peripheral ischemia. *Am J Surg* 134:604-607, 1977.
18. Burgess EM, Matsen FA: Determining amputation levels in peripheral vascular disease. *J Bone Joint Surg* 63A:1493-1497, 1981.
19. Moore WS: Amputation level determination. In Rutherford RB (ed): *Vascular Surgery*. Philadelphia, WB Saunders, 1984, pp 1307-1310.
20. Wagner FW: Transcutaneous Doppler ultrasound in the prediction of healing and the selection of surgical level for dysvascular lesions of the toes and forefoot. *Clin Orthop* 142:110-114, 1979.
21. Cederberg PA, Pritchard DJ, Joyce JW: Doppler-determined segmental pressures and wound-healing in amputations for vascular disease. *J Bone Joint Surg* 65A:363-365, 1983.
22. Pollack SB, Ernst CB: Use of Doppler pressure measurements in predicting success of amputation of the leg. *Am J Surg* 139:303-306, 1980.
23. Malone JM, Lalka SG: Amputation level selection by Doppler assessment. In Moore WS, Malone JW (eds): *Lower Extremity Amputations*. Philadelphia, WB Saunders, 1989, pp 32-37.
24. Barnes RW, Thornhill B, Nix L: Prediction of amputation wound healing: Roles of Doppler ultrasound and digit photoplethysmography. *Arch Surg* 116:80-83, 1981.
25. Gibbons GW, Campbell DR: Noninvasive diagnostic studies. In Kozak GP, Hoar CS, Rowbatham JL, Wheelock EC, Gibbons, Campbell DR: *Management of Diabetic Foot Problems*. Philadelphia, WB Saunders, 1984, pp 91-96.
26. Apelgvist J, Castenfors J, Larsson J: Prognostic value of systolic ankle and toe blood pressure levels in outcome of diabetic foot ulcers. *Diabetes Care* 12:373-378, 1989.
27. Rutherford RB, Lowenstein DH, Klein MF: Combining segmental systolic pressures and plethysmography to diagnose arterial occlusive disease of the legs. *Am J Surg* 136:211-218, 1979.
28. Moore WS, Ahn SS: Amputation level selection by isotope clearance techniques. In Moore WS, Malone JW (eds): *Lower Extremity Amputations*. Philadelphia, WB Saunders, 1989, pp 38-43.
29. Golbranson F, Yv E, Gelberman R: The use of skin temperature determinations in lower extremity amputation level selection. *Foot Ankle* 3:170-172, 1982.
30. Golbranson F: Amputation level selection by skin temperature measurement. In Moore WS, Malone JW (eds): *Lower Extremity Amputations*. Philadelphia, WB Saunders, 1989, pp 69-73.
31. Oishi CS, Fronek A, Golbranson FL: The role of noninvasive vascular studies in determining levels of amputation. *J Bone Joint Surg* 70A:1520-1523, 1988.
32. Wagner WH, Keagy BA, Kotb MM: Noninvasive determination of healing of major lower extremity amputation: the continued role of clinical judgement. *J Vasc Surg*, 8:703-709, 1988.
33. White RA, Klein SR: Amputation level selection by transcutaneous oxygen pressure determination. In Moore WS, Malone JW (eds): *Lower Extremity Amputations*. Philadelphia, WB Saunders, 1989, pp 44-49.
34. Burgess EM, Wyss CR, Matsen FA, Simmons CW: Transcutaneous oxygen tension measurements on limbs of diabetic and nondiabetic patients with peripheral vascular disease. *Surgery* 95:339-345, 1984.
35. Wyss CR, Harrington RM, Burgess EM, Matsen FA: Transcutaneous oxygen tension as a predictor of success after an amputation. *J Bone Joint Surg* 70A:203-207, 1988.
36. Dickhaut SC, DeLee J, Page CP: Nutritional status: importance in predicting wound healing after amputations. *J Bone Joint Surg* 66A:71-75, 1984.

37. Bailey MJ, Johnston CJP, Yates C: Preoperative haemoglobin as predictor of outcome of diabetic amputations. *Lancet* 2:168-170, 1979.
38. Silverman DG: Amputation level selection by skin fluorescence. In Moore WS, Malone JW (eds): *Lower Extremity Amputations*. Philadelphia, WB Saunders, 1989, pp 50-62.
39. Holloway, GA: Amputation level selection by laser Doppler flowmetry. In Moore WS, Malone JW (eds): *Lower Extremity Amputations*. Philadelphia, WB Saunders, 1989, pp 64-68.
40. Hartshorne MF, Peters VJ: Nuclear medicine applications for the diabetic foot. *Clin Podiatr Med Surg* 4:361-375, 1987.
41. Wheelock EC, Rowbotham JL, Hoar CS: Amputation. In Kozak GP, Hoar CS, Rowbatham JL, Wheelock EC, Gibbons GW, Campbell DR (eds): *Management of Diabetic Foot Problems*. Philadelphia, WB Saunders, 1984, pp 188-207.
42. Kosinski EJ, Pippin JJ, Kozak GP: Preoperative evaluation of the diabetic patient. In Kozak GP, Hoar CS, Rowbatham JL, Wheelock EC, Gibbons GW, Campbell DR (eds): *Management of Diabetic Foot Problems*. Philadelphia, WB Saunders,1984, pp 133-144.
43. Gallo JA, Brown BR: Anesthesia considerations for the amputation patient. In Moore WS, Malone JW (eds): *Lower Extremity Amputations*. Philadelphia, WB Saunders, 1989, pp 74-91.
44. Burgess EM: General principles of amputation surgery. *Instruc Course Lect* 37:14-16, 1980.
45. Sizer JS, Wheelock FC: Digital amputations in diabetics. *Surgery* 72:980-989, 1972.
46. Poppen NK, Mann RA, O'Konski M, Buncke HJ: Amputation of the great toe. *Foot Ankle* 1:333-337, 1981.
47. Sanders LJ: Amputations in the diabetic foot. *Clin Podiatr Med Surg* 4:481-501, 1987.
48. Selignan RS, Trepal MJ, Giorgini RJ: Hallux valgus secondary to amputation of the second toe. *J Am Podiatr Med Assoc* 76:89-92, 1986.
49. Gianfortune P, Pulla RJ, Sage R: Ray resection in the insensitive dysvascular foot: a critical review. *J Foot Surg* 24:103-107, 1985.
50. Wagner WF: Amputations of the foot and ankle: current status. *Clin Orthop* 122:62-69, 1977.
51. McKittrick LS, McKittrick JB, Risley TS: Transmetatarsal amputation for infection or gangrene in patients with diabetes mellitus. *Ann Surg* 130:826-842, 1949.
52. Schwindt CD, Lulloff RS, Rogers SC: Transmetatarsal amputations. *Orthop Clin North Am* 4:31-42, 1973.
53. Pinzur M, Kaminsky M, Sage R, Cronin R, Osterman H: Amputations at the middle level of the foot: a retrospective and prospective review. *J Bone Joint Surg* 68A:1061-1064, 1986.
54. Roach JJ, Deutsch A, McFarlane DS: Resurrection of the amputations of LisFranc and Chopart for diabetic gangrene. *Arch Surg* 122:931-934, 1987.
55. Syme J: Amputation at the ankle joint. *Monthly J Med Sci* 2:93-96, 1843.
56. Harris RI: Syme amputation: the technical details essential for success. *J Bone Joint Surg* 38B:614-617, 1956.
57. Spittler AW, Brenner JJ, Payne JW: Syme amputation performed in two stages. *J Bone Joint Surg* 36A:37-42, 1954.
58. Jany RS, Burkus K: Long-term follow-up of Syme amputations for peripheral vascular disease associated with diabetes mellitus. *Foot Ankle* 9:107-110, 1988.

Trauma of the Foot and Leg

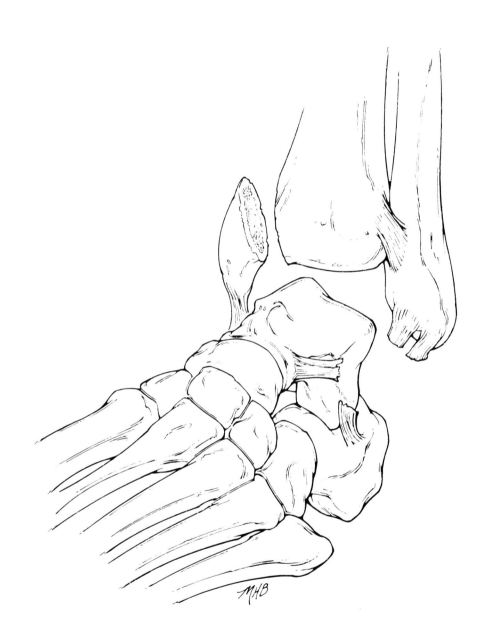

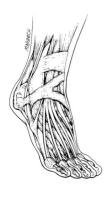

CHAPTER **56**

Nonosseous Injuries of the Foot

Barry L. Scurran, D.P.M.
Brian D. Gale, D.P.M.

SOFT TISSUE INJURIES

Nonosseous pedal trauma can cause a complex combination of macroscopic and microscopic injuries. These may range from simple, clean, surgical lacerations to massive traumatic losses of skin, with the muscular and neurovascular components contained within. The trauma may be associated with concomitant osseous involvement, that is, fracture or osteotomy, and may require rigid internal or external fixation or plaster immobilization. These factors may contribute to the difficulties in dealing with soft tissue compromise.

Assuming the patient is medically stable, one should evaluate the wound for further definitive treatment. Accurate diagnosis depends on a detailed history of the injury with specific regard to the nature and time of the offending trauma. Minor soft tissue trauma may respond to simple treatment with ice, elevation, and compression (1). More serious and complex pedal trauma may necessitate multiple procedures until definitive reconstruction is accomplished.

The current literature is replete with attempts to classify these injuries, ranging from simple to complex (1-3). No detailed classification scheme is presented here, but rather various types of pedal injuries are discussed along with a rational approach for understanding the multiple treatment options available.

Wounds are often described by their effect or action on the skin. Perhaps the simplest form of nonosseous trauma is the contusion or abrasion (Fig. 56.1). A contusion is considered a blunt or direct blow without integumentary interruption. A simple injury with an associated superficial partial-thickness skin loss is said to be an abrasion. A full-thickness skin cut may be considered a laceration or an incision (Fig. 56.2). These injuries may appear minor at first, but vascular or neurological damage may manifest later in the healing process. Extensive skin loss may be a late complication in a small percentage of so-called simple injuries or surgical procedures. When the skin is undermined or elevated through the subcutaneous plane, a shearing injury with potential degloving is said to be present (Fig. 56.3).

Tetanus and antibiotic prophylaxis against the most likely offending organism may be indicated (4). Physical examination includes immediate notation of vascular, neurological, and integumentary status. A more detailed inspection of the wound may require local anesthesia to adequately explore all tissue planes. Care should be taken to use the

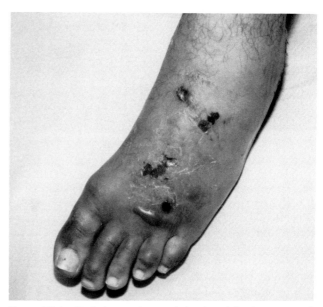

Figure 56.1. Typical contusions and abrasions following motorcycle trauma.

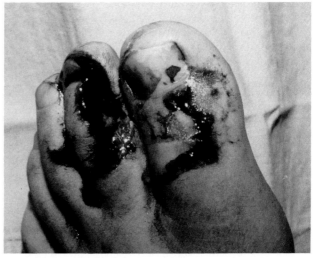

Figure 56.2. Full-thickness laceration following lawn mower trauma.

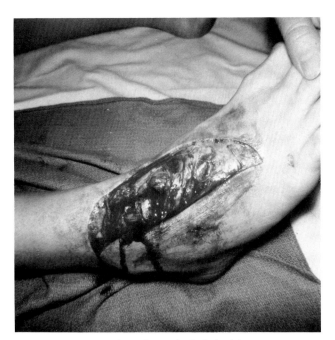

Figure 56.3. Traumatic degloving injury.

Table 56.1.
Wound Classification.

TIDY WOUND
   Surgical incision, laceration
UNTIDY WOUND
   Crush, avulsion, abrasion
WOUND WITH TISSUE LOSS
   Excision, burn, ulcer, avulsion
INFECTED WOUND
   Established (cellulitis, lymphangitis, abscess, burn, vasculitis)
   Incipient (burn, contaminated wound, abrasion)

From Noe JM, Kalish S: *Wound Care*. Greenwich, CT, Chesebrough-Pond's Inc, 1975; with permission.

smallest volume of local anesthetic without epinephrine so as not to increase the potential for vascular compromise. Generally a nerve block or infiltration proximal to the injury itself is preferred to the injection of a large volume of fluid into a closed traumatized space. Sedation of the patient may be indicated to allow an accurate and detailed inspection of the wound. Gentle cleansing of the skin with mild soap is usually necessary before attempting inspection of deeper tissue planes. Care should be taken to avoid the use of undiluted antiseptic scrub solutions because damage to deeper structures may result (5). Although these solutions may be bacteriocidal, they may also be toxic to healthy tissue. Musculoskeletal evaluations for range of motion, strength, and deformity are undertaken when possible. Additional studies, including radiographs and a complete blood cell count, are undertaken when indicated.

The primary objective of initial wound treatment is to remove all foreign debris and devitalized tissue (6). To do so, hemostasis must be optimal. Direct pressure or short-term use of a tourniquet proximal to the injury site may be necessary. Bleeding vessels, once visualized, may be clamped and ligated or cauterized. Thorough and copious flushing with sterile saline or lactated Ringer's solution aids in debridement, keeps the wound moist, and lowers potential for bacterial contamination.

Atraumatic tissue handling is essential to avoid further damage to already tenuous tissues (7). Skin is best retracted gently with sharp instruments rather than blunt forceps or clamps. If used improperly, these instruments may crush fragile tissue, causing further and irreparable damage. Any tissue that is clearly viable or questionably viable is better left intact until the wound has demarcated. Hematoma should be evacuated and its recurrence prevented by use of

drains or carefully applied pressure dressings. The importance of mechanical pressure cannot be overstated (8). Extravasated blood not only delays appropriate wound healing but has proved to be an excellent bacterial culture medium. Hematoma in and of itself is essentially avascular and should be debrided. The couplets of Sir James Learmonth are as valid today as when first written many years ago:

   Of the edge of the skin
   Take a piece very thin.
   The tighter the fascia
   The more you should slash'er.
   And muscle much more
   'Til you see fresh gore.
   And bundles contract
   at the least impact.
   Leave alone the bone
   except bits quite done.

After appropriate initial evaluation and debridement one attempts to classify the wound as to the feasibility for closure. Rank (9) and Thompson (10) have proposed four categories: tidy wounds, untidy wounds, wounds with tissue loss, and infected wounds (Table 56.1).

Wounds

To be considered tidy, a wound must be clean with minimal soft tissue loss or damage. These wounds should have low bacterial contamination (Fig. 56.4). An untidy wound is characterized by increased soft tissue damage, both superficial and deep (e.g., crush wounds or abrasions) (Fig. 56.5). These wounds have a greater propensity for bacterial contamination, complicating treatment alternatives. Rank's third classification includes wounds with a greater degree of tissue loss (e.g., ulceration or degloving) (Fig. 56.6). Neurovascular, as well as osseous, structures may be involved as injuries become deeper and more complex. The fourth category refers to the infected wound, either established or incipient—those that, if not already infected, are likely to become so.

If this classification seems rigid, one should realize the treatment alternatives are far less so. The multiplicity of factors involved in the selection of treatment modes makes the final therapeutic choice a dynamic, changing process rather than one that is static or fixed.

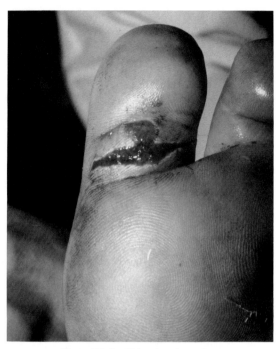

Figure 56.4. Tidy, clean laceration.

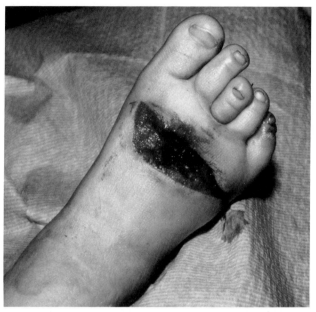

Figure 56.6. Lawn mower laceration with associated tissue loss in a 22-month-old male.

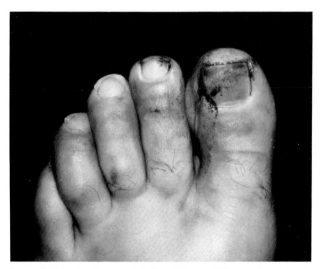

Figure 56.5. Crush wound inflicted by a 200-pound weight that dropped on the first and second digits.

WOUND HEALING

A basic understanding of wound healing concepts is necessary to appreciate the complexities of treatment choices. Healing starts immediately after injury, beginning with the exudative phase when capillary permeability is greatly increased, resulting in increased tissue perfusion. Leukotactic substance is released from traumatized tissue, which summons polymorphonuclear leukocytes to the area to aid in phagocytosis. The host-immunological response lags by 4 to 5 days. During this phase of so-called natural separation,

all nonviable tissue is removed or separated by phagocytosis or enzymatic digestion. Hoover and Ivins (5) noted that "surgical removal of all nonviable material will greatly expedite the process of separation and the success of surgical removal will depend upon the completeness with which it is done." The exudative phase is prolonged by poor tissue handling, hematoma, and failure to keep the wound moist, which results in tissue desiccation.

During the proliferative phase, beginning approximately 5 days after injury, granulation tissue develops initially to cover the wound and protect it from the hostility of the external environment. However, granulation tissue represents the body's response to bacteria (11). In an aseptic wound, granulation tissue does not form, although such a wound rarely exists in clinical practice. Granulation begets fibrosis, which contracts until epithelialization has occurred.

The final phase of healing, contracture, progresses slowly. In traumatic wounds left untended, scarring may limit the range of motion and function of the part. The principal cause of delayed healing in traumatic wounds is infection (11). The infection may be introduced directly into the wound at the time of injury or by the inadvertent introduction of organisms at a later date.

Experimental staphylococcal wounds have shown that antibiotics are ineffective if given later than 3 hours after the initial contamination (12). Antibiotics showed maximum effectiveness when administered before bacteria were introduced to the wound (i.e., preoperatively). Krizek (13) indicated that 7.5% of all surgical procedures became infected. Burke (12) notes two somewhat obvious factors involved in bacterial infection, namely the bacteria and the host. Capillary permeability in the first 3 to 5 hours of the exudative phase of wound healing is the fundamental delivery system for the host's early antibacterial response. This response serves as the main defense against primary bacterial infection. Although host defenses may be increased by the appropriate use of antibiotics, it may be extrapolated from the foregoing discussion that antibiotics have little or no place in the prevention of primary infection after the 3- to 5-hour golden period (14).

What determines if a wound may be safely closed? All wounds are essentially contaminated, yet relatively few result in clinical infection. Quantitative bacteriology has shown that approximately 10^5 or 10^6 organisms per gram of tissue in a surgical wound can cause a clinical infection (11). Elek (15) demonstrated that 10^6 bacteria per gram of tissue are necessary to produce a clinical infection in human skin. He also demonstrated that one suture reduced the number of bacteria necessary to cause a clinical infection by 10,000 organisms per gram of tissue.

Wound irrigation generally decreases only surface contamination or inoculation of bacteria. Jet lavage has been shown to decrease bacteria in deeper tissues once the tissue has been exposed (13). Debridement remains the most effective method to reduce bacterial inoculum.

Table 56.2.
Schema for Treatment of Tidy Wounds

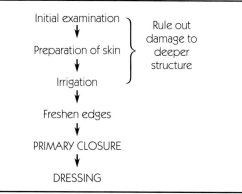

From Noe JM, Kalish S: *Wound Care*. Greenwich, CT, Chesebrough-Pond's Inc, 1975; with permission.

Table 56.3.
Schema for Treatment of Untidy Wounds

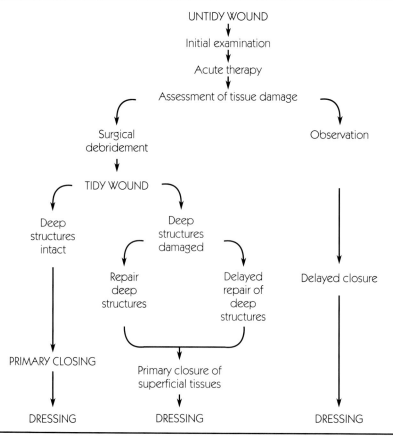

From Noe JM, Kalish S: *Wound Care*. Greenwich, CT, Chesebrough-Pond's Inc, 1975; with permission.

Table 56.4.
Schema for Treatment of Wounds with Tissue Loss

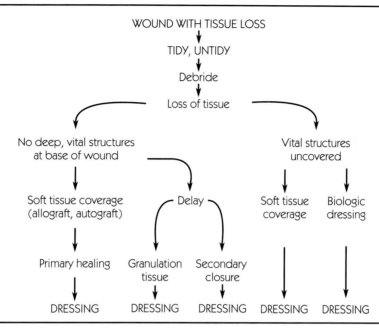

From Noe JM, Kalish S: *Wound Care*. Greenwich, CT, Chesebrough-Pond's Inc, 1975; with permission.

Tidy Wounds

Most tidy wounds, once debrided, may be closed after appropriate skin cleansing. Care should be taken to avoid strong antiseptics because local tissue destruction can be caused by these toxic solutions (5, 16). Wound edges may be freshened (i.e., a 1- to 2-mm debridement after copious flushing with sterile saline or lactated Ringer's solution). Deeper structures must still be inspected for occult damage. Once deeper damage has been noted or repaired, the skin may then be reapproximated without tension. Sutures placed with tension on skin edges only increase ischemia and may preclude successful wound closure (Table 56.2). Tables 56.2 through 56.4 denote Noe and Kalish's schematic treatment options (17) for the wounds described herein. Because the authors' monograph is oriented toward the importance of wound dressings, the final dressing option is noted in each table.

Untidy Wounds

Untidy wounds, or wounds with extensive tissue loss, present a more complex set of treatment alternatives. Deep damage must be assessed, and proper planning and timing of the repair must be calculated. The tissue-oriented examination of Weeks and Wray (18) provides a mental checklist and is useful in dealing with all wounds. First, neurovascular structures are identified and compromise is ruled out. Osseous damage is assessed and fractures stabilized by means of appropriate rigid internal or external fixation as indicated. Contamination only modifies appropriate osteo-

synthesis; it does not preclude it. Muscular damage and viability are assessed. A bluish or brown discoloration may not be the best criterion by which to assess muscle viability; rather, bleeding on debridement or contractility is better used. Skin closure, if possible, may then be addressed.

If viability cannot be ascertained, skin closure should be delayed until wound demarcation has progressed to the point where viability is reasonably ensured. Nonviable tissue must be debrided. Secondary closure or delayed primary closure may be indicated if untidy wounds cannot be converted by debridement to clean or tidy wounds. Swelling within closed compartments may indicate the need for the release of tight or damaged fascia or skin (i.e. fasciotomy or escharotomy). The resulting compartment syndrome may cause further ischemic damage unless decompressed in a timely fashion (Figs. 56.7 and 56.8).

Debridement and delayed primary closure are not recent concepts (5). As long ago as the thirteenth century Theodoric postulated that "if, at the beginning, you have made a suture, and if the wound has already been altered by air, then let the sides be refreshed [and] made bloody so that they may be better joined" (19). For best results debridement must be performed before contamination develops into an infection (5). Table 56.3 denotes Noe and Kalish's scheme for the treatment of the untidy wound.

Wounds With Tissue Loss

Wounds with tissue loss, whether superficial or deep, clean or contaminated, are more complex. Tissue loss creates

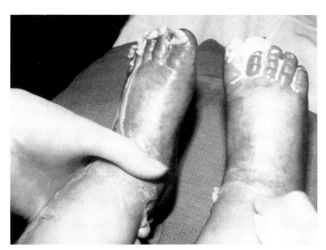

Figure 56.7. Eschar following bilateral pedal burns in 19-month-old female. Edema is contained by an inelastic eschar creating an associated compartment syndrome. Note the tautness of the skin.

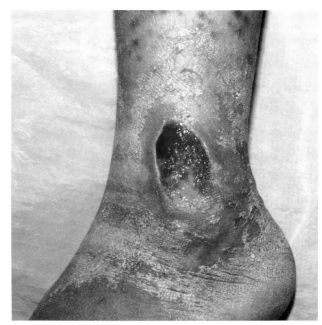

Figure 56.9. Full-thickness defect created when the malleolus was caught in a bicycle spoke.

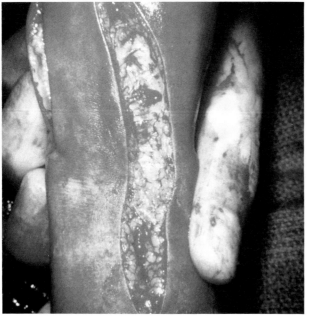

Figure 56.8. Explosive skin incision caused by the contained compartment pressure noted during the escharotomy.

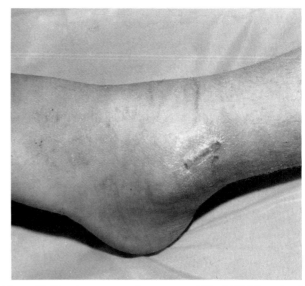

Figure 56.10. Appearance of same wound (Fig. 56.9) 2½ weeks after conservative treatment with Unna boot, changed at 5- to 7-day intervals.

voids with increased potential for hematoma and seroma, as well as potential secondary contamination with the loss of integumentary protection. If a wound is clean and the tissue lost is expendable, the wound may be closed. In most cases significant tissue loss prevents wound closure, and extensive drying of tissue becomes a hazard, as does the increased potential for contamination or infection. As noted in Table 56.4, exposed vital structures necessitate coverage to avoid both infection and desiccation. Local soft tissue (e.g., fat and fascia) may be used when appropriate. If available, biological dressings, such as allografts, porcine xeno-

grafts, and amniotic membranes, are also suitable to prevent drying and to decrease bacterial flora (20). If no deep structures are exposed, closure may be achieved in smaller defects by granulation (Figs. 56.9 and 56.10).

Infected Wounds

Table 56.5 denotes the scheme for treatment of the infected wound. It is a basic surgical principle that contaminated or

Table 56.5.
Schema for Treatment of Infected Wounds

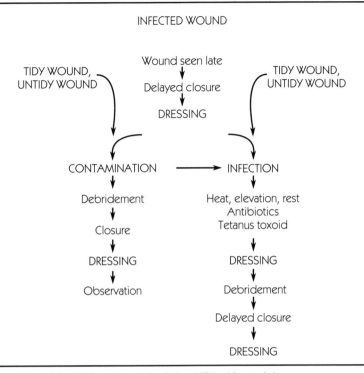

INFECTED WOUND

TIDY WOUND, UNTIDY WOUND

Wound seen late
↓
Delayed closure
↓
DRESSING

TIDY WOUND, UNTIDY WOUND

CONTAMINATION ⟶ INFECTION

Debridement

Heat, elevation, rest
Antibiotics
Tetanus toxoid

Closure

DRESSING

DRESSING

Debridement

Observation

Delayed closure

DRESSING

From Noe JM, Kalish S: *Wound Care.* Greenwich, CT, Chesebrough-Pond's Inc, 1975; with permission.

infected wounds are left open, that is, without primary closure. By consensus, infection is treated with rest and elevation, as well as appropriate antibiotics, tetanus prophylaxis, surgical debridement, and lavage. Burke and Morris (21) noted the importance of the "interface" between infection and surgical therapy. Any contaminated wound must first be converted to a clean wound before primary closure is considered. Debate exists as to the number of hours after injury that must elapse before a wound is considered contaminated. Even tidy, clean wounds, when seen more than 4 to 6 hours after injury, should be considered contaminated and attempts made to convert the wound to a clean wound before closure. Delayed closure may be performed later. Of note is that the immunological response to injury lags by 4 to 5 days. Closure before this time may not be in the patient's best interests.

In wounds in which contamination is suspected and closure is deemed necessary, then the procedure should be performed loosely over a drain. The drain should be removed or changed every 24 to 48 hours until the clinician is sure healing is progressing without infection or complication. Serial Gram's stains, as well as wound cultures, may be useful in evaluating wound flora. Careful debridement remains the most effective way to reduce local contamination.

Additional factors to be considered beyond the mechanism and source of injury and elapsed time from injury to initial treatment include the patient's biological status, for-

example, age, general health, and immune status. Once bacterial strains have been identified, the virulence of the organisms should be considered in selecting treatment options. For example, human bites contain 10^7 to 10^8 bacteria per milliliter of saliva, whereas dog bites contain 10^3 to 10^4 bacteria per milliliter. The organisms in human saliva tend to be more virulent than those of the dog; therefore, because of both the quantity and quality of bacterial organisms, human bites tend to become infected much more often than do dog bites. Our forefathers noted this empirically, thus the phrase "clean as a hound's tooth."

Once an infected wound has been converted to a clean wound by debridement and appropriate local and systemic treatment, it may then be safely closed. Very few circumstances necessitate closure of an infected wound. Implants used for osteosynthesis do not necessarily need to be removed if infection is noted, although external devices may be preferable to maintain osseous stability in the presence of established infection.

Case Reviews

CLEAN OR TIDY WOUND

A 12-year-old male novice karate student was attempting a phantom kicking maneuver in his shower when he slipped and kicked through the glass, lacerating the posterior surface of his ankle, including the Achilles tendon (Fig. 56.11).

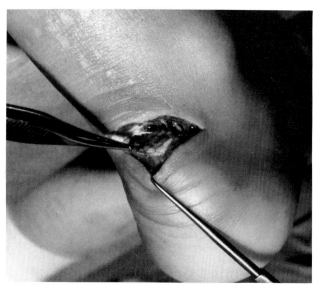

Figure 56.11. An Achilles tendon laceration sustained during a karate maneuver by a 12-year-old male who kicked through a glass enclosure in his shower.

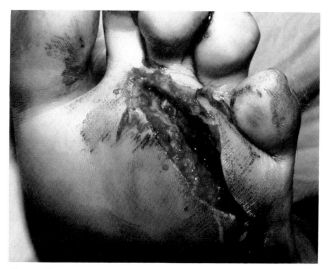

Figure 56.13. Contaminated plantar laceration sustained in an unusual lawn mower trauma.

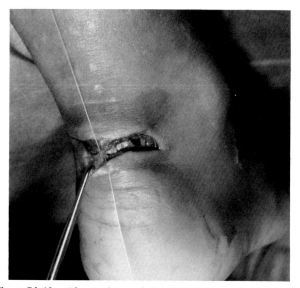

Figure 56.12. After tendon repair shown in Figure 56.11, the paratenon, if preserved, is appropriately closed.

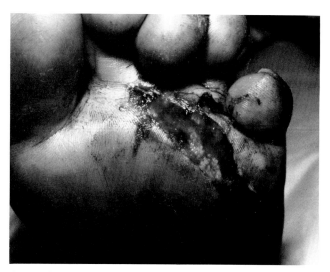

Figure 56.14. Six days after injury shown in Figure 56.13, no infection is noted.

After careful examination it was believed the wound was clean, and after appropriate cleaning and tendon repair the wound was closed primarily and healing progressed un-eventfully (Fig. 56.12).

UNTIDY OR CONTAMINATED WOUND

A 23-year-old male, who tripped while mowing his lawn, sustained an unusual plantar laceration (Fig. 56.13). It was believed that this contaminated wound could not be closed in its existent state. As discussed earlier, definitive treatment

for underlying fractures and tendon lacerations was not per-formed inasmuch as the initial efforts were directed at at-tempting to convert this contaminated wound into a clean wound. Despite copious flushing and debridement of the necrotic tissue, it was elected to treat this wound with de-layed primary closure. At 6 days after injury the wound appeared uninfected and stable enough for the surgeon to perform definitive repair of deeper structures and delayed primary repair of the skin (Figs. 56.14 to 56.16). The post-operative course was uneventful and uncomplicated.

WOUND WITH SKIN LOSS

A 32-year-old male, who was involved in a motorcycle ac-cident, sustained a degloving injury of the dorsum of the

Chapter 56: Nonosseous Injuries of the Foot **1419**

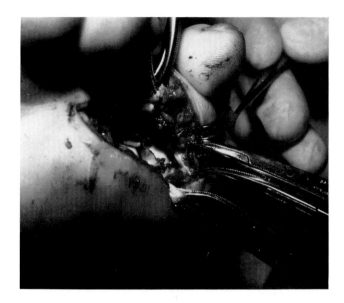

Figure 56.15. Definitive surgical repair of the involved osseus and soft tissue structures (e.g., tendon).

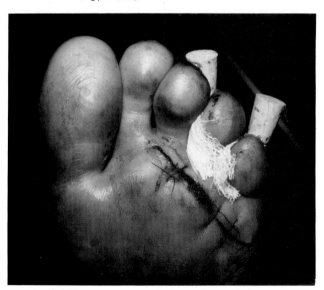

Figure 56.16. Seven days after surgery, uneventful healing.

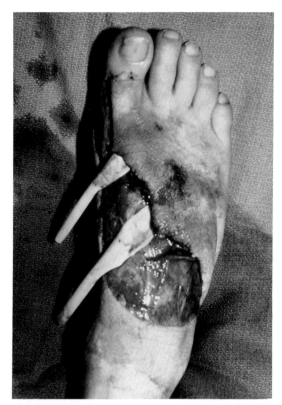

Figure 56.17. Degloving injury in 32-year-old male after motorcycle trauma.

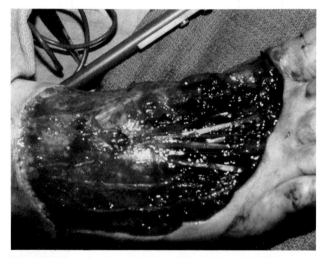

Figure 56.18. Nine days after injury; debridement of devitalized flap.

foot (Fig. 56.17). Initial treatment consisted of cleansing and debridement only because it was difficult to assess the amount of devitalized skin, as well as the degree of contamination. The wound was allowed to demarcate until it was obvious that the traumatized flap would not survive. At 9 days after injury the flap was debrided and a split-thickness skin graft was applied (Figs. 56.18 to 56.20). This wound progressed satisfactorily until the patient's discharge 25 days after injury.

INFECTED WOUND

A 29-year-old male sustained a laceration to the plantar surface of the hallux with a contaminated instrument (Fig.

56.21). Despite appropriate initial debridement and antibiotic therapy at approximately 6 hours after injury, the wound became red, warm, and swollen. Serial cultures revealed *Staphylococcus aureus*. After 10 days of appropriate local and systemic wound care and antibiotics, the wound was deemed satisfactory for attempted primary closure (Fig. 56.22). The wound healed uneventfully with small gaps clos-

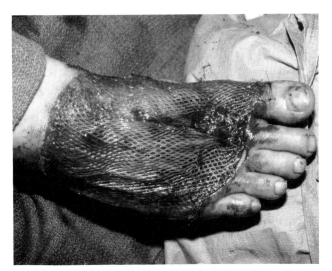

Figure 56.19. A split-thickness, meshed skin graft is applied.

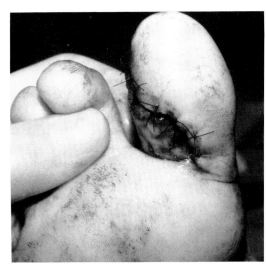

Figure 56.22. Loose delayed primary closure after control of an associated infection.

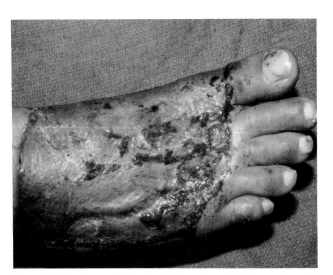

Figure 56.20. Uneventful healing 10 days after split-thickness skin graft.

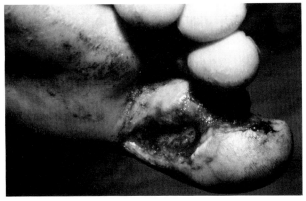

Figure 56.21. Grossly contaminated laceration in a 29-year-old male.

ing by secondary intention. Infected wounds, as noted previously, are usually not closed until the infection has been controlled by debridement and appropriate systemic and local wound care.

Bite Wounds

Soft tissue trauma in the form of bite wounds is common. In fact, 50% of the population will encounter such an incident during a lifetime (22). Approximately 1 to 2 million bite wounds occur per year, and this type injury accounts for an estimated 1% of emergency room visits. Of the different animal species, the most common bite wounds are associated with dogs. Cats account for approximately 400,000 bite wounds per year and snakes approximately 45,000 reported incidences (23, 24). Complications from these injuries include osteomyelitis, septic arthritis, amputations, sepsis, and occasionally death. Bite wounds in general peak in the spring and early summer and are also more common on weekends. Although the most common complication associated with bite wounds is bacterial infection, several other serious consequences should be considered, including the transmission of hepatitis B, syphilis, tuberculosis, actinomycosis, and tetanus.

Human Bites

Human bites are the third most frequently encountered wound after dog and cat bites. However, these injuries are very rare in the lower extremity. There are two specific types of bite wounds (25). The first is an occlusion bite in which the mouth or teeth are clenched onto the soft tissue. The second is the clenched fist injury in which the knuckles usually come in contact with the teeth and result in a sharper penetrating injury. These injuries are obviously related to aggressive acts such as fights and sports. Human bite injuries may be related to child abuse and sex-related crimes, with more than one wound occurring (26).

Prior to the advent of antibiotics, anaerobic and aerobic infections were both prevalent (27-29). Anaerobic infections were more severe; 10% of infections after bite wounds resulted in amputations if the patient was seen for medical treatment within 1 hour of the injury. If more than 1 hour elapsed before the patient was seen, a 33% amputation rate was noted. Joint stiffness was the most commonly reported complication. Death was not uncommon.

Rank (9) reported a 50% infection rate. Of these infections 16% resulted in osteomyelitis, 12% resulted in septic arthritis, tenosynovitis occurred in 22%, and amputations occurred in 6%. Approximately 50% of the time anaerobes were isolated (30-33).

The clenched fist-type human bite injury is the more serious of the two, occurring most commonly in young males. The possible inoculation of bacteria into a joint should be considered. Karate kicks to the mouth area may cause this injury in the feet.

The bacteria most commonly seen in this type of injury is *Eikenella corrodens*. This injury may result in a chronic infection, partially from resistance to first-generation cephalosporins (34-37). Because of the ineffectiveness of antibiotics or limited wound cleansing, secondary debridement is often necessary (38).

The role of hyperbaric oxygen in the treatment of this type wound is controversial (39). Empiric antimicrobial therapy should include coverage for *S. aureus*, *E. corrodens*, *Haemophilus* species, and anaerobic bacteria. Possible complications and disability from injuries, as discussed previously, include abscesses, tendonitis, tendon rupture after infection, joint stiffness, and osteomyelitis.

DOG AND CAT BITES

Both dog and cat bites are susceptible to infection because of the direct inoculation of bacteria from the animals into the bite wound. In addition to tearing tissue, dogs may produce enough force (150 to 450 pounds per square inch) to produce a significant crush injury. Cats produce a more characteristic puncture wound that has a greater tendency to become infected than dog bites. More than likely this is due to the difficulty in adequately cleansing and debriding this type of wound. The area traumatized varies as follows: face 25%, upper extremity 22%, hands 43%, trunk 7%, and lower extremity 21% (40, 41)(Fig. 56.23).

Up to 85% of patients with bite wounds who seek immediate medical attention have been noted to harbor bacteria (42-44). This indicates that aggressive therapy should be undertaken initially. Because the earliest signs of infection do not occur until approximately 8 hours after injury, it is not often possible to assess the quantity of the inoculum or the necessary extent of the debridement. It is estimated that 2% to 20% of bite wounds develop an infection (45-47).

A broad spectrum of bacteria may be isolated following animal bites. The presence of *Pasteurella multocida* as an

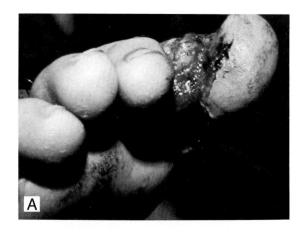

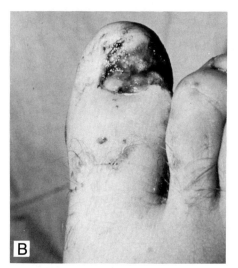

Figure 56.23. **A** and **B.** A dog bite to the hallux that was treated locally and that granulated without sequalae. The nail plate was removed to adequately clean the wound. (From Silvani SH: Animal bites. In Scurran BL (ed): *Foot and Ankle Trauma.* New York, Churchill Livingstone, 1989, p 134.)

infectious agent has probably been overemphasized following dog and cat bites; 20% to 25% of dog bites and approximately 50% of cat bites resulting in infection have been correlated with this infectious agent, which indicates that other infectious pathogens must also be considered. An increase in the severity of infection has been associated with anaerobic processes (48-50); 10% to 15% of culture results are negative for bacterial growth. The same bacteria have been cultured whether or not the patients are seen within the first 8 hours following injury. This suggests that it may not be possible to predict the development of an infection on the basis of an immediate Gram's stain (43, 44). Other authors note that there is no correlation between initial culture and sensitivity results and the development of a clinical infection (24, 51, 52). When multibacterial infections are present, it may be difficult to ascertain which ones are truly pathological.

A number of bacteria have been cultured from the oral cavity of dogs. Although early authors focused upon the presence of *P. multocida*, a more recent study found this to be present in only 25% of dog bite wounds (53). In another study 50% of those patients who developed infection demonstrated multiple pathogenic organisms. The predominant bacteria were of the family Enterobacteriaceae, as well as *Pseudomonas* organisms, *Staphylococcus aureus*, *Bacillus subtilis*, and beta streptococcus. *Pasteurella* organisms were not isolated from a single wound despite efforts to identify them (54).

In cats the primary organism implicated in the development of subsequent infection is *P. multocida*. This gram-negative bacillus may be isolated from the oropharynx of 50% to 74% of healthy cats (53). Cat scratches may also inoculate this organism because of the routine cleaning habits of felines. Infections resulting from this organism usually occur fairly soon after the injury. Other organisms commonly encountered following cat bites include *S. aureus*, *Streptococcus*, and *Staphylococcus epidermidis*.

The management of infection begins with a detailed history. Prior splenectomy or mastectomy may increase the risk of infection. Wounds should be well documented for clinical as well as medicolegal purposes, either in the form of drawings or photographs. The condition of all soft tissue and osseous structures should be documented. Culture and sensitivity testing prior to irrigation or debridement is usually performed (33, 43, 44). Some authors believe that cultures of contaminated wounds provide little clinical information because of the multiplicity of bacteria present and the absence of established infection. However, culture results may help to identify the flora involved in later infection of the wound.

Radiographs of all involved structures should be obtained initially to rule out fracture. Aggressive and thorough debridement and irrigation are required. Irrigation procedures vary greatly. Normal saline, lactated Ringer's solution, or dilutions of povidone-iodine have been used with manual and mechanical lavage systems. Lack of initial aggressive therapy may result in the occurrence of infectious processes in many of these wounds. If the foot is involved, elevation and immobilization in the position of function (with the ankle at 90°) and the use of a compressive dressing within a splint are most suitable. If the clinical presentation improves over 72 hours, the authors suggest early range of motion and adjunctive physical therapy to prevent residual stiffness and potential disability.

The decision to suture a bite wound within the first 12 hours (following irrigation) is controversial. Some clinicians favor suturing on the basis of the observation that 2.9% of sutured versus 25% of wounds treated open become infected (45, 55). Others recommend initial approximation with adhesive strips and delayed closure when indicated. More recently, Callaham (56) noted that dog bites could be safely sutured, with an infection rate of only 5% to 10%, which is comparable with the rate of infection for clean, nonbite lacerations. The authors prefer to leave any poten-

tially contaminated wound open for 4 to 6 days; at that time, if the wound is clean and without redness or swelling, it is reasonably safe to perform a primary closure. Clean, uncomplicated wounds may be closed at the initial presentation.

The use of prophylactic antibiotics for bite wounds is still a subject of debate. If administered, these agents should provide adequate coverage for the most likely organisms to precipitate an infection. However, one should recognize that no single antibiotic will be effective against all pathogenic bacteria. Callaham (56) states that dicloxacillin or cephalexin should be adequate for most dog bites. In one study 95% of patients with clinically infected wounds following dog bites were treated successfully with cephradine (54). Erythromycin is usually prescribed for patients with a penicillin allergy (56).

In cat bites penicillin or dicloxacillin is recommended, with erythromycin being selected on an alternate basis (56). Clinically erythromycin has been found to be effective against *Pasteurella* organisms, despite in vitro evidence to suggest otherwise. One small study found oxacillin to be a suitable agent for prophylaxis following cat bites (57). However, this agent was not found to be effective as a prophylactic agent for dog bites (49). If resistance to treatment occurs, culture specimens should be obtained and consideration given to the use of tetracycline, except for pregnant women and children (56).

Another possible concern in dog and cat bites is that of rabies. Specific geographical areas show varying rates of rabies infection in animals. The health department should be contacted for local epidemiological information. Of rabid animals 85% are wild versus 15% domesticated. Rabies vaccine is prophylactic rather than therapeutic. Once clinical infection occurs, survival in humans is rare (58, 59). Rabies immunoglobulin is administered on the first, third, seventh, fourteenth, and twenty-eighth days. Routine boosters after vaccination are not indicated because of potential side effects. In the mid-Atlantic regions raccoons have been the cause of reported rabies infections (58), whereas skunks and bats are usually the most frequent carriers in most other areas. In the United States more rabid cats than dogs have been reported annually since 1981.

Insect Stings

More than 1 million species are included in the class Insecta. The most common insect order involved in human contacts are Hymenoptera, which consist of ants, bees, and wasps. According to the American Association of Poison Control Centers no deaths have been reported as a result of stings, but anaphylactic reactions may be life-threatening. Because anaphylaxis is often reported as cause of death rather than the sting, statistics may be misleading. Older data suggest 40 to 100 deaths per year (60, 61). Delayed immune complex disorders have also been reported (62, 63). Signs of acute immune hypersensitivity include facial and laryngeal edema, urticarial rash, bronchospasm, hypotension, and smooth muscle spasm in the bowel and uterus.

Ant Bites

Ants (63, 64) both bite and sting depending on the specific species. The sting of fire ants, *Enopsis invicta*, causes severe pain and irritation. A painful wheal initially forms, followed by a small pustule. A small, scarred area is noted several days later. Although the venom is not a significant systemic toxin, the presence of alkaloids produces a local reaction that may resemble an early cellulitis. Field ants, genus *Formica*, inject formic acid, which produces a toxic reaction that results in local irritation.

Wasp Bites

Wasps (64) kill their prey by injecting toxin with a stinger that can be inserted repeatedly because it lacks barbs. Their bites are life threatening only if sensitivity to immunoglobulins (IgE) are encountered.

Bee Stings

Bees (64) sting for defense as opposed to wasps, which sting for food. Some (honeybees) have barbed stingers that, after stinging, are left behind, resulting in the death of the bee. Squeezing the skin to remove the stinger may release more venom into the surrounding soft tissue. Squeezing the stinger also may introduce more venom. Therefore, retained stingers should be wiped or flicked with a fingernail rather than squeezed to remove them from the skin.

When bees attack in a swarm, the first stinger releases a pheromone that triggers attack behavior by other bees in the hive. The victim should immediately leave the area of the nest. The African bee subspecies, *Apis mellifera adansonii*, which was brought from South Africa to Brazil, has since 1956 established colonies traveling north into Panama and Central America. This bee is aggressive and attacks in groups of up to 1000; death may result from the amount of envenomation.

Treatment of Insect Stings

Treatment of insect stings is usually symptomatic and consists of local measures such as ice, combined with systemic antipruritic agents to reduce irritation and itching.

Thermal Injuries

COLD INJURIES

Injuries that result from exposure to cold may be divided into localized injury to specific body parts, a generalized cooling of the entire body, or a combination thereof. Historically, soldiers have been most vulnerable because of potential exposure to extreme environmental conditions for 30% or more of each day (65, 66).

The amount of heat dissipation caused by exposure to cold is proportional to the temperature difference between the body and the environment (67). The body temperature may fall as a result of heat loss incurred by radiation, conduction, convection, and evaporation. The amount of heat loss may vary depending on the amount of exposed body surface area and also the position of the individual. For example, the head is an important source of radiant heat. At 4° C (39° F) the consequence of uncovering the head is loss of approximately one half of the total heat production.

Conduction is the transfer of thermal energy through direct contact. The conduction of heat from the body to air is self-limited unless the heated air moves away from the body so that new unheated air is continually brought in contact with skin, a process called heat loss by convection.

When the body is exposed to a layer of wind, the air immediately adjacent to the skin is replaced by new air much more rapidly than under still conditions, and heat loss by convection increases accordingly. Clothing traps air next to the skin and thereby decreases the flow of convection air currents. A typical suit of clothes decreases the rate of heat loss to about half that of an unclothed body, whereas arctic clothing may decrease the heat loss to as little as one sixth that of an unclothed body. However, the effect of clothing in preventing heat loss is almost completely lost when it becomes wet.

Opposing the loss of body heat are the mechanisms of heat conservation and gain. In general these mechanisms are controlled by a thermostat located in the hypothalamus. This usually maintains the body temperature very close to 37° C (98° F). When sympathetic nerves are excited, they cause the blood vessels in the skin to constrict markedly. The flow of warm blood from the core to the skin is depressed, thereby reducing the transfer of heat to the body surface. This reduction of blood flow in the skin is the prime physiological regulator of heat loss from the body. Stimulation of sympathetic nerves also causes the secretion of epinephrine and norepinephrine by the adrenal medullae. The hormones increase the metabolic rate of all cells, enhancing heat production. Impulses from the preoptic hypothalamus also activate the primary motor center for shivering, which in turn increases the tone of the muscles. The resulting increase of muscle metabolism may raise heat production by as much as 500% (68).

FROSTNIP

The mildest form of local cold injury is frostnip, which tends to occur in apical structures (nose, ears, hands, feet) where blood flow is most variable because of the richly innervated arterial venous anastomoses. Frostnip is most often seen in skiers exposed to fast-moving, very cold air. Simple warming either by the friction of a warm hand or by placing the hand in the axilla is sufficient treatment.

More consequential local cold injuries may be divided into freezing (frostbite) and nonfreezing (immersion foot) injuries. The diagnosis of freezing and nonfreezing injuries may be made on the basis of history and clinical evaluation.

IMMERSION FOOT

Immersion foot or trench foot stimulates both sympathetic nerves and blood vessels in the feet, as observed in survivors of shipwreck or in soldiers whose feet have been wet, in nonfreezing temperatures for prolonged periods (69). This condition may occur at ambient temperatures near or slightly above freezing and is usually associated with dependency and immobilization of the lower extremities and with constriction of the limb by shoes and clothing. Immediate symptoms include tingling, pain, and itching, progressing to leg cramps and complete numbness. The skin is initially red, later becoming progressively pale and then gray to blue.

The first stage is a prehyperemic phase, lasting a few hours to several days. The leg is cold, slightly swollen, and discolored and may be numb. Pulses are barely palpable. The second or hyperemic phase lasts from 2 to 6 weeks. It is characterized by bounding pulsatile circulation in a red, swollen foot. The third or posthyperemic phase lasts for weeks to months. The limb may be warm, with increased sensitivity to cold. The injury often produces a superficial moist, local gangrene, quite similar to the dry, mummification gangrene that occurs with severe frostbite.

Management involves washing and drying of the feet, gentle rewarming, and slight elevation of the extremity. Early physical therapy is essential. The patient should be warned that subsequent exposure to cool temperatures will affect the previously injured area significantly.

FROSTBITE

Several days after the injury, frostbite may be classified into four degrees of severity (Fig. 56.24). In first-degree frostbite, hyperemia and edema are evident. Second-degree frostbite is characterized by similar hyperemia and edema, with large clear blisters that may extend the entire length of the digit. Third-degree frostbite is characterized by hyperemia, edema, and vesicles filled with hemorrhagic fluid. These vesicles are usually smaller than in second-degree frostbite and do not extend onto the tip of the involved digit. Fourth-degree frostbite, the most severe, involves complete necrosis, with gangrene and loss of the affected part. The patient experiences pain in the tissues that are frozen. On examination the frozen tissue is white and anesthetic because of intense vasoconstriction.

Several factors predispose an individual to this cold injury. Clinical experience suggests that frostbite occurs at lower temperatures and in patients with preexisting arterial disease (70). It has also been demonstrated repeatedly that a person who previously suffered frostbite is more prone to develop this cold injury in the same body parts than an individual with no history of such a cold injury.

The treatment of frostbite has been universally accepted (70). The patient must be removed from the cold environment. A person may walk some distance on the affected extremity without seriously injuring the feet. However, once the rewarming process has begun, weight bearing on the affected part is almost certain to result in additional injury.

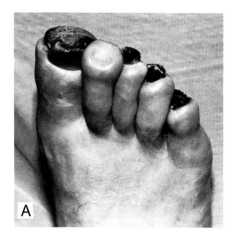

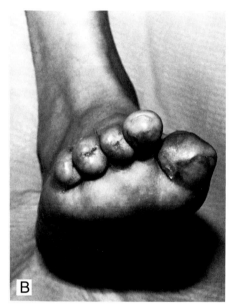

Figure 56.24.   **A.** Necrotic digits after cold injury, which have been allowed to demarcate over a period of weeks. **B.** Autoamputation occurred at the third, fourth, and fifth toes with surgical amputation of the hallux. (From Tuerk D: Burns and frostbite. In Scurran BL (ed): *Foot and Ankle Trauma.* New York, Churchill Livingstone, 1989, p 164.)

Normal body temperature should be restored before treating the local injury. Rapid rewarming in a water bath at a temperature of 39° to 42° C (102° to 108° F) is preferred. Strict aseptic technique (i.e., mask, gloves) should be employed by all personnel during the warming procedure and during subsequent wound treatments. Rewarming is continued until the affected tissue has a flushed appearance, demonstrating that the normal circulation has been reestablished. This rewarming procedure usually lasts 30 to 45 minutes. Because rewarming is quite painful, narcotics are often required to relieve the pain. A fine-pore cell sponge should be used to gently wash the skin after rewarming.

The difficulty in determining the depth of tissue destruction has led to a conservative approach in caring for local cold injuries. As a general rule, amputation and surgical debridement should be delayed for 60 to 90 days unless severe infection with sepsis develops.

A part that suffers frostbite seldom recovers completely. Some degree of cold sensitivity and hyperhidrosis is common. Neuropathies, decreased nail and hair growth, and persistent Raynaud's phenomenon often are noted.

Burns

A burn injury of the foot may be potentially disabling. The most important aspects of management include accurate assessment and early, appropriate treatment. Rapid rehabilitation is necessary to prevent permanent disability (71).

Four important principles are to be followed in the treatment of foot burns, including (a) accurate evaluation of the extent of the injury, (b) immediate institution of measures to reduce the burn process, (c) closure or coverage of the wound as soon as possible, and (d) early, aggressive rehabilitation.

Burn injuries may be caused by thermal agents, chemicals, electricity, or radiation. The intensity of the injuring agent and the duration of its contact with the skin determine the severity of the burn. Other factors, including the age of the patient and the presence of underlying diseases such as diabetes or arteriosclerosis, may influence the severity as well as morbidity of burn wounds.

THERMAL BURNS

Thermal burns usually occur from fire, scalding, or contact with hot objects. Specific flame burns of the feet are uncommon and usually occur only in patients with extremely

widespread injury (72). Children with burns, especially symmetrical scalding of the feet, may be victims of child abuse.

The depth of a burn may be termed a first-, second-, or third-degree wound. However, it is more accurate to express the depth of injury as partial thickness or full thickness. Partial-thickness burns involve the epidermis and varying amounts of the dermis, whereas full-thickness burns involve the epidermis, dermis, and subcutaneous tissue. The initial determination of burn depth may be difficult unless there is obvious necrosis of the wound. Dye studies with use of Evans blue (73) and fluorescein (74), thermography (75), and ultrasound (76) have been attempted to assess the depth of burns, but results have not been conclusive. The final degree of depth is also difficult to ascertain because a burn injury may be progressive (77, 78). The fact that the thermal injury is dynamic emphasizes the need for immediate cooling of the wound to limit any progressive damage to the tissues after the heating source is removed.

Three zones of injury have been described in the burn wound: the zone of hyperemia, the zone of stasis, and the zone of coagulation. The most peripheral zone is termed the zone of hyperemia. This zone is red and blanches on pressure until it is epithelialzed in approximately 7 days. The next circumferential zone consists of stasis, which also is initially red and then blanches on pressure after burning. However, the capillary blood flow stops after some minutes or hours, completely ceasing at 24 hours. After stasis of the capillary circulation develops, the zone will stay red, yet no longer blanche on pressure. Histological examination of this tissue shows the capillaries to be dilated and filled with red blood cells. Over the next 4 days the zone of stasis becomes red and white. It may develop petechial hemorrhages and,

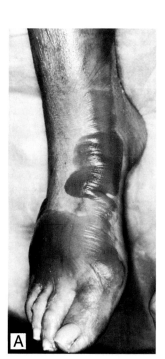
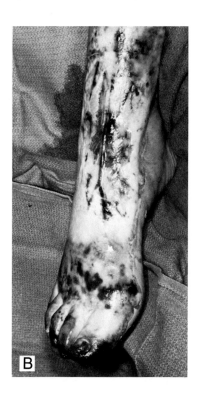

Figure 56.25. **A.** Early bleb formation demonstrates the difficulty often encountered in the assessment of wound depth. **B.** After demarcation this full-thickness burn is characterized by a white to dark, leathery appearance with thrombosed blood vessels. The wound is anesthetic. (From Tuerk D: Burns and frostbite. In Scurran BL (ed): *Foot and Ankle Trauma*. New York, Churchill Livingstone, 1989, p 155.)

because of hemolysis, appear pink before it becomes white and indistinguishable from the central zone.

The third zone, the central zone of coagulation, appears white initially, and the capillaries are contracted and devoid of red blood cells as if they had been coagulated in a state of spasm. In approximately 4 days, zones two and three are both white and indistinguishable from each other (79).

ASSESSMENT AND MANAGEMENT OF THE ACUTE BURN

The initial management of the acute burn involves careful assessment of the injury site, an accurate history of the type of inciting injury, and the duration of contact with the body. The extent and location of the burn, the surface area diameter, and the presence of any other injuries should be noted (Fig. 56.25). The depth of the wound may be difficult to ascertain, but an estimate should be obtained for treatment planning. Testing for sensation by pinprick will provide information in helping to assess the depth and degree of the injury inasmuch as fullthickness burns are generally insensate.

Upon initial examination it is critical to evaluate the circulatory status of the foot. The foot or other involved part should be compared with the opposite side when possible. An eschar over one of the extremities may become a constricting band. Edema may also occlude blood vessels and, unless relieved, can result in gangrene of the part of the body distal to the edema. If there is no pulse or sign of blood flow distally, especially in a hand or foot, there is significant danger of not being able to salvage the body part unless aggressive procedures are undertaken. Antibiotic therapy should be administered both systemically and topically (79). Systemic antibiotics should be considered initially for gram-positive and later for gram-negative organisms. Topical antibiotic therapy is used daily with dressing changes and debridement as indicated. Appropriate tetanus prophylaxis should be instituted.

Substances used to cover burn wounds have specific requirements, including low toxicity, minimal metabolic effects, and ease of application and removal. The covering should reduce bacterial colonization of the wound and the risk of infection. Agents commonly used in the treatment of burn wounds are silver nitrate, mafenide acetate (Sulfamylon) and silver sulfadiazine (Silvadene).

The objectives in burn wound care are (*a*) to prevent progression of the injury, (*b*) to prevent infection, and (*c*) to provide an environment to aid rapid healing. Progression of the injury may be slowed by cooling the area. Placing the burned area in cooled water at a temperature of approximately 25° C (77° F) for approximately 30 to 45 minutes produces the appropriate cooling (80). Progression of injury may also be decreased or slowed by maintaining a moist wound environment (81, 82). Blisters should be left intact or aspirated but not debrided. If the wound is a superficial, partial-thickness injury, covering it with gauze impregnated with petrolatum or an antiseptic in a petrolatum base (Xeroform) may provide a protective covering (Fig. 56.26). The use of a biological dressing such as a porcine xenograft or

homograft may decrease the progression of the ischemia within the dermis and promote an optimal environment for wound healing (83). If the burn injury has resulted in full-thickness necrosis, special attention must be paid to protection from bacterial contamination.

Small burns of the foot are treated in a manner similar to that of extensive wounds if evidence of healing does not appear within 8 to 10 days. This treatment involves debridement and grafting once the wound bed is clean and vascularity is sufficient to support a graft. After debridement the wound must be protected from desiccation or further eschar will develop. A biological dressing provides the best protection for a freshly debrided wound. *Epigard* and other semisynthetic skin coverings may prove useful toward that end.

Ungrafted wounds that heal by contraction and epithelization over a long period of time result in unstable scars and are subject to repeated breakdown (83). In these cases rehabilitation is often delayed and permanent deformities may develop. Serial wound culture specimens should be obtained before surgery and, when possible, quantitative culture specimens should be obtained before grafting procedures to ascertain bacterial counts less than 10^6.

ELECTRICAL BURNS

Electrical burns of the extremities, which can be classified as low- or high-tension injuries, occur from one of two mechanisms (84). The first involves a passage of a current through the limb; the second involves arcing. Burns do not occur from the electricity but rather result when the electrical energy is converted to heat upon meeting resistance. The current type, whether alternating (AC) or direct (DC), the amperage and voltage, the area of the body through which the current passes, the duration of exposure, and resistance of the body structures all influence the magnitude of the injury.

The more destructive type of current is AC because of the resultant tetanic muscle contractions and continued contact between the victim and the source of the current. A low tension-type injury occurs when the voltage is less than 1000 volts; it is characteristically seen in the household situation. High-tension injury, caused by voltage in excess of 1000 volts, usually occurs when there is contact with a power line.

The arc-type injury results from the current leaping from one conductor to the other. Typically this occurs between a source of electricity and the part of the body. The arc results from ionization of the air between the conductors. Intense heat is generated, usually in the area of 4000° F.

CHEMICAL BURNS

Chemical burns of the skin are considered to be more appropriately labeled as chemical injuries (85). The most important causative factors in chemical injuries are coagulation of protein by oxidation, reduction, salt formation, corrosion, protoplasmic poisoning, metabolic competitive inhibition, desiccation, and vesicant activity. The severity of chemical

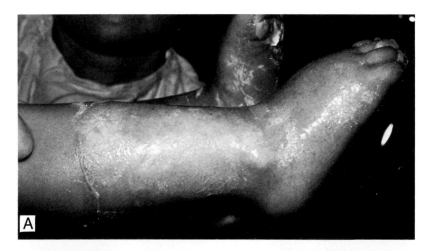

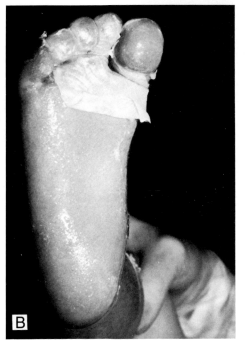

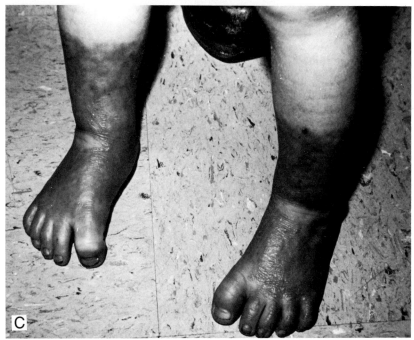

Figure 56.26. **A.** A child with second-degree scald burns of both legs and feet after immersion in a bathtub. The blisters have broken and have been debrided in the whirlpool. Note the edema of the dorsum of the foot, requiring continuing assessment of the distal circulation. **B.** View of the plantar surface of the foot. Because the plantar skin is thicker than the skin of the instep, injuries that result in third-degree burns of the instep may cause only second-degree burns of the sole. **C.** Two months after the injury. The second-degree burns have healed with the daily whirlpool and silver sulfadiazine cream dressings. After healing, the child is measured for individually fitted pressure garments that are worn continuously to prevent burn scar hypertrophy. (From Scurran BL: *Foot and Ankle Trauma.* New York, Churchill Livingstone, 1989, pp 157, 158.)

injuries is influenced by the concentration or pH of the solution, the mode of action of the agent, the vehicle, the volume, and the duration of contact. The most important aspect in the emergency treatment of a chemical injury is knowing the agent involved and the appropriate neutralization. In most chemical injuries all clothing should be removed and copious water should be immediately applied. This may be best performed by use of a continuous stream of water, either tap water or some type of irrigation equipment. This process will dilute as well as remove the chemical,

reducing the rate of reaction and restoring the pH level of the wound to normal.

Chemical injury caused by hydrofluoric acid and phosphorus should not be irrigated with water. A boric acid or sodium bicarbonate ($NaHCO_3$) wash is used after exposure to hydrofluoric acid, and a 2% copper sulfate ($CuSO_4$) solution is used for injuries caused by white phosphorus. Immediate removal of phosphorus particles is mandatory. These may be identified by use of the copper sulfate solution.

After emergency treatment of the chemical injury, management of the wound is similar to that of a thermal burn.

RADIATION BURNS

Alpha, beta, and gamma particles are the most common types of radiation that cause burns (86). The damage is determined by the type of radiation and the amount and duration of exposure. Radiation burns may also be described as acute or chronic.

Acute changes may subside completely, and a period of years or months may elapse before the chronic lesions appear. These late effects, radiodermatitis and radionecrosis, are of the greatest concern to the surgeon. Three distinct characteristics of these lesions are noted: endarteritis obliterans, excessive fibrosis of the tissue, and cellular changes that occur at the chromosomal level and adversely affect cellular replication.

Chronic ulcerations as a result of radionecrosis that affects the extremities may be managed by several different techniques. Skin grafts may be adequate when the necrosis is superficial. The requirements for skin grafts in this type of wound are the same as for other types of recipient beds. For deeper wounds involving tendon, muscle, and bone, flap coverage must be considered. The options include local flaps or distant flaps. Because of radiation injury to the vasculature, distant flaps such as island or free flaps may not be possible.

References

1. Hirata I: Soft tissue injuries. *College Health* 23:215-218, 1975.
2. Grossman JA: The repair of surface trauma. *Emerg Med* 12:220-235, 1982.
3. Milholland AV, Cowley RA: Anatomical injury code. *Am Surg* 45:93-100, 1979.
4. Rakel RE: *Family Practice*. Philadelphia, WB Saunders, 1978, pp 532-533.
5. Hoover NW, Ivins JC: Wound debridement. *Arch Surg* 79:701-710, 1959.
6. Bulletin of the American College of Surgeons, Committee on Trauma: *A Guide to Initial Therapy of Soft Tissue Wounds*. Chicago, American College of Surgeons, June 1974.
7. Converse JM: Plastic reconstructive surgery. *Plast Reconstr Surg* 1:9-13, 1964.
8. Blair VP: The influence of mechanical pressure on wound healing. *IMJ* 46:229, 1924.
9. Rank BK: *Surgery of Repair As Applied to Hand Injuries*, ed 3. Baltimore, Williams & Wilkins, 1968, pp 88-90.
10. Thompson RVS: *Primary Repair of Soft Tissue Injuries*. Melbourne, Australia, Melbourne University Press, 1969, Chapter 1.
11. Krizek TJ, Robson MC: Biology of surgical infection. *Surg Clin North Am* 55:1261-1267, 1975.
12. Burke JF: The effective period of preventative antibiotic action in experimental incisions and dermal lesions. *Surgery* 50:161-168, 1961.
13. Krizek TJ: Local factors influencing incidence of wound sepsis. *Contemp Surg* 10:45-50, 1977.
14. Burke JF: Elements affecting susceptibility to infection. *Contemp Surg* 10:38-41, 1977.
15. Elek SD: Experimental staphylococcal infections in the skin of man. *Ann NY Acad Sci* 65:85, 1956.
16. Branemark PI: Local tissue effect of wound disinfectants. *Acta Chir Scand* (suppl) 357:166, 1966.
17. Noe JM, Kalish S: *Wound Care*. Greenwich, CT, Chesebrough-Ponds, 1975.
18. Weeks PM, Wray RC: *Management of Acute Hand Injuries*. St Louis, CV Mosby, 1973, p 109.
19. Campbell E, Colton JB: Theodoric: master surgeon of the 13th century. *NY State J Med* 54:191-193, 1954.
20. Robson MC, Krizek TJ, Koss N: Amniotic membranes as a temporary wound dressing. *Surg Gynecol Obstet* 136:904-906, 1973.
21. Burke JF, Morris PJ: Recent trends in surgical bacteriology. *J Surg Res* 7:95-103, 1967.
22. Ellie JC, Goldstein, MA: Management of human and animal bite wounds. *J Am Acad Dermatol* 21:1275-1279, 1989.
23. Douglas LG: Bite wounds. *Am Fam Physician* 11:93-99, 1975.
24. Callaham M: Prophylactic antibiotics in common dog bite wounds: a controlled study. *Ann Emerg Med* 9:140-144, 1980.
25. Marr JS, Beck AM, Lugo JA Jr: An epidemiologic study of the human bite. *Public Health Rep* 94:514-521, 1979.
26. Vale GL, Norgueli TT: Anatomic distribution of human bite marks in a series of 67 cases. *J Forensic Sci* 28:61-69, 1983.
27. Welch CE: Human bite infections of the hand. *N Engl J Med* 215:901-908, 1936.
28. Barnes MN, Bibby BG: A summary of reports and a bacteriologic study of infections caused by human tooth wounds. *J Am Dent Assoc* 26:1163-1170, 1939.
29. Boland FK: Morsus humanus: sixty cases of human bites in Negroes. *JAMA* 116:127-131, 1941.
30. Farmer CB, Mann RJ: Human bite infections of the hand. *South Med J* 59:515-518, 1966.
31. Goldstein EJC, Citron AM: Comparative activities of cefuroxime, amoxicillin-culanic acid, ciprofloxacin, enoxacin and ofloxacin against aerobic and anaerobic bacteria isolated from bite wounds. *Antimicrob Agents Chemother* 32:1143-1148, 1980.
32. Goldstein EJC, Citron DM, Vagvolgyi AE: Susceptibility of bite wound bacteria to seven oral antimicrobial agents, including RV-985, a new erythromycin: considerations in choosing empiric therapy. *Antimicrob Agents Chemother* 29:556-559, 1986.
33. Brook I: Microbiology of human and animal bite wounds in children. *Pediatr Infect Dis J* 6:29-32, 1987.
34. Goldstein EJC, Miller TA, Citron DM: Infections following clench-fist injury: a new perspective. *J Hand Surg* 3:445-447, 1978.
35. Goldstein EJC, Barones MF, Miller TA: *Eikenella corrodens* in hand infections. *J Hand Surg* 8:563-567, 1983.
36. Schmidt AR, Heckman JA: *Eikenella corrodens* in human bite infections of the hand. *J Trauma* 23:478-482, 1983.
37. Bilos AJ, Kucharchuka A, Metzger W: *Eikenella corrodens* in human bites. *Clin Orthop* 134:320-324, 1978.
38. Chuinard RG, D'Ambrosia D: Human bite infections of the hand. *J Bone Joint Surg* 59A:416-418, 1977.
39. Lehman WC Jr, Jones WW, Allo MA: Human bite infections of the hand: adjunct treatment with hyperbaric oxygen. *Infect Surg* 4:460-465, 1985.
40. Harris D, Imperato PJ, Oken B: Dog bites: an unrecognized epidemic. *Bull NY Acad Med* 50:981-1000, 1974.
41. Goldstein EJC, Citron DM, Fine SM: Dog bite wounds and infections: a prospective clinical study. *Ann Emerg Med* 9:508-512, 1980.
42. Goldstein EJC, Reinhardt JF, Murray PM: Outpatient therapy of bite wounds: demographic data, bacteriology and a prospective randomized trial of amoxicillin/clavulanic acid versus penicillin + dicloxacillin. *Int J Dermatol* 26:123-127, 1987.
43. Lee MLH, Buhr AJ: Dog bites and local infection with Pasteurella septica. *Br Med J* 1:169-171, 1960.
44. Zook EG, Mier M, Van Beek AL: Successful treatment protocol for canine fang injuries. *J Trauma* 20:243-247, 1980.
45. Graham WP, Calabretta AM, Mier SH: Dog bites. *Am Fam Physician* 15:132-137, 1977.
46. Brook I: Microbiology of human and animal bite wounds in children. *Pediatr Infect Dis J* 6:29-32, 1987.
47. Goldstein EJC, Citron DM, Finegold SM: Role of anaerobic bacteria in bite wound infections. *Rev Infect Dis* (suppl 1) 6:177-183, 1984.
48. Feder HM Jr, Shanley JD, Barbara JA: Review of 59 patients hospitalized with animal bites. *Pediatr Infect Dis J* 6:24-28, 1987.
49. Elenbaas RM, McNabney WK, Robinson WA: Prophylactic oxacillin in dog bite wounds. *Ann Emerg Med* 11:248-251, 1982.

50. Rabies vaccine failures [editorial]. *Lancet* 1:917-918, 1988.
51. Immunization Practices Advisory Committee (ACIP): Rabies prevention: United States—1984. *MMWR* 33:393-408, 1984.
52. Rabies vaccine absorbed: a new rabies vaccine for use in humans. *MMWR* 37:217-223, 1988.
53. Goldstein EJC, Richwald GA: Human and animal bite wounds. *Am Fam Physician* 36:101-109, 1987.
54. Ordog GJ: The bacteriology of dog bite wounds on initial presentation. *Ann Emerg Med* 15:1324-1329, 1986.
55. Callaham MC: Treatment of common dog bites; infection risk factors. *JACEP* 7:83-87, 1978.
56. Callaham MC: Controversies in antibiotic choices for bite wounds. *Ann Emerg Med* 17:1321-1330, 1988.
57. Elenbaas RM, McNabney WK, Robinson WA: Evaluation of prophylactic oxacillin in cat bite wounds. *Ann Emerg Med* 13:155-157, 1984.
58. Callaham, M: Dog bite wounds. *JAMA* 44:2327-2328, 1980.
59. Goldstein EJC, Citron DM: Comparative activities of cefuroxime, amoxicillin-clavulanic acid, ciprofloxacin, enoxacin, and ofloxacin against aerobic and anaerobic bacteria isolated from bite wounds. *Antimicrob Agents Chemother* 32:1143-1148, 1988.
60. Parish HM: Analysis of 460 fatalities from venomous animals in the United States. *Am J Med Sci* 245:129, 1973.
61. Banard JH: Studies of 400 hymenoptera sting deaths in the United States. *J Allergy Clin Immunol* 52:259, 1987.
62. Banks BEC: The composition of hymenoptera venoms with particular reference to the venom of the honey bee. In Kornalik F, Mebs I: *Proceedings of the Seventh European Symposium on Animal, Plant and Microbial Toxins.* Prague, 1986, pp 41-59.
63. Light WC, Reisman RE: Stinging insect allergy. *Postgrad Med* 59:153, 1976.
64. Smith RL: *Venomous Animals of Arizona.* (Cooperative Extension Services College of Agriculture Bull. No. 8245.) University of Arizona, 1982.
65. Hanson HE, Goldman RF: Cold injury in man: a review of its etiology and discussion of its prediction. *Milit Med* 134:1307-1316, 1969.
66. Benzinger TR: Heat regulations: homeostasis of central temperature in man. *Physiol Rev* 40:672-759, 1969.
67. Iampietro PF, Vaughan JA, Goldman RF: Heat production from shivering. *J Appl Physiol* 15:632-634, 1960.
68. Weyman AE, Greenbaum DM, Grace WJ: Accidental hypothermia in an alcoholic population. *Am I Med* 56:13-21, 1974.
69. Ungley CC, Blackwood W: Peripheral vasoneuropathy, after chilling. "Immersion foot and immersion hand." Lancet 2:447-451, 1942.
70. Lapp NL, Juergens JL: Frostbite. *Mayo Clin Proc* 40:932-948, 1965.
71. Jahss M: *Disorders of the Foot,* vol 2. Philadelphia, WB Saunders Company, 1982, pp 1689-1702.
72. Artz CP, Moncrief JA: *The Treatment of Burns,* ed 2. Philadelphia, WB Saunders Co, 1969.
73. Goulian D Jr: Early differentiation between necrotic and viable tissue in burns. Review of the problem and development of a new clinical approach. *Plast Reconstr Surg* 27:359, 1961.
74. Bechtold F, Lipin RJ: Differentiation of full thickness and partial thickness burn with the aid of fluorescein. *Am J Surg* 109:436, 1965.
75. Mladick R, Georgiade H, Thorne F: Clinical evaluation of thermography in determining degree of injury. *Plast Reconstr Surg* 38:512, 1966.
76. Goans RE: Ultrasonic pulse-echo determination of thermal injury in deep dermal burns. *Med Phys* 4:259, 1977.
77. Hinshaw RJ: Early changes in the depth of burns. *Ann NY Acad Sci* 150:548, 1968.
78. Jackson DM: The diagnosis of depth of burning. *Br J Surg* 40:588, 1953.
79. Nathan P, Law EJ, Murphy DF, MacMillan BG: Laboratory method for selection of topical antimicrobial agents to treat infection burn wounds. *Burns* 4:177, 1977-78.
80. Epstein MF, Crawford JD: Cooling in the emergency treatment of burns. *Pediatrics* 52:430, 1973.
81. Zawacki BE: Reversal of capillary stasis and prevention of necrosis in burns. *Ann Surg* 180:98, 1974.
82. Forage, AV: The effects of removing the epidermis from burnt skin. *Lancet* 2:690, 1962.
83. Miller TA, Switzer WE, Foly FD, Moncrief JA: Early homografting of second degree burns. *Plast Reconstr Surg* 40:117, 1967.
84. Skoog T: Electrical injuries. *J Trauma* 10:816, 1970.
85. Jeleuko C III: Chemicals that "burn." *J Trauma* 14:65, 1974.
86. Robinson DW: Surgical problems in the excision and repair of radiated tissue. *Plast Reconstr Surg* 55:41, 1975.

Additional References

Brown PW: The prevention of infection in open wounds. *Clin Orthop* 96:42-50, 1973.
Clancey GJ, Hansen ST Jr: Open fractures of the tibia: a review of one hundred and two cases. *J Bone Joint Surg* 60A:118-122, 1978.
Scurran BL: *Foot and Ankle Trauma.* New York, Churchill-Livingstone, 1989.
Shaftan GW, Gardner B: *Surgical Emergencies.* Philadelphia, JB Lippincott, 1974.
Zuidema GD: *The Management of Trauma,* ed 3. Philadelphia, WB Saunders, 1979.

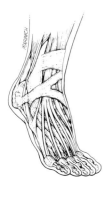

CHAPTER **57**

Puncture Wounds

Kieran T. Mahan, M.S., D.P.M., F.A.C.F.S.
Jeffrey A. Marks, D.P.M.

Puncture wounds of the foot are a common occurrence in the hospital emergency room, particularly during the warmer months when outdoor activity is more frequent and many persons are barefoot. Pedal puncture wounds account for 5.12% of all emergency room visits to Saint Joseph's Hospital in Philadelphia (Table 57.1). A similar study by Reinherz and associates (1) found an incidence of 7.4% at Zion Hospital in Illinois. A study by Fitzgerald and Cowan (2) noted 887 patients with puncture wounds from a total of 108,648 emergency room visits by children. Most injuries occurred between May and October. Nails accounted for 98% of the puncture wounds (Fig. 57.1), but other penetrating objects included wood, rocks, pieces of metal such as wire, sewing needles, and glass.

Although the injury is quite common, treatment is often inadequate, which may result in serious complications. Most hospital emergency rooms respond to these often small and innocuous wounds with superficial and incomplete treatment. Usually treatment consists of an inadequate history, topical cleansing, soaks, tetanus toxoid, occasionally oral antibiotics, and poor physician follow-up. Serious complications may result, including soft tissue infections, osteomyelitis, septic arthritis, foreign body granuloma, premature epiphyseal closure, joint degeneration, and residual deformity (1-3).

Soft tissue infections occurring after a puncture wound may include cellulitis and/or abscess formation. Houston and associates (3) reported 2583 puncture wounds of which some 10% developed infections. Most had a cellulitis that cleared overnight following appropriate treatment. Of the group that had initially appeared with clean wounds 2% later developed infections (Fig. 57.2). In Fitzgerald and Cowan's series (2), 8.4% of the patients who were seen within the first 24 hours after injury had cellulitis or developed it within 4 days. Cellulitis or localized soft tissue infection developed in 57% of the patients who were seen 1 to 7 days after the puncture wound (Fig. 57.3). The organism isolated in more than 50% of these early infections is *Staphylococcus aureus*. Alpha-hemolytic streptococcus, *Staphylococcus epidermidis*, *Escherichia coli*, and *Proteus* and *Klebsiella* organisms have also been reported (2, 4, 5). Puncture wounds sustained in swimming pools, lakes, or oceans can become infected with unusual organisms such as *Aeromonas hydrophila*, *Mycobacterium marinum*, and *Vibrio* species (6).

Of the complications following puncture wounds, the most difficult to manage is osteomyelitis (Fig. 57.4). Osteomyelitis occurs in 0.6 to 1.8% of all puncture wounds, and

Table 57.1.
Summary of Emergency Room Log, Saint Joseph Hospital, January 1989 to June 1990, Podiatric Surgical Service

Injury	No. of Cases	Total (%)
Lacerations	73	5.85
Puncture wounds	64	5.12
Foreign bodies	12	.96
Gunshot wounds	14	1.12
Burns	5	.4
Frostbite	8	.64
Animal bites	1	.08
Insect bites	1	.08
Nail injuries	22	1.76
Infections	28	2.24
Gout	17	1.36
Fractures	276	22.1
Sprains/ligament ruptures	364	29.1
Miscellaneous soft tissue	364	29.1
Total No. of patients treated	1249	

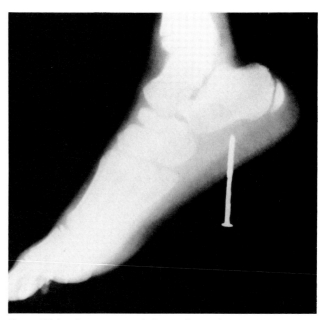

Figure 57.1. Puncture wounds from nails may frequently penetrate the deep fascia and cause infection in deep structures.

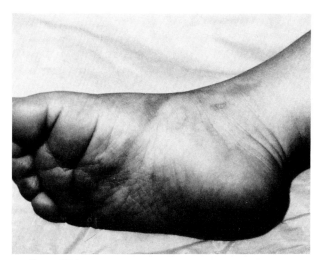

Figure 57.2. Lymphangitis from 3-day-old puncture wound.

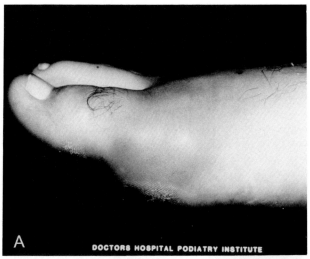

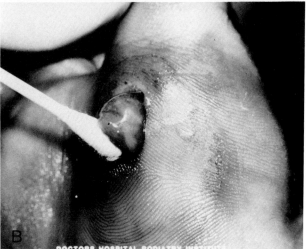

Figure 57.3. **A.** Clinical appearance of first metatarsophalangeal joint before treatment. **B.** Drainage of abscess following puncture wound.

Pseudomonas aeruginosa is isolated in 93% of these cases (2, 7, 8). In 1968, Johanson (9) first reported osteomyelitis caused by *P. aeruginosa* in children after puncture wounds. Since that time other authors have noted the particular predilection of *Pseudomonas* as a causative organism in children (2, 5, 8, 10-18). Recently, Baltimore and Jenson reported osteochondritis in the foot caused by *Pseudomonas maltophilia* (19). Johanson suggested that *Pseudomonas* osteomyelitis in children is common because of its preference for cartilage (9). Following osteomyelitis, premature epiphyseal closure and residual deformity may result (Fig. 57.5). Miller and Semian (7) were the first to document *Pseudomonas* osteomyelitis in adults. However other gram-negative organisms have been isolated (20, 21).

The course of osteomyelitis after puncture wounds of the foot is often slow and indolent. Typically, the patient is seen 2 to 5 days after a puncture wound, with increasing pain, swelling, and erythema. At this time treatment often consists of cleansing, soaks, tetanus toxoid, and occasionally oral antibiotics. This may partially relieve the symptoms without curing the infection. Johanson (9) reported an average delay of 3 weeks and Brand and Black (11) a delay of 23 days before osteomyelitis is diagnosed. Lang and Peterson (5) showed that patients may be free of symptoms for several months before the recognition of osteomyelitis. The diagnosis is made more difficult by the lack of systemic signs. Symptoms include an absent or low-grade fever, no leukocytosis, and a normal to slightly elevated sedimentation rate. Local signs and symptoms provide the key for diagnosis.

Early diagnosis of osteomyelitis after a puncture wound is critical to prevent or minimize permanent disability (Fig. 57.6). Green and Bruno (13) described three classes of clinical responses to *Pseudomonas* infections in children that depend upon the diagnosis time and treatment regimen:

Type I. Early diagnosis with surgical drainage and debridement with appropriate antibiotic coverage resulted in complete healing with no sequelae.

Type II. A delay in diagnosis from 9 to 14 days. Surgical debridement and appropriate antibiotic coverage will eradicate the infection; however, there may be residual bone or joint deformity.

Type III. A delay in diagnosis for more than 3 weeks results in chronic infection, necessitating bone resection.

Identification of the etiological organism in osteomyelitis after a puncture wound is often difficult and complicated by the antecedent use of broad-spectrum antibiotics. Determining whether a pathological organism or a contaminant has been isolated is difficult, and use of broad-spectrum antibiotics may also encourage opportunistic flora such as *Serratia marcescens* to become pathogenic (4). Minnefor and associates (17) postulated that the initial use of antibiotics is aimed at gram-positive organisms and may facilitate a gram-negative infection.

Once a diagnosis of osteomyelitis is established, treatment must be swift and aggressive. Gram-negative osteomyelitis requires surgical intervention to debride infected bone and

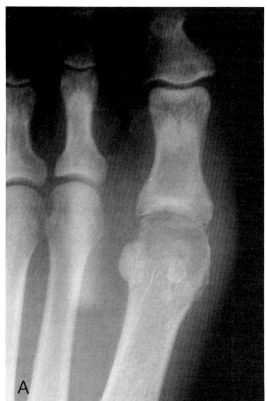 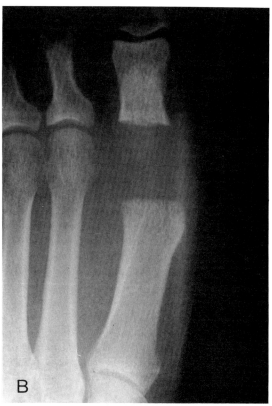

Figure 57.4. **A.** Preoperative dorsoplantar roentgenogram of left foot of patient with osteomyelitis 3 weeks after puncture wound. Note fragmentation of tibial sesamoid, lytic areas in first metatarsal head and base of proximal phalanx, and narrowing of first metatarsophalangeal joint space. **B.** Postoperative dorsoplantar roentgenogram demonstrating large area of infected bone that had to be removed. Note that both sesamoids had to be removed.

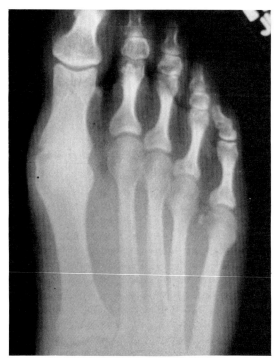

Figure 57.5.   Autofusion of first metatarsophalangeal joint 3 years after puncture-wound induced septic arthritis.

remove foreign bodies. Intravenous antipseudomonal antibiotics are required for several weeks. Jacobs and associates (15) recommend surgical debridement of infected bone in *Pseudomonas* osteomyelitis, followed by 10 to 14 days of antipseudomonal antibiotic therapy. Crosby and Powell (14) recommend at least 3 weeks of antipseudomonal antibiotic therapy. They also suggest following the sedimentation rate to monitor the progress of treatment. Failure to demonstrate a decline of approximately 1 mm/day in the sedimentation rate may be an indication for a change in antibiotic therapy or surgical intervention, or both.

INITIAL WOUND EVALUATION AND TREATMENT

The goals of treatment in puncture wounds are twofold: (*a*) conversion of a contaminated or dirty wound to a clean wound, thereby preventing osteomyelitis, and (*b*) prevention of tetanus.

History is extremely important in puncture wound evaluation, including the foot gear and clothing worn. Foreign bodies, including pieces of footwear and clothing, may be introduced into the wound. The history should also reveal the condition and type of penetrating material, time of injury, and the environment in which the wound occurred.

Evaluation of the wound should include radiographs or the use of xeroradiography in order to rule out the presence

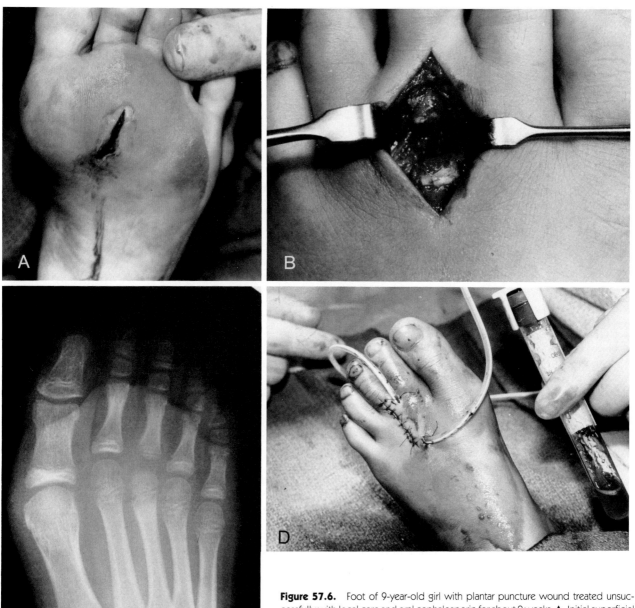

Figure 57.6. Foot of 9-year-old girl with plantar puncture wound treated unsuccessfully with local care and oral cephalosporin for about 2 weeks. **A.** Initial superficial incision and drainage; culture grew *Pseudomonas aeruginosa*. **B.** After 2 weeks of gentamicin therapy, condition continues to worsen. Infected third metatarsophalangeal joint debrided. **C.** Roentgenogram demonstrating bone resection. **D.** In-and-out closed suction irrigation drainage. Rapid improvement occurred after adequate bone debridement.

of a radiopaque foreign body. Trauma to neurovascular supply or damage to osseous structures must be carefully evaluated (Fig. 57.7). Adjacent muscle and tendon function should be thoroughly examined. Figure 57.8 demonstrates treatment techniques.

Cleansing of the wound with a bactericidal solution such as povidone-iodine diluted in sterile salaine is essential. Deep irrigation should be performed because *Pseudomonas* organisms have been recovered from nonsterile water (12).

Debridement and exploration of puncture wounds should be performed in the emergency room or office, and local an-

esthesia is often necessary. The local anesthetic should not be infiltrated in the immediate area of the wound but should be used proximally to achieve anesthesia without risk of spreading contamination. The wound can be explored with a blunt probe under sterile conditions to check for penetration of the deep fascia. If the deep fascia has been penetrated, a more aggressive debridement must be performed to prevent osteomyelitis. In any event, debridement must remove all devitalized tissue and retained foreign bodies with minimal damage to healthy tissue. Prolonged attempts to remove difficult-to-reach foreign bodies should be

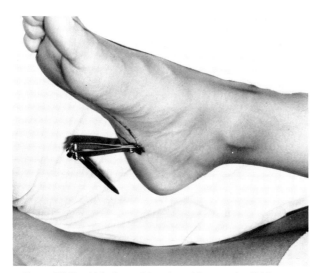

Figure 57.7. Nail clipper lying alongside posterior tibial artery.

avoided in the emergency room or office setting. Culture specimens should be obtained from deep punctures regardless of wound age. Excising epidermal edges around the wound can facilitate deeper inspection and cleansing, as well as decrease the risk of epidermal inclusion cyst formation (1, 3, 22). In general, puncture wounds should not be closed primarily, particularly when the wound has penetrated to deep fascia or when there is gross contamination. The wound should be packed open or closed over a drain.

The use of *antibiotics* is a controversial topic in the initial treatment of puncture wounds. Fitzgerald and Cowan (2) reported a study of 465 patients with puncture wounds who were not treated with antibiotics. Only two patients developed complications requiring incision and drainage. Antibiotics cannot compensate for improper wound care and may both mask infections without curing them and promote the growth of nonsusceptible opportunistic flora. Antibiotics are less effective in the presence of a retained foreign body. However, in grossly contaminated wounds or those penetrating a bone or joint, semisynthetic penicillinase-resistant penicillins have been recommended until results of cultures and sensitivity tests have been reported (18, 22, 23).

Local wound care is an important adjunct to treatment. Rest, elevation, and limited weight bearing on the affected foot are vital parts of the treatment plan. Soaks can encourage drainage; however, improper application could facilitate an infection (12). Careful monitoring of the patient is essential to detect any change in symptoms.

TETANUS PROPHYLAXIS

A puncture wound is the classical tetanus-prone wound. Prophylaxis for tetanus involves individualizing therapy for each wound with four components: wound care, tetanus toxoid, immunoglobulin, and antibiotics. Basic active immunization for tetanus is acquired by means of three injections of absorbed tetanus toxoid. The first two are admin-

istered 4 to 6 weeks apart, and the third injection is given 6 to 12 months after the second. A booster injection is then required every 10 years (24). Tetanus toxoid is a highly effective antigen, and a completed primary series generally induces protective levels of serum antitoxin that persist for 10 or more years (24). A careful history should be taken from patients regarding their immunization status. One study revealed that 20% of children in the United States younger than 13 years of age are not adequately immunized (25). Limited surveys performed since 1977 demonstrate that the protective levels of circulating antitoxin decreases with increasing age. An estimated 40% of persons 60 years of age or older lack protective levels of antitoxin (24). For individuals with an indeterminate number of toxoid injections, many physicians recommend a booster whenever a patient's last injection was more than 1 year earlier and their wound is tetanus prone (24, 26, 27). For non-tetanus-prone wounds, an interval of 5 years or less is satisfactory (26). Antitoxin antibodies develop rapidly in persons who have previously received at least two doses of tetanus toxoid.

Consideration for passive immunization with tetanus immunoglobulin should also be evaluated on an individual basis depending on the wound. If needed, the human tetanus immunoglobulin is preferred because it provides longer protection than the animal form, with fewer adverse reactions. The current recommendation for tetanus-prone wounds in patients with questionable immunization is 250 units intramuscularly. However, 500 units is suggested for severe, neglected, or old (more than 24 hours) tetanus-prone wounds (24, 26).

Wound care for the prophylaxis of tetanus involves removing *Clostridium tetani* organisms and nonviable tissue. Debridement of necrotic tissue must be aggressive and thorough. Correspondingly, handling of viable tissue must be gentle to encourage survival. The wound should be vigorously irrigated with copious amounts of saline or dilute bactericidal solution. The wound should be left open by means of a drain or packing if there is any question as to the presence of anaerobic bacteria in the wound, which in a closed wound can exhaust the oxygen supply and facilitate anaerobic bacterial growth (4).

Antibiotic prophylaxis for tetanus has not been demonstrated to be effective against toxin. Penicillin can be effective against the vegetative organism. If used to prevent infection from organisms that have not been surgically removed, penicillin must be given over at least a 5-day period (24).

BITE WOUNDS

Bite wounds consist of punctures, lacerations, and scratches of various depth. Approximately 0.7% to 1% of all emergency room visits are attributed to bite wounds (28, 29). Saint Joseph Hospital reports a 0.16% incidence of pedal bite wounds. By far, dog bites are most common, followed by cat and human bites (27, 30-33). Approximately 1 to 2 million Americans are bitten by dogs and 400,000 by cats annually (28, 34, 35). Bite wounds to the lower extremities

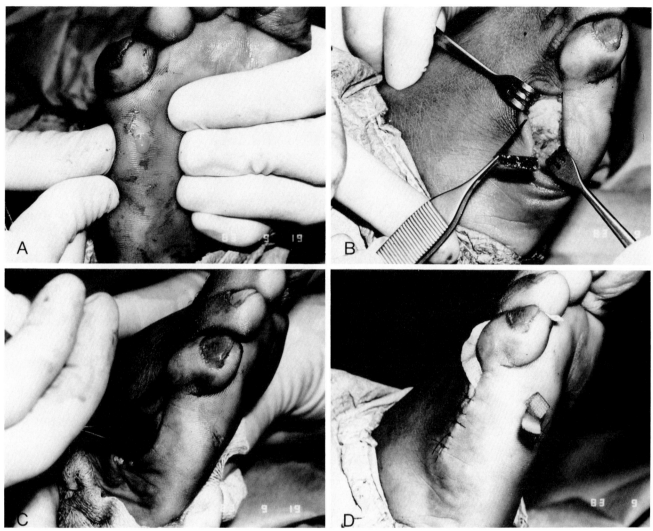

Figure 57.8. Foot of 40-year-old female with chronic pain and drainage after she tripped on wooden stairs. **A.** Initial plantar incision with drainage of abscess. **B.** Dorsal incision required for removal of large fragment of wood. Patient had reported that she had not felt any splinter. **C.** Thorough irrigation with dilute iodophor solution. **D.** Closure over drain.

are most common in the warmer months, March through August, when only minimal protective clothing and shoes are worn. Bite wounds, like puncture wounds, are often inadequately evaluated and treated. The rate of complications secondary to bite wounds is between 25% to 50% (32, 33). Bacteria isolated from infected wounds may originate from the victim's skin flora or the environment but most commonly comes from the flora of the biting animal (27). Bite wound infections may develop septic arthritis, tenosynovitis, and osteomyelitis, resulting in long-term disability.

The extremities account for over 70% of all bite wounds (27). Approximately 3% of all dog bites affect the foot (30, 36). Human bites largely affect the upper extremity and specifically the hand, usually secondary to a clenched-fist blow to the oral area. A study by Marr and associates (31) reported that only 3.7% of human bites affect the lower extremity and only 0.2% affect the foot. The location and depth of the wound are extremely important because of the various closed spaces of the foot that may provide for deeper extension of the infection.

Microbiological Factors

Oral cavities harbor a great supply and variety of organisms that may become pathogenic in poorly treated wounds. Human bites are considerably more virulent than are animal bites. The human oral cavity may contain 10^8 bacteria per milliliter, representing as many as 42 species (33). The most common isolate within infected human bite wounds appears to be alpha-hemolytic streptococcus followed closely by *S. aureus* (6, 27, 30, 32, 37). Anaerobic bacteria are also a predominant oral flora isolated in 50% of infected wounds, with *Bacteroides* being the most common genus found. *Eikenella corrodens*, a gram-negative capnophilic rod found in dental plaques, has been isolated in 20% of infected human bite wounds (27, 32). Rare cases of *Treponema pallidum* have also been documented in the literature (33).

Dog and cat bite wound infection isolates strongly correlate with the normal oral flora (27, 30). The incidence of *Pasteurella multocida* in dog bite wounds is 20% to 25%. Long considered the most important pathogen, recent studies have demonstrated *Streptococcus* to be the most commonly isolated bacteria, followed by *S. aureus* and various anaerobes such as *Bacteroides* and *Fusobacterium* (30, 37). Dogs may also transmit tetanus, rabies, tularemia, blastomycosis, and mycobacteriosis (27, 30, 38).

Cat bite wound infections are most frequently caused by *P. multocida*, which may be isolated in 50% to 80% of infected wounds. *S. aureus*, alpha-hemolytic streptococcus, and anaerobic bacteria may also be present. Quenzer and associates (39) reported a case of cat bite-induced tularemia. Tetanus, rabies, and plaque have also been transmitted by cat bites (28, 40).

Management

A study by Goldstein and co-workers (30) found that patients seen at the emergency room for treatment of bite wounds 12 or more hours following the injury usually had an established infection. Wounds less than 8 hours old seldom developed infection. Early and aggressive treatment is essential in the prevention of adverse sequelae in bite wounds.

History should include the location and time the attack occurred, as well as the behavior and appearance of the animal. Unprovoked attacks should be noted. In dealing with human bites an attempt should be made to determine the presence of infectious diseases such as acquired immune deficiency syndrome (AIDS), hepatitis, or herpes. Tetanus immunization history must be elicited because all bite wounds are tetanus prone.

Evaluation of the wound should include radiographs to rule out fracture or a retained foreign body such as a broken tooth. Injury to tendons and neurovascular structures must be assessed.

Cleansing, debridement, and exploration should be performed as outlined in the puncture wound section. Aerobic and anaerobic culture specimens should be obtained after proper superficial surface decontamination and before irrigation. Several studies, however, suggest that culture results of fresh bite wounds often correlate poorly with those of the same site once infected (27, 30, 37, 41).

Antibiotic usage for prophylaxis in patients without established infections is a controversial topic (6, 28, 32, 37). Antibiotics cannot make up for improper wound care. Antibiotic therapy in infected wounds should be based on the culture results. Extensive and grossly contaminated wounds should receive empiric therapy on the basis of the animal involved and its usual spectrum of oral pathogens (6, 30). The empiric therapy should include agents that are effective against *Streptococcus* organisms, *S. aureus*, *P. multocida*, and

in human bites *E. corrodens*. Wounds should be reevaluated again within 24 to 48 hours.

Rabies Prophylaxis

Rabies is a viral infection of warm-blooded animals, which causes acute encephalomyelitis and progresses to coma and death in humans within 14 days of onset. In North America rabies is primarily a disease of wildlife, (e.g., raccoons, skunks, bats, foxes, coyotes, and bobcats). The incidence of rabies is increasing, and exposure to domesticated animals is becoming more frequent. Rabies is endemic in dogs, which continue to be the most important source of human bites (42).

The decision to administer postexposure prophylaxis is based on the risk of the specific animal involved in the incident. The best protection against rabies is adequate local wound treatment followed by rabies immunoglobulin (RIG) and human diploid cell rabies vaccine (HDCV). The current recommendations from the Centers for Disease Control are based on the species and condition of the attacking animal. Dog and cat bites are not treated when the offending animal is healthy and can be observed for 10 days. However, bites from rabid or suspected rabid or escaped animals are treated with RIG and HDCV. The skunk, raccoon, bat, fox, coyote, and bobcat are regarded as rabid unless the animal is submitted for analysis and determined to be rabies free. Again, RIG and HDCV are administered. Livestock, rodents, and rabbits vary regionally, and consultation with local public health officials is recommended (43).

FOREIGN BODIES

Foreign bodies in the foot are common following puncture wounds. Approximately 1% of emergency room visits to Saint Joseph Hospital involve patients with retained pedal foreign bodies. Metal fragments, broken glass, and wooden splinters account for 95% of all foreign bodies commonly seen (44). Rocks, clothing, insect stingers, hair, and liquid foreign bodies such as lubricating grease, paint, and molten plastic have also been reported (37, 45-47). A needle or pin is considered the most common pedal foreign body, usually found embedded in carpet pile (48). Miller and Semian (7) reported that 60% of patients with infected puncture wounds who did not respond to intravenous antibiotics were found to have a retained foreign body. Small fragments may not produce symptoms, but serious complications such as inclusion cyst formation, abscess formation, septic arthritis, and osteomyelitis can lead to permanent deformity and disability (49-51) (Figs. 57.9 and 57.10).

Diagnosis

The diagnosis of a retained foreign body is often a difficult one and may ultimately be made only after the symptoms of infection manifest. A careful history of the initial puncture wound can help determine whether a portion of the

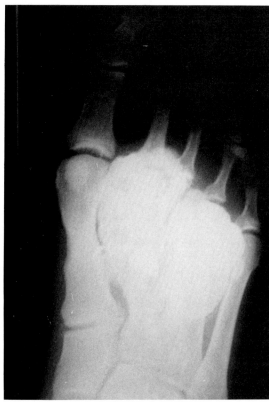

Figure 57.9. Foreign body granuloma 4 years after bullet wound. Retained bullet was later excised along with granuloma and involved portion of second metatarsal head.

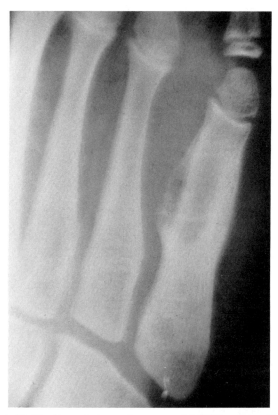

Figure 57.10. Dorsoplantar roentgenogram of right fifth metatarsal in 8-year-old girl, showing periosteal reaction along shaft. Patient had stepped on wooden splinter 2 months earlier. Retained wooden foreign bodies may often cause osteoblastic or osteolytic reactions, creating an interesting differential diagnosis.

offending object was retained. In addition to a history, radiographical examination is the best diagnostic tool available. Anderson and co-workers (44) reported that a lack of such examination was responsible for 38% of missed foreign bodies.

All metal fragments are visible on standard radiographs (44, 47, 52, 53), and approximately 96% of glass fragments are visible. A common misconception about glass is that it must be leaded to be radiopaque. Felman and Fisher (54) demonstrated that all glass is visible radiographically because the density of the glass is greater than that of the surrounding tissue. Tandberg (55) confirmed this finding by testing 66 types of glass and concluded that the presence of heavy metals or pigments was not required for radiopacity. He was able to discern fragments as small as 2 mm when superimposed on bone and 0.5 mm when unobscured.

Wooden foreign bodies are difficult to detect on standard radiographs. A study by Woesner and Sanders (56) compared the use of standard radiography and xeroradiography and concluded that xeroradiography was superior for the detection of wooden foreign bodies imaged in the positive mode. Charney and associates (52) demonstrated that xerography was not superior to standard radiography in the detection of wooden foreign bodies. The position of the fragment was determined to be most important for visual-

ization. Transversely oriented wooden fragments were more easily seen than the longitudinally oriented fragments. Wood stains and iron oxide paints did not significantly change the radiographic appearance. Kuhns (53) compared the use of standard radiography, xeroradiography, and computed tomography for the detection of wooden foreign bodies. He allowed the fragments to become water-logged so that their density was similar to the surrounding tissues. Only computed tomography could detect the wooden fragment embedded into cadaver limbs. Plastics are similar to wood and may not be viewed on standard radiographs (52, 57).

The use of ultrasonography for the detection of foreign bodies has been suggested (58). Foreign material is hyperechoic and is characterized by a comet-tail artifact. However, only the proximal surface of metallic objects can be visualized (58, 59). Magnetic resonance imaging (MRI) has had limited use in the detection of foreign bodies. Preliminary work suggests MRI is an excellent tool for the detection of nonmetallic material such as wood. The inflammatory capsule that wood induces is easily demonstrated in T2-weighted images (60).

References

1. Reinherz PR, Hong DT, Tisa LM, Winters GJ, Beneson DE, Schecter VA, DeRose DA, Lizerbram R: Management of puncture wound in the foot. *J Foot Surg* 24:288-292, 1985.
2. Fitzgerald R, Cowan J: Puncture wounds of the foot. *Orthop Clin North Am* 6:965-972, 1975.
3. Houston A, Roy W, Faust R, Ewin D: Tetanus prophylaxis in the treatment of puncture wounds of patients in the deep South. *J Trauma* 2:439-446, 1962.
4. Abramson C: Normal "opportunistic" flora of the lower extremity related to postoperative surgical wound infections. *J Am Podiatry Assoc* 67:9-27, 1977.
5. Lang A, Peterson HA: Osteomyelitis following puncture wounds of the foot in children. *J Trauma* 16:993-999, 1976.
6. Joseph WS: *Handbook of Lower Extremity Infections.* New York, Churchill Livingstone, 1990, pp 65-83.
7. Miller E, Semian DW: Gram negative osteomyelitis following puncture wounds in the foot. *J Bone Joint Surg* 57A:535-537, 1975.
8. Chusid MJ, Jacobs WM, Sty JR: Pseudomonas arthritis following puncture wounds in the foot. *J Pediatr* 94:429-431, 1979.
9. Johanson RH: Pseudomonas infections of the foot following puncture wounds. *JAMA* 204:170-172, 1968.
10. Das De S, McAllister T: Pseudomonas osteomyelitis following puncture wound of the foot in children. *Injury* 12:334-339, 1980.
11. Brand R, Black H: Pseudomonas osteomyelitis following puncture wounds in children. *J Bone Joint Surg* 56A:1637-1640, 1974.
12. Hagler D: Pseudomonas osteomyelitis: puncture wounds of the feet [letter]. *Pediatrics* 48:672, 1971.
13. Green N, Bruno J: Pseudomonas infection of the foot after puncture wounds. *South Med J* 73:146-149, 1980.
14. Crosby LA, Powell DA: The potential value of the sedimentation rate in monitoring treatment out-come in puncture wound related pseudomonas osteomyelitis. *Clin Orthop* 188:168-172, 1984.
15. Jacobs RF, McCarthy RE, Elser JM: Pseudomonas osteochondritis complicating puncture wounds of the foot in children: a 10-year evaluation. *J Infect Dis* 160:657-661, 1989.
16. Collins BS, Karlin JM, Silvani SH, Scurran BL: Pseudomonas pyarthrosis and osteomyelitis from a puncture wound of the foot. *J Am Podiatr Med Assoc* 75:316-320, 1985.
17. Minnefor AB, Olson MI, Carver DH: Pseudomonas osteomyelitis following puncture wounds of the foot. *Pediatrics* 47:598-601, 1971.
18. Riegler HF, Routson GW: Complications of deep puncture wounds of the foot. *J Trauma* 19:18-22, 1979.
19. Baltimore RS, Jenson HB: Puncture wound osteochondritis of the foot caused by *Pseudomonas maltophilia. Pediatr Infect Dis J* 9:143-144, 1990.
20. Congeni B, Weiner D, Izsak E: Expanded spectrum of organisms causing osteomyelitis after puncture wounds of the foot. *Orthopedics* 4:531-533, 1981.
21. Mahan DT, Kalish ST: Complication following puncture wound of the foot. *J Am Podiatry Assoc* 72:497-504, 1982.
22. Chrisholm CD, Schlesser JF: Plantar puncture wounds controversies and treatment recommendation. *Ann Emerg Med* 18:1352-1357, 1989.
23. Joseph WS, LeFrock JL: Infections complicating puncture wounds of the foot. *J Foot Surg* 26:S30, 1987.
24. Centers for Disease Control: Recommendation of the Immunization Practices Advisory Committee: Diphtheria, tetanus, and pertussis: guidelines for vaccine prophylaxis and other preventive measures. *Ann Intern Med* 103:896-905, 1985.
25. Krugman S, Katz S: Childhood immunization procedures. *JAMA* 237:2228, 1979.
26. Lindsey D: Tetanus prophylaxsis—do our guidelines assure protection? *J Trauma* 24:1063-1064, 1984.
27. Mandell GL, Douglas RG, Bennett JE: *Principles and Practice of Infectious Disease,* ed 3. New York, Churchill Livingstone, 1990. pp 825-837.
28. Goldstein EJC: Infectious complications and therapy of bite wounds. *J Am Podiatr Med Assoc* 79:486-491, 1989.
29. Aghababian RV, Conte JE: Mammalian bite wounds. *Am Emerg Med* 9:79, 1980.
30. Goldstein EJ, Citron DM, Wield B, Blachman U, Sutter VL, Miller TA, Finegold SM: Bacteriology of human and animal bite wounds. *J Clin Microbiol* 8:667-672. 1978.
31. Marr JS, Beck AM, Lugo JA: An epidemiologic study of the human bite. *Public Health Rep* 94:514-521, 1979.
32. Martin LT: Human bites—guidelines for prompt evaluation and treatment. *Postgrad Med J* 81:221-224, 1987.
33. Peebles E, Boswick JA, Scott FA: Wounds of the hand contaminated by human or animal saliva. *J Trauma* 20:383-389, 1980.
34. Douglas LG: Bite wounds. *Am Fam Physician* 11:93, 1975.
35. Elenbaas RM, McNabney WK, Robinson WA: Evaluation of prophylactic oxacillin in cat bite wounds. *Ann Emerg Med* 13:155, 1984.
36. Callaham ML: Prophylactic antibiotics in common dog bite wounds: a controlled study. *Ann Emerg Med* 9:410, 1980.
37. Scurran BL: *Foot and Ankle Trauma.* New York, Churchill Livingstone, 1989, pp 95-152.
38. Fiala M, Bauer H, Khaleeli M, Giorgio A: Dog bite Bacteroides infection, coagulopathy, renal microangiopathy. *Ann Intern Med* 87:248-249, 1977.
39. Quenzer RW, Mostow SR, Emerson JK: Cat-bite tularemia. *JAMA* 238:1845, 1977.
40. Werner SB, Weidmer LE, Nelson BC: Primary plaque pneumonia contracted from a domestic cat at South Lake Tahoe, California. *JAMA* 251:929, 1989.
41. Feder HM, Shanley JD, Barbera JA: A review of 59 patients hospitalized with animal bite. *Pediatr Infect Dis* 6:27, 1987.
42. Anderson LJ, Nicholson KG, Tauxe RV: Human rabies in the United States 1960-1979. Epidemiology, diagnosis and prevention. *Ann Intern Med* 100:728, 1984.
43. Recommendations of the Immunization Practices Advisory Committee. Rabies prevention—United States. *MMWR* 33:393, 1984.
44. Anderson MA, Newmeyer WL, Kilgore ES: Diagnosis and treatment of retained foreign bodies in the hand. *Am J Surg* 144:63-67, 1982.
45. Byron TJ: Foreign bodies found in the foot. *J Am Podiatry Assoc* 71:30-35, 1981.
46. Puhl RW, Altman MI, Seto JE, Nelson GA: The use of fluoroscopy in the detection and excision of foreign bodies in the foot. *J Am Podiatry Assoc* 73:514-517, 1983.
47. Rickoff SE, Bauder T, Kerman BL: Foreign body and localization and retrieval in the foot. *J Foot Surg* 20:33-34, 1981.
48. Gilsdorf IR: A needle in the sole of the foot. *Surg Gynecol Obstet* 163:573-574, 1986.
49. Alfred RH, Jacobs R: Occult foreign bodies of the foot. *Foot Ankle* 4:209-211, 1984.
50. Dowling GL: Foreign body: a review of two cases. *J Foot Surg* 21:70-72, 1982.
51. Rhydderch A: Chronic septic arthritis caused by foreign bodies. *J Bone Joint Surg* 42B:405, 1960.
52. Charney DB, Manzi JA, Turlik MT, Young M: Nonmetallic foreign bodies in the foot: radiography versus Xero radiography. *J Foot Surg* 25:44-49, 1986.
53. Kuhns LR: Technical notes: an in-vitro comparison of computed tomography, xeroradiography and radiography in detection of soft tissue foreign bodies. *Radiology* 132:218-219, 1979.
54. Felman AH, Fisher MS: The radiographic detection of glass in soft tissues. *Radiology* 92:1529-1531, 1969.
55. Tandberg D: Glass in the hand and foot. *JAMA* 248:1872-1874, 1982.
56. Woesner ME, Sanders I: Xeroradiography: significant modality in the detection of nonmetallic foreign bodies in soft tissue. *Am J Radiol* 115:636, 1972.
57. Jeffery JI: Surgical excision of foreign bodies. *J Am Podiatry Assoc* 74:229-232, 1984.
58. Fornage BD: *Ultrasonography of Muscles and Tendons: Examination Technique and Atlas of Normal Anatomy of the Extremities.* New York, Springer-Verlag, 1989, pp 38-39.
59. Bernardino ME, Jing BS, Thomas JL, Marvin MM, Zornoza J: The extremity soft-tissue lesion: a comparative study of ultrasound, computed tomography, and xerography. *Radiology* 139:53-59, 1981.
60. Stoller DW: *Magnetic Resonance Imaging in Orthopedics and Rheumatology.* Philadelphia, JB Lippincott Co, 1989, pp 77-78.

Additional References

Cracchiolo A: Wooden foreign bodies in the foot. *Am J Surg* 140:585-587, 1980.

Faust R, Roy W, Ewin D, Espenan P, Brown J: Management and tetanus prophylaxis in the treatment of puncture wounds. *Am Surg* 69:1484-1485, 1976.

Fordham S: The detection of glass foreign bodies. *South Med J* 69:1484-1485, 1976.

Fritz R: Concerning the source of *Pseudomonas* osteomyelitis of the foot [letter]. *J Pediatr* 91:161-162, 1977.

Hikes D, Manoli A: Wound botulism. *J Trauma* 21:68-71, 1981.

Lindsey D: Tetanus prophylaxis—do our guidelines assure protection? [editorial]. *J Trauma* 24:1063-1064, 1984.

Uhren R, Curtis P: Calcaneal osteomyelitis of the newborn: a case report. *J Fam Pract* 11:809-810, 1980.

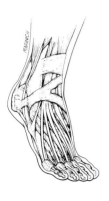

CHAPTER 58

Trauma to the Nail
and Associated Structures

D. Scot Malay, D.P.M.

Injuries involving the nail plate and associated structures are quite common. Acute toenail injuries are most frequently caused by dropping heavy objects on the toes or stubbing the toe into a solid object. Other mechanisms of acute injury include puncture wounds, as well as lacerations caused from lawn mower blades, axes, and other power tools or industrial machinery (1). Chronic nail trauma is usually associated with digital deformities and pressure from shoe gear. Nail bed reconstruction and secondary procedures for perionychial repair commonly produce less than satisfactory results. Therefore it is important that appropriate acute care of nail injuries be provided.

NAIL ANATOMY, PHYSIOLOGY, AND FUNCTION

The perionychium consists of the paronychium (proximal nail fold, medial and lateral nail grooves), the nail matrix, and the nail bed (2) (Fig. 58.1). The proximal end of the nail plate rests in the proximal nail groove, with the proximal nail fold situated dorsally. The stratum corneum of the proximal nail fold forms the cuticle, which adheres to the dorsal surface of the nail plate. The nail plate consists of specialized keratin formed from the matrix cells located beneath the proximal nail fold and extending distally to the level corresponding to the distal margin of the lunula. The lunula is the whitish semilunar area of matrix extending distal to the proximal nail fold and cuticle. The nail bed consists of epithelial cells that do not add to the ventral surface of the nail plate but form a relatively smooth, faintly furrowed (longitudinally) plateau on which the nail plate glides as it grows distally (3, 4). It takes at least 5 to 6 months to grow a new toenail in a healthy adult.

The subcutaneous region deep to the nail bed is highly vascularized, and the nail bed and matrix are situated almost immediately adjacent to the periosteum of the distal phalanx of the toe. In essence the nail bed anchors the nail plate to the distal phalanx. At least 5 mm of healthy nail bed distal to the lunula is necessary for nail plate stability (5).

The plantar toe pulp consists primarily of subcutaneous tissue providing a firm yet elastic pad for contact with the weight-bearing surface. Afferent nerves terminating in the toe conduct touch and temperature sensations, allowing proprioception, nocioception, and balance, whereas digital vascular structures (subungual plexus, glomus) permit ef-

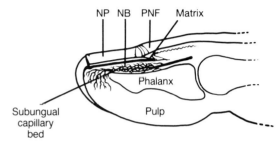

Figure 58.1. Nail anatomy and associated structures (*NP*, nail plate; *NB*, nail bed; *PNF*, proximal nail fold).

fective peripheral temperature regulation. The resilient nail plate protects these underlying structures from injury and combines with the distal phalanx to provide a stable support for the toe pulp as it contacts the substrate.

The sequelae of toenail injuries can cause both functional and cosmetic problems. Nail matrix and bed damage can result in poor nail plate adherence and malalignment. Onycholysis, onychocryptosis, and a predisposition to onychomycosis or bacterial infection may develop following injury. Hypertrophic, dystrophic, and deformed nails with ridges, split-nail (canaliformis) changes, discolorations including streaking and loss of normal nail plate sheen, and pterygium formation (permanent adherence of the proximal nail fold ventral epithelium to the dorsal surface of the nail plate) may occur after perionychial injuries. It has been reported that distal growth of the nail plate is delayed for up to 21 days following trauma, with a resultant thickening of the nail plate proximal to the site of injury (6). The thickening results from an approximately 50-day period of increased matrix activity. During the last 30 days distal progression of the nail plate occurs. Following the period of increased matrix activity (nail plate production), there is an approximately 30-day period of decreased activity before normal matrix activity resumes. Therefore approximately 100 days of abnormal nail plate production can be expected following trauma. The nail plate will typically reveal a transverse groove, or Beau's line, after such an injury (Fig. 58.2).

The nail plate and perionychium are subject to a variety of injuries ranging from minor contusions to trauma causing severe tissue loss and the need for either acute or delayed surgical reconstruction. Such injuries include primary (id-

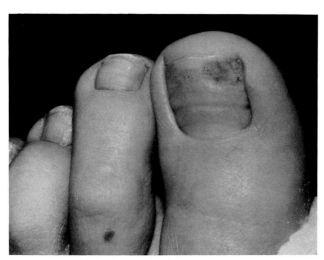

Figure 58.2. Dystrophic nail plate with Beau's line approximately 4½ months following stubbing injury. Note new well-formed nail growth proximally and residual distomedial subungual hematoma.

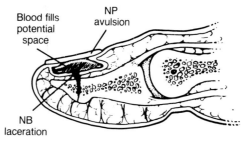

Figure 58.3. Subungual hematoma.

iopathic) onycholysis, subungual hematoma, simple nail bed lacerations, complex (crushing, stellate) nail bed lacerations, nail bed lacerations with distal phalangeal fracture, and a variety of nail bed and toe tip avulsions, amputations, and degloving injuries. Patients with such injuries may seek medical attention at the hospital emergency room or the local podiatrist's office. Accurate initial diagnosis of the extent of injury and proper initial treatment will greatly enhance the chance that posttraumatic sequelae will not develop. The guideline to remember for the acute care of the traumatized nail is to preserve the unity of the toe tip: nail plate, nail bed and matrix, proximal nail fold and lateral grooves, distal phalanx, and toe pulp.

MECHANICAL ONYCHOLYSIS

Mechanical onycholysis is not considered an emergency situation. However, a distinction between chronic mechanical nail injury and pathogenic onychomycosis should be made so that appropriate therapy can be rendered (7). Separation of the nail plate from the underlying nail bed effects a change in the nail plate's refractive index of light, and the lesion appears as a small white blotch in the nail plate. Mechanically induced separation of the distal margin and/or edges of the nail plate from the nail bed often occurs in conjunction with hammertoe deformities and wearing of tight-fitting or high-heeled shoes. Such a separation frequently affects the hallux or longest toe. The lesion may become secondarily infected with dermatophytes or yeast. In addition, the shallow toe boxes of many of today's shoes cause friction of the shoe against the nail, resulting in onycholysis. Associated minor subungual hematoma may also be present, especially in athletes. Treatment is aimed at alleviating the cause of the chronic mechanical trauma and providing appropriate antimicrobial therapy if necessary.

SUBUNGUAL HEMATOMA

A potential space exists between the nail plate and the underlying nail bed and matrix (Fig. 58.3). Digital injuries frequently cause nail bed damage, with resultant subungual hematoma. Unless subungual hematoma is suspected, it may be overlooked because the condition is hidden by the overlying nail plate. When a patient is seen with a swollen toe and reports throbbing pain following a digital injury, nail bed damage and subungual hematoma should be suspected. Subungual pressure secondary to hemorrhage can damage matrix cells and the surrounding healthy nail bed, especially if not relieved within 6 to 12 hours after the initial trauma. Hemorrhagic nail plate discoloration, which appears reddish-blue initially and brownish-black after 5 to 7 days, confirms the diagnosis of a disrupted nail bed. Radiographs of the digit should always be obtained during the initial evaluation of a subungual hematoma, because approximately 19% to 25% of these lesions are associated with an underlying phalangeal fracture (8).

Treatment of subungual hematoma involves draining the blood to reduce subungual pressure. If the hematoma involves an area less than 25% of the visible nail plate, drainage can be obtained through the nail plate with the use of an 18-gauge needle, a No. 11 blade scalpel, a heated paper clip, a hand cautery unit, or the podiatry drill with appropriate small ball bur (2, 8) (Fig. 58.4). The status of the patient's tetanus prophylaxis should always be ascertained and the nail plate cleansed before penetrating it. Although there is no definite guideline, the author recommends that appropriate antibiotic therapy be initiated prior to nail plate penetration. Once the plate is penetrated, blood is expressed and pressure released. A water-soluble disinfectant and a dry sterile dressing with appropriate splinting are then applied. The patient is normally seen for follow-up evaluation in 3 days. If the subungual hematoma involves greater than 25% of the visible nail plate and/or the nail plate has been avulsed into or through the proximal nail fold or lateral nail folds, then a significant nail bed laceration should be suspected and direct visualization of the nail bed is recommended (2) (Fig. 58.5).

SIMPLE NAIL BED LACERATION

When a significant nail bed laceration is suspected, the nail plate is avulsed following digital block and a surgical scrub

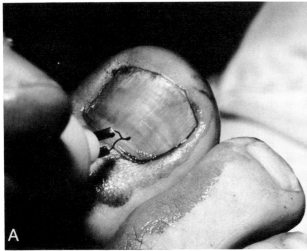

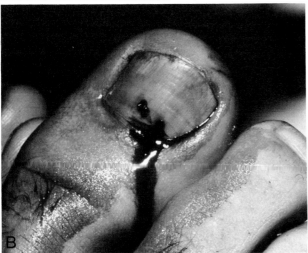

Figure 58.4. **A.** Hand cautery unit used to penetrate the nail plate. **B.** Hemorrhage is expressed through nail plate, with relief of pressure.

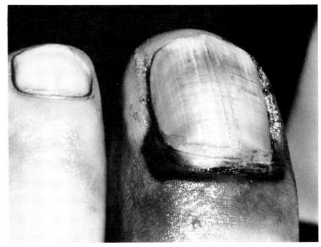

Figure 58.5. Crush injury, with 100% subungual hematoma. Note the dissecting hematoma separating the proximal nail fold epidermis from the underlying dermis.

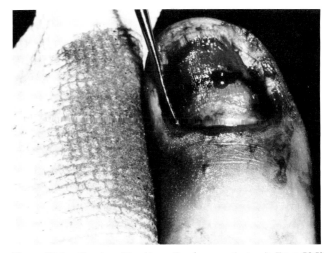

Figure 58.6. Simple nail bed laceration (same patient as in Figure 58.5) after nail plate removal and lavage.

and draping. Tetanus prophylaxis and appropriate antibiotics are initiated. If indicated, a Penrose digital tourniquet may be used for hemostasis. If the toe is too edematous for further fluid injection, a more proximal regional block (Mayo block) is employed and the digital tourniquet is not used.

Once the nail plate has been removed, dilute povidone-iodine irrigation is used to flush away hematoma and debris, and the nail bed is inspected (Fig. 58.6). Because of the friable nature of the tissue, nail bed debridement is kept to a minimum. The margins of the laceration are then meticulously reapproximated with the use of a 5-0 or 6-0 absorbable suture on an atraumatic needle in a simple interrupted fashion. Suturing can be difficult because the nail bed is very friable and intimately adherent to the periosteum of the underlying phalanx. Lacerations of the proximal and lateral nail folds are repaired with 4-0 or 5-0 nonabsorbable simple interrupted sutures on a reverse cutting needle. Care must be taken to avoid driving the needle through the nail matrix. Primary repair of the nail bed can be attempted up

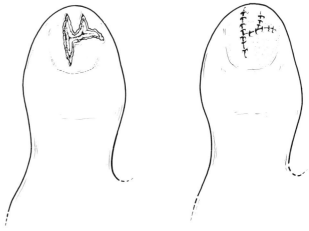

Figure 58.7. Complex (stellate) nail bed laceration. The laceration may occur in any irregular configuration.

to 7 days following laceration, after which time wound contraction and granulation are typically too advanced for accurate nail bed reapproximation (2).

After the nail bed has been repaired, attention should be directed toward preserving or repairing the proximal nail groove and overlying proximal nail fold. Initially it is important to maintain the cul-de-sac nature of the proximal nail groove inasmuch as epidermal epithelization and dermal contraction occur in the proximal nail fold and underlying nail bed. This will prevent posttraumatic adherence of the proximal nail fold to the nail bed and subsequently

will allow the new nail plate to grow out from the matrix without scar tissue impedance (3, 4, 9, 10). It is also desirable to splint or mold the repaired nail bed so that it will provide a smooth surface for the newly formed nail as it grows distalward.

Controversy exists as to what method best preserves the proximal nail groove and the contour of the nail bed. One method, espoused by Schiller (11), involves cleansing and trimming the patient's avulsed nail plate and placing it over the nail bed and into the proximal groove. A small hole may be made in the nail plate to facilitate drainage. The nail

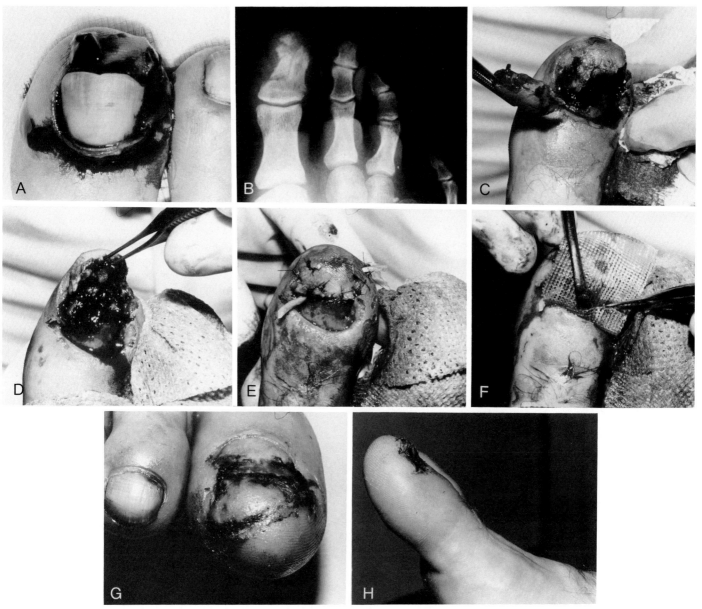

Figure 58.8. **A.** Crushed hallux with subungual hemorrhage, displaced nail plate, and extensive proximal nail fold and pulp injury. **B.** The radiograph reveals a comminuted distal phalangeal fracture. **C.** Removal of the nail plate reveals a complex nail bed laceration. **D.** Displaced bony fragments are excised. **E.** The nail bed and paronychium are reapproximated and a rubber-band drain employed. **F.** Nonadherent gauze is placed under the proximal nail fold and over the nail bed. **G** and **H.** Follow-up at 14 days revealed intact sensation and an even nail bed and toe pulp contour.

plate is anchored with two simple 4-0 nonabsorbable sutures through the nail bed and lateral nail folds, one on each side of the nail plate. If the patient's own nail plate is lost or too damaged, a 0.02-inch thickness of silicone polymer cut to fit over the nail bed and into the proximal groove may be used. The silicone sheet is anchored in the same way that the nail plate would have been anchored. Nonadherent gauze (Adaptic, Xeroform) may also be used, and it has been shown that no significant difference exists between results obtained using the patient's own nail plate, a silicone template, or nonadherent gauze during the acute care of the injured nail bed (12).

If the trimmed and cleansed nail plate or the silicone template is used, a nonadherent gauze is applied atop the nail plate or silicone. This is followed by the application of a single saline-moistened dressing sponge and a dry sterile dressing. A digital splint may be indicated, and the patient may abstain from weight bearing on the affected side. The first redressing is performed 3 to 5 days later. Nonabsorbable sutures used to repair lateral or proximal nail fold injuries are removed after 10 to 14 days, and those used to anchor nail plate or silicone to the nail bed are removed after 3 weeks. The old nail plate or silicone template is usually pushed off the nail bed by the initial growth of the new nail plate, at about 3 or 4 months after injury.

NAIL BED LACERATIONS

Crushing (Stellate) Injuries

Crushing nail bed lacerations are managed in the same way as simple nail bed lacerations; however, the degree of tissue disruption is greater (Fig. 58.7). Accurate reapproximation of wound margins may be difficult, and posttraumatic sequelae caused by nail bed scarification are common. Stellate lacerations of the nail bed frequently propagate through the nail folds, thereby producing large segments of unstable tissue, and concomitant underlying phalangeal fractures are almost always present.

Fractures

Distal phalangeal fractures, simple and comminuted, frequently result from crush injuries to the toe (Fig. 58.8). When the nail bed or surrounding nail folds are disrupted, these injuries represent open fractures and require appropriate local wound care, tetanus prophylaxis, and antibiotic therapy. Small fragments of bone that are exposed to the outside environment should be debrided. If the wound is obviously infected or heavily contaminated, further surgical debridement and delayed closure should be considered. Otherwise, fragments that are in good alignment with minimal displacement can usually be reduced and stabilized by reapproximating the nail bed and splinting with replaced nail plate, a silicone nail bed template, or a surgical bandage. The spontaneous reduction of the distal phalangeal fracture occurs because of the intimate proximity of the nail bed to the periosteum of the phalanx. Large fragments that remain

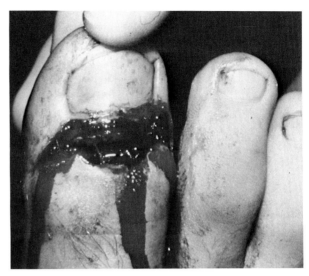

Figure 58.9. Distal phalangeal physeal fracture with proximal nail fold laceration after stubbing injury in a 14-year-old male. Appearance in the emergency room revealed the nail plate to be firmly attached to the nail bed.

grossly unstable can be reduced with a single axial Kirschner wire (K-wire) if necessary.

In young persons the status of the distal phalangeal physis should be assessed. The proximal center of ossification appears in the distal phalanx between 3 and 6 years of age, and the two centers are usually fused by 18 years of age. Severe stubbing or plantarflexory injuries can create a laceration and fracture that propagate along the dorsal surface of the nail plate into the proximal nail fold and through the physeal plate of the distal phalanx (13) (Fig. 58.9). More often this type of injury occurs with the nail plate avulsed from the proximal nail fold. At least the proximal portion of the nail plate should be removed to allow for adequate inspection and cleansing. Lacerations may require primary repair. After a thorough cleansing and debridement, the phalanx can be readily realigned simply by splinting the toe in hyperextension and applying a surgical bandage. Splinting and a surgical shoe are used for 3 to 4 weeks. Antibiotic therapy should be administered, and the wound should be closely monitored for signs of infection. If drainage or other signs of infection develop, further debridement should be performed.

NAIL BED AVULSIONS, AMPUTATIONS, AND DEGLOVING OF THE DIGITS

The chances of a good functional and cosmetic result following acute care decrease substantially with nail bed avulsion injuries and partial digital amputations. Treatment of such injuries varies with the level and direction of the tissue loss (Fig. 58.10). Rosenthal classifies these injuries according to level and direction (5). There are three levels of injury (Fig. 58.11):

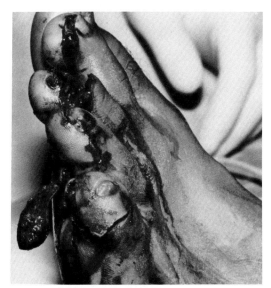

Figure 58.10. Lawn mower injury revealing multiple incomplete digital amputations and severe perionychial tissue loss.

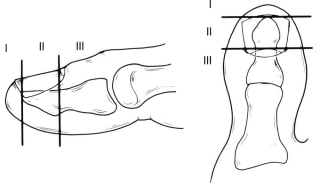

Figure 58.11. Level of tissue loss: zone I, distal to bony phalanx; zone II, distal to lunula; zone III, proximal to distal end of lunula.

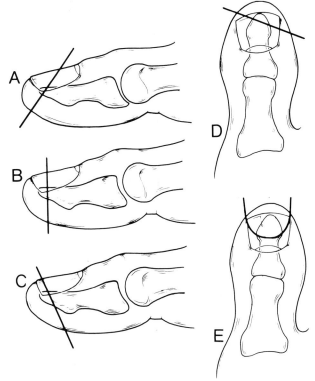

Figure 58.12. Direction (plane) of tissue loss. **A.** Dorsal (oblique). **B.** Transverse. **C.** Plantar (oblique). **D.** Axial (tibial or fibular oblique). **E.** Central (gouging).

Zone I Distal to bony phalanx
Zone II Distal to lunula
Zone III Proximal to distal end of lunula

The directions (planes) of tissue loss (Fig. 58.12) are as follows:

Dorsal (oblique)
Transverse
Plantar (oblique)
Axial (tibial or fibular oblique)
Central (gouge)

Distal digital injuries with nail bed defects within zone I, without exposed bone, can usually be allowed to granulate closed by secondary intention (Fig. 58.13). The injury is cleansed, mildly debrided, dressed with a povidone-iodine–soaked dressing, and the patient is allowed to ambulate to tolerance in a surgical shoe. Redressing is in 3 to 5 days.

If the zone I tissue loss is greater than 1 cm², skin grafting

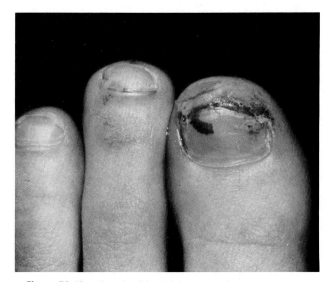

Figure 58.13. Zone I nail bed defect secondary to crush injury.

on an acute or delayed basis should be considered. Newmeyer and Kilgore (14) advocated using a split-thickness skin graft (STSG) on an acute care basis, and they developed a simple and effective one-person method easily performed in the office or emergency room. This technique can also be useful in the repair of chronic superficial nail bed lesions

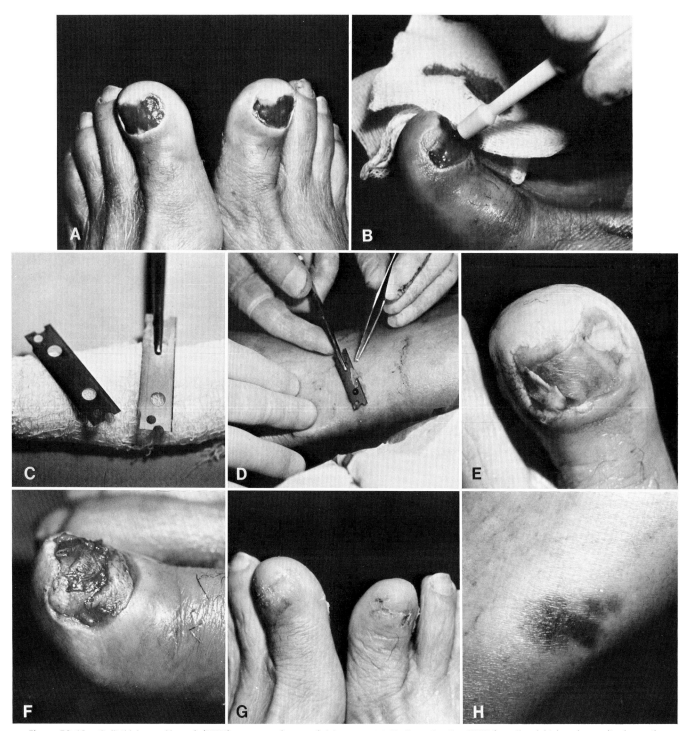

Figure 58.14. Split-thickness skin graft (STSG) coverage of a superficial nail bed defect. **A.** Chronic granulating, nonepithelializing nail beds in an elderly male. **B.** Punch biopsy (4 mm) of the nail bed, performed bilaterally, with resultant diagnosis of chronic granulation tissue. **C.** Makeshift dermatome consisting of sterilized straight-edge razor blade and a hemostat. **D.** Procuring the STSG from the right leg donor site, harvesting enough graft to cover both hallux defects. **E** and **F.** Left and right, hallux nail bed recipient sites following graft application. **G** and **H.** Fully-healed recipient and donor sites, respectively, several months following graft application.

(Fig. 58.14). Newmeyer and Kilgore recommended the use of the STSG on fingertips; however, the use of such grafts for weight-bearing or contact-area toe-tip injuries may lead to poor graft durability. Moreover, excessive contraction of a STSG may require secondary surgical reconstruction (2, 5). For these reasons the author recommends that strong consideration be given to the application of a full-thickness skin graft (FTSG) for digital-tip injuries that display tissue loss of greater than 1 cm², especially in the repair of hallucal defects.

Clayburgh and associates (15) recommended reverse dermal grafts for filling large nail bed avulsion defects and believed that the newly formed nail plate would adhere better to a dermal graft than would a graft covered with skin epithelium. Donor sites for a STSG include the dorsum of the foot, calf, thigh, buttocks, or volar surface of the arm. The FTSG is best procured from the groin; reverse dermal grafts can be obtained from the calf, thigh, buttocks, or volar surface of the forearm. The use of a skin graft requires intact periosteum upon which the graft is placed. Avulsed or amputated portions of adjacent digits too severely injured to be salvaged may be used as autogenous graft sources. Except for emergency coverage of a large defect with a STSG as described by Newmeyer, skin grafting is best performed on a delayed basis in the operating room.

Zone II injuries are complicated by exposed bone and substantial nail bed loss. In the toes, local (adjacent) pedicle flaps are used for both acute and delayed repair of such injuries. The direction, or plane of the amputation, dictates the type of flap to be used. The Atasoy-type plantar (16) (Fig. 58.15) or Kutler-type biaxial (17) (Fig. 58.16) neurovascular V-Y advancement flaps are best suited for toe reconstruction. These procedures can be readily performed in the emergency room or office. A small amount of bone reduction may be necessary to allow the flaps to cover the defect. Nail bed augmentation is best performed by means of the Atasoy-type plantar advancement flap after dorsal-oblique tissue loss. Central gouging zone II defects typically require significant distal phalangeal reduction in order to create adequate plantar soft tissue flaps for wound coverage and proximal nail bed preservation (Fig. 58.17).

The use of distant pedicle flaps is not typically feasible in partial amputations of the toes, unless the contralateral foot or leg is being considered as the donor site. In fingertip

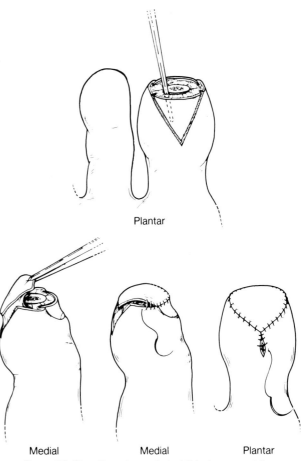

Plantar

Medial   Medial   Plantar

Figure 58.15. Atasoy-type plantar V-Y advancement flap.

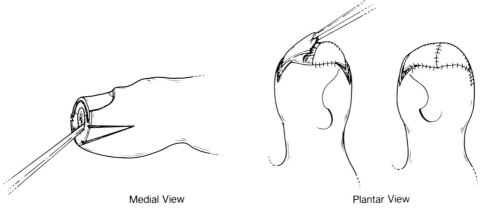

Medial View   Plantar View

Figure 58.16. Kutler-type bi-axial V-Y advancement flap.

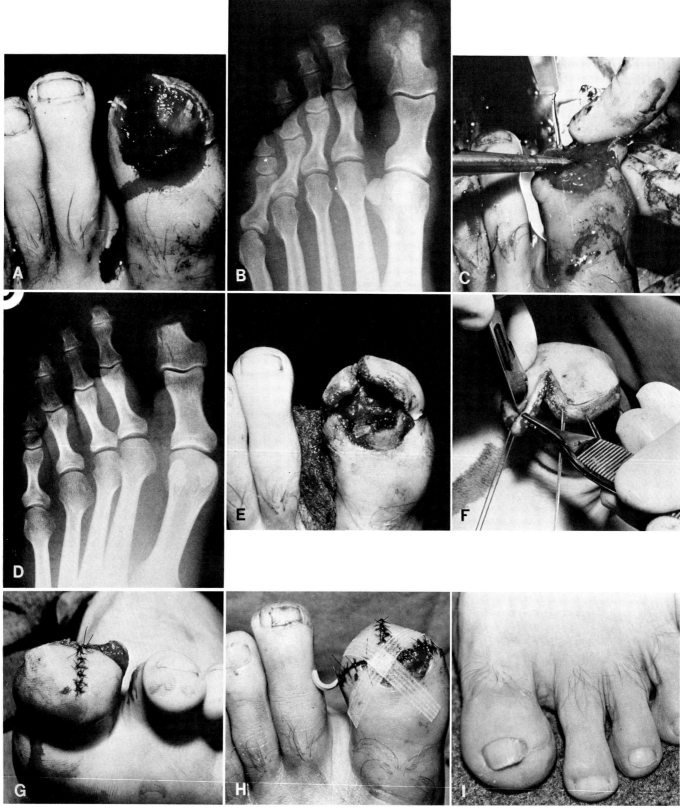

Figure 58.17. Zone II central gouging defect secondary to an axe injury through shoe gear. **A.** Initial appearance almost 12 hours after injury. **B.** Radiograph showing comminuted distal phalangeal open fracture. **C.** Initial surgical debridement in the operating room after procurement of soft tissue and bone specimens for bacteriological and pathological evaluation. **D.** Immediate postoperative radiograph. **E.** Appearance after several days of local care and systemic antibiotics. Note preservation of plantar soft tissue flaps and the degree of osseous reduction. **F** to **H.** Definitive surgical repair of redundant tissues and delayed primary closure, after identification of negative bacteriology results and good wound appearance. **I.** Excellent functional result at 1-year follow-up reveals a mild loss of nail plate sheen. (Courtesy of Thomas D. Cain, DPM)

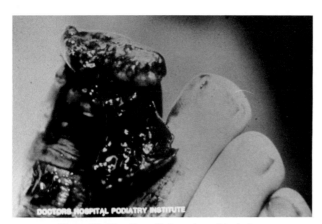

Figure 58.18. Zone III tissue loss, right hallux.

injuries, cross-finger and thenar distant pedicle flaps are commonly used. Because of the short length of the toes, distant pedicle grafts using the ipsilateral foot or toes are not possible.

Nail bed augmentation can also be performed using salvaged nail bed fragments procured from the plantar surface of the avulsed nail plate. These autogenous nail bed fragments are placed in a jigsaw fashion over the exposed periosteum of the distal phalanx. Reattachment of the amputated distal digit as a free composite toe-tip graft is not recommended because results are predictably unfavorable. If too much of the nail bed has been lost (proximal zone II injury) and subsequent nail plate instability is anticipated, then consideration should be given to ablation of the inadequate residual nail bed.

Zone III injuries in the toes are generally not considered amenable to nail bed reconstruction (Fig. 58.18). Proximal nail fold and groove damage is usually irreparable, and ter-

minal ablation of the perionychium at an appropriate level is recommended. Primary amputation is usually performed in the operating room. Preservation of the distal interphalangeal joint and digital tendon function is attempted.

REFERENCES

1. Bornstein B, Profera B: Lawn mower injury: the surgical management of a hallux amputation. *J Am Podiatry Assoc* 70:478-480, 1980.
2. Zook EG: The perionychium: anatomy, physiology, and care of injuries. *Clin Plast Surg* 8:21-31, 1981.
3. Zaias N: Embryology of the nail. *Arch Dermatol* 87:37-53, 1963.
4. Zaias N, Alvarez J: The formation of the primate nail plate. An autoradiographic study in squirrel monkey. *J Invest Dermatol* 51:120-136, 1968.
5. Rosenthal EA: Treatment of fingertip and nail bed injuries. *Orthop Clin North Am* 14:675-697, 1983.
6. Baden HP: Regeneration of the nail. *Arch Dermatol* 91:619-620, 1965.
7. Baran R, Badillet G: Primary onycholysis of the big toenails: a review of 113 cases. *Br J Dermatol* 106:529-534, 1982.
8. Farrington GH: Subungual hematoma: an evaluation of treatment. *Br Med J* 21:742-744, 1964.
9. Kligman AM: Why do nails grow out instead of up? *Arch Dermatol* 84:313-315, 1961.
10. Baran R: Nail growth direction revisited. *J Am Acad Dermatol* 4:78-83, 1981.
11. Schiller C: Nail replacement in fingertip injuries. *Plast Reconstr Surg* 19:521-530, 1957.
12. Zook EG, Guy RJ, Russell RC: A study of nail bed injuries: causes, treatment, and prognosis. *J Hand Surg* 9A:247-252, 1984.
13. Banks AS, Cain TD, Ruch JA: Physeal fractures of the distal phalanx of the hallux. *J Am Podiatr Med Assoc* 78:310-313, 1989.
14. Newmeyer WL, Kilgore ES: Fingertip injuries: a simple, effective method of treatment. *J Trauma* 14:58-64, 1974.
15. Clayburgh RH, Wood MB, Cooney WP: Nail bed repair and reconstruction by reverse dermal grafts. *J Hand Surg* 8:594-599, 1983.
16. Atasoy E, Iokimidis E, Kasdan ML, Kutz JE, Kleinert HE: Reconstruction of the amputated fingertip with a triangular volar flap. *J Bone Joint Surg* 52A:921-926, 1970.
17. Kutler W: A new method for fingertip amputation. *JAMA* 133:29-30, 1947.

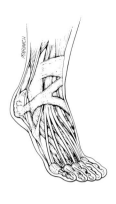

CHAPTER **59**

Management of Acute Tendon Trauma

Stephen Silvani, D.P.M.

There are eleven muscles that originate in the leg and 14 tendons that cross the ankle joint. Many more muscles and tendinous structures originate and insert within the foot. All of these serve to maintain the structural and functional integrity of the foot and are necessary for normal biomechanical performance. Tendon injuries about the foot and ankle are less common, but no less important, than bone or ligamentous trauma. Tendon injuries can result in decreased function, prolonged disability, and subsequent joint destruction if not diagnosed immediately and treated appropriately.

Before a discussion of specific ruptures, dislocations, and lacerations, a few comments on tendon anatomy, types of injuries, and diagnostic modalities are pertinent.

TENDON ANATOMY

Tendons are integral parts of muscles, largely composed of collagen fibers, which run parallel to the long axis of the muscle and concentrate or extend the muscle's action. These cross-linked collagen fibers allow flexibility while maintaining extreme tensile strength. This anatomical arrangement allows tendons to be angulated around bony trochleae or to be restrained beneath retinacula. The combination of elasticity and tensile strength allows tendons to resist or transmit linear forces and produce torque around joint axes, thereby producing body movement and function.

Tendons appear white because of their inherent low density of vascular networks. The blood supply to tendons is provided by a few small arterioles that run longitudinally from the adjacent muscular tissue. These are augmented by vessels from surrounding areolar tissue, paratenon, mesotenon, and vincula. At the osteotendinous junction, periosteal vessels anastomose with the interfascicular vessels. Peacock (1) demonstrated that blood vessels entering from the muscular origin and the periosteal insertion nourish the proximal and distal one third of the tendon, respectively. Vessels entering through the paratenon nourish the middle one third. Tendon metabolism is generally low except in response to injury or infection, when increased blood supply occurs by neovascularization through adhesions to surrounding tissue during the repair process.

The anatomical arrangement of vessels creates certain areas of poor blood supply, especially in longer tendons. These undernourished areas show a correlation with common areas of rupture. In the Achilles tendon, microangiographical studies demonstrate a decrease in vascularity 2 to 6 cm proximal to the calcaneal insertion (2, 3). This area of relatively poor oxygenation undergoes local micronecrosis and is more susceptible to injury from repetitive microtrauma. Areas of better blood supply, the myotendinous and tendo-osseous junctions, are injured less frequently. The vascularity of certain tendons has been shown to decrease with increasing age (4). The clinical correlation of increasing rupture as age progresses lends credence to this observation. Therefore a knowledge of the tendinous blood supply helps the clinician understand and predict certain injury patterns.

The nerve supply to tendons is afferent, with specialized receptors called neurotendinous endings at the myotendinous junction. These monitors stretch and contract, ensuring smooth muscle response. The nerve fibers proceeding centrally are carried partly in the muscular motor nerves and also in small branches to the nearby peripheral nerves. The Golgi tendon organ is located within the tendon itself and is stimulated by either stretch or contraction of the muscle. At certain lengths of stretch, the organ will inhibit the stretch response and provide complete muscular relaxation. This is a means of protection against rupture.

A tendon that runs a straight course from its muscle belly to its insertion without running under retinacula or over bony prominences is covered with a paratenon. A paratenon consists of multiple layers of loose fibrous elastic tissues and vessels that move with the tendon during contraction. Tendon synovial sheaths occur where tendons are subject to pressure, such as under retinacula, through fascial slips, or fibro-osseous tunnels. The sheath consists of a double-walled cylinder: the internal visceral layer that is attached to the tendon by loose areolar tissue and the external parietal layer that attaches to the surrounding connective tissue or periosteum. Synovial fluid lubricates the tendon as it glides within these two layers, thus providing smooth function. These tissue structures must be protected, preserved, or repaired during tendon surgery to avoid adhesions and tendon dysfunction.

The goal of repairing traumatized tendons is to produce a union of adequate tensile strength and to restore gliding function as quickly as possible. (The reader is referred to the chapter on tendon surgery and repair.) A thorough

Table 59.1.
Classification of Muscle and Tendon Injuries

Type	Cause
Direct injury	Laceration (open)
	Crush (closed)
	Puncture/gunshot
Indirect injury	Stretching force applied to contracting muscle
	Extremely forceful contraction
	Avulsion from osseous insertion
Spontaneous rupture	Posttraumatic (single or repetitive injury)
	Pathological (tendon disease)
	Degenerative
Subluxation/dislocation	Acute
	Chronic
Iatrogenic injury	Corticosteroid injection
	Intraoperative complication

understanding of these principles is mandatory before undertaking such surgical correction and explains why certain techniques are favored over others. Atraumatic technique is a primary principle of traumatology. Above all the surgeon must avoid adding extra surgical trauma upon an already traumatized area.

GENERAL PRINCIPLES

Tendon injuries consist of direct trauma, such as laceration or crushing; indirect trauma, such as a stretching force applied to the contracting muscle or an unusually forceful contraction with possible avulsion of the tendinous insertion; spontaneous rupture; subluxation; and complete dislocation and iatrogenic injury (Table 59.1).

The diagnosis of acute tendon injury is primarily made through a thorough history and clinical examination, along with imaging studies. A working knowledge of muscle and tendon anatomy, innervation, function, and topographical relationships is mandatory. The clinician must maintain a high index of suspicion for tendon injury in evaluating the traumatized foot and ankle, regardless of how minor the injury may appear. All muscle function must be evaluated and accounted for in a systematic manner before the patient is sedated, injected with a local anesthetic, or operated upon for fracture fixation or wound toilet. During debridement, all lacerations must be thoroughly examined, with special care taken to evaluate the tendon competence and appearance, especially in seemingly innocuous digital lacerations or deep puncture wounds. Surprisingly, superficial tendon lacerations are frequently missed or neglected in emergency departments and urgent care centers (Fig. 59.1). This leads to future, more complicated reconstructive procedures and decreased function, with increased patient morbidity.

Radiographs are mandatory to rule out not only concomitant or occult fractures but avulsion of the tendinous insertion or injuries to sesamoid bones within tendons (Fig. 59.2). Radiographs also rule out osseous subluxation and fractures that may entrap tendons and are necessary to eval-

uate Kager's triangle (Fig. 59.3). Swelling of the soft tissue or other disturbances may be seen.

Xerography, because of its excellent soft tissue imaging, can confirm the diagnosis of tendon injury. As a result of its current limited availability and its replacement with superior modalities, however, its use is slowly becoming obsolete.

Tenography is the indirect visualization of tendons within their sheaths through the injection of a radiopaque dye. Frank ruptures, partial tears, stenosis, and lesions may be visualized on radiographs. However, this procedure is invasive, technically difficult, and involves potential side effects. False normal results can occur when dye is injected into adjacent tendon sheaths that are read as intact (e.g., dye into the flexor digitorum longus in a search for posterior tibialis rupture). False-positive readings occur when the dye is deposited outside a tendon sheath, causing the misinterpretation of a rupture. For these reasons, tenography is less favored than other imaging techniques that offer superior resolution and ease of use.

Sonography is a nonradiating, noninvasive modality that can image tendons in real time and also provide hard-copy documentation of tears, complete ruptures, and intratendinous changes. It was initially used in examination of the Achilles tendon (5-8), but with the availability of high-resolution techniques, all types of soft tissue trauma have been examined (9-12). Sonography is also useful for following the healing tissue after either open or closed repair of tendon ruptures and for judging the apposition of tendon ends in closed management (e.g., the amount of equinus needed in closed Achilles treatment).

Real-time machines are preferred over B-mode static equipment because they allow quicker identification of the involved tendon, the optimal scan plane, and dynamic examination during contraction and relaxation of the muscle. Linear array transducers are preferred because their beams are perpendicular to the superficial structures (8). A stand-off pad is necessary to improve the contact between the probe and the varying anatomical structures. This also allows visualization of the skin and the immediate subcutaneous tissue and places the tendon in the optimal focal zone (13). Because most tendons and soft tissue structures in the foot and ankle are quite superficial, a very high-frequency probe is used (7.5 or 10 MHz). These probes, which have a short depth of field (3 to 4 cm), give excellent spacial and contrast resolution.

A combination of longitudinal and transverse scans is necessary for three-dimensional localization and visualization of tendinous lesions (Fig. 59.4). Tendon echogenicity and fibrillar texture are easily seen, especially in the large Achilles tendon. Two echogenic lines surround the tendon, representing the peritenon.

Tendon tears, either partial or total, are represented by discontinuity of fibers and the presence of hematoma, which usually appears hyperechogenic. Swollen portions of tendons, usually near the rupture site, will be observed. However, false-negative sonogram results can occur because of the similar echogenic properties of the tendon and the he-

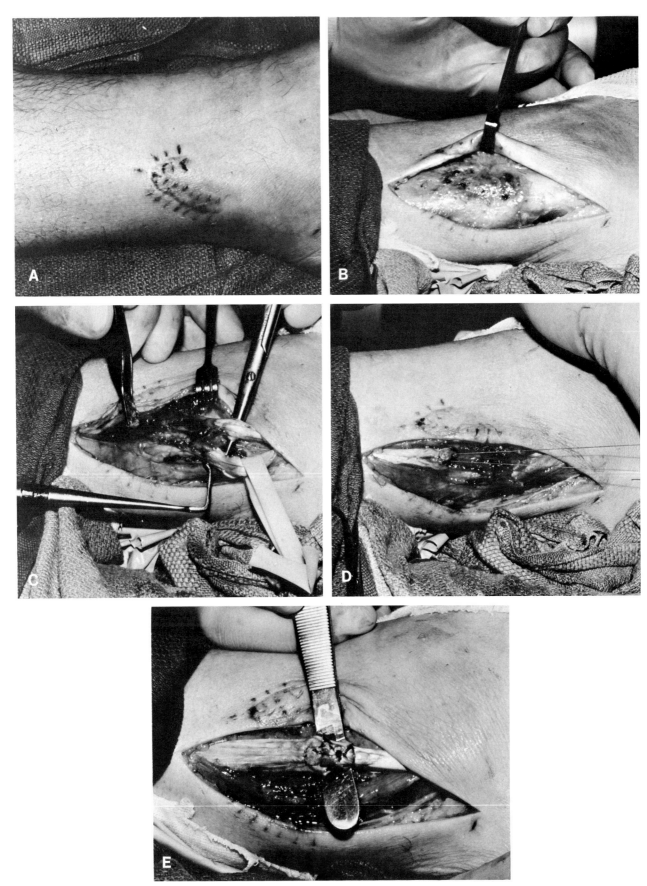

Figure 59.1.   A-E.

Figure 59.1. **A.** A patient suffered a trap-door type of laceration to the lateral leg and was treated at an urgent care center. Three weeks later, he reported difficulty in everting his foot and lateral leg pain. The healed, sutured laceration is shown here. **B.** The hematoma within the peroneal tendon sheath. **C.** A complete laceration of the peroneus brevis is ap-parent. The distal stump (scissors is under) is adhered to deep tissue. The proximal stump (forceps) is retracted. **D.** Modified Bunnell stitch placed in the proximal stump. **E.** The completed tendon repair, before sheath closure.

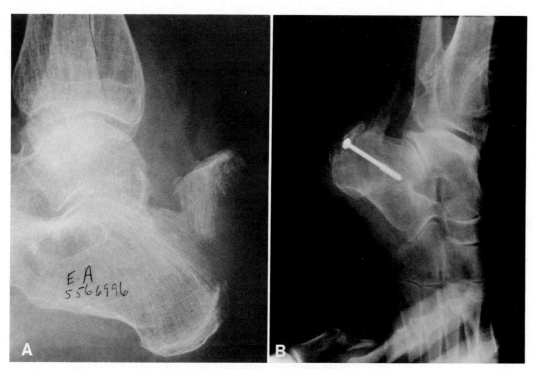

Figure 59.2. **A.** An Achilles tendon avulsion at its calcaneal insertion. **B.** Repair of a similar injury with use of a 4.0-mm cancellous screw reattachment of the tendon to the calcaneus.

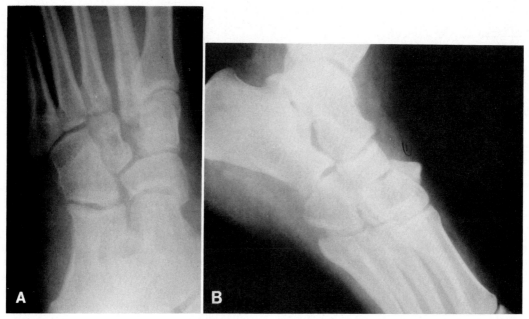

Figure 59.3. **A** and **B.** An osseous dislocation that is irreducible by appropriate closed technique should alert the physician to the possibility of an entrapped tendon or soft tissue. Here the dislocation of the second cuneiform has been maintained by an entrapped extensor tendon to the second digit.

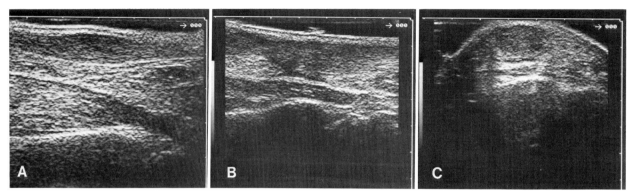

Figure 59.4. **A.** A longitudinal sonogram of the Achilles tendon showing echogenic paratenon and intratendinous swelling of chronic tendonitis. **B.** A healed Achilles tendon rupture at 14 weeks. **C.** A transverse view showing the healing section of Achilles tendon and its echo pattern.

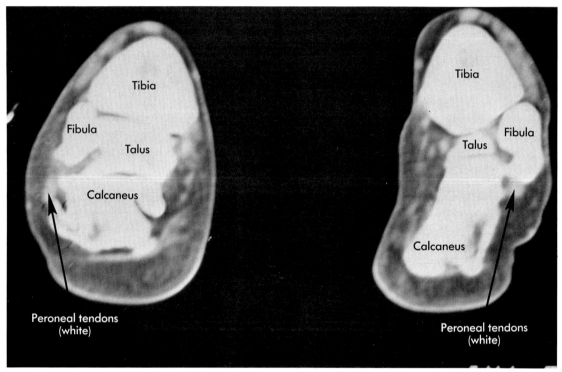

Figure 59.5. CT scan demonstrates the peroneal tendon impingement in a healed, untreated calcaneal fracture.

matoma, especially in neglected ruptures or late examinations when the organization of the hematoma is occurring (14).

Sonograms are useful in diagnosing incomplete ruptures and determining the amount of equinus necessary for closed Achilles tendon treatment. This technique allows the clinician to directly observe the tendon as it functions during contraction and relaxation of the muscle. Thus, partial tears may be observed and recurrent subluxations evaluated.

Obviously, the technical ability of the sonographer and the interpretation of the results can be variable and confusing and are directly dependent upon experience. Only

with continued experimentation will this useful and cost-efficient diagnostic aid advance to its fullest extent.

Computerized tomography (CT) is useful in visualizing the osseous and soft tissue relationships of trauma. An example of this is the CT imaging of the impingement of the peroneal tendons in fresh or healed calcaneal fractures as seen in the frontal plane (Fig. 59.5). Tendons are discretely visualized and calcifications within their structures can be seen, which may be predisposing factors in tendon ruptures. CT is much more applicable for osseous trauma.

The ultimate diagnostic tool for soft tissue visualization is the magnetic resonance image (MRI). MRI shows soft tissue directly and will demonstrate tears, ruptures (either partial or complete), dislocations, subluxations, tendonitis, tenosynovitis, and internal derangements of tendons. The literature is filled with instructive, descriptive, and pictorial articles to which the reader is referred (15-19). An MRI allows superior soft tissue imaging, especially in the delineation of small anatomical structures, excellent contrast resolution, adequate spatial resolution, noninvasiveness, and absence of ionizing radiation. These characteristics make it invaluable in the diagnosis and management of tendon trauma. It behooves the physician treating the lower extremity to become familiar with a local imaging facility that has the necessary technology for extremity visualization and has the interpretive skills required for meaningful foot and ankle studies.

No imaging technique can replace the astute practitioner who, through a high index of suspicion and sound anatomical knowledge, makes a diagnosis of tendon trauma by clinical examination. Scans are adjunctive and must be ordered accordingly.

LACERATIONS

A complete history and physical examination with specific attention to the type of trauma, when it occurred, concomitant injuries, and the state of tetanus immunization are mandatory in the treatment of lacerations. It will be assumed for this discussion that the patient is stable, is a candidate for surgery, and has been provided with antibiotic prophylaxis as necessary. Wound toilet will have been performed as discussed elsewhere.

Many tendon disruptions are treated by surgical repair and postoperative immobilization. Suture selection and application are extremely important because for the first 10 postoperative days, the tensile strength of the repaired tendon relies exclusively on the suture material and technique (20). The sutured tendon can tolerate a little stress after 2 weeks, and limited passive motion can be instituted 3 weeks after repair. A gradual return to full active function and the discontinuance of immobilization are allowed at 4 weeks as the tendon continues to heal.

The purpose of the suture is to hold the tendon ends in close apposition so that primary healing can occur. The clinician must ensure that a tendon does not become encircled or strangled by the suture, thus interfering with the blood supply and prolonging the healing process or promoting necrosis of the tendon ends. Viable tissue must be present at each end of the tendon. If this is not possible following a thorough debridement, secondary or delayed repair is indicated. The grace period for primary repair of tendon lacerations is considered 6 to 8 hours; if longer than that, secondary repair is recommended. If any doubt exists about the tissue viability or wound cleanliness, it is necessary to wait and perform a delayed tendon repair. It is better for the patient to undergo a secondary repair and closure than to develop an infection after a primary repair.

Crush wounds as a reuslt of blunt or oblique trauma ex-

hibit a greater degree of soft tissue damage (Fig. 59.6). Necrosis may not become evident for several days and multiple debridements may be necessary. Usually the surgeon employs skin grafting to achieve final wound closure, making sure that the tendons are first covered with tissue to prevent adhesions (Fig. 59.7).

To ensure strength and healing, nonabsorbable sutures are required for tendon repair. Stainless steel is the strongest and least reactive suture, but its difficulty in handling, its brittleness, and its loss of tensile strength through electrolysis after 3 weeks lead the surgeon to other types of sutures. Supramid is the strongest synthetic nonabsorbable suture before and after knotting (21). It is composed of caprolactam and has good handling characteristics and lack of memory. A braided polyester suture (Tevdek and Ticron) has great strength and resists disruptive forces after 3 weeks better than either nylon or polypropylene (22). Absorbable sutures, such as polyglactin 910 (Vicryl), polyglycolic acid (Dexon), and polydioxanone (PDS), may also provide strength long enough for repair and are useful in reinforcing other primary sutures.

An ideal suturing technique apposes the tendon ends and allows some early passive motion without gaping. The various suture techniques are discussed in detail in the chapter on tendon surgery. Aftercare in most cases of tendon lacerations consists of a cast for 3 to 4 weeks while the collagen fibers are formed, realigned, and gain strength. Passive motion may be initiated at 3 weeks through bivalving the cast or splint. In cases of avulsion of the tendon from its osseous insertion or surrounding fracture, further immobilization is necessary until 6 weeks after injury.

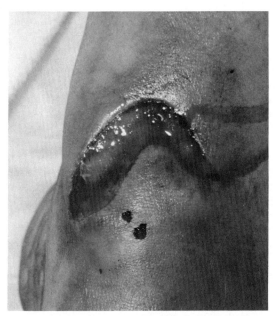

Figure 59.6. An oblique blow to the foot by a falling piece of masonry caused a tibialis anterior tendon laceration and skin damage. This wound (over 8 hours old) should not be closed until sterility and viability of wound margins are determined.

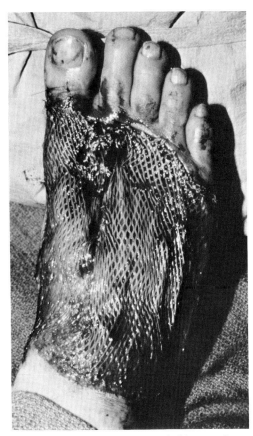

Figure 59.7. A dorsal degloving motorcycle injury requires a delayed skin graft once the extensor tendons are surrounded by granulation tissue. This prevents future tendon adhesions.

TENDON RUPTURE

Tendons are the strongest part of the musculotendinous unit (23). Usually sound tendons do not rupture, but injury occurs at their insertion into bone, through the muscle belly, or at their origin in response to sudden strain. Disease processes of tendons predispose them to injury. Biomechanical abnormalities of the lower extremity, age, decreased blood supply, underlying medical conditions, infections, arthritis, tendonitis, tenosynovitis, calcifications, or cortisone injections all predispose tendon to rupture. When the elasticity of the tendon collagen is overstretched repeatedly, damage will occur, leading to frank rupture.

Tibialis Anterior

The tibialis anterior is a strong dorsiflexor of the ankle and an invertor of the subtalar and midtarsal joints. It is restrained at the ankle by the superior and inferior extensor retinacula. Rupture of the tendon is caused by a plantarflexory force that suddenly stretches the contracted muscle. Tendon rupture usually occurs just proximal (1 to 2 cm) to the insertion (24, 25). The proximal stump may retract and form a palpable bulbous enlargement above the anterior

medial ankle. Rarely, a fracture of the medial cuneiform secondary to tendon avulsion occurs.

Pain and swelling occur along the anterior course of the tendon. Active dorsiflexion is diminished, and no bulge of the tendon will be visualized anteriorly. Dorsiflexion of the foot may be accomplished by the extensors; foot drop and a steppage gait may be observed. Electromyography (EMG) and ultrasound may confirm the diagnosis. Because of the extreme superficial prominence of the tendon, MRI is seldom needed.

Conservative treatment consists of a below-knee, non-weight-bearing cast, with the foot dorsiflexed and inverted for 4 to 6 weeks. Operative repair is recommended for the active young and middle-aged patient. End-to-end repair with nonabsorbable suture is usually achievable if performed early and after freshening the tendon ends. If this is not possible or a gap exists between the ends, a free tendon graft from the extensor digitorum longus or a split portion of the tibialis anterior may be used (26). The extensor hallucis longus may be transferred to the anterior tibial stump at the cuneiform if necessary. The distal portion of the extensor hallucis longus tendon can then be anastomosed side-by-side to the extensor digitorum longus tendon to the second digit for continued function. Any of these repairs require a below-knee non-weight-bearing cast for 6 weeks, followed by a walking cast for an additional 2 weeks.

Extensor Hallucis Longus

The extensor hallucis longus dorsiflexes the great toe and to a lesser degree the ankle joint. Lacerations are common as a result of sharp objects impacting on the relatively unprotected course of the tendon on the dorsum of the foot. Ruptures are rare but may occur as a result of a sudden plantarflexory force applied to the extended hallux, such as stubbing the great toe in a hole while running barefoot. Occasionally, emergency room physicians will suture a skin laceration and not perform muscle testing, thus missing this injury (Fig. 59.8A). A strong extensor hallucis brevis can mimic the tendon's function but will not extend the hallux at the interphalangeal joint (Fig. 59.8B).

Diagnosis of extensor hallucis longus dysfunction is made by clinical examination consisting of active dorsiflexion of the hallux at the interphalangeal joint against resistance. Palpation of the severed stump may be possible if no edema is present. One may notice the loss of the tented appearance of the skin at the first metatarsophalangeal joint because extensor hood function is absent. Caution must be used to ensure that the extensor hallucis brevis is not responsible for dorsiflexing the hallux.

Usually end-to-end anastomosis is possible with use of nonabsorbable suture. The distal stump is easily located; the proximal stump may have retracted within the extensor sheath or lie underneath the retinaculum. A tendon-passing instrument is introduced proximally into the sheath and the stump may be drawn distally. Sometimes various stab incisions may be necessary to locate the proximal end, particularly beneath the retinaculum.

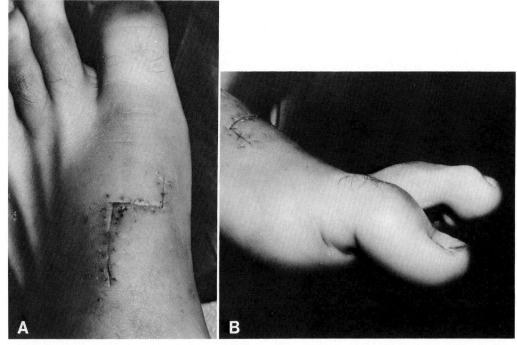

Figure 59.8. **A.** A laceration caused by a piece of sheet metal was sutured without appreciating the lacerated extensor hallucis longus (EHL). Note the skin is not tented as one normally expects when the tendon is intact. **B.** Interphalangeal joint extension is lacking, but the metatarsophalangeal joint will dorsiflex because of the EHB.

In cases of extensive retraction or delayed repair, a free tendon graft of the extensor hallucis brevis may be used. An end-to-end or a side-to-side repair may be used. A short-leg non-weight-bearing cast with the ankle at 90° and the hallux in neutral position is used for 4 weeks.

Extensor Digitorum Longus

Ruptures of the lesser toe extensors are rare. This injury is usually managed conservatively in a below-knee cast for 4 weeks. Surgical intervention is usually not indicated. The severed extensor tendon ends will send out multiple fibrous projections from the epitenon in an attempt to repair themselves. It has been postulated that these fibers adhere to surrounding structures and contract, producing a functioning tendon unit.

Tibialis Posterior

The tibialis posterior muscle plantarflexes the foot at the ankle and supinates the midtarsal and subtalar joints. This tendon courses posterior to the medial malleolus and inserts into the navicular tuberosity with multiple slips into the plantar aspect of most of the tarsal bones (the sustentaculum tali, the cuneiforms, and the metatarsal bases).

True spontaneous rupture is very rare. It was documented in only three cases of a series of 1014 tendon ruptures (27). Most commonly the tendon rupture is due to chronic or acute stress on an already degenerated tendon. Chronic tenosynovitis, pes valgo planus, collagen vascular disease, gout, gonococcal infection, or repeated corticosteroid injections are associated with tibialis posterior ruptures (28). The watershed region of low vascularity is located behind the medial malleolus and is a common site for rupture.

When the tibialis posterior tendon is ruptured, the talus plantarflexes, adducts, moves anteriorly, and is prolapsed at the navicular articulation. The longitudinal arch collapses, the medial spring ligament is stretched, Chopart's joint abducts, and the calcaneus everts. A callus may be present over the subluxed navicular tuberosity or the medial head of the talus in chronic cases. A severe pes valgo planus foot with arch pain may be the presenting complaint after a tibialis posterior rupture.

The early diagnosis of tibialis posterior tendon rupture is often missed. Only two patients were correctly diagnosed in a series of 19 nonrheumatoid patients with this rupture. The average time between injury and referral was 43 months (29). In the acute injury, the rupture may not cause a noticeable deformity and is usually misdiagnosed as a medial ankle sprain. The inciting injury is usually not recalled. Activity and weight bearing increase the pain, which is poorly localized. The patient may notice a progressive flattening of the arch, which prompts seeking attention.

Pain and swelling occur inferior to the medial malleolus. The patient has a loss of forceful inversion, especially when the foot is held in plantarflexion. The tendon will not be palpable as it courses behind the malleolus to its navicular insertion. A functioning posterior tibialis will invert the heel during tiptoe gait; a ruptured one will not.

This diagnosis is more subtle in a patient with rheumatoid

arthritis. These patients routinely experience pain and swelling in the rearfoot and midfoot joints and walk with an apropulsive shuffle. The incident may be diagnosed as an arthritic flare and treated medically. A higher index of suspicion for this rupture in a patient with rheumatoid arthritis may prevent the sequelae of irreversible pes valgo planus.

Imaging techniques may help greatly in establishing an adequate diagnosis. Plain radiographs will reveal a unilateral flatfoot with an increased talocalcaneal angle on both the lateral and anteroposterior projections. Tenography has been replaced by MRI and sonography. Sagittal T1-weighted images are best for visualization of the tendon because they show it longitudinally along its course, and its absence when ruptured is easily identified. Axial images, although harder to interpret for complete ruptures because only cross-sections are shown, are better for longitudinal tears and synovial fluid accumulations. Technical problems may arise if the tendon runs in more than one radiographical plane, and consecutive rather than stepped images may be necessary to distinguish a true rupture from tangential, partial-volume sectioning of a normal tendon. As previously mentioned, an experienced radiologist of the foot and ankle will be invaluable in establishing the correct MRI diagnosis.

Sonography offers an excellent visualization of the tendon in both static and dynamic testing. As compared with the contralateral normal side, ultrasound demonstrates a lack of tendon and a fluid density within the sheath.

Thus far, however, no preoperative visualization techniques accurately diagnose the exact type of the variety of lesions seen during surgery. The four types of ruptured tibialis posterior lesions are avulsion of the tendon, usually 1 to 2 cm proximal to the navicular insertion (Group 1); midsubstance tears about the medial malleolus (Group 2); in-continuity longitudinal tear without complete rupture (Group 3); and tenosynovitis without visible disruption (Group 4) (30) (Table 59.2).

Conservative treatment consists of a below-knee non-weight-bearing cast with the foot in plantarflexion, adductus, and inversion for 6 weeks. A below-knee weight-bearing cast with the foot in neutral position is applied for another 2 to 4 weeks. Extensive physical therapy is used in the post-cast period to regain muscle strength and reduce adhesions. This treatment is best for the sedentary older patient who may not be an optimal surgical candidate.

Surgical repair techniques depend upon the location and type of lesion, as well as the timing. Avulsion injuries are treated with reattachment of the tendon to the navicular using nonabsorbable sutures through drill holes and placing the inverted foot in the below-knee non-weight-bearing cast for 6 weeks. Midsubstance ruptures are rarely correctable by primary repair, and an interposition of the flexor digitorum tendon is used. The flexor digitorum longus tendon is transected at the height of the navicular and either anastomosed to the remaining tibialis posterior stump or sutured by drill holes into the navicular. Side-to-side anastomosis may be performed behind the medial malleolus between the flexor digitorum longus and the tibialis posterior tendon for

Table 59.2.
Lesion Types of Ruptured Posterior Tibialis

Group 1	Insertion avulsion
Group 2	Midsubstance tear about malleolus
Group 3	In-continuity longitudinal tear without complete rupture
Group 4	Tenosynovitis without visible disruption

added strength. The distal stump of the flexor digitorum longus may be anastomosed to the flexor hallucis longus for function. The foot is casted plantarflexed, inverted, and adducted for 6 weeks in a non-weight-bearing below-knee cast.

Longitudinal, in-continuity tears without complete rupture are treated with debridement and synovectomy. Patients who demonstrate synovitis without a visible tear or disruption are treated with synovectomy and sheath decompression alone.

Most patients who underwent the flexor digitorum longus transfer for a midsubstance tear or had synovectomies did well and were pleased with their results (29-31). Patients with the avulsion-type injuries did not do as well. It is noted that none of the flatfoot appearance resolved, but the symptoms did improve in some cases.

When these soft tissue procedures fail to adequately resolve symptoms, when deformity is severe, when significant structural problems exist, or when there is joint arthrodesis, a triple arthrodesis will provide structural alignment and improve the function of the remaining tendons about the foot and ankle.

Flexor Hallucis Longus

The tendon of the flexor hallucis longus arises in the distal posterior part of the leg and courses behind the posterior process of the talus. It then passes under the sustentaculum tali and inserts into the proximal aspect of the base of the distal phalanx of the great toe. This tendon flexes the hallux interphalangeal joint in open kinetic chain. In closed kinetic chain, it plantarflexes the metatarsophalangeal joint, supinates the subtalar joint, and helps plantarflex the ankle joint.

Ruptures of the flexor hallucis longus tendon are rare. The few cases reported in the literature describe a strong dorsiflexory force of the ankle or foot and the metatarsophalangeal joint that injures the tendon (32-34). Traumatic lacerations are more common.

The patient usually reports minimal symptoms. Active hallux interphalangeal joint stabilization is lost during muscle testing. A fusiform enlargement of the tendon may occur with a central rupture of the tendon. Occasionally, a popping sensation or triggering of the hallux is seen.

Plain radiographs are necessary to rule out osseous avulsion at the distal phalangeal level. MRI is difficult to interpret, especially if the tendon rupture is in the rearfoot. Dynamic sonography results will demonstrate the patency of the tendon with flexion and extension of the first metatarsophalangeal joint, but clinical confusion with the flexor digitorum longus is common. Localization of the tendon stump may be achieved with this technique, which is necessary for surgical repair and incision planning.

If primary repair is possible by means of a modified Bunnell-type stitch of nonabsorbable material, the foot is placed into a non-weight-bearing cast for 3 to 4 weeks. Active range of motion is instituted after this period, with eventual return to full weight bearing.

The flexor hallucis longus is very susceptible to iatrogenic laceration during elective or exploratory surgery. Unfortunately, this occurs often during fibular sesamoid removal or apparatus release during hallux valgus repair. It also may occur during tibial sesamoid excision for osteochondrosis or a fracture, particularly from a medial approach. If it is not noticed and repaired, a weak, apropulsive hallux during push-off or hallux extensus (i.e., cock-up toe) will occur. This tendon is also vulnerable to laceration during posterior ankle and subtalar joint release for equinus and during the removal of an os trigonum. Iatrogenic injury must be recognized, repaired, and casted for normal function to resume.

Peroneal Tendons

The peroneus brevis tendon lies adjacent to bone in the groove in the fibula as the tendon passes laterally into the foot. It then inserts into the styloid process of the fifth metatarsal base and serves as an evertor of the foot. The peroneus longus tendon runs in the peroneal groove of the cuboid, crosses under the foot, and inserts into the base of the first metatarsal and the medial cuneiform. The retrofibular sulcus is very shallow and barely contains the peroneus brevis tendon. The peroneus longus is attached via a common synovial sheath, which is anchored by the osteofibrous tunnel of the superior peroneal retinaculum. Distally on the calcaneus, the inferior peroneal retinaculum holds the tendons against bone. Both tendons are weak plantarflexors of the foot and strong pronators of the subtalar joint, and the peroneus longus additionally stabilizes the first ray.

Ruptures of one or both of these tendons are rare and usually are due to strong tendon contractions against an actively inverting foot. Longitudinal tendon rupture occurs when the peroneus brevis splits the longus tendon as it gets caught between the malleolus and the cuboid during forced dorsiflexion (35). The longus tendon has been reported to be torn by a large peroneal tubercle during violent inversion (36) and with fractures of the os peroneus (37). Impingement from fracture fragments of severe calcaneal injuries may cause closed microlacerations or impingement with tenosynovitis that may lead to eventual rupture (Fig. 59.9).

Presenting pain in these injuries is variable, ranging from minimal to severe, and may be located from behind the malleolus to the lateral cuboid region. Careful clinical examination usually differentiates which tendon is ruptured. Many acute anterior dislocations about the malleoli will spontaneously reduce, but the patient may be able to recreate the snapping dislocations by moving the ankle or toes.

Radiographs may demonstrate calcaneal fracture impingements, retrofibular fractures (38), an enlarged peroneal tubercle, or a fractured os peroneum. CT scans in the coronal plane are especially useful in assessing this tendon in relationship to the widened calcaneal body seen in intra-articular compression fractures. Sonography or MRI will demonstrate tears of the tendons or discontinuities.

Conservative treatment consists of a below-knee weight-bearing cast with the foot in a neutral and slightly everted position for 6 to 8 weeks. Surgical repair of lacerations, if possible, is recommended for active young patients with

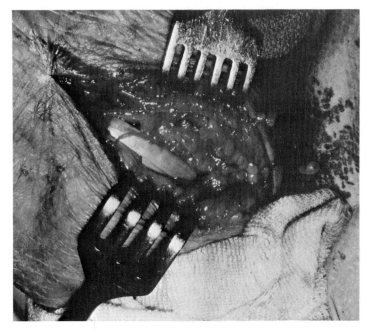

Figure 59.9. The exploded lateral wall of a calcaneal fracture of the left foot (toes are on the left) impinged on the peroneal tendons, which led to chronic tenosynovitis and partial longus rupture 3 years after injury.

primary tendon anastomosis. If not, the remaining tendon stump is sutured to the other intact peroneal tendon to preserve function.

Acute traumatic dislocations occur during violent dorsiflexory forces to the foot. The peroneus brevis tendon subluxes primarily from its shallow sulcus and pulls the longus tendon with it because of the shared synovial sheath. These acute dislocations reduce easily (sometimes spontaneously) and need only a below-knee weight-bearing cast for 4 to 6 weeks to scar down the tendon behind the malleolus. However, the correction is difficult to maintain and most proceed to chronic subluxations. If these cause symptoms, numerous reconstructive operations have been described to restrain the tendons in their shallow retrofibular sulcus and are discussed elsewhere in this text.

Achilles Tendon

The medial and lateral heads of the gastrocnemius and the soleus muscles unite to form separate aponeuroses that eventually form the Achilles tendon. This myotendinous unit crosses the knee, ankle, and subtalar joints. The variably present plantaris muscle and its tendon inserts on the medial aspect of the posterior calcaneus. The Achilles tendon is the most powerful ankle plantarflexor and is necessary for normal propulsion and gait.

This tendon is not encased in a true synovial sheath; a layer of deep fascia overlies a blood-rich mesotenon, which covers a filmy layer that is separate from the epitenon. As previously discussed, the region of poorest blood supply is 2 to 6 cm proximal to the calcaneal insertion and is an important etiological factor of these ruptures.

The sural nerve is located lateral to the tendo Achillis and runs in the superficial subcutaneous layer. It is a sensory nerve and supplies the posterior and lateral aspects of the leg and the dorsolateral aspect of the foot. It is usually visualized during surgery to repair the Achilles tendon and must be protected.

It is commonly accepted in the literature that a degenerative process is necessary to weaken the tendon before it is ruptured. Many investigators have shown the extreme force that the normal Achilles tendon can withstand (39, 40). Therefore the muscle belly, myotendinous junction, or osseous attachment should be disrupted before the tendon substance tears when the leg is subjected to extreme forces. This assumed degeneration of the tendon substance has been proved by several investigators studying the histological changes seen in ruptured tendons (41-43). Chronic inflammation with chronic micronecrosis and chronic repair processes, particularly in the area of chronic microischemia from poor blood supply, predisposes the Achilles tendon to rupture.

Injected corticosteroids have been shown to weaken the collagen cross-linking in tendon and thus predispose it to rupture (44-46). This is in relation to the dosage, type, and frequency of the steroid injection. The fact that cortisone was necessary in the first place implies some underlying pathological condition or degenerative process

of tendon that also predisposes to rupture. Oral steroid use has been shown to increase the chance of tendo Achillis ruptures (47-49).

The Achilles tendon is ruptured when the applied force exceeds the tensile strength of the tendon fibers (whether or not they are degenerated). This occurs with either excessive stretch or contraction, or both. Stretch occurs when the knee is forcefully extended with the foot and ankle fixed in dorsiflexion or the foot is forcefully dorsiflexed with the knee fully extended. The exact joint positions of the ankle, subtalar, and midtarsal joints at the moment of stretch influence the amount of tension or laxity present in the kinetic chain and therefore affect the likelihood of injury. Sudden, very forceful contractions of the muscle may also cause rupture. This is seen in basketball, racquetball, tennis, and other sport injuries or results from patients pushing or lifting heavy loads. The injury often occurs in the sedentary patient who, without proper training, conditioning, or warm-ups, becomes active (weekend athletes or "do-it-yourselfers"). This may also lend credence to the degenerative tendon predisposition to rupture.

The posterior fibers of the Achilles tendon rupture first inasmuch as they are most taut because of their position further out on the calcaneal lever arm. Anterior fibers are frequently not torn, as seen in partial ruptures. Also, the plantaris tendon is less frequently ruptured because of its anterior insertion on the calcaneus, which puts this tendon under less stretch.

Patients generally remember the precipitating trauma and report a feeling of being shot in the calf or hearing a loud pop at that time. Pain is typically not severe initially, and a patient commonly reports finishing the game or tennis set. The resultant weakness, swelling, and unremitting, increasing pain usually cause the patient to seek medical help.

Physical examination reveals a periankle edema and ecchymosis. A palpable gap in the Achilles tendon is usually seen even in the presence of edema (Fig. 59.10). In the case of neglected rupture, this gap may not be seen because of an organized hematoma. The patient is best examined in the prone position with the feet hanging off the end of the examining table. With relaxation, as a result of the tendon discontinuity, less equinus is seen on the injured side. The Thompson-Doherty (or Thompson) test (50) is a reliable diagnostic procedure. It consists of squeezing the calf muscle and watching the foot response. Plantarflexion of the foot is considered a normal response or a negative Thompson-Doherty test result, which indicates integrity of the tendon. Absence of plantarflexion movement denotes a positive Thompson-Doherty test result and indicates severe rupture of the Achilles tendon. Partial tears cannot be fully differentiated from total ruptures, and false-negative results may occur. Patients can actively plantarflex the foot with the posterior and lateral muscle groups even with a total rupture of the Achilles tendon. It is important to examine the amount of equinus on the contralateral, uninjured side. This becomes particularly important during conservative casting.

The detailed history and physical examination usually provide adequate data for a diagnosis, but certain diagnostic

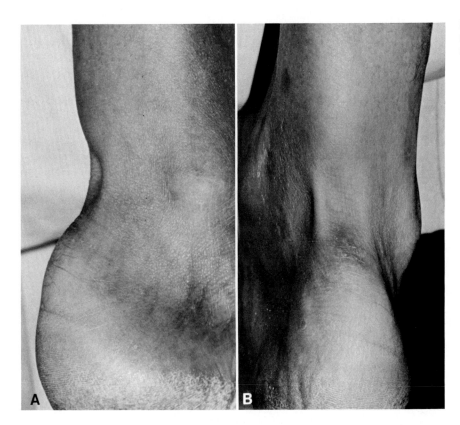

Figure 59.10. **A.** A large visible and palpable defect is present with a total Achilles tendon rupture. **B.** Intact plantaris tendon, medially.

tests are useful. Standard radiographs will rule out any concomitant osseous injury or avulsion fracture of the calcaneal insertion. These radiographs will also demonstrate intratendinous calcifications that may have contributed to the rupture. Kager's triangle will appear blunted superiorly because of the retraction of the proximal stump. Soft tissue swelling and hematoma may also change the appearance of Kager's triangle as compared with the contralateral side.

Sonography, as previously discussed, is an excellent and safe way to visualize the large and superficial Achilles tendon. If a total rupture has occurred, the tendon's continuity and movement are not visualized. The echoes are disorganized within the tendon sheath at the rupture site because the site is full of blood. This makes the site echo-poor as compared with the normal tendon. A dyshomogeneous echogenicity (usually hyperechogenic) of the fat-filled Kager's triangle is seen with a rupture of the Achilles tendon as compared with the normal side.

Acute partial tears give a similar sonographical appearance, but the tendon continuity is preserved with dynamic examination. Neglected tears are not easy to identify because of the organization of the hematoma, which has an echogenicity similar to that of normal tendon. In the conservative treatment of a total rupture, sonography provides an excellent resource to evaluate how much equinus must be used to appose the tendon ends. MRI allows easy visualization of the tendon and helps differentiate partial versus neglected total ruptures.

Much controversy exists regarding surgical versus con-

servative care for acute Achilles tendon ruptures. Either way, the most important goal is to prevent the tendon from healing with significant equinus. Residual equinus will stress the tendon during normal function and contribute to the frequent complication of rerupture seen after either surgical or conservative treatment.

Unless the patient is extremely active or very physically fit, conservative care may be tried in those patients over 50 years old. Primary surgical repair should be considered in the younger or very athletic patient. However, acceptable results have been reported with either method, and conservative care may avoid inherent surgical and anesthetic risks (51-55).

Lea and Smith (56, 57) popularized the below-knee weight-bearing cast with the foot in gravity equinus was used for 8 weeks. No manipulation was performed, and they reported a minimal rerupture rate. The preferred conservative method for the less athletic or elderly patient with an Achilles rupture is a below-knee non-weight-bearing cast for 8 to 10 weeks with a progressive reduction in equinus. The cast is changed every 2 weeks to reduce the amount of equinus. This is followed by 2 to 4 weeks in a weight-bearing cast with the ankle in neutral position. The total casting time is 12 weeks. The amount of initial equinus necessary to bring the tendon ends together may be determined sonographically. Avoidance of residual equinus is the goal; however, further treatment may be necessary if this occurs.

In the conservative cast care of a more physically demanding patient, the amount of ankle equinus needed for apposition of the tendon ends is measured sonographically with the knee flexed approximately 30°. The patient is then casted in an above-knee non-weight-bearing cast for 4 weeks. This initially allows more dorsiflexion and therefore increased tendon length during the casting period. It protects the healing tendon ends better because of the immobilization of both the knee and the ankle joints. This approach more successfully avoids posthealing equinus which significantly increases the chance of rerupture. The initial cast is kept intact for 4 weeks and then is changed, with minimal dorsiflexion of the foot, for another 2 weeks in an above-knee cast. At 6 weeks after casting, a below-knee non-weight-bearing cast with less equinus is used for 2 weeks. This is changed and the ankle placed in neutral position for another 2 weeks non-weight-bearing followed by a weight-bearing below-knee cast for an additional 2 weeks. Usually the total casting period is 10 to 12 weeks followed by vigorous physical therapy and rehabilitation, which are necessary to regain strength and flexibility. Superior results are provided by this method because less equinus is used during the healing, the tendon ends can be initially apposed in good position, and the gastrocnemius muscle belly is not firing during healing, thus not stressing the early tendon union.

Surgical repair for the ruptured Achilles tendon is offered to motivated athletic and healthy patients. With the patient in the prone position under general anesthesia and tourniquet control, a large S-shaped incision is created over the defect. This incision runs from proximal and lateral to distal and medial. The skin and subcutaneous tissue are dissected in one layer and retracted carefully. Meticulous hemostasis is used, and care is taken to protect and retract the laterally located sural nerve and lesser saphenous vein. The covering over the tendon is sharply incised and retracted medially and laterally. After hematoma removal, the ruptured tendon ends are inspected and freshened if necessary. The plantaris tendon should be located and inspected.

The foot is plantarflexed and the tendon ends placed together with use of two modified Kessler or Bunnell sutures of large-gauge nonabsorbable material. These are tied to avoid tendon tissue strangulation and placed medially and laterally to prevent knot irritation with function.

After copious amounts of irrigation, extreme care is used to completely close the paratendon to ensure postoperative neovascularity and to prevent adhesions with the surrounding tissue. The deep fascia and subcutaneous layer are closed independently with small-gauge absorbable suture. The skin is then closed with absorbable or nonabsorbable suture and technique of choice.

With the wound dressed, the foot is casted in gravity equinus and placed into an above-knee cast with the knee flexed 20° to 30°. The patient totally abstains from weight bearing for 10 weeks after repair. The cast is first changed at approximately 2 weeks after surgery, the sutures are removed, and the ankle equinus is reduced slightly, with the foot being dorsiflexed to resistance. A similar above-knee cast is applied for another 2 weeks. At 6 weeks this cast is changed to a below-knee cast, with the foot still in equinus. At 8 weeks the cast is changed with the ankle joint dorsi-

flexed to neutral. At 10 weeks after repair the ankle is maintained in neutral position, and the patient is allowed to walk for another 2 weeks in this cast. Finally, the cast is removed and vigorous physical therapy is instituted. The patient must wear a half-inch heel lift bilaterally for approximately 2 months. This may be reduced to a quarter-inch heel lift for the following 6 to 8 weeks, at which time all heel lifts are discontinued.

During the initial evaluation of the patient with a tendo Achillis rupture, the amount of equinus on the normal side is evaluated. It is recommended that the equinus should be minimized on the operated side to reduce the development of increased stretch across the susceptible healed scar portion of the tendon, which is predisposed to rerupture. Kuwada and Schuberth (55) recommend an intraoperative lengthening procedure as part of the acute repair if preoperative equinus is present. A gastrocnemius recession is preferred because it does not disrupt the primary blood supply of the tissue being mobilized and it uses direct suturing of analogous tissue. The tongue-and-groove recession of Fulp and McGlamry is used most frequently (58). Other techniques for gastrocnemius recession may be used. The goal is to mobilize the proximal portion of the tendon and the aponeurosis to reduce the gap created at the ruptured site when the foot is placed in the desired position of dorsiflexion. It is advisable to perform the tendon rupture repair first and then the gastrocnemius recession in order to adequately ascertain how much additional length is needed. The postoperative management is the same as that described for the primary tendon repair.

Old, neglected, or initially missed ruptures of the tendo Achillis present unusual challenges for the reconstruction of a tendon that will sustain the forces of weight bearing and provide adequate propulsion.

References

1. Peacock EE: Research in tendon healing. In Tubiana R (ed): *The Hand*. Philadelphia, WB Saunders, 1981.
2. Arner O, Lindholm A, Orell SR: Histologic changes in subcutaneous rupture of the Achilles tendon. A study of 74 cases. *Acta Chir Scand* 116:484-491, 1959.
3. Lagergren C, Lindholm A: Vascular distribution in Achilles tendon. An arteriographic and microangiographic study. *Acta Chir Scand* 116:491-493, 1959.
4. Hastad K, Larsson HG, Lindholm A: Clearance of radiosodium after local deposit in the Achilles tendon. *Acta Chir Scand* 116:251-253, 1959.
5. Mathieson JR, Connell DG, Cooperberg PL, Lloyd-Smith DR: Sonographic of Achilles tendon and adjacent bursa. *Am J Radiol* 151:127-131, 1988.
6. Leekam RN, Salsberg BB, Bugoch E, Shankar L: Sonographic diagnosis of partial Achilles tendon rupture and healing. *J Ultrasound Med* 5:115-116, 1986.
7. Maffuli N, Dymond NP, Capasso G: Ultrasonographic findings in subcutaneous rupture of Achilles tendon. *J Sports Med* 29:365-368, 1989.
8. Fornage BD: Achilles tendon: Ultrasound examination. *Radiology* 159:759-764, 1986.
9. Fornage BD, Rifkin MD. Ultrasound examination of tendons. *Radiol Clin North Am* 1:87-107, 1988.
10. Fornage BD, Touche DH, Segal P, Rifkin M: Ultrasonography in evaluation of muscular trauma. *J Ultrasound Med* 2:549, 1983.

11. Vincent LM: Ultrasound of soft tissue abnormalities of the extremities. *Radiol Clin North Am* 1:131-144, 1988.

12. Pathria MN, Zlatkin M, Sartoris DJ, Scheibel W, Resnick D: Ultrasonography of the popliteal fossa and lower extremities. *Radiol Clin North Am* 1:77-85, 1988.

13. Fornage BD, Touche DH, Rifkin DH: Small parts real time sonography: a new "water-path." *J Ultrasound Med* 3:355-357,1984.

14. Fornage BD: The hypoechoic normal tendon: a pitfall. *J Ultrasound Med* 6:19-22, 1987.

15. Sartoris CJ, Resnick D: Magnetic resonance imaging of podiatric disorders: a pictorial essay. *J Foot Surg* 26:336-350, 1987.

16. Sartoris DJ, Resnick D: Magnetic resonance imaging of the foot: technical aspects. *J Foot Surg* 26:351-358, 1987.

17. Hajek PC, Baker LL, Bjorkengren A, Sartoris DJ, Resnick D: High-resolution magnetic resonance imaging of the ankle: normal anatomy. *Skeletal Radiol* 15:536-540, 1986.

18. Daffner RE, Riemer BL, Lupetin AR, Dash N: Magnetic resonance imaging in acute tendon ruptures. *Skeletal Radiol* 15:619-621, 1986.

19. Ziess J, Saddemi SR, Ebraheim NA: MR imaging of the peroneal tunnel. *J Comput Assist Tomogr* 13:840-844, 1989.

20. Ketchum LD, Martin NL, Knappel DA: Experimental evaluation of factors affecting the strength of tendon repairs. *Plast Reconst Surg* 59:708-719, 1977.

21. Ketchum LD: Suture materials and suture techniques used in tendon repair. *Hand Clin* 1:43-53, 1985.

22. Urbaniak J: Tendon suturing methods: analysis of tensile strength. In *AAOS Symposium of Tendon Surgery of the Hand*. St Louis, 1975, CV Mosby, p 70.

23. McMaster EE: Tendon and muscle ruptures. *J Bone Joint Surg* 15:705-718, 1933.

24. Scheller ID, Kasser JR, Quigley TB: Tendon injuries about the ankle. *Orthop Clin North Am* 2:801-811, 1980.

25. Meyr MA: Closed rupture of the anterior tibial tendon. *Clin Orthop* 113:154-157, 1975.

26. Lipscomb PR: Injuries to the extensor tendons in the distal part of the leg and ankle. *J Bone Joint Surg* 37A:1206-1219, 1955.

27. Anzel SH, Covey KW, Lipscomb PR: Disruption of muscles and tendons. An analysis of 1,014 cases. *Surgery* 45:406-409, 1959.

28. McMaster PE: Tendon and muscle ruptures: clinical and experimental studies of the causes and location of subcutaneous ruptures. *J Bone Joint Surg* 15:705-721, 1933.

29. Mann RA, Thompson FM: Rupture of the posterior tibial tendon causing flat foot. *J Bone Joint Surg* 67A:556-561, 1985.

30. Funk DA, Cass JR, Johnson KA: Acquired adult flat foot secondary to posterior tibial tendon pathology. *J Bone Joint Surg* 68A:95-102, 1986.

31. Jahss MH: Spontaneous rupture of the posterior tibialis: cinical findings, tenographic studies and a new technique of repair. *Foot Ankle* 3:158-166, 1982.

32. Krackow KA: Acute traumatic rupture of the flexor hallucis longus tendon. *Clin Orthop* 150:261-262, 1980.

33. Frenett JP, Jackson DW: Laceration of the flexor hallucis longus in the young athlete. *J Bone Joint Surg* S9A:673-676, 1977.

34. Sammarco GJ, Miller EH: Partial rupture of the flexor hallucis longus tendon in classical ballet. *J Bone Joint Surg* 61A:149-150, 1979.

35. Munk RL, Davis PH: Longitudinal rupture of the peroneus brevis tendon. *J Trauma* 16:804-806, 1976.

36. Burman M: Subcutaneous tear of the tendon of the peroneus longus. *Arch Surg* 73:216-219, 1956.

37. Peacock KC, Resnick EJ, Thoder JJ: Fracture of the os peroneum with rupture of the peroneus longus tendon. *Clin Orthop* 202:223-225, 1936.

38. Murr Z: Dislocation of the peroneal tendons with marginal fracture of the lateral malleolus. *J Bone Joint Surg* 43B:563-566, 1961.

39. Cronkite AE: The tensile strength of human tendon. *Anat Rec* 64:173-180, 1935.

40. McMaster EE: Tendon and muscle ruptures; clinical and experimental study on the causes and locations of subcutaneous ruptures. *J Bone Joint Surg* 15:705-711, 1933.

41. Davidsson L, Salo M: Pathogenesis of subcutaneous tendon ruptures. *Acta Chir Scand* 135:209-212, 1969.

42. Clancy WG, Niedbart D, Brand RL: Achilles tendonitis in runners. A report of five cases. *Am J Sports Med* 4:46-57, 1976.

43. Fox JM, Blazina ME, Jobe FW, Kerlan RK, Carter RS, Shields CL, Carlson G: Degeneration and rupture of the Achilles tendon. *Clin Orthop* 107:221-224, 1975.

44. Kapetanos G: The effect of the local corticosteroids on healing and biomechanical properties of the partially injured tendon. *Clin Orthop* 163:170-174, 1982.

45. Balasubramaniam P, Prathaop K: The effect of injection of hydrocortisone into rabbit calcaneal tendons. *J Bone Joint Surg* 54B:729-734, 1972.

46. Mackie JW, Goldin B, Foss MC, Cockrell JL: Mechanical properties of rabbit tendon after repeated anti-inflammatory steroid injections. *Med Sci Sports Exerc* 6:198, 1974.

47. Schuberth JM: Management of Achilles tendon trauma. In Scurran BL (ed): *Foot and Ankle Trauma*. New York, Churchill Livingston, 1989, pp 191-217.

48. Melmed EP: Spontaneous rupture of the calcaneal tendon during steroid therapy. *J Bone Joint Surg* 47B:104-105, 1965.

49. Haines JF: Bilateral rupture of the Achilles tendon in patients on steroid therapy. *Ann Rheum Dis* 42:652-654, 1983.

50. Thompson IC, Doherty JG: Spontaneous rupture of the tendon of Achilles: a new clinical diagnostic test. *J Trauma* 2:126-131, 1962.

51. Beskin JC, Sanders RA, Hunter SC: Surgical repair of Achilles tendon rupture. *Am J Sports Med* 15:1-8, 1987.

52. Gillies H, Chalmers J: The management of fresh ruptures of the tendo Achilles. *J Bone Joint Surg* 52A:337-343, 1970.

53. Inglis AE, Scott WN, Patterson AH: Ruptures of the tendo Achilles: an objective assessment of surgical and nonsurgical treatment. *J Bone Joint Surg* 58A:990-993, 1976.

54. Nistor L: Surgical and non-surgical treatment of Achilles tendon rupture. A prospective randomized study. *J Bone Joint Surg* 63A:394-399, 1981.

55. Kuwada GT, Schuberth JM: Evaluation of Achilles tendon reruptures. *J Foot Surg* 23:340-343, 1984.

56. Lea RB, Smith L: Rupture of the Achilles tendon. Nonsurgical treatment. *Clin Orthop* 60:115-118, 1968.

57. Lea RB, Smith L: Non-surgical treatment of tendo Achilles rupture. *J Bone Joint Surg* 54A:1398-1407, 1972.

58. Fulp MJ, McGlamry ED: Gastrocnemius tendon recession: tongue and groove procedure to lengthen gastrocnemius tendon. *J Am Podiatry Assoc* 64:161-173, 1971.

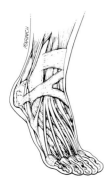

CHAPTER 60

Dislocations

Thomas F. Smith, D.P.M.

Dislocations represent injuries to the anatomical structures that bind joints together. The soft tissue structures about joints provide strength for stability and yet permit freedom for motion. These soft tissues are prone to a multitude of injuries and injury patterns in the various joints of the foot. Their discussion and review constitute a complex study of joint function and anatomy. The disruption of bony continuity in fractures may be obvious radiographically, but the ligamentous damage that is present with dislocation must be extrapolated from the radiographs. This extrapolation is based on a knowledge of local anatomy. Joint damage may vary from a simple sprain to occult joint subluxation. All may represent a significant degree of ligamentous compromise, depending on the pedal joint involved. An understanding of all soft tissues that surround the specific joints is therefore vital to the discussion of specific pedal dislocations.

GENERAL CONSIDERATIONS

As in all trauma patients, a careful history must be taken, and a physical examination must be performed to establish the overall health status of the patient. Both healthy and compromised persons are susceptible to injury. Medications and treatment programs must be tailored to the needs of each individual patient. Coordination of efforts among health care professionals will be mandated by the degree of trauma and the health status of the patient.

A careful and thorough history of the injury should be obtained. Especially in the patient with a pedal dislocation, the how, where, and when of the trauma will help in the assessment of the more subtle dislocations. The history of the injury will aid in determining the mechanism of the injury. Knowledge of the mechanism of injury is of paramount importance in the planning of reduction and evaluation for associated fracture-dislocation injury patterns.

The diagnosis of the dislocation begins with careful palpation of the involved joint area. Subtleties in pedal malalignment may be initially detected in this manner. Careful evaluation of the neurovascular status is paramount to establishing the survival potential of the extremity. Pedal dislocations may imply tremendous force and resultant damage not only to the neurovascular structures but also to the tendons about the area. Loss of tendon function may imply entrapment of the tendon with resultant irreducibility of the dislocation. Breaks in the continuity of the skin must be carefully examined. An open joint injury requires immediate attention and drastically alters the postreduction treatment program.

A minimum of three radiographs of the foot are usually necessary for assessment of pedal joint injury. Significant pedal injuries may warrant ankle radiographs and vice versa to rule out associated injuries. The presence of associated injuries may be the only clue of subtle dislocation possibilities of the foot or ankle. The malalignments associated with dislocations may be very subtle. Main and Jowett (1) reported that a delay in diagnosis in 30 of 73 cases of midtarsal dislocation was related to inadequate radiographs. Fractures may accompany dislocations, and all pedal and ankle osseous structures must be carefully evaluated. The normal joint alignment in all planes must be understood.

Once all these factors have been gathered, the mechanism of the injury begins to unfold. Establishing the mechanism of the injury is important for two reasons. The reduction maneuvers of dislocations are primarily, first, an exaggeration and then a reversal of the original injury pattern. Further, associated injuries about the joint may be evaluated more logically if the mechanism of injury can be determined. Some injury patterns are predictable, and the components should not be missed if a pattern of injury is established.

Once the injury has been assessed and the mechanism identified, reduction maneuvers may be planned and executed. Postreduction radiographs should be carefully evaluated for fractures or dislocations hidden by osseous overlap and malalignment in the prereduction films. According to the specific injury, certain sequelae are predictable complications of the injury. The patient must be informed of the potential complications of these injuries. Postreduction dislocation radiographs without fracture appear normal; however, the extra-articular damages can have a devastating prognosis, even in a properly managed patient. There is no substitute for a well-informed patient. These factors will be reviewed under the discussion of specific pedal joints.

SUBTALAR JOINT DISLOCATION

According to Shands (2), the first case involving subtalar joint dislocation was reported in the literature in 1811 by Judey and Dufaurest. The incidence of this dislocation is estimated to be approximately 1% of all dislocations (3, 4). Subtalar dislocations have appeared in the medical literature under many names including luxatio pedis sub talo, subastragalar dislocation, and peritalar dislocation (5).

Talocalcaneonavicular joint dislocation is probably the

most descriptive heading. The injury actually involves not only the subtalar joint but the talonavicular joint as well (6). Currently the term most used is *subtalar dislocation*. The injury is categorized according to the direction the foot takes in relation to the talus after the injury. In medial subtalar dislocation the calcaneus is medial to the talus. In a lateral subtalar dislocation the foot and calcaneus are lateral to the talus. In anterior dislocation the foot is anterior to the talus. In posterior subtalar dislocation the foot is posterior to the talus.

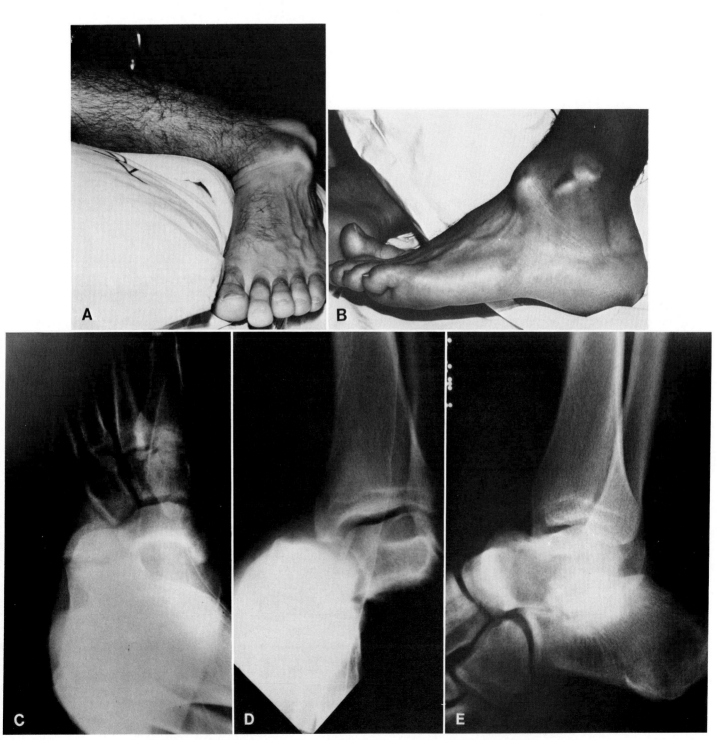

Figure 60.1.   Medial subtalar dislocation. **A** and **B.** Clinical presentation. **C** to **E.** Radiographic presentation.

Figure 60.2. Associated fractures and sub-talar dislocation. **A.** Medial subtalar dislocation with inversion force. **B.** Lateral subtalar dislocation with eversion force.

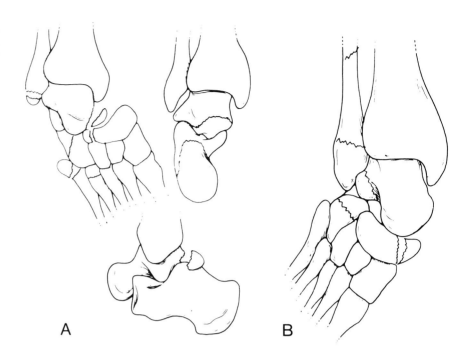

CLASSIFICATION

The most common dislocation pattern reported in the medical literature is the medial subtalar dislocation (2, 3, 7-9). The appearance and incidence have prompted some authors to describe the injury as basketball foot or the acquired clubfoot (10-12). Larsen (11) described the mechanism of medial subtalar joint dislocation as a forceful inversion of the foot. The sustentaculum tali acts as a fulcrum for the posterior body of the talus to produce the dislocation (Fig. 60.1). Two anatomically distinct joints are disrupted in this injury. It is important to note the sequence of disruption. The talonavicular joint is dislocated first. A rotary subluxation of the subtalar joint then occurs as the calcaneus proceeds medially under the talus. Leitner (13) believed that subtalar dislocation represented the primary stage of a total dislocation of the tarsus and ankle. The ankle is already weakened by this injury, and further inversion force could produce gross ankle dislocation. Inversion-type ankle fractures may accompany this injury. The medial swivel dislocation of the midtarsal joint described by Main and Jowett (1) may actually be the first stage of this injury that has not progressed through the subtalar joint. This force of inversion may produce predictable injuries at remote sites in the foot as well. The associated injuries and their incidence were summarized by Christensen and associates (8). With the force of inversion, lateral column avulsion and rupture injuries may occur along with medial column crush-type injuries of the respective osseous and soft tissues. Fracture of either the lateral navicular or dorsomedial head of the talus and fracture of the posterior process of the talus are the most common (Fig. 60.2).

Lateral subtalar dislocation results from forced eversion of the tarsus. The anterior calcaneal process acts as a fulcrum for the anterolateral corner of the talus (14). The joint disruptions of this injury also follow a sequential pattern. First the head of the talus is forced through the talonavicular joint capsule medially. The subtalar joint itself is disrupted as the calcaneus is forced laterally beneath the talus and the leg (Fig. 60.3).

The talus in both medial and lateral subtalar joint dislocations can be considered fixed in the ankle as part of the leg. The foot, including the calcaneus, is disrupted from the leg about the talar articulations with the navicular and the calcaneus. The calcaneocuboid joint remains congruous.

ANATOMIC CONSIDERATIONS

The ligaments that normally support these joints are disrupted. The subtalar joint is reinforced by a joint capsule. Thickenings within the capsule known as the medial and lateral talocalcaneal ligaments help bind the joint medially and laterally. The sinus tarsi contains the interosseous talocalcaneal ligament. It is composed of thickenings of the anterior aspect of the subtalar joint and the posterior aspect of the talocalcaneonavicular joint capsules. The ligamentum cervicis lies at the lateral aspect of the sinus tarsi attached to the neck of the talus and below to the calcaneus (15). These ligaments are all disrupted after subtalar joint dislocations.

The talocalcaneonavicular joint complex is supported by its joint capsule or by the talonavicular ligament. The ligament surrounds the joint and blends into the deltoid ligament as the two main supporting structures of the joint. The talar head punctures this ligament medially and dorsally as the first phase of a subtalar dislocation (Fig. 60.4). The bifurcate ligament and the spring ligament are the only ligaments of the subtalar and talonavicular joints that are not disrupted in this injury. Their attachments do not include the talus directly. They remain intact within the foot, whether medial or lateral dislocations of the subtalar joint occur. The calcaneocuboid and navicular relationships and ligaments remain intact.

A very important consideration is that ankle ligaments are also involved in this injury. Buckingham (14) created medial and lateral subtalar dislocations in cadavers in an effort to assess ankle ligamentous injury. He found that the ankle ligament injury was the same in both medial and lateral dislocations. The deep portions of both the deltoid and the calcaneofibular ligaments were torn. This is understandable since both ligaments cross the subtalar joint, binding the calcaneus to the ankle. The deltoid ligament inserts along the sustentaculum tali of the calcaneus from the tibia. The calcaneofibular ligament attaches to the midportion of the lateral surface of the calcaneus from the fibula (15). Ankle instability, stiffness, and pain are potential sequelae of subtalar dislocation.

DIAGNOSIS

Clinical assessment of medial subtalar dislocations demonstrate the head of the talus palpable on the dorsum of the foot. Anatomically, the talar head is disarticulated, lying between the extensor hallucis longus and the extensor digitorum longus. It actually rests dorsally on the navicular or cuboid. The skin overlying the talar head may be tight and blanched. Skin necrosis and loss are possible if reduction is delayed. The heel is displaced medially with respect to the leg. The medial border of the foot appears shortened, while the lateral border appears lengthened. The digits may appear dorsiflexed. The lateral process of the talus is easily

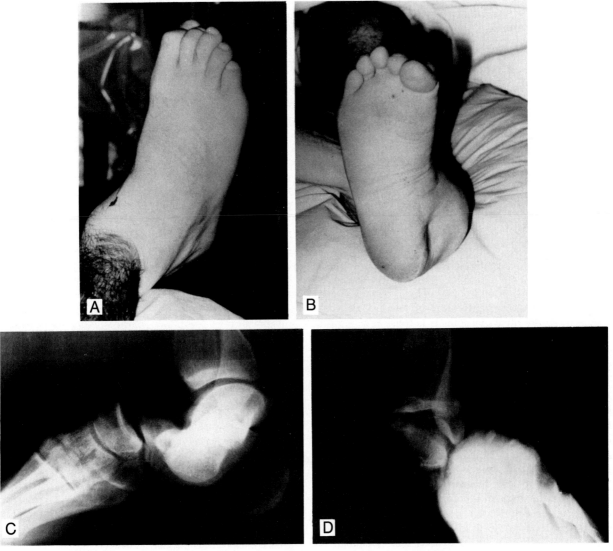

Figure 60.3. Lateral subtalar dislocation. **A** and **B.** Clinical presentation. **C** and **D.** Radiographic presentation.

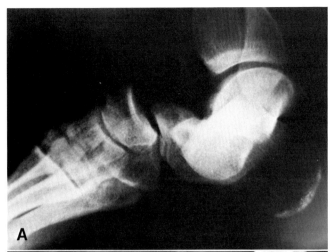

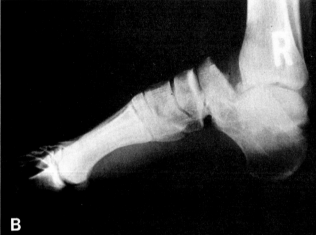

Figure 60.4. **A.** Classic subtalar dislocation with disruption of talonavicular and subtalar joints. **B.** Hawkins II talar neck fracture and subtalar joint disruption. This may be a radiographic but not necessarily a clinical diagnosis.

palpable. Medially, the sustentaculum tali and navicular are palpable, while the tibial malleolus is not visible (Fig. 60.1 A and B).

Radiographic examination of a medial subtalar dislocation should include ankle and foot studies. The presence of inversion-type ankle fracture patterns should be looked for along with the associated foot fractures mentioned previously. Ankle injuries may require fixation and alter the postreduction treatment programs. The anterior ankle radiograph shows the foot displaced medially through the subtalar joint with the talus intact in the ankle mortise. Lateral radiographs of the foot and ankle will demonstrate overlap of the talus with the tarsal bones and no clear subtalar joint. Depending on the angle of the x-ray tube, the head of the talus may be visible dorsal to the midtarsal bones. The foot appears more as it would in an oblique radiograph. The calcaneocuboid joint remains congruous. The dorsoplantar radiograph exhibits a medially displaced navicular with a nonarticular talonavicular joint. Kite's angle is negative (Fig. 60.1 C to E).

Clinically, the lateral subtalar dislocation shows the foot laterally displaced to the leg. The lateral border appears shortened, whereas the medial border appears lengthened. The digits appear plantarflexed because of the stretch of tarsal canal structures. The talar head is palpable medially, and the fibular malleolus is not visible laterally (Fig. 60.3 A and B).

Radiographic evaluation of lateral subtalar dislocation should include studies of both the ankle and the foot. Associated eversion-type ankle injuries are possible. Foot fractures remote from and about the dislocation should also be ruled out. As in medial subtalar dislocations, lateral radiographs demonstrate overlap of the tarsal bones without a demonstrable subtalar joint. Anterior ankle radiographs reveal an intact ankle mortise and talus with the foot laterally displaced. The calcaneocuboid joint remains congruous, and the navicular is laterally displaced from the talus in the anteroposterior foot radiograph. Lateral dislocations seem more likely to be associated with fractures than medial dislocations (7) (Fig. 60.2).

TREATMENT

Reduction of these dislocations requires an understanding of the mechanism of the injury. Generally reduction is a procedure that requires general or spinal anesthesia. Intravenous muscle relaxants may be needed to relax muscle spasms and splinting about the tarsal joints and ankle. Reduction of the dislocation should proceed as quickly as possible to relieve pressure on vital structures and relax skin tension over the bony prominences created by the injury. The reduction maneuvers are based on the mechanism of injury and the sequence of events involved in the dislocation. The reduction is accomplished by first exaggerating the existing deformity and then reversing the forces that produced the dislocation (15).

Initially, distal traction is applied to the heel and countertraction is applied to a flexed knee. This helps relax the gastrocnemius muscle to facilitate reduction. Relocation of the talocalcaneal component of the subtalar joint dislocation is accomplished by forced inversion, which is followed by a return to the neutral position of the calcaneus while the distal traction force is maintained. The talonavicular component may then be reduced by downward pressure on the head of the talus while the foot is plantarflexed. Dorsiflexing and pronating the subtalar and midtarsal joints about the talus then relocate the head of the talus with the navicular. Certain obstacles may prevent a successful closed reduction. These obstacles include impaction of the navicular with the talar head, talar head buttonholing of the extensor retinaculum, peroneal tendons about the talar head, and talar head buttonholing of the extensor digitorum brevis muscle belly (3). Leitner (3) has suggested closed reduction maneuvers that help overcome these obstacles.

Open reduction may be indicated in resistant cases to release the talar head from entrapment in local soft tissue or osseous structures. The incision is placed laterally over the head of the talus and oriented proximal to distal. Any structures that bind the head of the talus may then be released, permitting reduction.

The maneuvers for reduction of lateral subtalar dislocations follow the same principles as those for medial dislocations. Distal traction is applied to the calcaneus about a flexed knee. Relocation of the talocalcaneal joint is accomplished first because this phase of the injury occurred last. The foot is forcefully everted, and this is followed by inversion about the talus to a neutral position. The talonavicular joint is reduced by pressure on the head of the talus with the foot held pronated. The tibialis posterior tendon (3, 16), long flexor tendon (6), or impaction fracture of the navicular and talus (14) may prevent closed reduction. Open reduction is carried out through an incision lateral to the head of the talus oriented proximal to distal. Structures that may be binding the head of the talus may be released, and compromise of medial skin is thus avoided.

After reduction, bulky compression dressings are applied. These dressings are maintained and vascular status is monitored until swelling is controlled. Generally, these dressings are maintained for 3 to 5 days. Internal fixation or percutaneous wire fixation is generally not indicated for subtalar dislocation alone. Fixation may be indicated for fractures associated with the injury. Kenwright and Taylor (17) reported an unstable reduction of the subtalar joint requiring fixation associated with a fracture of the sustentaculum tali. Postreduction radiographs are mandatory for assessment of the adequacy of reduction. Examination for fractures near or remote from the dislocation should be repeated. Hidden fractures may be more evident now than with the overlap of osseous structures in the radiographs taken before reduction.

As devastating as these injuries may seem, the long-term disabilities and complications have not been reported to be severe (5, 7-9, 11, 14, 17, 18). Skin necrosis is the most immediate complication encountered. Christensen and associates (8) reported skin necrosis in 3 of 30 patients, one requiring grafting. Sharit and Cole (19) pointed to the importance of monitoring skin blisters.

The long-term complications resulting from this injury include postural deformations, ankle instability, avascular necrosis of the talus, arthritis, and pain (8). Avascular necrosis of the talus is not considered a common complication of subtalar dislocation as an isolated injury (8, 9, 18). In 1944 Plewes and McKelvey (20) first reported the absence of this complication. Two cases have appeared in the literature with associated fractures of the posterior process of the talus (7, 8). Damage to the posterior talus may compromise a circulation already affected by damage to the vessels of the sinus tarsi. This appears to increase the risk of avascular necrosis. If posterior process fracture is present, careful monitoring of the talus is indicated. Subtalar dislocations associated with ankle dislocations have a poor prognosis, with avascular necrosis of the talus a strong possibility.

Stiffness of the subtalar joint has been consistently noted. A limited range of motion is not necessarily related to dis-

ability and pain (7, 9, 14). Radiographic changes in the posterior facet of the subtalar joint appear most frequently. Monson and Ryan (9) noted pain about the talonavicular joint when tarsal pain existed after this injury. They did not note significant subtalar joint pain.

These injuries have traditionally been treated with non-weight-bearing below-the-knee cast immobilization for 4 to 6 weeks. An interesting finding has been that subjective long-term pain is greater when associated injuries have required prolonged immobilization (8, 14). Current trends in treatment are to promote early ambulation with the protection of a below-the-knee cast. Guarded weight-bearing cast support has been used as initial treatment in these cases. Minimal residual pain has been noted. A reduction in range of motion was noted in all cases. Physical therapy modalities, including whirlpool and range of motion exercises, were continued for an average of 3 to 4 months. Early results after an average of 2 years have been encouraging. This bears out McKeever's findings in 1963 that early guarded ambulation helps prevent subtalar stiffness and pain (21).

The recommended treatment includes 2 weeks of non-weight-bearing immobilization followed by 4 weeks of guarded weight bearing in a cast. Aggressive physical therapy is then instituted for a minimum of 3 months. Occasionally, persistent stiffness and pain may be alleviated by manipulation with the use of general anesthesia. Those who do not respond may require triple arthrodesis. Subtalar fusion alone has not proved adequate to eliminate pain.

ANTERIOR AND POSTERIOR DISLOCATIONS

Anterior and posterior dislocations of the subtalar joint have been reported but are extremely rare (10). Posterior dislocations result from falls from a height on an outstretched foot in a plantarflexed position (11). Clinically, the longitudinal axis of the foot appears normal. The forefoot appears shortened, with the heel protruding posteriorly (Fig. 60.5). Reduction is carried out by reversal of the mechanism of injury. Heel traction is first applied to disengage the dislocation for reduction while the patient is under general anesthesia. The foot then is dorsiflexed on the talus (22).

Anterior dislocation results from a fall from a height onto a dorsiflexed foot. Clinically, the foot appears lengthened longitudinally with a flattened heel (11). Reduction is carried out by reversal of the mechanism of injury while the patient is under general anesthesia. The foot is first distracted distally with heel traction. It is then forcefully directed backward under the talus (22).

Both injuries involve a disruption of the talonavicular and subtalar joints. Postreduction management is as for closed reduction of medial or lateral subtalar dislocations.

MIDTARSAL JOINT DISLOCATIONS

Trauma to the midtarsal or Chopart's joint is a relatively common foot injury and is frequently overlooked. Main and Jowett (1) reported that in 30 of 73 cases, diagnosis was delayed because of inadequate radiographs. They recommend anteroposterior, lateral, and oblique views for diagnosis and postreduction assessment. The distinguishing factor in differentiating this injury from a subtalar dislocation is the relatively intact talocalcaneal relationship. Both injuries may involve a talonavicular dislocation.

Main and Jowett (1) proposed a classification system based on the mechanism of injury. They defined midtarsal joint injuries according to the direction of force producing the dislocation. For example, medial force injury is defined by a force directed against the lateral aspect of the foot in a medial direction. The forces that produce these injuries make up the basis for the classification system. The classification includes medial force injury, longitudinal force injury, compression force injury, lateral force injury, plantar force injury, and crush force injury. They also proposed a

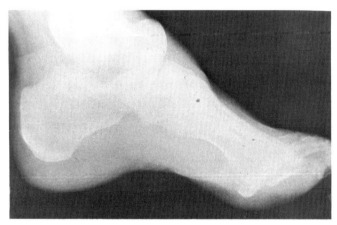

Figure 60.5.   Posterior subtalar dislocation.

new classification that includes swivel injury or tarsal rotation injury. This dislocation may occur within either medial or lateral force injury classifications. Main and Jowett noted no incidence in pure dorsal injury. They agreed with Wilson (23) and Wiley (24) that such force will produce injury, primarily at Lisfranc's joint. Radiographs and clinical appearance will be used to highlight these injuries and demonstrate their objective findings.

Medial force results in three grades of injury. The first type—fracture sprain—may demonstrate only flake fractures of the talus or navicular dorsally and avulsion fractures of the calcaneus and cuboid laterally (Fig. 60.6). The second type is fracture subluxations or dislocations. They are evidenced by a medially displaced forefoot and a normal talocalcaneal relationship. The third or swivel dislocation may be considered similar to the first step of a subtalar dislocation. The mechanism appears to be a rotation of the midtarsal joint about an axis that corresponds to the interosseous talocalcaneal joint. The calcaneocuboid joint remains intact (Fig. 60.7). The subtalar joint is subtly subluxed and deviated, not totally disrupted.

Longitudinal forces result in navicular fractures of varying degrees, depending on where compression of the navicular occurs between the talus and cuneiforms. This is a serious injury to the articular portions of the navicular both proximally and distally (Fig. 60.8).

Lateral forces or forces directed to the medial foot in a lateral direction, demonstrate three grades of injury similar to medial force injuries. Fracture sprains are clinically demonstrated by pull-off fractures of the navicular tuberosity, flake fractures over the dorsal talus or navicular, and/or impaction fractures of the cuboid (Fig. 60.9). Fracture subluxations occur from greater force and may result in a talo-

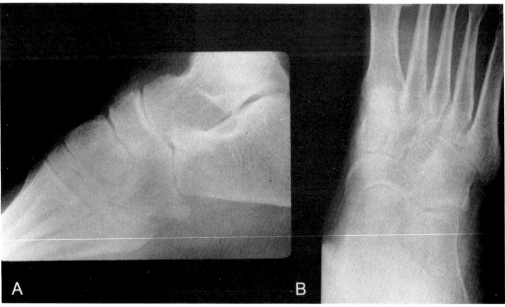

Figure 60.6.   Medial force midtarsal fracture sprain. **A.** Dorsal talonavicular joint flake fractures. **B.** Calcaneocuboid joint avulsion fracture.

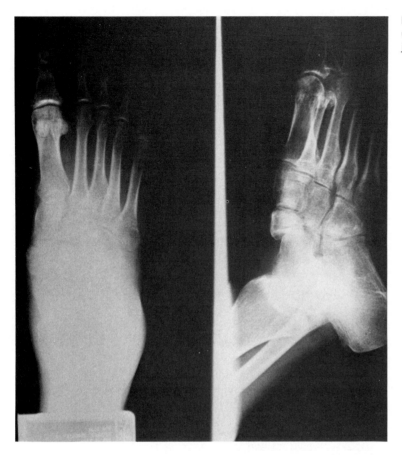

Figure 60.7. Medial swivel dislocation of the talonavicular joint (diagnosis missed 6 months). Note talonavicular joint incongruity with subtalar joint congruity.

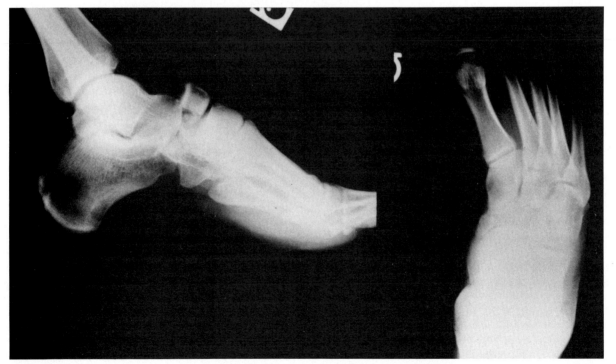

Figure 60.8. Longitudinal compression injury of the midtarsal joint. Note fractures of the navicular and the adductus attitude of the foot.

Figure 60.9. Lateral force midtarsal fracture sprain. Note the avulsion fracture and edema of the local soft tissues about the navicular tuberosity, left foot. This possibly represents a disruption of a type II accessory navicular.

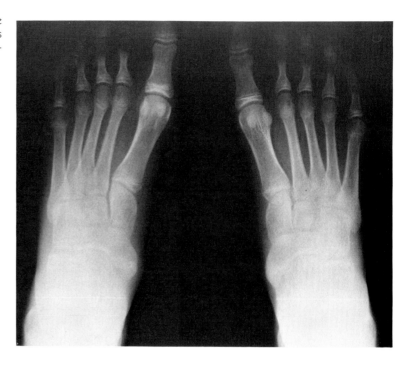

navicular lateral subluxation combined with cuboid crush injury. Hermel and Gershon-Cohen's (25) nutcracker cuboid fracture and the cuboid extrusion injury of Drummond and Hastings (26) fall into this category. Swivel injuries result in a laterally displaced talus from the navicular and an intact calcaneocuboid joint.

Plantar forces result in a dorsally dislocated talus and calcaneus on the navicular and cuboid. The talocalcaneal relationship is intact. Fracture sprains are demonstrated by dorsal talonavicular flake fractures. Impaction fractures or bifurcate ligament avulsion fractures of the anterior superior calcaneus may be noted (Fig. 60.10).

Crush injuries are of a varying nature with variable patterns. They are usually associated with open wounds. Contusion to soft tissues may result in serious vascular compromise and loss of tissue (Fig. 60.11).

Medial injuries are reduced by traction and reversal of the mechanism of injury. A wide variety of treatment programs have been attempted, from strapping to casting with weight bearing permitted or avoided. The most satisfactory treatment for medial fracture sprain and fracture subluxation has been a compression dressing, no weight bearing for 1 to 2 weeks, followed by use of a weight-bearing cast for 4 to 6 weeks. Persistent midtarsal pain has accompanied immediate weight bearing, with or without a cast. Patients tolerate the well-molded weight-bearing cast well. Chronic pain is noted to be substantially minimized. Early identification and treatment are essential. Similar methods are applied to the plantar and lateral injuries of similar types.

Lateral injuries are potentially the most serious (27). This is believed to be caused by disruption of the rigid lateral column needed for normal ambulation. Calcaneocuboid fu-

sion is recommended for persistent symptoms. For persistent problems after medial or lateral injury, triple arthrodesis is traditionally recommended over talonavicular fusion alone. Recurrent midtarsal joint subluxations have also been reported (28).

Swivel dislocation injuries to the midtarsal joint represent severe tarsal malalignment mandating immediate reduction. Delay in reduction of these injuries due to misdiagnosis results in devastating destruction to the tarsal joints (Fig. 60.12). The subtleties of talonavicular and talocalcaneal radiographic assessment must be carefully understood by the practitioner (Fig. 60.13). Triple arthrodesis affords the only surgical solution to aid in the persistent pain if the diagnosis is missed and reduction is not effected (29).

TARSOMETATARSAL JOINT DISLOCATION

Lisfranc's joint or the tarsometatarsal joints form a bony arc from medial to lateral across the midfoot region. The anatomy of the articulating surfaces appears as a stone arch with wide dorsal and narrow plantar contours. This osseous configuration, along with the strong ligaments and recessed second metatarsal base, provides the stability for this joint complex. Dislocations of these joints are rare, less than 1% of fracture dislocations reported (30-36). The severity may range from occult subluxation to subtle malalignment (37, 38).

The diagnosis has reportedly been missed in 20% of the cases (39). The chance for morbidity after this injury is great, whether reduction is open or closed. Damage to the perforating vessels in this area and arterial spasm or significant

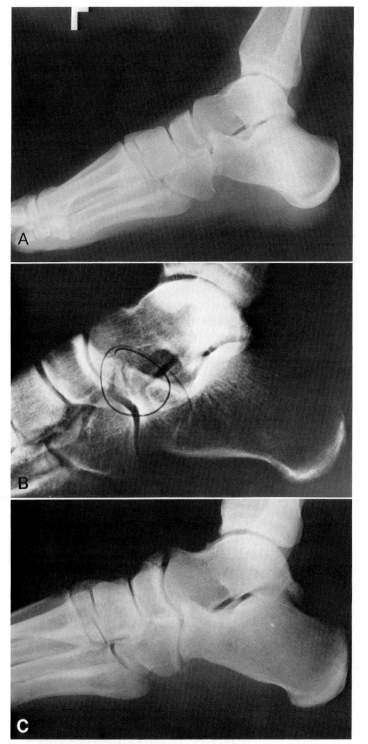

Figure 60.10. Plantar force midtarsal dislocation. **A.** Talonavicular joint congruity with plantarflexory disruption of calcaneocuboid joint. **B.** Avulsion fracture of anterior process of calcaneus. **C.** Avulsion fracture of dorsal talonavicular joint.

hematoma may compromise distal tissue blood supplies. Amputations may be necessary, depending on the degree of necrosis produced (40). These injuries represent medical emergencies. Control of edema and careful monitoring of the peripheral vascular status by ultrasonic or plethysmo-graphic methods are essential. This injury is classically considered an equestrian injury that occurs as the foot is caught in a stirrup by a falling rider (41). At present industrial injuries and motor vehicle accidents comprise the majority of cases (33, 35, 38).

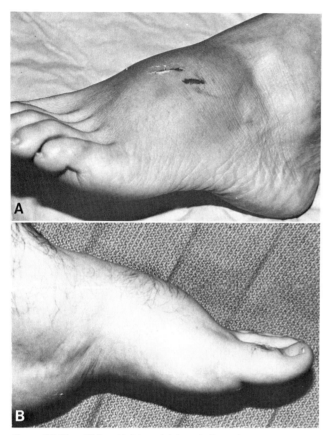

Figure 60.11. Midtarsal joint crush injury. **A.** Contusions and lacerations about the midtarsal joint in a crush injury. **B.** Edema about the midtarsal joint without contusion in noncrush injury of the midtarsal joint.

ANATOMIC CONSIDERATIONS

The principles essential to understanding the Lisfranc's dislocation are centered on the structural anatomy of this joint complex. The mechanism of the injury, subsequent injury patterns, and reduction maneuvers are dependent on the osseous relationships and the ligaments that not only bind the metatarsals together but also bind them to the midtarsus (Fig. 60.14). The metatarsals are bound to one another by the transverse dorsal and plantar ligaments (42, 43). There is no ligament joining the first metatarsal to the lesser metatarsals proximally at the base. This anatomical fact produces injury patterns in which the four lesser metatarsals generally dislocate as a unit (44). The first metatarsal may or may not dislocate with them. The first metatarsal pattern of dislocation is independent of the lesser metatarsals (40, 45). The intermetatarsal ligaments are not necessarily disrupted in the dislocation, and their integrity is used during reduction.

The ligaments that tether the metatarsus to the lesser tarsus are disrupted during this injury. The ligaments are stronger plantarly than dorsally. The dorsal medial ligament attaching the medial cuneiform to the first metatarsal is the largest ligament at this level. During open repairs of this injury, it is often possible to repair this ligament primarily (46). Probably the most significant ligament of the tarsometatarsal joint is the interosseous ligament that attaches the medial cuneiform to the second metatarsal base. This structure is commonly designated the Lisfranc's ligament and is responsible for the production of an avulsion fracture of the medial aspect of the second metatarsal (Fig. 60.15). The remaining ligaments are either disrupted or avulsed from their attachments, creating multiple small flake fractures.

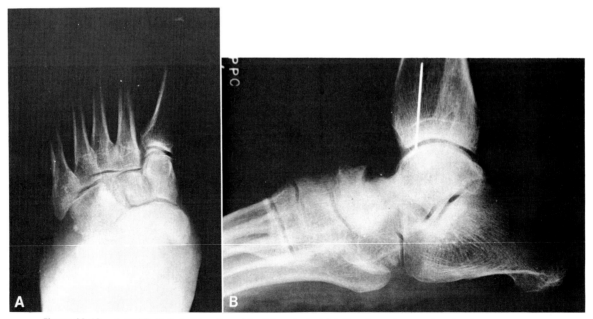

Figure 60.12. **A** and **B.** Swivel dislocation of the talonavicular joint; the diagnosis was missed at the time of injury. Note internal fixation of the ankle fracture, which was reduced.

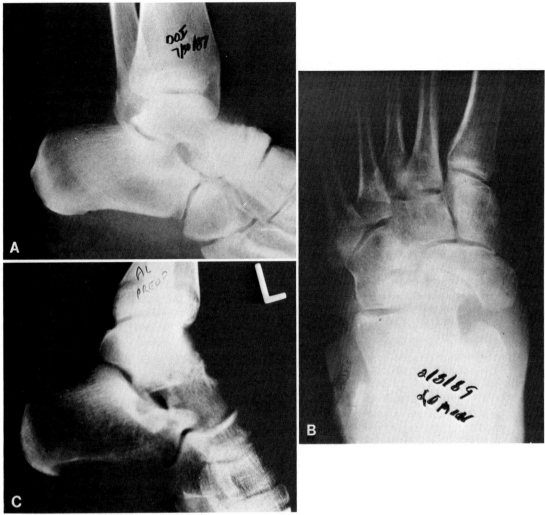

Figure 60.13.   A and **B.** Swivel dislocation of the talonavicular joint with an intact subtalar joint (diagnosis missed for 20 months). **C.** Hawkins I talar neck fracture with an intact subtalar joint. Note the subtle incongruity of the anterior and posterior facets of subtalar joint in each.

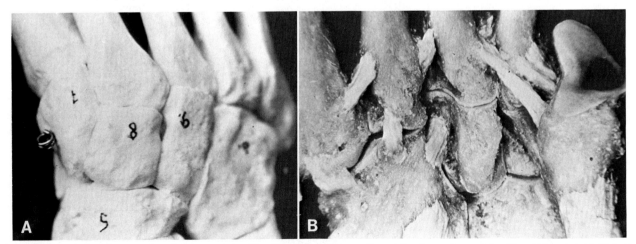

Figure 60.14.   A. Dorsal perspective of osseous relationships, Lisfranc's joint. Note the recessed position of the second metatarsal. **B.** Plantar perspective of the ligamentous relationships, Lisfranc's joint. Note the absence of ligaments to the first metatarsal from the second metatarsal.

The inherent osseous stability of the tarsometatarsal joint was previously mentioned. The convex shape formed by the metatarsal-lesser tarsus articulations from medial to lateral, combined with the dorsal to plantar wedged shape of the articulations, creates added stability in both the transverse and the sagittal planes.

CLASSIFICATION

Many classification systems have been proposed and have been based on the mechanism of injury (42, 44, 47-49), the way force was applied (34), and the resultant injury patterns (23, 35, 50). Each has merit in attempts to identify particular aspects of the injury. Hardcastle and associates (35) point out, however, that no system aids in treatment selection and prognosis. They reported that the pattern of the metatarsal displacement will influence the degree of fixation and prognosis. The classification system of Hardcastle and associates (35) is simple and is based on the radiographic presentation of the injury. This classification system does not necessarily truly represent the injury evidenced on static radiographs. Stress radiography may greatly influence the determination of the degree of injury to the joint (Fig. 60.16).

Type A—total: Total incongruity of the entire tarsometatarsal joint. The displacement may occur in the sagittal or transverse planes.

Type B—partial: Partial incongruity of the joint complex in either the sagittal plane, transverse plane, or both. Partial injuries may exist and are of two types:

Medial displacement affects the first metatarsal, either in isolation or combined with displacement of one or more of the second, third, or fourth metatarsals.

Lateral displacement involves one or more of the four lesser metatarsals, while the first is unaffected.

Type C—divergent: There may be partial or total incongruity of the joint. The first metatarsal is displaced medially, and any combination of the lateral four metatarsals is displaced laterally in either the sagittal or transverse planes or both.

DIAGNOSIS

The diagnosis of tarsometatarsal fracture dislocation requires little insight with obvious clinical and radiographic evidence. This is contrasted to the diagnosis of an occult, reduced fracture-dislocation that requires a high index of clinical suspicion because of the long-term sequelae of a missed diagnosis. Often the patient recalls an audible snap or pop after experiencing a forced plantarflexion or direct injury mechanism. The patient may relate stepping off a curb, slipping on the stairs, or stepping in a hole. The history most commonly includes a motor vehicle accident as opposed to a fall from a horse. The plantarflexed foot sustains a longitudinal force against a fixed surface.

Clinically, the foot appears grossly edematous about the midfoot region. It may appear shortened when compared with the opposite extremity. The forefoot may appear abducted or adducted on the rearfoot. Dorsiflexion and plan-

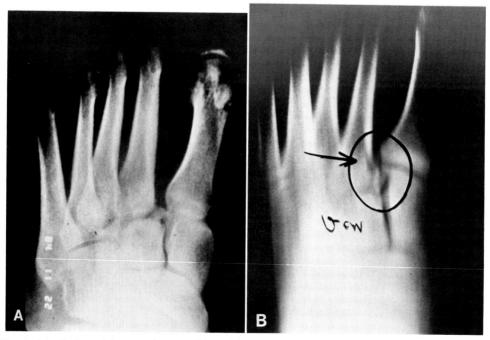

Figure 60.15.   Avulsion fracture of the second metatarsal from Lisfranc's ligament. Radiographic **(A)** and tomographic **(B)** representations.

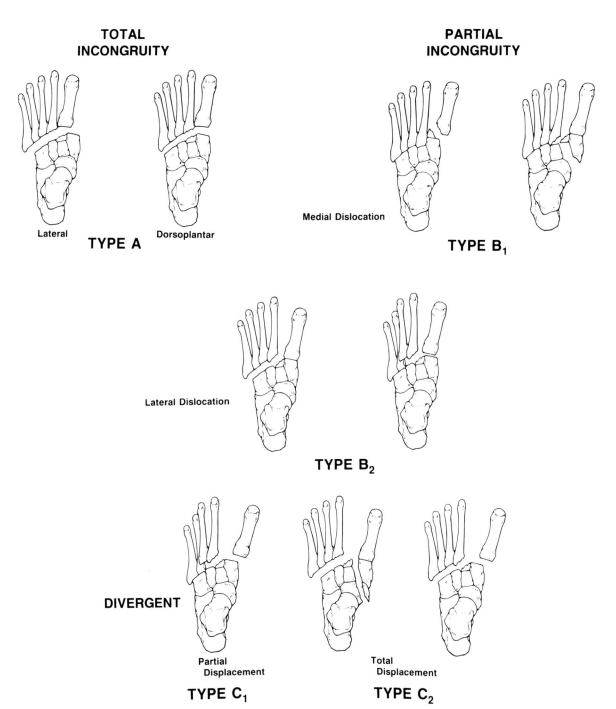

TOTAL INCONGRUITY

Lateral   Dorsoplantar

TYPE A

PARTIAL INCONGRUITY

Medial Dislocation

TYPE B₁

Lateral Dislocation

TYPE B₂

DIVERGENT

Partial Displacement

TYPE C₁

Total Displacement

TYPE C₂

Figure 60.16. Classification system of Hardcastle and associates (35) for Lisfranc's joint injuries. (From Dinapoli DR, Cain TD: Lisfranc's fracture-dislocation: Update 1988. In McGlamry ED (ed): *Reconstructive Surgery of the Foot and Leg, Update '88*. Tucker, GA, Podiatry Institute Publishing Co, 1988, p 200.)

tar flexion attitudes are also possible for the forefoot on the rearfoot. Pain is elicited about the joint area. Palpation may reveal the dorsal or plantar deviation of the second metatarsal base from its even contour with the cuneiforms dorsally (Fig. 60.17). Identification of pedal pulses is paramount. If the dorsalis pedis and the posterior tibial artery cannot be palpated, a Doppler ultrasound must be used. Excessive range of motion at Lisfranc's joint may be present. The only clue of a dislocation may be subtle radiographic changes. Cases in which the diagnosis was missed have been reported (39, 51).

Radiographs in three planes are an essential part of the

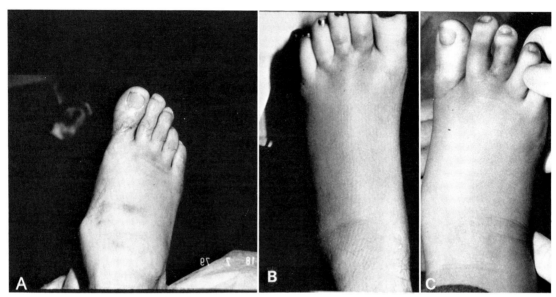

Figure 60.17. Clinical presentation of dislocations of Lisfranc's joint. **A.** Gross obvious severe injury. **B.** Subtle injury with edema, no malalignment. **C.** Posttraumatic hypermobility with abductory stress.

diagnostic evaluation. Comparison views of the uninvolved extremity may be helpful for diagnosis and postreduction assessment. Lateral radiographs of the foot may demonstrate the uneven dorsal contour of Lisfranc's joint. Normally there is an uneven curvature of metatarsals and cuneiforms dorsally. With Lisfranc's dislocation, the second metatarsal base is generally deviated dorsally from the cuneiforms in stairstep fashion. The first metatarsal may likewise show deviation in the lateral radiograph (Fig. 60.18).

Foster and Foster (38) studied Lisfranc's joint and the difficulties in evaluating this joint radiographically. They found the most consistent relationship to be the medial edge of the base of the second metatarsal and the medial edge of the second cuneiform. There was only one exception to this alignment in the 200 radiographs they reviewed. The space between the first and second metatarsals was not considered significant unless a step effect existed between the second metatarsal and the second cuneiform. The first metatarsal usually aligns laterally with the first cuneiform. Other alignments were noted but were not found to be consistent. Comparison radiographs were suggested to confirm alignment in the remaining metatarsals. Norfray and associates (37), in their studies, did note a consistent alignment of the lateral margin of the third metatarsocuneiform joint 72% of the time. The fourth metatarsocuboid joint aligns medially in the oblique and anteroposterior projections. A notch in the base of the fifth metatarsal aligns with the lateral cuboid in 80% of the cases studied. Because of the range of motion in the fourth and fifth metatarsocuboid joints, offsets of up to 3 mm are considered normal. Offsets in the first, second, and third metatarsals never occur normally (38). Goossens and DeStoop (39) recommend stress pronation and supination radiographs in cases in which dislocation is clinically suspected. They demonstrated pathological laxity

of the joint in an otherwise normal-appearing radiograph. This procedure may have to be performed with the patient under general anesthesia (Fig. 60.19). Fractures at the Lisfranc's joint level are present in most cases, even if they are too small to be detected on the radiograph (48, 52).

The radiographs should be examined for injuries known to occur in association with Lisfranc's dislocation. Fractures of the metatarsal shafts and metatarsophalangeal joint dislocations have been observed. Compression fractures of the navicular or cuboid are possible, depending on the direction of the dislocation (33, 35, 38, 53, 54). Cuneometatarsal disruption or intercuneiform injury may likewise be present (55). If these injuries are present, a more unstable situation is present after reduction and must be considered (42). Radiographic evaluation of the ankle should also be considered.

MECHANISM OF INJURY

Mechanisms of these injuries are poorly understood. The recessed articulation of the second metatarsal provides the stability to this joint. The remaining metatarsals are not as interdigitated as the second. The second metatarsal must be disrupted first, whether by fracture or by dorsal dislocation, to permit total disruption to proceed. With the release of the second metatarsal, the remaining metatarsals may be easily dislocated. Two mechanisms of tarsometatarsal joint injury have been postulated: direct and indirect.

Aiken and Paulson (34) examined these injuries according to how the force was applied to the joint to create the dislocation. A direct injury is described as occurring when the foot is struck by an object. For example, a weight dropped from above causes a plantar Lisfranc's dislocation if the second metatarsal is fractured. Plantar dislocation of the second metatarsal is unlikely. Variable dislocations and fractures may occur at the base of the lesser metatarsals. Direct dorsal dislocation has been shown to be impossible (42, 44, 48). Injury from such a force occurs elsewhere within the foot or ankle.

The indirect mechanism is the least understood and the most variable. Wiley (42), in 1971, performed cadaver studies and proposed that there were two main forces associated with the indirect mechanism: forefoot abduction and forced forefoot plantar flexion. The foot is usually injured while in a plantarflexed or equinus-type position. A traumatic abductory force applied to the forefoot produces an exces-

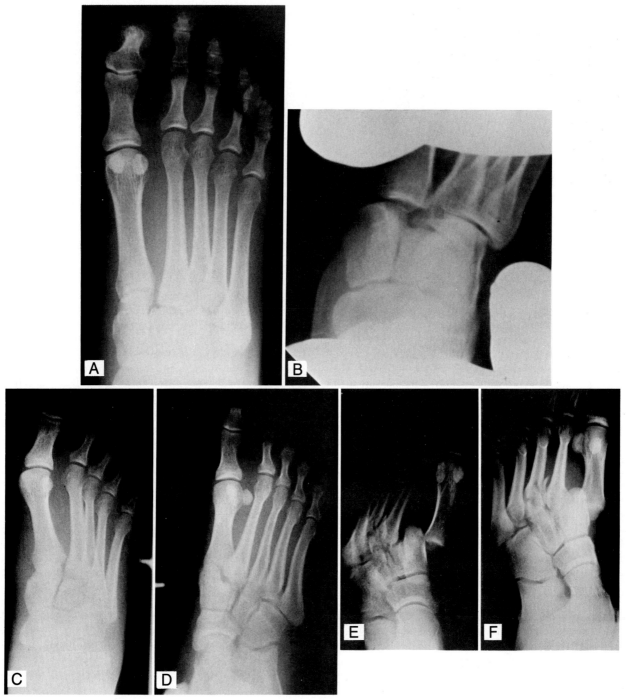

Figure 60.18. Radiographic presentations of dislocations of Lisfranc's joint. **A** and **B.** Type A demonstrated with abductory stress. **C** and **D.** Type B with intact fourth and fifth cuboid area. **E** and **F.** Type C divergent dislocation.

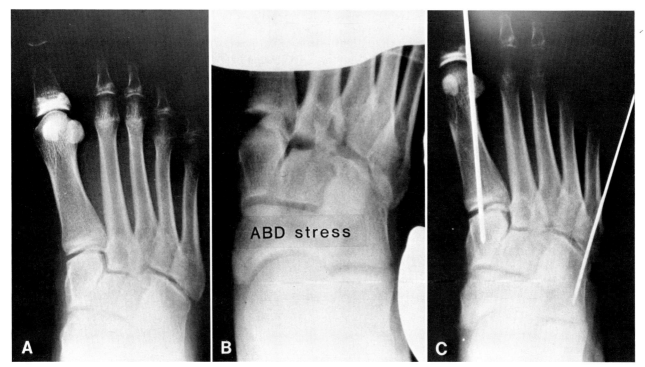

Figure 60.19. Subtle Lisfranc's dislocation. **A.** Unremarkable postinjury radiograph. **B.** Abductory stress radiograph demonstrating disruption of Lisfranc's joint. **C.** Postreduction radiograph with fixation.

sive amount of shear stress at the second metatarsal base. This results in either a transverse base fracture of the second metatarsal or an avulsion fracture of the medial aspect of the second metatarsal base. The avulsion fragment is usually attached to the Lisfranc ligament. If the abduction force continues, the lesser metatarsals may shift laterally as the lateral tarsometatarsal ligaments fail and rupture. Occasionally the severe adductory force will result in a distal cuboid compression fracture. Indirect injuries occur as the result of falls. It is generally believed that torsional force is necessary first to unlock the second metatarsal. The remaining metatarsals may then deviate medially, laterally, dorsally, or plantarly, depending on the directing force. The most common force is a pronatory one that produces a dorsal lateral deviation of the lateral metatarsals. Plantar dislocation of the metatarsal bases has been reported (39, 56).

TREATMENT

The literature concerning appropriate treatment tends to combine all injuries under the heading of Lisfranc's dislocation and to evaluate their management regardless of the injury pattern. Some authors have noted differences in the injury pattern and appropriateness of treatment (35). Accurate anatomical reduction, whether open or closed, has consistently provided better functional results (33, 34, 48, 52, 57). Anatomic reduction is certainly not a guarantee of a satisfactory result, and cases of resistant nonsymptomatic

subluxation have been reported (34). Brunett and Wiley (51) found no correlation between radiographic assessment and the patient's symptoms or between type of fracture dislocation and treatment on subsequent function. Wire fixation has proved helpful in maintaining alignment after reduction to prevent recurrence in unstable joints (33, 35). Internal temporary screw stabilization of accurate anatomic reduction has been found to work suitably (58-60). Casting of unstable joints without fixation has not proved effective (33, 35, 39). Conservative casting of the injury without reduction or fixation is also ineffective (35, 39). Primary arthrodesis is rarely used (52), although it may be indicated where there is significant loss of articular surfaces. Secondary arthrodesis is always a possibility (58).

The approach to management of these injuries follows that of Wilson (48). Closed reduction may be attempted first (34, 35, 57, 61-63). Anesthesia, either general or regional, combined with muscle-paralyzing agents, may be required. Distal forefoot traction is applied against countertraction on the heel. The forefoot is suspended from the operating room table by tape or digital finger traps distal to the injury. Countertraction weights may be suspended from the leg once adequate relaxation has been achieved. Manipulation may then be attempted to engage the second metatarsal base between the cuneiforms. A pronating type of force is required if the metatarsals are dorsally dislocated. The lesser metatarsals will follow the reduction maneuver consistent with the Vassal phenomenon and the intact intermetatarsal ligaments. The first metatarsal is reduced individually in divergent type C injuries. Once relocation is verified radiographically, percutaneous wire stabilization is employed. Open reduction permits visual assurance of adequate anatomic reduction.

Soft tissue interposition and bony fragments may prevent closed reduction. The tibialis anterior tendon has been noted to become lodged in the medial-intermediate cuneiform articulation, preventing reduction (44, 62-65). The avulsed fracture fragment of Lisfranc's ligament from the second metatarsal may become interposed and prevent reduction (41, 61). In cases in which closed reduction is difficult, careful inspection of this area directly through open reduction may be necessary. Closed reduction can be and is obstructed until interposed soft tissues are released or interposed bony fragments are removed.

If closed reduction methods fail, open reduction is necessary. Open reduction is indicated to inspect pedal blood vessels when vascular compromise is evident (35, 40). Incisions are placed longitudinally to help prevent further vascular compromise. Two incisions are generally used: one medially for the first and second related bases and one laterally for the fourth and fifth metatarsal bases (34). The first metatarsal is relocated and fixated first. All interposed soft tissues and bony fragments should be excised. The lesser metatarsals may then be relocated anatomically under direct visualization. Closure may need to be delayed if severe edema or blunt trauma to soft tissue is present.

When open or closed reduction is effected and the joint remains unstable, percutaneous wire fixation is indicated. The wiring technique required, based on the type of injury present, was thoroughly evaluated by Hardcastle and associates in terms of long-term results (35). Type A injuries are best fixated with two wires, one medially through the first metatarsocuneiform joint and one laterally through the fifth metatarsocuboid joint. Type B injuries of the medial variety are very unstable, and two wires are suggested for the first metatarsal. Lateral type B injuries require only one wire through the fifth metatarsocuboid joint. Type C injuries require two wires medially and one wire laterally. This injury is also unstable, as are medial type B injuries.

Stress radiography may greatly affect the classification of an injury and can affect the degree of fixation chosen. Stress radiography is not only important in the diagnosis of the injury present but aids in classification for fixation purposes. After radiographic confirmation of alignment, soft tissue repair is completed. Recent experience with this injury has shown that primary repair of the dorsomedial ligament of the first metatarsocuneiform joint and its capsule is quite possible.

The need for delayed closure may exist if severe edema or extensive trauma to the soft tissues exists. Compression dressings are applied after reduction until edema and the vascular status have stabilized. The time interval may vary depending on the extent of the injury and associated injuries. Generally 5 to 14 days is required. Below-the-knee casting is then maintained for 6 to 12 weeks. Pins may be removed at 6 to 8 weeks. Weight-bearing ambulation has been initiated as early as 2 weeks (35). Careful monitoring for redislocation is very important. Once the cast is removed and the joint is assessed as stable, supportive footwear is instituted.

COMPLICATIONS

Redislocation and circulatory compromise, the most important short-term complications, have been discussed. Arthritis and Sudeck's atrophy are possible long-term complications. Goossens and DeStoop (39) noted Sudeck's atrophy in patients in whom the diagnosis had been missed and inappropriate treatment administered. They also noted its occurrence in cases in which unsatisfactory alignment was achieved after reduction. Arthrosis is an almost inevitable sequela of this injury (33, 44). Radiographic changes, however, do not always correlate with clinical findings. Accuracy of reduction definitely plays a role in symptomatic arthritis. Resection of painful prominences in patients with a history of Lisfranc's dislocation generally has not proved satisfactory in relieving symptoms. Arthrodesis of Lisfranc's joint has generally provided a more stable, symptom-free result. Arthrodesis as a primary procedure has been advocated after this injury (49, 52). Currently it is not recommended unless there is severe comminution of the joints.

SUMMARY

Fracture-dislocation of the Lisfranc joint complex is a relatively uncommon injury. Diagnosis of occult dislocations with obvious radiographic changes is not difficult. The subtle disruption of this joint complex requires a high index of suspicion. Accurate anatomic reduction at initial presentation has produced the most satisfactory results. Surgical intervention in acute and chronic cases may be warranted.

FIRST METATARSOPHALANGEAL JOINTS

Dislocations of the first metatarsophalangeal joint are rare (62, 63). Jahss reported seeing only two such cases among 25,000 foot patients in 18 years (66). This injury has been given renewed attention in the literature because of its association with athletic endeavors (67). With the advent of artificial playing surfaces, hyperextension injuries to the great toe have become more commonplace (68). Trauma texts do not contain thorough reviews of the pathomechanics of this injury. Dislocation of the first metatarsophalangeal joint, although a rare occurrence, represents an interesting anatomical and pathomechanical study. The first metatarsophalangeal joint is a complex structure in both design and function. A multitude of soft tissues, including ligaments, tendons, and joint capsule, not only bind the osseous components but permit motion for ambulatory function. A review of this dislocation and of methods of treating it is presented. This review is based on The Podiatry Institute experience and current trends in the literature.

The injury occurs primarily as a result of motor vehicle accidents (66, 69-72). Falls from heights account for a secondary number of cases (73-75). Two cases of pathological dislocation have been recorded. One case was associated with spina bifida (76). A second case associated with insulin-dependent diabetes mellitus and Charcot joint disease has been recorded (77) (Fig. 60.20). Sports injuries represent an increasing number of cases of first metatarsophalangeal joint disruptions.

Hyperextension is believed to be the force that creates the injury. The clinical presentation supports this mechanism. The hallux is dorsally subluxed at the metatarsophalangeal joint. A prominence of the first metatarsal head is noted plantarly. Pain is elicited on attempted range of motion and palpation of the involved joint. The extensor apparatus is in a contracted state. The flexor apparatus is tightened because of the direction of the dislocation. A flexion attitude of the interphalangeal joint of the hallux may be present. The deformity may be subtle because of masking caused by the swelling that follows the injury.

The complex soft tissue anatomy surrounding this joint figures strongly in the ease of reduction of the dislocation. The soft tissue injuries may be extrapolated from the radiographs. Jahss (66), in his review, noted two distinct radiographic patterns based on sesamoid position after the injury. The sesamoid position correlated well with the ease of reduction.

The two dislocation types show displacement of the base of the proximal phalanx above the first metatarsal. The sesamoid position of one in relation to the other is variable and defines the type of dislocation present. In type I dislocations the intersesamoidal ligament remains intact (66). The sesamoids are unfractured. The sesamoids remain normally apposed one to the other but not necessarily to the base of the proximal phalanx (Fig. 60.21). Their position relative to the first metatarsal and proximal phalanx is variable. The sesamoids generally remain apposed to the prox-

imal phalangeal base and come to lie dorsal to the metatarsal head. Giannikas and associates (69) reported a case in which the sesamoids remained plantar to the first metatarsal and the intersesamoidal ligament appeared to remain intact. Daniel and associates (72) and most reports in the literature describe cases in which the sesamoids came to lie dorsal to the first metatarsal. Immediate closed reduction is generally unsuccessful and open reduction is necessary (69, 72, 73). In most cases reported, closed reduction failed to reduce the deformity. This may be attributed to the locked position of the metatarsal beneath the proximal phalanx and joint capsule. The first metatarsal is reigned in medially by the abductor hallucis tendon and laterally by the adductor hallucis tendon and the flexor hallucis longus. The collateral ligaments remain intact and reinforce the position of the deformity (66). The presence of an intact flexor hallucis brevis to maintain this fixed position may not be required.

If dislocation occurs and the sesamoids remain plantarly, the short flexor must be disrupted. Jahss (66) demonstrated their constant position relative to the proximal phalanx in flexion and extension. The excursion or stretch within the short flexor apparatus to permit joint motion occurs proximal to the sesamoids within the muscle mass. The flexor hallucis brevis may or may not be ruptured, depending on the sesamoid position. Results at follow-up in these cases showed no difference in hallux position or function based on type I dorsal or plantar sesamoid position. In this respect, the analysis may be only academic, but the soft tissue injury is not similar (78).

Open reduction through a dorsal longitudinal incision has been described by Daniel (72). Adequate exposure of all soft tissue structures was noted. A plantar approach has also been described (75, 79). This permits exposure to the plantar first metatarsophalangeal joint and associated structures.

Figure 60.20. Pathological dislocation of the first metatarsophalangeal joint. **A.** Spina bifida. **B.** Charcot joint disease.

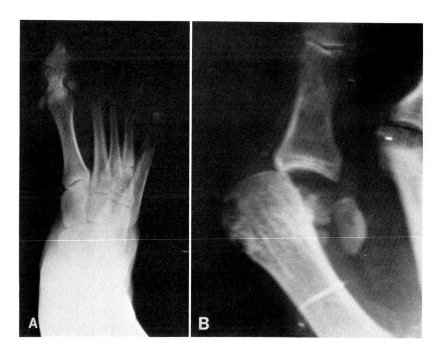

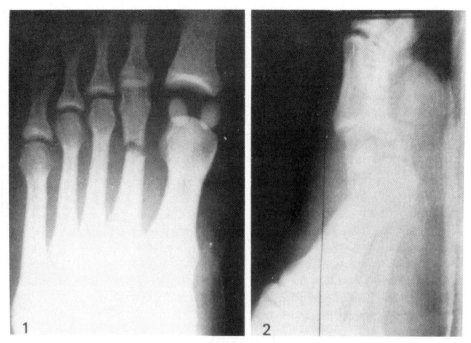

Figure 60.21. Type I dislocation of the first metatarsophalangeal joint with associated fracture of the second metatarsal.

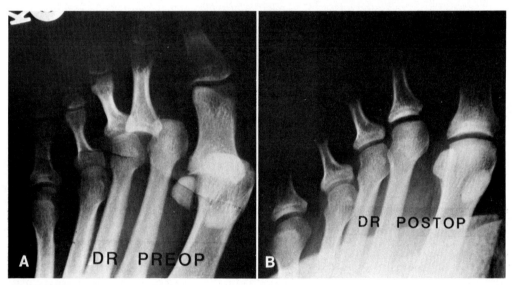

Figure 60.22. Type II-A dislocation of the first metatarsophalangeal joint. Prereduction **(A)** and postreduction **(B)** radiographs. Note the associated dorsal dislocation of the second metatarsophalangeal joint.

The dorsal linear incision as advocated by Daniel (72) is recommended in most cases of dislocation of the first metatarsophalangeal joint that require open reduction. Splinting or below-knee casting is recommended for 3 to 4 weeks to permit adequate healing of soft tissues. Ambulation as tolerated in a stiff-soled shoe may then be encouraged.

Type II injuries demonstrate a disruption in the intersesamoidal apparatus. The sesamoids no longer remain ap-

posed one to the other (66). This disruption may occur in two ways. In type II-A dislocations the sesamoids are not fractured. The intersesamoidal ligament is ruptured. The sesamoids come to lie widely separated medially and laterally, respectively, about the first metatarsal head (Fig. 60.22). Type II-B dislocations demonstrate a transverse fracture of one of the sesamoids. This fracture is an avulsion type caused by further hyperextension force (Fig. 60.23). Crush-

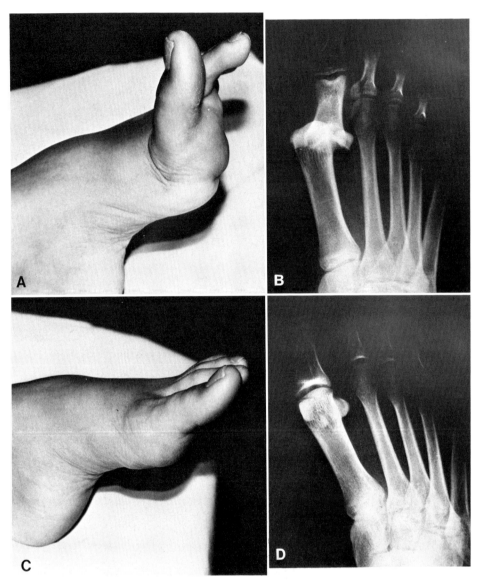

Figure 60.23. Type II-B dislocation of the first metatarsophalangeal joint. Prereduction clinical **(A)** and radiographic **(B)** presentation. Postreduction clinical **(C)** and radiographic **(D)** presentation.

ing may also fracture the sesamoid as in falls from a height (75). The proximal fragment remains apposed to the opposite sesamoid through the intact intersesamoidal ligament and the distal fragment remains apposed to the base of the proximal phalanx. Brown (73) reported a case in which this fracture healed uneventfully. Generally, the distal fragment must be excised (71, 74). It acts as a loose body and produces pain that is relieved on excision. Crushing may also fracture the sesamoids, as in falls from heights (75). Generally the tibial sesamoid is implicated in this injury with variable fracture patterns. The avulsion injury associated with first metatarsophalangeal joint dislocations generally involves the fibular sesamoid and is transverse in orientation.

Type II injuries may be reduced by closed manipulation (69, 71, 73, 74). Distal traction is effected across the joint

with a plantarflexory force. The soft tissue buttressing effect appears to be slacked enough to permit reduction in patients with disruption of the intersesamoidal apparatus.

First metatarsophalangeal joint dislocations have not usually resulted in long-term disability. The foot is maintained in compression dressings for 2 to 3 weeks. Ambulation is then encouraged as tolerated by the patient. No positional deformities or arthroses have been reported. Recurrent dislocations have been reported, and careful monitoring is required as part of treatment (80).

When dislocations are left unreduced for extended periods arthroplastic surgery is generally required to permit reduction. Giannikas and associates (69) reported a case in which extensive internal injuries and unsuccessful closed reduction resulted in delay of open reduction for 3 weeks.

A Keller type of arthroplasty was required to effect correction. The chronic pathological dislocation reported by Schlefman and associates (76) likewise required Keller-type arthroplasty. The sesamoids were excised because of a chronic ulcer, and an interphalangeal joint fusion was employed to assist with hallux stabilization.

Mullis and Miller (81) reported a case of instability of the great toe in a patient after a jump during a basketball game. No occult dislocation was present. Persistent pain and instability prompted stress radiographs of the first metatarsophalangeal joint. Varus excursion of the involved joint was far greater than the opposite extremity. Repair of the torn conjoined adductor tendon, collateral ligament, and lateral joint capsule relieved symptoms and provided stability to the toe. Disruption of the first metatarsophalangeal joint may occur about any plane (67, 81, 82). Disruptions should be suspected in the presence of persistent joint pain, especially in the active athletic person.

Clanton and colleagues (67) discussed the association of athletic injuries and the first metatarsophalangeal joint. They describe injuries from mild sprains to severe tearing of the capsule ligamentous complex including avulsion fractures of the sesamoids. They recommend stiffening of the forefoot in athletic shoes or the use of orthotic devices within shoes to prevent these injuries in patients who participate in sports on athletic fields with artificial turf. The flexible nature of shoes that evolved with the transition of athletic endeavors from grass to artificial turf is implicated in the increased incidence of these injuries. Stiffening of the forefoot in athletic shoes will likely reduce the incidence of this injury and its long-term potential sequela.

LESSER METATARSOPHALANGEAL JOINTS

Lesser metatarsophalangeal joint dislocations are rare injuries (83, 84). They may be associated with other more obvious lower extremity trauma and should not be overlooked. They have been described as involving multiple metatarsophalangeal joints (84) or, although extremely rare, as isolated dislocations (83). Lesser metatarsophalangeal joint dislocation has been reported associated with Lisfranc's dislocation (85). Reduction here may not be possible until the Lisfranc's dislocation is reduced. Pathological dislocations of the lesser metatarsophalangeal joints may be found in patients who have chronic problems with arthritis. Significant pain and discomfort may be noted by the patient, without a history of trauma.

Anatomy

Hyperextension appears to be the mechanism for this injury (69, 83, 84, 86). As the proximal phalanx dorsiflexes, the metatarsal head may be forced plantarly through the fibrocartilaginous volar or flexor plate. The metatarsal becomes prominent and palpable plantarly. The digit is dorsally displaced. Pain is elicited on palpation of the joint and attempted range of motion. The metatarsal head may become trapped by the fibrocartilaginous plate plantarly and by the

deep transverse intermetatarsal ligament and dorsal capsule dorsally. The flexor tendon may become laterally displaced. Soft tissue entrapment may necessitate open reduction.

Radiographic evaluation will demonstrate either overlap or widening of the joint margins on the anteroposterior view with lateral deviation of the digit (Fig. 60.22). The lateral view will reveal an isolated proximal phalanx that is not superimposed with the other digits of the foot. The oblique foot radiograph may be helpful in subtle injury presentations. Radiographic variance may exist depending on the mechanism of injury. Associated injuries, such as fractures of the metatarsals and phalanges, should be carefully evaluated in the patient with dislocation of a lesser metatarsophalangeal joint.

Management

Historically, closed reduction has proved to be a satisfactory means of treatment in the acute dislocation (86). After reduction, padded metal splinting may be used (87). Casting may also be employed for 3 or 4 weeks of immobilization in a weight-bearing attitude. Ambulation in a stiff-soled shoe is followed with an increase in activity as tolerated. Careful monitoring for recurrence of the dislocation should be considered.

The long-term sequelae of chronic dislocation include claw digit or hammer toe deformity as well as painful plantar keratomas and metatarsalgia. Undiagnosed or improperly treated dislocations may be analogous to amputation of a digit, with resultant transverse plane deformity of the adjacent digits caused by loss of the buttressing effect of the involved toe. Degenerative changes in the involved joint can occur necessitating resection procedures to aid in management of chronic pain.

Occasionally these injuries may not be reduced by closed manipulation. Open reduction by Roa and Manuel (84) showed the head of the metatarsal trapped within the fibrocartilaginous flexor plate plantarly, the dorsal capsule and deep transverse metatarsal ligament dorsally, and the flexor tendon medially with the lumbricales tendon laterally. Reduction could be accomplished only after release of the fibrocartilaginous flexor plate, deep transverse metatarsal ligament, and dorsal capsule. Murphy (83) reported a case in which the fibrocartilaginous plate also acted as an obstacle to closed reduction. The literature generally reports favorable results of closed and open reduction of lesser metatarsophalangeal joint dislocations without resultant digital deformity or discomfort. The prognosis for this type of dislocation is satisfactory.

Chronic dislocations generally are not reducible. Patients with rheumatoid arthritis or significant osteoarthritis may have chronic dislocations of the lesser metatarsophalangeal joints. Generally, reduction may be effected only by arthroplastic techniques with resection of a portion of the joint to permit reduction of the digit to a more normal anatomic alignment (Fig. 60.24). Medial and lateral dislocations are possible when an object is forced between the digits. These injuries are unstable because of rupture of the collateral

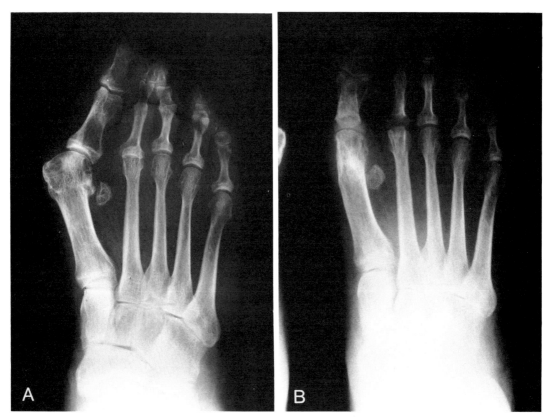

Figure 60.24.   Prereduction **(A)** and 18-month postoperative **(B)** radiographs of a chronic dislocation of the second metatarsophalangeal joint with joint implant.

ligaments on one side of the joint (85). Giannestras and Sammarco (87) recommend percutaneous pinning. Experience with this type of injury shows subtle recurrence of the malalignment of the digit to be more the exception than the rule. Lesser digit transverse plane instability may be extremely difficult to correct, and recurrence of the malalignment is likely.

INTERPHALANGEAL JOINTS

Dislocations of the interphalangeal joints of the digits are rare injuries but may prove difficult to reduce and to maintain after reduction. The hallux interphalangeal joint is the most common interphalangeal dislocation, followed by the second digit (45, 83, 88). Interphalangeal dislocations are commonly associated with other pedal injuries. Careful radiographic evaluation of the periarticular structures for possible fracture is necessary. Open interphalangeal dislocation injuries are possible and represent significant destruction of the periarticular structures (77).

Dorsal dislocation of the distal phalanx in hyperextension is the most common injury pattern (Fig. 60.25). Abductory and adductory injuries as well as plantar flexion are possible depending on the mechanism of injury. Subtle injury may be missed or relocation of occult dislocation may be overlooked if clinical and radiographic findings are not subjected to careful scrutiny.

Anatomy

The interphalangeal joints of the digits are ginglymus or hinge joints in which the trochlear surface of the phalangeal head articulates with the inversely shaped proximal phalangeal base. The joint is reinforced and surrounded by a capsule. Two collateral ligaments—one medial and one lateral—reinforce the joint for dorsiflexory and plantarflexory hingelike motion.

The plantar capsule is thickened to form a firm fibrous plate known as the volar or plantar plate. It has also been termed the plantar ligament. Masaki (89) found an interphalangeal sesamoid bone in 56.3% of 958 radiograms of ambulatory patients. The incidence of interphalangeal sesamoids increased to 93% when a one-quarter sensitivity-intensifying radiographic film was used. The sesamoid bone was found in 95.5% of 144 feet of 73 adult cadavers by macroscopic observation. Most adults then can be said to have an interphalangeal sesamoid bone of the great toe that is not always demonstrated radiographically. The presence of the interphalangeal sesamoid and flexor plate apparatus plays a critical role in irreducible dislocations of the interphalangeal joints of the digits.

Management

Interphalangeal joint dislocations may almost always be reduced by closed reduction (84, 90). Multiple case studies

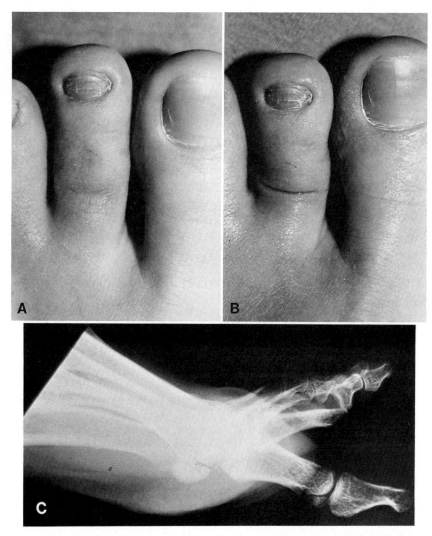

Figure 60.25. Proximal interphalangeal joint dislocation of a second digit. Prereduction **(A)** and postreduction clinical **(B)** presentation. **C.** Prereduction radiograph.

have demonstrated that irreducible dislocations are possible, especially of the interphalangeal joint of the great toe (88, 91-94). Entrapment of the volar plate and interphalangeal sesamoid within the interphalangeal joint is blamed for preventing reduction. Miki (88) discusses two types of injury pattern that correlate well with clinical findings of irreducible dislocations. Type I is a subtle injury with interposition of the volar plate without gross malalignment of the interphalangeal joint. Widening of the joint space is noted radiographically. Elongation of the digit is clinically noted without gross malalignment. Type II interphalangeal joint dislocations demonstrate hyperextension injury of the distal phalanx on the proximal phalanx. The interphalangeal sesamoid and volar plate are luxated dorsally onto the proximal phalanx. Radiographically, malalignment and dorsal positioning of the distal phalanx are noted. Clinically, an obvious hyperextension attitude of the joint is noted with dimpling of the dorsal skin on the digit.

Closed reduction of the hyperextension injury may gen-

erally be effected by application of an extension force, followed by traction, and finally a plantarflexory relocation force to the dislocated joint. Most dislocations are easily reduced in this fashion. Careful evaluation for instability is carried out to ensure maintenance of reduction. Radiographic evaluation is necessary to ensure adequacy of reduction of the interphalangeal joint to a normal joint space. Contralateral radiographs may be helpful in assessing the degree of joint space present within the interphalangeal joint.

Irreducible dislocations may be of either the type I or the type II variety. Type II dislocations may relocate to produce a type I dislocation. This is still an unsatisfactory reduction, since soft tissue interposition and resultant instability of the interphalangeal joint still exist. Reduction is effectively accomplished only when a normal radiographic joint space is observed. Clinical alignment may not be a satisfactory basis on which to judge adequacy of reduction.

Stability of the reduction should be evaluated critically. If

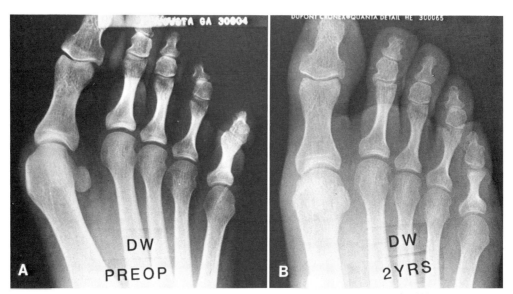

Figure 60.26. Unstable dislocation of a proximal interphalangeal joint, fifth digit. Preoperative **(A)** and postoperative **(B)** views of proximal phalangeal arthroplasty of fifth digit and syndactyly of fourth and fifth digits.

satisfactory stability exists, a splint and surgical shoe or a below-the-knee weight-bearing cast may be used to maintain reduction for 3 to 4 weeks. This is followed by splinting and a return to normal activities as tolerated. If instability of the interphalangeal joint exists, careful scrutiny of the radiographs for possible soft tissue interposition is suggested. If adequate reduction of the interphalangeal joint is noted, percutaneous pinning of the joint may be necessary to maintain alignment through the early phases of joint healing. Splinting and casting are then used for 3 to 4 weeks as noted previously.

Irreducible dislocations require open reduction and fixation of the dislocated interphalangeal joint. Generally, a transverse dorsal approach to the interphalangeal joint is used (91). A medial approach to the joint has been described (92), as well as a lateral approach (94). The goal of the open reduction is to relocate the flexor plate and sesamoid apparatus of the interphalangeal joint to its normal plantar attitude. Excision of the sesamoid or any small fracture fragments may be necessary to permit open reduction. Percutaneous pinning of the joint and casting or splinting techniques are used for 4 to 6 weeks after the open reduction. Return to activity may then be initiated as tolerated.

Interphalangeal joint dislocations of the lesser digits may generally be reduced by closed means. Katayama and associates (90) presented a case of irreducible dislocation of the distal interphalangeal joint of the second digit. Their findings on open reduction were very similar to those of the interphalangeal joint of the great toe. Interposition of the small flexor plate within the interphalangeal joint of the lesser digit prevented reduction. Reduction was easily effected through a dorsal transverse incision and repositioning of the flexor plate inferior to the interphalangeal joint. Buddy taping or splinting techniques are generally used for 3 to 4 weeks to maintain alignment until satisfactory healing

and stability of the joint are present. Instability or pain is a possible complication after reduction of dislocations of the interphalangeal joints of the lesser digits (77). Digital surgical procedures such as joint resection, arthrodesis, and syndactyly are effective techniques for managing chronic problems associated with a history of digital interphalangeal joint dislocation (Fig. 60.26).

References

1. Main BJ, Jowett RL: Injuries of the midtarsal joint. *J Bone Joint Surg* 57B:89, 1975.
2. Shands AR Jr: The incidence of subastraguloid dislocation of the foot with a report of one case of the inward type. *J Bone Joint Surg* 10:306, 1928.
3. Leitner B: Obstacles to reduction in subtalar dislocation. *J Bone Joint Surg* 36A:299, 1954.
4. Smith H: Subastragalar dislocation. *J Bone Joint Surg* 19:373, 1937.
5. Barber JR, Bricker JD, Haliburton RA: Peritalar dislocation of the foot. *Can J Surg* 4:205, 1961.
6. Fahey JJ, Murphy JL: Dislocations and fractures of the talus. *Surg Clin North Am* 45:79, 1965.
7. Heppenstall RB, Farahvar H, Balderston R, Lotke P: Evaluation and management of subtalar dislocations. *J Trauma* 20:494, 1980.
8. Christensen SB, Lorentzen JE, Krogsoe O, Sneppen O: Subtalar dislocation. *Acta Orthop Scand* 48:707, 1977.
9. Monson ST, Ryan JR: Subtalar dislocation. *J Bone Joint Surg* 63A:1156, 1981.
10. Grantham SA: Medial subtalar dislocation: five cases with a common etiology. *J Trauma* 4:845, 1964.
11. Larsen HW: Subastragalar dislocation (luxatio pedis sub talo). *Acta Chir Scand* 113:380, 1957.
12. Straus DC: Subtalar dislocation of the foot. *J Bone Joint Surg* 30:427, 1935.
13. Leitner B: Mechanism of total dislocation of the talus. *J Bone Joint Surg* 37A:89, 1955.
14. Buckingham WW: Subtalar dislocation of the foot. *J Trauma* 13:753, 1973.
15. Ganel A, Ahronson F, Heim M, Pritch M, Chechick A: Subtalar dislocations. *J Foot Surg* 20:142, 1981.

16. Mulroy RD: The tibialis posterior tendon as an obstacle to reduction of a lateral anterior subtalar dislocation. *J Bone Joint Surg* 37A:859, 1955.

17. Kenwright J, Taylor RG: Major injuries of the talus. *J Bone Joint Surg* 52B:36, 1970.

18. Mindell ER, Cisek EE, Kartalian G, Dziob M: Late results of injuries to the talus. *J Bone Joint Surg* 45A:221, 1963.

19. Sharit FE, Cole LF: Subtalar dislocations. *J Am Podiatry Assoc* 74:386, 1984.

20. Plewes LW, McKelvey KG: Subtalar dislocation. *J Bone Joint Surg* 26:585, 1944.

21. McKeever FM: Treatment of complications of fractures and dislocations of the talus. *Clin Orthop* 30:45, 1963.

22. Jahss MH (ed): *Disorders of the Foot*, Philadelphia, WB Saunders, 1982.

23. Wilson DW: Injuries of the tarso-metatarsal joints. *J Bone Joint Surg* 54B:677, 1972.

24. Wiley JJ: The mechanism of tarso-metatarsal joints. *J Bone Joint Surg* 53B:474, 1971.

25. Hermel MB, Gershon-Cohen J: The nutcracker fracture of the cuboid by indirect violence. *Radiology* 60:850, 1953.

26. Drummond DS, Hastings DE: Total dislocation of the cuboid bone. *J Bone Joint Surg* 51B:716, 1969.

27. Dewar FP, Evans DC: Occult fracture-subluxation of midtarsal joint. *J Bone Joint Surg* 50B:386, 1968.

28. Hooper G, McMaster MJ: Recurrent bilateral midtarsal subluxations. *J Bone Joint Surg* 61A:617, 1979.

29. Smith TF: Subtle tarsal dislocations. In DiNapoli DR (ed): *Reconstructive Surgery of the Foot and Leg, Update '90*. Tucker, GA, Podiatry Institute Publishing Co, 1990, pp 9-15.

30. Maerschalk P: Luxationsfracturen im Lisfrancschen Gelenk. *Unfallchirurgie* 8:112, 1982.

31. English TA: Dislocations of the metatarsal bone and adjacent toe. *J Bone Joint Surg* 46B:700, 1964.

32. Leitner B: Behandlung und Behandlungserge-bnisse von 42 frischen Fallen von luxatio pedis sub talo im Unfallkrankenhaus in Wien in der Jahren 1925-1940. *Ergebn Chir Orthop* 37:501, 1952.

33. Hesp WLEM, Van Der Werken C, Goris RJA: Lisfranc dislocations: fractures and/or dislocations through the tarso-metatarsal joints. *Injury* 15:261, 1984.

34. Aiken AP, Poulson D: Dislocation of the tarsometatarsal joint. *J Bone Joint Surg* 45A:246, 1963.

35. Hardcastle PH, Reschauer R, Kutscha-Lissberg E, Schoffman W: Injuries to the tarsometatarsal joint: incidence, classification and treatment. *J Bone Joint Surg* 64B:349, 1982.

36. Easton ER: Two rare dislocations of the metatarsal at Lisfranc's joint. *J Bone Joint Surg* 20:1053, 1938.

37. Norfray JF, Geline RA, Steinberg RI, Galinski AW, Giluca LA: Subtleties of Lisfranc fracture dislocations. *Am J Roentgenology* 137:1151, 1981.

38. Foster SC, Foster RR: Lisfranc's tarsometatarsal fracture-dislocation. *Radiology* 120:79, 1976.

39. Goossens M, DeStoop N: Lisfranc's fracture-dislocations: etiology, radiology, and results of treatment. *Clin Orthop* 176:154, 1983.

40. Gissane W: A dangerous type of fracture of the foot. *J Bone Joint Surg* 33B:535, 1951.

41. Del Sel JM: The surgical treatment of tarso-metatarsal fracture-dislocations. *J Bone Joint Surg* 46B:203, 1955.

42. Wiley JJ: The mechanism of tarso-metatarsal joint injuries. *J Bone Joint Surg* 53B:474, 1971.

43. Romanes GJ (ed): *Cunningham's Textbook of Anatomy*, ed 11. New York, Oxford University Press, 1972.

44. Jeffreys TE: Lisfranc's fracture-dislocation: a clinical and experimental study of tarso-metatarsal dislocations and fracture-dislocations. *J Bone Joint Surg* 45B:546, 1963.

45. Ashhurts APC: Divergent dislocation of the metatarsus. *Ann Surg* 83:132, 1926.

46. DiNapoli DR, Cain TD: Lisfranc fracture-dislocation update 1988. In McGlamry Ed (ed): *Reconstructive Surgery of the Foot and Leg, Update '88*. Tucker GA, Podiatry Institute Publishing Co, 1988, pp 198-204.

47. Francesconi F: Sopra un caso di lussanzione di Lisfranc. *Chir Organi Mov* 9:589, 1925.

48. Wilson DW: Injuries of the tarso-metatarsal joints. *J Bone Joint Surg* 54B:677, 1972.

49. Bonnel F, Barthelemy M: Traumatismes de l'articulation de Lisfranc: entroses graves, luxations, fractures: etude de 39 observations personnelle et classification biomecanique. *J Chir* (Paris) 111:573, 1963.

50. Quenu E, Kuss G: Etude sur les luxations du metatarse du diastasis entre le 1er et le 2e metatarsien. *Rev Chir* 39:281, 720, 1093; 1909.

51. Brunett JA, Wiley JJ: The late results of tarsometatarsal joint injuries. *J Bone Joint Surg* 69B:437, 1987.

52. Granberry WM, Lipscomb PR: Dislocations of the tarso-metatarsal joints. *Surg Gynecol Obstet* 114:467, 1962.

53. Cain PR, Seligson D: Lisfranc's fracture-dislocation with intercuneiform dislocation: presentation of two cases and a plan for treatment. *Foot Ankle* 2:156, 1981.

54. Cook JM, Galorenzo R, Gold RH: Lisfranc's joint dislocation: a review and case report. *J Am Podiatry Assoc* 71:611-617, 1981.

55. Wargon CA, Goldman FD: LisFranc fracture dislocation. *J Am Podiatr Med Assoc* 76:466-468, 1986.

56. Biyani A, Sharma JD, Mathur NC: Plantar panmetatarsophalangeal dislocation—a hyperflexion injury. *J Trauma* 28:868, 1988.

57. Bassett FH: Dislocations of the tarsometatarsal joints. *South Med J* 57:1294, 1964.

58. Arntz CT, Veith RG, Hansen ST: Fractures and fracture-dislocations of the tarsometatarsal joint. *J Bone Joint Surg* 70A:173, 1988.

59. Arntz CT, Hansen ST: Dislocations and fracture dislocations of the tarsometatarsal joints. *Orthop Clin North Am* 18:105, 1987.

60. Myerson M: The diagnosis and treatment of injuries to the LisFranc joint complex. *Orthop Clin North Am* 20:655, 1989.

61. Lenczner EM, Waddell JP, Graham JD: Tarsal-metatarsal (Lisfranc) dislocation. *J Trauma* 14:1012, 1974.

62. Holstein A, Joldersma RD: Dislocation of first cuneiform in tarsometatarsal fractures dislocations. *J Bone Joint Surg* 32:419, 1950.

63. Lowe J, Yosipovitch Z: Tarsometatarsal dislocation: a mechanism blocking manipulative reduction. *J Bone Joint Surg* 58:1029, 1976.

64. De Benedette MJ, Evanski PM, Waugh TR: The unreducible Lisfranc fracture. *Clin Orthop* 136:238, 1978.

65. Blair WF: Irreducible tarsometatarsal fracture dislocation. *J Trauma* 21:988, 1981.

66. Jahss MH: Traumatic dislocations of the first metatarsophalangeal joint. *Foot Ankle* 1:15, 1980.

67. Clanton TO, Butler JE, Eggert LA: Injuries to the metatarsophalangeal joints in athletes. *Foot Ankle* 7:162, 1986.

68. Bowers KD, Martin RB: Turf-toe: a shoe surface related football injury. *Med Sci Sports* 8:81, 1976.

69. Giannikas AC, Papachristou G, Papavasilou N, Nikifordis P, Hartofilak-idis-Garofalidis G: Dorsal dislocation of the first metatarso-phalangeal joint. *J Bone Joint Surg* 57B:384, 1975.

70. Salamon PB, Gelberman RH, Huffer JM: Dorsal dislocation of the metatarsophalangeal joint of the great toe. *J Bone Joint Surg* 56A:1073, 1974.

71. DeLuca FN, Kenmore PI: Bilateral dorsal dislocations of the metatarsophalangeal joints of the great toes with a loose body in one of the metatarsophalangeal joints. *J Trauma* 15:737, 1975.

72. Daniel WL, Beck EL, Duggar GE: Traumatic dislocation of the first metatarsophalangeal joint. *J Am Podiatry Assoc* 66:97-100, 1976.

73. Brown TIS: Avulsion fracture of the fibular sesamoid in association with dorsal dislocation of the metatarsophalangeal joint of the hallux. *Clin Orthop* 149:229, 1980.

74. Konkel KF, Muehlstein JH: Unusual fracture-dislocation of the great toe. *J Trauma* 15:733, 1975.

75. Mouchet A: Deux cas de luxation dorsale complete du gros orteil avec lesions des sesamoides. *Rev Orthop* 18:221, 1931.

76. Schlefman BS, McGlamry ED, Hilkemann RJ: First metatarsophalangeal joint dislocation in spina bifida. *J Am Podiatry Assoc* 74:147-152, 1984.

77. Smith TF, Cain T, DiNapoli RD: Dislocation injuries of the foot. In Scurran BL (ed): *Foot and Ankle Trauma*. New York, Churchill Livingstone, 1989, pp 271-308.

78. Smith TF: Pedal dislocations: an overview. *Clinics in Podiatry* 2:349-364, 1985.

79. Sage R, Holloway PW: Type I dorsal dislocation of the first metatarsophalangeal joint. *J Am Podiatric Med Assoc* 75:215-217, 1985.

80. Burns MJ: Recurrent dislocation of first metatarsophalangeal joint. *J Foot Surg* 15:118, 1976.

81. Mullis DL, Miller WE: A disabling sports injury of the great toe. *Foot Ankle* 1:22, 1980.

82. Coker TP, Arnold JA, Weber DL: Traumatic lesions of the metatarsalphalangeal joint of the great toe in athletes. *Am J Sports Med* 6:326, 1978.

83. Murphy JL: Isolated dorsal dislocation of the second metatarsophalangeal joint. *Foot Ankle* 1:30, 1980.

84. Roa JP, Manuel TB: Irreducible dislocation of the metatarsophalangeal joints of the foot. *Clin Orthop* 145:224, 1979.

85. English TA: Dislocation of the metatarsal bone and adjacent toe. *J Bone Joint Surg* 46B:700, 1964.

86. Anderson LD: Injuries of the forefoot. *Clin Orthop* 122:18, 1977.

87. Giannestras NJ, Sammarco GJ: Fractures and dislocations in the foot. In Rockwood CA, Green DP (eds): *Fractures.* Philadelphia, JP Lippincott, 1975, p 1488.

88. Miki T, Yamamurot, Kitai T: An irreducible dislocation of the great toe. *Clin Orthop* 230: 200, 1988.

89. Masaki T: An anatomical study of the interphalangeal sesamoid bone on the hallux. *Nippon Seikeigeka Gakkai Zasshi* 58: 419, 1984.

90. Katayama M, Murakami, Y, Takahashi, H: Irreducible dorsal dislocations of the toe. *J Bone Joint Surg* 70A:769, 1988.

91. Nelson TL, Uggen W: Irreducible dorsal dislocation of the interphalangeal joint of the great toe. *Clin Orthop* 157: 110, 1981.

92. Kursunoglu S, Resnick D, Goergen T: Traumatic dislocation with sesamoid entrapment in the interphalangeal joint of the great toe. *J Trauma* 27:959, 1987.

93. Noonan R, Thurber NB: Irreducible dorsal dislocation of the hallucal interphalangeal joint. *J Am Podiatr Med Assoc* 77:98-101, 1987.

94. Muller G: Dislocation of sesamoid hallux. *Lancet* 1: 789, 1948.

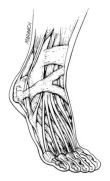

CHAPTER **61**

Digital and Sesamoidal Fractures

Michael S. Downey, D.P.M.

Although not generally considered to be serious injuries, fractures of the phalanges and sesamoids, if mistreated, can result in serious functional limitations and sequelae. As with all fractures, certain criteria for treatment must be remembered. These include (*a*) early recognition of the fracture(s) and reduction as soon as possible; (*b*) accurate anatomical reduction of the fracture fragments with restoration of any joint surfaces involved, if possible; (*c*) appropriate maintenance of the fracture fragments in the proper alignment during the healing period; and (*d*) early restoration of motion in any joints involved. Furthermore, a thorough understanding of the anatomy involved, as well as the principles of closed and open reduction, is a prerequisite to the proper treatment of these injuries (Fig. 61.1). If the digital nail is involved, an understanding of nail anatomy and care is needed (Fig. 61.2). Finally, if the fractures are associated with severe comminution, dislocation, or open injury, the clinician must be particularly attentive to these principles or the digit(s) involved may be lost.

DIGITAL FRACTURES

Etiology

As with any injury, the pathological forces that cause digital fracture(s) may be directed in any one of the cardinal body planes (frontal, sagittal, or transverse plane) or in a combination of these planes. Although the majority of injuries involve a combination of forces from varying body planes, a predominant plane of force can usually be identified. Certain fracture patterns are more frequently observed and can be related to these injury mechanisms. Identification of the pattern or mechanism of injury in this manner will afford the clinician easier reduction and realignment of the fracture fragments regardless of whether closed or open reduction is performed.

SAGITTAL PLANE

The predominant plane of injury most frequently observed in digital fractures is the sagittal plane. The most common examples of this injury are those that result from direct trauma and those that are secondary to hyperextension or hyperflexion of the involved digit(s) and digital joint(s).

Direct trauma caused by dropping a heavy object on the toes often results in a crushing injury to the soft tissues and nail(s) and a fracture of a phalanx or phalanges (Fig. 61.3). Occasionally the injury will compromise the neurovascular supply to the involved digits. Initial assessment of the neurovascular status and immediate treatment of the compromised structures are mandatory. With crushing injuries there often are associated subungual hematomas that must be assessed (Fig. 61.4). Subungual pressure secondary to hemorrhage can damage matrix cells and the surrounding nail bed if not relieved within the first 6 to 12 hours after the injury. Simple decompression can be afforded to small subungual hematomas. If the hematoma involves more than 25% of the visible nail plate, however, it is generally recommended that the nail involved be avulsed and the nail

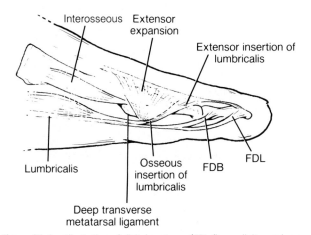

Figure 61.1. Illustration of digital anatomy. (*FDL*, flexor digitorum longus; *FDB*, flexor digitorum brevis.)

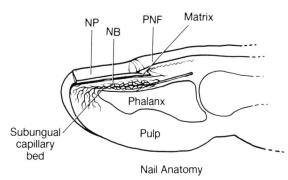

Figure 61.2. Illustration of nail anatomy. (*NP*, nail plate; *NB*, nail bed; *PNF*, proximal nail fold.)

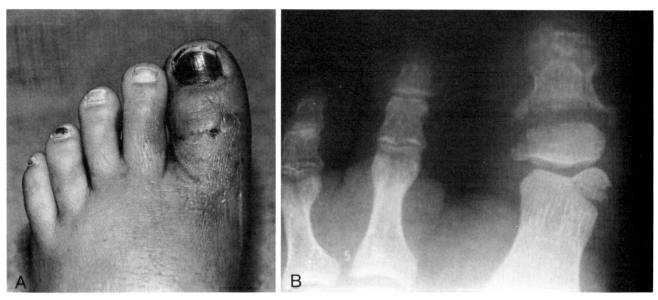

Figure 61.3. **A** and **B.** Direct trauma and crush injury to the hallux secondary to dropping a scuba tank on the foot. Note the clinical appearance of edema with associated subungual hematoma and severe comminution.

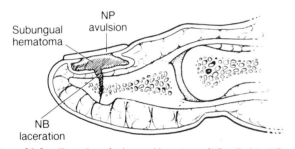

Figure 61.4.   Illustration of subungual hematoma. (*NP*, nail plate; *NB*, nail bed.)

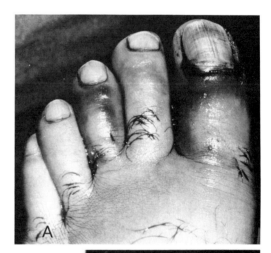

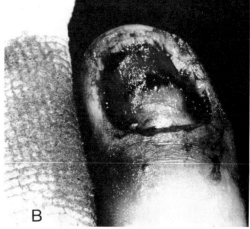

Figure 61.5. **A** and **B.** Subungual hematoma with a nail bed laceration evident on nail avulsion.

bed examined (1-3). If a nail bed laceration is discovered, the injury must be treated as if it were open (Fig. 61.5). The digital fractures seen in direct traumatic injuries are frequently comminuted and most commonly involve the phalanges of the hallux and the middle and distal phalanges of the lesser digits.

Another frequently observed sagittal plane injury is that caused by hyperextension or hyperflexion of the joints of the digit(s) involved. This injury is commonly known as the stubbed toe and, as one's childhood experiences would support, the hallux is most often involved. Dislocation of involved joints and open injuries are frequent with these fractures (Fig. 61.6).

TRANSVERSE PLANE

The predominantly transverse plane injury is another frequent mechanism of digital fracture. These injuries are caused by abduction-adduction forces and generally result in transverse or short oblique fractures of the proximal phalanges. The most notorious example of this injury has been termed the "bedroom fracture" because it often results from striking the fifth digit against a bedpost while walking in the dark. These fractures are often amenable to closed reduction if the fracture is transverse in nature and does not involve articular surfaces. Although the proximal phalanx of the fifth digit is most frequently involved, other phalanges and digits may suffer similar injuries (Fig. 61.7).

FRONTAL PLANE

The least frequent predominant pathological force in digital fractures is that caused by rotation and occurring in the frontal plane. Rotational or inversion-eversion injuries generally are secondary components associated with predominantly transverse or sagittal plane fractures. When spiral fractures of the phalanges occur, closed reduction will be more difficult.

Clinical Presentation

The symptoms associated with digital fracture(s) consist of acute pain, discomfort in wearing a shoe, and difficulty in walking. Generally any movement of the digit produces pain. Ecchymosis and edema usually develop within 2 to 3

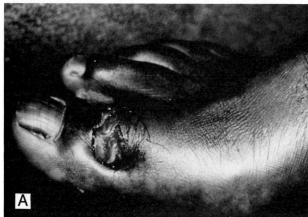
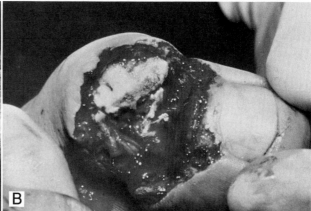

Figure 61.6. Two examples of hyperflexion injuries of the hallux with open fracture of the interphalangeal joint area. **A.** Injury secondary to stubbing of the hallux. **B.** Injury secondary to hyperflexion while jumping on a trampoline.

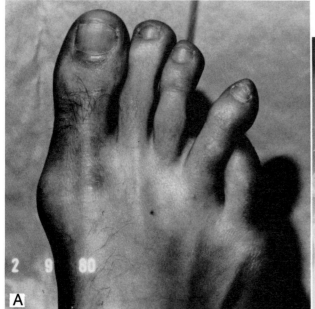
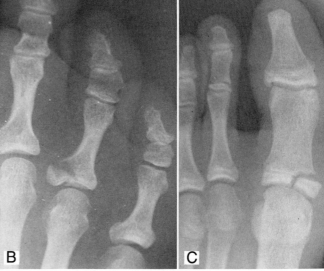

Figure 61.7. Examples of predominantly transverse plane injuries. **A.** Abduction injury of fourth digit with fracture of proximal phalanx. The injury occurred after striking an object between the third and fourth toes. **B.** Small avulsion fracture of the second plantar interosseus muscle from medial aspect of fourth toe proximal phalangeal base. The patient had abducted the toe when kicking a door. **C.** Salter-Harris type III injury to the physis of the proximal phalanx of the hallux. The patient suffered the abduction injury when kicking a soccer ball.

hours after injury (Fig. 61.8). Thus the profound edema associated with most digital fractures must be anticipated when immediate care is provided. A splint or bandage must not constrict the digit as this edema ensues. Often, especially in crush injuries caused by direct trauma, there is an associated subungual hematoma that must be treated.

Treatment

CLOSED INJURIES

When a digital fracture is suspected, a thorough history and physical examination, including radiographs, should be obtained. The physical examination should direct particular attention to the neurovascular status of any structures involved. Radiographs should include three views (dorsoplantar, lateral, and oblique), and attempts should be made to isolate the injury. As stated earlier, a thorough understanding of the anatomy of the digit is necessary for the occasionally difficult diagnosis. In addition, if the injury occurs in a juvenile patient, an understanding of the digital ossification centers and physeal injuries will be needed (4). As with most acute injuries, initial treatment should include rest, ice, and elevation of the injured area.

The treatment of closed digital fracture(s) can be categorized into methods based on several factors, including (*a*) alignment of the fracture fragments (*b*) if malaligned, the

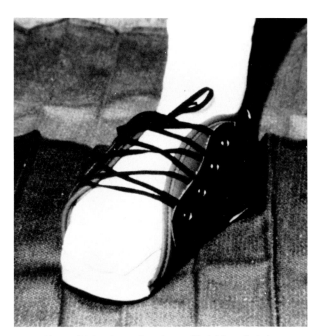

Figure 61.9.   Protection alone with rigid surgical shoe.

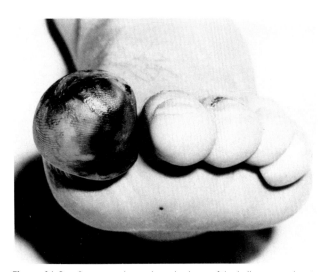

Figure 61.8.   Severe ecchymosis and edema of the hallux secondary to crush injury and fracture.

Table 61.1.
Methods of Treatment for Digital Fractures

Protection alone
Immobilization
Closed reduction/immobilization
Closed reduction/external fixation
Open reduction/internal fixation
Excision of fracture fragment(s)

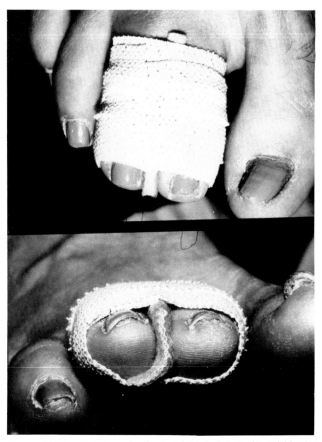

Figure 61.10.   Splinting of a fractured third digit to the neighboring second digit with felt and tape.

possibility that the fragments can be anatomically realigned with closed reduction, and (*c*) the possibility that alignment can be maintained once the fragments are reduced. The treatment methods, therefore, range from protection alone to surgical reduction or excision of all or some of the fracture fragments (Table 61.1).

Protection alone is simply alleviation of the usual forces applied to the injured bone. It is indicated for undisplaced, very stable fractures (e.g., incomplete fracture or hairline-type fracture). It also may be used after apparent clinical union resulting from another mode of treatment but before a full return to activity. Protection alone will generally consist of maintaining the injured part with no weight bearing or, if desired, in a rigid surgical shoe (Fig. 61.9). Often protection alone will not be adequate and further treatment will be necessary.

Immobilization by external splinting (without reduction)

can be added to any protective regimen. It is indicated for nondisplaced, fairly stable fractures. These fractures require simple maintenance of the alignment of the fracture fragments. Lesser digital fractures may be immobilized by splinting the injured digit(s) to the neighboring digit(s). With the use of tape, felt, silicone molds, urethane molds, or other similar materials, an effective splint can be created (Fig. 61.10). Alternatively, prefabricated digital splints are available and may be used (Fig. 61.11). For phalangeal fracture of the hallux, a splint of rigid material can be formed with the hallux incorporated into a dressing and secured to the splint along the medial aspect of the foot (Figs. 61.12 and 61.13). The injured foot with appropriate splintage can then be additionally protected with a rigid shoe or non-weight-bearing attitude.

If the fracture fragments are not properly aligned, either closed or open reduction should be considered. A thorough

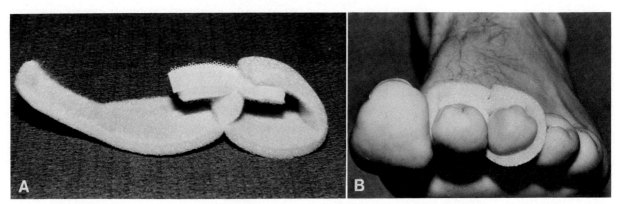

Figure 61.11.   A and **B.** Prefabricated splints with hook and loop (Velcro) fasteners can be used in digital fractures. These devices are generally less conforming but do allow easy removal for bathing.

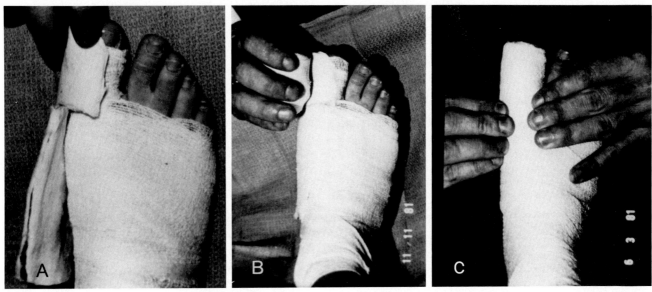

Figure 61.12.   A to **C.** Bandaging of the hallux to a Celastic splint along the medial aspect of the foot in a patient with a hallux fracture. Note that the splint should not completely surround and constrict the hallux if edema is anticipated.

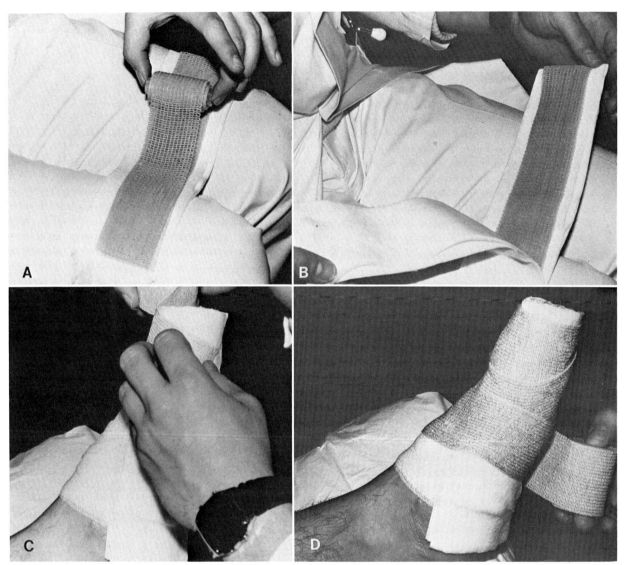

Figure 61.13. Immobilization of hallux fracture with a splint of cast material. **A** and **B.** Splint made by sandwiching a layer of cast material (e.g., 2- or 3-inch synthetic cast material) between layers of cast padding.

C and **D.** Splint applied along medial aspect of first ray and hallux. Immobilization will be afforded when the splint hardens.

understanding of the principles of closed and open reduction, as well as the anatomy and mechanism of injury, is a prerequisite to any reduction attempt. In the nonoperative or closed management of fractures, the actual bone fragments are considered to be of secondary importance. The primary structures necessary for successful realignment and maintenance of reduction of the fracture fragments are the intact and ruptured soft tissues associated with the fracture itself. The mechanism of injury of most fractures creates rupture of soft tissue structures (e.g., periosteum, ligaments, fascia) on the convex side of the fracture deformity and leaves the soft tissue structures on the concave side of the deformity intact. Reduction of the fracture becomes depen-

dent on these intact soft tissues, as they are used as a hinge or guide for realignment. It is these intact soft tissues that will prevent overcorrection when the fracture is reduced by closed reduction. Before one can take advantage of this soft tissue hinge, an accurate mental image of the predominant plane of force that created the injury must be formulated. Traction, along with the corresponding tension on the soft tissue hinge, followed by manipulative reversal of the predominant planal pathological force will usually result in adequate reduction.

Once successful reduction has been achieved, maintenance of the reduction becomes the foremost concern. The ability to maintain the reduction is dependent on the intrinsic stability of the fracture configuration. Intrinsic stability is the ability of the reduced fracture to withstand telescoping forces (e.g., muscle tension or edema) that would tend to displace and shorten the fractured segment. Fractures may be classified as stable, potentially stable, or unstable on the basis of their configuration.

The stable fracture is one that, after reduction, is completely able to withstand telescoping forces. These fractures are generally transverse in orientation to the longitudinal axis of the bone. Likewise, the potentially stable fracture is one that needs only protective support to aid in withstanding telescoping forces. The short oblique phalangeal fracture is a common example of a potentially stable fracture. Closed reduction followed by immobilization is indicated for stable and potentially stable displaced fractures that can be reduced (Figs. 61.14 and 61.15). Once realigned, the

fractures are easily maintained in reduction. After closed reduction, stable fractures and potentially stable fractures can be treated with immobilization as described earlier. Proper immobilization should support the fracture not only against shortening forces but also against angular forces.

The unstable fracture has minimal intrinsic ability to withstand shortening. These injuries are classically long oblique, spiral, or comminuted fractures. Often these unstable fractures will require additional support by external fixation or may necessitate open reduction with appropriate fixation. Therefore closed reduction with external fixation or with percutaneous pinning can be used for unstable fractures. Kirschner wires (K-wires) can be inserted percutaneously to maintain a realigned fracture (Fig. 61.16). This may be done with serial radiographs or fluoroscopy if necessary. Proper

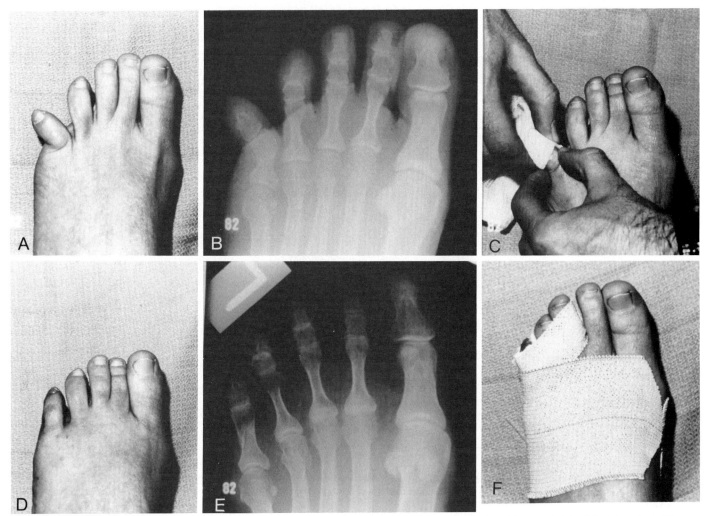

Figure 61.14. Demonstration of closed reduction of a potentially stable fracture of the proximal phalanx of the fifth digit. **A** and **B.** Prereduction clinical and radiographic appearance. **C.** Attempted closed reduction stabilizing the proximal segment and reducing the distal segment. Intact soft tissue hinge is on the lateral (concave) side of the injury. **D** and **E.** Postreduction clinical and radiographic appearance. **F.** Immobilization of the fifth digit by splinting to the neighboring third and fourth digits.

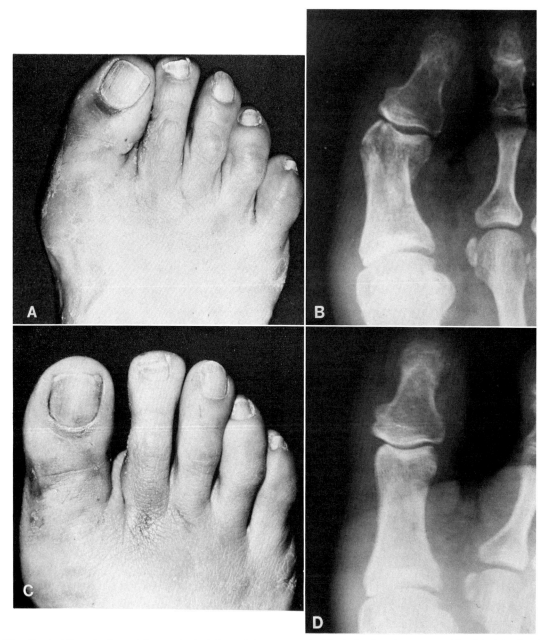

Figure 61.15.   Short oblique fracture of the proximal phalanx of the hallux. **A** and **B.** Prereduction clinical and radiographic appearance. Since this is an abduction injury, the intact soft tissues are along the lateral aspect of the hallux (i.e., the concave side of the injury) and can be used as a soft tissue hinge when closed reduction is performed. **C** and **D.** Postreduction clinical and radiographic appearance.

sterile precautions must be used to decrease the chances of postoperative pin tract infection.

If a fracture is unstable, nonreducible, intra-articular, or associated with concomitant injury (e.g., neurovascular injury), open reduction may be considered. As with any surgical procedure after trauma, proper precautions, including evaluation of edema and risk of infection, must be observed. Once the fragments are reduced, fixation may be achieved with K-wires (Fig. 61.17), screws (Fig. 61.18), or other forms

of fixation (e.g., Bilos pin). Intra-articular fractures of the hallux have a significant potential to develop posttraumatic arthritis, and frequently open reduction should be considered (Fig. 61.19)(5).

Occasionally, digital fractures will result in small fracture fragments that, because of their size, are not amenable to closed or open reduction. These fragments may be excised if open treatment is performed immediately, but more commonly they are excised only if they are causing symptoms after a course of conservative treatment (Fig. 61.20). If, after conservative treatment, an angulational malunion or painful arthrosis persists, resection arthroplasty of the involved joint may be necessary (6).

In most cases of digital fracture(s), clinical stabilization will occur within 4 to 8 weeks of initial immobilization. Radiographic evidence of fracture healing may occur within the same time frame, but it is not unusual to visualize digital fracture lines for several months. Thus the clinician need not wait for complete osseous consolidation but should temper the radiographic appearance of healing with the clinical examination. Once clinically stable and free of symptoms, a patient may be returned to normal shoes and rehabilitative physical therapy may be instituted.

Unfortunately, even with appropriate treatment, posttraumatic sequelae may occur after digital fractures. Included in the potential long-term problems are delayed union or nonunion of the fractured segments, malunion, and posttraumatic intra-articular arthrosis. In these instances, surgical intervention, possibly including revisional or salvage procedures such as arthroplasty or arthrodesis, may be necessary to obtain pain relief for the patient (5-8).

OPEN INJURIES

Open injuries frequently represent a surgical emergency, and a thorough history and physical examination are imperative. Examination should immediately address the neurovascular status of the injured part as well as the extent of any soft tissue loss (Fig. 61.21). As with closed injuries, initial treatment should consist of rest and elevation of the injured part. Ice can be applied proximal to the injured area if the neurovascular status is not compromised. In addition,

proper tetanus prophylaxis should be administered. In dirty wounds, a Gram's stain and cultures (aerobic and anaerobic) can be taken. Appropriate antibiotics may be instituted if deemed appropriate. Radiographs taken in three views should be evaluated (Fig. 61.22). Fundamentally, open injuries differ in many respects from closed injuries. The soft tissue injury is of primary concern in most open injuries. Once the soft tissue injury has been appropriately treated, the fracture may be addressed in a fashion similar to that used for the aforementioned closed injury (Fig. 61.23).

SESAMOID FRACTURES

Etiology

Similar to digital fractures, sesamoid fractures are most frequently caused by sagittal plane injuries that crush the ses-

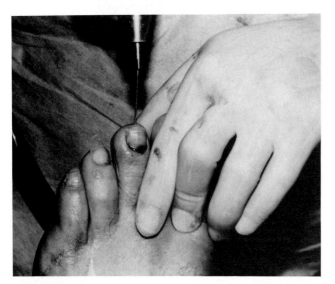

Figure 61.16. Percutaneous pinning with a K-wire of fractured third digit. The unstable fracture is treated with closed reduction and maintained manually while the K-wire is inserted. The percutaneous K-wire then maintains the reduction.

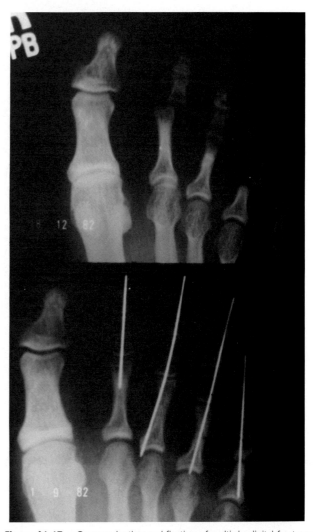

Figure 61.17. Open reduction and fixation of multiple digital fractures and dislocations using K-wires.

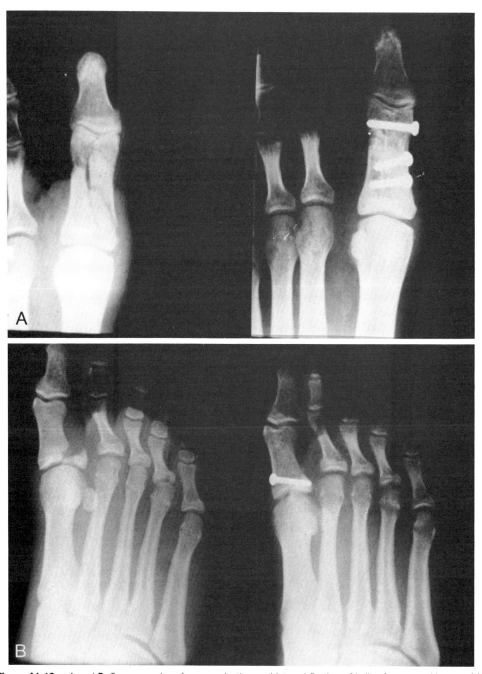

Figure 61.18. **A** and **B.** Two examples of open reduction and internal fixation of hallux fractures with screw(s).

amoid between the first metatarsal bone and the supporting surface. With the increasing popularity of active sports programs, such as aerobics, jogging, long-distance running, and accelerated or race walking, these injuries have become more common. Many sesamoid injuries are insidious in onset, with the patient unable to recall any single, acute traumatic event. Since the sesamoids of the first metatarsophalangeal joint receive the weight-bearing forces carried by

the first metatarsal head, they have a supportive role comparable to that of the lesser metatarsal heads (9, 10). Therefore it should be noted that sesamoid fractures can occur after repetitive sagittal plane trauma with no identifiable precipitating event (11). Certain biomechanical derangements and foot types (e.g., the cavus foot or the foot with metatarsus primus equinus) are predisposed to chronic repetitive sesamoid trauma and possible fracture (Fig. 61.24).

In addition, hyperflexion injuries may result in an avulsion fracture of a sesamoid or disruption of a multipartite sesamoid. Again, repetitive flexion trauma, frequently associated with active sports (e.g., aerobics, tennis, basketball), can be responsible for the subacute fracture of a sesamoid or the disruption of a multipartite sesamoid with no history of a single traumatic event (12, 13).

Clinical Presentation

Typically, the patient with a sesamoid fracture has acute or chronic pain beneath the first metatarsal area. In more acute cases, the pain will be severe and the patient may guard against any weight bearing and dorsiflexion of the first metatarsophalangeal joint. Obviously, edema and ecchymosis may accompany the injury. More chronic fractures may have reduced or no edema and may feel more like a bruise to the patient. The pain may increase with activity, dorsiflexion of the first metatarsophalangeal joint, or in certain shoes

(e.g., high-heeled shoes). In more chronic cases, the patient may or may not recall a specific acute traumatic event. If the onset was sudden but the patient did not seek immediate professional help, the time elapsed since the traumatic incident will be of assistance in developing the prognosis with conservative management.

On physical examination, localized pain is elicited with direct palpation of the injured sesamoid(s). The pain may shift with the position of the sesamoids as the first metatarsophalangeal joint is taken through its range of motion. In addition, pain may be found with passive flexion, abduction, or adduction of the hallux at the metatarsophalangeal joint (14).

Treatment

When a sesamoid fracture is suspected, radiographs should be performed. At least three radiographic views should be obtained, including a sesamoid axial view if possible. The

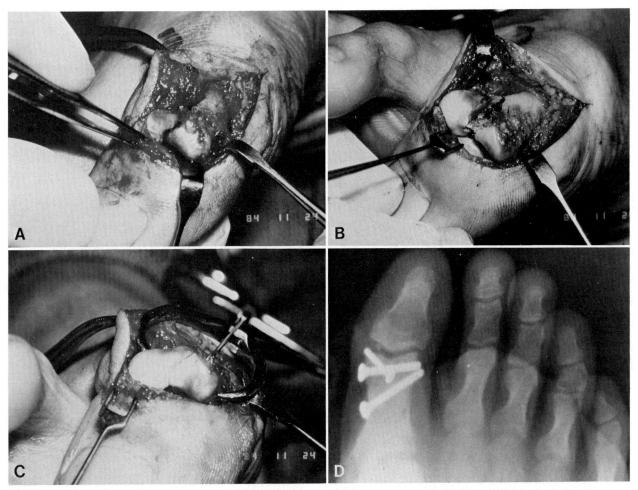

Figure 61.19. **A** and **B.** Intraoperative clinical appearance of an intra-articular fracture of hallux with fracture extension into the interphalangeal joint. **C.** Intraoperative clinical appearance after reduction and fixation. **D.** Postoperative radiograph demonstrating reduction of fracture with internal fixation.

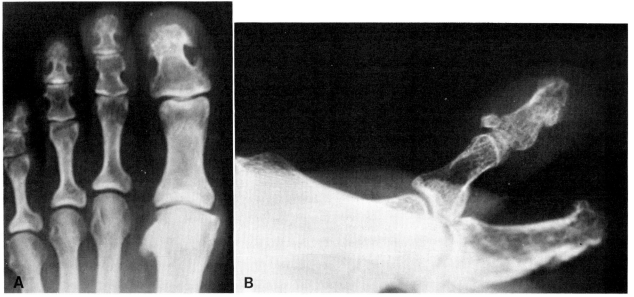

Figure 61.20. **A** and **B.** Radiographic appearance of small dorsal intra-articular fracture fragment of the distal interphalangeal joint of the second toe. The fragment was still causing pain with joint motion 4 months after injury and was excised. Note that the fragment is readily visible only on an isolated lateral view of the second toe.

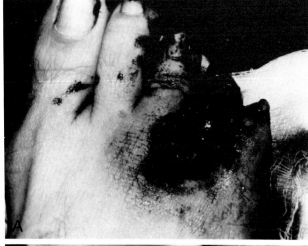

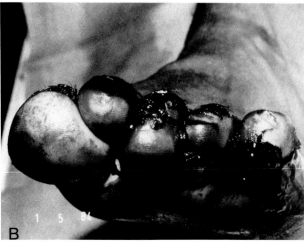

Figure 61.21. Examples of soft tissue injuries associated with digital fractures. **A.** A gunshot injury to the fourth toe. **B.** A lawn mower injury to the lesser digits.

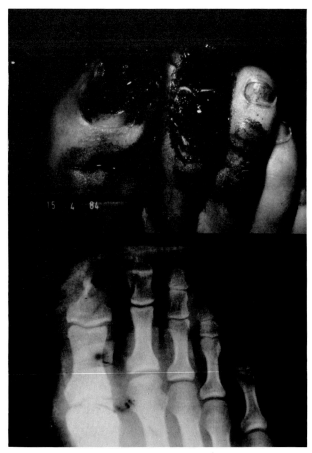

Figure 61.22. Soft tissue injury and associated fractures after a lawn mower accident. Correlation of clinical and radiographic appearance is important in planning a sound surgical approach.

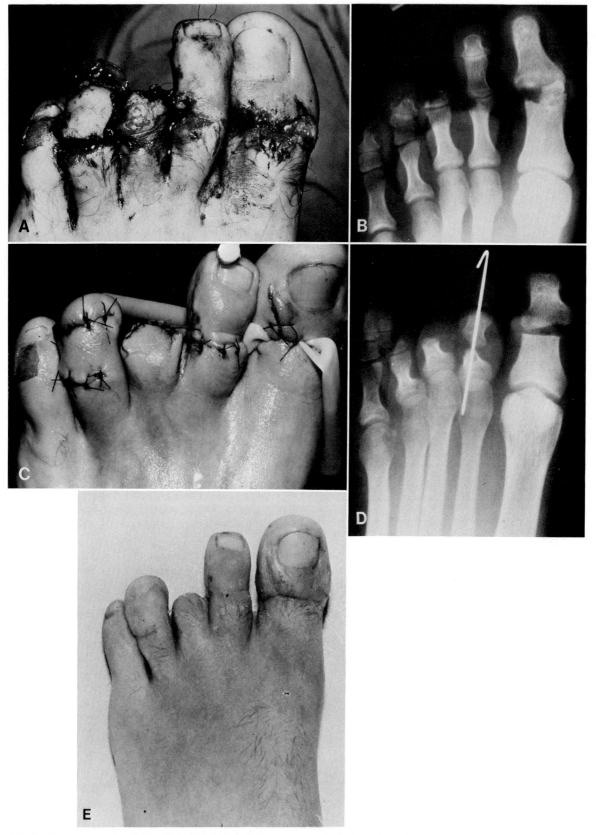

Figure 61.23. Severe open injury to the digits after a motorcycle accident. **A** and **B.** Initial clinical and radiographic presentation. Immediate treatment is oriented at treating the wounds and preventing infection. **C** and **D.** After stabilization of the soft tissues, surgical treatment and management of the fractures are completed. **E.** Clinical appearance 6 months after injury.

Figure 61.24. Fractured fibular sesamoid in a patient with metatarsus primus equinus. There is no history of trauma, but the patient does participate in high-impact aerobics.

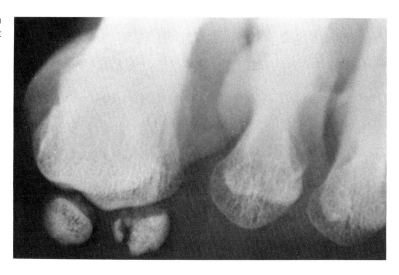

Table 61.2.

Radiographic Criteria Suggestive of a Fracture in Attempted Differentiation of a Sesamoid Fracture From a Partite Sesamoid

No evidence of fracture on previous/earlier radiographs
Irregular, serrated, jagged line(s) of separation
Longitudinally or obliquely oriented division lines
Absence of similar findings in contralateral foot
Injured sesamoid similar in size to neighboring sesamoid
Exaggerated space of fragment separations
Anatomically abnormal fragment positions
Multiple irregular fragments
Interrupted peripheral cortices
Bone callous formation

tibial sesamoid is more commonly fractured because of its increased load in closed kinetic chain gait. Rarely, both sesamoids of the same metatarsal may be fractured (15).

Differentiation of a sesamoid fracture from a bipartite or multipartite sesamoid can be a diagnostic challenge. Usually, a sesamoid fracture is transverse or comminuted, and the line of separation is more jagged, irregular, and uneven. Although transverse separation is most common, if the line of division is longitudinally or obliquely oriented, or if the space between the fragments is particularly large, a sesamoid fracture is likely. Contralateral views may be helpful, as the finding of partite sesamoids in an uninjured foot may suggest a similar congenital partition in the traumatized foot. In addition, bipartite or tripartite sesamoids are usually larger than a normal sesamoid. This knowledge may provide support to a tentative diagnosis (Table 61.2). If radiographs are equivocal or if additional diagnostic information is needed, technetium 99 bone scans, dorsiflexion stress radiographs of the metatarsophalangeal joint, computed tomography (CT), or magnetic resonance imaging (MRI) may be considered (Fig. 61.25). In any case, if the radiographs suggest a possible fracture and the patient has symptoms, the injury must be treated as a fracture.

Treatment of sesamoid fractures is directed toward relieving direct and indirect pressure to the injured bone(s). Direct pressure is eliminated by keeping the first metatarsal from weight bearing. This may be accomplished by placing the foot in a non-weight-bearing attitude or cast or by padding the foot to prevent first metatarsal contact with the weight-bearing surface (e.g., use of a walking cast or surgical shoe with a dancer's pad or a pad with the area under the first metatarsal removed). Indirect pressure is applied to the sesamoids by tension on the intrinsic muscular attachments to the sesamoids with sagittal plane dorsiflexion or transverse plane motion. Relief of this pressure may be achieved by limitation of dorsiflexion, adduction, or abduction of the first metatarsophalangeal joint. The limitation of dorsiflexion is most important, and the first metatarsophalangeal joint may even be splinted in plantarflexion to prevent this indirect pressure. In most sesamoid fractures, conservative treatment should be aggressive. Conservative measures frequently fail if the treatment is delayed or inadequate. Thus the author prefers a non-weight-bearing below-knee cast that extends to the end of the hallux. The cast padding and material are applied to maintain the first metatarsophalangeal joint slightly plantarflexed, and the cast is extended to the end of the hallux to prevent joint motion. The non-weight-bearing cast is maintained for a minimum of 4 weeks.

In more chronic injuries or in fractures that are seen several months after an acute traumatic event, a technetium-99 bone scan or magnetic resonance imaging study may be helpful in determining the vascularity of the injured osseous fragments and their potential to heal with conservative management. The author prefers to use the accommodative weight-bearing devices mentioned above only after a course of non-weight-bearing immobilization or when the injury is not a fracture but sesamoiditis.

When conservative treatment fails, surgical intervention may be considered. Nonunion, malunion, and intra-articular arthritis of the first metatarso-sesamoidal articulation may result after a sesamoid fracture. Blake (16) has stated

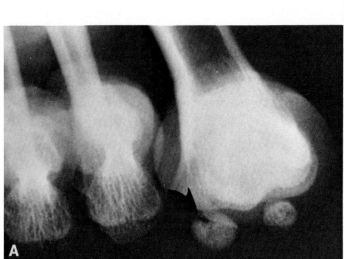 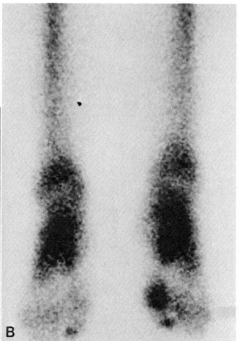

Figure 61.25. Suspected fracture of the fibular sesamoid of the left foot. **A.** Sesamoid axial view demonstrating suspected fibular sesamoid fracture (arrow). **B.** Third phase of technetium 99 bone scan of foot. Note increased activity in the area of the fibular sesamoid of the left foot, strongly suggesting a fracture.

that more than 30% of all sesamoid fractures will eventually require surgery. Although this percentage may be high, it reiterates the importance of early and aggressive conservative management. Generally, excision of the injured sesamoid is performed.

A fractured tibial sesamoid is removed through a plantarmedial approach (Fig. 61.26). A 3 to 6 cm incision is made, extending from the first metatarsophalangeal joint proximally. The incision is deepened with care to prevent damage to the proper digital branches of the medial plantar and medial dorsocutaneous nerves. The first metatarsophalangeal joint capsule is then incised along the dorsomedial margin of the sesamoid. This capsular approach allows the sesamoid to be shelled from its attachments to the intrinsic tendoligamentous complex while minimizing damage to these structures. If the attachments of the medial head of the flexor hallucis brevis or abductor hallucis muscles are significantly damaged during removal of the sesamoid, they should be repaired or reattached.

Marcinko and Elleby (8) have suggested removal of only the distal fragment of a fractured tibial sesamoid with retention of the proximal fragment. Although their results have been promising, as they have noted, additional long-term evaluation of this technique is needed. After excision of the sesamoid, layer closure of the capsule, superficial fascia, and skin may be accomplished. Postoperatively, the foot is immobilized in a non-weight-bearing cast or guarded weight bearing is allowed for approximately 3 weeks with a subsequent gradual return to full weight bearing.

Removal of a fractured fibular sesamoid is best accomplished from a dorsal approach over the first intermetatarsal space. Alternatively, a direct plantar approach may be considered, but the increased risk of a plantar weight-bearing scar must be recognized. The dorsal approach involves a 3 to 6 cm incision extending from the web space proximally. The incision is carried deep, and the extensor expansion is incised. Once the sesamoid is identified, it is clamped or skewered with a K-wire or the Vogen sesamoid clamp. The sesamoid is then freed from its soft tissue attachments and excised. Care must be taken to avoid damage to the flexor hallucis longus tendon and to minimize damage to the intrinsic tendoligamentous complex. With the clamp or wire and plantarflexion of the first metatarsophalangeal joint, the sesamoid may be removed in an unlabored fashion. In addition, by sequential release from its attachments (first, release of lateral capsule and tendon investment; second, release of proximal attachments; third, release of distal attachments; fourth, release of the intersesamoidal ligament), layer closure is then performed.

Postoperatively, immobilization in a non-weight-bearing cast or weight bearing in a guarded fashion is indicated for the first 3 weeks. This is followed by a gradual return to full activity.

After extirpation of a fractured sesamoid, dynamic imbalance of the remaining musculoligamentous complex must be one's primary concern. Although rare, hallux valgus may occur after tibial sesamoid removal and hallux varus may occur after fibular sesamoid removal. Long-term man-

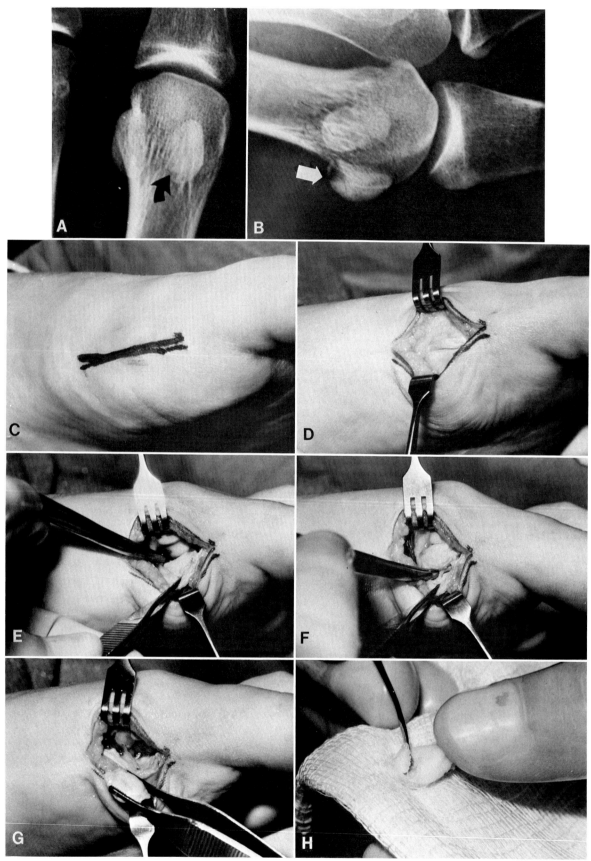

Figure 61.26. Nonunion after fracture of the tibial sesamoid of the left foot. Surgical approach to the removal of the sesamoid. **A** and **B.** Dorsoplantar and oblique views of injured tibial sesamoid. **C.** Plantar-medial incision at the level of the first metatarsal-sesamoid articulation. **D.** Incision deepened to the level of the joint capsule. Care is taken to avoid the proper digital branches of the medial dorsocutaneous nerve and medial plantar nerve. **E.** Capsular incision at the dorsomedial aspect of the tibial sesamoid. Note that the plantar aspect of the first metatarsal head (identified by end of Metzenbaum scissors) and the dorsal portion of the sesamoid (just above forceps) are clearly visible. **F.** The tibial sesamoid is carefully freed from intrinsic attachments. **G.** Fractured tibial sesamoid removed in toto. **H.** On removal, fracture fragments and nonunion of the tibial sesamoid are easily separated and visualized.

agement with functional orthoses or a hallux splint may decrease the likelihood of these potential problems.

If both sesamoids are removed, the flexor apparatus may be overpowered and a hallux malleus deformity frequently results. Thus, if both sesamoids are to be removed, an interphalangeal joint arthrodesis, possibly combined with a Jones' tenosuspension of the extensor hallucis longus, should be considered at the time of sesamoid removal. Alternatively, joint destructive procedures such as a Keller arthroplasty, with or without an implant, or an arthrodesis of the first metatarsophalangeal joint may be indicated in certain situations or arthritic conditions (17).

SUMMARY

A complete overview of the etiology, clinical presentation, and treatment for digital and sesamoidal fractures has been presented. As can be noted from the text, significant attention and care are required for these seemingly unimportant and innocent injuries. Casual, inappropriate, or inadequate treatment of these fractures may result in debilitating sequelae. The physician treating the lower extremity must continuously stress and reinforce the proper and thorough management of these common fractures.

REFERENCES

1. Malay DS: Trauma to the nail and associated structures. In McGlamry ED (ed): *Comprehensive Textbook of Foot Surgery.* Baltimore, Williams & Wilkins, 1987, pp 996-1002.
2. Zook EG: The perionychium: anatomy, physiology, and care of injuries. *Clin Plast Surg* 8:21-31, 1981.
3. Farrington GH: Subungual hematoma—an evaluation of treatment. *Br Med J* 21:742-744, 1964.
4. Banks AS, Cain TD, Ruch JR: Physeal fractures of the distal phalanx of the hallux. *J Am Podiatr Med Assoc* 78:310-313, 1988.
5. Jahss MH: Stubbing injuries to the hallux. *Foot Ankle* 1:327-332, 1980.
6. Elleby DH, Marcinko DE: Digital fractures and dislocations: diagnosis and treatment. *Clin Podiatry* 2:233-245, 1985.
7. Heim U, Pfeiffer KM: *Internal Fixation of Small Fractures: Technique Recommended by the AO-ASIF Group,* ed 3. New York, Springer-Verlag, 1988, p 371.
8. Marcinko DE, Elleby DH: Digital fractures and dislocations. In Scurran BL (ed): *Foot and Ankle Trauma.* New York, Churchill Livingstone, 1989, pp 309-322.
9. Jahss MH: The sesamoids of the hallux. *Clin Orthop* 157:88-97, 1981.
10. David RD, Delagoutte JP, Renard MM: Anatomical study of the sesamoid bones of the first metatarsal. *J Am Podiatr Med Assoc* 79:536-544, 1989.
11. Speed K: Injuries of the great toe sesamoids. *Ann Surg* 60:478-480, 1914.
12. Goldman F: Ipsilateral dual sesamoid injury: a case report. *J Am Podiatr Med Assoc* 74:187-191, 1984.
13. Frankel JP, Harrington J: Symptomatic bipartite sesamoids. *J Foot Surg* 29:318-323, 1990.
14. Bizarro AH: On the traumatology of the sesamoid structures. *Ann Surg* 74:783-791, 1921.
15. Abraham M, Sage R, Lorenz M: Tibial and fibular sesamoid fractures on the same metatarsal: a review of two cases. *J Foot Surg* 28:308-311, 1989.
16. Blake RL: Athletic injuries: orthoses versus surgery. In Jay RM (ed):

Current Therapy in Podiatric Surgery. Philadelphia, BC Decker, 1989, pp 296-301.
17. Stroh KI, Altman MI, Yee DYS: First metatarsophalangeal joint arthrodesis: treatment for sesamoid fractures. *J Am Podiatr Med Assoc* 80:595-599, 1990.

Additional References

Bartis JR: Uncommon phalangeal fracture, a case report. *J Am Podiatr Assoc* 54:410, 1964.
Brown TIS: Avulsion fracture of the fibular sesamoid in association with dorsal dislocation of the metatarsophalangeal joint of the hallux: report of a case and review of the literature. *Clin Orthop* 149:229-231, 1980.
Christensen SE, Cetti R, Niebuhr-Jorgensen U: Fracture of the fibular sesamoid of the hallux. *Br J Sports Med* 17:177-179, 1983.
Cobey JC: Treatment of undisplaced toe fractures with a metatarsal bar made from tongue blades. *Clin Orthop* 103:56, 1974.
Connolly JF: Fractures of the toes. In *DePalma's The Management of Fractures and Dislocations: An Atlas,* ed 3. Philadelphia, WB Saunders, 1981, vol 2, pp 2073-2077.
Dennis KJ, McKinney S: Sesamoids and accessory bones of the foot. *Clin Podiatr Med Surg* 7:717-723, 1990.
Dix R: Fractured sesamoid, a case report. *J Am Podiatr Assoc* 53:663, 1963.
Dobas DC, Slavitt JA: Impact fractures of the lesser digits: a clinical description with a case history. *J Am Podiatr Assoc* 67:571-573, 1977.
Dobas DC, Silvers MD: The frequency of partite sesamoids of the first metatarsophalangeal joint. *J Am Podiatr Assoc* 67:880-882, 1977.
Giannestras NJ, Sammarco GJ: Fractures and dislocations in the foot. In Rockwood CA Jr, Green DP (eds): *Fractures,* Philadelphia, JB Lippincott, 1975, vol 2, pp 1400-1495.
Gilchrist AK: Surgical care of the traumatized foot. *J Am Podiatry Assoc* 65:816-824, 1975.
Glass B: Fractured fibular sesamoid: a case report. *J Foot Surg* 19:19-21, 1980.
Green DP, Anderson JR: Closed reduction and percutaneous pin fixation of fractured phalanges. *J Bone Joint Surg* 55A:1651-1654, 1973.
Heckman JD: Fractures and dislocations of the foot. In Rockwood CA Jr, Green DP (eds): *Fractures in Adults,* ed 2. Philadelphia, JB Lippincott, 1984, vol 2, pp 1703-1832.
Heppenstall RB: *Fracture Treatment and Healing.* Philadelphia, WB Saunders, 1980, pp 878-880.
Hobart MH: Fracture of sesamoid bones of the foot: with report of a case. *J Bone Joint Surg* 11:298-302, 1929.
Hulkko A, Orava S, Pellinen P, Puranen J: Stress fractures of the sesamoid bones of the first metatarsophalangeal joint in athletes. *Arch Orthop Trauma Surg* 104:113-117, 1985.
Orr TG: Fracture of great toe sesamoid bones. *Ann Surg* 67:609-612, 1918.
Parra G: Stress fractures of the sesamoids of the foot. *Clin Orthop* 18:281-285, 1960.
Pinckney LE, Currarino G, Kennedy LA: The stubbed great toe: a cause of occult compound fracture and infection. *Radiology* 138:375-377, 1981.
Richardson EG: Injuries to the hallucal sesamoids in the athlete. *Foot Ankle* 7:229-244, 1987.
Seder JI: Sesamoiditis. *J Am Podiatr Assoc* 64:444-446, 1974.
Siegel N, Cutler S: Fractured tibial sesamoids: a case report and clinical review. *J Am Podiatr Assoc* 66:702-705, 1976.
Tobin GR: Closure of contaminated wounds: biologic and technical considerations. *Surg Clin North Am* 64:639-652, 1984.

Van Hal ME, Keene JS, Lange TA, Clancy WG Jr: Stress fractures of the great toe sesamoids. *Am J Sports Med* 10:122-128, 1982.
Vranes R: Hallux sesamoids: a divided issue. *J Am Podiatr Assoc* 66:687-698, 1976.
Zacher JB: Management of injuries of the distal phalanx. *Surg Clin North Am* 64:747-760, 1984.
Zinman H, Keret D, Reis ND: Fracture of the medial sesamoid bone of the hallux. *J Trauma* 21:581-582, 1981.

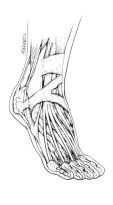

CHAPTER **62**

Metatarsal Fractures

George R. Vito, D.P.M.
Stanley R. Kalish, D.P.M.
*Jerry R. Maxwell, D.P.M.**

Fractures of the metatarsals are common conditions seen by all practitioners. Metatarsal fractures are most often a result of direct trauma, typically due to a heavy object having been dropped on the foot. The second, third, and fourth metatarsals are affected most frequently. Indirect trauma may result in these injuries if the forefoot is fixed and a medial or lateral torque is applied (1). Metatarsal fractures may be undertreated, and there may be inadequate follow-up in many instances (2). A working knowledge of anatomical and mechanical relationships of the foot is needed to manage the fracture most appropriately.

The patient's general health, age, occupation, and ambulatory status prior to the injury may all influence the treatment plan. If possible, the mechanism of injury should be determined and consideration should be given to additional injuries that may have occurred concomitantly. The neurovascular status should always be assessed, as marked edema may lead to vascular compromise resulting in a possible compartment syndrome. Although rare, compartment syndrome of the foot has been reported after metatarsal fractures (3, 4). If a compartment syndrome is suspected, early decompression of the fascial spaces is recommended.

Radiographic evaluation should include at least two views oriented at 90 degrees to one another (5). Preferably, three images, including the dorsoplantar, lateral oblique, and lateral projections, should be taken. The dorsoplantar view demonstrates the amount of transverse plane displacement, metatarsal shortening, and changes in the parabolic curve of the metatarsals. The oblique view assists in determining the relationship of the fracture fragments in both the sagittal and transverse planes. The lateral view assesses sagittal plane displacement but can be misleading because of the inherent overlap of the segments in this view. If proper anatomic position is in question, a plantar axial or sesamoid axial view may be considered. The axial radiograph may reveal the relative positions of the metatarsal heads in the sagittal plane.

The major goal of fracture treatment is to return the injured part to full function. Restoration of the normal weight-bearing alignment of the metatarsal heads is ideal.

Immediate and appropriate treatment is optimized if the patient is evaluated within a relatively short period of time after the injury. Ideally, open reduction should be performed within the first 6 to 12 hours after the fracture; otherwise, reactive edema ensues and increases the risk of postoperative wound complications. Depending on the nature of the injury, surgical intervention may have to be delayed to allow reduction of posttraumatic edema and to stabilize any associated skin damage. Closed reduction of metatarsal fractures is also compromised by severe edema. The swelling must be controlled initially, and temporary immobilization must be instituted.

Whether closed or open techniques are considered, a total conceptualization of the fracture type, potential complications, and secondary functional problems is necessary. For example, displaced metatarsal neck fractures are notoriously difficult to reduce and maintain in alignment by closed means.

When all of these elements are properly understood and evaluated and correct treatment is instituted at the right time, patients with traumatic injuries will have the best chance for early and complete recovery.

CLOSED REDUCTION TECHNIQUES

Generally speaking, anatomic closed reduction of most metatarsal fractures cannot be achieved if there is significant displacement. With certain guidelines and manipulative techniques, however, closed reduction of specific fractures can be achieved. Guidelines for any closed reduction procedure include *(a)* prereduction films to study the extent and direction of the fracture, *(b)* an anesthetic agent, either general or local, depending on the severity of the injury, *(c)* traction and countertraction during the manipulative maneuvers, and *(d)* postreduction films to assess the alignment.

Displaced transverse neck fractures are especially difficult to reduce. Closed reduction techniques involve distal traction of the toes at the metatarsophalangeal joint. Often a traction finger splint is employed. Flexion or extension of the metatarsophalangeal joint and plantarflexion or dorsiflexion of the forefoot (depending on the direction of the metatarsal head displacement) is then executed.

Oblique fractures are usually located at the metatarsal neck or midshaft. Closed reduction traction and countertraction techniques in the latter circumstance are at times

Appreciation is expressed to Jerry R. Maxwell, D.P.M., who wrote this chapter in the first edition.

difficult because of the location of the fracture, as traction tends to be less effective than with more distal injuries. Key radiographic points include the degree of shortening of the affected metatarsal (overriding of the fragments), metatarsophalangeal joint congruity, and transverse and sagittal plane alignment on the weight-bearing plane.

OPEN REDUCTION TECHNIQUES

Open reduction and internal fixation of metatarsal fractures should be considered if the advantages outweigh those of closed reduction. Implementation of the principles of atraumatic technique, rigid fixation, and early motion of the adjacent soft tissues provide optimum recovery. These techniques provide the surgeon with a sophisticated approach to operative fracture treatment, which allows for the best functional end result.

ANATOMICAL FRACTURE TYPES

Fractures of the First Metatarsal

Generally, first metatarsal fractures should be treated more aggressively than those that involve the lesser metatarsals because of the role of the first ray in locomotion. Simple fractures of the shaft of the first metatarsal that are well aligned may be treated by immobilization with no weight bearing for 6 to 8 weeks. Displaced fractures of the shaft of the first metatarsal are generally reduced and fixated. Short

oblique fractures may be fixated with one or two cortical screws. However, long oblique fractures and more transverse fractures may incorporate a combination of interfragmental screws and/or a neutralization plate. With the use of internal fixation, no weight bearing is allowed for a period of 6 to 8 weeks.

Intra-articular fractures of the first metatarsophalangeal joint are generally treated by open reduction and internal fixation techniques. LaPorta (6) suggests that fixation of an intra-articular fragment should be performed when one fifth to one fourth of the articular surface is involved.

First metatarsal base fractures not associated with Lisfranc's joint dislocation are infrequent because of the inherent stability of the associated osseous and ligamentous structures and because the stresses applied to the medial side of the foot are generally not as great as those applied laterally (7). Avulsion fractures of the anterior tibial or peroneus longus tendons may occur as either intra-articular or extra-articular injuries (Fig. 62.1).

Fractures of the Lesser Metatarsal Heads

Fractures of the metatarsal heads, if intra-articular, should be surgically reduced to restore anatomic alignment of the articular surface (Figs. 62.2 and 62.3). If the fragments are too small, closed manipulative reduction may be performed. The use of a rigid-soled shoe or an orthosis with early range of motion may be instituted. Fractures of the distal metaphyseal area are usually transverse in nature and can be

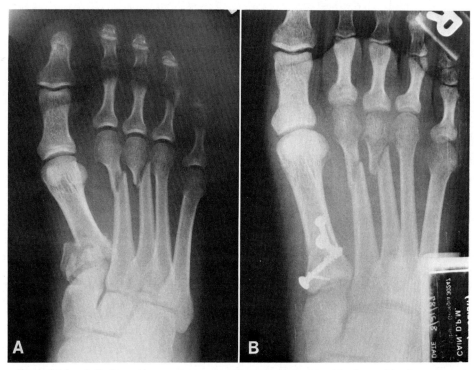

Figure 62.1.   **A.** Radiographic appearance of an intra-articular fracture of the base of the first metatarsal.
B. After open reduction with internal fixation.

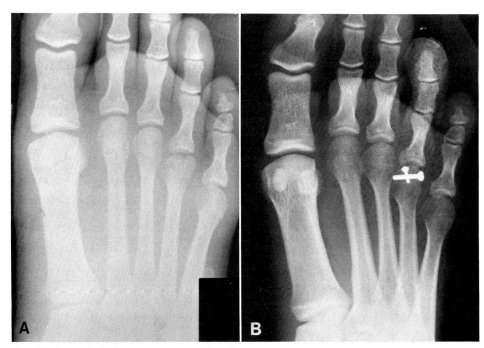

Figure 62.2. **A** and **B.** Intra-articular fracture of the head of the fourth metatarsal reduced and fixated with 2.0 mm and 1.5 mm screws.

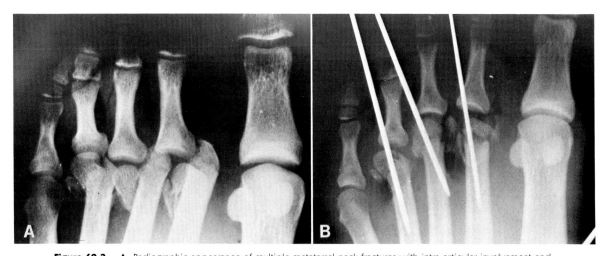

Figure 62.3. **A.** Radiographic appearance of multiple metatarsal neck fractures with intra-articular involvement and displacement. **B.** Multiple K-wire fixation.

treated with closed casting techniques. If displaced, open reduction may be employed with either wires, screws, or a small T-plate. Freiberg's infraction or aseptic necrosis of the metatarsal head has been noted after this type of injury (8).

Fractures of the Lesser Metatarsal Necks

Fractures of metatarsal necks are common because the traumatic force is often perpendicular to the long axis of the metatarsal. The fracture configuration is usually oblique, although transverse, spiral, and comminuted injuries may

occur. If the fracture is not displaced, a well-molded, non-weight-bearing cast may suffice. If the fracture is displaced, significant shortening may occur with resultant loss of the metatarsal parabola and possible metatarsalgia. Closed reduction may be attempted with the patient under anesthesia, followed by cast immobilization if successful. Soft tissue edema and muscle contracture frequently prevent the maintenance of satisfactory reduction. Failure to achieve satisfactory reduction with moderate displacement may result in a primary painful plantar foot with or without callosities and a secondary floating toe deformity with clawing of the

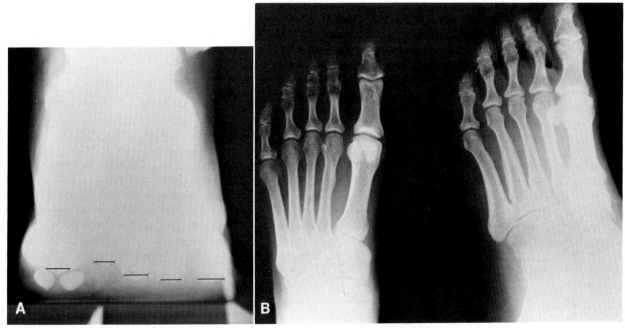

Figure 62.4. **A** and **B.** After an oblique second metatarsal fracture with shortening and elevation, with symptoms now experienced plantar to the first and third metatarsals. Healing alone should not be used as a criterion for success after metatarsal fractures.

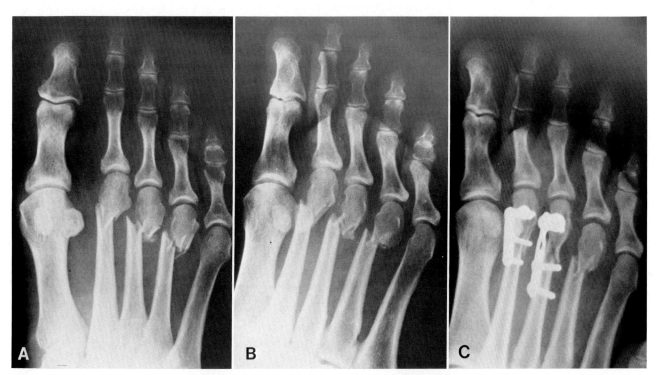

Figure 62.5. **A** and **B.** Preoperative radiographs of a patient with displaced metatarsal neck fractures. Not only is there malalignment, but, with multiple injuries, the stabilizing effect of the deep transverse intermetatarsal ligament is lost. **C.** After ORIF.

adjacent toes. Surgery is often needed later to alleviate metatarsalgia associated with malunited neck fractures (2)(Fig. 62.4).

Oblique fractures are amenable to a variety of fixation techniques, including intramedullary pinning with Kirschner wires (K-wires) and interfragmental compression by the lag screw technique or plate fixation (Fig. 62.5). The cerclage wiring technique, as described by Smith and Green (9), resulted in minimal difficulty in healing. The only deterrent was the period of immobilization required. This form of fixation provides limited stability compared to other forms of fixation and may be disrupted more easily. However, difficult comminuted fractures of the internal metatarsals may be treated in this manner (5, 10).

Transverse fractures of the epiphysis with displacement may also require open reduction and internal fixation. Smooth Kirschner wires offer the best form of fixation, as they may be placed across the physis without encouraging growth arrest (Fig. 62.6).

If more than one of the internal metatarsal heads are fractured, the most unstable fracture should be fixated first. The more stable fractures may frequently be treated with lesser forms of fixation, although at times they will reduce spontaneously. This is due to the Vassal principle of fracture fixation. Stabilization of the dominant fracture by rigid means will enhance the alignment of the lesser fractures because of the common soft tissue elements. The soft tissue structure that acts as a primary stabilizer in many metatarsal

fractures is the deep transverse intermetatarsal ligament. With realignment of a dislocated fracture, this ligament tethers the remaining metatarsals and tends to pull them into a more anatomic position.

Lesser Metatarsal Neck Fractures With Joint Dislocation

Metatarsal neck fractures with dislocation are uncommon. Closed restoration of joint alignment is almost always unsuccessful. The mechanism of the fracture/dislocation is one of excessive dorsiflexion (hyperextension) of the proximal phalanx over the metatarsal head. A retrograde plantarflexory force against the metatarsal head results. This drives the head through the fibrocartilaginous plantar joint plate so that it becomes literally trapped beneath the plantar, medial, and lateral structures (11). These structures form a noose around the metatarsal head, making closed reduction impossible (Fig. 62.7).

Midshaft Fractures

Fractures that occur in the shaft or diaphyseal area of the metatarsal are oblique for the most part, although transverse, spiral, and comminuted patterns occur as well (Fig. 62.8). These injuries are usually caused by direct trauma or a twisting injury to the foot. If the fracture is nondisplaced, use of a well-molded, non-weight-bearing cast for 4 to 6

Figure 62.6. A and **B.** Preoperative and postoperative radiographs of a displaced fourth metatarsal neck fracture just proximal to the physis.

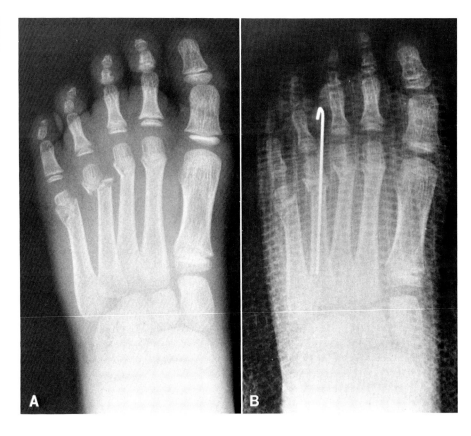

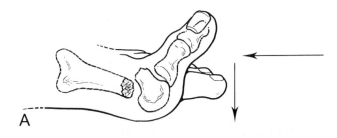

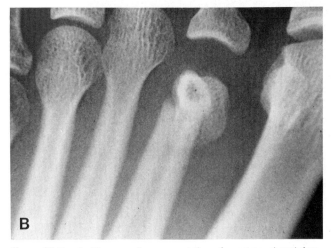

Figure 62.7. **A.** Diagrammatic representation of a metatarsal neck fracture with joint dislocation. **B.** Radiographic appearance of the same.

weeks is adequate. Displaced metatarsal shaft fractures, with separation of the fragments, have been treated conservatively with acceptable results (2).

Oblique diaphyseal fractures may present further difficulty if displaced in the sagittal plane. If significant shortening occurs from proximal displacement of the distal fragment, then the metatarsal parabola is disrupted and later metatarsalgia may result. Such fractures should be openly reduced and fixated by one of several techniques, including cerclage wiring, intramedullary pinning with a K-wire, or interfragmentary compression with a lag screw.

Comminuted fractures of the diaphysis of an internal metatarsal may be successfully fixated with cerclage wire, K-wires, lag screw technique, buttress plating, or a combination of the aforementioned methods.

Metatarsal Base Fractures

Fractures at the metatarsal bases are usually transverse and typically develop 1 cm distal to the articular surface (Fig. 62.9). It is important to assess Lisfranc joint congruity when one is evaluating base fractures, as dislocation may have occurred with the injury to other segments. Provided the tarsometatarsal joint is intact and there are no signs of intraarticular fracture, conservative casting and immobilization usually provide a good functional result.

Fifth Metatarsal Fractures

Fractures of the fifth metatarsal are common and may pose many problems. Unique injuries of the fifth metatarsal include the proximal diaphyseal fracture or Jones fracture, as

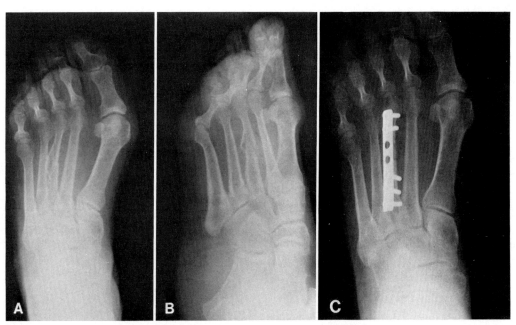

Figure 62.8. **A** and **B.** Preoperative radiographs of a midshaft third metatarsal fracture. **C.** Postoperative appearance. The shattered fragments precluded interfragmental compression, and stabilization was achieved with a plate alone.

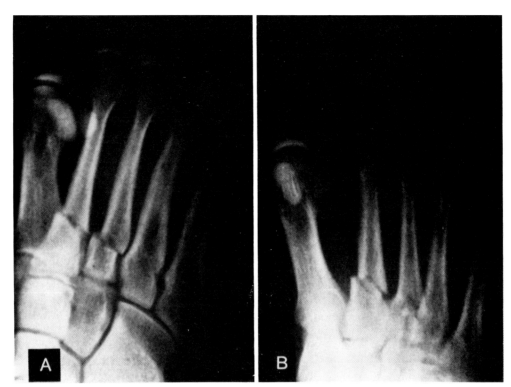

Figure 62.9. **A** and **B.** Base fractures of the second, third, and fourth metatarsals. (From Spector FC, Karlin JM, Scurran BL, Silvani SL: Lesser metatarsal fractures. *J Am Podiatry Assoc* 74:263, 1984, with permission.)

well as the more common avulsion type of injury involving the tuberosity of the fifth metatarsal. In addition, head and neck fractures may occur as a result of direct trauma, and midshaft and base fractures can occur from indirect violence or from muscle and tendinous traction.

Fractures of the Fifth Metatarsal Head

The majority of intra-articular fractures of the fifth metatarsal head should be reduced to restore normal function of the joint and minimize the development of degenerative arthritis. Small fragments may be excised if symptomatic, followed by early gentle, passive range-of-motion exercises of the joint and soft tissues. Impaction fractures, intra-articular fractures, and isolated fifth metatarsal head fractures are relatively uncommon.

Fractures of the Fifth Metatarsal Neck

Fifth metatarsal neck fractures are more common than injuries to the metatarsal head. These fractures should be reduced only if there is abnormal angulation or displacement. If malaligned, they may require open reduction since the alignment directly affects the weight-bearing load on the fifth metatarsal head. Methods of fixation for transverse fractures include intramedullary wire fixation, monofilament wire, and small L or T plates with axial compression. Oblique or spiral fractures may be reduced by means of

intramedullary wire, cerclage wire, interfragmentary compression with lag screw fixation and/or a neutralization plate (Figs. 62.10 and 62.11).

Fractures of the Fifth Metatarsal Shaft

Shaft fractures are most often oblique or spiral oblique. The mechanism of injury is straightforward and easily understood if the biomechanics and anatomical structures are considered. The soft tissue structures, including musculotendinous attachments at the base, stabilize and lock the fifth metatarsal with the cuboid and the base of the fourth metatarsal. This relationship allows the shaft of the fifth metatarsal to fracture in the following manner. A powerful ground force is exerted at the head and neck. The axis of motion of the fifth metatarsal is primarily dorsiflexion-plantarflexion and inversion-eversion, with very little abduction-adduction available (12, 13). The reactive forces of gravity act distally against a stable proximal base. A triplane torque is produced, and if the forces are severe enough, a comminuted oblique fracture with a small butterfly fragment occurs.

These may be inherently unstable, even if they are not comminuted, because of the length of the fracture, the independent axis of motion for the fifth ray, the fairly long lever arm through which motion may disrupt the fracture interface, and the fact that the fifth metatarsal derives adjacent stability only from its medial side.

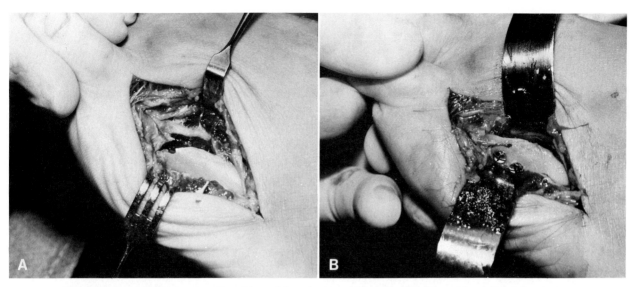

Figure 62.10. **A.** Clinical presentation of long oblique fracture of the shaft of the fifth metatarsal. **B.** Interfragmentary compression with two 2.0 mm cortical screws.

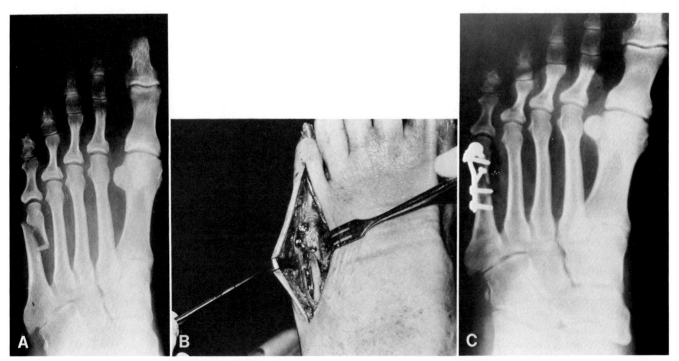

Figure 62.11. **A.** Preoperative radiographic appearance of long oblique fracture of the fifth metatarsal. **B.** Clinical appearance after plate fixation with interfragmentary compression. **C.** Postoperative radiographic appearance.

Fifth Metatarsal Base Fractures

Fractures of the base of the fifth metatarsal are considered one of the most common foot fractures (1, 12, 14). Two classifications are described—the Jones fracture and the base-avulsion fracture.

JONES FRACTURE

The Jones fracture occurs in the proximal diaphysis of the fifth metatarsal approximately 1.5 to 3.0 cm distal to the tuberosity or just distal to the articulation of the fourth and fifth metatarsals (Fig. 62.12). This injury is not nearly as

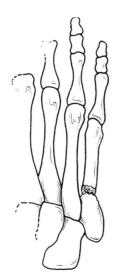

Figure 62.12. Diagrammatic representation of a Jones fracture.

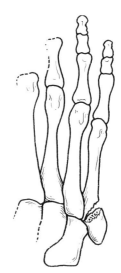

Figure 62.13. Diagrammatic representation of an avulsion fracture of the base of the fifth metatarsal.

common as the avulsion fracture of the metatarsal base (15). Robert Jones (16) was the first to describe this fracture pattern, having sustained the injury himself.

Devas (17) described the fracture as being a stress-related injury. Kavanaugh and associates (18) agreed with this premise and noted the highest incidence in healthy young male athletes. These authors also described the mechanism of injury as vertical and mediolateral forces acting on a fixed foot that cannot be inverted.

Treatment has classically consisted of some form of weight-bearing immobilization. However, several authors began to notice delayed union or nonunion of the fracture. Dameron (14) recommended conservative measures, although he admitted that healing occurred slowly. Early bone grafting was recommended for serious or professional athletes. Kavanaugh and associates (18) noted a 66.7% incidence of delayed union with conservative treatment; prolonged immobilization was required for those who did heal successfully. They recommended screw fixation of the fracture site for those patients who were serious athletes. Nonathletes were treated conservatively. Zelko and associates (19) also instituted conservative measures initially and yet employed bone grafting of the fracture site in patients who sustained reinjury.

Arangio (20) used percutaneous crossed wires for stabilization of two Jones fractures. DeLee and associates (21) reported screw fixation as a successful means of treating this injury in the athlete.

Torg and co-workers (22) provided a classification for Jones fractures based on radiographic appearance. Acute injuries demonstrated a narrow fracture line without intramedullary sclerosis. Patients with delayed union had evidence of intramedullary sclerosis with a widened fracture interface. Patients with nonunion demonstrated complete sclerotic obliteration of the medullary canal.

In their series patients with acute injuries healed 100% of the time with the use of a non-weight-bearing cast. De-

layed unions similarly healed with a non-weight-bearing cast, albeit over a prolonged period. Medullary curettage with an inlay graft from the distal tibia was recommended for patients with nonunion and for athletes with delayed union. The purpose of surgery was to restore the continuity of the medullary canal and to facilitate healing with the bone graft. This treatment approach has subsequently been advocated by others (23, 24).

The grading system instituted by Torg and associates (22) is still quite applicable for guiding the treatment of Jones fractures. Generally, acute injuries should heal quite will with a below-knee non-weight-bearing cast. Prolonged healing of these injuries has been attributed to intrinsic muscle attachments to the area, which increase the stress at the fracture site (20, 22). A reduced blood supply to this area of the cortex has also been implicated (15, 25).

Previous authors have generally ignored the specific mechanical relationships of the fifth metatarsal. Injuries at this level have an inherent instability because of the long lever arm of the distal metatarsal through which motion may introduce stress to the fracture, the independent axis of motion of the fifth ray, and the fact that the fifth metatarsal derives adjacent stability only on its medial side. Abstinence from weight bearing is more effective in eliminating these mechanical factors, which act upon the fracture, thereby explaining the success of previous authors employing this approach (22-24).

Surgical stabilization may be indicated in the serious athlete for whom the most rapid recovery is required. Screw fixation has generally proved suitable, but there may be chronic irritation from the screw head when activity is resumed (21, 23). Other forms of stabilization, including wire fixation (20) and plates, may also be applicable, especially in patients with delayed union. Grafting with plate fixation of fractures progressing to nonunion seems prudent.

FRACTURES OF THE BASE OF THE FIFTH METATARSAL TUBEROSITY

Fractures of the base of the fifth metatarsal are among the most common of all skeletal injuries of the foot (26). Despite their common occurrence, there has been considerable confusion in the literature, at times equating the avulsion injury to that of a Jones fracture. These fractures are generally oriented perpendicular to the applied force (Fig. 62.13).

The mechanism of injury is primarily that of inversion of the foot. Two mechanisms have been described to explain the fracture of the fifth metatarsal tuberosity. The first is an avulsion fracture that is produced by a sudden pull of the peroneus brevis muscle that inserts into the base of the metatarsal. This occurs with acute supination and results in a small displaced fragment. This type of avulsion is quite common with lateral ankle sprains. The second fracture is produced by excessive weight bearing on the lateral aspect of the foot. Fractures may also be produced by direct trauma, although the fracture is generally larger and may be comminuted.

Richli and Rosenthal (27) have suggested that the lateral cord of the plantar aponeurosis, which attaches to the base of the metatarsal, may also create an avulsion fracture with inversion and plantarflexion of the forefoot.

Treatment by closed reduction with casting is usually adequate. When closed reduction is unsuccessful, open reduction may be required (1, 13, 18, 22, 28). Open reduction may also be considered if the fracture compromises the fifth metatarsocuboid articulation. If the bone is completely avulsed, closed reduction is extremely difficult because of the traction of the peroneus brevis tendon. If smaller fragments are present, multiple small, crossed K-wires or ten-sion-band wiring may be used (Fig. 62.14). If the fragment is larger, intramedullary screw fixation may be employed (23)(Fig. 62.15).

STRESS FRACTURES

Stress fractures develop in a bone without acute trauma. Repeated, and usually submaximal, strain results in fatigue of the osseous structure. Typically, the fracture is limited to one side of the cortex; if untreated, however, it may involve the entire cortical margin (29). Stress fractures are generally considered to be exercise-related conditions that characteristically occur in normal bone. Persons most commonly afflicted are athletes and military recruits (30). In other groups, however, stress fractures due to a recent increase or change in work load have also been reported (31). McBryde (32) suggests that stress fractures may account for as many as 10% of all sports injuries.

Wilson and Katq (33) presented a retrospective analysis of 250 stress fractures and suggested that the initial radiographic features could be categorized into one of four basic patterns:

Type 1—Fracture line only demonstrable, with no evidence of endosteal callus or periosteal reaction.
Type 2—Focal sclerosis of bone and the formation of endosteal callus.
Type 3—Periosteal reaction and external callus.
Type 4—Mixed combinations of the above.

Type 1 stress fractures of the metatarsal invariably progressed to the stage of periosteal reaction and external callus formation.

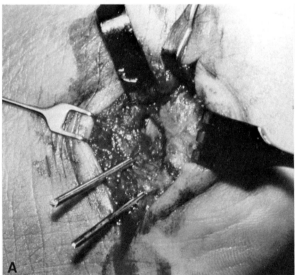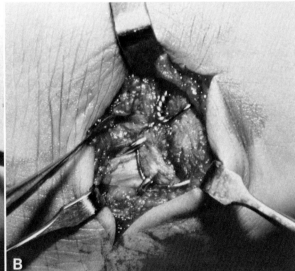

Figure 62.14. **A.** Intraoperative appearance of fifth metatarsal base avulsion fracture with two K-wires in place for tension band fixation. Note the fracture site. **B.** After completion of the fixation. The fracture line is now compressed and is no longer visualized.

Figure 62.15. **A.** Displaced intra-articular fracture of the fifth metatarsal base. **B.** Fixation with a 4.0 mm cancellous screw and washer.

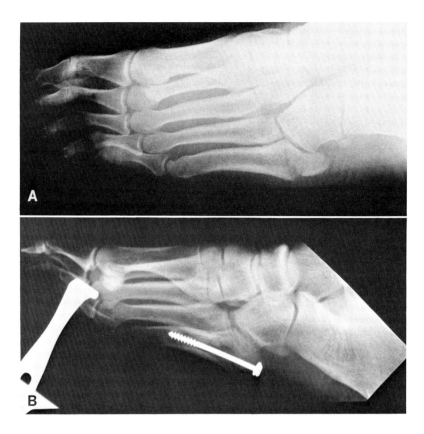

Type 2 stress fractures are characteristic of calcaneal and medial tibial plateau fractures, and almost invariably there are areas of focal sclerosis.

Type 3 is the most typical pattern. This may require caution in interpretation. Especially in long bones, the presence of apparently unexplained periosteal reaction in a young patient may initially raise the question of a possible malignant bone tumor. The problem is usually resolved by the demonstration of a radiolucent fracture line within otherwise normal cortical bone. Multiple projections or even mammography film may be necessary to completely exclude the possibility of pathologic fracture within an area of diseased bone.

Wilson and Katq (33) suggested that in 17% of the patients radiographs are initially negative. The importance of this observation is that repeat radiographs are indicated in patients whose symptoms continue despite initially negative findings. It may be 1 to 3 weeks before positive radiographic findings are evident. Technetium 99 bone scanning techniques may be employed to identify possible lesions before standard radiographs are taken. The technetium 99 bone scan is a sensitive test that enables the diagnosis to be confirmed long before plain x-ray changes are evident. Taunton and associates (34), in a study of 62 runners with stress fractures, showed that initial radiographs were positive in 47.2% of the cases whereas bone scans were positive in 95.8%.

The treatment of stress fractures is usually conservative, with the emphasis on early return to normal function. The majority of metatarsal stress fractures respond favorably to limited weight bearing, but more severe and symptomatic fractures may require complete immobilization with casting.

Stress fractures of the first metatarsal are rare (35, 36). However, they should be considered in the differential diagnosis of acute arch pain when there is no history of gross trauma. Most stress fractures of the first metatarsal will occur at the base.

Stress fractures of the lesser metatarsals are quite common, with the second metatarsal being involved most frequently (35). Displaced fractures of the second metatarsal are most common in runners (36).

The third metatarsal is less commonly fractured than the second (35); yet it shows a higher percentage of involvement in multiple stress fractures (37). If the patient has a third metatarsal stress fracture, then 50% of the time he or she will have additional stress fractures of the remaining lesser metatarsals.

Stress fractures of the fourth metatarsal are rare and are usually seen only in conjunction with multiple injuries (35). Stress fractures of the fifth metatarsal are divided into two types. The stress fracture at the metatarsal base appears on the lateral cortex oriented transversely across the bone and is often complete. It is usually noticed in conjunction with a fracture of the second or third metatarsal. Stress fractures of the shaft are rare and occur in conjunction with other metatarsal stress fractures. When multiple stress fractures are seen, they occur first in the more medial metatarsal bone and progress to the more lateral structures (35).

Most authors agree that immobilization, be it by strapping, a surgical shoe, or a cast, is the treatment of choice for stress fractures. Most patients will do well with a surgical shoe in which a liner material is cut out under the fractured metatarsal to alleviate stress. Compression may help to alleviate symptoms and may be applied by means of a compressive stocking, tape dressings, or other modalities.

References

1. Giannestras NJ, Sammarco GJ: Fractures and dislocations in the foot. In Rockwood CA, Green DP (ed): *Fractures*, Philadelphia, JP Lippincott, 1975, p 1478.
2. Maxwell J: Open or closed treatment of metatarsal fractures. *J Am Podiatry Assoc* 73:100-107,1983.
3. Bonutti P, Bell G: Compartment syndrome of the foot: a case report. *J Bone Joint Surg* 68A:1449-1450, 1986.
4. Goldman FD, Dayton PD, Hansen CJ: Compartment syndrome of the foot. *J Foot Surg* 29:37-43, 1990.
5. Kirchwehm WW, Figura MA, Binning TA, Leis SB: Fractures of the internal metatarsals. In Scurran B (ed): *Foot and Ankle Trauma*. New York, Churchill Livingstone, 1989, p 347.
6. LaPorta G: Fractures of the first metatarsal. In Scurran B (ed): *Foot and Ankle Trauma*. New York, Churchill Livingstone, 1989, p 323.
7. O'Donoghue DH: *Treatment of Injuries to Athletes*. Philadelphia, WB Saunders, 1976, p 769.
8. Harrison M: Fractures of the metatarsal head. *Can J Surg* 11:511-514, 1968.
9. Smith GH, Green AL: Cerclage wiring of metatarsal fracture; a case report. *J Am Podiatry Assoc* 73:25-27, 1983.
10. Dorfman GR: Reduction of comminuted metatarsal fractures utilizing cerclage wire fixation. *J Foot Surg* 15:99-103, 1976.
11. Rao JP, Banzon MT: Irreducible dislocation of the metatarsophalangeal joints of the foot. *Clin Orthop* 145:224-226, 1979.
12. Laurich LJ, Witt CS, Zielsdarf LM: Treatment of fractures of the fifth metatarsal bone. *J Foot Surg* 22:207-211, 1983.
13. Root ML, Orien WP, Weed JH: *Normal and Abnormal Function of the Foot*. Los Angeles, Clinical Biomechanics Corp, 1977, vol 2, pg 219-221.
14. Dameron TB Jr: Fractures and anatomical variations of the proximal portions of the fifth metatarsal. *J Bone Joint Surg* 57A: 788-792, 1975.
15. Kirchwehm W: Fractures of the fifth metatarsal. In Scurran B, (ed): *Foot and Ankle Trauma*. New York, Churchill Livingstone, 1989, pp 363-375.
16. Jones R: Fractures of the base of the fifth metatarsal bone by indirect violence. *Ann Surg* 35:697, 1902.
17. Devas M: *Stress Fractures*. Edinburgh, Churchill Livingstone, 1975, pp 1, 163, 230.
18. Kavanaugh JH, Brower TD, Mann RV: The Jones fracture revisited. *J Bone Joint Surg* 60A:776-782, 1978.
19. Zelko RR, Torg JS, Rachun A: Proximal diaphyseal fractures of the fifth metatarsal—treatment of the fractures and their complications in athletes. *Am J Sports Med* 7:95-101, 1979.
20. Arangio GA: Proximal diaphyseal fractures of the fifth metatarsal (Jones' fracture): two cases treated by cross-pinning with review of 106 cases. *Foot Ankle* 3:293-296, 1983.
21. DeLee JC, Evans JP, Julian J: Stress fracture of the fifth metatarsal. *Am J Sports Med* 11:349-353, 1983.
22. Torg J, Balduini F, Zelko R, Pavlov H, Peff TC, Das M: Fractures of the base of the fifth metatarsal distal to the tuberosity. *J Bone Joint Surg* 66A:209-214, 1984.
23. Lehman R, Torg J, Helene P, DeLee J: Fractures of the base of the fifth metatarsal distal to the tuberosity: a review. *Foot Ankle* 7:245-252, 1987.
24. Zogby RG, Baker BE: A review of nonoperative treatment of Jones' fracture. *Am J Sports Med* 15:304-307, 1987.
25. Key J, Conwell H: *The Management of Fractures, Dislocation and Sprains*. St Louis, CV Mosby, 1934, p 1116.
26. Rockwood CA, Green DP: *Fractures*. Philadelphia, JB Lippincott, 1975, pp 1482-1483.
27. Richli WR, Rosenthal DI: Avulsion fracture of the fifth metatarsal: experimental study of pathomechanics. *AJR* 143:889-891, 1984.
28. Joplin R: Injuries of the foot. In Cave E, Burk J, Boyed T (eds): *Trauma Management*. Chicago, Year Book Medical Publishers, 1974, p 851.
29. Orava S: Stress fractures. *Br J Sports Med* 14:40-44, 1980.
30. Slowik AJ: Stress fracture of the first metatarsal. *J Am Podiatry Assoc* 59:333-335, 1969.
31. Daffner RH, Martinez S, Gehweifer JA: Stress fractures in runners. *JAMA* 247:1039-1041, 1982.
32. McBryde AM: Stress fractures in athletes. *J Sports Med* 3:212-17, 1975.
33. Wilson E, Katq F: Stress fractures: an analysis of 250 consecutive cases. *Radiology* 92:481-486, 1969.
34. Taunton JE, Clement DB, Webber D: Lower extremity stress fracture in athletes. *Physicians Sports Med* 9:77-83, 1981.
35. Mann RA: *DuVries Surgery of the Foot*, ed 4. St Louis, CV Mosby, 1978, p 261.
36. Montalbano M, Hugar D: Metatarsal stress fractures in runners. *J Am Podiatry Assoc* 72:581-583, 1982.
37. Morris JM, Blickenstaff LD: *Fatigue Fractures*. Springfield, IL, Charles C Thomas, 1978, p 439.

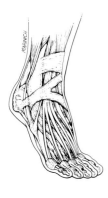

CHAPTER **63**

Midfoot Fractures

Flair D. Goldman, D.P.M.

Most injuries involving the midfoot consist of either small avulsion fractures, stress fractures, or nondisplaced body fractures. Treatment of these injuries is generally nonoperative and consists of rest, elevation, and immobilization. Occasionally severe fracture dislocations and severe compression injuries will occur. Management of these conditions may require more aggressive measures, such as closed reduction and percutaneous fixation, open reduction and internal fixation, or primary fusion.

The specific treatment of any given injury depends upon (*a*) the type of injury, (*b*) the surgeon's experience and skill, and (*c*) the patient's overall medical status and functional needs. The basic principle of anatomic reduction is especially important, when one considers that each midfoot bone articulates with at least four adjacent bones. Furthermore, each of these joints is subjected to weight-bearing stress. Accordingly, even small articular incongruities may lead to later degenerative changes and pain.

Nonunion of midfoot fractures is extremely rare because of the numerous radially penetrating vessels that perfuse each bone (1) (Fig. 63.1). Therefore it is difficult to completely interrupt the blood supply to any segment. The exception to this is the central portion of the tarsal navicular (2)(Fig. 63.2). Despite appropriate treatment, many midfoot

fractures and fracture dislocations may heal with residual stiffness and edema of the foot.

The identification of midfoot fractures requires a high index of suspicion on the part of the clinician. This is true in cases of overt trauma as well as in instances involving more subtle stress fractures and trabecular compression injuries. Midfoot fractures may be complicated by other injuries of the foot or by serious bodily trauma and, therefore, may be initially overlooked. If the patient experiences a loss of consciousness, these fractures may be discovered only after the patient resumes ambulation. Many times midfoot fractures are not considered as a part of the differential diagnosis of vague midfoot pain in the absence of major trauma. This is especially true of stress fractures, small nondisplaced injuries, and osteochondral fractures.

Radiographs of the midfoot are often difficult to evaluate because of the multiple overlapping irregular bones, which create double densities on standard views. In addition, there exists the possibility of misinterpreting accessory bones, vascular and ligamentous calcification, and epiphyseal variations as chip or avulsion fractures.

Normal anteroposterior radiographs should demonstrate the navicular shadow overlapping all the cuneiforms equally. In the lateral view all the cuneiforms should overlap

Figure 63.1. The ossified specimen from a 19-year-old showing the blood supply to the navicular. Note numerous radially penetrating arteries. (From Waugh W: Deossification and vascularization of the tarsal navicular and their relation to Kohler's disease. *J Bone Joint Surg* 40B: 765, 1958, by permission.)

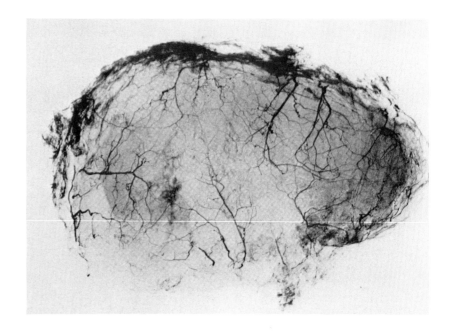

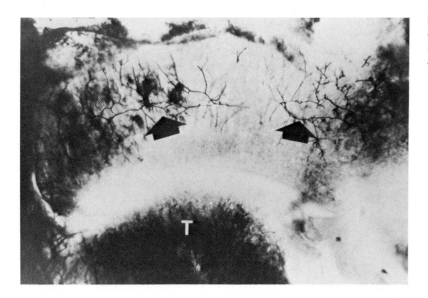

Figure 63.2. Note the relatively avascular area in the central third of this fully matured navicular. (From Torg JS et al: Stress fracture of the tarsal navicular. *J Bone Joint Surg* 64A:700, 1982, by permission.)

each other and should lie directly in line with the navicular (3). Simple techniques that help in the diagnosis of midfoot fractures include comparison views of the opposite foot, magnification views, spot views, and the use of high-resolution radiographic film. Other techniques that have proved helpful include tomograms, bone scans, computerized tomography (CT) scans, and magnetic resonance imaging (MRI). The general approach to these studies is to first obtain a technetium-99 bone scan to identify and localize an osseous source of pathology, and a follow-up with additional imaging modalities as indicated (4). Using such an algorithm, one may at times have patients with positive bone scans but negative tomograms or CT scans. In these instances treatment is dictated by physical examination findings, symptoms, and clinical experience. When one is faced with this scenario, immobilization in a walking cast for 4 to 6 weeks usually allows for clinical resolution of the problem. An MRI scan may help to identify some patients with diminished signal intensity, which is consistent with trabecular compression injury. This confirms what many investigators have previously proposed: with a high index of suspicion, a thorough history, and careful physical examination, many midfoot injuries will be recognized as specific fractures (2, 5-10).

FRACTURES OF THE TARSAL NAVICULAR

Tarsal navicular fractures are the most common midfoot fractures, comprising 62% of all such injuries and 0.37% of all fractures. Ten out of every twelve navicular fractures occur in patients between the ages of 20 and 50 years (11).

Wilson (11), Watson-Jones (12), DePalma (13), and Rockwood and Green (14) have all provided classifications for navicular fractures. However, the author prefers the following system: (*a*) dorsal avulsion fractures, (*b*) tuberosity fractures, (*c*) body fractures, (*d*) displaced fractures, and (*e*) osteochondral fractures.

Dorsal Avulsion Fractures

The dorsal avulsion fracture is the most common navicular fracture, representing 47% of the reported cases. These injuries are sometimes referred to as cortical avulsion fractures (15). The mechanism of injury is plantar displacement of the foot, followed by either inversion or eversion. During plantarflexion and eversion the dorsal tibionavicular ligament (part of the deltoid ligament) becomes taut and avulses part of the dorsal cortex of the navicular at its insertion. During plantarflexion and inversion the talonavicular ligament becomes stressed and acts in a similar manner. The avulsed fragment usually contains a portion of articular cartilage and is best viewed on a lateral radiograph (Fig. 63.3).

Examination of the patient will demonstrate tenderness and edema at the fracture site. Open reduction and internal fixation are generally not necessary. If the fracture is significantly displaced, the position may be improved by application of direct pressure over the fracture. Since the region may be extremely edematous and the fracture does not have interdigitating fragments, the reduction is typically unstable and complete anatomic reduction by closed means is virtually impossible. At times a modest improvement in alignment may be achieved.

Acute fractures are treated in a short leg cast for 4 to 6 weeks, with the foot in a neutral position relative to inversion and eversion and the ankle joint dorsiflexed if possible. Casting generally provides patients with good symptomatic relief and better function than would be permitted with lesser forms of immobilization. However, some patients may not be candidates for casting. These might include older patients with balance problems or pre-existing hip or knee symptoms. In such cases symptomatic treatment with an Ace bandage and a wooden-soled shoe may be appropriate.

Some authors have recommended open reduction and internal fixation for fractures that involve more than 20% of the articular cartilage (15). Observation of these fractures reveals that as edema subsides and healing progresses fracture position usually improves. When fully healed, it is common to have an irregular dorsal navicular surface that is prominent. This is best appreciated on a lateral radiograph (Fig. 63.4). Occasionally the dorsal exostosis will become symptomatic, or a nonunion may develop. In either circumstance, excision of the fracture fragment is indicated.

Fractures of the Navicular Tuberosity

Fractures of the navicular tuberosity are relatively common, representing 24% of all navicular fractures in one series (15).

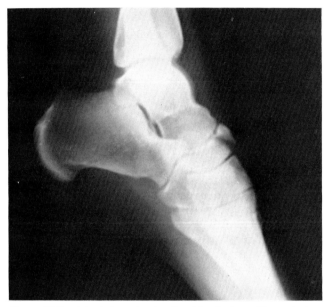

Figure 63.3. Lateral view of a dorsal avulsion fracture of the navicular. (From Goldman FD: Fractures of the midfoot. *Clin Podiatr* 2:259, 1985, by permission.)

The size and shape of the navicular tuberosity varies greatly. A random sampling of radiographs will demonstrate an accessory navicular between 2% and 12% of the time. This ossicle may articulate with the true navicular by either fibrous union or a true synovial joint (16-18). The accessory navicular has been classified into two types (19). Type 1 is small, round, and discrete from the main body. Type 2 is closely related to the body but is separated by dense fibrocartilage (Fig. 63.5). Type 2 is more common and may be confused with a fracture. In one study of 14 children, the accessory navicular totally fused to the main body in five of the children, partially fused in three, and remained independent in six children (18).

Most tuberosity fractures occur as avulsion injuries (Fig. 63.6). The tendon of the posterior tibial muscle is the only tendon that inserts into the navicular and exerts force on the navicular tuberosity when the foot is forcibly everted. The fracture is demonstrated well on oblique and anteroposterior radiographs. It has been suggested that stress on the calcaneal navicular ligament and the deltoid ligament may also produce this injury (15). These fractures are generally nondisplaced by virtue of the multiple ligamentous attachments to the navicular and the broad insertion of the posterior tibial tendon (Fig. 63.7). Many authors have indicated the need to distinguish fractures of the tuberosity from an accessory navicular (13, 20-22). As previously mentioned, a type 2 accessory navicular may be very difficult to distinguish from fractures of the tuberosity. Radiographically, the classic differentiation is based on three criteria: (*a*) the accessory navicular is usually bilateral, (*b*) fractures are usually sharp with jagged edges, and (*c*) the os tibiale externum usually has smooth, rounded edges. However, traumatic disruption of a fibrous union or synovial joint between an accessory and true navicular may be as symptomatic and disabling as a true avulsion fracture. Although treatment is similar in both injuries, osseous healing will never occur in cases of a disrupted accessory navicular.

Figure 63.4. Lateral view. Note the healed dorsal avulsion fracture of the navicular.

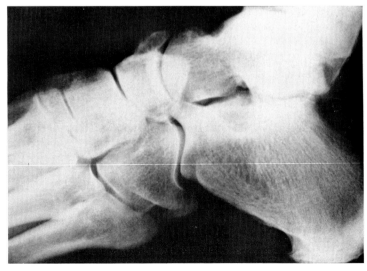

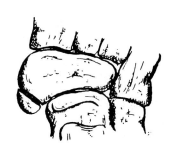

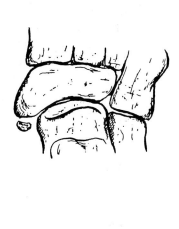

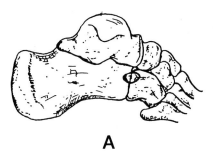

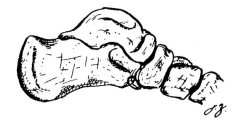

A

B

Figure 63.5. **A.** Anteroposterior and lateral views of a type 1 accessory navicular. **B.** Anteroposterior and lateral views of a type 2 accessory navicular. (From MacNicol MF, Voutsians S: Surgical treatment of the symp- tomatic accessory navicular. *J Bone Joint Surg* 66B: 218, 1984, by per- mission.)

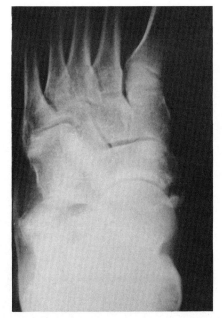

Figure 63.6. Anteroposterior view. Note the avulsion fracture of the tuberosity of the navicular as well as the crush fracture of the cuboid after a severe abduction injury. (From Goldman F: Foot and ankle trauma. Mid- foot fractures. In Scurran BL (ed): *Foot and Ankle Trauma*, New York, Churchill Livingstone, 1989, by permission.)

TREATMENT

Initial treatment consists of elevation and a compression dressing as indicated, along with no weight bearing for the first 24 to 72 hours. However, edema is generally not a problem. A short leg walking cast is later applied with a well-molded arch. The foot is held in a neutral position or slightly plantarflexed and inverted for 6 to 8 weeks. Some clinicians may prefer a more cavalier approach, such as use of an Ace bandage and a postoperative shoe or a multitude of other noncasting techniques. These often prove unsatisfactory, both in the immediate control of symptoms and in the overall patient-management scheme. Patients generally achieve greater initial comfort and mobility with a snug, below-the-knee walking cast.

Casting for more than 2 months is generally not indicated, even when radiographs do not show osseous union. Many of these cases may represent a disrupted fibrous union or synovial joint as opposed to a true fracture. Even with proper diagnosis and immobilization, a significant number of these injuries remain symptomatic and may require surgical treatment. If pain persists with mild, occasional activity, orthotic devices may help alleviate symptoms. When more significant pain is present and function is compromised, surgical excision of the fragment is indicated.

Surgery is performed through a medial longitudinal incision centered over the tuberosity. The capsule is incised and the posterior tibial tendon is reflected. The fragment is identified and removed completely, with care taken to

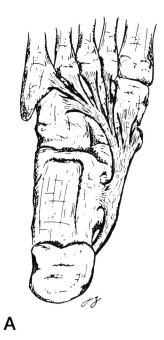

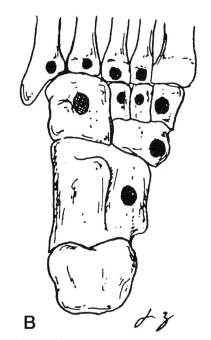

A

B

Figure 63.7. **A** and **B.** Note the multiple points of insertion of the tibialis posterior tendon. (From MacNicol MF, Voutsians S: Surgical treatment of the symptomatic accessory navicular. *J Bone Joint Surg* 66B: 218, 1984, by permission.)

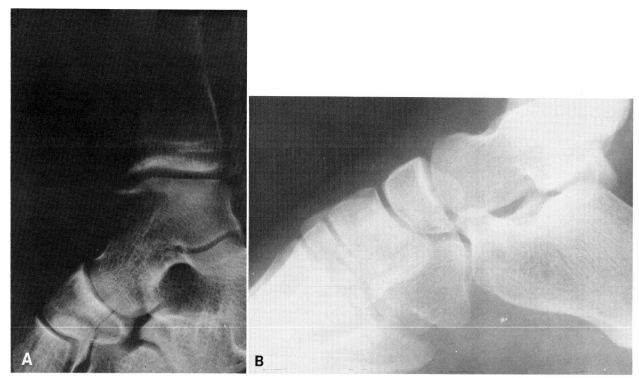

Figure 63.8. **A.** Oblique view showing a nondisplaced fracture of the navicular in the interval between the second and third facets. (From Goldman FD: Fractures of the midfoot. *Clin Podiatr* 2: 259, 1985, by permission.) **B.** Lateral view showing a nondisplaced fracture through the navicular. (From Goldman F: Midfoot fractures. In Scurran BL (ed): *Foot and Ankle Trauma*, New York, Churchill Livingstone, 1989, by permission.)

smooth any remaining rough edges. At times the fragment will clinically appear united and may be difficult to identify. In such cases an osteotome of the appropriate size may be used as if one were excising an enlarged navicular tuberosity. Invariably this will separate the fragment from the body of the navicular, revealing the fibrous union. Care must be taken not to remove so much of the navicular that the head of the talus will be significantly exposed when the foot is maximally pronated. The capsulotendinous flap is re-approximated and secured to the undersurface of the navicular or spring ligament. After wound closure a short leg walking cast is applied for approximately 4 to 6 weeks. Follow-up with orthotic devices may be indicated.

Fractures of the Body of the Navicular

Fractures of the body represent 29% of all fractures of the navicular (15). These injuries may be classified as either nondisplaced vertical or horizontal, crush, stress, or displaced fractures. The nondisplaced vertical or horizontal fracture is the most common (Fig. 63.8). These injuries usually remain nondisplaced as the result of multiple tendinous and ligamentous investments and the buttressing of surrounding bones.

NONDISPLACED FRACTURES OF THE BODY OF THE NAVICULAR

Nondisplaced fractures may occur by a variety of mechanisms, including falls with the foot striking the ground in plantarflexion (11, 23) or plantarflexion and abduction at the midtarsal joint (24, 25). Heck attributes this fracture pattern to forced dorsiflexion (26). Eichenholtz and Levine state that a twisting injury may produce such a fracture from "stress applied from the bone by opposite rotatory forces from the short dorsal and plantar talonavicular and naviculocuneiform ligaments"(15). In these instances the navicular becomes compressed between the talar head proximally and the cuneiforms distally. Fractures are usually evident on oblique and lateral radiographs. Often the ver-

tical fracture will show a fracture line passing between the second and third cuneiforms. This seems to suggest that the interval between the cuneiforms and the three facets on the anterior surface of the navicular act as a stress riser (Fig. 63.8).

Conditions considered in the differential diagnosis of navicular body fracture include bipartite tarsal navicular (27) or lithiasis of the navicular (28) (Fig. 63.9).

TREATMENT

Nondisplaced vertical or horizontal fractures of the navicular are treated with a short leg walking cast for 6 to 8 weeks. These injuries will generally heal without adverse sequelae. After discontinuation of the cast, treatment should be symptomatic, and vigorous activities such as athletics may have to be curtailed. The foot may be protected with an orthosis to eliminate excessive subtalar and talonavicular motion as indicated.

Fractures of the Body of the Navicular With Displacement

Fractures of the body of the navicular with displacement occur when the foot strikes the ground in a plantarflexed position with subsequent buckling of the midfoot. Stress is applied in the region of the dorsal capsular and ligamentous tissues by the bones of the forefoot and rearfoot, which act as lever arms against the midfoot. The navicular is thus wedged between the cuneiforms distally and the talar head proximally. This results in dorsal extrusion of the navicular, once the soft tissues have failed. The mechanism is similar to dislocations of the cuneiforms and cuboid and has been likened to the splitting of a pod and the resultant ejection of a pea (14) (Fig. 63.10). Plantarflexion and adduction of the foot have been said to produce fracture dislocation in a similar manner (25). Nyska and associates described the medial fragment as dislocating dorsomedially (29). During reduction the smaller lateral fragment is most often visible under the head of the talus.

Figure 63.9. Lateral view showing bipartite navicular. (From Goldman FD: Fractures of the midfoot. *Clin Podiatr* 2:259, 1985, by permission.)

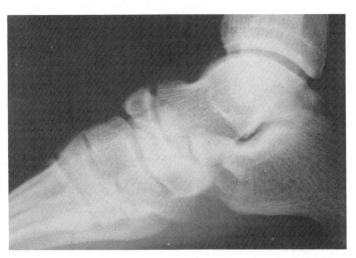

Figure 63.10. Axial loading of the foot allowing dislocation dorsally of the midfoot bones during plantarflexion. (From Wargon C, Goldman FD: Lisfranc's fracture dislocation: a variation. *J Am Podiatr Med Assoc* 76: 466, 1986, by permission.)

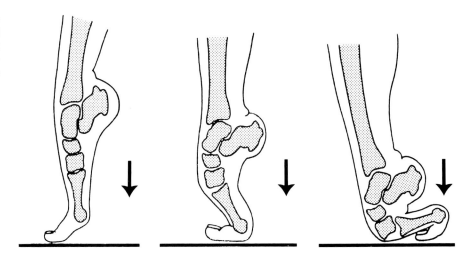

Plantar extrusion of the main fracture fragments is unlikely since the dorsal capsular and ligamentous structures are much weaker than the plantar structures. Plantarly, the foot is reinforced by strong ligaments, muscular origins, and tendinous insertions. Even so, complete isolated plantar dislocation of the navicular has been reported and a proposed mechanism has been described (30) (Fig. 63.11).

The displaced dorsomedial fragment has been prone to develop aseptic necrosis (13). Sangeorzan et al. reported an incidence of 28.5%, with avascular necrosis occurring in 6 of 21 patients (31). Radiographic signs included increased density, with or without fragmentation. The entire navicular was involved in two patients, and only part of the bone in four. Two patients in whom avascular necrosis of the entire navicular developed demonstrated subsequent collapse of the bone. Of the four patients with partial avascular necrosis, three had a good result.

Fractures of the body of the navicular have been subclassified (31). In type 1 the fracture line is transverse, with the dorsal fragment consisting of less than 50% of the body and without disruption of the medial border of the foot on the anteroposterior radiograph. Type 2 is described as the most common variant, with the fracture running transversely from dorsolateral and plantarmedial across the body of the navicular. The major fragment is dorsomedial and the smaller, often comminuted fracture is plantar lateral. The cuneonavicular joint is usually not disrupted, but the dorsal talonavicular ligament is often torn. A type 3 injury includes fractures with central or lateral comminution. The major fragment is usually medial, and the medial border of the foot is disrupted at the naviculocuneiform joint. Type 3 injuries demonstrate lateral displacement of the foot with some disruption of the calcaneocuboid joint.

Nyska and associates have reported what they described as a "simple, practical classification" (29). In type 1 vertical fractures with two main fragments evident, open reduction with internal fixation is indicated. For type 2 injuries exhibiting severe comminution of the navicular, primary talonavicular-cuneiform arthrodesis is recommended.

TREATMENT

Closed reduction for displaced body fractures of the navicular has been described as improbable, and open reduction has been recommended (23). However, some reports have advocated closed reduction. Bohler, in 1958, recommended the use of skeletal traction through the calcaneus (32). Wilson recommended forced plantarflexion of the forefoot with pressure on the dorsal surface of the fracture to achieve closed reduction. In fractures that were more than 8 days old, or if complete reduction was not accomplished, Wilson recommended talonavicular arthrodesis (11). Day suggested that initial manipulation should be attempted and indicated that Henderson found considerable force was required to reduce the fragments. Day reviewed cases by Penhalo and Lehman, who claimed to have achieved good early results with manipulation, but cautioned that later review may show degenerative changes. Day also thought that isolated talonavicular fusion would be inadequate and suggested a triple arthrodesis combined with a naviculocuneiform arthrodesis in selected cases (25). Eichenholtz and Levine concluded that the treatment of these fracture dislocations is controversial. They suggested that closed reduction should be attempted but also cautioned that redislocation or partial redislocation occurs frequently enough to make this method uncertain (15). DePalma advocated manipulation followed by the application of a short leg cast and the use of crutches (13). Eftekhar and co-workers believed that anatomic reduction by whatever method chosen was important (24). Chapman noted that there was no consensus in the treatment of this injury and recommended open reduction and internal fixation with pins or screws (20). Giannestras suggested that closed reduction be attempted but admitted that open reduction with internal fixation would usually be necessary (21). Rockwood and Green noted that closed reduction was usually ineffective and that open reduction and internal fixation would be necessary to maintain reduction (14)(Fig. 63.12). Carr and associates realized that open reduction and internal fixation could be difficult and recommended various forms of distraction of the midfoot, usu-

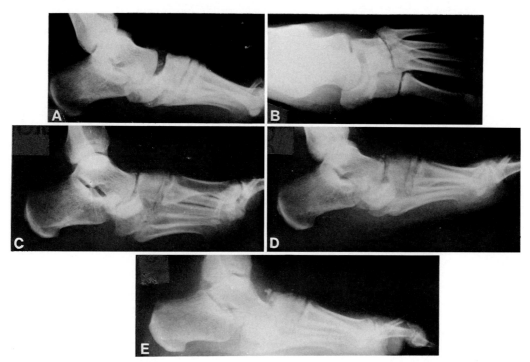

Figure 63.11. **A** to **E.** Complete isolated plantar dislocation of the navicular and subsequent retraction of the foot. (From Goldman FD: Iden-tification, treatment and prognosis of Charcot joint in diabetes mellitus. *J Am Podiatry Assoc* 72: 485, 1982, by permission.)

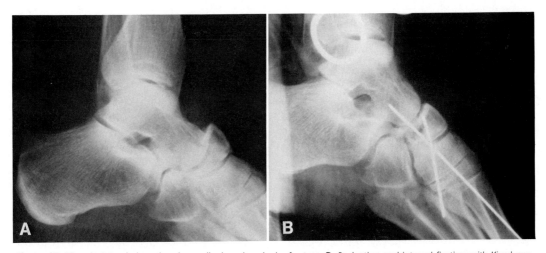

Figure 63.12. **A.** Lateral view showing a displaced navicular fracture. **B.** Reduction and internal fixation with Kirschner wires. (From Goldman FD: Fractures of the midfoot. *Clin Podiatr* 2: 259, 1985, by permission.)

ally with pins in the forefoot/midfoot and calcaneus/tibia to achieve the necessary soft tissue traction (33).

The surgical approach has been described as a dorso-medial longitudinal incision lateral to the anterior tibial ten-don and extending from the talus to the cuneiforms (13, 14, 24, 34). An alternative approach has also been described, with the incision in the interval between the tendons of the tibialis anterior and the tibialis posterior, beginning just dis-tal to the medial malleolus (31). After open reduction and

internal fixation patients are immobilized in a non-weight-bearing short leg cast until osseous union is apparent, usu-ally in about 8 weeks.

Ashurst and Crossan reported several cases in which open reduction was impossible in old cases of navicular fracture that were missed and recommended excision of the navic-ular (23). In selected cases of severe comminution, DeLee recommended the use of Kirschner wires through the frac-ture fragments and into surrounding bones to preserve the

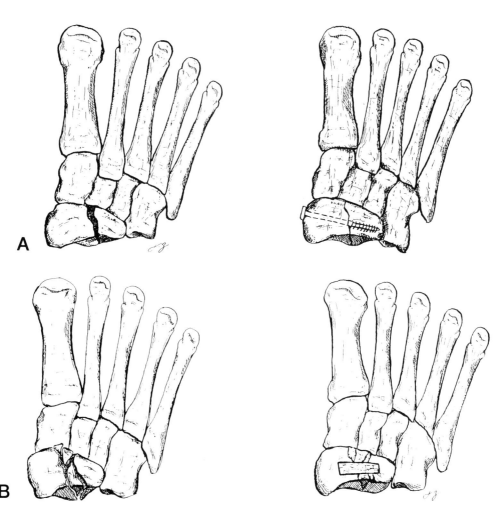

Figure 63.13. **A.** Displaced navicular fracture. Diagram of anteroposterior view with open reduction internal fixation using screw fixation. **B.** Comminuted fracture of the navicular with inlaid bone graft. Note preserved medial column length and architecture. (From Goldman F: Midfoot fractures. In Scurran BL (ed): *Foot and Ankle Trauma.* New York, Churchill Livingstone, 1989, by permission.)

architecture of the navicular and the arch (35)(Fig. 63.12). He also noted that in cases of collapse, reconstruction with elevation of the depressed fragments by means of bone grafts should be considered. Later degenerative changes might require arthrodesis (35)(Fig. 63.13). In cases of severe comminution of the navicular, talus, or cuneiform, primary arthrodesis has been recommended (21, 24, 29). Although precise open reduction and internal fixation may appear favored, surgical management may not be preferred in less active, elderly patients (14).

Stress Fractures of the Tarsal Navicular

Stress fractures of the navicular were first described in greyhounds by Bateman (36). In human beings, this fracture typically involves the middle third of the body of the navicular. In one study no trend was found with respect to anatomic differences in foot type or with respect to loading pattern in controls versus patients with stress fractures. It was concluded that excessive pronation and pronation velocity may play a role in the development of these injuries (37). Stress fractures of the navicular have been described as either complete or incomplete (Figs. 63.14 and 63.15). Complete fractures may result in subsequent dislocation if allowed to progress untreated (2).

This fracture has been described as being underdiagnosed and requires a high index of suspicion. These injuries occur most often in young male athletes, and symptoms may range from weeks to years in duration, with an average delay in diagnosis of 7.2 months (9). The pain is poorly localized to the dorsum of the foot and the medial longitudinal arch. It is described as having an insidious onset. Direct palpation of the area elicits pain. Characteristically, there is little swelling. As with all stress fractures, the symptoms are exacerbated by activity and are relieved with rest. This is just the opposite of what one would expect to find with a soft tissue

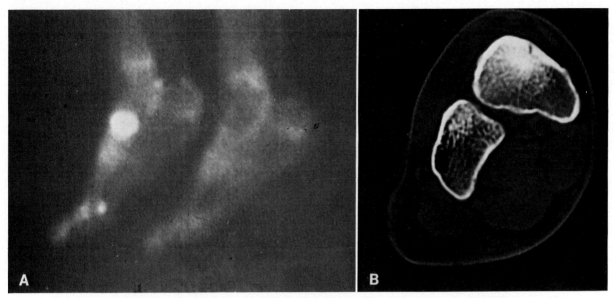

Figure 63.14. **A.** Positive technetium scan in the navicular region. **B.** CT scan showing incomplete stress fracture of the navicular. (Courtesy Dr. L. Oloff.)

strain or tendinitis where symptoms will typically improve during activity, once past muscle-warm-up stages, but then will become more painful once the activity has ceased. Routine radiographs will generally fail to adequately penetrate the central third of the navicular and, therefore, may fail to reveal the fracture. In one study anteroposterior radiographs revealed the fracture in only 9 of 23 cases, and the fracture was never evident on oblique or lateral views (9). In suspected cases of stress fracture, a technetium-99 bone scan should be considered (Fig. 63.14A). Once a positive bone scan is obtained, a tomogram or CT scan should be ordered (Figs. 63.14B). When ordering tomograms, it is important to specify an anatomic tomogram of the navicular, since normal tomograms may fail to show the lesion. The difference between the standard tomogram and the anatomic tomogram is the position of the foot. For an anatomical tomogram, the foot is positioned in slight supination, similar to that necessary for a lateral oblique radiograph. This aligns the central third of the navicular more perpendicular to the film (2). In one study, anatomic tomograms demonstrated the lesion in 17 of 23 cases, whereas standard tomograms were definitive in only 1 of 23 cases (2).

TREATMENT

Failure to treat these fractures may precipitate delayed union or nonunion. In one report, all uncomplicated fractures treated with a non-weight-bearing cast for 4 to 6 weeks healed. Full activity was resumed in 3 to 6 months, with an average of 3.8 months (9). Fractures with displacement and nonunions require surgical treatment (Fig. 63.15).

Osteochondritis Dissecans of the Navicular

Osteochondral fracture of the navicular has been reported only once (38). The diagnosis was made by tomograms guided by a bone scan and plane radiographs. Treatment consisted of excision of the fragment and drilling of the cavity. Limited follow-up revealed a good course. The authors recommended a trial of conservative treatment before surgical intervention.

FRACTURES OF THE CUNEIFORMS AND CUBOID

Collectively, fractures of the cuneiforms and cuboid constitute 8.4% of all tarsal fractures and 0.24% of all fractures. The diagnosis of cuboid and cuneiform fractures is sometimes obvious, frequently difficult, occasionally elusive, and surprisingly not rare. Furthermore, these fractures are often neglected, usually unsuspected, frequently undiagnosed, and occasionally mismanaged (15).

Fractures of the Cuneiforms

Cuneiform fractures represent 4.2% of tarsal fractures; 1.7% are isolated injuries and 2.5% are associated with other foot and ankle trauma (11). Fractures of the cuneiforms are classified as avulsion, body, fracture dislocation, and osteochondral fractures. Body fractures are further classified as simple, comminuted, and crush types.

Avulsion fractures may occur on the medial side of the first cuneiform and are usually the result of traction applied by the anterior tibial tendon.

Fractures of the body may be caused by direct trauma or by axial and rotational forces transmitted through the

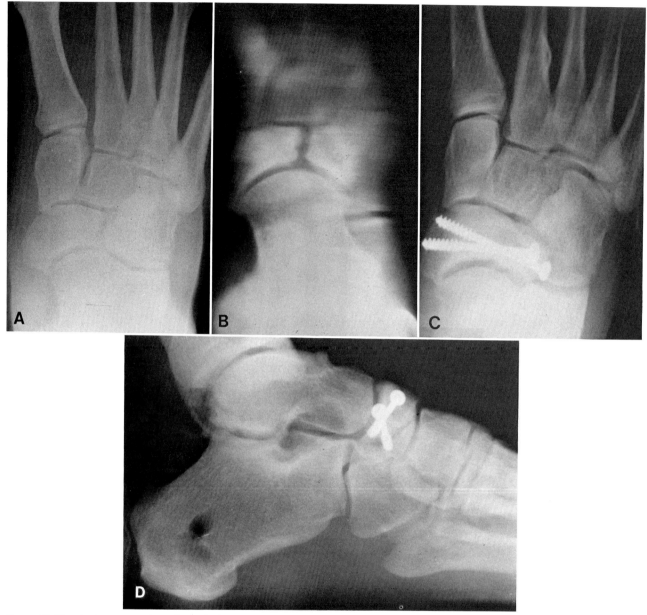

Figure 63.15. **A.** Anteroposterior radiograph showing nondisplaced nonunion of a navicular stress fracture. **B.** Tomogram of the same. **C.** Open reduction, internal fixation, and bone grafting with screws directed from lateral to medial. Anteroposterior view. **D.** Lateral view showing results of open reduction internal fixation. Note bone graft donor site in the calcaneus. (Courtesy Dr. E. D. McGlamry.)

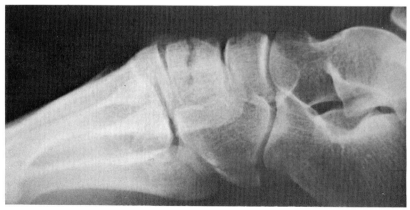

Figure 63.16. Nondisplaced fracture of the medial cuneiform, lateral view.

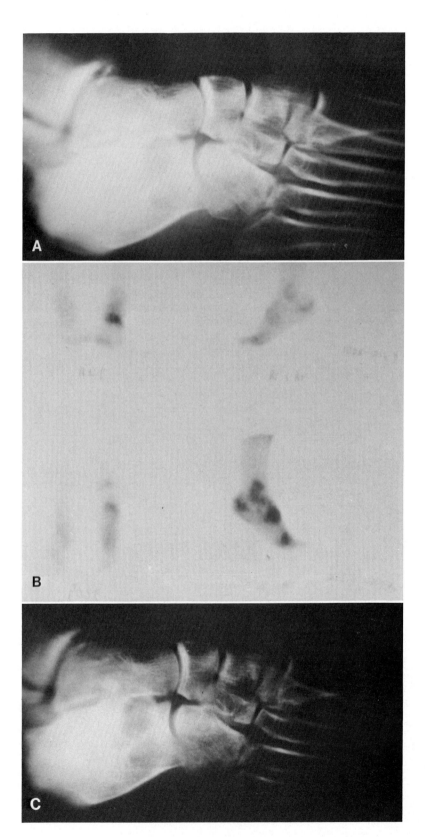

Figure 63.17. **A.** Radiograph showing a stress fracture of the third cuneiform. **B.** Technetium bone scan of the same. **C.** Tomogram of the same. (Courtesy Dr. V. Mandracchia.)

foot. Isolated fractures rarely show displacement, since they are strongly bound by intertarsal ligaments and surrounding bones (Fig. 63.16). Generally these fractures will heal readily if immobilized for 6 to 8 weeks in a short leg walking cast. After removal of the cast, patients may benefit from the use of supportive shoes or orthotic devices to help limit motion and reduce stress to the area. Injuries caused by a direct blow should be observed for edema, and compression dressings may be necessary before casts are applied. In addition, the condition of the skin must be assessed (21).

Stress fractures of the cuneiforms have been described (6, 7)(Fig. 63.17). As with other midfoot stress fractures, a high index of suspicion is necessary for diagnosis of this condition. In suspect cases bone scans should be performed, with the results of the bone scan directing tomographic or CT studies (Fig. 63.18). If tomograms and CT scans are negative, an MRI scan may be considered. MRI can detect trabecular compression injuries that may not be revealed with other modalities.

Cuneiform fractures are frequently associated with midtarsal and tarsometatarsal dislocations (13, 21, 39-41). Generally, with such fracture dislocations, axial force is applied as the foot strikes the ground in a plantarflexed attitude, similar to that seen with navicular fractures. Thus the long bones of the forefoot and rearfoot act as levers, wedging the midfoot and causing fracture and dislocation. Generally, the metatarsals will dislocate dorsally and laterally (Fig. 63.19). Dorsal dislocation predominates, as the dorsal cap-

sular ligamentous structures are weaker than the plantar structures and because the anatomy of the medial longitudinal arch buckles the foot in a dorsal direction. Dislocation occurs laterally because the tarsometatarsal joint is angulated from distal to proximal as it progresses from the second to the fifth metatarsals. The second metatarsal is recessed between the first and third cuneiforms, and therefore it is the most stable. Generally either fracture or dislocation of the second metatarsal base must occur before the other metatarsals can dislocate. A variation of this in which the second cuneiform dislocated and the second metatarsal remained intact has been described (37). The stability of the second metatarsal depends upon Lisfranc's ligament between the first cuneiform and the base of the second metatarsal. Once this ligament is ruptured, not only are the metatarsals at risk of dislocation, but so is the first cuneiform.

TREATMENT

In reducing these fracture dislocations, there are two fundamentals. First, the foot needs to be distracted to relax the soft tissues. Usually this is accomplished by using finger traps and hanging the foot from an intravenous pole. Additional traction is obtained by draping a cervical collar over the lower leg and applying weights as necessary (Figs. 63.20 and 63.21). At times the toes may be so swollen that finger traps will not fit and a heavy percutaneous pin is placed through the involved metatarsals to apply traction (Fig.

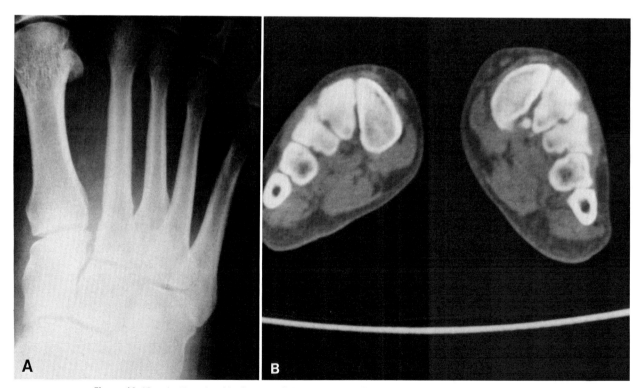

Figure 63.18. A. Note the chip fracture off the medial cuneiform distal laterally. **B.** CT scan of the same.

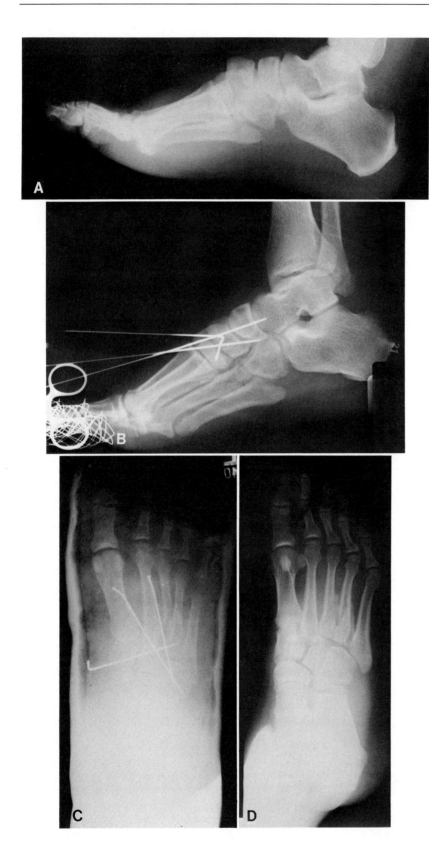

Figure 63.19. **A.** Lateral view. Note the dislocation of the medial cuneiform. **B.** Axial traction applied through finger traps with reduction and fixation using K-wires. **C.** Postreduction anteroposterior view. **D.** Long-term follow-up and healing of associated metatarsal fractures.

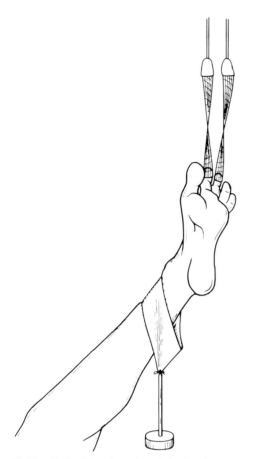

Figure 63.20. Method for distraction of the foot by means of finger traps and counterweight with cervical collar and weights about distal leg. (From Wargon C, Goldman FD: Lisfranc's fracture dislocation: a variation. *J Am Podiatr Med Assoc* 76:466, 1986, by permission.)

63.22). Visualization by C-arm fluoroscopy is helpful for pin placement. To obtain adequate reduction, complete muscular relaxation and analgesia are necessary, usually requiring general or spinal anesthesia. The keystone effect of the second metatarsal is only as good as the mortise that the cuneiforms create for fitting. Therefore, anatomic reduction of the cuneiforms with secure fixation is necessary.

Fractures of the Cuboid

Isolated fractures of the cuboid may occur, but they are usually associated with other injuries; these most often involve the lateral column, including the calcaneus or the fifth metatarsal. Fractures of the navicular may also be noted (Fig. 63.6). As with other fractures in the midfoot, displacement of cuboid fractures is rare. These injuries may be classified as either avulsion fractures or body fractures, which are further classified as simple, stress, comminuted, crush, or fracture dislocation. Avulsion fractures of the cuboid most often occur on the lateral surface (25). They have been attributed to the pull of the inferior calcaneocuboid

ligament. The lateral calcaneocuboid ligament may also cause an avulsion fracture as the cuboid is adducted on the calcaneus.

Simple body fractures of the cuboid usually occur when the foot strikes the ground in a plantarflexed position with axial and rotatory forces directed up the rigid lateral column of the foot. The force transmitted from the fifth metatarsal then produces a crescent-shaped fracture (Fig. 63.23). These fractures are intra-articular, and less than anatomic reduction may lead to degenerative changes (Figs. 63.24 and 63.25). Direct trauma is another common cause of simple body fractures. The soft tissues and skin should be monitored initially for any evidence of impending compromise. Avulsion fractures and nondisplaced body fractures generally heal well when placed in a short leg walking cast for 6 to 8 weeks. Crush fractures of the cuboid generally occur from the mechanisms of injury previously described but require more force. Hermel and Gershon-Cohen describe a nutcracker fracture of the cuboid in which the cuboid is "caught like a nut in a nutcracker between the base of the fourth and fifth metatarsal in the calcaneus"(42). These fractures occur with severe abduction of the forefoot and are often associated with an avulsion fracture of the navicular. Figure 63.6 shows a variation in which the navicular has an avulsion fracture and, instead of sustaining a cuboid fracture, the anterior calcaneus collapsed at the calcaneocuboid joint. In cases of severe comminution and articular damage, primary arthrodesis of the involved joint surfaces may be indicated (Fig. 63.26).

Total dislocations of the cuboid are rare but have been reported (43). Fracture dislocation is also rare and requires open reduction with internal fixation if closed reduction is not successful (Fig. 63.27). Open reduction with internal fixation has been recommended for depressed fractures, with bone grafting as required. Positive bone scans suggesting stress fractures of the cuboid have been reported (44)(Fig. 63.28). However, confirmation with a tomogram was lacking. More recently positive bone scans followed by MRI have demonstrated decreased signal intensity suggesting trabecular compression injury.

Other sources of pain in the cuboid region are (*a*) subluxed cuboid, (*b*) peroneus longus tendinitis, (*c*) degenerative changes of the os perineum, (*d*) calcaneocuboid joint arthritis, (*e*) capsuloligamentous strain associated with cavus foot type, and (*f*) extensor digitorum brevis myositis.

NEUROPATHIC JOINT DISEASE

Asymptomatic swelling in the insensate patient should alert the clinician to the possibility of neuropathic joint disease (30). Often in such patients the condition is diagnosed as idiopathic edema, phlebitis, or cellulitis. The midfoot is the favored site for Charcot fracture dislocations. Diabetes is currently the most common cause of neuroarthropathy within the foot. Generally, patients have no symptoms although pain may be present at times. On examination, the foot is warm with bounding pulses, since patients with peripheral neuropathy and Charcot foot have sustained an

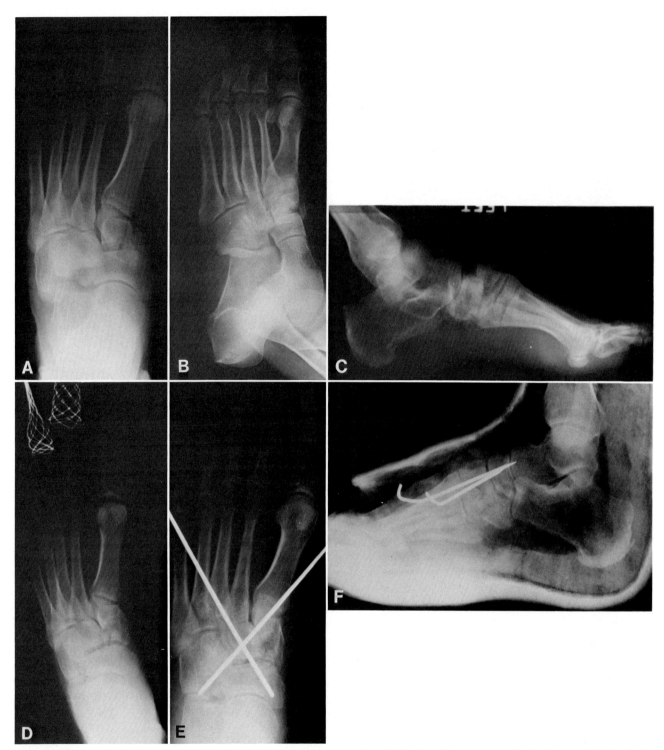

Figure 63.21. **A.** Anteroposterior view demonstrating a fracture dislocation of the medial cuneiform with dislocation of the lesser cuneiforms. **B.** Oblique view. **C.** Lateral view. **D.** Finger traps are employed to distract and bring the foot to length. Note reduction of the fractures and dislocations. **E.** Fixation with percutaneous K-wire placement. **F.** Lateral view after reduction. (From Goldman FD: Fractures of the midfoot. *Clin Podiatry* 2: 259, 1985, by permission.)

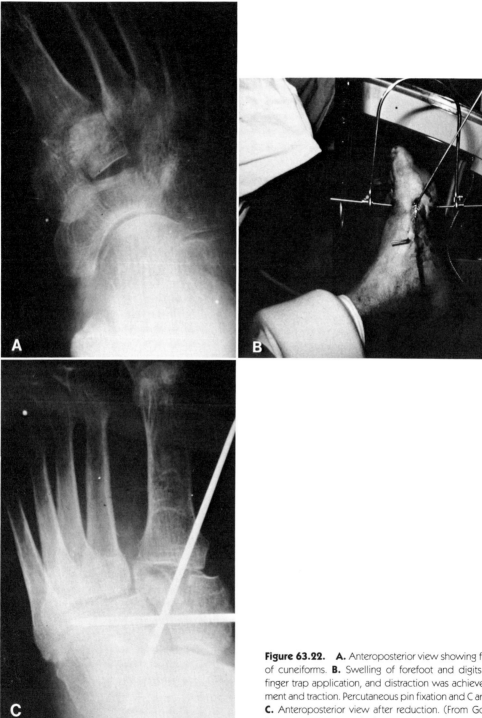

Figure 63.22.   A. Anteroposterior view showing fracture dislocation of cuneiforms. **B.** Swelling of forefoot and digits would not allow finger trap application, and distraction was achieved with pin placement and traction. Percutaneous pin fixation and C arm for visualization. **C.** Anteroposterior view after reduction. (From Goldman F: Midfoot fractures. In Scurran BL (ed): *Foot and Ankle Trauma.* New York, Churchill Livingstone, 1989, by permission.)

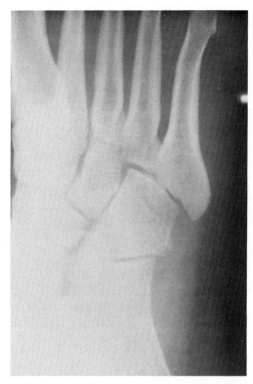

Figure 63.23. Oblique view showing crescent-shaped fracture of the cuboid secondary to axial loading of the lateral side of foot. (From Goldman F: Midfoot fractures. In Scurran BL (ed): *Foot and Ankle Trauma*. New York, Churchill Livingstone, 1989, by permission.)

autosympathectomy. Radiographs often show complete destruction of normal bony architecture and bony disintegration in later stages. Early stages may show more subtle fracture dislocations and periarticular bony fragmentation dorsally in the midfoot. Later changes may be confused radiographically with osteomyelitis. Recently several cases of moderately painful navicular fractures have been identified in diabetics with some degree of peripheral neuropathy. These patients do recall some minor trauma, such as a misstep or turning of the ankle (Fig. 63.29). This is representative of the first stage of a Charcot joint. Surgical treatment has met with some success, with early open reduction and internal fixation preventing destruction of bony architecture (Fig. 63.30).

TREATMENT

Treatment consists of elevation of the affected extremity and no weight bearing until the edema subsides and the erythema and fever of the part have resolved. Evidence of osseous consolidation should be present on radiographs prior to the resumption of weight bearing. Patients may then be treated with supportive and accommodative foot gear, including ankle-foot orthoses. When conservative measures fail, Banks and McGlamry have demonstrated good success with midfoot and rearfoot fusion in the patient with chronic osteoarthropathy (45).

As mentioned earlier, there is a subgroup of painful Charcot joint. Such patients have diminished sensation but still recognize pain and at times can remember a specific trau-

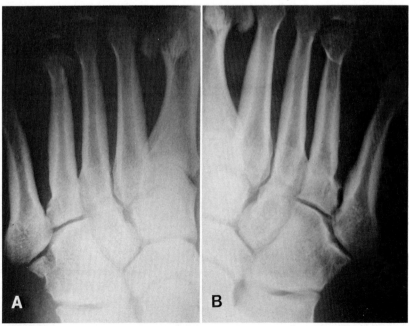

Figure 63.24. **A.** Oblique view demonstrating a small crescent-shaped fracture of the cuboid with displacement. **B.** Healed fracture with subsequent degenerative changes at the fifth metatarsal cuboid joint and between the fourth and fifth metatarsals. (From Goldman F: Midfoot fractures. In Scurran BL (ed): *Foot and Ankle Trauma*. New York, Churchill Livingstone, 1989, by permission.)

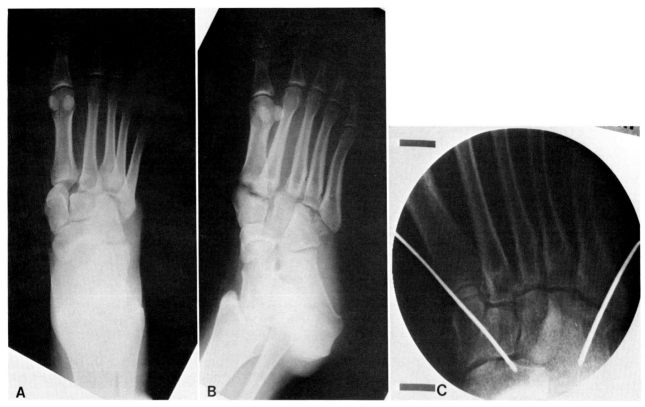

Figure 63.25. **A.** Lisfranc fracture dislocation. **B.** Note involvement of fifth metatarsal cuboid joint. **C.** Restoration of Lisfranc articulation as well as reduction of fifth metatarsal cuboid joint. (From Goldman F: Midfoot fractures. In Scurran BL (ed): *Foot and Ankle Trauma.* New York, Churchill Livingstone, 1989, by permission.)

Figure 63.26. Anteroposterior tomograms demonstrating central depression fracture of the cuboid. This was not appreciated on standard radiographs. (From Goldman FD: Fractures of the midfoot. *Clin Podiatr* 2:259, 1985, by permission.)

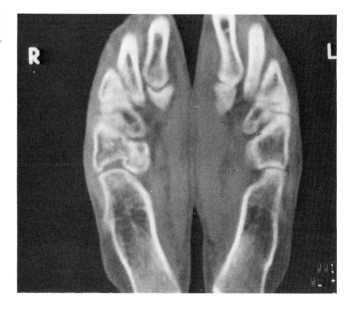

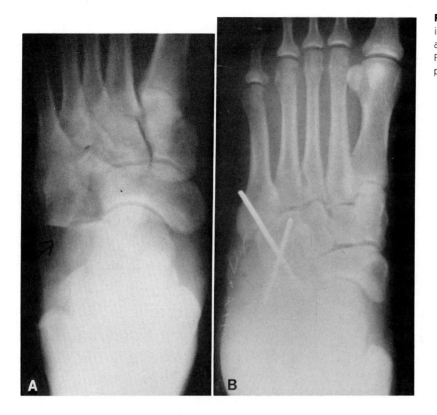

Figure 63.27. **A.** Anteroposterior view demonstrating a displaced fracture of the cuboid. **B.** Reduction and internal fixation with K-wires. (From Goldman FD: Fractures of the midfoot. *Clin Podiatr* 2:259, 1985, by permission.) (Courtesy of Dr. S. Silvani.)

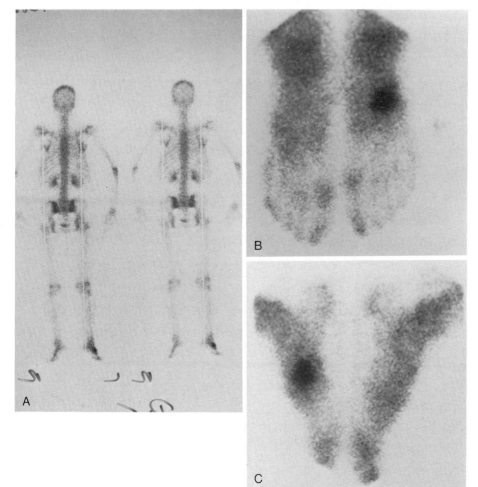

Figure 63.28. Technetium bone scan. **A.** Whole body. **B.** Anteroposterior foot. **C.** Lateral foot with increased uptake localized to the cuboid. (From Goldman FD: Fractures of the midfoot. *Clin Podiatry* 2: 259, 1985, by permission.)

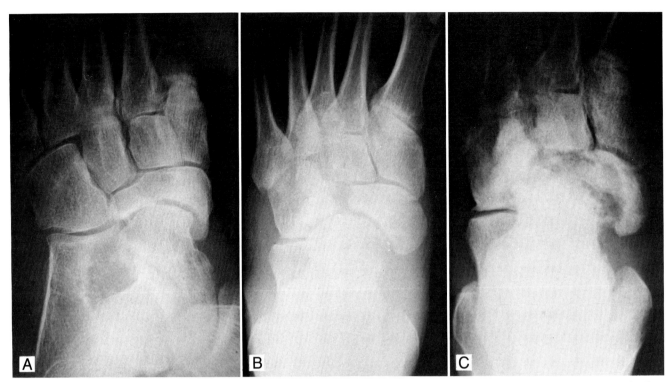

Figure 63.29. **A.** Oblique view showing minimal offset of articular congruity at the talonavicular joint. This was originally missed in the emergency room and on radiograph. **B.** Anteroposterior view showing a displaced fracture of the navicular 1 month later. **C.** The same patient 3 months after injury demonstrating complete collapse of the navicular with medial displacement.

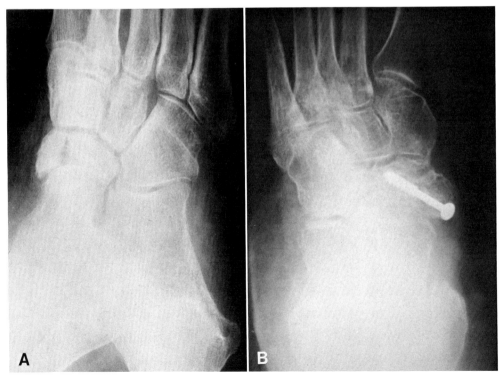

Figure 63.30. **A.** Oblique view showing mild minimally displaced fracture of the navicular approximately 2 weeks old. **B.** Anteroposterior view showing ORIF with screw fixation, 12 months postoperatively. Note maintenance of the architecture of the foot without collapse of the medial column but with some degenerative changes.

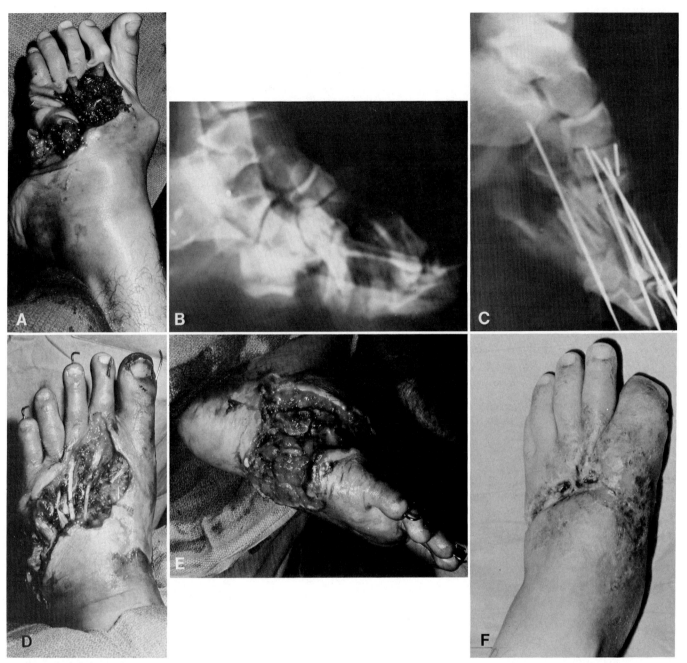

Figure 63.31. **A.** Open fractures involving the forefoot and midfoot. **B.** Lateral view with the foot splinted. **C.** Lateral view after open reduction and internal fixation. **D** and **E.** Clinical view within first postoperative week. **F.** Approximately 2½ months after injury. (From Goldman FD: Fractures of the midfoot. *Clin Podiatry* 2: 259, 1985, by permission.)

matic incident. Usually the trauma is minor in nature and the symptoms are initially minimal. It is only later, when edema and discomfort persist, that these patients seek medical attention. Again, a high index of suspicion is necessary for accurate diagnosis of these injuries.

OPEN AND CRUSH INJURIES

The principles guiding treatment of open midfoot fractures are essentially a combination of the tenets of open fracture treatment and midfoot fracture treatment. The treatment of open injuries is discussed elsewhere in this text.

Many severe midfoot injuries involve some degree of crushing or other major disruptive forces. Therefore the patient may be at risk of the development of a compartment syndrome. Tetanus status must be addressed as well.

Early surgical treatment should be aimed at the debridement of devitalized tissue and debris without hasty removal of viable tissue. The bony architecture should be re-established with internal fixation, keeping function in mind.

Early treatment should allow for maximum maintenance of foot structure. With use of a staged approach, ultimate repair will often require multiple revisions/debridements and may at times end in amputation (Fig. 63.31). Recently one-stage treatment of crush injuries of the foot with compartment syndrome has been described (46).

References

1. Waugh W: Deossification and vascularization of the tarsal navicular and their relation to Kohler's disease. *J Bone Joint Surg* 40B:765-777, 1958.
2. Torg JS, Pavlou H, Cooley LH, Bryant MH, Arowoczky S, Bergfeld J, Hunter LY: Stress fracture of the tarsal navicular. *J Bone Joint Surg* 64A:700-712, 1982.
3. Meschan I: *An Atlas of Normal Radiographic Anatomy.* Philadelphia, WB Saunders, 1951, pp 167-168.
4. Maurice HD, Newman JH, Watt I: Bone scanning of the foot for unexplained pain. *J Bone Joint Surg* 16B:448-452, 1987.
5. Hunter LY: Stress fracture of the tarsal navicular, more frequent than we realize. *Am J Sports Med* 9:217-219, 1981.
6. Marymount JH, Mills GQ, Merritt WD: Fracture of the lateral cuneiform bone in the absence of severe direct trauma: diagnosis by radionucleotide bone scan. *Am J Sports Med* 9:135-136, 1980.
7. Meurman KOA, Elfvings S: Stress fracture of the cuneiform bones. *Br J Radiol* 53:157-160, 1980.
8. Meurman KOA: Less common stress fractures in the foot. *Br J Radiol* 54:1-7, 1981.
9. Pavlou H, Torg J, Freiberger RH: Tarsal navicular stress fractures: radiographic evaluation. *Radiology* 148:641-645, 1983.
10. Towne LC, Blazina ME, Cozen LN: Fatigue fracture of tarsal navicular. *J Bone Joint Surg* 52A:376-378, 1970.
11. Wilson PD: Fractures and dislocations of the tarsal bones. *South Med J* 26:833-845, 1933.
12. Watson-Jones R: *Fractures and Joint Injuries,* ed 4. Baltimore, Williams & Wilkins, 1955, vol 2, pp 900-901.
13. DePalma AF: *The Management of Fractures and Dislocations,* ed 2. Philadelphia, WB Saunders, 1970, pp 1683-1694.
14. Rockwood CA, Green DP: *Fractures,* Philadelphia, JB Lippincott, 1975, pp 1465-1473.
15. Eichenholtz SN, Levine DB: Fractures of the tarsal navicular. *Clin Orthop* 34:142-157, 1964.
16. Wu K: *Surgery of the Foot.* Philadelphia, Lea & Febiger, 1986, pp 319-337.
17. Lemont H, Eravisano V, Lyman J: Accessory navicular: appearance of a synovial joint. *J Am Podiatry Assoc* 71:423-425, 1981.
18. Sarrafian SK: *Anatomy of the Foot and Ankle,* ed 1. Philadelphia, JB Lippincott, 1983, pp 65-68, 88.
19. MacNicol MF, Voutsians S.: Surgical treatment of the symptomatic accessory navicular. *J Bone Joint Surg* 66B:218-226, 1984.
20. Chapman MW: Fractures and fracture-dislocations of the ankle and foot. In Mann RA (ed): *DuVries' Surgery of the Foot,* ed 4. St Louis, CV Mosby, 1978, pp 177-183.
21. Giannestras NJ: *Foot Disorders, Medical and Surgical Management,* ed 2. Philadelphia, Lea & Febiger, 1976, pp 553-557.
22. Rogers L, Campbell R: Fractures and dislocations of the foot. *Semin Roentgenol* 131:157-166, 1978.
23. Ashurst APC, Crossan ET: Fractures of the tarsal scaphoid and the os calcis. *Surg Clin North Am* 10:1477-1487, 1930.
24. Eftekhar NM, Lyddon DW, Stevens J: An unusual fracture dislocation of the tarsal navicular. *J Bone Joint Surg* 51A:577-781, 1969.
25. Day MA: Treatment of injuries to the tarsal navicular. *J Bone Joint Surg* 29:359-366, 1947.
26. Heck CV: Fractures of the bones of the foot except the talus. *Surg Clin North Am* 45:103-116, 1965.
27. Wiley JJ, Brown DE: The bipartite tarsal scaphoid. *J Bone Joint Surg* 63B:583-586, 1981.
28. Wiley JJ, Brown D: Lithiasis of tarsal scaphoid. *J Bone Joint Surg* 56B:586, 1974.
29. Nyska M, Margulies JY, Barbarawi M, Mutchler W, Dekel S, Segal D: Fractures of the body of the tarsal navicular bone: case reports and literature review. *J Trauma* 29:1448-1451, 1989.
30. Goldman FD: Identification, treatment and prognosis of Charcot joint in diabetes mellitus. *J Am Podiatry Assoc* 72:485-490, 1982.
31. Sangeorzan BJ, Benirschke SK, Mosca V, Mayo K, Hansen S: Displaced intra-articular fractures of the tarsal navicular. *J Bone Joint Surg* 71A:1504-1510, 1989.
32. Bohler L. *The Treatment of Fractures,* ed 5. New York, Grune & Stratton, 1958, vol 3, pp 2120-2124.
33. Carr JB, Hansen, ST, Benirschke SK: Surgical treatment of foot and ankle trauma: Use of indirect reduction techniques. *Foot Ankle* 9:176-178, 1989.
34. Nadeau P, Templeton J: Vertical fracture dislocation of the tarsal navicular. *J Trauma* 16:669-671, 1976.
35. DeLee JC: Fractures of the midpart of the foot. In Mann RA, (ed): *Surgery of the Foot,* ed 5. St Louis, CV Mosby, 1986, pp 714-725.
36. Bateman J: Broken hock in the greyhound: repair methods and plastic scaphoid. *Vet Rec* 70:621-623, 1985.
37. Ting A, King W, Yocum L, Antonelli D, Moynes D, Kerlan R, Jobe F, Wong L, Bertolli J: Stress fractures of the tarsal navicular in long distance runners. *Clin Sports Med* 7:89-101, 1988.
38. Lehman R, Gregg JR: Osteochondritis dissecans of the mid foot. *Foot Ankle* 7:177-181, 1986.
39. Cain PR, Seligson D: Lisfranc's fracture dislocation with inter-cuneiform dislocation; presentation of two cases and a plan for treatment. *Foot Ankle* 2:156-160, 1981.
40. Gopal-Krishnan S: Dislocation of the medial cuneiform and injuries of the tarsometatarsal joints. *Int Surg* 38:805-806, 1973.
41. Schiller MG, Ray RD: Isolated dislocation of the medial cuneiform bone: a rare injury of the tarsus. *J Bone Joint Surg* 52A:1632-1636, 1970.
42. Hermel MB, Gershon-Cohen J: The nutcracker fracture of the cuboid by indirect violence. *Radiology* 60:850-854, 1953.
43. Drummond DS, Hastings DE: Total dislocation of the cuboid bone. *J Bone Joint Surg* 51B:716-718, 1969.
44. Goldman FD: Fractures of the midfoot. *Clin Podiatry* 2:259-285, 1985.
45. Banks AS, McGlamry ED: Charcot foot. *J Am Podiatr Med Assoc* 79:213-235, 1989.
46. Ziv I, Mosheiff R, Zelizowski A, Zyebergal M, Lowe J, Segal D: Crush injuries of the foot with compartment syndrome: immediate one-stage management foot and ankle. *Foot Ankle* 9:185-189, 1989.

Additional References

Bolognini N, Goldman FD: Management of major forefoot trauma. *J Foot Surg* 24:88-98, 1985.
Dayton P, Goldman F, Barton E: Compartment pressure in the foot: analysis of normal values and measurement technique. *J Am Podiatr Med Assoc* 80:521-525, 1990.
Goldman F: Midfoot fractures. In Scurran BL (ed): *Foot and Ankle Trauma.* New York, Churchill Livingstone, 1989, pp 377-403.
Wargon C, Goldman FD: Lisfranc's fracture dislocation: a variation. *J Am Podiatr Med Assoc* 76:466-468, 1986.

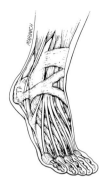

CHAPTER **64**

Calcaneal Fractures

John A. Ruch, D.P.M.
G. Clay Taylor, D.P.M.

Raymond G. Cavaliere, D.P.M.*

Calcaneal fractures, although representing only 2% of all fractures, are frequently associated with prolonged disability (1). These injuries have devastating potential, and as a result the literature is replete with information describing and promoting various classifications and treatment plans. This voluminous material often leads to general confusion regarding appropriate assessment and treatment.

The purpose of this chapter is to help the reader develop a clear understanding of all types of calcaneal fractures. In an effort to establish this understanding, the pertinent anatomy, a historical review, and the mechanism of the injuries will be explored. The authors will use this information, as well as clinical experience, to present a recommendation as to classification and preferred method of treatment. Both extra-articular and intra-articular calcaneal injuries are included.

*Appreciation is expressed to Raymond G. Cavaliere, D.P.M., author of this chapter in the first edition.

OS CALCIS FRACTURES

Although calcaneal fractures are relatively uncommon, they represent approximately 60% of all major tarsal injuries (2). Calcaneal fractures are frequently intra-articular and are more serious and disabling than extra-articular fractures. Based on a review of 241 calcaneal fractures, Essex-Lopresti (3) found 75% of these to be intra-articular. Other authors have agreed that the majority of calcaneal fractures are intra-articular (4-7). It is with this group of calcaneal fractures that considerable debate regarding classification, treatment, and prognosis exists.

Calcaneal fractures usually occur between the ages of 30 and 50 years, with a peak incidence at approximately 45 years of age. They are usually incurred by workers as a result of a fall (6-12) (Fig. 64.1), and men are affected five times as often as women (13, 14). It has been suggested that a fall from a height of approximately 12 feet is needed before an athletic human sustains such a fracture (15), although in a study by Lance et al. (6), calcaneal fractures occurred from

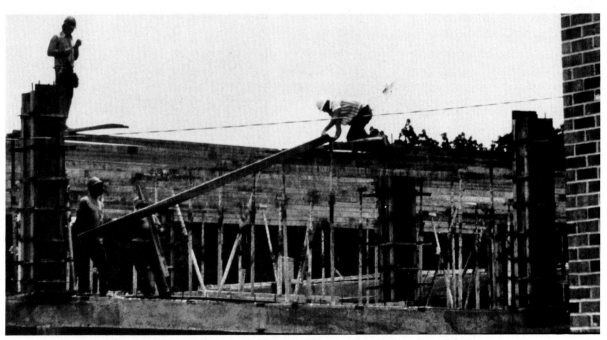

Figure 64.1. Occupations involving heights have highest incidence of calcaneal fractures.

heights ranging from 3 to 50 feet, with the average being 14 feet. Motor vehicle accidents are also common causes of this fracture.

Infrequent causes of calcaneal fractures include sudden forceful contraction of the triceps surae (12), sequelae of heel spur surgery (16), and stress-related injuries (17, 18) (Fig. 64.2). Communications with Perry of the Naval Hospital at Paris Island, South Carolina, reveal an 18.4% inci-

dence of calcaneal stress fractures involving female marine recruits (19). A stress fracture has also been reported in a 3-year old boy with cerebral palsy and no associated injury (20).

With tarsal injuries one must examine the patient thoroughly because of the high incidence of concomitant injuries. Related injuries include fractures of the spine, femur, tibia, fibula, malleoli, and talus and Colles' fractures

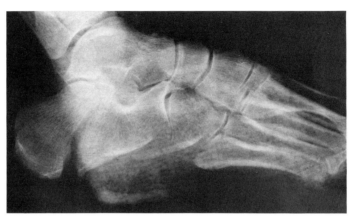

Figure 64.2.   Calcaneal fracture 3 days after heel spur resection.

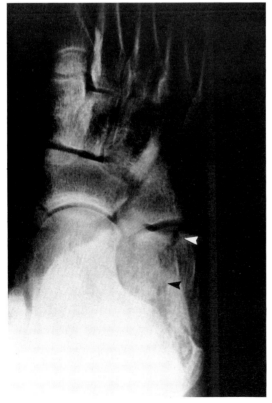

Figure 64.3.   Severe calcaneal injury in young woman secondary to automobile accident. Fracture is seen involving calcaneocuboid joint with associated navicular fracture.

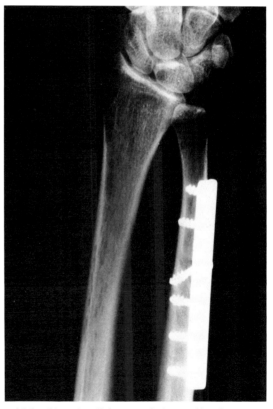

Figure 64.4.   "Associated" fracture of ulna resulting from automobile accident of same patient as in Figure 64.3.

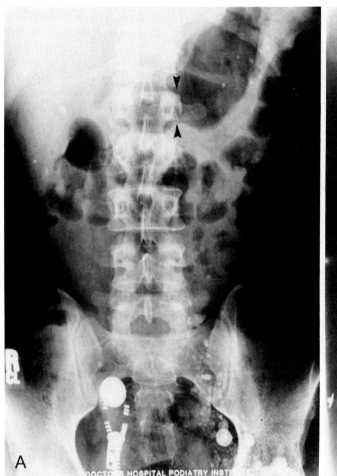

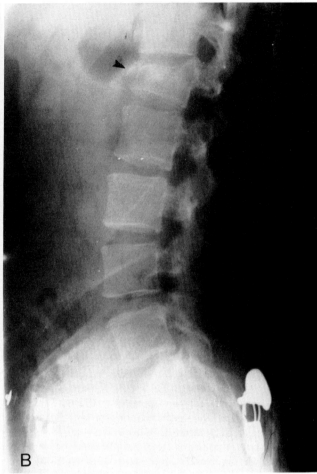

Figure 64.5. **A.** Anteroposterior (AP) projection of lumbar spine demonstrates compression fracture at L1 in young male who sustained comminuted joint depression-type calcaneal fracture as result of vertical fall.

B. Lateral projection of lumbar spine further demonstrates compression fracture at L1.

(2) (Figs. 64.3 and 64.4). Spinal injuries usually involve the dorsolumbar junction (T12 to L2, inclusively) and are usually compression fractures (21) (Fig. 64.5). L1 is the most frequently involved vertebra (22). The incidence of spinal fractures ranges from 10% as reported by Lance and associates to over 20% according to Wilson (5, 6, 13, 23).

Associated soft tissue injuries have been implicated as a source of continued pain and morbidity following calcaneal injury and therefore should not be overlooked. Related injuries include impingement to peroneal or flexor tendons, disruption of plantar fat pad, or compression of the tarsal canal leading to tarsal tunnel syndrome (7, 24-27).

ANATOMICAL CONSIDERATIONS

The calcaneus is the largest bone of the foot and has an internal architecture designed to withstand transmission of the entire body load to the weight-bearing surface. It is composed of a thin cortical shell enclosing soft cancellous

bone that contains traction trabeculae. These trabeculae radiate from the talar articular surface posteroinferiorly and anteroinferiorly to the calcaneal tuberosity and the calcaneocuboid articulation, respectively. This trabecular pattern represents the weight distribution through the calcaneus. A sparsely trabeculated area, the neutral triangle, is located just below the anterior edge of the posterior facet and is considered the weakest area of the calcaneus (1, 28) (Fig. 64.6). Essex-Lopresti theorized that a vertical fracture occurs through this location with compression of the talus onto the calcaneus (3).

On its superior surface, the calcaneus articulates with the talus via the anterior, middle, and posterior cartilaginous facets. The larger posterior facet is separated from the anterior and middle facets by a roughened groove called the sulcus calcaneus. This groove is narrow at its medial end and widens as it continues anterolaterally. When combined with the talus, the groove forms the canalis tarsus medially and the sinus tarsi at its widened lateral region. The sinus tarsi region of the calcaneus gives rise to the bifurcate lig-

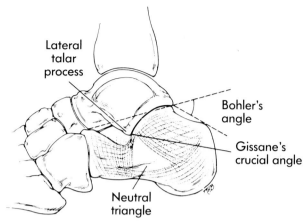

Figure 64.6. Lateral view of left calcaneus demonstrating Bohler's tuber joint angle, talocalcaneal articulation, and typical trabecular pattern directed to support articular facets. Other anatomical boundaries are highlighted.

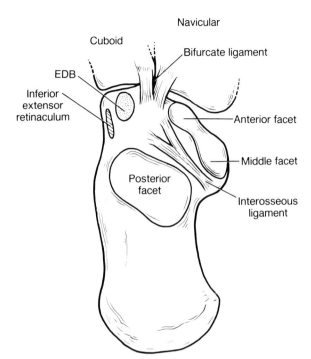

Figure 64.7. Superior aspect of left calcaneus demonstrating three articular facets, as well as integral soft tissue attachments. EDB, extensor digitorum brevis.

ament, the extensor digitorum brevis muscle, and the inferior extensor retinaculum (Fig. 64.7).

The medial side of the calcaneus has a shelflike projection supporting the middle facet called the sustentaculum tali. The sustentaculum tali is an important component of the initial stage of joint compression fractures inasmuch as it is sheared from the lateral main portion of the body of the calcaneus (29-31). The sustentaculum tali also forms the superior and lateral boundary of the tarsal tunnel; the flexor hallucis longus tendon runs inferior to the bony projection, and the flexor digitorum longus tendon travels along the edge.

Because the peroneal tendons are located along the lateral side of the calcaneus, their impingement frequently occurs with calcaneal fractures. The peroneus brevis and peroneus longus tendons course along the lateral calcaneus in grooves located above and below the peroneal trochlea, respectively. This trochlea is located along the central region of the lateral side. The calcaneofibular ligament also attaches to the posterior region of the lateral calcaneus.

The calcaneal tuberosity is present along the inferior surface of the calcaneus and is the posterior point of weight bearing in the foot. The tuberosity is divided into medial and lateral processes and gives origin to several intrinsic muscles of the foot. The flexor retinaculum and plantar aponeurosis also attach to the tuberosity. The calcaneus is protected inferiorly by a dense fibrofatty tissue designed to absorb impact.

The Achilles tendon inserts into the posterior calcaneus along the middle and the inferior two-thirds region. The anterior surface of the calcaneus articulates with the cuboid, forming a saddle-shaped joint.

RADIOGRAPHIC EXAMINATION

"The roentgenograms are not easily interpreted and often tell only part of the truth" (29). This statement was made

by Palmer in 1948 in reference to calcaneal fractures and remains true today. The authors have frequently found additional features of this injury at open reduction despite careful preoperative radiographic examination. Others have shared in this finding (32). Some factors clouding exact radiographic analysis include variations in the lateral roentgen projection with heel inversion and eversion as pointed out by Wilson (33), individual anatomical variations, and joint structure such as the lateral sloping convex surface of the posterior facet obscuring a portion of the joint surface on the lateral projection (29). Even though these variabilities exist and evaluation is not exact, proper radiographic analysis must be obtained.

Standard radiographs for a suspected calcaneal fracture include a dorsoplantar projection of the foot, lateral projection of the ankle and calcaneus, and a calcaneal axial view. A lateral calcaneal projection of the uninjured foot is sometimes useful for comparison (29). An anteroposterior projection of the ankle, as well as a lateral-oblique projection of the calcaneus (medial oblique view), are additional views that are used when deemed necessary (34). For further evaluation of the subtalar joint, additional views have been suggested by Anthonson, Broden, and Isherwood (35-37). Each describes special views that allow for evaluation of the posterior facet, but today, computerized tomography (CT) is readily available and consequently these special views are seldom used for calcaneal fractures.

In the anteroposterior projection of the ankle, injuries to the ankle are evaluated and one may visualize the lateral spread of the calcaneus evidenced by bulging, especially about the lateral malleolus. The lateral oblique projection of the os calcis helps visualize involvement of the articular surface of the calcaneus at the calcaneocuboid joint, as well as fractures of the anterior process. Some authors believe that views not taken to rule out involvement of the calcaneocuboid and/or talonavicular joints have been responsible for poor results encountered in the past with treatment other than triple arthrodesis (34). The dorsoplantar projection of the foot also reveals fractures involving the articular surface of the calcaneus at the calcaneocuboid joint, which frequently is associated with a lateral spreading displacement of the lateral cortex at the joint. In severely comminuted fractures, subluxation of the talar head at the talonavicular joint may be seen with this view.

The lateral view of the ankle and calcaneus allows visualization of the fracture lines involving the calcaneus, reveals ankle joint involvement, and allows interpretation of Bohler's angle. In 1931 Bohler (10) described the tuberosity joint angle, which is a measurement of the sagittal plane relationship between the talus and calcaneus. According to Bohler a line from the highest point on the posterior articular surface to the most superior portion of the calcaneal tuberosity intersects with a line from the highest point of the posterior articular surface and the highest point of the anterior process to create an angle of 30° to 35°. Stephenson (3) reports the normal range of this angle as 25° to 40°, with the average being 35°. This angle classically is more acute in the pes cavus deformity and in children's feet whereas it is flatter in the pes valgus deformity. This angle is used to assess the degree of intra-articular depression of the calcaneal; however, measurement of the injured foot should always be compared with the contralateral foot. Some have cautioned against too much dependence on the measurement of this angle, because gross distortion of the subtalar joints may result from a fracture without any measurable abnormality in Bohler's angle (21). In fractures of the os calcis this angle may become smaller, straight, or even reversed (Fig. 64.6).

The crucial angle described by Gissane (38) in 1947 is also visualized on the lateral projection. This angle is created by the subchondral bone of the posterior facet and the subchondral bone of the anterior and middle facets and subsequently gives some indication of the relationship of the posterior, middle, and anterior facets. The normal range is between 120° and 145° (31) and should be equal to that of the contralateral foot. The bone creating this angle supports the lateral process of the talus, which under compression acts as a wedge, creating the so-called primary fracture line in the calcaneus.

Last, the tangential view of the os calcis (calcaneal axial) allows visualization of the posterior articular facet, the sustentaculum tali, and the extent of the bulging of the calcaneus medially and laterally, as well as encroachment about the medial and lateral malleoli. This view also allows for evaluation of the base of the fifth metatarsal and the medial concave and lateral convex surfaces of the calcaneus.

The use of linear tomography may be helpful in evaluating the extent of involvement of the subtalar joint but is not recommended as a routine part of evaluation (Fig. 64.8). CT, however, is an extremely valuable tool for evaluating the extent of the injury. Frontal plan CT imaging clearly demonstrates the nature of the injury by showing the components involved, the extent of comminution, and the status of the articular segments (39, 40) (Fig. 64.9).

Recently the development of volumetric three-dimensional (3-D) CT has allowed further insight into calcaneal fractures. At present this 3-D reconstruction has limited ability to display the articular fractures but provides a readily recognizable image of the calcaneal extra-articular fracture anatomy. These images may enhance preoperative planning, as well as provide an additional teaching tool for this complex fracture (41)(Fig. 64.10)

CLINICAL DIAGNOSIS

Causative trauma of calcaneal fractures in children may be indistinguishable from the child's everyday activities; therefore these fractures are often overlooked and written off as

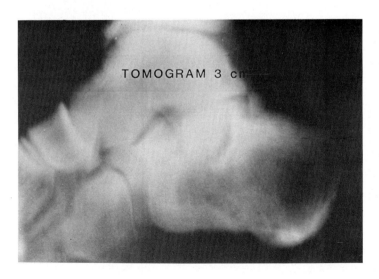

Figure 64.8. Tomography may be helpful in identifying suspected fractures when they are not readily discernable on routine radiographs. This calcaneal fracture is minimally displaced; however, its intra-articular involvement is clearly seen here.

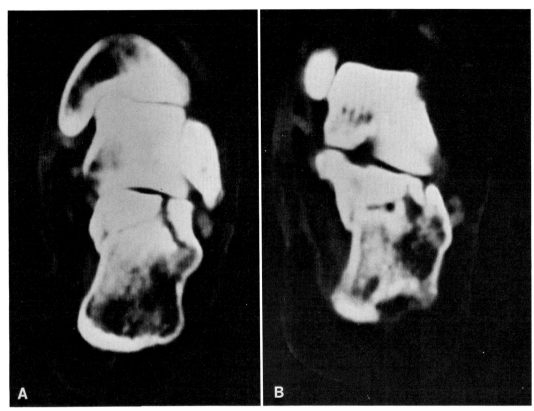

Figure 64.9. **A** and **B.** Same fracture as seen in Figure 64.8 is shown here on CT scans. Exact osseous involvement is seen: intra-articular involvement of posterior subtalar joint, large void within cancellous bone secondary to compression recoil, and bulging of lateral wall with impingement of peroneal tendons. All fracture fragments are identified.

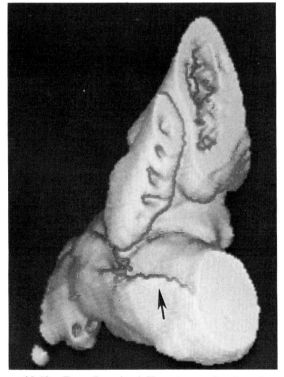

Figure 64.10. Three-dimensional CT: posteroanterior view of nondisplaced tongue-type fracture of the calcaneus (arrow).

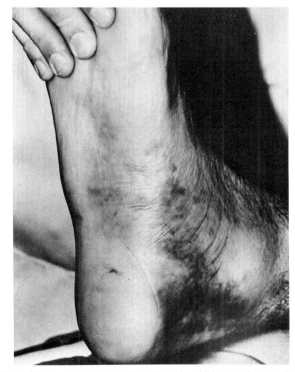

Figure 64.11. Hematoma and ecchymosis, which extends toward sole of foot, is often seen with calcaneal fractures. This sign is seldom found in ankle fractures.

a sprain (42-44). Tenderness on lateral compression of the calcaneus, as well as the characteristic posture of flexion of the knee and hip, and plantarflexion of the foot with refusal to bear weight on the heel should increase suspicion of a calcaneal fracture in a child (42).

In adults the history is obviously most important when one deals with possible calcaneal fractures. The history of a vertical fall on the heel from a height of several meters may suggest such a condition (10). An important diagnostic sign of calcaneal fractures is pain limited to the os calcis especially on medial to lateral compression. Other diagnostic signs include inability to bear weight on the heel, broadening and swelling about the involved area, and the hematoma that extends toward the sole of the foot, a sign seldom seen in ankle fractures (Fig. 64.11). If the fracture is intra-articular, pain may be present on subtalar joint range of motion.

With all calcaneal injuries, one should entertain the possibility of additional injuries to the extremities and spine. Proper clinical, as well as radiological, assessment should be performed.

CALCANEAL FRACTURES IN CHILDREN

Blount (45) stated that calcaneal fractures in children are rare. Matteri and Frynoyer (42), on the basis of a study of 53 calcaneal fractures from 1962 through 1971, reported a 6% incidence of calcaneal fractures in children. Schofield (16) reviewed 2025 fractures of the calcaneus, and his youngest patient was an 18-year-old boy. Zayer (47) included one 12-year-old patient in 110 cases. Essex-Lopresti (3) found 12 patients with this injury between the ages of 9 and 20 years in his analysis of 241 fractures of the calcaneus.

Fractures of the calcaneus in children are easily overlooked on routine foot and ankle roentgenograms because of the often minimal disturbance in the bony architecture and the higher percentage of cartilage present within the os calcis in the child. Starshak and associates (1984) found that only four of ten calcaneal fractures in children between the ages of 19 to 41 months were visible on the initial radiographs (48). Hahn and Stock (1984) recommended "repeat radiographs after 10 days if the clinical findings indicated a fracture and the initial radiographs are negative" (49). A common clinical diagnostic clue of calcaneal fractures in children is the characteristic posturing of hip and knee flexion and plantarflexion of the foot, with refusal to bear weight.

In contrast to adult calcaneal fractures, extra-articular fractures are more characteristic in children. Schmidt and Weiner (50) reviewed 59 fractures in children under 19 years of age and found a 63% incidence of extra-articular fractures in this group. They identified adult patterns of calcaneal fractures to occur in the older child, 15 years of age and older. This lower incidence of intra-articular fractures of children's calcanei is commonly attributed to its more elastic nature and greater cartilaginous composition, allowing more resistance to compressive forces, although this is disputable. In 1984 Wiley and Profitt (51) found an average fall height of 1 meter in fractures of children under 10 years old. Schantz and Rasmussen (49) also found an average fall

height of 1 meter with calcaneal fractures of children and subsequently concluded that the rarity of the fractures in children is more likely the result of less exposure to trauma and that the fractures may be overlooked.

Associated fractures of the extremities occur twice as frequently in children as in adults, whereas axial skeletal injuries are half as frequent as in adults. No mention is found in the literature regarding incongruent calcaneal growth deformities as a sequela to physeal injury. This has been supported by Schmidt and Weiner (50).

Because of the nature of this injury and the remodeling capability of the cartilaginous-filled calcaneus, one may expect a normal functioning calcaneus with minimal posttraumatic arthrosis after most calcaneal fractures in children. Generally, conservative treatment approaches have been advocated, with good prognosis.

CLASSIFICATION

In a review of the literature one finds many classification schemes, with much acclamation of each. The authors agree with King (52), who suggested that there is no one satisfactory radiological classification of these fractures. Many clinicians, including Essex-Lopresti, Watson-Jones, Nade and Monahan, Rowe, Campbell and DePalma, Thoren, Widen, and Gaul have classified calcaneal fractures. Kalish (19) in 1975 suggested the use of the Essex-Lopresti and DePalma methods for classifying calcaneal fractures as a comfortable and simple way to understand these complex injuries.

The fact that at least two types of fractures of the calcaneus occur was recognized by Malgaigne as long ago as 1843. Bohler in 1935 published his classification, which reflected appreciation of the relationship between the type of fracture and the prognosis. These two types are simply extra-articular and intra-articular calcaneal fractures. The authors suggest a classification to describe both groups of fractures more inclusively. The recommended classification is a combination of the classification of Rowe et al. (5) and Essex-Lopresti (3). The Rowe classification is shown in Figure 64.12; it is most inclusive regarding extra-articular calcaneal fracture types. The Essex-Lopresti classification (Figs. 64.13 and 64.14) is reserved for intra-articular fractures and is used in lieu of Rowe types IV and V fractures.

In severe fractures a combination of types will occur and classification will be extremely difficult, if not impossible. Warrick and Bremner (53) have prepared an excellent atlas illustrating the various types of calcaneal fractures. Palmer's description in 1948 similarly has provided great insight into understanding the mechanisms of these severe fractures.

Extra-Articular Calcaneal Fractures

FRACTURE OF THE CALCANEAL TUBEROSITY

Calcaneal tuberosity fractures, which represent Rowe type Ia fracture, usually result from a fall with the heel everted or inverted. As the heel strikes the ground, the medial or lateral prominence is separated from the tuberosity by a shearing force. Treatment depends on the amount of dis-

Rowe Classification

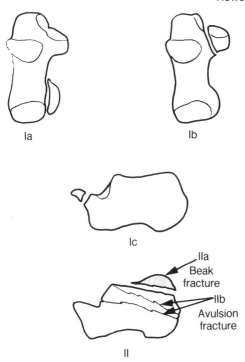

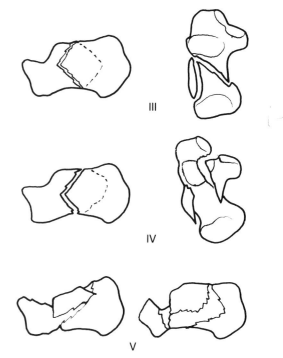

Figure 64.12. Rowe classification of calcaneal fractures, which is most inclusive regarding extra-articular calcaneal fracture types. Type Ia, fracture of tuberosity. Type Ib, fracture of sustentaculum tali. Type Ic, fracture of anterior process. Type IIa, beak fracture. Type IIb, avulsion fracture involving Achilles tendon insertion. Type III, oblique body fracture not involving subtalar joint. Type IV, body fracture involving subtalar joint. Type V, joint depression fracture with comminution.

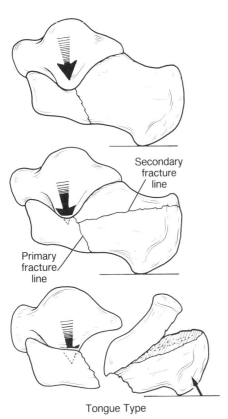

Tongue Type

Figure 64.13. Essex-Lopresti's drawing showing tongue-type fracture with its typical displacement. Primary and secondary fracture lines are shown.

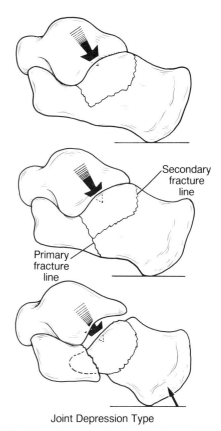

Joint Depression Type

Figure 64.14. Essex-Lopresti's drawing showing typical joint depression type of fracture with displacement of articular fragment inferiorly and upward displacement of tuberosity fragment. Primary and secondary fracture line are shown.

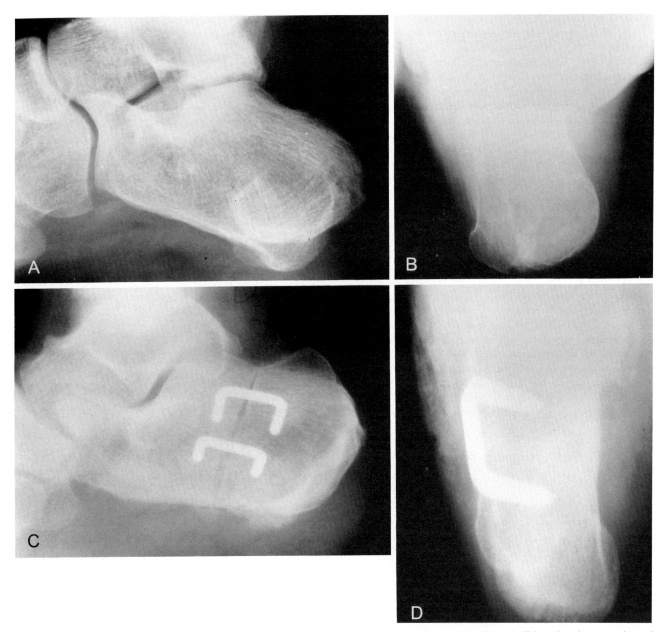

Figure 64.15.   Isolated, displaced posterolateral extra-articular calcaneal fracture involving calcaneal tuberosity. Treatment consisted of conservative casting for 4 to 6 weeks. Both lateral (**A**) and axial (**B**) calcaneal radiographs are needed to make accurate diagnosis. This patient later experienced pain on ambulation secondary to heel malposition. **C** and **D.** Dwyer calcaneal osteotomy, as well as exostectomy, were subsequently performed.

placement of the fracture, as well as the size of the fragment and the experience of the physician. Generally, all types of undisplaced fractures should be conservatively treated with immobilization for a period of 3 to 10 weeks, with an average casting time of 5 to 6 weeks (Fig. 64.15).

Posterior vertical (sagittal plane) fractures of the tuberosity with displacement causes splaying or widening of the calcaneus and may disrupt the normal peroneal tendon grooves. These fractures should be manipulated with thenar pressure and casted for 4 to 8 weeks in a below-the-knee cast. Open reduction is an alternative here. The prognosis is good because of sparing of the talocalcaneal joint.

FRACTURE OF THE SUSTENTACULUM TALI

A fracture of the sustentaculum tali is classified as a Rowe type Ib fracture; however, it is now recognized as the first stage of joint depression fractures. The fracture often occurs after a fall, with some type of twisting or torsional strain on a supinated foot. There is usually pain and swelling approximately 1 inch inferior to the tip of the medial malleolus. An important diagnostic test is flexion and extension of the hallux, which may cause pain inasmuch as the flexor tendon courses along the inferior surface of the sustentaculum tali (54, 55).

A posteroanterior roentgenogram of the heel (calcaneal axial view) will demonstrate this fracture best (Fig. 64.16). Treatment of the nondisplaced fracture consists of a below-the-knee walking cast for 4 to 6 weeks with the foot in mild inversion. Fractures with a considerable degree of displacement may be anatomically reduced by use of LAG screws. The overall prognosis for this isolated injury is good.

A synovitis of the anterior talocalcaneal joint and/or posterior tibial tendon sometimes occurs and may respond to anti-inflammatory medications as well as to supportive devices.

FRACTURE OF THE ANTERIOR PROCESS

A Rowe type Ic calcaneal fracture is a fracture of the anterior process and represents the most common type I injury (5, 14, 56). Of interest is that this fracture is the only one in which female patients predominate and is probably related to the wearing of high-heeled shoes (19). The most common mechanism reported is one of supination-plantarflexion of the foot in which the bifurcate ligament is put under tension and avulses bone at its origin on the calcaneus (Fig. 64.17A). Dachtler (57) was the first to describe fractures of the an-

terior portion of the calcaneus; however, he combined the anterior avulsion fractures with a more severe injury: a compression fracture of the anterior articular surface of the calcaneus. These compression type fractures are a separate entity, as first noted by Gellman (56), and have a completely different mechanism, as well as prognosis (Fig. 64.17B). Their mechanism is that of forced forefoot abduction or dorsiflexion eversion, and they are usually associated with an avulsion fracture of the tuberosity of the navicular (58, 59).

The typical history with anterior process fractures is a twisting injury of the foot, with complaints of pain and swelling midway between the tip of the lateral malleolus and the fifth metatarsal base in the area of the sinus tarsi. The medial oblique and lateral views of the foot show this fracture best (Fig. 64.18). If minimal displacement is present, it may be difficult to see radiographically and therefore may be misdiagnosed as an ankle sprain if a careful physical examination is not performed (Fig. 64.19). Figure 64.20 represents a suspected anterior beak fracture, which is clearly

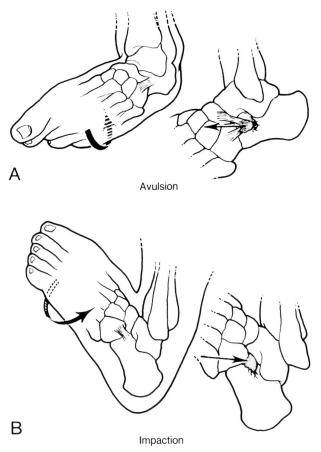

A

Avulsion

B

Impaction

Figure 64.17.   **A.** Inversion-plantarflexion is commonly reported mechanism resulting in anterior process fractures. **B.** Others include dorsiflexion-eversion mechanism, as well as forefoot abduction mechanism, both of which result in compression-type fractures—different in type and prognosis.

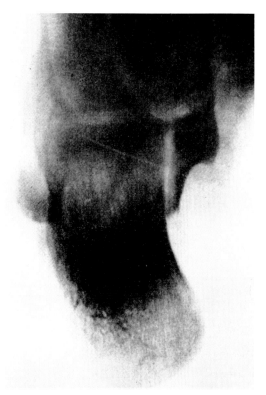

Figure 64.16.   Axial calcaneal view best demonstrates isolated sustentaculum tali fracture.

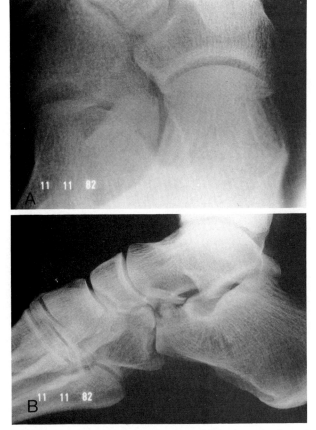

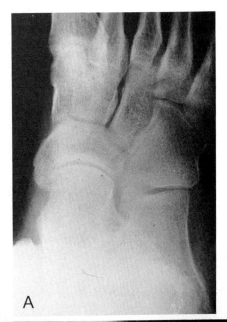

Figure 64.18. Medial oblique **(A)** and lateral **(B)** calcaneal radiographs demonstrating type III anterior process fracture that is large and displaced, and that involves calcaneocuboid joint. Initial conservative casting treatment resulted in painful fracture fragment nonunion.

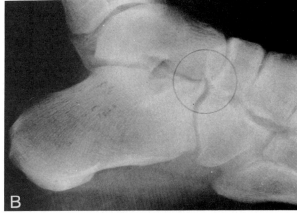

Figure 64.19. Anterior-process calcaneal fracture is suspected; however, it is barely visible in medial oblique **(A)** and lateral **(B)** calcaneal radiographs. Because mechanism involved in this type of injury is similar to that causing sprain of anterior talofibular ligament, many of these are misdiagnosed as ankle sprain.

visualized on tomogram, and results of the anterior drawer test were negative for anterior talofibular ligament rupture.

Treatment for anterior beak fractures ranges from physical therapy and weight bearing as tolerated (55) to the use of a below-the-knee cast. Persistent pain may necessitate total excision of the fracture fragment (Fig. 64.21). Degan and associates (60) first described three fracture types, with type III being a large displaced fragment that involved the calcaneocuboid joint. In their study, five of the seven patients who underwent surgical excision had type III fractures. One may conclude that large, displaced fracture fragments should be anatomically reduced by means of Swiss compression techniques (61).

Of interest is a common calcaneal avulsion fracture reported by Norfray and associates (62), which is often confused with an anterior calcaneal process fracture or os peroneum. The fracture is actually an avulsion fracture off the dorsolateral aspect of the calcaneus secondary to a pull-off mechanism by the extensor digitorum brevis muscle at its insertion during stressful inversion injuries. They reported a 10% incidence of these fractures in a review of all emergency room ankle trauma cases from 1978 through 1979.

The routine dorsoplantar foot film and/or the routine anteroposterior ankle view demonstrates this fracture well. Treatment here is conservative, with elevation, ice, supportive bandages, and early activity (Fig 64.22).

BEAK AND AVULSION FRACTURE OF THE POSTERIOR CALCANEUS

A beak or an avulsion fracture to the posterior calcaneus is a Rowe type II extra-articular fracture that may or may not involve the insertion of the Achilles tendon (Fig. 64.23). Most cases will involve the insertion of the Achilles tendon (14); however, this injury is rather rare (63). Bohler (64) suggested a clear distinction between the beak fracture and the avulsion fracture: the former does not affect the at-

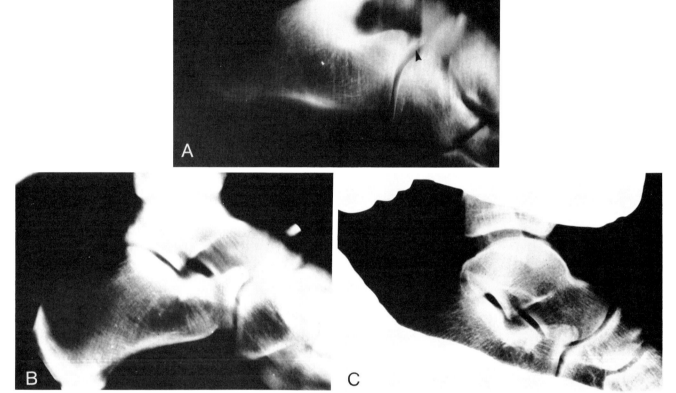

Figure 64.20. **A** and **B.** Tomogram was obtained in same case reported on in Figure 64.19. Suspected anterior-process fracture of the calcaneus is now clearly seen. **C.** During initial work-up in emergency room, anterior drawer test failed to show any ligamentous damage but clearly delineated true pathological nature of injury. Small and undisplaced fracture was treated by conservative non-weight-bearing casting.

tachment of the Achilles tendon, and the latter is associated with loosening of this attachment. Watson-Jones writes that the beak fracture is caused by direct trauma to the posterior surface of the calcaneus, as in falling down stairs, whereas the avulsion fracture is caused by strong pull from the Achilles tendon when under stress. The foot is often plantarflexed (13, 19, 55). These fractures commonly occur between the ages of 50 to 70 years in contrast with Achilles tendon ruptures, which occur between the ages of 30 and 50 years (65).

With type II fractures the patient reports tenderness over the posterior process of the calcaneus. A lateral roentgenogram is usually sufficient to demonstrate this fracture. If a true avulsion fracture (types IIb and IIc) exists, the patient may have weak plantarflexion and walk with an antalgic calcaneus gait. The avulsion injury is likened to an Achilles tendon rupture, and most authorities agree as to the need for anatomical reduction and proper fixation to avoid later calcaneal gait disability (13, 19, 55, 65-69) (Figs. 64.24 and 64.25). The limb is then placed in a non-weight-bearing

above-the-knee cast in gravity ankle equinus for 4 to 6 weeks, after which time the patient may be placed in a below-the-knee walking cast for 2 weeks or may begin non-weight-bearing exercises for 2 weeks and then start to ambulate gradually. Undisplaced fractures may be treated with a non-weight-bearing equinus cast for 6 weeks followed by either of the previously mentioned protocols.

Nondisplaced beak fractures may be treated by casting with the foot in plantarflexion for 6 weeks. If significant displacement exists or there is a threat to local skin circulation over the displaced fragment, then operative reduction and fixation are indicated (65, 69). The Achilles tendon usually inserts about the middle third of the calcaneal tuberosity; however, Heck (67), Lowry (68), and Protheroe (69) describe its insertion into the upper third. Because the insertion of the Achilles tendon has been shown to be variable and because x-ray studies do not give a definite indication as to the Achilles tendon insertion, an argument can be made for open assessment of some larger beak fractures (66, 68).

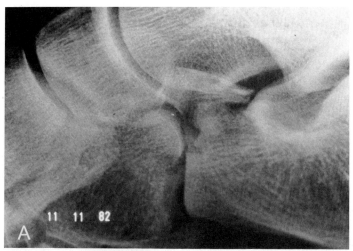

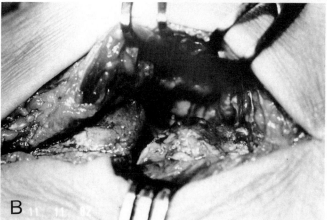

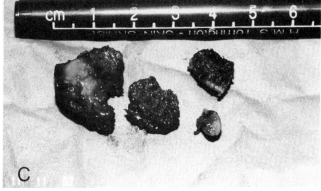

Figure 64.21. A to **C.** Same patient as in Figure 64.18, with large, displaced, and intra-articular anterior calcaneal process fracture. Initial treat-ment failed, requiring delayed excision of painful fracture fragment non-union. Patient is reportedly pain-free at present.

The overall prognosis for union and function following these fractures is excellent.

FRACTURE OF THE CALCANEAL BODY WITHOUT INVOLVEMENT OF THE TALOCALCANEAL JOINT

Extra-articular fractures to the body of the calcaneus are Rowe type III fractures and occur about one fourth as often as the intra-articular type of fracture. They comprise about 20% of all calcaneal fractures (5, 6). This type of fracture is the most common extra-articular fracture of the calcaneus and usually results from a fall with the heel in varus or valgus, forcing an edge of the talus into the calcaneus. If the force is great, comminution and displacement may occur, but this is usually not the case.

Treatment for these extra-articular fractures depends on the degree of displacement present at the fracture site. Occasionally, conservative treatment alone will suffice; an above-knee cast with the knee flexed approximately 35° is used to relax the pull of the triceps surae, and the foot is placed in a neutral position. Usually open reduction with internal fixation is required, and the patient is then placed in a below-the-knee cast and abstains from weight bearing for at least 4 to 6 weeks. Disability in this injury is usually not long-term because of sparing the talocalcaneal joint.

Intra-Articular Calcaneal Fractures

Intra-articular calcaneal fractures, classified by Essex-Lopresti, comprise the vast majority of calcaneal fractures. Essex-Lopresti types A and B (tongue type and joint depression type, respectively) are classically differentiated by the location of the secondary fracture line and the shape of the fragments (Figs. 64.13 and 64.14). In Essex-Lopresti's description, the primary or vertical fracture line is from superior to inferior, extending from the vertex of Gissane's crucial angle to the plantar aspect of the calcaneus, and it is the same for both fracture types (Fig. 64.26). The secondary fracture line is determined by the direction of force.

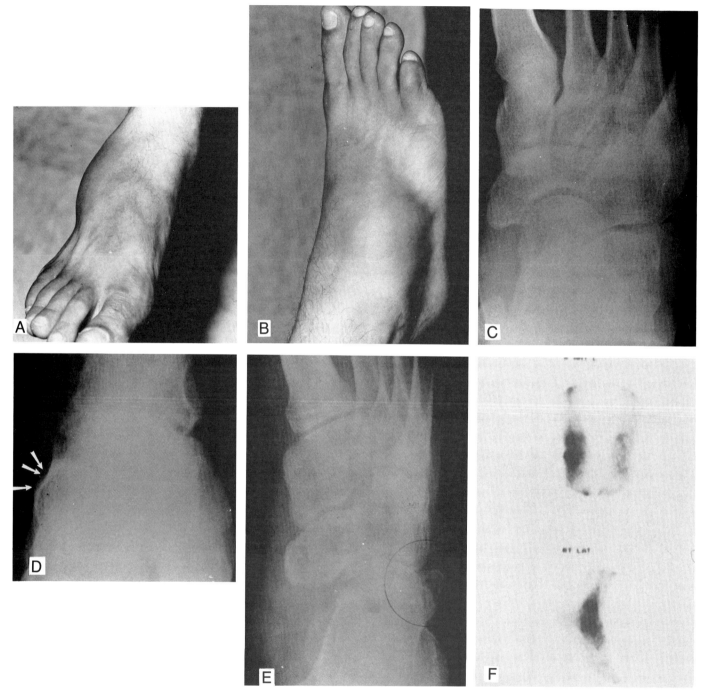

Figure 64.22. **A** and **B.** Clinical appearance of right foot following inversion injury. **C.** Dorsoplantar foot radiograph demonstrates rarely reported and rarely recognized common calcaneal avulsion fracture caused by severe inversion stress placed on extensor digitorum brevis muscle at its origin on anterosuperior surface of calcaneus. **D.** Anteroposterior ankle view demonstrates this injury; however, trained and suspicious eye is needed. Arrows have been added to highlight avulsion fracture fragments. **E.** Same fracture demonstrated on medial oblique foot radiograph. Note just how subtle findings can be. **F.** Bone scan demonstrates extent of injury and therefore need for initial accurate diagnosis and treatment.

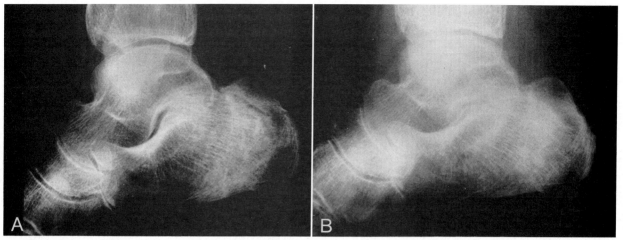

Figure 64.23. **A.** Calcaneal beak fracture well demonstrated on lateral radiograph. This fracture does not involve insertion of Achilles tendon. **B.** Six-week follow-up after below-knee conservative casting with foot plantarflexed. There is no further disability, and healing was uneventful.

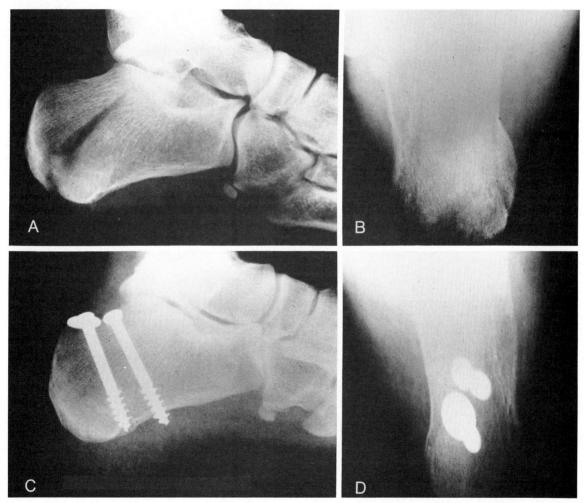

Figure 64.24. **A** and **B.** Lateral and axial calcaneal radiographs demonstrating true calcaneal avulsion fracture, which involves avulsion of the Achilles tendon. **C** and **D.** Postoperative lateral and axial calcaneal radiographs after open reduction with internal fixation was performed. Reduction is anatomical. **E.** Intraoperative incision is placed over fracture and courses just anterior to Achilles tendon and over superior calcaneal shelf. Further anterior placement of incision would provide less optimal surgical exposure and would encroach on sural nerve and lesser saphenous vein. **F.** Fracture is identified, reduced, and temporarily held with staple. **G.** Final fixation is accomplished with use of two 6.5-mm cancellous compression screws. **H.** Eight-month follow-up after screw removal shows maintenance of anatomical reduction with excellent surgical result.

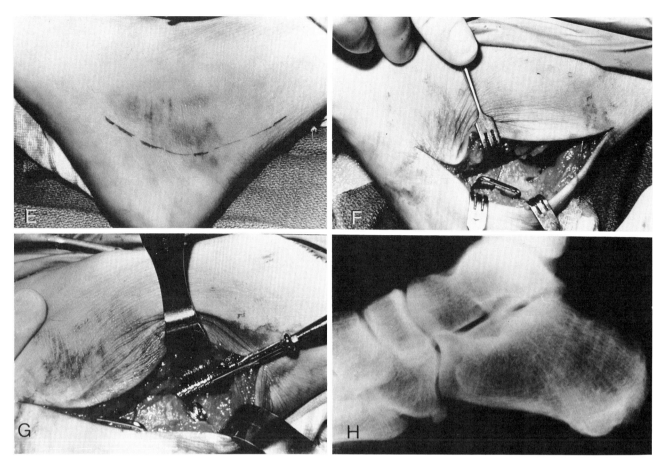

Figure 64.24. E-H.

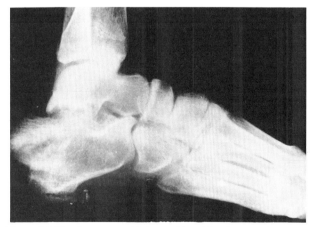

Figure 64.25. In contrast, this is an old avulsion fracture of calcaneus treated by conservative above-knee casting in gravity equinus. Obviously there is no anatomical reduction, and an antalgic calcaneus gait should be expected until strengthening of triceps occurs.

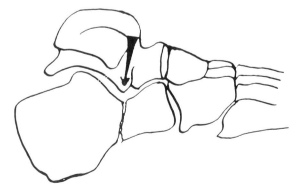

Figure 64.26. Primary fracture line is common to both types of intra-articular calcaneal fractures and is created by vertical process (spur) of talus under vertical compressive loads.

TONGUE FRACTURE VERSUS JOINT DEPRESSION FRACTURE

The tongue-type fracture occurs because a sagittal or longitudinal fracture line separates a major lateral portion of the posterior facet from the medial aspect of the calcaneus. As the fracture line progresses posteriorly, it takes on a more plantar-lateral orientation or more horizontal plane and includes the entire superior portion of the calcaneal tuber and lateral portion of the posterior facet as a solid and intact segment of the fracture. In many cases, this fracture pattern takes on the appearance of an avulsion fracture of the superior portion of the posterior segment of the calcaneus and does not appear to involve the subtalar joint (Fig. 64.27). This, however, according to Essex-Lopresti (3), Palmer (29), and Burdeaux (30), is not the case inasmuch as the tongue-

type fracture definitely is a compression and shear fracture that does involve the subtalar joint in its superior extension.

The classical joint depression type of fracture occurs when the lateral portion of the posterior facet, as an isolated segment, is depressed into the body of the calcaneus. A fracture line at the posterior rim of facet margin allows the lateral portion of the facet to separate from the proximal tuber and drive deep into the body of the calcaneus without proximal extension or the appearance of a tongue-type configuration (3, 29, 30).

The production of a tongue or a joint depression fracture is believed to depend on the sagittal plane position of the foot on impact. Thoren (70) clearly demonstrated, in cadaveric studies, the significance of foot position on the mechanism of injury and subsequent fracture pattern. He found that the tongue-type fracture was consistently reproduced when the foot was impacted while in a plantargrade or plantarflexed attitude. The joint depression type of fracture occurred when the impaction force struck the foot in a dorsiflexed position, driving the isolated segment of the posterior facet into the tuber of the os calcis.

Joint Depression Fractures

Essex-Lopresti's description of the joint depression fracture postulated a sequence of events in the mechanism pattern. He believed that the initial fracture line was the result of the lateral process of the talus being driven into the calcaneus (Fig. 64.26). He described this initial phase of the injury as a frontal plane fracture that begins superiorly at the crucial angle and extends to the plantar cortex, dividing the calcaneus into anterior and posterior segments. The level of the frontal plane fracture is most commonly seen at the anterior edge of the posterior facet.

Palmer, and later Burdeaux, although agreeing on the

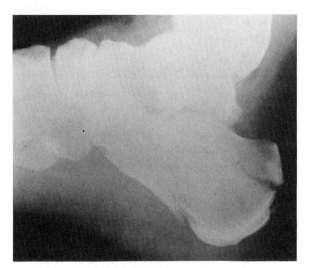

Figure 64.27. Failure to recognize this fracture as intra-articular involving posterior facet of os calcis may lead to inappropriate treatment of injury.

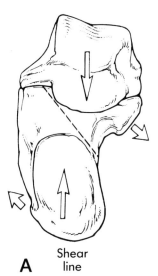

A

Shear line

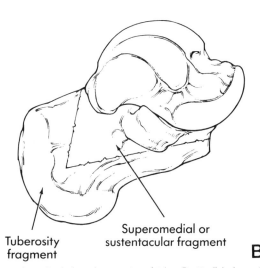

Tuberosity fragment

Superomedial or sustentacular fragment

B

Figure 64.28. **A.** Drawing of calcaneus from posterior (axial) view showing shear fracture line or primary fracture line. Note how center of calcaneal tuberosity is lateral to center of talus. **B.** Medial view of sagittal plane shear fracture. Exits inferiorly through the medial wall of the calcaneus.

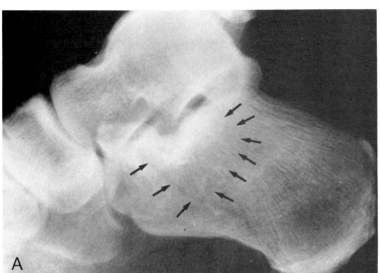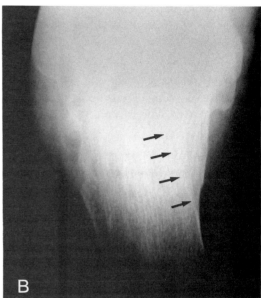

Figure 64.29. Lateral (**A**) and axial (**B**) calcaneal radiographs exhibiting the exact features of stage II intra-articular injury. Primary shearing fracture is readily apparent in both views and enters posterior facet laterally. There is significant downward displacement of medial sustentacular fragment, with no secondary compression of main lateral tuberosity fragment. As result of limited injury there is no lateral cortical wall injury nor is there any tongue or joint depression component.

constituent fracture lines, disagreed with the mechanism and sequence of the injury as postulated by Essex-Lopresti. According to Palmer and Burdeaux, the frontal plane fracture configuration, or crucial angle fracture, is not always seen. Palmer believed that the initial fracture line in the joint depression type of injury of the os calcis is a vertical shear fracture and is the primary fracture of this devastating injury. This sagittal plane fracture divides the calcaneus into medial and lateral components (Fig. 64.28A). The medial portion (sustentaculum fragment) includes the sustentaculum tali and a medial segment of the posterior facet. The lateral portion (tuberosity fragment) includes the lateral segment of the posterior facet and the remaining body of the calcaneus. The sagittal fracture exits inferiorly through the medial wall of the calcaneus (Fig. 64.28B). This primary sagittal plane fracture, which shears off the sustentaculum tali, is consistently seen in initial stages of all joint depression fractures of the os calcis (Fig. 64.29). Both Palmer and Burdeaux believed that the crucial angle fracture described by Essex-Lopresti was a secondary fracture, which explained its absence in a significant percentage of the cases examined. Burdeaux has proved this experimentally, and it is certainly logical when one carefully studies early drawings by Malgaigne, appreciates normal anatomy, and realizes the pathological force of the injury.

The last consistent portion of the intra-articular calcaneal fracture is the lateral wall blow-out. The lateral portion of the posterior facet of the subtalar joint becomes an isolated impaction fragment with progression of the joint depression injury (Fig. 64.30). The fragment has initially been created as the medial portion is sheared away with the primary

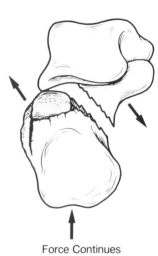

Force Continues

Figure 64.30. As injury progresses, tuberosity fragment is left in its superior and lateral position affixed to ground, whereas talar and sustentacular fragment continues its downward and medial movement. Note impaction of lateral part of posterior facet, as well as comminution of lateral calcaneal wall.

sagittal fracture line. The lateral portion of the posterior facet then further impacts into the body of the calcaneus with a combination of secondary fracture lines. An anterior defect may occur with the creation of the crucial angle fracture as the anterior edge of the posterior facet is depressed into the body of the calcaneus and separated from the neck portion of the calcaneus. Posteriorly, a secondary fracture

Intra-articular
Calcaneal Fracture Mechanism

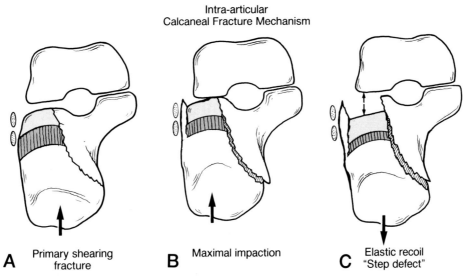

A Primary shearing
fracture

B Maximal impaction

C Elastic recoil
"Step defect"

Figure 64.31. Diagram showing mechanism of comminuted fracture of the calcaneus. **A.** Primary shearing fracture line. **B.** Maximal deformation at time of maximal deforming force. **C.** Step defect shown after elastic recoil. All main components of calcaneal fracture are shown.

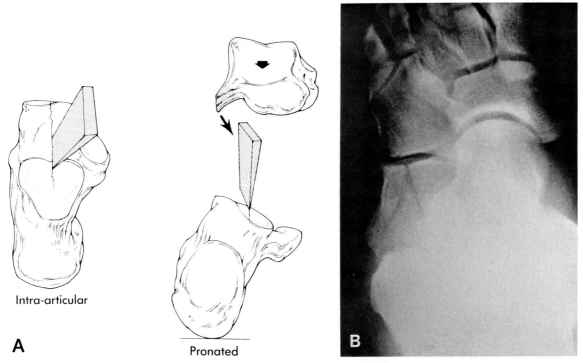

Intra-articular

A

Pronated

Figure 64.32. **A.** Posterior and superior schematic illustrations of the calcaneus and talus. A wedgelike action from the lateral process of the talus creates an intra-articular fracture of the calcaneocuboid joint while the foot is in a pronated position. The impacting force is directed inside the lateral wall. **B.** Dorsoplantar radiograph demonstrating intra-articular fracture of the calcaneocuboid joint.

line occurs around the rim of the facet and can allow the lateral facet fragment to separate from the calcaneal tuber. Finally, the isolated and free impaction fragment of the lateral portion of the posterior facet is created as a secondary lateral fracture occurs at the base of this major facet. This allows the complete separation and impaction of the isolated lateral portion of the posterior facet of the calcaneus to be depressed inside the lateral wall of the calcaneus and deep into the body itself (Fig. 64.31).

As the main body of the talus and the posterolateral portion of the posterior facet of the subtalar joint is driven into the trabecular substance of the body of the calcaneus, the body is expanded and osseous failure occurs as the outer wall of the calcaneus is exploded laterally. This medial to lateral expansion of the calcaneus results in another sagittal plane fracture line as the wedge action of the lateral segment of the posterior facet shears away the lateral wall of the calcaneus.

The sagittal plane fracture that creates the lateral wall blow-out may manifest as one of two basic configurations. The cortical type occurs when the fracture line extends distally and exits out the lateral wall of the calcaneus just proximal to the calcaneocuboid joint. An intra-articular configuration is created when the fracture line extends more longitudinally out into the calcaneocuboid joint, creating another intra-articular fracture.

It can be postulated that foot position may dictate the pattern of the lateral wall blow-out fracture. In a pronated foot, the apex of the lateral process of the talus and focus of the impacting force are directed inside the lateral wall of the body of the calcaneus. This results in a wedgelike action that splits the neck of the calcaneus and extends distally to terminate as an intra-articular fracture of the calcaneocuboid joint (Fig. 64.32).

In a slightly supinated foot, the lateral process of the talus and the direction of impaction force are directed externally to the lateral wall of the calcaneus, and the subsequent fracture line propagates out through the substance of the lateral

cortex of the body of the calcaneus (Fig. 64.33). In this type of lateral wall fracture, the distal exit of the lateral wall injury is proximal to the calcaneocuboid joint and may communicate directly with the frontal plane fracture line of the crucial angle fracture. It is this combination of fracture lines that makes the crucial angle fracture radiographically demonstrable (Fig. 64.34)(29-31, 71).

CT and intra-operative experience have greatly enhanced our knowledge of the components of the joint depression-type fracture of the os calcis. Although there is often significant and interesting variation of the actual fracture lines, the basic components of this severe injury fall into a predictable and logical pattern (Table 64.1).

HISTORICAL REVIEW OF TREATMENT

Treatment of intra-articular fractures of the calcaneus is an area of continued controversy. A review of the literature will give some insight into the various treatment methods used. These methods include (*a*) compression bandaging and early mobilization (nonreduction technique), (*b*) closed manipulation or semi-invasive manipulative techniques with traction spikes or pins, (*c*) open reduction with various methods of internal fixation, and (*d*) primary subtalar or triple arthrodesis. Other infrequent treatments have included excision of the calcaneus and amputation for chronic pain syndromes.

Many surgeons have favored conservative treatment

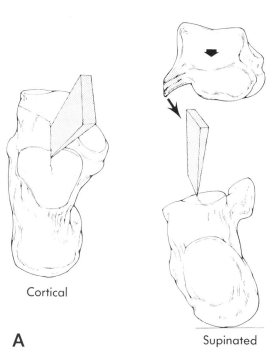

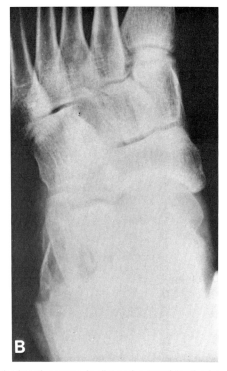

Figure 64.33. **A.** Posterior and superior schematic illustrations of the calcaneus and talus demonstrating lateral wall blow-out fracture with the foot in a supinated position. The distal exit of the lateral wall injury is proximal to the calcaneocuboid joint because the wedgelike action of the talar lateral process is directed external to the lateral wall of the calcaneus. **B.** Dorsoplantar radiograph of the foot demonstrating cortical-type fracture of the lateral wall of the calcaneus.

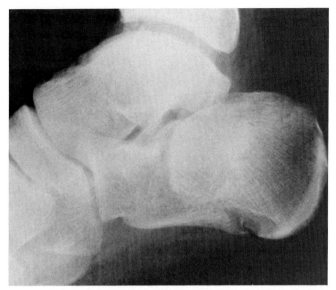

Figure 64.34. Crucial angle fracture becomes visible when lateral wall blow-out exits proximal to the calcaneocuboid joint and communicates with the frontal plane fracture.

Table 64.1.
Joint Depression Fracture of the Os Calcis

Primary Vertical Sagittal Plane Fracture

Creates the medial fragment, which includes the sustentaculum tali and a medial portion of the posterior facet of the subtalar joint.

Separation and Depression of the Posterior Facet

The main lateral portion of the subtalar joint's posterior facet is driven into the body of the calcaneus.

Lateral Wall Fracture

With either lateral cortical extension (crucial angle fracture) or distal intra-articular (calcaneocuboid joint) extention.

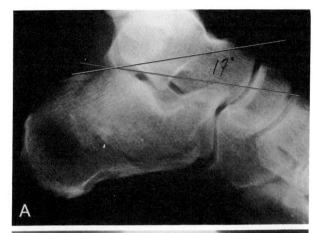

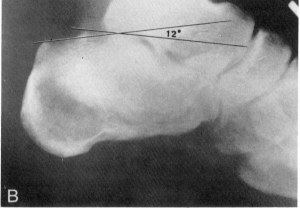

Figure 64.35. A. After joint depression intra-articular calcaneal fracture, measurement of Bohler's angle was approximately 17°. **B.** After 3 months of conservative casting treatment, during which time patient abstained from weight bearing, Bohler's angle decreased to approximately 12°. It is assumed that further collapse of fracture fragments has occurred secondary to gross instability.

methods consisting of no reduction, compression bandaging, and early mobilization. In this way they claim to avoid pin tract infections and stiff joints secondary to immobilization (72, 73). The aim of treatment is early return of function with minimal morbidity. Active range of motion of the ankle, toes, and foot follows as soon as tolerated, and in approximately 1 week the patient ambulates with partial weight bearing. In approximately 6 to 12 weeks, full weight bearing is begun depending on the degree of comminution. Pain reduction is not an indication for weight bearing because further depression of the fracture fragments may still occur (Fig. 64.35). Lance and associates (6, 74) favor early mobilization in os calcis fractures and denounce the use of pins or wires with skeletal traction or the use of plaster immobilization. They reported unacceptably high numbers of pin tract infections, as did Bohler (75) and Aars and Bie (76). Pretty (77) reported a 7% and Hermann (78) reported a 10% incidence of osteitis developing at pin sites in the os calcis.

Parkes (55) stated that "in my opinion, the safest and best management of intra-articular calcaneal fractures is early mobilization coupled with delayed weightbearing." He noted that "nonunion of the os calcis is unheard of" and that attempts at fixation would be like "nailing a custard pie to the wall." Lindsay and Dewar (7) personally studied 144 patients who sustained calcaneal fractures 10 to 11 years after injury. They compared results obtained through various methods and found equally good results with surgical treatment and conservative treatment. In addition, they identified a higher rate of complications with surgical intervention and reported an 11% incidence of pin tract infection.

Rowe and associates (5) studied 146 patients over 1 to 20 years and concluded that hand molding, supportive bandages, and early mobilization should be performed in type V calcaneal fractures. They found relatively no difference in good to excellent results when comparing those treated this way versus the Palmer open reduction method. Nade and Monahan (79) reviewed 203 fractures of the calcaneus occurring between 1961 and 1968 and stated that the results of nonoperative treatment were no worse than those of operative intervention; however, they concluded that these results are not good enough. Shannon and Murray (80) advocated early active range of motion exercises in most calcaneal fractures; however, they recognized the need for accurate anatomical reduction of joint surfaces in those with incongruous and squash-fractures.

Pozo and associates (1984) described a series of 21 patients who were treated conservatively for severely comminuted calcaneal fractures (81). The treatment consisted of compression bandaging and early range of motion of the ankle, subtalar, and midtarsal joints. Maximal recovery from the injury was noted at 2 to 3 years. The authors described good results in 76% of the cases with only minor symptoms that did not interfere with occupational or leisure activities.

Many others have advocated conservative treatment in these severe injuries and the list is never ending (13, 14, 24, 82-84).

Bohler (10), in 1931, recommended closed reduction with traction. His treatment consisted of reduction with use of the Bohler clamp followed by pin traction and plaster immobilization. This method was earlier used by many authors; however, today it is not used because of severe soft tissue injury as a result of the Bohler clamp and a high incidence of pin tract infection.

Essex-Lopresti (3) described his method in 1952. He stated that there are two very constant patterns of crush injury to the calcaneus, and only 4% are so smashed that reduction is impossible. He also drew attention to the fact that bad results were a direct result of poor reduction (as in any intra-articular fracture) and stressed the importance of exercise and motion after injury.

Essex-Lopresti advocated Gissane's technique of reduction. For the tongue-type intra-articular fracture, reduction was performed with the use of a Gissane spike or a heavy Steinmann pin inserted percutaneously into the tuberosity fragment in a longitudinal direction. The fragment was reduced by manipulation of the pin, and correction was then maintained through a plaster shoe incorporating the spike (Fig. 64.36). Lateral compression with the palms was also used to reduce broadening of the heel (1, 71, 85).

In joint depression calcaneal fractures, Essex-Lopresti recommended exposure of the depressed fragment by an open operation to elevate it into alignment under direct visualization and then, while exposed, to maintain it by use of the Gissane spike. Immediate range of motion of the ankle and subtalar joint was then carried out within the confines of the plaster shoe in both cases. The spike is removed in 4 to 6 weeks. No bone graft was believed necessary if the open reduction was performed early.

Essex-Lopresti stressed the value of understanding and classifying the injury pattern because postoperative results were directly related to the type of fracture and surgical approach used.

Aaron and Howat (86) reported the use of Essex-Lopresti's method in 41 patients, all working men. Their minimum follow-up time was 24 months, with an average of 56 months. Each patient was seen personally. They con-

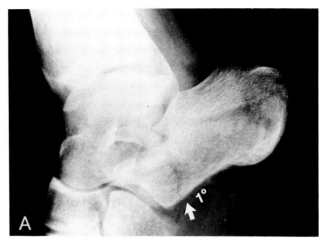
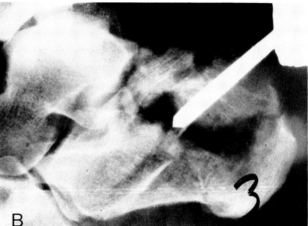

Figure 64.36. A. Lateral calcaneal radiograph clearly showing Essex-Lopresti type A fracture (tongue-type fracture). **B.** Proper use of Steinmann pin during closed reduction to elevate posterolateral tuberosity fragment, which contains posterior facet. After elevation of fragment is completed, note large void within cancellous bone of body of calcaneus secondary to compressive injury.

cluded that spike reduction was superior to conservative treatment and suggested that good subtalar joint range of motion was a valuable guide to the long-term prognosis. They also advocate early range of motion exercises of the subtalar joint, ankle, and midtarsal areas. Range of motion exercises are begun 1 day after surgery. Weight bearing is begun no sooner than 8 weeks after injury, and the slipper cast and spike are removed at 6 weeks. Postoperative emphasis remains on maintaining good range of motion of all joints and restoring full muscle power to the calf.

Arnesen (87) used traction with manipulation and reported ideal reduction in 22 of 36 intra-articular fractures. Omoto and associates (88) reported on 11 patients treated with manual reduction techniques, followed by early active range of motion exercises, and noted 10 satisfactory results. They advocate this reduction technique using the calcaneo-fibular and tibiocalcaneal ligaments for closed reduction manipulation because they state that these are rarely ruptured.

Early operative procedures in the United States consisted of early subtalar joint or triple arthrodesis. Gallie (89) published his classical description of his subtalar joint fusion via a posterior approach in 1943. Proponents of early arthrodesis claim that severe trauma to the articular facets creates irreparable damage to the articular cartilage, with resultant osteoarthritis and later disability. After the articular cartilage is removed, the fracture fragments are usually maintained by pins and the lateral cortex is manually reduced. The leg is placed in a below-the-knee cast, and the pins are left in place for approximately 4 weeks. The patient is allowed to bear weight at 8 weeks in a walking cast, and by 12 weeks the patient is usually at full weight bearing.

Conn (90) in 1935 suggested triple arthrodesis as "a plan of treatment more completely correcting the extensive anatomical distortion" that occurs secondary to severe calcaneal fracture. Thompson and Friesen (34) also believed that injury to the talocalcaneal joint was irreparable and stressed that undiagnosed injury to either the talonavicular or calcaneocuboid joint may be responsible for the poor results reported. They advocated primary triple arthrodesis as the procedure of choice at any age with such fractures. Hall and Pennal (91) reported on primary subtalar arthrodesis and in 1960 reported on 29 patients, 27 of whom returned to full employment in an average of 64 months; 25 of these returned to their original employment. Boon and Hanemaaijer (92) in 1968 reported on 19 patients treated with delayed triple arthrodesis 6 weeks after manual reduction. Fifteen patients in this study recovered without any residual disability. Noble and McQuillan (93) also advocate posterior subtalar joint fusion between 2 to 4 weeks after injury. They reviewed 47 fractures in 43 patients at an average of 7 years after operation and found 90% with excellent, good, or satisfactory results, with patients returning to similar work within 6 months of the injury.

Open reduction of calcaneal fractures is thought to have begun with a procedure described by Lenormant and Wilmoth in the French *Journal of Surgery* in 1932. The method remained in Europe for some years until Whittaker (94) in 1947 first reported open reduction without fusion in this country. Present-day open reduction theory is based almost exclusively on the work of Palmer of Sweden, who modified the original idea of Lenormant and Wilmoth. Palmer published his classical paper in 1948 (29) and at that time had insight into the complicated mechanism of calcaneal fractures as it has been presented here. He stated that "the depressed fragment bearing the articular surface was sharply outlined, firm and stable." By means of an elevator he was able to lever up the fragment and restore normal joint structure. He then inserted an autogenous iliac crest bone graft beneath the fragment to give the reduction stability. He indicated that no pins are needed. He reported on 23 cases and stated that the results were favorable, with all patients back to their previous work within 4 to 8 months, with all but two having 15° to 3° of painless supination-pronation of the subtalar joint. His postoperative course consisted of a short-leg non-weight-bearing cast for 12

weeks, followed by a zinc-paste stocking and a strong shoe with a longitudinal arch support.

Horn (32) in 1968 also advocated open reduction with stabilization by bone grafts, followed by active motion at 6 to 8 weeks and protected weight bearing in 8 to 12 weeks. In a series of 50 fractures treated by four methods he stated that this operative method gave the best results. His goals were to restore articular congruity, correct the widening of the calcaneus, and therefore restore normal width and height to the heel bone and achieve a painless and adequate subtalar joint and midtarsal range of motion. Hazlett (95) in 1969 described the cases of 22 consecutive patients with comminuted fractures and displaced subtalar facets of the calcaneus who were treated with open reduction and internal fixation consisting of screws and Kirschner wires (K-wires). The benefits of early active range of motion and static triceps surae exercises were discussed. Thirteen patients returned to work in less than 4 months, and 19 of the 22 returned to work in less than 8 months. Of the three failures, two had less than adequate reduction and one was said to lack motivation. Lanzetta and Meani (96) reported on 220 fractures of the calcaneus operated on between 1966 and 1975 in Milan, Italy. They reviewed 162 cases with a minimum follow-up of 1 year. They not only recognized the importance of accurate anatomical reconstruction and early active range of motion exercises but also discussed the importance of choosing the correct internal fixation devices to maintain rigid internal fixation of the reduced fracture fragments. Here they introduced three plate types that they applied to the lateral calcaneal wall affixed with screws that purchased the large sustentaculum tali fracture fragment. They reported good and very good results in 77% of their series. Weight bearing was begun approximately 10 to 12 weeks after reduction. It is important to note that they believed that bone grafting of the crushed calcaneal body is not necessary and that the void will rapidly fill in once reduction was obtained. Some have shared in this belief (3, 97, 98), whereas others continue to advocate bone grafting (29, 99).

In 1981, Hammesfahr and Fleming (72) described a series of patients treated with a variety of different techniques. Their findings included relatively poor results with percutaneous pinning of joint depression fractures and approximately 80% excellent or good results in their series of joint depression fractures after open reduction by the Palmer method. They identified a positive correlation between facet reduction and successful treatment results and concluded "treatment of intra-articular calcaneal fractures should follow the same guidelines as the treatment of any other intra-articular fracture; that is, reduction of the articular surface and restoration of joint congruity."

Stephenson (100) further supported the use of open reduction and internal fixation for the primary treatment of intra-articular fractures of the calcaneus. He described the primary approach to reduction of the calcaneal fracture from a lateral incision and combined a medial approach when necessary to ensure anatomical reduction of the medial shear fragment. Compression screw techniques were used as the primary fixation of the articular fragments. The primary fixation was supplemented when necessary with a buttressing staple to reinforce the lateral wall injury. Stephenson summarized his findings thus: "For optimum results in the treatment of displaced intra-articular fractures, the normal anatomy of the joint must be restored and motion of the joint must be started early." Other authors have held beliefs that accurate anatomical alignment of the subtalar joint complex (especially that of the posterior subtalar joint facet) correlates directly with satisfactory postinjury results and therefore have advocated open reduction with bone graft stabilization or other forms of fixation (8, 30, 101-104).

It is apparent, after this historical review, that treatment of intra-articular fractures of the os calcis has been anything but uniform. Surgical treatment was advised in the 1950s; however, this gradually gave way to conservative treatment as many authors boasted about their treatment success, with each study being difficult to compare with the others. Today the debate continues among the many supporters of conservative and nonoperative treatment, mainly because of their limited experience with open reduction.

AUTHORS' TREATMENT

The authors believe in the principles of open reduction and internal fixation of joint depression fractures of the os calcis. This is especially important in dealing with a major weight-bearing joint; however, the patient's age and general health have to be considered before surgical intervention. Knowledge of proper radiographic assessment of the injury and a thorough understanding of the normal and abnormal anatomy of these complex joint surfaces, as well as principles of applied rigid internal fixation, are all fundamental prerequisites to open reduction. One must be aware that intraoperative findings are generally, if not always, more extensive than those seen on initial radiographs.

Initial treatment begins with the application of a Jones compression dressing and icing of the foot and ankle to combat swelling. Maximum elevation of the extremity is maintained before surgical intervention. Open reduction is attempted as early as possible before the onset of severe swelling. The appearance of trauma blisters are a direct contraindication to surgical intervention. Early operative intervention before the onset of traumatic swelling is optimal because displaced fracture fragments directly contribute to and maintain edema (98).

Operative Technique

INCISION PLANNING

Proper placement of the surgical incision is critical in the successful repair of the joint depression fracture of the calcaneus. Unrestricted exposure of the underlying osseous fragments or target structures is predicated on accurate placement of the skin incision. Because of the severe depression of the posterior facet of the calcaneus, the normal po-

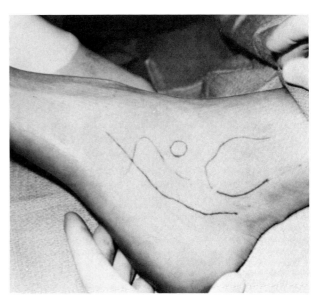

Figure 64.37. Incision used in exposing calcaneal fracture is placed laterally. Landmarks for its course include dorsolateral margin of calcaneocuboid joint, tip of fibular malleolus, and superolateral margin of calcaneal tuber.

sitional relationships of the lateral aspect of the foot and ankle are significantly altered. Great care must be taken to clearly identify the critical landmarks for plotting of the surgical incision (Fig. 64.37).

The key landmarks for placement of the incision include the dorsolateral margin of the calcaneocuboid joint, the tip of the fibular malleolus, and the superolateral margin of the calcaneal tuber.

The incision should cross each of these specified landmarks to provide direct access to the critical components of the fracture complex, even in the presence of severe positional distortion. As the incision courses proximally, it is directed linearly toward the superolateral margin of the calcaneus rather than curving around the tip of the fibular malleolus as commonly performed in other similar surgical approaches to the subtalar joint. This variation allows for direct evaluation of the posterior exit of the tuber fracture and accurate restoration of the posterior margin of the posterior facet to the calcaneal tuber. Care must be taken to avoid laceration of, or traction injury to, the sural nerve and lesser saphenous vein that will be directly exposed (Fig. 64.38).

SOFT TISSUE DISSECTION

Dissection is carried through the soft tissues over the lateral side of the foot for exposure of the subtalar joint and fracture fragments. Although the procedure is similar to that of an elective approach, it is complicated significantly by distortion of key landmark relationships created by the joint depression fracture. The lateral process of the talus, which is a key targeting landmark in the clean approach to the

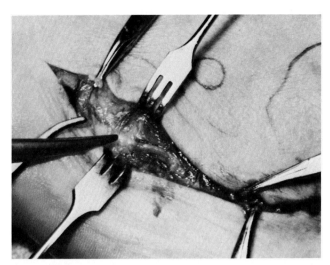

Figure 64.38. Sural nerve is directly exposed during dissection for calcaneal joint depression fracture repair. Careful dissection and retraction of nerve will help prevent injury and entrapment.

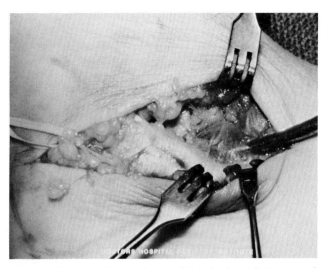

Figure 64.39. Deep fascia is shown as it is incised superior to peroneal tendons.

subtalar joint, is usually so severely depressed into the body of the calcaneus that it is not even palpable and therefore cannot be used as a guide into the sinus tarsi or the posterior facet of the subtalar joint. The soft tissues must be used as the initial guide to the deeper levels of the fracture.

Meticulous dissection is needed to identify the displaced osseous components of the fracture while preserving the integrity of the soft tissues and vital blood supply.

Once the skin incision has been made, the standard techniques of anatomical dissection are used to separate the superficial fascial layer from the deep fascia over the lateral aspect of the foot and ankle. The deep fascia is most readily identified over the extensor digitorum brevis muscle belly and over the tip of the fibular malleolus. These two initial areas are exposed to facilitate separation of the superficial layers from the deeper layers over the area of the sinus tarsi and the posterolateral aspect of the calcaneus.

The technique of separation is critical behind the fibular malleolus. Here the dissection plane along the deep fascia must cleanly lift the superficial tissues away from the peroneal retinaculum and along the dorsolateral margin of the calcaneus without actual incision through superficial tissues. The sural nerve and lesser saphenous vein course posteriorly around the fibular malleolus and can be preserved and protected by undermining and elevating this intact tissue layer and retracting it from the field of operation.

The next step in the sequence involves incision of the deep fascia along the inferior border of the extensor digitorum brevis muscle. The fascia is solely incised and the muscle belly is separated from the superior margin of the peroneal tendons (Fig. 64.39) to give direct access to the periosteum and capsular tissue: over the lateral wall of the calcaneus and the region of the calcaneocuboid joint. The superior margin of the lateral wall blow-out fracture is usually encountered with this manipulation.

At this point, the lateral wall fracture is explored and the

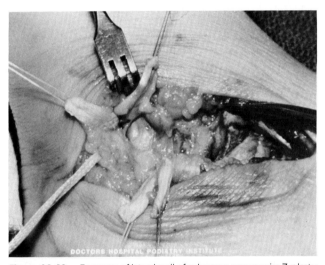

Figure 64.40. Exposure of lateral wall of calcaneus may require Z-plasty transection of peroneal tendons. Colored suture material will aid in identification of opposing tendon ends during wound closure.

extent of joint depression is evaluated to determine the need for possible transection of the peroneal tendons. When there is significant depression of the major portion of the posterior facet into the body of the calcaneus, open reduction is greatly facilitated by Z-plasty or transection of the peroneal tendons (Fig. 64.40) to give free and unrestricted access to the lateral aspect of the calcaneus and subtalar joint region. If the degree of joint depression is less severe, open reduction may be accomplished without the need for transection of the peroneal tendons. Although transection of the peroneal tendons may greatly facilitate the procedure, a significant degree of limitation of subtalar joint motion is commonly experienced because of fibrosis and loss of gliding function of these tendons through the surgical area.

This is one area for which the classical axiom "one wound, one scar" seems to hold true. The primary motion lost is in the direction of inversion and may be an acceptable consequence for successful anatomical restoration of the subtalar joint itself.

The extent of joint depression is specifically evaluated by exposing the area of the crucial angle fracture. Periosteum and muscle tissue are cleanly lifted from the dorsal surface of the neck of the calcaneus. This dissection plane is followed proximally into the area of the crucial angle fracture and the once easily identified anterior margin of the posterior facet of the subtalar joint. Typically, as the crucial angle fracture is appreciated, an unfamiliar mass of bone blocks further proximal progression into the anticipated region of the sinus tarsi. This obstruction is actually the superior and anterior aspect of the lateral process of the talus. This critical distortion must be appreciated before proper orientation of the relationships of the key fragments of the fracture may be identified.

The lateral process of the talus has been driven deep into the body of the calcaneus and the level of the posterior facet may not even be visible. That is, the lateral facet fragment may have been recessed within the confines of the lateral wall fragment of the body of the calcaneus.

At this point the soft tissues must be meticulously dissected from the key components of the joint depression fracture. The two critical areas to cleanly expose include the region of the sinus tarsi and the lateral aspect of the subtalar joint and calcaneus itself.

Exposure of the sinus tarsi began with elevation of the soft tissues from the dorsal surface of the neck of the calcaneus. The capsular tissues from the anterior surface of the lateral process are also cleanly reflected as dissection is carried medially across the calcaneus at the level of the crucial angle fracture. Evacuation of the tissues of the sinus

tarsi is usually necessary with resection of the fibrofatty plug and the intertarsal ligament for full visualization of the neck of the calcaneus, the entrance to the sinus tarsi, and the level of the middle facet of the subtalar joint. These bony surfaces must be cleanly exposed for complete identification of the fracture lines that have disrupted the integrity of the calcaneal platform of the subtalar joint (Fig. 64.41).

Once a determination is made with respect to transection of the peroneal tendons, the lateral wall fracture must be identified and its margins determined. With the peroneal tendons reflected, the calcaneofibular ligament is primarily transected and the superior edge of the lateral fracture is exposed. Minimal periosteal reflection is carried along the superior edge of the lateral wall plate to define its margins and to identify its distal and proximal exit points. It is important to attempt to leave periosteum and ligamentous attachments to the major portion of the lateral wall fragments to preserve blood supply and maintain alignment if significant comminution has occurred.

MANIPULATION AND TEMPORARY FIXATION

The key to reduction of the joint depression fracture of the calcaneus is elevation of the lateral segment of the posterior facet of the subtalar joint. The lateral wall of the calcaneus is folded laterally, and the full extent of depression of the lateral segment of the calcaneal portion of the posterior facet is visualized. A Sayer elevator is useful in the reduction sequence. The elevator is inserted beneath the main fracture fragment and used to apply an upward pressure on the lateral segment of the calcaneal facet. The fragment is usually totally separated anteriorly from the neck of the calcaneus at the level of the crucial angle fracture but may be hinged at its proximal aspect along the fracture line that separates it from the calcaneal tuber. The lateral portion of the facet must be elevated and retracted laterally to more fully explore and evaluate the internal fracture lines of the calcaneus, specifically the primary sagittal fracture line that has separated the sustentaculum tali from the lateral portion of the calcaneus. Additional secondary fracture lines may be present that even divide the medial aspect of the posterior facet from the sustentacular tali as well. This multiple comminution pattern may significantly complicate the reduction and fixation process and can also represent more extensive damage to the primary posterior facet of the subtalar joint.

With the fracture fully opened, copious lavage and removal of clot material and small fracture fragments must be performed to fully expose all surfaces of the fracture fragments and allow clean anatomical reduction of the main components of the fracture.

The primary guideline in the reduction sequence is the restoration of the subchondral bone plate pattern of the posterior facet of the subtalar joint. The middle facet is intact and pinnacled as the medial apex of the reconstruction scheme. The primary structural fragment of the middle facet is the sustentaculum tali, and the subtalar joint is actually rebuilt by realigning the sequential fracture fragments to the medial sustentacular fragment of the calcaneus.

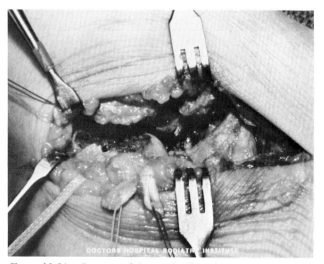

Figure 64.41. Exposure of sinus tarsi will require complete evacuation of fibrous and fatty tissue located in area. Middle facet and calcaneal neck are easily seen once this dissection is performed.

The subchondral bone pattern of the medial fragment of the calcaneus is clearly visualized, and the main lateral fragment is reduced by realigning the articular relationship of the posterior facet to the main medial fragment. When this final goal is accomplished, the anterior margin of the posterior facet will be elevated to produce reduction of the crucial angle fracture.

Similarly, the posterior fracture line across the calcaneal tuber should be restored to its anatomical contour to confirm complete anatomical restoration of the calcaneal platform of the subtalar joint.

The primary lateral fragment of the posterior facet now becomes the pinnacle for reduction of the calcaneal fracture. Its anatomical relationship to the medial fracture fragments must be temporarily maintained for completion of the reduction and fixation process. Two 0.062-inch K-wires are driven from lateral to medial to provide temporary fixation and a guide for permanent fixation (Fig. 64.42A).

The fracture line that is being temporarily fixated is actually a sagittal fracture line running down the middle of the posterior facet. The direction of the K-wires is essentially lateral to medial, but at least one of these wires should be aimed at the focal prominence of the sustentaculum tali to establish complete medial to lateral transfixion of the calcaneus. Permanent fixation directed along this path from the main lateral fragment of the posterior facet to the main medial fragment of the sustentaculum tali will be accomplished with a small cancellous bone screw. This fixation device will actually act as an internal Bohler's clamp and also securely maintain restoration of the calcaneal contour of the facets of the subtalar joint.

Intra-operative radiographs should be taken once temporary fixation has been achieved (Fig. 64.42B). A lateral projection will demonstrate the restoration of the normal facet pattern of the subtalar joint, with elevation of the previously depressed posterior facet and a normal angular relationship between the middle and posterior facets. The axial view will reveal the remaining incongruity of the calcaneal tuber to the superior segment of the calcaneus, which includes the anatomically restored articular facets of the subtalar joint. The calcaneal tuber is usually in a varus angulation and still apparently impacted.

FINAL FIXATION

Once satisfactory restoration of the subtalar joint is determined, small cancellous bone screws are introduced for permanent fixation. Typically, one of the K-wires is removed and its guide hole is used for the thread hole of the compression bone screw (Fig. 64.43A). A standard technique is followed for insertion of the compression screws. If the alignment or position of the temporary K-wire was unsatisfactory, a new thread hole may be used for insertion of the fixation screws. The main lateral fragment of the posterior facet is usually fixated to the main medial fragments of the calcaneus with two compression screws and the remainder of the fixation process is continued (Fig. 64.43B).

REDUCTION OF THE CALCANEAL TUBER AND LATERAL WALL FRACTURE

The calcaneal tuber is actually reduced by classical closed reduction technique. The tuber is manipulated into a varus position, and then distal tension is applied. The heel is then forcibly everted to realign the medial wall fragments and restore the anatomical position of the main body of the

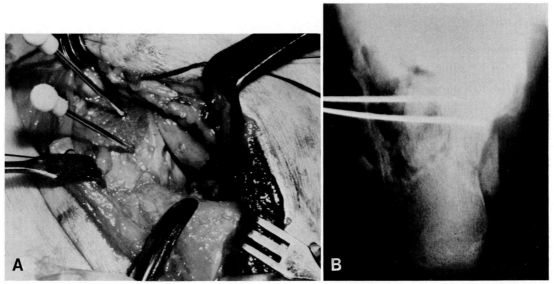

Figure 64.42. **A.** Two 0.062-inch K-wires provide temporary fixation of posterior facet fragment to medial aspect of calcaneus. **B.** Intraoperative radiographs verify restoration of normal facet alignment; 0.062-inch K-wires also act to provide a guide for placement of permanent fixation.

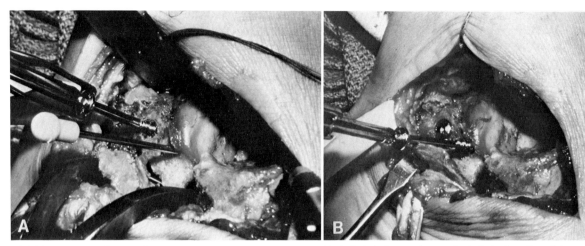

Figure 64.43. Permanent fixation of the lateral fragment of the posterior facet is usually fixated to the main medial fragments of the calcaneus with small cancellous screws. **A.** One temporary K-wire has been removed with its hole being used as a pilot hole for insertion of the compression bone screw. **B.** Second K-wire now removed with insertion of second cancellous screw.

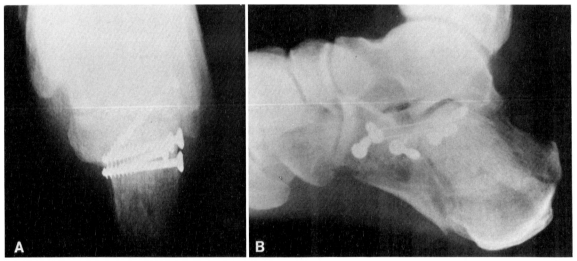

Figure 64.44. **A.** Intra-operative radiographs are used to confirm proper screw placement and adequate fracture reduction. **B.** Compression screws were also used to fixate large intra-articular fracture of calcaneocuboid joint in this tongue-type calcaneal fracture.

calcaneus beneath the subtalar facets. Successful reduction may be confirmed with a second intra-operative axial view of the calcaneus (Fig. 64.44A). The internal substance of the calcaneus should now be inspected, and any significant defect within the body is packed with cancellous graft. Cancellous bone chips may be inserted if significant loss of bone has occurred. At this point, reduction of the lateral wall blow-out fracture is all that remains (Fig. 64.44B).

The two basic patterns of lateral blow-out fracture may be encountered. If the intra-articular pattern has occurred, restoration of the calcaneocuboid articulation becomes as important as the primary reduction of the subtalar joint facets. Lateral to medial compression screws are usually employed to fixate the intra-articular fracture, which extends through the neck of the calcaneus and into the calcaneocuboid joint (Fig. 64.32A).

The cortical type of lateral blow-out fracture may require a variety of different types of fixation. Comminution and fragile cortical bone may make solid and rigid fixation impossible. Lateral to medial fixation, however, is attempted, with at least one compression screw directed into the main substance of the sustentaculum tali. A laterally applied plate, staples, or even variations of tension band wire may be used to maintain reduction of the lateral wall fragments.

The key reduction, however, remains the restoration of the articular facets of the subtalar joint and realignment of the calcaneal tuber. A smooth and relatively normal range of motion may be attained once the alignment of the subtalar joint has been accomplished. Successful salvage of this joint is then dictated by appropriate postoperative management and maintenance of the initial fracture reduction.

Wound Closure and Management

Repair of soft tissues follows standard technique. Each tissue layer is closed separately, and transected ligament and tendon are repaired primarily. A closed suction drain apparatus is routinely employed for evacuation of postoperative hemorrhage. A surgical dressing is applied, and the extremity is incorporated in a Jones compression dressing and splint.

Postoperative management includes strict abstinence from weight bearing. The extremity is immobilized for several weeks, and early range of motion with extensive physical therapy is initiated as soon as possible. Partial weight bearing may be initiated within 2 to 3 months after surgery if radiographs show adequate fracture healing. The most significant complication the authors have encountered involves wound dehiscence and full-thickness skin slough along the incision line (Fig. 64.45). Its incidence is related to the severity of the injury, amount of edema and hematoma before and after the surgery, tissue handling, and other perisurgical factors.

The authors continue to advocate this procedure only in the hands of the skillful surgeon who has a complete knowledge of anatomy and calcaneal fracture pathology. It is only with this observance that the prognosis of intra-articular calcaneal fractures will improve. This is surgery in which the exactness of technique decides the outcome.

POSTINJURY COMPLICATIONS

Most postinjury complications of calcaneal fractures are seen with intra-articular fractures. Pain beneath the lateral

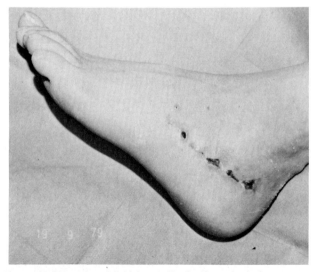

Figure 64.45. Minor full-thickness skin slough resulted after open reduction and internal fixation of this patient's calcaneal fracture. Condition eventually healed quite satisfactorily.

malleolus is the most common site and is thought to occur secondary to ligamentous injury about the ankle joint and/or tenosynovitis of the peroneal tendons caused by a narrowing of the space as they pass beneath the fibular malleolus. Conn (90) reviewed 72 such intra-articular os calcis fractures and stated that "peroneal spasm was a constant finding." Pain beneath the medial malleolus has also been reported and is often related to unrecognized damage to the ankle joint, combined with prolonged immobilization and subsequent stiffness and arthrofibrosis.

Painful heels may occur secondary to direct soft tissue injury or exostosis formation (24, 74). Subtalar or midtarsal arthritis is a very real consideration following injury. Abnormal function as a result of an unreduced fracture may cause pain. Reversal of the tuber angle resulting from an unreduced fracture may cause pressure pain anterior to the calcaneal tuberosity; it also causes a relative lengthening of the Achilles tendon, resulting in a flatfooted, abnormal, and diminished propulsive gait. Among other postinjury complications are nerve entrapment, infection, and gout. One complication rarely reported is nonunion.

Most authors suggest that a period of 2 years is needed before patients can view their disability with objectivity.

SUMMARY

Calcaneal fractures are divided into two main categories: intraarticular and extra-articular. The mechanisms, classification, and management of extra-articular calcaneal fractures are, for the most part, uniformly accepted. The prognosis is good to excellent. Unfortunately the classification of mechanism and treatment of intra-articular calcaneal fractures is still an issue of much debate. The prognosis for these fractires, although reported by some to be good to excellent, is still poor.

A historical review of intra-articular calcaneal fractures and their management found only the nature of the fracture fragments to be uniformly acknowledged. On this anatomical basis the authors have presented a sound mechanism of injury and have suggested a useful classification. Abiding by the accepted principle of intra-articular fracture management, the authors have continued to promote open reduction and internal fixation of such fractures in the hands of the skillful surgeon. The authors agree that the prognosis of calcaneal fractures will vary according to the extent and location of the injury; however, a good functional result is directly correlated with anatomical reduction and stable fixation, which allows early postoperative range of motion exercises.

If surgical restoration of the talocalcaneal joint fails, then a triple arthrodesis or subtalar fusion may be recommended as a last resort. Accomplishments at this point would still include restoration of calcaneal height and width, therefore avoiding further associated conditions. It is widely accepted that a period of 2 years is needed before accepting a particular treatment regimen as a failure. Most patients will continue to improve over this period of time.

Intra-articular calcaneal fractures need not have a poor

prognosis. The prognosis depends on the surgeon's understanding of the pathological anatomy, proper radiographical analysis, classification, the proper choice of surgical approach and fixation, and finally the clinician's surgical skills.

References

1. Burns AE: Fractures of the calcaneus. *Clin Podiatr Med Surg* 2:311-324, 1985.
2. Chapman MW: Fractures and fracture-dislocations of the ankle and foot. In Inman VT (ed): *DuVries' Surgery of the Foot*, ed 4. St. Louis, CV Mosby, 1978, p 168.
3. Essex-Lopresti P: The mechanism, reduction technique, and results in fractures of the os calcis. *Br J Surg* 39:395-419, 1952.
4. Garcia A, Parkes JC: Fractures of the foot. In Giannestras NJ (ed): *Foot Disorders: Medical and Surgical Management*, ed 2. Philadelphia, Lea & Febiger, 1976, p 528.
5. Rowe CR, Schellarides HR, Freeman PA, Sorbie C: Fractures of the os calcis: a long term follow-up study of 146 patients. *JAMA* 184:98-101, 1963.
6. Lance EM, Carey EJ, Wade PA: Fractures os the os calcis: a followup study. *J Trauma* 4:15-56, 1964.
7. Lindsay WRN, Dewar FP: Fractures of the os calcis. *Am J Surg* 95:555-576, 1958.
8. Slatis P, Kiviluoto O, Santavirta S, Laasonen EM. Fractures of the calcaneum. *J Trauma* 19:939-943, 1979.
9. Aaron D, Howat TW: Intra-articular fractures of the calcaneum. *Injury* 7:205-211, 1975.
10. Bohler L: Diagnosis, pathology, and treatment of fractures of the os calcis. *J Bone Joint Surg* 13:75-89, 1931.
11. Widen A: Fractures of the calcaneus. *Acta Chir Scand* 188 (Suppl):1-119, 1954.
12. Magnuson P: Mechanics of fractures of the os calcis. *Pedic Items* 7:48, 1917.
13. Spector, EE: Fractures of the calcaneus. *J Am Podiatry Assoc* 65:789-801, 1975.
14. Clisham MW, Berlin SJ: The diagnosis and conservative treatment of calcaneal fractures—a review. *J Foot Surg* 20:28-32, 1981.
15. Wells C: Fracture of the heel bones in early prehistoric times. *Practitioner* 217:294-298, 1976.
16. Donohue T, Sorkin B, Kanat IO: Postoperative fracture of os calcis and treatment. *J Foot Surg* 26:261-265, 1987.
17. Hullinger CW: Insufficiency fracture of the calcaneus. Similar to march fracture of the metatarsal. *J Bone Joint Surg* 26:751-757, 1944.
18. Winfield AC, Dennis JM: Stress fractures of the calcaneus. *Radiology* 72:415-418, 1959.
19. Kalish SR: The conservative and surgical treatment of calcaneal fractures. *J Am Podiatry Assoc* 65:912-926, 1975.
20. Stein MD, Stelling FH: Stress fracture of the calcaneus in a child with cerebral palsy. *J Bone Joint Surg* 59A:131, 1977.
21. Edward CP: Fractured os calcis and lumbar vertebra. *Trauma Rounds* 103:177-179, 1970.
22. Wong PCN: Vertebral column and os calcis fracture patterns in a confined community (Singapore). *Acta Orthop Scand* 37:357-366, 1966.
23. Wilson DW: Functional capacity following fractures of the os calcis. *Can Med Assoc J* 95:908-911, 1966.
24. Miller WE: Pain and impairment considerations following treatment of disruptive os calcis fractures. *Clin Orthop* 177:82-86, 1983.
25. Miller WE: The heel pad. *Am J Sports Med* 10:19-24, 1982.
26. Miller WE, Lichtblau PO: The smashed heel. *South Med J* 58:1229-1237, 1965.
27. Day FG: Treatment of fractures of the os calcis. *Can Med Assoc J* 63:373-377, 1950.
28. Nahmias MC, Dudzinski RT: Intra-articular comminuted calcaneal fractures, a brief review and case presentation. *J Am Podiatr Med Assoc* 78:87-91, 1988.
29. Palmer I: The mechanism and treatment of fractures of the calcaneus. *J Bone Joint Surg* 30A:2-8, 1948.
30. Burdeaux BD: Reduction of calcaneal fractures by the McReynolds medical approach technique and its experimental basis. *Clin Orthop* 177:87-103, 1983.
31. Stephenson JR: Displaced fractures of the os calcis involving the subtalar joint: a key role of the superomedial fragment. *Foot Ankle* 4:91-101, 1983.
32. Horn CE: Fractures of the calcaneus. *Calif Med* 108:209-215, 1968.
33. Wilson GE: Fractures of the calcaneus. *J Bone Joint Surg* 32A:59-70, 1950.
34. Thompson KR, Friesen CM: Treatment of comminuted fractures of the calcaneus by primary triple arthrodesis. *J Bone Joint Surg* 41A:1423-1436, 1959.
35. Anthonsen W: An oblique projection for roentgen examination of the talo-calcaneal joint, particularly regarding intra-articular fracture of the calcaneus. *Acta Radiol* 24:306-310, 1943.
36. Broden B: Roentgen examination of the subtaloid joint in fractures of the calcaneus. *Acta Radiol* 31:85-91, 1949.
37. Isherwood I: A radiological approach to the subtalar joint. *J Bone Joint Surg* 43B:566-574, 1961.
38. Gissane W: News notes: the British Orthopaedic Association. *J Bone Joint Surg* 29:254-255, 1947.
39. Rosenberg ZS, Feldman F, Singson RD: Intra-articular calcaneal fractures: computed tomographic analysis. *Skeletal Radiol* 16:105-113, 1987.
40. Gilmer PW, Herzenberg J, Frank JL, Silverman P, Martinez S, Goldner JL: Computerized tomographic analysis of acute calcaneal fractures. *Foot Ankle* 6:184-193, 1986.
41. Carr JB, Noto AM, Stevenson S: Volumetric three-dimensional computed tomography for acute calcaneal fractures: preliminary report. *J Orthop Trauma* 4:346-348, 1990.
42. Matteri RE, Frymoyer JW: Fractures of the calcaneus in young children. *J Bone Joint Surg* 55A:1091-1094, 1973.
43. Watson-Jones R: *Fractures and Joint Injuries*, ed 4. Baltimore, Williams & Wilkins, 1960, p 862.
44. Richman JD, Barre PS: The plantar ecchymosis sign in fractures of the calcaneus. *Clin Orthop* 207:122-125, 1986.
45. Blount WP: *Fractures in children*. Baltimore, Williams & Wilkins, 1955, p 196.
46. Schofield RO: Fractures of the os calcis. *J Bone Joint Surg* 18:566-580, 1936.
47. Zayer M: Fracture of the calcaneus, a review of 110 fractures. *Acta Orthop Scand* 40:530-542, 1969.
48. Starshak RJ, Simons GW, Sty JR: Occult fracture of the calcaneus—another toddler's fracture. *Pediatr Radiol* 14:37-40, 1984.
49. Schantz K, Rasmussen F: Calcaneus fracture in the child. *Acta Orthop Scand* 58:507-509, 1987.
50. Schmidt T, Weiner DJ: Calcaneal fractures in children. *Clin Orthop* 171:150-155, 1982.
51. Wiley JJ, Profitt A: Fractures of the os calcis in children. *Clin Orthop* 188:131-138, 1984.
52. King R: Axial pin fixation of fractures of the os calcis (method of Essex-Lopresti). *Orthop Clin North Am* 4:185-188, 1973.
53. Warrick CK, Bremner AE: Fractures of the calcaneum with an atlas illustrating various types of fractures. *J Bone Joint Surg* 35B:33-45, 1953.
54. Gudas C: Traumatic fractures and dislocations of the foot and ankle. In *The Seventh Annual Northlake Surgical Seminar*. Chicago, Northlake Podiatry Department, 1977, p 84.
55. Parkes JC: Injuries of the hindfoot. *Clin Orthop* 122:28-36, 1977.
56. Gellman M: Fractures of the anterior process of the calcaneus. *J Bone Joint Surg* 33A:382-386, 1951.
57. Dachtler HW: Fractures of the anterior superior portion of the os calcis due to indirect violence. *AJR* 25:629, 1931.
58. Wisotsky L: Compression fracture of the anterior articular surface of the calcaneus associated with avulsion fracture of the tuberosity of the navicular. *Arch Podiatr Med Foot Surg* 4:3-12, 1977.
59. Hunt DD: Compression fracture of the anterior articular surface of the calcaneus. *J Bone Joint Surg* 52A:1637-1642, 1970.
60. Degan TJ, Morrey BF, Braun DP: Surgical excision for anterior-process fractures of the calcaneus. *J Bone Joint Surg* 64A:519-524, 1982.
61. Heim U, Pfeiffer KM: *Internal Fixation of Small Fractures*, ed 3. Berlin, Springer-Verlag, 1988, p 31.

62. Norfray JF, Rogers LF, Adamo GP, Groves HC, Heiser WJ: Common calcaneal avulsion fracture. *AJR* 134:119-123, 1980.

63. Bierwag K: Avulsion fracture of the calcaneus. *Int Surg* 54:424-427, 1970.

64. Bohler L: *The Treatment of Fractures*, ed 4. New York, Grune & Stratton, 1958, p 2047.

65. Buhr AJ: Calcaneal tuberosity fractures. *Nova Scotia Med Bull* December:188-189, 1969.

66. Lyngstadaas S: Treatment of avulsion fractures of the tuber calcanei. *Acta Chir Scand* 137:579-581, 1971.

67. Heck CV: Fractures of the bones of the foot. *Surg Clin North Am* 45:103-117, 1965.

68. Lowry M: Avulsion fractures of the calcaneus. *J Bone Joint Surg* 51B:494-497, 1969.

69. Protheroe K: Avulsion fractures of the calcaneus. *J Bone Joint Surg* 51B:118-122, 1969.

70. Thoren O: Os calcis fractures. *Acta Orthop Scand* (suppl) 70:11-29, 1964.

71. Hammesfahr R: Surgical treatment of calcaneal fractures. *Orthop Clin North Am* 20:679-689, 1989.

72. Hammesfahr R, Fleming LL: Calcaneal fractures: a good prognosis. *Foot Ankle* 2:161-171, 1981.

73. O'Connell F, Mital MA, Rowe CR: Evaluation of modern management of fractures of the os calcis. *Clin Orthop* 83:214-223, 1972.

74. Lance EM, Carey EJ, Wade PA: Fractures of the os calcis: treatment by early mobilization. *Clin Orthop* 30:76-90, 1963.

75. Bohler L: *The Treatment of Fractures*, ed 5, vol 3. New York, Grune & Stratton, 1958, vol 3, pp 2045-2114.

76. Aars H, Bie K: Fractures of the calcaneus, late results after treatment by Arnesen's method. *Acta Chir Scand* 121:67-81, 1960.

77. Pretty HG: Conservative treatment for fracture of the os calcis. *Can Med Assoc J* 41:40-45, 1939.

78. Hermann OJ: Conservative therapy for fracture of the os calcis. *J Bone Joint Surg* 19:709-718, 1937.

79. Nade S, Monahan PRW: Fracture of the calcaneus: a study of the long term prognosis. *Injury* 4:201-207, 1973.

80. Shannon FT, Murray AM: Os calcis fractures treated by non-weight-bearing exercises. A review of 65 patients. *J R Coll Surg Edinb* 23:355-361, 1978.

81. Pozo JL, Kirwan E, Jackson AM: The long term results of conservative management of severely displaced fractures of the calcaneus. *J Bone Joint Surg* 66B:386-390, 1984.

82. Evans JD: Conservative management of os calcis fractures. *J R Coll Surg Edinb* 12:40-45, 1966.

83. Barnard L, Odegard JK: Conservative approach in the treatment of fractures of the calcaneus. *J Bone Joint Surg* 52A:1689, 1970.

84. Benamara RS, Weissman SL: Functional treatment of intra-articular fractures of the calcaneus. *Clin Orthop* 115:236-240, 1976.

85. Colburn MW, Karlin JM, Scurran BL, Silvani SH: Intra-articular fractures of the calcaneus: a review. *J Foot Surg* 28:249-254, 1989.

86. Aaron DAR, Howat TW: Intra-articular fractures of the calcaneum. *Injury* 7:205-211, 1976.

87. Arnesen A: Treatment of fracture of the os calcis with traction manipulation. *Acta Chir Scand* 132:566-573, 1966.

88. Omoto H, Kazuyuki S, Mototsugu S, Nakamura K: A new method of manual reduction for intra-articular fracture of the calcaneus. *Clin Orthop* 177:104-111, 1983.

89. Gallie WE: Subastragalar arthrodesis in fractures of the os calcis. *J Bone Joint Surg* 25:731-736, 1943.

90. Conn HR: The treatment of fractures of the os calcis. *J Bone Joint Surg* 17:392-405, 1935.

91. Hall M, Pennal G: Primary subtalar arthrodesis in the treatment of severe fractures of the calcaneum. *J Bone Joint Surg* 42B:336-343, 1960.

92. Boon JG, Hanemaaijer R: Experiences with a method devised by Ehalt for the treatment of fractures of the calcaneus with intra-articular involvement. *Arch Chirurg Neerlandicum* 22:95-102, 1968.

93. Noble J, McQuillan WM: Early posterior subtalar fusion in the treatment of fractures of the os calcis. *J Bone Joint Surg* 61B:90-93, 1979.

94. Whittaker AN: Treatment of fractures of the os calcis with open reduction and internal fixation. *Am J Surg* 74:687-696, 1947.

95. Hazlett JW: Open reduction of fractures of the calcaneum. *Can J Surg* 12:310-317, 1969.

96. Lanzetta A, Meani E: Operative indications in fractures of the calcaneus: problems of reduction and fixation. *Ital J Orthop Traumatol* 4:31-35, 1978.

97. Soeur R, Remy R: Fractures of the calcaneus with displacement of the thalamic portion. *J Bone Joint Surg* 57B:413-421, 1975.

98. Morita S, Oda H: Treatment of the fractures of the calcaneus involving the subtalar joint. *Nippon Geka Hokan* 36:509-518, 1967.

99. Vestad E: Fractures of the calcaneum. *Acta Chir Scand* 134:617-625, 1968.

100. Stephenson JR: Treatment of displaced intra-articular fractures of the calcaneus using medial and lateral approaches, internal fixation, and early motion. *J Bone Joint Surg* 69A:115-129, 1987.

101. Pennal GF, Yadav MP: Operative treatment of comminuted fractures of the os calcis. *Orthop Clin North Am* 4:197-211, 1973.

102. Romash MM: Calcaneal fractures: three-dimensional treatment. *Foot Ankle* 8:180-197, 1988.

103. Melcher G, Bereiter H, Leutenegger A, Ruedi T: Results of operative treatment for intra-articular fractures of the calcaneus. *J Trauma* 31:234-238, 1991.

104. Sclamberg EL, Davenport K: Operative treatment of displaced intra-articular fractures of the calcaneus. *J Trauma* 28:510-1516, 1988.

Additional References

Brindley HH: Fractures of the os calcis. A review of 107 fractures in 95 patients. *South Med J* 59:843-847, 1966.

Burghele N, Serban N: Reappraisal of the treatment of fractures of the calcaneus involving the subtalar joint. *Ital J Orthop Traumatol* 2:273-279, 1976.

Castellano BD, Cain TD, Kalish SR, Ruch JA: Calcaneal fractures: what could be. In McGlamry ED (ed): *Reconstructive Surgery of the Foot and Leg—'88*. Tucker, GA, The Podiatry Institute, 1988, pp 155-170.

Cotton FJ, Henderson FF: Results of fracture of the os calcis. *Am J Orthop Surg* 14:290-298, 1916.

Crosby LA, Fitzgibbons T: Computerized tomography scanning of acute intra-articular fractures of the calcaneus. *J Bone Joint Surg* 72A:852-859, 1990.

Duddy R, Donahue W, Cavolo D: Anterior calcaneal process fractures. Recognition and treatment. *J Am Podiatry Assoc* 74:398-401, 1984.

Gaul JS Jr, Greenberg BG: Calcaneal fractures involving the subtalar joint. A clinical and statistical survey of 98 cases. *South Med J* 59:605-613, 1966.

Jarvholm U, Korner L, Thoren O, Wiklund L: Fractures of the calcaneus. A comparison of open and closed treatment. *Acta Orthop Scand* 55:652-656, 1984.

King J, Hammer A: A simple measure to reduce and hold a depressed fracture of the calcaneum. *Arch Orthop Trauma Surg* 100:33-35, 1982.

Malgaigne JF: Memoir sur la fracture. *J Chir* 1:2, 1843.

Paley D, Hall H: Calcaneal fracture controversies—can we put Humpty Dumpty together again? *Orthop Clin North Am* 20:665-677, 1989.

Parkes JC II: The nonreductive treatment for fractures of the os calcis. *Orthop Clin North Am* 4:193-194, 1973.

Pelletier JP, Kanat IO: Avulsion fracture of the calcaneus at the origin of the abductor hallucis muscle. *J Foot Surg* 29:268-271, 1990.

Reich RS: Fractures of the calcaneus [editorial]. *Milit Med* 140:491-492, 1975.

Sidlow CJ, Frankel SL, Chioros PG: Essex-Lopresti type II joint depression calcaneal fracture from a fall of eighteen inches. *J Foot Surg* 27:206-210, 1988.

Watson-Jones R: *Fractures and Joint Injuries*, ed 4. Edinburgh, Churchill-Livingstone, 1962, p 902.

Zayer M: Fracture of the calcaneus. A review of 110 fractures. *Acta Orthop Scand* 40:530-542, 1969.

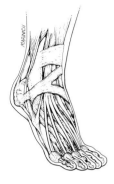

CHAPTER **65**

Talar Fractures

Raymond G. Cavaliere, D.P.M.

Fractures of the talus are second in frequency of all tarsal bone injuries. Most are chip and avulsion fractures representing pull-off fractures at the site of ligamentous attachments (1). Major fractures and dislocations in the region of the talus are uncommon and are often associated with ankle mortise injuries. These facts underscore the secure anatomical positioning of the talus within the ankle mortise (2)—its functional significance as well as the significance of injury.

As a group, talar fractures represent approximately 0.1% to 0.85% of all fractures in general (3). The mechanism of fracture is varied, but impact and forced twisting play a major role. Injury may result in arterial compromise because of the tenuous blood supply to the talar body. Treatment is based on a thorough understanding of the injury and its functional significance. The prognosis after talar injury is usually good provided that early recognition occurs and proper treatment is instituted.

ANATOMY

Anatomy is the key to understanding the delicate function and blood supply of the talus. Prompt recognition of the injury and appropriate initiation of treatment are based on this understanding.

The talus is the second largest tarsal bone, with more than one half of its surface being articular cartilage. Its superior body is widest anteriorly and therefore more secure within the ankle mortise when it is in the position of dorsiflexion. The medial wall is straight and the lateral wall curves posteriorly so that they meet at the posterior tubercle. Each of its surfaces is articular, and its three main parts are the body, head, and neck. The neck of the talus deviates medially approximately 15° to 20° in the adult and is the most vulnerable area of the bone (4).

The talus has no musculature or tendinous attachments and is strengthened by articular capsule and synovial soft tissues only. Ligaments bind the talus to the ankle mortise, the calcaneus, and the navicular and provide stability while allowing motion. The tendon of flexor hallucis longus lies within a groove on the posterior talar tubercle and is held by a retinacular ligament. The spring ligament lies inferior to the talar head whereas the deltoid ligament is medial and inferomedial. Inferiorly, three facets are present: the posterior, middle, and anterior, corresponding to articular facets of the calcaneus. Between the posterior and middle facets is a transverse groove, which, with a similar groove on the

dorsum of the calcaneus, forms the tarsal canal that exits laterally into a cone-shaped space, the tarsal sinus. The tarsal canal is located just below and behind the tip of the medial malleolus. One may think of these two anatomical regions as a funnel: the tarsal sinus is the cone and the tarsal canal is the tube.

Because blood vessels reach the talus through its surrounding soft tissues, injury resulting only in capsular disruption may be complicated by vascular compromise to the talus.

BLOOD SUPPLY TO THE TALUS

Many have described the exact vascular supply of the talus. In 1925, Sneed (5) concluded that the talus was supplied by numerous small vessels without a main nutrient artery. Watson-Jones (6) and Kleiger (7) both supported this theory, whereas Phemister (8) believed that the major arterial supply to the talus was the dorsalis pedis artery and its branches. In 1943, McKeever (9) described the anterior tibial artery and its branches as the sole arterial supply, entering from the dorsomedial surface of the talar neck. In 1948, on the basis of clinical observations alone, Kleiger (7) hypothesized that other vessels existed.

Wildenauer (10) was the first to correctly describe the blood supply to the talus in detail. Haliburton and associates (11) then supported these findings through microscopic and gross dissection studies on cadaver limbs. In 1970, Mulfinger and Trueta (12) provided a more complete description of the blood supply to the talus. They described both an intraosseous and extraosseous arterial circulation. In the main this description supported the earlier findings of Haliburton.

Only two fifths of the talus can be perforated by vessels, the other three fifths being covered by cartilage. The extraosseous blood supply of the talus comes from three main arteries and their branches. These arteries, in order of significance, are the posterior tibial artery, the anterior tibial artery, and the perforating peroneal artery. In addition, the artery of the tarsal sinus (a branch of the perforating peroneal) and the artery of the tarsal canal (a branch of the posterior tibial artery) are two discrete vessels that form an anastomotic sling inferior to the talus from which branches arise and enter the talar neck area. The main supply to the talus is through the artery of the tarsal canal, which gives off an additional branch that penetrates the deltoid ligament and supplies the medial talar wall. The main artery provides branches to the inferior talar neck, thereby supplying most of the talar body. Therefore, most of the talar body is supplied by branches of the artery of the tarsal canal, whereas the head and neck are supplied by the dorsalis pedis and the artery of the tarsal sinus. The posterior part of the talus is supplied by branches of the posterior tibial artery through calcaneal branches that enter through the posterior tubercle. In 1974, Peterson and associates (12) reported on an additional artery crossing from the tibia to the talus within the joint capsule. An excellent in-depth description of this fine anastomotic network of blood vessels to the talus can be found in an article by McNerney (13). Injury to the osseous structure of the talus or its surrounding soft tissues can therefore have equally devastating consequences. A satisfactory prognosis after injury is best ensured on the basis of intact talar blood supply and measures aimed at restoring it.

CLASSIFICATION

Many authors have attempted to classify talar fractures. As with calcaneal fractures, but with less confusion, few authors have agreed on any one classification. Bonnin (14) recommended that fractures and dislocations be divided into single, double, or triple dislocations. Coltart (15) and Mindell and associates (16) divided the injuries into fracture, dislocation, and fracture-dislocation. Rijbosch (17) divided the fractures into avulsion and flake, transverse, multiple and longitudinal, and fractures of the head. In 1963, Pennel (18) published his classification of talar fractures that dealt with the type of injury. DuVries (19) and Giannestras (20) classified talar fractures according to three and five major categories, respectively, depending on the area of the talus involved. Watson-Jones (6) used a system of classification based on the mechanism of injury, as developed so effectively for ankle injuries. Dimon (21) classified fractures of the posterior facet of the body according to the mechanism of injury, as did Hawkins (22) in 1965 in addressing fractures of the lateral talar process. In 1970, Hawkins (1) published his classical paper on talar neck fractures and presented a simple classification. Kleiger and Ahmed (23) used the mechanism of injury in dealing with each type of talar fracture.

The author will review talar fractures according to type and anatomical site of injury. The possible mechanism of injury will be discussed as well.

ASEPTIC NECROSIS OF BONE

Fractures and fracture-dislocation of the talus are frequently complicated by an aseptic form of bone necrosis similar to that which occurs with fractures of the scaphoid bone and the femoral head under certain conditions of injury. This is caused by interruption of the blood supply to the involved portion of the talus, and its occurrence is usually related to the location and extent of injury. The incidence of this complication after fractures and dislocations of the talus, as reported in different series, varies from 15% to 71% (24).

When two thirds or more of the vascular channels to the injured talus are destroyed, avascular necrosis of the part almost always follows (15). The incidence of avascular necrosis for each talar fracture type will be discussed later in the text.

Aseptic necrosis of the talus is not always easily recognized. Hawkins indicates that the opportune time to recognize its presence is between the sixth and eighth weeks after fracture-dislocation. However, it may occur anytime between 4 weeks and 6 months (13), manifesting as a relative sclerosis or opacity of the involved bone. This is caused by the washing out of the neighboring bones of the foot with intact blood supply during the period of non-weight-bearing and disuse atrophy. An anteroposterior (AP) radiograph of

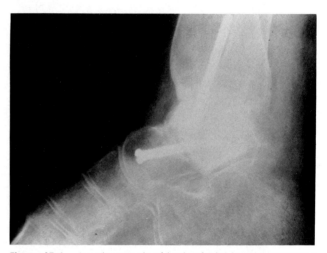

Figure 65.1. Aseptic necrosis of body of talus is quite apparent 3 months following open reduction. Patient will remain non-weight bearing until revascularization occurs.

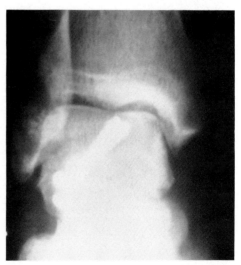

Figure 65.2. Subchondral atrophy in dome of talus 6 weeks after reduction. This optimistic prognostic sign excludes development of aseptic necrosis.

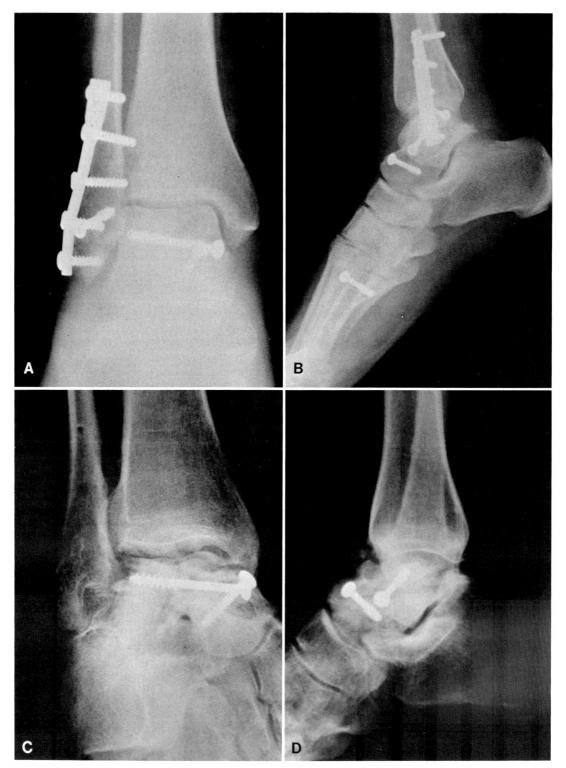

Figure 65.3. **A** and **B.** Early repair of a severely comminuted sagittal talar fracture with fracture of the lateral malleolus. **C** and **D.** The post-operative course is complicated by aseptic necrosis of the talar body, with fragmentation and collapse of the repair.

the ankle is the best view for diagnosis because a lateral ankle view is deceiving as a result of the superimposition of the malleoli and the body of the talus. As time progresses, this relative sclerosis becomes more apparent even on the lateral view because of the continued surrounding bone atrophy (Fig. 65.1). Hawkins (1) stated that the presence of subchondral atrophy in the dome of the talus, recognized in an AP radiograph of the ankle, out of a cast, between weeks 6 and 8 excludes the occurrence of aseptic necrosis. This appears to be useful as an objective prognostic sign (Fig. 65.2). When necessary, a film of the normal side taken at the same exposure should be available for comparison.

McKeever (9) states that the first sign of aseptic necrosis after injury is intractable pain. When aseptic necrosis is suspected, the clinician must be prepared to deal with the subsequent collapse or fragmentation of the involved talus if the patient is allowed to bear weight on the extremity. Over a period of time, deformity, malalignment, and narrowing of the cartilaginous surfaces with ensuing posttraumatic arthritis may occur.

Treatment of avascular necrosis is controversial (Fig. 65.3), with most authors today following the principle of non-weight-bearing conservative treatment. In this way the fracture is allowed to heal in an anatomical position in a

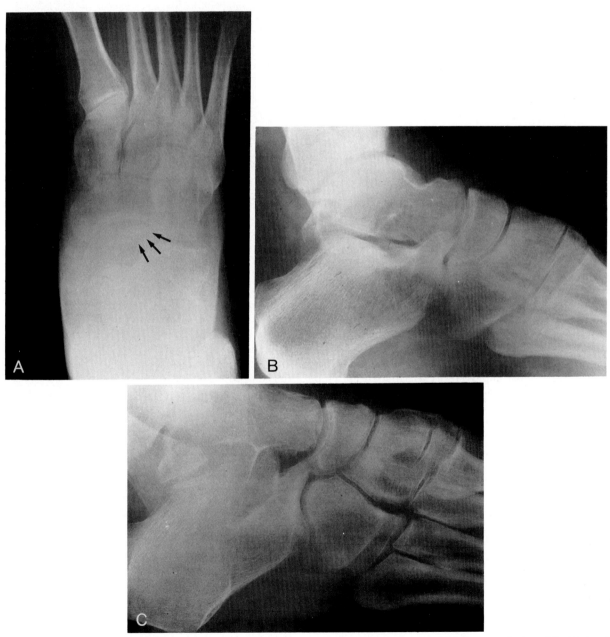

Figure 65.4. AP **(A)**, lateral **(B)**, and oblique **(C)** views of right foot of patient reporting severe pain about talonavicular joint region. No history of significant trauma was available; however, fracture of the talar head was suspected (arrows).

non-weight-bearing plaster dressing. Replacement of necrotic bone within the body of the talus may take several years; however, it will almost always occur with time. Removal of dead bone occurs through the process of creeping substitution. As necrotic bone is slowly replaced, new bone is laid down and revascularization occurs in a slow but exact process. A patellar-tendon weight-bearing brace may be used after adequate bone replacement has occurred. In 15 cases conservatively treated, Coltart (15) found that necrotic bone regeneration occurred over an average time of 24 weeks. Hawkins (1) found no single treatment for avascular necrosis that was superior to others and therefore advocates conservative treatment.

Other modalities have been recommended in the treatment of avascular necrosis. Talectomy as recommended by Fabricius in 1608 and by Syme in the early nineteenth century totally eliminated the complication of aseptic necrosis (25). In an effort to increase talar revascularization, McKeever (2) advocated triple arthrodesis when this complication was first diagnosed. However, this view has been attacked by other authors who believe that avascular necrosis of the talus is an established complication of triple arthrodesis itself. Kelly and Sullivan (26) reported a 6% incidence following 274 triple arthrodeses, whereas Marek and Schein (27) also reported its occurrence. Other treatment modalities may include such procedures as subtalar arthrodesis (7), pantalar arthrodesis, Blair ankle fusions (28), tibiocalcaneal fusion, and even below-the-knee amputation after repeated failed attempts at surgical fusion. Bone grafting was used by many as a means to accelerate union. Hawkins (1) found no accelerated fusion after grafting, whereas others such as DePalma and associates (24) advocate its use.

Other complications after talar fracture-dislocation include nonunion (rare), local skin necrosis, traumatic osteoarthritis (ankle and subtalar joint), malunion, infection, pseudarthrosis, and late collapse.

The incidence of aseptic necrosis following talar injury is most often predictable and is directly related to the location and extent of injury and degree of interruption of the blood supply to the body of the talus. The physician can alert the patient concerning the possibility of avascular necrosis of the talus and alternative treatment plans if aseptic necrosis develops. Most authors continue to support conservative treatment in a non-weight-bearing below-the-knee cast until revascularization occurs (15, 16, 29).

TALAR INJURIES

Fractures of the Talar Head

Talar head fractures are rarely mentioned in the literature. Coltart (15), in his review of 228 talar head injuries, identified only a 5% incidence of talar head injuries caused by a compressive force. Most of these resulted from flying accidents. Kenwright and Taylor (30) reviewed 58 talar injuries and found an approximate 3% incidence of talar head injury, whereas Pennel (18) reported approximately a 10%

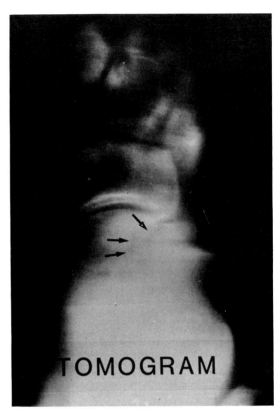

Figure 65.5. AP tomogram of same foot shown in Figure 65.4 verifies comminuted, nondisplaced fracture of talar head (arrows).

incidence among all fracture-dislocations involving the talus.

The mechanism of injury according to Coltart consisted of a fully plantarflexed foot with a sudden dorsiflexory force as in an airplane crash, therefore imparting a compressive force through the talar head. Another mechanism is presumed to be impact on a completely extended foot, resulting in compression of the talar head against the anterior tibial cortex.

The patient usually gives a history of a traumatic fall and reports pain about the talonavicular joint region. Swelling and ecchymosis may be present, along with painful talonavicular joint motion. Radiographs of the foot in the AP, lateral, and oblique views are usually adequate for diagnosis; however, tomograms may occasionally be needed (Figs. 65.4 to 65.6). Although the fracture is occasionally comminuted, significant displacement is rare.

Treatment consists of initial rest, ice, elevation, and compression, followed by the application of a short-leg cast. Immobilization for 6 to 8 weeks is recommended, and the patient should abstain from weight bearing. Open reduction and internal fixation are occasionally necessary in dealing with larger fragments with a small degree of comminution or in cases of nonunion or delayed union. Fragments that do not unite or that cause limitation of joint motion or pain should be excised.

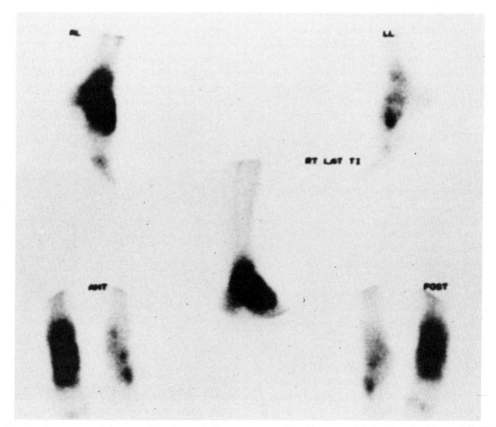

Figure 65.6. Technetium bone scan of the same foot shown in Figure 65.4 reveals intense uptake that tends to substantiate diagnosis. Patient was placed in non-weight-bearing short-leg cast for 5 weeks and is now free of symptoms.

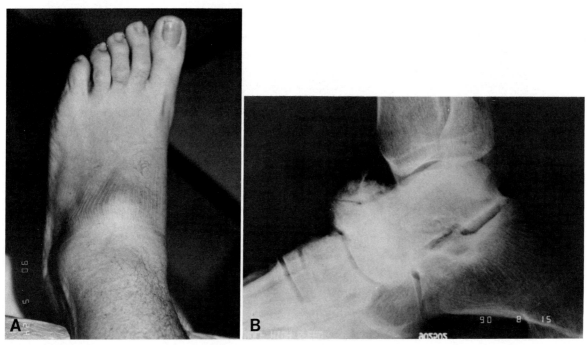

Figure 65.7. **A.** Clinical appearance of a large and painful talar exostosis 21 years after compressive football injury treated with conservative casting. **B.** Radiograph delineated extent of injury to include extensive proliferative bone formation, degeneration of the talonavicular joint space, and impingement of ankle and subtalar joint motion.

The prognosis is reported as good as long as severe comminution is not present (30). Obvious sequelae include post-traumatic osteoarthritis, which may be effectively treated with orthoses and steroid injections or may require later talonavicular joint arthrodesis or triple arthrodesis (Fig. 65.7).

Chip and Avulsion Fractures of the Talus

Chip and avulsion fractures occur on various areas of the talus: the superior surface of the neck and the medial, lateral, or posterior aspects of the body at points of ligamentous attachments.

Fractures involving the superior surface of the talar neck are usually attributed to a longitudinal compressive force combined with forced plantarflexion of the foot and ankle. Treatment and prognosis are the same as for fractures of the talar head (Fig. 65.8).

Medial avulsion fractures of the talar body usually result from stress placed on the talus by the deltoid ligament fibers at their insertion into bone (Figs. 65.9 and 65.10). Fabrikant and Hlavac (31) described a case of a fractured medial talar process secondary to closed chain pronation in a runner. A similar injury has been described by Dimon (21), with a slightly different mechanism of dorsiflexion and slight external rotation of the foot. Cedell (32) in 1974 described this injury occurring in four Swedish athletes secondary to dorsal extension and pronation of the foot, which caused

the posterior talotibial ligament to pull off bone at its insertion into the posteromedial talar process. Large avulsion fractures may extend posteriorly to involve the medial portion of the groove for the flexor hallucis longus tendon. These fragments, if painful, may require later excision. Initial treatment, however, consists of casting in a short-leg cast with abstinence from weight bearing for 4 to 6 weeks. If the

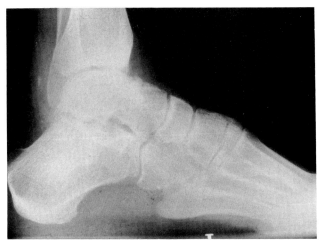

Figure 65.8.   Small avulsion fracture involving superior surface of talar neck. Treatment consisted of conservative casting until fragment united.

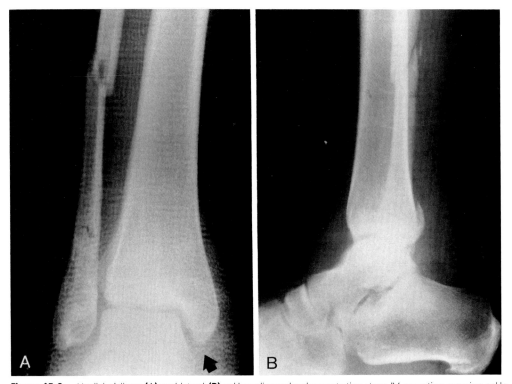

Figure 65.9.   Medial oblique **(A)** and lateral **(B)** ankle radiographs demonstrating stage IV pronation-eversion ankle fracture. Large medial avulsion fracture of talar body is present but obscured by cast material (arrow).

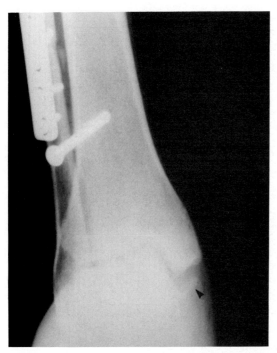

Figure 65.10. After reduction with internal stabilization of fibular fracture and interosseous membrane, avulsion fracture fragment of talus is evident (arrow). Deltoid ligament is intact.

fragment is larger than 0.5 cm and is displaced, then primary surgical excision may be entertained. Larger fragments should be reduced and fixated with small cortical screws or internal Kirschner wires (K-wires) (Figs. 65.11 and 65.12).

Fractures of the Lateral Talar Process

Fracture of the lateral process of the talus is a common injury. However, it is often missed in the initial diagnosis of ankle trauma. The lateral process of the talus is the portion of the body that is most lateral and extends from the lower margin of the vertical articular surface for the fibula to the posterior inferior surface of the talus. It has both articular and nonarticular surfaces and therefore the fracture is an intra-articular fracture involving both the subtalar joint and talofibular joints. If it is treated improperly, posttraumatic arthritis develops or nonunion or malunion may occur (Fig. 65.13). Thus inadequate treatment may cause a very disabling complication.

Thirteen fractures of this type, which constitutes the second most common fracture of this bone, were reported by Hawkins (22) in a review of 50 fractures of the talus. The initial diagnosis was frequently missed in this series, resulting in surgical exploration 6 months later in 6 of the initial 13 cases. Treatment at that time consisted of surgical excision of an ununited fracture fragment or subtalar joint arthrodesis (Figs. 65.14 and 65.15). The mechanism of injury is thought to be forced dorsiflexion of the foot with

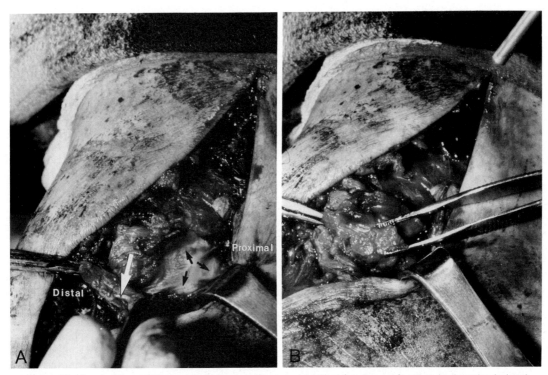

Figure 65.11. **A.** Intraoperatively, deltoid ligament fibers are identified (small arrows) and avulsed portion isolated (large arrow). **B.** Avulsed fracture fragment is shown being grasped by surgical forceps.

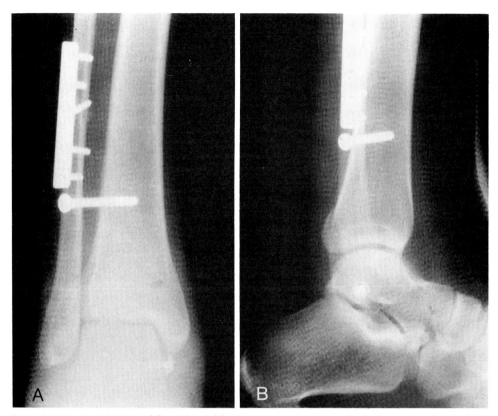

Figure 65.12.   Medial oblique **(A)** and lateral **(B)** ankle roentgenograms showing final repair. Medial talar fracture fragment has been anatomically reduced with use of small cortical screw and polyacetyl washer.

associated inversion, usually in young men, as a result of a fall or automobile accident. Mukherjee and associates (33) reported on 13 cases collected over 13 months from approximately 1500 cases of ankle sprains and fractures (an incidence of 0.86%). The cases were identified after anatomical and clinical study supported the occurrence of the mechanism of injury proposed by Hawkins. Fjeldborg (34) proposed a similar mechanism of a supinated, dorsally flexed foot. He was first to describe three stages of the fracture, consisting of fissure (stage I), fracture with displacement of the lateral process (stage II), and fracture with subtalar dislocation (stage III). Before Hawkin's paper only 21 cases of this injury had been reported. Marottoli (1942) appears to be credited with the first reported cases. Other reports include those of Kleiger (1948) (7), Bonnin (1950) (14), Cummino (1963) (35), and Pennel (1963) (18).

This potentially disabling injury should be suspected and investigated in any traumatic ankle joint injury, especially one involving dorsiflexion and inversion of the foot at the time of injury. Initially the clinical picture may be masked by soft tissue injury; however, a helpful sign is acute local tenderness over the lateral process of the talus, just below the tip of the lateral malleolus (Fig. 65.16). AP and lateral ankle views are suggested for initial evaluation, together with a medial oblique ankle view, with the ankle at 0° of

dorsiflexion and the leg rotated inward 10° to 20° (Fig. 65.17). Chronic, unexplained, and persistent pain, especially on motion, are clues to this fracture diagnosis.

The fracture is usually reported as comminuted or displaced. Complications generally develop after misdiagnosis or substandard treatment and include malunion, nonunion, or painful degenerative arthritis. Early treatment has been found to give the best results, with most authors agreeing that open reduction with internal fixation of large single fragments should be performed, whereas smaller or comminuted fragments should be initially removed (Figs. 65.18 and 65.19).

Fractures of the Posterior Talar Process

The posterior tubercle of the talus is also vulnerable to injury. This injury, reported by Lapidus (36) in 1975 and by Ihle and Cochran in 1982 (37), is known as fracture of the fused os trigonum. The os trigonum is an accessory bone located in the posterior aspect of the talus, behind the posterior tubercle, and it may appear either as a separate ossicle or fused to the talus. It may be unilateral or bilateral; fused to the talus or calcaneus, or both; or bipartite or connected by fibrous tissue. These possible findings may present a diagnostic dilemma; however, one should note that they are

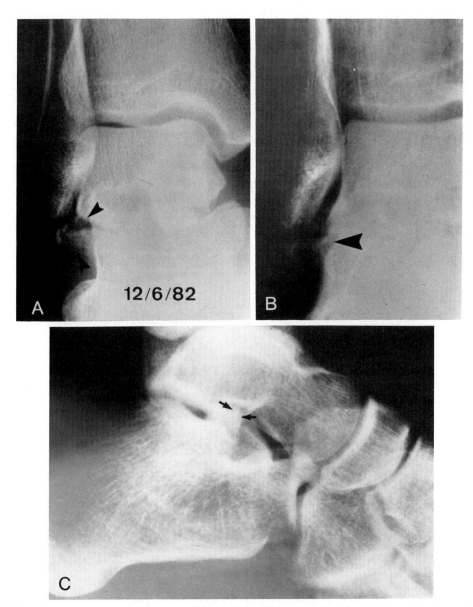

Figure 65.13. AP **(A)**, oblique **(B)**, and lateral **(C)** ankle radiographs demonstrating improperly treated lateral talar process fracture. Malunion has occurred with subsequent symptomatic degenerative osteoarthritis about talofibular and subtalar joints.

found more often in the fused versus the free state. This has been substantiated by Burman and Lapidus (38) and by Shands and Durham (39). The incidence of this fracture is low, as reported by Meisenbach (40), Lapidus (36), and Shands and Durham (39).

The os trigonum appears radiographically between the eighth and tenth years of life, whereas the body of the talus appears at about 7 months. McDougall (41) states that this secondary ossification center will unite with the talar body within 1 year of its appearance. Rosenmuller (42) was first to describe the os trigonum, and in 1882 Shepherd (43) reported on three cases that he believed to be fractures,

rejecting the possibility of a secondary ossification center with failure to unite to the main talar body. Turner (44) later rebutted Shepherd and first stated that the os trigonum was indeed a secondary center of ossification.

The mechanism of fracture is thought to be sudden violent plantarflexion or repeated extreme plantarflexion (41) (Fig. 65.20). Kleiger and Ahmed (23) have described a mechanism of inversion and medial subtalar joint dislocation; however, this is less conclusive. Clinically the patient will be seen with the foot in equinus and valgus and will report pain about the ankle. Pain may be exaggerated by weight bearing and plantarflexion and also by movement of the

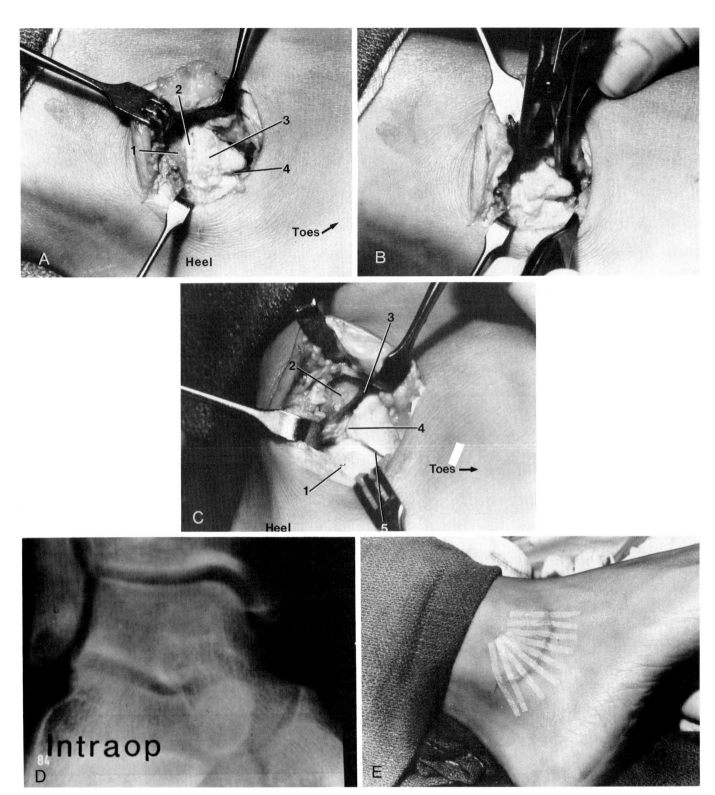

Figure 65.14. Same patient as shown in Figure 65.11 1 year after initial injury. **A.** Arthrotomy was performed through curvilinear incision just inferior to lateral malleolus exposing talofibular (*2*) and subtalar (*4*) joints. *1*, Fibula; *3*, degenerative hypertrophic bone. **B.** Arthroplasty is performed removing all hypertrophic bone. **C.** All joint surfaces are now free of degenerative bony changes. Note articular surfaces of subtalar (*5*) joint and talofibular (*3*) joint. *1*, Calcaneus; *2*, fibula; *4*, lateral process of talus. **D.** Intraoperative ankle radiograph demonstrating clean joint surfaces. **E.** Appearance at closure.

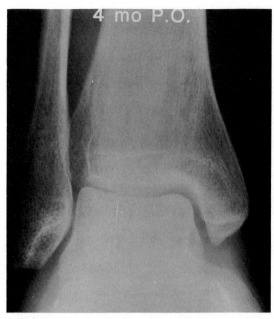

Figure 65.15. Four months after surgery patient shown in Figure 65.11 is free of all symptoms and radiographs continue to show clean joint surfaces. Arthroplasty has proved to be viable alternative to subtalar joint arthrodesis in selected patients.

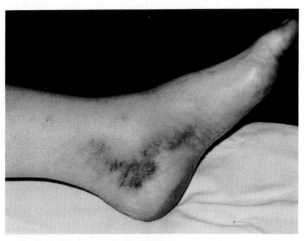

Figure 65.16. Patient seen in emergency room reporting pain medially about deltoid ligament secondary to an ankle sprain. Ecchymosis and severe pain to palpation suggested deltoid ligament rupture; however, patient also had pain just inferior to tip of lateral malleolus. Mechanism was determined to be dorsiflexion-eversion injury.

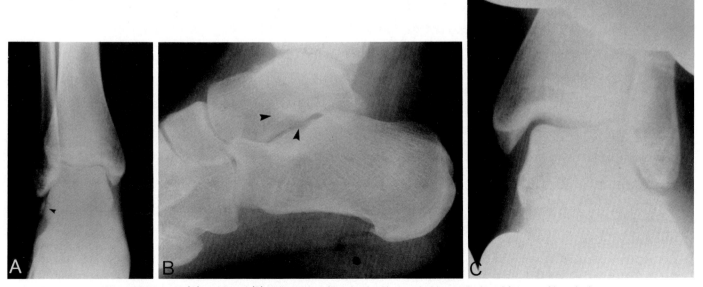

Figure 65.17. AP **(A)** and lateral **(B)** radiographs of involved ankle revealed large, displaced fracture of lateral talar process (arrows). **C.** Medial stress views documented deltoid ligament rupture.

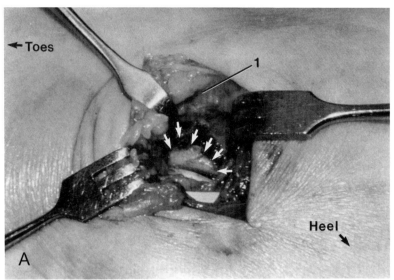

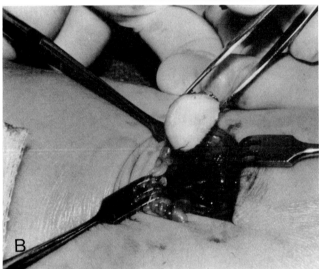

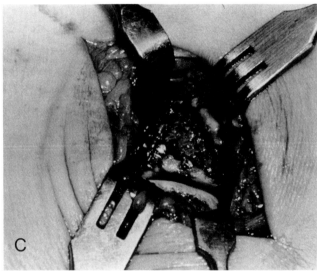

Figure 65.18. **A.** Displaced intra-articular fracture fragment (arrows) was identified through curvilinear incision just inferior to lateral malleolus (*1*). **B.** Fracture fragment is removed temporarily. Note large inferior articular surface for articulation with calcaneal facet. **C.** Fracture fragment is anatomically reduced and fixated with small cortical screw and K-wire.

hallux in dorsiflexion because of the flexor hallucis longus tendon coursing within its groove at the posterior talar surface. Muscle spasm may restrict ankle range of motion, crepitation may be felt, and local ecchymosis may be present anterior and lateral to the Achilles tendon insertion.

The differential diagnosis should include fracture of the tibia, talus, or calcaneus. Because of the variability of the os trigonum, lateral radiographs should be taken of both ankles. An unfused ossicle may not represent fracture, and clinical correlation is needed. It has been stated that the free os trigonum is usually round and smooth, whereas a fracture of a fused os trigonum may be seen radiographically as serrated and rough. A delayed diagnosis is easily made if healing later occurs after treatment; however, these fractures often fail to unite (36, 37).

Initial treatment of a suspected fracture includes a short-leg walking cast for 6 weeks. If pain still persists after this time and other conservative measures fail, then operative removal is needed. A posterolateral approach is used, and postoperative disability is usually minimal (Fig. 65.21).

Fractures of the Talar Body

Fractures of the body of the talus are the third most common type of reported talar fractures. These fractures may be either simple vertical or horizontal fractures through the body, with little displacement, or they may be associated with dislocation of the body or subtalar joint. Various degrees of comminution can be present (Fig. 65.22). The

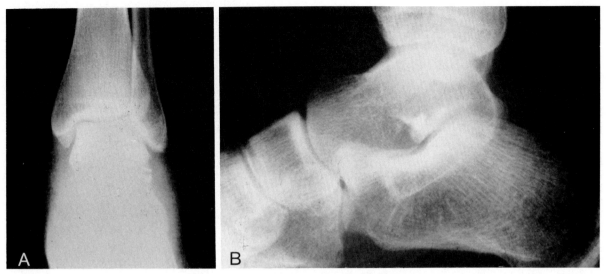

Figure 65.19. AP **(A)** and lateral **(B)** radiographs reveal reduction of lateral talar process. Deltoid ligament was not primarily repaired.

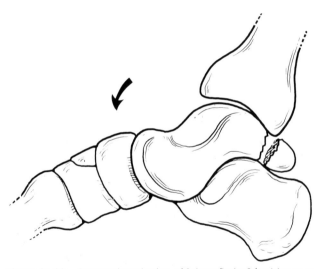

Figure 65.20. Proposed mechanism of "plantarflexion" (sudden or repeated) in fracture of fused os trigonum.

mechanism of injury is usually severe dorsiflexion force, with or without compression.

Kleiger (7) reported an incidence of 38% of talar body fractures among talar fractures in parachuters during wartime. In his series of simple linear fractures through the body, close to its juncture with the head, all had healed within 8 weeks after plaster immobilization without any reported incidence of aseptic necrosis. Coltart (15) reported an incidence of 6.5%, Kenwright and Taylor (30) less than 7%, and Mindell and associates (16) approximately 7.5%. In the Kleiger's series, union of the nondisplaced fracture occurred uniformly within 6 to 8 weeks after plaster immobilization, with good to excellent functional results. Each

author reported cases of fracture-dislocation with subtalar joint dislocation or posterior dislocation of the body. These injuries are more severe with considerable disruption of the talar blood supply (Fig. 65.23). If anatomical closed reduction with stable immobilization fails, then open reduction with internal fixation should be immediately performed. Mindell and associates reported an incidence of 50% avascular necrosis of the talar body. Failure of closed reduction may occur secondary to posterior displacement of the talar body, behind the tibia, and between the tendons of flexor hallucis longus and flexor digitorum longus, as demonstrated by Gibson and Inkster (45). Comminution of the talar body is almost always complicated by avascular necrosis (30).

Clinically the patient is in intense pain, unable to move the ankle joint or to bear weight. Gross swelling of the foot with or without ecchymosis is obvious (Fig. 65.24). On examination marked tenderness is elicited about the ankle joint and subtalar joint with decreased range of motion and possibly crepitus. A history of a fall from a height or forced loading injury, such as an automobile injury, may be elicited. The physician is obligated to examine for other associated injuries, especially involving the thoracolumbar spine.

Radiographic assessment consists of AP, lateral, and medial oblique views of the ankle (Fig. 65.25). Contralateral views may be needed for comparison if no gross dislocation is present.

Treatment of a nondisplaced stable fracture of the talar body consists of a non-weight-bearing below-the-knee cast until union is complete. Displaced fractures or fracture-dislocations may be treated by closed reduction with casting; however, attempts at closed reduction usually fail, requiring open reduction with internal fixation (Fig. 65.26).

Prognosis is good only in cases of perfect anatomical reduction, which is maintained until union is complete, with

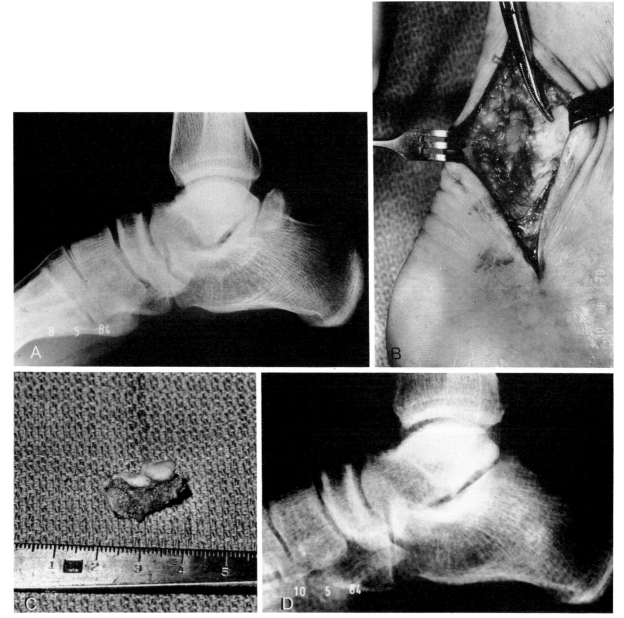

Figure 65.21. **A.** Large displaced fracture of fused os trigonum. Patient reported chronic ankle pain. **B.** Curvilinear approach is used midway between Achilles tendon and lateral malleolus. During operative dissection, care should be taken to avoid damage to flexor hallucis longus tendon, posterior facet of subtalar joint, and sural nerve. **C.** Fracture fragment is removed. Note articular cartilage that provided smooth gliding surface for flexor hallucis longus tendon. **D.** Postoperative radiograph demonstrates total removal of fracture fragment.

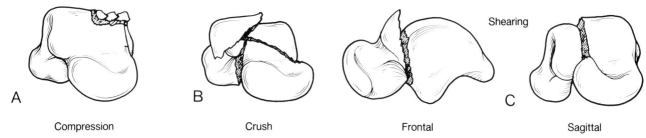

Figure 65.22. Fractures of talar body may be those of compression **(A),** crush **(B),** or shearing **(C).** Shearing fractures can be either frontal or sagittal in direction.

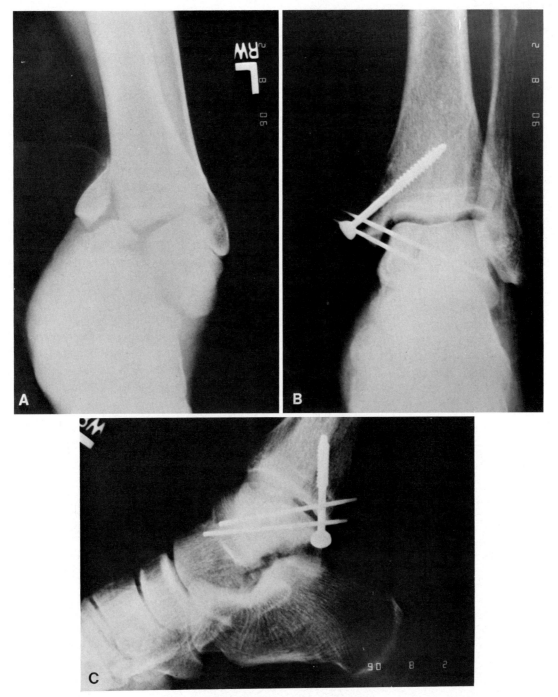

Figure 65.23. **A.** Sagittal fracture of the talar body with gross displacement and rotation of the fragments. Note associated vertical fracture through the medial malleolus. **B.** Anatomical restoration of the ankle mortise and talar body with use of malleolar screw and multiple K-wires. **C.** Lateral postreduction radiograph. Without open reduction with internal fixation (ORIF) function would be compromised and aseptic necrosis inevitable.

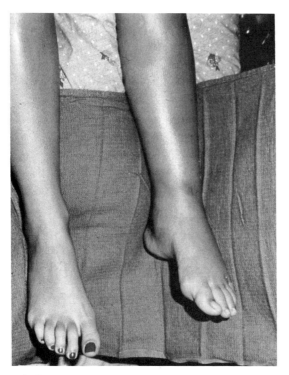

Figure 65.24. Clinical appearance of gross swelling of left foot and leg with minimal ecchymosis. Patient was unable to move her ankle or subtalar joint without excruciating pain.

the patient abstaining from weight bearing (Fig. 65.27). As stated earlier, long-term results are less encouraging after serious injury; however, the principles of anatomical and stable reduction remain the same. If stable reduction is maintained, then early active range of motion is allowed without weight bearing (Fig. 65.28). In this way muscle atrophy is reduced.

COMMINUTED FRACTURES

Fortunately comminuted fractures of the talar body are rare. Initial therapy consists of treatment of the soft tissue injury with Jones compression dressings, elevation, ice, and complete bed rest. When the swelling has decreased the treatment depends on the degree of comminution and the skills of the surgeon. Open reduction with internal fixation is certainly a possibility; however, care must be taken during operative dissection to avoid violating the remaining blood supply by poor tissue dissection. Kenwright and Taylor (30) reported on one case with talar body comminution that developed avascular necrosis. However, revascularization occurred after 7 months with treatment by restricted weight bearing. Others recommend secondary pantalar arthrodesis in the neutral position in both the frontal and sagittal planes (4), whereas Pennel (18) recommends early tibiocalcaneal fusion at 3 to 4 weeks after injury. Another possibility is fusion as described by Blair (28).

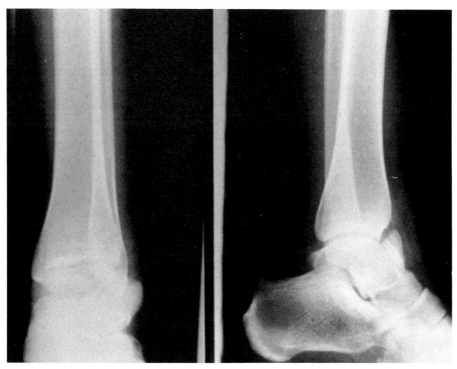

Figure 65.25.   Lateral oblique and lateral ankle radiographs demonstrating frontal plane shearing fracture of talar body with anterolateral displacement and minimal subtalar joint dislocation.

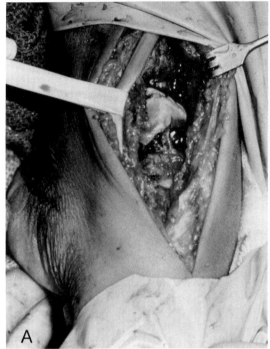

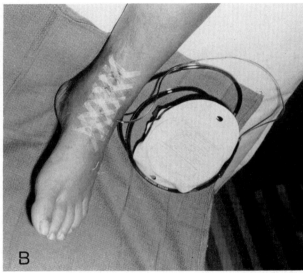

Figure 65.26. **A.** Gross appearance of fracture during open reduction and internal fixation with use of lag screws. Anatomical alignment with rigid compressive fixation is therefore achieved. Tibialis anterior tendon is retracted medially. **B.** Surgical drain is employed postoperatively.

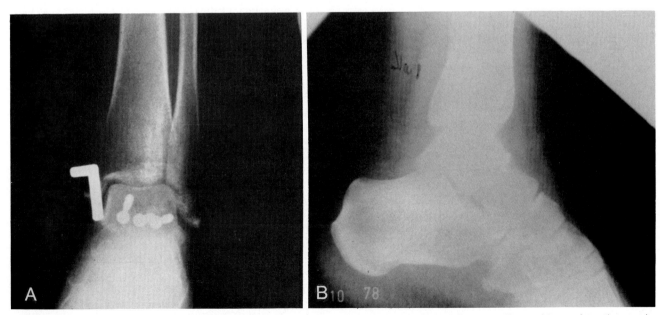

Figure 65.27. AP **(A)** and lateral **(B)** radiographs 11 weeks after surgery show maintained anatomical alignment with no evidence of aseptic necrosis.

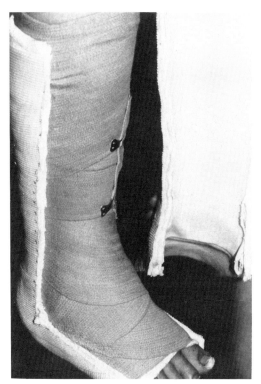

Figure 65.28. Bivalved cast allows for early return to function of part when patient is at home. During ambulation cast provides additional protection.

The author believes that if open reduction with internal fixation is not possible, then conservative treatment should be used until revascularization of the talus is achieved. Procedures such as tibiocalcaneal fusion leave the patient with an awkward gait resulting from loss of motion and also cause problems in shoe fitting because of a shortened and widened foot. Prognosis in this type of injury is guarded, with complications being almost inevitable (Fig. 65.29).

Compression fractures of the talar dome are less severe injuries compared with the crush or comminuted talar body fractures. Compression fractures result in depression of the subchondral bone plate and fragmentation or destruction of the articular cartilage (Fig. 65.30). Treatment may be either open or closed and is dependent on the size and position of the fracture fragments (Fig. 65.31). Prognosis is variable and depends on the severity of the injury, as well as the appropriateness of the rendered treatment.

Crush fractures of the talus are fortunately rare injuries that are caused by tremendous vertical loading forces transmitted through the hindfoot as a result of a fall from a height or an automobile or airplane accident. These injuries may be open and usually occur with associated injuries such as calcaneal fracture and lower thoracic and lumbar column injury. Prognosis is uniformly poor (Fig. 65.32).

Open Fractures

Open fractures complicate matters just one step further. These are surgical emergencies and must be treated immediately regardless of the type of fracture or fracture-dislocation sustained. Intravenous antibiotics are started in the emergency room with coverage for both gram-positive and gram-negative organisms. A culture specimen may be obtained in the emergency room; however, this may complicate matters later and the author recommends that cultures be taken in the operating room after proper debridement is performed. Tetanus prophylaxis and/or human immunoglobulin are administered when appropriate.

Initially, in the operating room, debridement is performed preserving all viable tissue. Sterile saline or an antibacterial irrigation is used vigorously. At least 2 L of irrigant should be used. The instruments are then discarded, and the surgeon should don clean gloves and gown. A decision is made as to the utilization of internal fixation devices (if possible) and whether to close the wound. Wounds open for short periods of time (usually less than 6 hours) and not grossly contaminated may sometimes be closed; however, this remains a topic of controversy. If internal fixation of the fracture and closure of the wound is initially performed, a drain should be employed for future culturing. Antibiotics should be continued intravenously for 2 weeks. If the wound was left open and packed, then further treatment depends on future debridements and negative culture results. A skin graft may be necessary in cases in which there is soft tissue loss.

Other complications are also possible and depend on the location and severity of the fracture. Osteomyelitis is always a real concern.

Total Talar Dislocation

Total dislocation of the talus (triple dislocation) is a serious and rare injury that many times is open, with the talus being extruded from the wound. Most injuries of this kind are caused by severe trauma, the mechanism thought to be severe forced plantarflexion of the foot associated with a compressive force that literally pops the talus out of the ankle joint. This produces complete rupture of the anterior, medial, and lateral capsular and ligamentous structures, and the talus assumes a position anterior and lateral to its mortise after rupture of the talocalcaneal ligaments. If the injury is closed, the skin is immediately in danger of necrosis; however, many are open injuries.

Of 11 dislocations reported by Mindell and associates (16), three (27%) were total talar dislocations. All three were open injuries that were treated by open reduction and immobilization. One result was good after 13 months of non-weight bearing to treat aseptic necrosis. Complete replacement of necrotic bone occurred with only moderate arthritic change. In another case the viability of bone could not be determined, and the third resulted in amputation as a result of low-grade infection and causalgia. Coltart (15) reported nine cases of total talar dislocation among 228 talar injuries (4%),

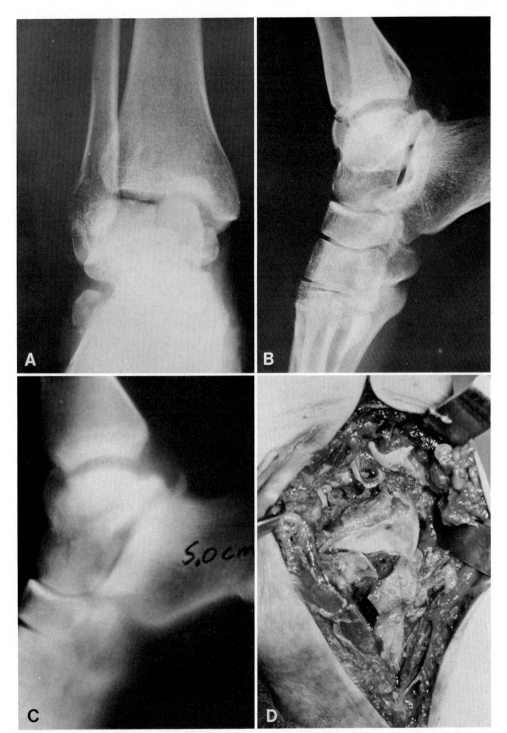

Figure 65.29. **A** and **B.** Initial radiographic assessment clearly demonstrating a comminuted sagittal injury of the talar body. **C.** Lateral tomogram demonstrates additional medial talar fragments displaced anteroposteriorly, as well as transverse and linear extension of secondary fracture lines. **D.** Intraoperative findings show the degree of comminution. Decision making in cases such as these is difficult during all phases of management. See Figure 65.3 for initial management.

Figure 65.30. Intraoperative view of a talar dome compression fracture seen from an anteromedial position across dorsal surface of talus. Note degree of cartilage fragmentation and destruction.

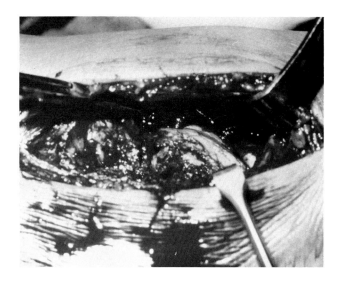

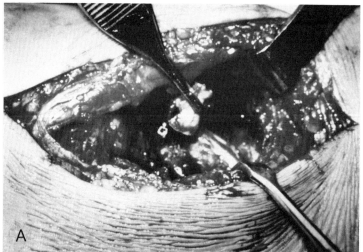

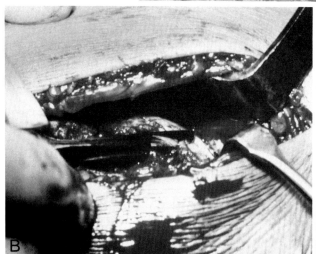

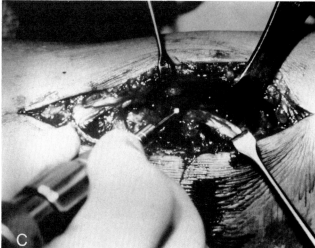

Figure 65.31. **A.** Completely detached fracture fragment is being removed from dorsomedial surface of talar dome. **B.** Remaining cartilaginous surfaces are being skived smooth with sharp surgical blade. **C.** Remaining defects are smoothed with power bur and drilled to promote fibrocartilage proliferation.

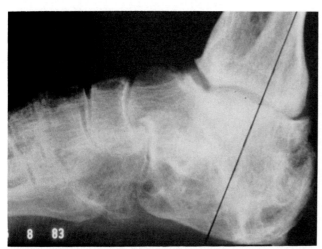

Figure 65.32. Lateral radiograph of hindfoot and ankle revealing old crush injury of talus with associated calcaneal fracture. No aseptic necrosis of talar body occurred; however, patient's gait and ankle joint range of motion are poor.

all of which occurred in flying accidents and six of which were open fractures. Treatment consisted of removal of the talus; however, the author stresses the difficulty in manipulative reduction and the urgency with which the skin tension must be relieved to reduce sloughing and infection.

Bonnin (46) reported a single case in which the extruded talus was operatively reduced with good results. Kenwright and Taylor (30) reported two such injuries out of 58 (less than 4%); in which one was successfully close reduced and was maintained in plaster with the foot plantarflexed at the ankle. The other patient had additional injuries to the talar head and posterior talar tubercle in which a K-wire was needed to maintain reduction. Both patients abstained from weight bearing for 12 weeks. Surprisingly, none of these cases developed avascular necrosis and satisfactory results were achieved; one patient examined 11 years after injury was found to have normal anatomy and minimal symptoms.

Clinically the patient is first seen in intense pain, and if the injury is not open, the physician will see tenting and blanching of the skin over the underlying displaced talus. Swelling of the foot and ankle may be severe. The remainder of the foot lies in a medial position.

Three views of the ankle are needed for proper radiographic evaluation of this injury. The talus is seen dislocated out of the ankle mortise in an anterolateral position and may be rotated in one or two planes (4, 15). The talus lies anterior to the lateral malleolus, and in the lateral view the calcaneus is in close proximity to the tibia and the talus is seen superimposed over the distal tibia and fibula. Associated malleolar fractures may be present, and the foot is seen medially displaced along with the navicular.

Treatment of closed injuries of this type represent an emergency situation. The patient should be taken to the operating room and a K-wire passed through the calcaneus for use in distraction and relocation of the talus within the ankle mortise. The patient is then placed in a long-leg cast for 4 to 6 weeks before the initiation of protected weight bearing or range of motion exercises with continued nonweight-bearing for an additional 2 weeks. If closed reduction fails, then open reduction is immediately performed. Open injuries are treated as previously discussed.

The prognosis is poor; however, avascular necrosis is not inevitable, as shown in this literature review. The patient should, however, be informed about the nature of the injury and the possibility of future disability, prolonged nonweight bearing, infection, and possible additional surgery.

Isolated peritalar dislocation, also known as subtalar joint dislocation (without any associated talar fracture), has been discussed in detail in the chapter dealing with dislocations.

Fractures of the Talar Neck

Talar neck fractures are the second most common talar injury, second only to chip and avulsion fractures of the talus (15, 16). In 1919 Anderson (47) reported on 18 cases of fracture-dislocation of the talus and coined the term *aviator's astragalus.* He was the first to emphasize the mechanism of injury, forced dorsiflexion of the foot and ankle (extension). This force causes impingement of the neck of the talus against the anterior tibial crest, which produces the typical vertical fracture. In a study by Hawkins (1), 26% of his patients had associated fractures of the medial malleolus, and in the study by Canale and Kelly (48), 15% had associated fractures of the medial and lateral malleoli (ten medial and one lateral). This suggests that, in addition to dorsiflexion, there may be external rotation and adduction (an additional rotary component), and these forces are responsible for the associated fractures and displacement of the talus. Talar neck fractures are of such a magnitude that Hawkins reported 64% of his patients had other fractures as well; 21% had open fractures.

Improvement in the overall management of these fractures has occurred since Anderson described the mechanism of injury. Miller and Baker (1939) (49) emphasized the importance of early recognition and reduction, and Boyd and Knight (1942) (29) insisted on early open reduction when closed reduction failed. Today this thinking still prevails (1, 3, 4, 7, 15, 16, 25, 30, 48) in dealing with displaced dislocated fractures that can neither undergo closed reduction nor be held in a stable position after successful closed reduction. Mindell and associates (10) stated that "the late results were best when reduction was very nearly perfect." Santavirta and associates (3) reviewed 35 talar fractures over a mean period of 8 years and stressed "immediate and satisfactory reduction" with use of compression screw osteosynthesis for severely dislocated fractures. They found a significant correlation between long-term follow-up disability and the grade of dislocation both before and after reduction. This method of treatment is also advocated by DeLee and Curtis (50) because of similar findings. These authors believe that the complications of fractures of the talus are probably partly the result of the rather conservative treatment practiced earlier (1). Of interest is the observation by Slatis and associates (51) that patients who were treated by them at the same time for fractures of the calcaneus along with the talar fractures did better.

One dreaded complication of these fractures involving the talar neck is avascular necrosis, which was discussed in detail earlier in this chapter. Its overall incidence in these fractures has been reported as 58% by Hawkins (1), 35% by Mindell and associates (16), and 52% by Canale and Kelly (48). Other complications identified were delayed union, nonunion, traumatic arthritis, malunion, and infection. Infection is such an alarming complication in traumatic talar fractures because the principal content of the talus is cancellous bone and its blood supply is relatively deficient after major injury. An established osteomyelitis of the talus may be resistant to treatment, as suggested by McKeever (2). Repeated sequestrectomy or attempted excision of draining sinus tracts is not indicated in a case of established osteomyelitis of the talus. Canale and Kelly (48) suggest talectomy followed by tibiocalcaneal fusion as the preferred method of treatment. Mindell and associates (16) agree that surgical excision is recommended in cases of established osteomyelitis and report on one case requiring amputation.

Fractures of the neck of the talus are generally divided into three groups according to severity and prognosis. Although classifications offered by Coltart (15) in 1952, Watson-Jones (52) in 1960, and Pennel (18) in 1963 included these three principal groups, Hawkins (1) has been given recognition for the classification of talar neck fractures. Because the prognosis is different in each group, Hawkins' classical paper outlined a classification that could be used for initial treatment purposes. He also discussed the recognition and incidence of avascular necrosis of the body of the talus following talar neck injuries.

Hawkins' classification for vertical fractures of the neck of the talus is based on the roentgenographic appearance at the time of injury. Group I vertical fractures of the neck of the talus are undisplaced (Fig. 65.33). The fracture line enters the subtalar joint between the middle and posterior facets, and frequently the fracture line may enter the body of the talus and therefore involve the posterior facet of the subtalar joint or the anteriormost portion of the trochlea tali. The talus remains anatomically within the ankle and the subtalar joint. Only one of the three major blood supply sources is disrupted in this injury, the one entering through the neck. This explains why there is a low incidence of avascular necrosis following this injury. In the series reported by Hawkins (3), Kenwright and Taylor (30), and Coltart (15), no cases of avascular necrosis were reported. Canale and Kelly (48) reported a 13% incidence of avascular necrosis; however, all of these had excellent results after prolonged treatment. Treatment of these fractures consists of a non-weight-bearing below-the-knee cast for 6 to 12 weeks. The cast is then removed, and the patient abstains from weight bearing for an additional 2 to 5 months while range of motion ankle exercises are encouraged. The prognosis for this injury is good to excellent.

Group II talar neck fractures consist of a vertical fracture of the neck of the talus with displacement. There is dis-

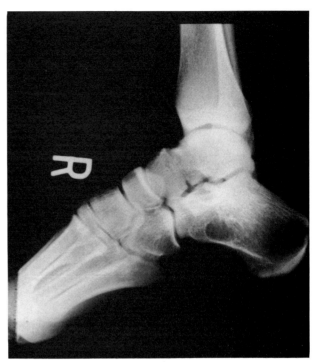

Figure 65.33. Vertical fracture of neck of talus without displacement (Hawkins type I). Treatment consisted of conservative non-weight-bearing casting for 8 weeks, with good results.

placement of the foot, about the talar body, and through the subtalar joint and fracture line. The body of the talus remains anatomically located in the ankle mortise. The ankle joint is normal (Fig. 65.34). The fracture line may frequently enter a portion of the body and posterior facet of the talus. In the 24 cases reported by Hawkins (1), the posterior facet of the body of the talus dislocated posteriorly in 10 fractures, thus leaving the remainder of the foot to assume an equinus position (Fig. 65.35). Most of the remaining cases had a medial subtalar dislocation of the posterior calcaneal facet, leaving the foot and calcaneus displaced medially. Two of the main sources of blood supply are interrupted in this injury: the vessels entering the neck and proceeding proximally to the body and the blood entering the foramina in the sinus tarsi and tarsal canal. The third source of blood supply that enters through the foramina in the medial surface of the body may at times also be injured but is usually preserved as a result of the anatomical positioning of the talar body within the ankle joint mortise. Hawkins (1) identified avascular necrosis in 42% of these fractures, with subsequent fracture union occurring in all. Canale and Kelly (48) identified 50% avascular necrosis in their series, whereas Kenwright and Taylor (30) and Coltart (15) identified 14% and 31.5%, respectively. One now can appreciate the usefulness of such a classification and how it predicts very accurately posttraumatic avascular necrosis.

Treatment of type II fractures is reported as closed reduction with below-the-knee non-weight-bearing casting

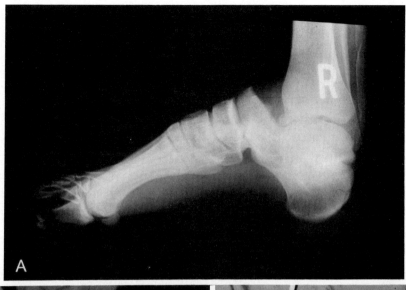

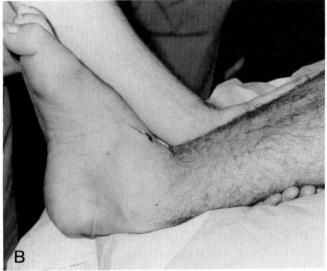

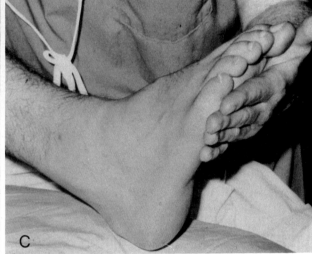

Figure 65.34. **A.** Displaced, vertical fracture of neck of talus with lateral subtalar joint dislocation (Hawkins type II). The foot and calcaneus are displaced laterally. **B.** Clinical photograph showing initial appearance of limb in emergency room. Note "tenting" of skin medially over talar body just inferior to medial malleolus. Hallux is plantarflexed, which alerts cli- nician of possibility of neurovascular compromise of foot secondary to talar body impingement in tarsal tunnel. Fracture is "open." **C.** Clinical appearance after closed reduction in emergency room. This patient un- derwent casting and remained non-weight bearing with good results.

until evidence of union has occurred. As earlier reported, early and anatomical open reduction with internal fixation should be employed when closed reduction techniques fail or the original reduction is unstable. Operative reduction may be carried out through an anteromedial or anterolateral approach with use of K-wires or lag compression screws (Figs. 65.36 and 65.37). The latter offer a more rigid and stable compressive fixation that ultimately results in better fixation. If during operative exposure there is a need to divide the deltoid ligament or to perform an osteotomy of the medial malleolus for reduction of the talar body, Pan- tazopoulos and associates (53) recommend the latter because

it interferes less with the arterial supply through the deltoid ligament. Theoretically a posterior approach may cause less trauma to the vascular supply of the talus than is the case with conventional operative approaches (54).

Prognosis in group II injuries is related to the develop- ment of avascular necrosis. If avascular necrosis does not complicate the treatment, then a good to excellent result may be anticipated. In cases complicated by avascular ne- crosis Canale and Kelly (48) found a high percentage of fair and poor results, with a loss of ankle and subtalar joint motion, aching pain with fatigue, and calf muscle atrophy reported. Similar findings are reported in other studies.

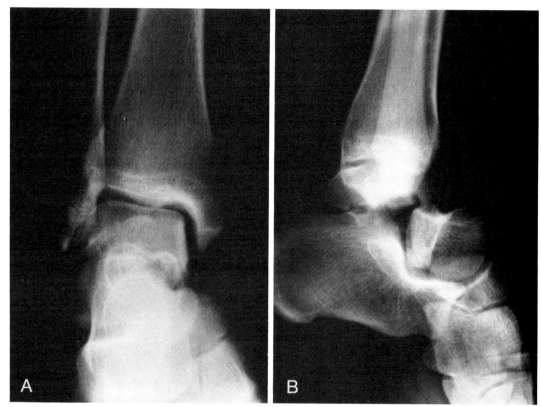

Figure 65.35. AP **(A)** and lateral **(B)** radiographs of another Hawkins type II talar neck fracture with posterior dislocation of talar body from subtalar joint. Foot now assumes position of equinus.

Group III injury is a vertical fracture of the neck of the talus, with displacement of the talar body from the ankle and subtalar joints (Fig. 65.38). The fracture line may enter the body of the talus. Hawkins identified 27 such fractures and found the body of the talus to extrude posteriorly and medially, being located between the posterior surface of the tibia and the Achilles tendon. The body of the talus may rotate within the ankle mortise; however, the head of the talus usually remains aligned with the navicular. All three sources of blood supply to the talus are usually disrupted in this injury, and Hawkins reported a 91% incidence of avascular necrosis, with nonunion requiring talectomy in three of the 27 reported cases. Avascular necrosis was reported in 16 of 19 patients (84%) identified in the study by Canale and Kelly (48), whereas Coltart (15) and Kenwright and Taylor (30) reported an incidence of 45% and 75%, respectively.

Treatment of these fractures should be by open reduction with internal fixation. Accurate anatomical reduction must be achieved to increase the chances of a favorable outcome. A below-the-knee cast should then be applied for at least 3 to 4 months.

Prognosis in this particular injury is fair to poor as a rule and again is very much related to the development of avascular necrosis. It is safe to assume that many of these patients will require additional surgery for relief of pain or fracture union. It should be noted that arthrodesis procedures give better results as a secondary procedure than talectomy alone (1, 15, 48). Every effort should be made to preserve the talus when possible.

In 1978 Canale and Kelly (48) described a type IV injury, previously unreported. In this type of injury, in addition to dislocation of the talar body from the ankle and subtalar joints, there is an additional dislocation or subluxation of the head of the talus from the talonavicular joint (Fig. 65.39). The incidence of this type of fracture was 4.2% (3 of 71 talar fractures reported). The authors stated that "the significance of this fracture, with the talar head subluxated or dislocated from the talonavicular joint, is unknown." They reported unsatisfactory long-term results in 100% of these patients and indicate that "avascular necrosis is likely and the prognosis is poor."

Physical examination in all four types of talar neck injury usually reveals significant swelling of the forefoot and midfoot. Gross deformity is present, depending on the amount of displacement of the fracture fragments. Motion and palpation are usually extremely painful, and there usually is a history of a fall or an accident resulting in a severe dorsiflexory force to the foot (airplane crash, automobile or motorcycle accidents). The physician should assess the neu-

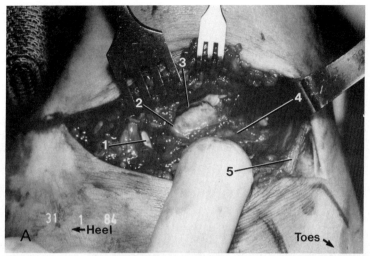

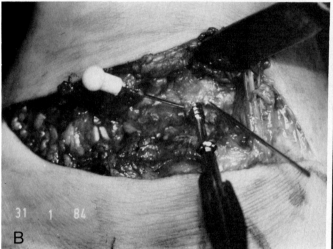

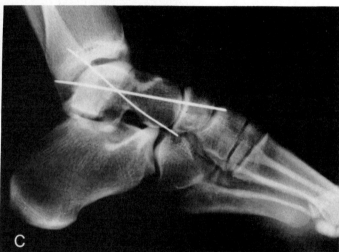

Figure 65.36. **A.** Anterolateral approach was chosen because fracture approaches lateral talar process, which would serve as landmark during reduction. Fracture line is evident, and appropriate landmarks are outlined. *1,* Peroneal tendons; *2,* lateral talar process; *3,* fracture line; *4,* talar neck area; *5,* intermediate dorsal cutaneous nerve. **B.** Temporary K-wire fixation is used, and fracture is ultimately stabilized with cancellous compression screws. **C.** Intraoperative radiograph confirms alignment before final fracture fixation.

rovascular status of the foot, as well as the local neurovascular status of the skin over and about the fracture area. If any compromise of function is noted, closed reduction should be attempted if operative treatment is delayed. One should always keep in mind that early anatomical reduction in displaced/dislocated talar fractures yields the most favorable long-term results. The fractures may manifest as open fractures, which will further complicate treatment.

Roentgenographic examination consists of at least three views of the ankle with radiographs taken of any and all areas suspected of concomitant injury. One should not overlook injury to the lumbosacral area.

Although talar fractures are not unusual in the adult, most physicians regard this as a very uncommon injury in the skeletally immature because of cartilage resiliency. Letts and Gibeault (55) reviewed the literature in 1980 and found only

35 reported cases of talar neck fractures in children. They reported on 13 group I (undisplaced) fractures of the talar neck treated by closed methods, of which three developed avascular necrosis of the talar body. In two of these cases the fractures were recognized only after avascular necrosis could be established radiographically. Because the initial fracture is often diagnosed clinically rather than radiographically, it is recommended that those who see children keep in mind the diagnosis of talar neck fracture. The patient should therefore abstain from weight bearing until the diagnosis is ruled out by repeat radiographic studies 7 to 10 days following injury. Fortunately revascularization of the talar body occurs more rapidly and completely in children (55). The foot should be casted while the child abstains from weight bearing until the avascular segment heals. Spak (56) in 1954 and Sullivan and Jackson (57) in 1958 contended

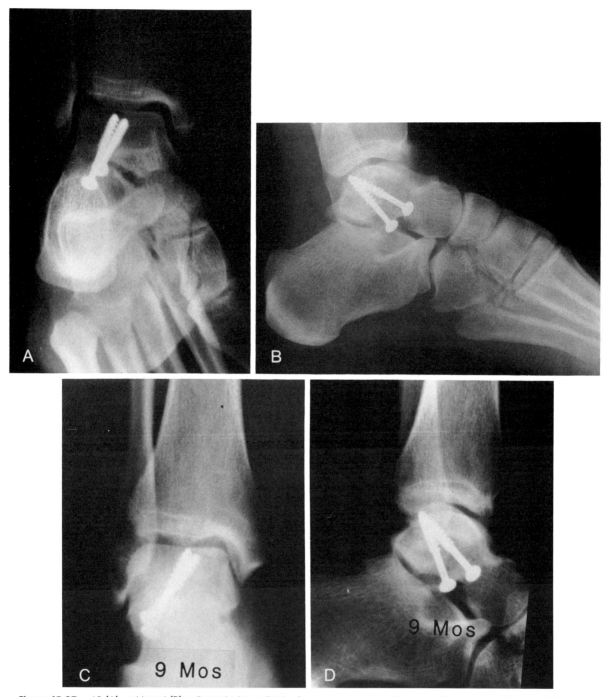

Figure 65.37.   AP **(A)** and lateral **(B)** radiographs immediately after open reduction with internal fixation and at 9-month follow-up **(C** and **D),** which reveals excellent result without any complications. Patient is doing well and is free of symptoms.

that there is no essential difference between injuries of the talus in children and adults, with the outcome being approximately 50% unsatisfactory in both. Blount (58), on the other hand, stated that fractures in children, in contrast to those in adults, heal satisfactorily without serious residual effects from avascular necrosis.

Osteochondral Lesions of the Talus

The incidence of osteochondral talar dome injuries is about 0.9% of all fractures and approximately 0.1% of all talar fractures (59). They usually accompany an inversion ankle sprain but are often missed in the initial assessment and diagnosis of injury. As suggested by others, the true inci-

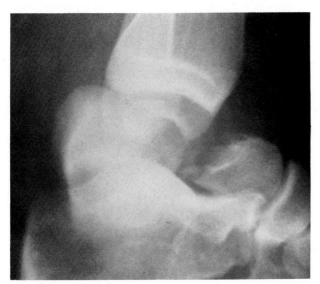

Figure 65.38. Displaced, vertical fracture of neck of talus with posterior dislocation of talar body from subtalar and ankle joints (Hawkins type III).

dence of this lesion may be greater because of the frequency of missed diagnosis (60).

Historical descriptions surrounding these lesions are many and varied, which no doubt has added to the confusion surrounding the injury. Much of this controversy has evolved because of differences in understanding of the etiological factors of the lesion. The first loose body removed from the ankle was reported by Munro in 1856 (61). In 1888 Konig (62) observed loose bodies in the knee joint and referred to them as corpora mobile. He theorized that they were a result of spontaneous necrosis of bone without any supporting evidence. Konig therefore coined the term *osteochondritis dissecans*, which is frequently used today. Kappis (63), in 1922, was the first to apply this term to similar lesions in the ankle joint. In 1932, Rendu (64) reported a case of "intra-articular fragmentary fracture of the talus," which, after study, appeared to be the same type of lesion as earlier reported by Monro and Kappis. Other confusing terms used to describe this lesion included "osteocartilaginous body," "joint mice," "chip fracture," "flake fracture," and "loose bodies."

The etiological history of talar dome injuries is equally as colorful as terms used to describe them. A hereditary factor was favored by Wagoner and Cohn (65), Gardiner (66), Pick

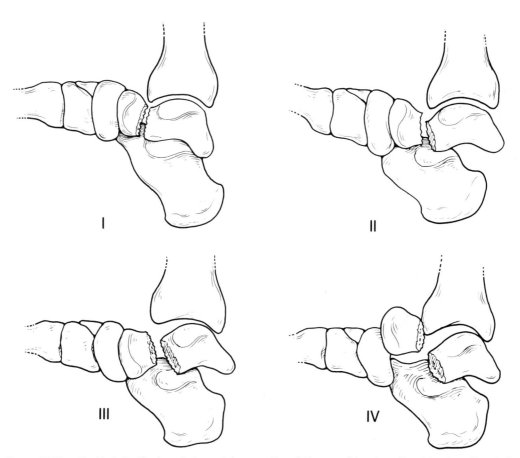

I

II

III

IV

Figure 65.39. Hawkins' classification of talar neck fractures. Type IV fracture dislocation with subluxation of head of talus from talonavicular joint, as described by Canale and Kelly in 1978, is also shown.

(67), and Hanley and associates (68). Other proposed causes have included embolic phenomenon, endocrine disorders, and accessory ossicle formation (69).

Trauma was proposed by Roden and associates in 1953 (70) as a causative factor. These authors reported on 55 osteochondritis dissecans-like lesions of the talus and concluded that all but one were caused by trauma. In 1959 Berndt and Harty (71) were to be credited with accurately describing the etiology and the lesion. They performed fresh cadaver studies and were able to reproduce these lesions traumatically. They described these lesions correctly as transchondral fracture. This term is accurate both from etiological and anatomical standpoints. By descriptive definition, the term describes a fracture through articular cartilage of the talus to include the subchondral trabeculae of the underlying cancellous bone.

Since the study of Berndt and Harty (71), many others have upheld trauma as the etiological factor in these fractures. These authors include O'Donoghue (72), Davidson and associates (73), and Naumetz and Schweigel (74). In 1980 Canale and Belding (75) reported both traumatic and nontraumatic cases of transchondral talar dome fractures in 29 patients with 31 ankle lesions. Of these lesions, trauma was an etiological factor in 25 cases, whereas the remaining 6 had no such reported cause. Although more unusual, atraumatic transchondral talar dome injuries are possible and may represent lesions that are secondary to repeated microtrauma, overuse, or faulty biomechanics or a combination of these factors. Naumetz and Schweigel (74), as well as Flick and Gould (76), have also reported transchondral fractures occurring without any evidence of any direct, documented injury.

CLASSIFICATION AND MECHANISM OF INJURY

Berndt and Harty (71) are recognized for classifying talar dome lesions into stages. They described four such stages (Fig. 65.40): stage I, a small area of compression of subchondral bone; stage II, a partially detached osteochondral fragment; stage III, a completely detached osteochondral fracture fragment remaining in the defect; and stage IV, a displaced osteochondral fracture fragment. They found approximately 44% of the lesions laterally and anteriorly, whereas approximately 56% were found medially and posteriorly on the talar dome (Fig. 65.41). Berndt and Harty, using refrigerated and fresh lower extremity specimens, reproduced both medial and lateral talar dome lesions. In both medial and lateral lesions, they indicated that the principal force that caused injury was torsional impaction. Lateral lesions involving the central or middle third of the lateral border were reproduced by inversion and a strong dorsiflexory force of the foot at the ankle (Fig. 65.42). As the mechanism of injury continues, rupture of the lateral collateral ligaments eventually occurs, and with increased shearing forces, the lesion may progress through more involved stages. Medial talar dome lesions involving the posterior third of the talus were reproduced by inversion and plantarflexory ankle forces, with concomitant lateral rota-

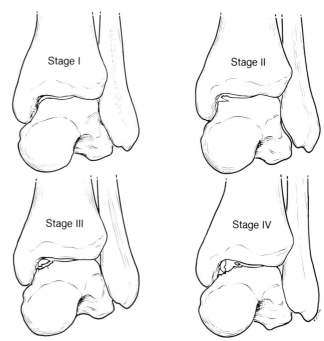

Figure 65.40. Four stages of osteochondral talar lesions according to classification of Berndt and Harty.

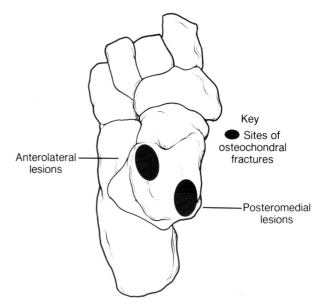

Figure 65.41. Usual sites of transchondral talar dome lesions according to Berndt and Harty. Posteromedial lesions are more stable and therefore less symptomatic than are anterolateral ones.

tion of the tibia on the talus (Fig. 65.43). As the force continues, eventually fibers of the deltoid or lateral collateral ligament will tear and the injury continues to a more severe stage.

Other authors have supported the mechanism of injury proposed by Berndt and Harty with identification of the location and pattern of injury. Davidson and associates (73)

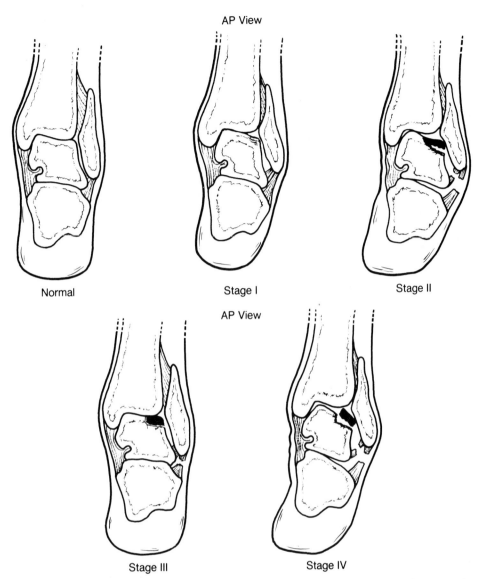

Figure 65.42. Mechanism of lateral transchondral talar dome lesions according to Berndt and Harty. Stage I is compression of lateral talar dome against fibula as the foot is inverted and dorsiflexed on the leg. Lateral collateral ligament remains intact. Further progression of "inversion sprain" ruptures lateral collateral ligament and leads to further progression of lesion (stages II to IV).

identified 10 lateral and 11 medial transchondral talar dome fractures. Canale and Belding (75) reported on 31 osteochondral lesions: 14 medial, 15 lateral, and 2 central.

DIAGNOSIS

The examiner's index of suspicion in cases of possible inversion ankle sprain must remain high. One should remember that stage I lesions accompanying mild sprains are initially asymptomatic because of the absence of sensory nerves within cartilage and the maintenance of ligamentous integrity. This absence of clinical findings, coupled with the difficulty in diagnosing a stage I injury radiographically, is no doubt responsible for such a low reported incidence of these lesions (60, 71, 73-81) (Fig. 65.44). Stage I injuries are often missed because of this lack of identifiable clinical findings after a grade I ankle sprain. In addition, there are "no symptoms that are pathognomonic for transchondral fractures of the ankle" (71). Often radiographic findings are minimal or absent. Ankle range of motion is usually full, unrestricted, and painless. Viability of the cartilage is good. These injuries are often labeled as an ankle sprain. In Thompson and Loomer's retrospective review of patients with osteochondral lesions, only 3 of 11 were initially diagnosed (77). Flick and Gould (76) reported on a group of patients, 43% of whom were erroneously diagnosed as having an ankle sprain.

Repeat radiographs should be taken after an inversion

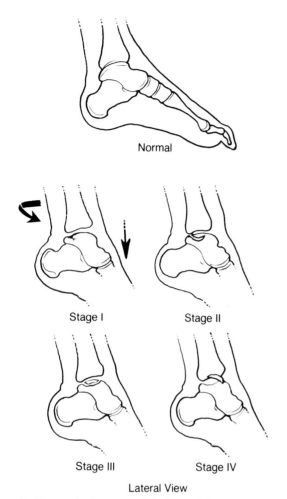

Normal

Stage I   Stage II

Stage III   Stage IV

Lateral View

Figure 65.43. Mechanism responsible for medial transchondral talar dome lesions as proposed by Berndt and Harty. Plantarflexion of inverted foot, followed by rotation of tibia on talus, results in posteromedial area of compression (stage I injury). As plantarflexory force continues to drive upturned medial margin of talus into inferior lip of tibia, lesion progresses through its stages (stages II to IV). Rupture of posterior fibers of deltoid ligament or anterior fibers of lateral collateral ligament usually occurs in stage II.

ankle injury if the patient reports persistent swelling, exercise related pain, or clicking or catching of the ankle. The total range of motion of the ankle may be full or restricted. Repeat studies should be performed approximately 2 weeks after initial radiographs when clinical suspicion remains high; however, confirmation of the lesion may occur as long as 5 months after the initial injury. If plain film radiographic findings are negative, then tomogram studies, nuclear magnetic resonance imaging, or computerized axial tomography (CAT) scanning may be appropriate. Should the lesion appear chronic, then a bone scan may provide additional useful information. At times arthrography and even ankle arthroscopy may be needed for proper diagnosis.

On a theoretical basis, early lesions may progress to more severe lesions over time because of a process of posttrau-

matic resorption and avascular necrosis of the initial fracture fragment, coupled with repeated microtrauma (76).

Stage 2 lesions, as well as stage III and stage IV lesions, are painful as a result of associated ligamentous injury, as well as subchondral injury. The symptoms of osteochondral lesions are either acute or chronic. In lateral dome lesions, in the acute phase, there is pain over the lateral collateral ligaments, whereas in acute medial dome lesions, there is pain over the deltoid ligament. There may be a history of appropriate injury, which may lead one to suspect osteochondral damage. Other acute phase symptoms may include swelling, ecchymosis, and perhaps limited ankle passive or active range of motion because of traumatic synovitis. Acute phase symptoms may continue for approximately 3 to 6 weeks (60) but can be present for several months. The duration of initial symptoms is dependent upon the severity of the initial injury.

The chronic phase begins as the acute phase ends, and its severity depends on the initial treatment of the ankle injury and the extent of the fracture. Symptoms now include those of degenerative osteoarthritis, pain and swelling during and after activity, stiffness, crepitation, aching, limited motion, and possibly feelings of ankle instability. Other clinical findings may include joint locking and documented instability of the collateral ankle ligament. In anterolateral lesions, the examiner may find tenderness localized over the intrasyndesmotic space between the talus and tibiofibular syndesmosis. This chronic phase may last indefinitely without proper treatment. Lesion progression can also occur during this time.

The acute phase signs and symptoms are usually proportional to the degree of ligamentous disruption and fracture degree and size. Chronic phase signs and symptoms are also related to the fracture stage and to the size and degree of degenerative changes of the ankle mortise.

Initial diagnosis is usually made by an astute and intuitive clinician upon initial examination of an "ankle sprain." Standard three-view radiographs of the ankle are usually sufficient for proper diagnosis. Should the initial findings be negative and clinical suspicion remain high, then radiographs should be repeated in approximately 10 days to 2 weeks. Repeat radiographs will usually show the lesion, and treatment should initially be tailored to the situation.

The AP ankle view will show the medial talar dome clearly, although in this view the lateral dome is obscured by the superimposition of the lateral malleolus (Fig. 65.45). A medial oblique view of the ankle will provide a clearer view of the lateral margin of the talus. This is accomplished by rotating the ankle approximately 10° medially, which will place the transmalleolar axis parallel with the plate and therefore open up the talofibular and tibiotalar joint spaces (Fig. 65.46). The lateral view, which will show the size of the lesion and indicate whether the lesion is anterior or posterior, will help guide the surgical approach. One must remember that in the lateral view, part of the talar trochlear surface is obscured by superimposition of the malleoli upon one another (Fig. 65.47). At times, multiple radiographs in a lateral projection with the foot in neutral position, plan-

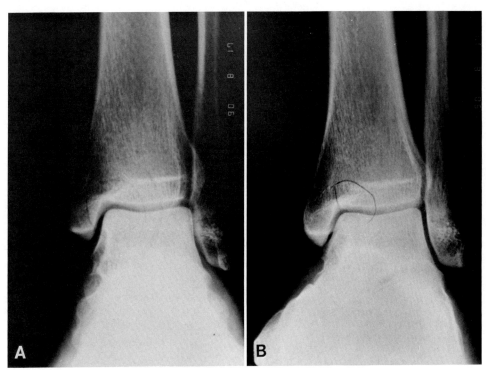

Figure 65.44. **A** and **B.** Initial radiographs of this left ankle were taken following a strong inversion ankle injury. No ligamentous injury was diagnosed; however, the patient reported persistent pain and swelling over the medial ankle. These views suggest impaction medial talar dome injury stage I. Magnetic resonance imaging documented subchondral edema with intact articular surfaces.

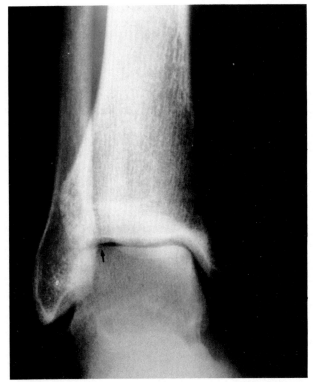

Figure 65.45. In this AP ankle radiograph, lateral malleolus almost completely obscures stage III lateral osteochondral lesion (arrow).

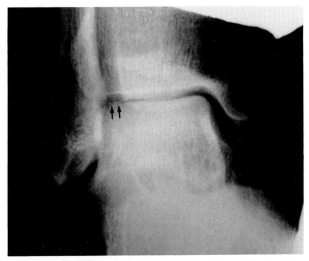

Figure 65.46. Medial oblique ankle radiograph more clearly demonstrates stage III lateral osteochondral lesion (arrows).

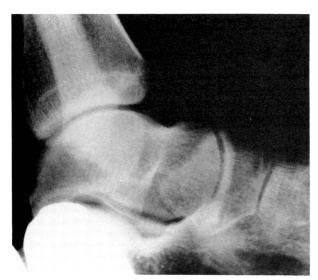

Figure 65.47. Even with close scrutiny, lesion shown in Figures 65.45 and 65.46 cannot be located on this lateral ankle radiograph. Note how superimposition of malleoli may hinder study of various portions of talar dome (especially posteriorly).

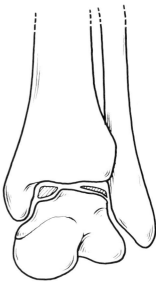

Figure 65.48. Findings of Canale and Belding regarding morphological appearance of lateral versus medial osteochondral lesions. Medial lesion is deep and cup-shaped whereas lateral lesion is shallow and wafer-shaped.

tarflexed, and dorsiflexed will help locate a suspected osteochondral fragment. This maneuver may also be helpful from an AP projection as well.

TREATMENT

Berndt and Harty described the pathogenesis and progression involving the osteochondral fracture fragment. The sequence of events begins with trauma leading to fracture, followed by disruption of blood supply to the osteochondral fragment. The cartilaginous portion of the fractured fragment remains viable to synovial nutrition of the chondrocytes, which have low metabolic demand. The osseous portion, however, becomes avascular because of interruption in its vascular supply; therefore it becomes necrotic and undergoes avascular necrosis. The fracture has been described as a "dead prisoner in a sterile cell." Subsequent healing of the osteochondral fracture fragment is accomplished through a process known as creeping substitution. In this process, capillaries invade the fracture fragment through the underlying subchondral bone. Absolute immobilization is necessary throughout this process to ensure healing without shearing forces and subsequent disruption of the fine capillary network. Should motion occur and capillary ingrowth be destroyed, then sequestration or avascular necrosis and nonunion of the fracture fragment will result. This healing process is possible only in stage I, II, and III lesions. Stage IV lesions, being totally separated from their nutrient bed and possibly rotated in their position, do not have this potential to heal in a conservative manner.

Canale and Belding (75) reported significant morphological differences in medial versus lateral talar dome lesions. These authors found that lateral lesions were mor-

phologically shallow and wafer-shaped, whereas the medial lesions were morphologically deep and cup-shaped (Fig. 65.48). This reported morphological difference, in which the lateral lesions had a greater width than depth, is thought to be responsible for the greater degree of displacement and symptoms found with lateral lesions. In addition, this may explain why lateral lesions have a greater potential to worsen without proper treatment. The medial lesions, being deep and therefore having a greater depth than width, are more stable. They therefore have less frequency of displacement.

Treatment of these lesions is generally conservative. However, the treatment can be surgical, depending on the stage, size, and location of the lesion. In general, most authors treat stage I and stage II lesions conservatively regardless of their location. This is also true for medial stage III lesions. Should medial stage III lesions fail to resolve upon initial nonoperative treatment and symptoms persist, then surgical intervention would be appropriate. All lateral stage III lesions, as well as stage IV lesions, should be treated by early operative intervention (75). However, it has been found that a delay in surgical treatment for several months to a year fails to adversely affect the surgical results. If surgery is indicated in any lesion that does not respond to conservative care, it should be performed prior to 1 year's duration.

Conservative measures include the application of a short-leg cast with the patient remaining either weight bearing or non-weight bearing and for various reported periods of time. Other conservative measures include rest, physical therapy, ankle corsets, arch supports, patellar-tendon weight-bearing braces, supportive dressings, and supportive stockings. Regarding cast immobilization, there has been no reported optimal length of time for casting, although some evidence does exist that short periods of immobilization are associated with poor results. In a review of casting times correlated with good results, Flick and Gould reported that longer periods of casting gave better results. It is therefore prudent to consider casting for periods from 3 to 4 months for the most optimal results. This would ensure revascularization of the fracture fragment. The goal of cast immobilization is the relief of symptoms, and one should not expect to eliminate the lesion from the radiograph. This rarely occurs with conservative treatment (75).

Cameron reported a period of 7.5 months prior to radiographic evidence of healing and stated that immobilization was the only effective means to achieve union before the onset of nonunion (81).

In a review of the literature there is sufficient evidence to demonstrate that operable lesions do better with early operation than with conservative care. Berndt and Harty (71) reported superior results in adults and children who were treated surgically compared with those treated conservatively. Davidson and associates (73) supported these findings that operative intervention produces superior results. They also advocated a lateral ankle stabilization during surgical intervention in those cases with documented lateral ankle instability. Other proponents of early operative intervention include Alexander and Lichtman (80), Blom and Strijk (82), and O'Farrell and Costello (60). O'Farrell and Costello concluded that early operation gives the best results with 12 months being the critical delay time. They suggested that the location of the defect is of little significance and

that the defect should be drilled for improved results. This allows mesenchymal cells to infiltrate the defect area with fibrocartilage regeneration. Filling of the defect by fibrous tissue will appear in the radiographs long after the surgical procedure. Burr (83) reported that this radiographic change took 7 years. In 31 cases that failed to respond to nonoperative treatment, Naumetz and Schweigel (74) reported that good results were provided in 63% and fair results in 30% of their patient population after lesion excision and curettage of the base of the lesion.

Operative approaches vary and are dependent upon lesion location, size, and anticipated surgical procedure. The operative approach for an anterolateral talar lesion is through a linear anterolateral arthrotomy, which usually provides adequate surgical access (Fig. 65.49). Typically, small osteochondral fractures are easily located and excised. The remaining cartilage is then sharply demarcated with a sharp blade applied perpendicular to the articular surface. The defect is therefore circumferentially debrided. The remaining defect is then drilled multiple times, with a small K-wire or drill bit to encourage fibrocartilaginous ingrowth to resurface the defect. Small curettes may also be used during resurfacing. Filling of the defect by fibrous tissue occurs over months and years, and has been reported to take as long as 7 years before full radiographic resurfacing is noted (82). With enlarged anterolateral osteochondral lesions, replacement of the fracture fragment must be attempted. The surgical approach is identical to identification

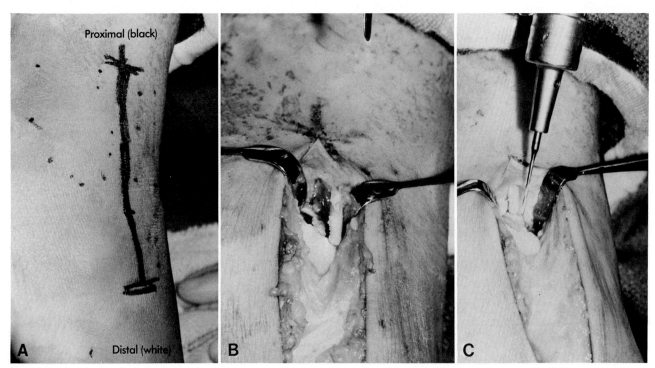

Figure 65.49. **A.** Anterolateral approach for osteochondral injury with incision just medial to crest of fibula. Avoiding the superficial peroneal nerve is crucial. **B.** Lesions are usually easily accessible, and small lesions are excised and discarded. **C.** Drilling of the subchondral bone plate will open up vascular channels and allow ingrowth of fibrocartilage through mesenchymal cell migration. This resurfacing of the joint will allow for smooth and nonpainful ankle motion.

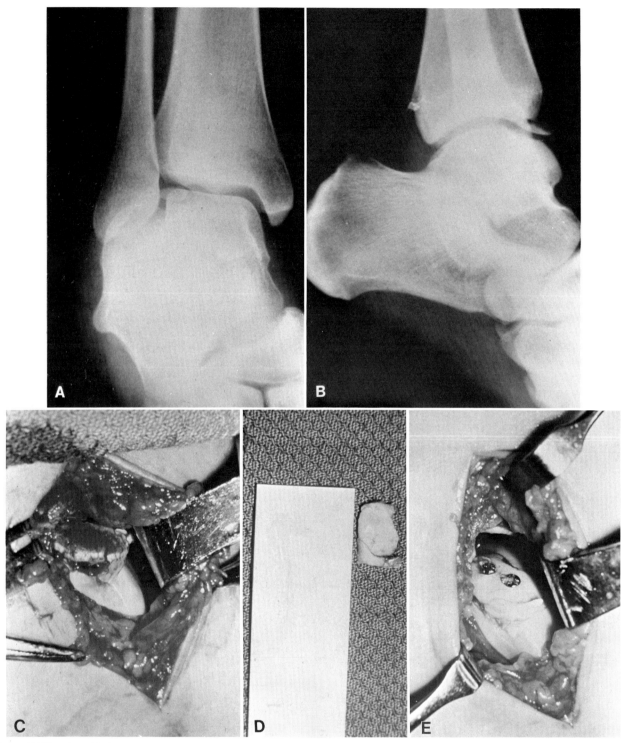

Figure 65.50. **A** and **B.** Preoperative medial oblique and lateral radiographs of an operative anterolateral stage III osteochondral injury. **C.** By means of an anterolateral linear arthrotomy, adequate exposure and identification of the fracture fragment are obtained. **D.** Note the extensive size of the fracture that must be replaced. **E.** Anatomical reduction using small cortical bone screws. **F** and **G.** Postoperative radiographs confirm anatomical alignment and stable reduction.

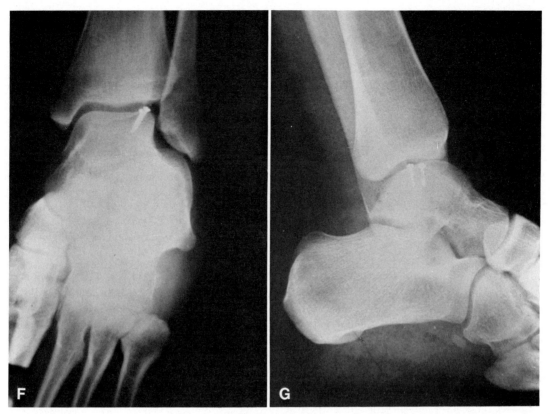

Figure 65.50. F-G.

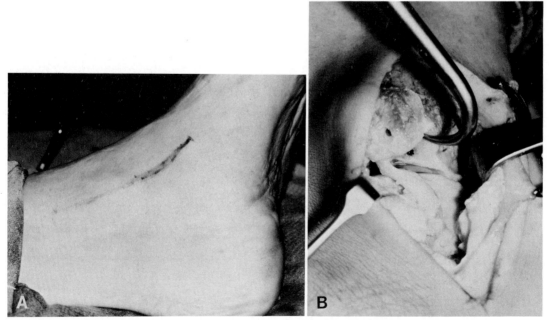

Figure 65.51. **A.** Excisional approach for a posterior medial transchondral dome fracture. The greater saphenous vein is retracted anteriorly. **B.** Medial malleolar osteotomy provides direct access to posteromedial talar dome fractures and to talofibular joint space lesions. Note deltoid ligament attachment, as well as fixation holes in place.

and curettage of the defect and fracture fragment. The fracture fragment is then anatomically replaced in the defect and secured with minifragment cortical screws that are recessed beneath the cartilaginous surface to compress the fragment rigidly (Fig. 65.50).

One may also consider the use of absorbable fixation pins, which are currently available for this indication. On occasion, the surgeon may need to divide the anterior talofibular ligament and forcibly invert the ankle joint to gain access to more central lesions. The lateral-collateral ligament is primarily repaired. Rarely is there a need for a lateral-malleolar osteotomy or syndesmotomy.

Medial osteochondral injuries are often approached through a medial malleolar osteotomy because of their posterior location on the talar surface. A curvilinear incision is centered anteriorly over the medial malleolus, and an anteromedial arthrotomy is performed into the ankle joint. Prior to medial malleolar osteotomy, care should be taken to identify the ankle joint mortise so as to avoid inadvertent osteotomy into the dome of the talus. Before the osteotomy, final fixation screws should be secured through the medial malleolus and then retracted so that the osteotomy can be performed and the medial malleolus subsequently reflected. The osteochondral lesions can then be approached and the medial malleolus firmly and accurately reattached by advancing the internal fixation screws. Two screws should be used to prevent rotation of the fragment (Fig. 65.51).

In all operative lesions, the importance of early and active range of motion exercises cannot be overemphasized. Motion is imperative for healthy joint resurfacing, as well as

for nutrition of the chondrocytes and stress loading of the subchondral trabecular bone. Even in cases of conservative care with short-leg casting, exercises such as quadriceps strengthening and toe flexing not only will prevent deep vein thrombophlebitis but also will limit the amount of muscular atrophy and subsequent cast disease.

Thompson and Loomer (77) use a procedure different from medial malleolar osteotomy in their approach to medial transchondral dome fractures. They described a 10-cm incision curved convex posteriorly, posterior to the medial malleolus, exposing the medial capsule through which the entire medial trochlear surface of the talus could be reached. A 2-cm longitudinal anterior medial ankle arthrotomy is performed, and the anterior one half to one third of the superior rim of the talus is inspected with maximal plantarflexion of the foot at the ankle (Fig. 65.52). If adequate exposure is not possible, then an incision is placed over the tibialis posterior tendon sheath posteriorly, the tendon is retraced anteriorly, and the remainder of the neurovascular bundle and tarsal tunnel is gently retracted in a posterior direction. A posterior medial arthrotomy is then performed by incising the deep surface of the flexor retinaculum. In this way the posterior one half of the talus is exposed. With maximal ankle dorsiflexion, the posterior and medial transchondral lesion can be examined and treated (Fig. 65.53).

Anterior medial ankle lesions that are not too posterior may be reached from an anterior medial ankle arthrotomy. The surgical approach involves curvilinear incision placed just lateral to the tibialis anterior tendon. The tibialis anterior tendon sheath is incised, and the tendon is retraced

Figure 65.52. Through an anteromedial ankle arthrotomy and with minimal ankle plantarflexion, many transchondral talar dome lesions may be reached.

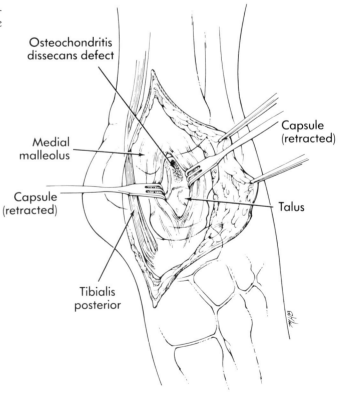

Osteochondritis dissecans defect

Medial malleolus

Capsule (retracted)

Tibialis posterior

Capsule (retracted)

Talus

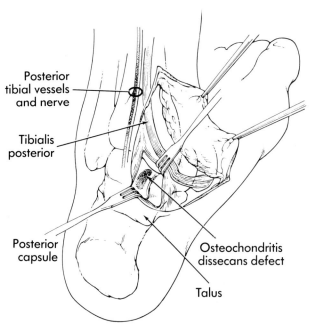

Posterior tibial vessels and nerve

Tibialis posterior

Posterior capsule

Osteochondritis dissecans defect

Talus

Figure 65.53. Through a posteromedial arthrotomy with anterior retraction of the tibialis posterior tendon and maximal ankle dorsiflexion, many posterior medial transchondral talar dome lesions can be examined and treated.

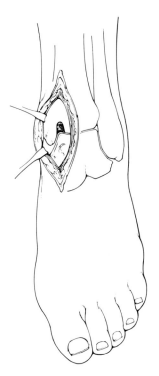

Figure 65.54. Groove technique may allow exposure of anterior medial or central transchondral lesions without the need for medial malleolar osteotomy.

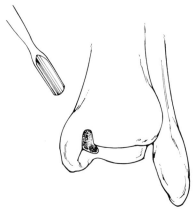

Figure 65.55. A small sharp gouge is used to gain exposure to talar lesions.

in a medial direction. All venous and arterial structures are carefully identified and retracted, or adequate hemostasis is accomplished to avoid postoperative hematoma and potential loss of skin. The arthrotomy is then performed deep to the tibialis anterior tendon, which exposes the medial and anterior portion of the talar dome. Through forced plantarflexion of the foot at the ankle, many anterior and central talar transchondral lesions may be exposed and treated.

In the event that plantarflexion of the ankle does not allow for adequate exposure of a more posteriorly located central or medial talar dome lesion, then a small gouge can be used about the articular surface of the tibia overlying the suspected lesion. This procedure in which a small groove is formed within the distal tibia was first described by Gould (84) and later by Flick and Gould (76). The defect created in the distal tibial articular surface is approximately 5 to 6 mm in width and 6 to 8 mm in total depth. Through this small grove, the osteochondral lesion can be reached and treated (Figs. 65.54 and 65.55). The defect created in the distal tibial articular surface is removed but not replaced. Early active and aggressive range of motion ankle exercises are quickly instituted. Flick and Gould reported no increase in radiographic or clinical evidence of ankle arthrosis at 2 years in six of eight patients requiring this approach (76). The author does not advocate this approach except in very rare instances in which there is a clear benefit to gouging articular cartilage over other more standard and less destructive techniques.

CONCLUSION

There is a vast array of talar fractures. These fractures range from simple chip and avulsion fractures to severe fracture-dislocation with concomitant injury to other areas of the skeleton. Classification and treatment are uniform and easily determined following accurate diagnosis. The prognosis, in most cases, is dependent not only on the extent of injury but also on the accuracy of initial diagnosis and appropriateness of the initial injury management.

It is the intent of this chapter to familiarize the reader with all talar fractures so that proper recognition and early treatment may be effected. In this way, future morbidity resulting from talar injury will be greatly reduced.

References

1. Hawkins L: Fractures of the neck of the talus. *J Bone Joint Surg* 52A:991-1002, 1970.
2. McKeever F: Treatment of complications of fractures and dislocations of the talus. *Clin Orthop* 30:45-52, 1963.
3. Santavirta S, Seitsalo S, Kiviluoto O, Myllynen P: Fractures of the talus. *J Trauma* 24:986-989, 1984.
4. Rockwood CA Jr: Fractures and dislocations of the talus. In Rockwood CA Jr, Green DP (eds): *Fractures*. Philadelphia, JP Lippincott, 1975, p 1444.
5. Sneed WL: The astragalus: a case of dislocation, excision and replacement: an attempt to demonstrate circulation in this bone. *J Bone Joint Surg* 7:384, 1925.
6. Watson-Jones R: *Fractures and Joint Injuries*, ed 5, vol 2. Baltimore, Williams & Wilkins, 1976, p 1196.
7. Kleiger B: Fractures of talus. *J Bone Joint Surg* 30A:735, 1948.
8. Phemister DB: Changes in bones of joints resulting from interruption of the circulation. *Arch Surg* 41:436, 1940.
9. McKeever FM: Fractures of the neck of the astragalus. *Arch Surg* 46:720, 1943.
10. Wildenauer E: Die Blutversorgung des Talus. *Z Anat Entwicklungsgesch* 115:32, 1950.
11. Haliburton R, Sullivan R, Kelly P, Peterson L: The extra-osseous and intra-osseous blood supply of the talus. *J Bone Joint Surg* 40A:1115-1120, 1958.
12. Peterson L, Goldie I, Lindell D: The arterial supply of the talus. *Acta Orthop Scand* 45:260, 1974.
13. McNerney JE: The incidence of aseptic necrosis of the talus following traumatic injuries: a review of the literature. *J Foot Surg* 17:137-143, 1978.
14. Bonnin JG: *Injuries to the Ankle*. New York, Grune & Stratton, 1950.
15. Coltart WD: Aviator's astragalus. *J Bone Joint Surg* 34B:545, 1952.
16. Mindell EB, Cisek EE, Kartalian G, Dziob JM: Late results of injuries to the talus. *J Bone Joint Surg* 45A:221, 1963.
17. Rijbosch JKC: Fractures of the talus. *Arch Chir Neerl* 8:163, 1956.
18. Pennel GF: Fractures of the talus. *Clin Orthop* 30:53, 1963.
19. DuVries H: *Surgery of the Foot*, ed 2. St Louis, CV Mosby, 1965, pp 369-377.
20. Giannestras NJ: *Foot Disorders, Medical and Surgical Management*. Philadelphia, Lea & Febiger, 1967, pp 392-399.
21. Dimon JH III: Isolated displaced fracture of the posterior facet of the talus. *J Bone Joint Surg* 43A:275-281, 1961.
22. Hawkins LG: Fracture of the lateral process of the talus. A review of thirteen cases. *J Bone Joint Surg* 47A:1170-1175, 1965.
23. Kleiger B, Ahmed M: Injuries of the talus and its joints. *Clin Orthop* 121:243-262, 1976.
24. DePalma AF, Ahmad I, Flannery G, Gandhi OP: Aseptic necrosis of the talus. Revascularization after bone grafting. *Clin Orthop* 101:232-235, 1974.
25. Laughlin JE: Injuries to the talus: a review of the literature and case presentation. *J Am Osteopath Assoc* 71:334-380, 1971.
26. Kelly PJ, Sullivan CR: Blood supply to the talus. *Clin Orthop* 30:37-43, 1963.
27. Marek FM, Schein AJ: Aseptic necrosis of the astragalus following arthrodesing procedures of the tarsus. *J Bone Joint Surg* 27:587-594, 1945.
28. Blair HC: Comminuted fractures and dislocations of the body of the astragalus; operative treatment. *Am J Surg* 59:37, 1943.
29. Boyd HB, Knight RA: Fractures of the astragalus. *South Med J* 35:160, 1942.
30. Kenwright J, Taylor RG: Major injuries of the talus. *J Bone Joint Surg* 52B:36-48, 1970.
31. Fabrikant JM, Hlavac HF: Fracture of the posterior process of the talus in runners. A case report. *J Am Podiatry Assoc* 69:329-332, 1979.
32. Cedell C: Rupture of the posterior talotibial ligament with the avulsion of a bone fragment from the talus. *Acta Orthop Scand* 45:454, 1974.
33. Mukherjee SK, Pringle RM, Baxter AO: Fracture of the lateral process of the talus, a report of thirteen cases. *J Bone Joint Surg* 56B:263-273, 1974.
34. Fjeldborg O: Fracture of the lateral process of the talus. Supination-dorsal flexion fracture. *Acta Orthop Scand* 39:407-412, 1968.
35. Cummino CV: Fracture of the lateral process of the talus. *Am J Roentgenol* 90:1277-1280, 1963.
36. Lapidus PW: A note on the fracture of os trigonum. Report of a case. *Bull Hosp Jt Dis* 33:150-154, 1975.
37. Ihle CL, Cochran RM: Fracture of the fused os trigonum. *Am J Sports Med* 10:47-50, 1982.
38. Burman MS, Lapidus PW: The functional disturbances caused by the inconstant bones and sesamoids of the foot. *Arch Surg* 22:936-975, 1931.
39. Shands AR Jr, Durham NC: The accessory bones of the foot: an x-ray study of the feet of 1,054 patients. *South Med Surg* 326-334, 1931.
40. Meisenbach R: Fracture of the os trigonum: report of two cases. *JAMA* 89:199-200, 1927.
41. McDougall A: The os trigonum. *J Bone Joint Surg* 37B:257-265, 1955.
42. Rosenmuller (quoted in Holland CT): On rarer ossifications seen during x-ray examination. *J Anat* 55:235-268, 1921.
43. Shepherd RJ: A hitherto undescribed fracture of the astragalus. *J Anat Physiol* 17:79-81, 1882.
44. Turner W: A secondary astragalus in the human foot. *J Anat Physiol* 17:82, 1882.
45. Gibson A, Inkster RG: Fractures of the talus. *J Can Med Assoc* NS31:357, 1934.
46. Bonnin JG: Dislocations and fracture-dislocations of the talus. *Br J Surg* 28:88, 1940.
47. Anderson HG: *Medical and Surgical Aspects of Aviation*. London, Oxford Medical Publications, 1919.
48. Canale TS, Kelly FB: Fracture of the neck of the talus. Long-term evaluation of seventy-one cases. *J Bone Joint Surg* 60A:143-156, 1978.
49. Miller OL, Baker LD: Fracture and fracture-dislocation of the astragalus. *South Med J* 32:125-136, 1939.
50. DeLee JC, Curtis R: Subtalar dislocation of the foot. *J Bone Joint Surg* 64A:433-437, 1982.
51. Slatis P, Kiviluoto O, Santavirta S: Fractures of the calcaneum. *J Trauma* 19:939-943, 1979.
52. Watson-Jones R: *Fractures and Joint Injuries*, ed 4, vol 2. Edinburgh, ES Livingstone, 1960.
53. Pantazopoulos T, Galanos P, Vayanos E, Mitsou A, Hartofilakidis-Garofalidis G: Fractures of the neck of the talus. *Acta Orthop Scand* 45:296-306, 1974.
54. Lemaire RG, Bustin W: Screw fixation of fractures of the talus using a posterior approach. *J Trauma* 20:669-673, 1980.
55. Letts RM, Gibeault D: Fractures of the neck of the talus in children. *Foot Ankle* 1:74-77, 1980.
56. Spak I: Fractures of the talus in children. *Acta Chir Scand* 107:553-556, 1954.
57. Sullivan CR, Jackson SC: Fracture dislocations of the astragalus in children: a clinical study and survey of the literature. *Acta Orthop Scand* 27:302-309, 1958.
58. Blount WP: *Fractures in Children*. Baltimore, Williams & Wilkins, 1955, pp 195-196.
59. Lindholm TS, Osterman E: Osteochondritis dissecans of the elbow, ankle and hip: a comparison survey. *Clin Orthop* 148:245, 1980.
60. O'Farrell TA, Costello BG: Osteochondritis dissecans of the talus. *J Bone Joint Surg* 64B:494-497, 1982.
61. Phemister DB: The causes and changes in loose bodies arising from the articular surface of the joint. *J Bone Joint Surg* 6:278-315, 1924.
62. Konig F: Uber freie Korper in den Gelenken. *Dtsch Z Chir* 27:90, 1888.
63. Kappis M: Weitere Beitrage zur traumatisch-mechanischen entstehung der "spontanen" Knorpelablosungen (sogennante osteochondritis dissecans). *Dtsch Z Chir* 171:13, 1922.
64. Rendu A: Fracture intra-articulaire parcellaire de la poulie astraglienne. *Lyon Med* 150:220-222, 1932.
65. Wagoner G, Cohn BNE: Osteochondritis dissecans. A resume of the theories of etiology and the consideration of heredity as an etiologic factor. *Arch Surg* 23:1-24, 1931.

66. Gardiner TB: Osteochondritis dissecans in three members of one family. *J Bone Joint Surg* 37B:139-141, 1955.

67. Pick MP: Familial osteochondritis dissecans. *J Bone Joint Surg* 37B:142-145, 1955.

68. Hanley WB, McKusick VA, Barranco FT: Osteochondritis dissecans with associated malformation in two brothers. *J Bone Joint Surg* 49A:925, 1967.

69. Arcomano JP, Kamhi E, Karas S, Moriarty VJ: Transchondral fracture and osteochondritis dissecans of talus. *NY State J Med* 78:2183-2189, 1978.

70. Roden S, Tillegard P, Unander-Scharin L: Osteochondritis dissecans and similar lesions of the talus. *Acta Orthop Scand* 23:51-66, 1953.

71. Berndt A, Harty M: Transchondral fractures (osteochondritis dissecans) of the talus. *J Bone Joint Surg* 41A:988-1020, 1959.

72. O'Donoghue DM: Chondral and osteochondral fractures. *J Trauma* 6:469-481, 1966.

73. Davidson AM, Steele HD, Mac Kenzie DA, Penny JA: A review of twenty-one cases of transchondral fracture of the talus. *J Trauma* 7:378-415, 1967.

74. Naumetz VA, Schweigel JF: Osteocartilaginous lesions of the talar dome. *J Trauma* 20:924-927, 1980.

75. Canale T, Belding R: Osteochondral lesions of the talus. *J Bone Joint Surg* 62A:97-102, 1980.

76. Flick AB, Gould N: Osteochondritis dissecans of the talus (transchondral fractures of the talus): a review of the literature and new surgical approach for medial dome lesions. *Foot Ankle* 5:165, 1985.

77. Thompson JP, Loomer RL: Osteochondral lesions of the talus in a sports medicine clinic. *Am J Sports Med* 12:460-463, 1984.

78. Newberg AH: Osteochondral fractures of the dome of the talus. *Br J Radiol* 52:105-109, 1979.

79. Rynn M, Fazekas EA, Hecker RL: Osteochondral lesions of the talus. *J Foot Surg* 22:155-158, 1983.

80. Alexander AH, Lichtman DM: Surgical treatment of transchondral talar-dome fractures. *J Bone Joint Surg* 62A:646-652, 1980.

81. Cameron BM: Osteochondritis dissecans of the ankle joint. A report of a case simulating a fracture of the talus. *J Bone Joint Surg* 38A: 857, 1956.

82. Blom JMH, Strijk SP: Lesions of the trochlea tali: osteochondral fractures and osteochondritis dissecans of the trochlea tali. *Radiol Clin* (Basel) 44:387-396, 1975.

83. Burr RC: Osteochondritis dissecans. *Can Med Assoc J* 41:232-235, 1939.

84. Gould N: Technique tips. *Foot Ankle* 3:184, 1982.

Additional References

Dennis DM, Tullos HS: Blair tibiotalar arthrodesis for injuries to the talus. *J Bone Joint Surg* 62A:103-107, 1980.

Dobas DC, Bruscia RJ: Transchondral fractures of the talar dome. A review and case report. *J Am Podiatry Assoc* 68:182-190, 1978.

Dobas DC, Shadle JH: Fractures of the talus and associated complications: A review. *Arch Podiatr Med Foot Surg* 4:23-31, 1977.

Giannestras NJ, Sammarco GJ: Fractures and dislocations in the foot. In Rockwood CA, Green DP (eds): *Fractures*. Philadelphia, JB Lippincott, 1975, pp 1443-1465.

Heppenstall BR: Injuries of the foot. In Heppenstall BR (ed): *Fracture Treatment and Healing*. Philadelphia, WB Saunders, 1980, pp 839-861.

Kenny CH: Inverted osteochondral fracture of the talus diagnosed by tomography. *J Bone Joint Surg* 63A:1020-1022, 1981.

Lieberg OU, Henke JA, Bailey RW: Avascular necrosis of the head of the talus without death of the body: report of an unusual case. *J Trauma* 15:926-928, 1975.

Lorentzen JE, Christensen SB, Krogsoe O, Sneppen O: Fractures of the neck of the talus. *Acta Orthop Scand* 48:115-120, 1977.

Mensor MC, Melody GF: Osteochondritis dissecans of the ankle joint. *J Bone Joint Surg* 23:903-909, 1941.

Miskew DBW, Goldflies ML: Atraumatic avascular necrosis of the talus associated with hyperuricemia. *Clin Orthop* 148:156-159, 1980.

Monkman G, Johnson KA, Duncan DM: Fractures of the neck of the talus. *Minn Med* 58:335-340, 1975.

Morris HD: Aseptic necrosis of the talus following injury. *Orthop Clin North Am* 5:177-189, 1974.

Mukherjee SK, Young AB: Dome fracture of the talus. A report of ten cases. *J Bone Joint Surg* 55B:319-326, 1973.

Nyari T, Kazar GY, Frenyo S, Balla I: The role of intraosseous phlebography in the prognosis of injuries of the talus. *Injury* 13:317-323, 1982.

O'Brien ET: Injuries of the talus. *Am Fam Physician* 12:95-105, 1975.

Pantazopoulos T, Kapetsis P, Soucacos P, Gianakis E: Unusual fracture-dislocation of the talus. *Clin Orthop* 83:232-234, 1972.

Pathi KM: Fracture neck of talus in children. *J Indian Med Assoc* 63:157-158, 1974.

Penny NJ, Davis LA: Fractures and fracture-dislocations of the neck of the talus. *J Trauma* 20:1029-1037, 1980.

Percy EC: Open fracture of the talus. *Can Med Assoc J* 101:91-92, 1969.

Perry RD, O'Toole ED: Stress fracture of the talar neck and distal calcaneus. *J Am Podiatry Assoc* 71:637-638, 1981.

Peterson L, Goldie IF: The arterial supply of the talus. *Acta Orthop Scand* 46:1026-1034, 1975.

Peterson L, Goldie IF, Irstam L: Fracture of the neck of the talus. *Acta Orthop Scand* 48:696-706, 1977.

Peterson L, Romanus B: Fracture of the collum tali—an experimental study. *J Biomech* 9:277-279, 1976.

Petrie PWR: Aetiology of osteochondritis dissecans. *J Bone Joint Surg* 59B:366-367, 1977.

Ray RB, Coughlin EJ Jr: Osteochondritis dissecans of the talus. *J Bone Joint Surg* 29:697-706, 710, 1947.

Reckling FW: Early tibiocalcaneal fusion in the treatment of severe injuries of the talus. *J Trauma* 12:390-396, 1972.

Shafa MH, Fernandez-Ulloa M, Rost RC, Nyquist SR: Diagnosis of aseptic necrosis of the talus by bone scintigraphy. Case report. *Clin Nucl Med* 8:50-53, 1983.

Sneppen O, Buhl O: Fracture of the talus. *Acta Orthop Scand* 45:307-320, 1974.

Sneppen O, Christensen SB, Krogsoe O, Lorentzen J: Fracture of the body of the talus. *Acta Orthop Scand* 48:317-324, 1977.

Weinstein SL, Bonfiglio M: Unusual accessory (bipartite) talus simulating fracture. *J Bone Joint Surg* 57A:1161-1163, 1975.

Wray DG, Muddu BN: Lateral dome fracture of the talus. *J Trauma* 21:818-819, 1981.

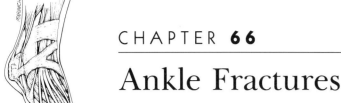

CHAPTER **66**

Ankle Fractures

Michael S. Downey, D.P.M.
D. Scot Malay, D.P.M.
John A. Ruch, D.P.M.

The primary goal in the treatment of ankle fractures is to encourage the return of normal function to the injured lower extremity. Such restoration may be accomplished only with a full understanding and appreciation of the fracture, the concomitant soft tissue injuries, the pathological mechanism by which the injury occurred, and the mechanical demands of the joint(s) involved. In 1931 Bohler (1) stated that "every incongruity even the smallest visible displacement on x-ray, or faulty axis position may cause permanent complaints at the articular surfaces. The joints that are no longer congruent are therefore abraded. With time, the greater the displacement, the more pronounced the arthritic changes. The ankle joint remains permanently painful."

ANATOMY

Although the anatomy of the ankle is described in other anatomy texts, certain points are worth emphasizing. The inferior tibiofibular joint is the area between the rough, convex surface of the medial side of the distal portion of the fibula and the rough, concave surface of the fibular notch of the tibia (2). It extends proximally 2.5 cm from the ankle mortise. The joint is supported anteriorly by the anterior inferior tibiofibular ligament, which is quite thick and strong. The ligament is located obliquely between the distal fibula and the anterolateral margin of the tibia. Wagstaffe (3) was the first to describe avulsion fractures of the distal fibula by the anterior inferior tibiofibular ligament. A fracture of the fibula in this area has since been termed a Wagstaffe fracture (4). The anterolateral margin of the distal tibia is often referred to as the tubercle of Tillaux-Chaput. In 1872 Tillaux (5) described fractures of this tubercle, implicating the anterior inferior tibiofibular ligament in relation to the injury. In 1907 Chaput (6) was the first to demonstrate the avulsion fracture of this tubercle radiographically. The anterior joint capsule is relatively thick as compared with the thin posterior joint capsule and directly overlies the anterior inferior tibiofibular ligament.

Posteriorly, the even stronger posterior inferior tibiofibular ligament joins the distal fibula and tibia. In 1828 Earle (7) described the fracture of the posterior tibia, which is also known as the posterior malleolus. This anatomical segment of the tibia is sometimes referred to as Volkmann's triangle, and fractures in this area often bear his name (8). The lower

and deeper portion of the posterior inferior tibiofibular ligament forms the inferior transverse ligament. This portion of the ligament blends with the posterior ankle joint capsule.

Extending proximally between the tibia and the fibula is the tibiofibular interosseous membrane. Disruption of the distal ligamentous and capsular structures will make the interosseous membrane susceptible to rupture. If the interosseous membrane is torn, diastasis between the tibia and the fibula may occur.

In many ankle injuries both ligamentous and osseous injuries occur. Often radiographs will reveal a fracture with no obvious hint of ligamentous injury. A ligament can either tear through its body, in which case no radiographic evidence may be present, or avulse from its insertion to a bone, in which case a small avulsion fragment may be seen on radiographs. These avulsion fragments vary in size and are generally perpendicular in orientation to the ligamentous course coinciding with its insertion. Helpful signs in determining ligamentous injury are palpable tenderness overlying the ligament, visualization of radiographic distraction between the osseous structures that the ligament binds (i.e., development of clear space), and a thorough understanding of the mechanism of injury. If a ligamentous injury is suspected but not visualized on radiographs, a stress radiographic view may be obtained. The clinician will apply tension along the normal course of the ligament and attempt to distract the osseous structures that are normally bound together.

Finally, a thorough understanding of the Dias and Tachdjian (9) classification system of physeal ankle injuries is necessary when one is treating ankle fractures in children and adolescents (see chapter on epiphyseal injuries). The classification system may be directly related to the mechanisms that follow.

MECHANISMS OF ANKLE INJURY

Before treating an ankle injury or fracture, one must have a thorough working knowledge of the pathological mechanisms involved. With this knowledge, the practitioner may fully evaluate both soft tissue and osseous derangement. Furthermore, this will facilitate accurate anatomical joint restoration. However, one must be aware that not all ankle injuries may be categorized. Certain atypical injuries do occur, and the astute practitioner must be flexible in the application of any classification system.

Throughout the medical literature there have been many different attempts to provide a systematic method for the evaluation of ankle injury and fracture. The earliest descriptions were purely anatomical, listing fractures as malleolar, bimalleolar, and trimalleolar. No attempt was made to correlate the ankle injury with its causal mechanism. In 1922 Ashurst and Bromer (10) were the first to attempt a classification of ankle fractures based on the mechanism of injury. They divided fractures into three main groups: external rotation, abduction, and adduction.

In 1950, by fixing fresh cadaver feet to boards and subjecting them to different stresses, Lauge-Hansen (11) devised a classification of ankle injuries based on the position of the foot and the deforming force at the time of injury. After the fracture had been created by a specific mechanism, the pathological anatomy of the fracture and ligamentous injury was determined by dissection. Later, radiographs were used to support the findings and to assist in classifying the fractures into appropriate categories. Lauge-Hansen's experimental work has been widely accepted, and his classification serves as a basis for evaluation of ankle injuries. Although this system is somewhat cumbersome, it is well worth mastering because it takes into account both fractures and ligamentous injuries (12, 13).

Lauge-Hansen Classification

Despite the fact that the Lauge-Hansen classification is based on cadaver experiments, investigators have shown that more than 95% of ankle fractures conform to the system (14). Lauge-Hansen (11) described four main patterns of injury based on the position of the foot at the time of impact and the direction of the injuring force—supination-adduction, pronation-abduction, supination-eversion, and pronation-eversion. Each pattern of injury was further subdivided into specific sequential stages. Later stages could not occur without the earlier stages having previously developed. This makes the Lauge-Hansen system particularly useful in determining soft tissue injury.

The first word of the system describes the foot position at the time of injury and the second word describes the overall motion of the foot (i.e., talus) through the injury. The actual terminology used by Lauge-Hansen is very misleading and may cause confusion when taken in a strict anatomical sense.

Supination-Adduction

The mechanism of the supination-adduction injury is relatively simple. It occurs with essentially pure inversion of the heel, inverting the talus through the ankle joint. The supinated foot is forced into inversion or adduction in relation to the cardinal plane of the body. Thus the Lauge-Hansen term *supination-adduction*. The talus is the primary agent delivering the pathological force through the ankle as vertical displacement of body weight occurs (Fig. 66.1).

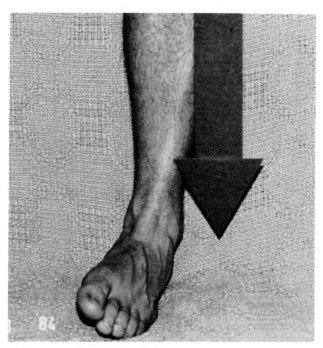

Figure 66.1. Position of foot and leg just before a supination-adduction injury. The arrow demonstrates the vertical displacement of body weight, which is the pathological force.

Direct inversion of the foot in this manner will cause some degree of rupture of the lateral collateral ligaments of the ankle or the classic avulsion fracture of the distal portion of the fibular malleolus (Figs. 66.2 and 66.3). This is a transverse fracture of the fibular malleolus at or below the level of the ankle joint. If the mechanism of injury continues, the talus will impact upon the medial malleolus, creating the classic vertical fracture (Fig. 66.4). The inferior tibiofibular syndesmosis and tibiofibular interosseous membrane remain intact in this injury pattern. A step-by-step sequence of injury is as follows.

STAGE 1

The first component of injury is failure of the lateral structures (Figs. 66.2 and 66.3). This may occur by partial or whole rupture of the lateral collateral ligaments or by an avulsion fracture of the lateral collateral ligaments from the distal fibula. The various grades of lateral ankle ligamentous sprains are subdivisions of this injury. When the fracture occurs, a varying portion of the lateral ligamentous structure must remain intact to create the avulsion of the distal fibula. This fibular fracture is a hallmark of this injury pattern (i.e., transverse fractures of the fibula at or below the ankle joint occur only in supination-adduction injuries). The fracture need not be present, however, and complete disruption of the lateral collateral ligaments may represent stage 1 of the injury instead.

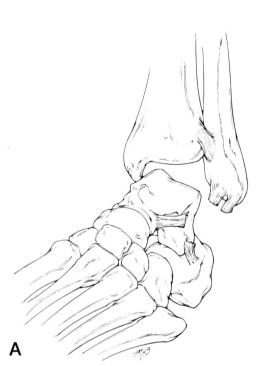

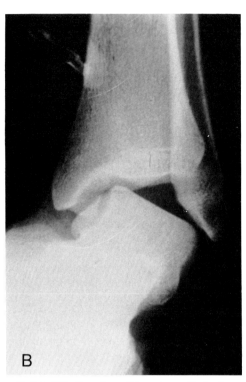

Figure 66.2. **A.** Supination-adduction stage 1 injury with disruption of the lateral collateral ankle ligaments. **B.** Lateral ankle stress radiograph (ankle stress inversion radiograph) revealing significant talar tilt. This finding sug-gests complete disruption of the calcaneofibular ligament and possible disruption of other lateral ligaments.

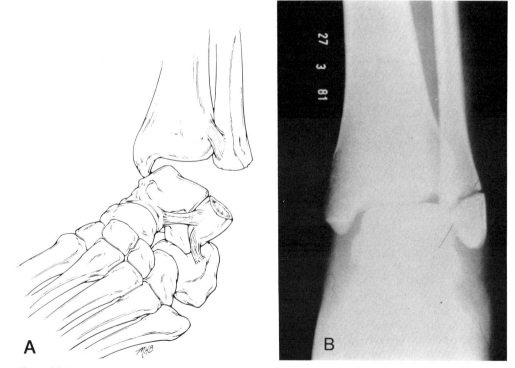

Figure 66.3. **A** and **B.** Supination-adduction stage 1 injury exhibiting a classic avulsion fracture of the fibular malleolus. Note that the lateral collateral ligaments remain intact.

STAGE 2

If the inversion force and motion continue, the talus pushes through the medial malleolus, creating the classic fracture with the fracture line somewhere between the horizontal and the vertical (Fig. 66.4). This fracture, like the distal transverse fibular fracture mentioned earlier, is seen only in supination-adduction injuries. This fracture only follows previous lateral injury as described in stage 1. Therefore, if an isolated vertical fracture of the medial malleolus is observed, complete disruption of the lateral collateral ligaments may be presumed. (Confirmation of this fact can be accomplished with lateral ankle stress radiographs.)

Pronation-Abduction

The second pattern of injury in the Lauge-Hansen classification system is also rather simple, occurring with pure eversion of the foot through the ankle mortise. The foot is in a pronated position at the time of impact. The lateral force of injury creates eversion or abduction of the foot away from the midline of the body. The vertical force of body weight is delivered through the ankle and everts the talus through the ankle joint mortise (Fig. 66.5).

The first injury will be either a complete disruption of the deltoid ligament or a transverse avulsion fracture of the medial malleolus (Figs. 66.6 and 66.7). If the pathological force continues, disruption of the inferior tibiofibular ligamentous complex occurs followed by a classic short oblique fracture of the fibular malleolus at the level of the ankle joint (Fig. 66.8). The stages of injury are as follows.

STAGE 1

The injury begins with partial or total disruption of the deltoid ligament or an avulsion fracture of the deltoid ligament from the medial malleolus (Figs. 66.6 and 66.7). The medial malleolar fracture in this injury is transverse (horizontal) and generally occurs at or below the tibiotalar articulation.

STAGE 2

Partial or complete disruption of the anterior and posterior inferior tibiofibular ligaments then occurs. As the everting talus contacts the fibular malleolus, the ligaments that bind the distal aspect of the fibula and tibia are torn. The anterior and posterior inferior tibiofibular ligaments may avulse small fragments of bone from the distal fibula and tibia instead of disrupting. Complete disruption of both ligamentous structures by either tearing through the body of the ligament or avulsion must occur for the injury pattern to progress to the next stage. The interosseous tibiofibular membrane remains intact in this injury.

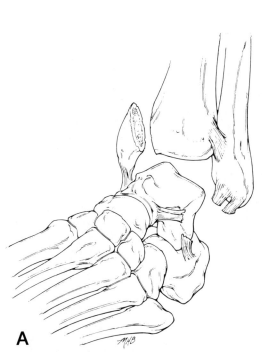
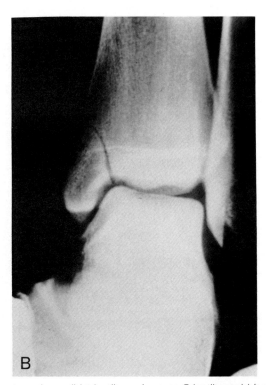

Figure 66.4. **A** and **B.** Supination-adduction stage 2 injury with disruption of the lateral collateral ligaments (stage 1) and a classic vertical fracture of medial malleolus (stage 2). Although the radiograph is not a stress view, mild talar tilt can be seen. Talar tilt would become more pronounced with lateral stress radiographs.

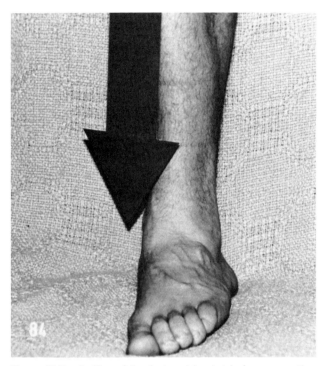

Figure 66.5. Position of the foot and leg just before a pronation-abduction injury. The arrow demonstrates the vertical displacement of body weight, which is the pathological force.

STAGE 3

The final injury in this pattern is a classic short fibular fracture occurring at the level of the tibiotalar joint line (Fig. 66.8). The hallmark appearance is confirmed on radiographic evaluation of the ankle as the anteroposterior view demonstrates a short oblique fracture and the lateral view demonstrates a transverse appearance of the fracture (Fig. 66.9). Frequently lateral comminution or a butterfly fragment may be visualized. No other injury pattern creates a fracture of the fibula at this level with this appearance. If this classical fibular fracture is visualized without apparent medial malleolar fracture, then complete deltoid ligament disruption may be presumed (confirmation can be obtained with medial ankle stress radiographs if desired).

Supination-Eversion

Supination-eversion and pronation-eversion are actually misnomers as eversion in this instance refers to external, outward, or lateral rotation. The primary motion is a transverse plane external rotation of the talus out of the ankle mortise. The key to the differentiation of supination-eversion and pronation-eversion injuries is the direction in which the talus pivots as it rotates through the ankle mortise.

Lauge-Hansen (11) described the foot as being in a supinated attitude at the time of impact. The forefoot is actually inverted in relationship to the leg with the foot being

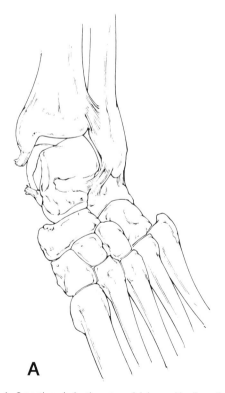

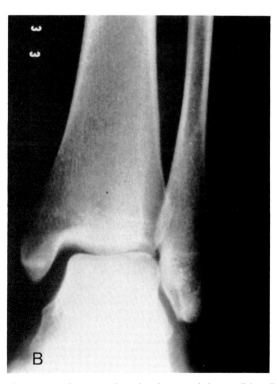

Figure 66.6. **A.** Pronation-abduction stage 1 injury with disruption of the medial collateral ankle (deltoid) ligaments. **B.** Note the medial clear space between the talar dome and the medial malleolus, suggesting medial ligamentous disruption.

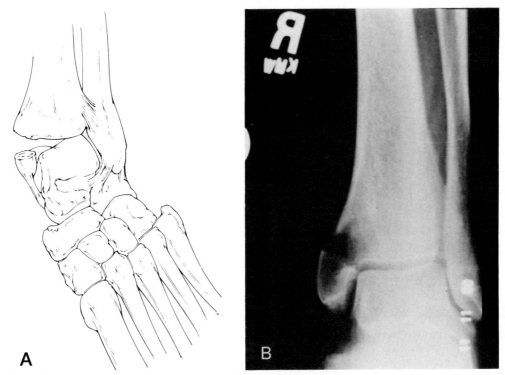

A

Figure 66.7. **A** and **B.** Pronation-abduction stage 1 injury demonstrating an avulsion fracture of the tibial malleolus. Note that the medial ligamentous structures remain intact when this avulsion fracture occurs.

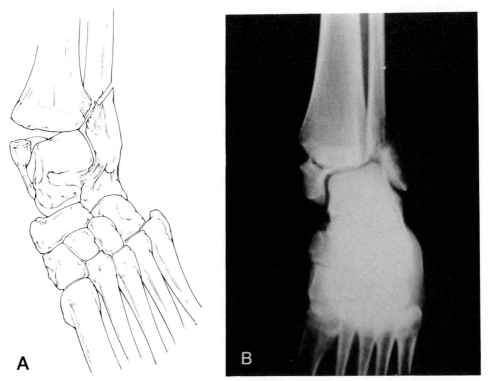

A

Figure 66.8. **A** and **B.** Pronation-abduction stage 3 injury with avulsion fracture of the medial malleolus (stage 1), disruption of the inferior tibio-fibular ligamentous complex (stage 2), and a classic short oblique fracture of the lateral malleolus (stage 3).

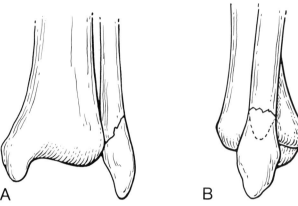

Figure 66.9. **A.** Fibular fracture of a pronation-abduction stage 3 injury in an anteroposterior view. Note that the fracture line is oblique (short spiral) in appearance. **B.** Fibular fracture of pronation-abduction stage 3 injury in a lateral view. Note that the fracture is transverse in appearance in the lateral view because of the absence of a rotational component in the pathological force.

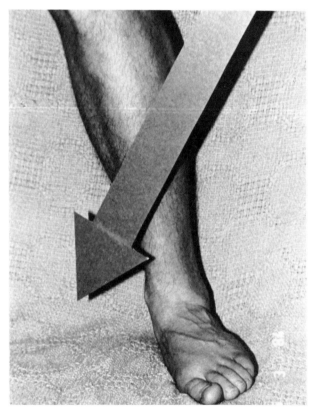

Figure 66.10. Position of the foot and leg just before a supination-eversion injury. The arrow indicates the direction of the pathological force.

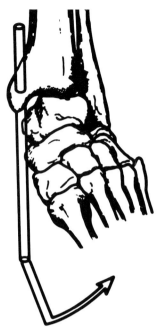

Figure 66.11. Medial pivot point in a supination-eversion injury pattern. External rotation occurs about this medial axis.

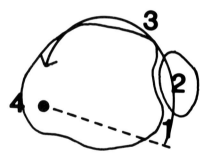

Figure 66.12. Transverse plane schematic of a supination-eversion injury pattern showing stages of the injury.

firmly planted on the ground. He then described the direction of injury as eversion. As stated earlier, this is a misnomer and the motion is really external rotation. In actuality the injury occurs as the knee is flexed and the leg rotates inwardly. The talus creates pressure against the fibular mal-

leolus and there is a slight moment of dorsiflexion of the foot at the ankle as the knee buckles (Fig. 66.10). Thus eversion describes the external rotation of the talus out of the ankle joint mortise.

In the supination-eversion injury pattern the talus pivots around the medial malleolus with the medial malleolus and deltoid ligament acting as the axis of rotation (Fig. 66.11). As the talus pivots externally about the medial malleolar axis anterior injury occurs first. The talus contacts the fibula and the anterior inferior tibiofibular ligament is either disrupted or avulsed from the tibia (Tillaux-Chaput fragment) or fibula (Wagstaffe fracture). Next a classical spiral fracture of the fibula beginning at the tibiotalar syndesmosis is created. The injury then continues posteriorly, disrupting the posterior inferior tibiofibular ligament or avulsing it from the tibia (Volkmann's fracture) or fibula. Finally the axis itself is disrupted and either the deltoid is torn or an avulsion fracture of the medial malleolus is created (Fig. 66.12). The stages of this injury in sequence are as follows.

STAGE 1

Partial or complete disruption of the anterior inferior tibiofibular ligament. The ligament may also avulse from the anterior inferior tibia or the anterior inferior fibula as opposed to a midbody rupture. Complete disruption or avulsion must occur for the injury to progress to the next stage.

STAGE 2

A classical spiral fracture of the fibular malleolus develops beginning at the tibiofibular syndesmosis and extending

proximally (Fig. 66.13). The fracture begins at the anterior aspect of the ankle joint, and as the talus externally rotates the fracture progresses laterally and proximally to the posterior aspect of the fibula. The spiral fracture of the fibular malleolus beginning at the joint line only occurs in this pattern of injury.

STAGE 3

With disruption of the fibula, the next structure to be encountered is the posterior inferior tibiofibular ligament. Par-

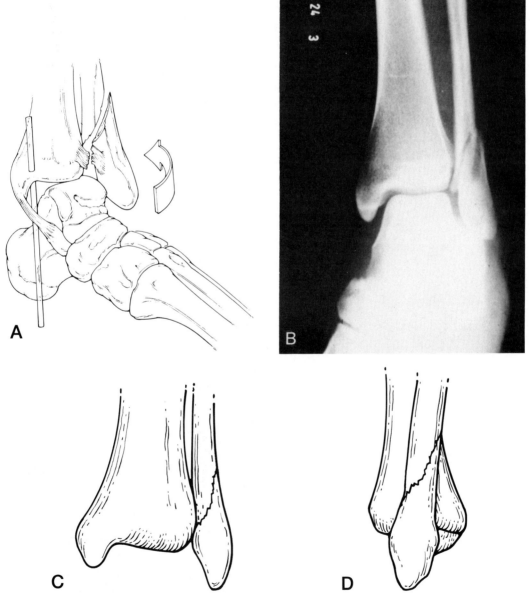

Figure 66.13. **A** and **B.** Supination-eversion stage 2 injury with disruption of the anterior inferior tibiofibular ligament (stage 1) and classic spiral fracture of fibular malleolus (stage 2). **C** and **D.** Note the fibular fracture line in this injury is spiral in appearance in both the anteroposterior and lateral ankle views.

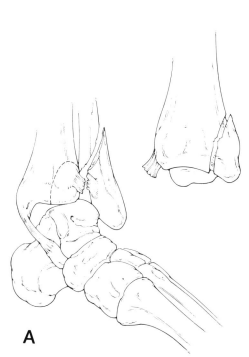

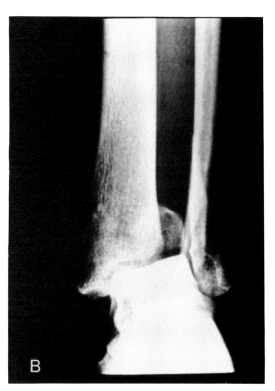

Figure 66.14. **A** and **B.** Supination-eversion stage 3 injury with disruption of the anterior inferior tibiofibular ligament (stage 1), classic spiral fracture of lateral malleolus (stage 2), and avulsion fracture of posterior inferior portion of the tibia (stage 3).

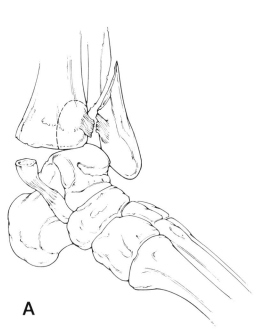

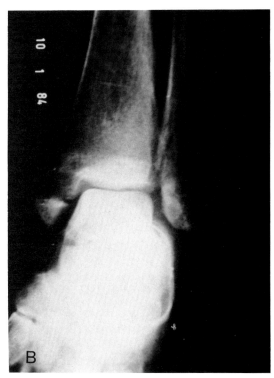

Figure 66.15. **A** and **B.** Supination-eversion stage 4 injury demonstrating disruption of the anterior inferior tibiofibular ligament (stage 1), the classic spiral fracture of the lateral malleolus (stage 2), disruption of the posterior inferior tibiofibular ligament (stage 3), and an avulsion fracture of the medial malleolus (stage 4).

tial or complete disruption of this ligament may occur. Alternatively, the ligament may avulse the posterior inferior portion of the tibia from Volkmann's triangle or the posterior inferior fibula (Fig. 66.14).

STAGE 4

If the force of injury continues the ankle will dislocate, and finally disruption of the deltoid ligament or a transverse avulsion fracture of the medial malleolus will occur (Fig. 66.15).

Pronation-Eversion

Like the supination-eversion pattern, this mechanism involves an external rotation of the talus out of the ankle joint mortise. However, this time the talus pivots around the fibula and lateral collateral ligaments (Fig. 66.16). Lauge-Hansen (11) describes the foot position at the time of injury as being pronated with the motion occurring as eversion. The foot is in a pronated attitude as the rotational torque of the talus creates the fracture pattern. There is a slight moment of plantarflexion of the foot as it is pulled laterally out of the ankle joint (Fig. 66.17).

This establishes immediate tension on the deltoid ligament and the medial structures are the first to fail. Disruption of the deltoid ligament or a transverse avulsion fracture of the medial malleolus occurs first. The injury then con-

tinues anteriorly and the anterior inferior tibiofibular ligament is disrupted or avulsed from the anterior inferior tibia (fragment of Tillaux-Chaput) or anterior inferior fibula (Wagstaffe fracture). The injury progresses up the tibiofibular interosseous membrane and fibular fracture above the tibiofibular syndesmosis is created. Finally, the injury continues posteriorly, and the posterior inferior tibiofibular ligament is disrupted or avulsed from the posterior inferior tibia (Volkmann's fracture) or posterior inferior fibula (Fig. 66.18). The stages of the injury are as follows.

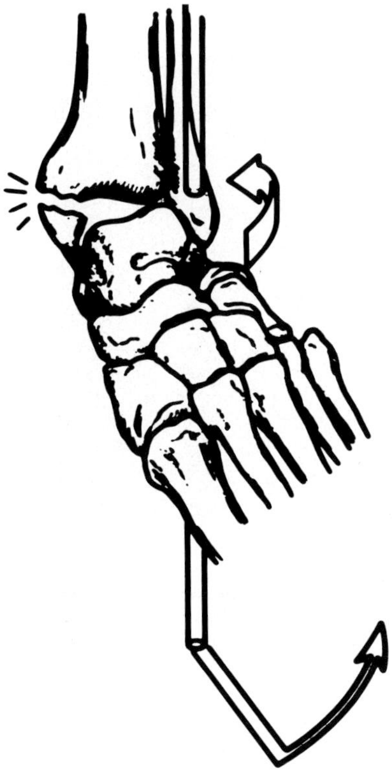

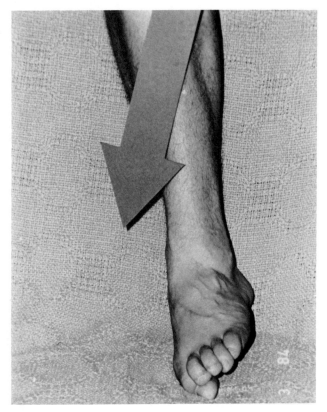

Figure 66.17. Position of the foot and leg just before a pronation-eversion injury. The arrow indicates the direction of the pathological force.

Figure 66.16. Lateral pivot point in pronation-eversion injury pattern. External rotation occurs about this lateral axis.

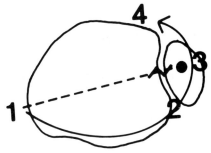

Figure 66.18. Transverse plane demonstration of a pronation-eversion injury pattern showing stages of the injury.

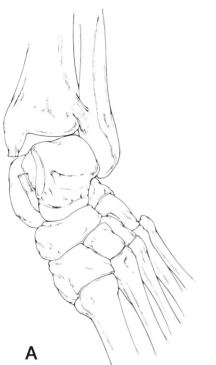

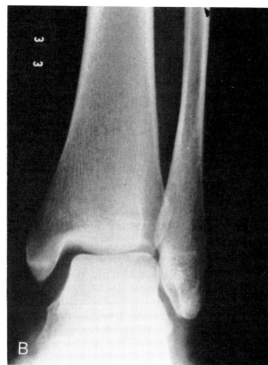

Figure 66.19. **A.** Pronation-eversion stage 1 injury demonstrating disruption of the medial collateral (deltoid) ligaments. **B.** Anteroposterior view of the ankle exhibiting a medial clear space suggesting medial ligamentous disruption.

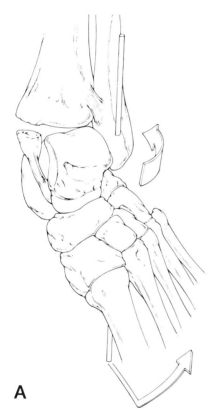

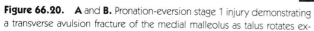

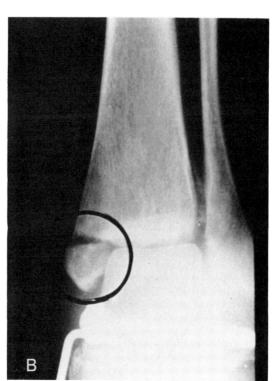

Figure 66.20. **A** and **B.** Pronation-eversion stage 1 injury demonstrating a transverse avulsion fracture of the medial malleolus as talus rotates externally about a lateral pivot. Note in this avulsion fracture that the medial ligaments remain intact.

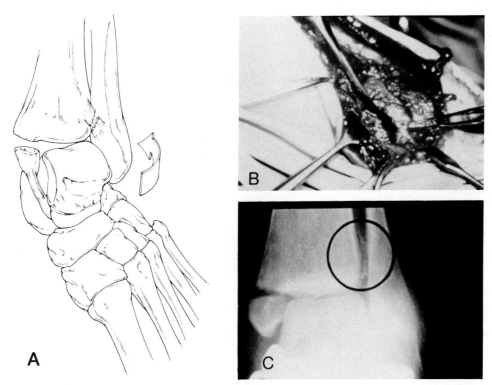

Figure 66.21. **A.** Pronation-eversion stage 2 injury with an avulsion fracture of the medial malleolus (stage 1) and disruption of the anterior inferior tibiofibular ligament (stage 2) as talus rotates externally about a lateral point. **B** and **C.** Radiographic and surgical evidence of diastasis between the tibia and fibula.

STAGE 1

The first stage is a partial or complete disruption of the deltoid ligament (Fig. 66.19). Instead of completely tearing, the ligament may create a transverse avulsion fracture of the medial malleolus (Fig. 66.20). Complete disruption of the ligament or an avulsion fracture must occur for the injury to progress to the next stage.

STAGE 2

With further external rotation, the anterior inferior tibiofibular ligament is disrupted or avulsed from the anterior inferior tibial tubercle of Chaput or the anterior inferior fibula (Fig. 66.21). After this disruption the injury will continue proximally between the tibia and the fibula with rupture of the tibiofibular interosseous membrane.

STAGE 3

The tibiofibular interosseous membrane is torn a varying distance proximally until a classical fibular fracture occurs somewhere above the tibiofibular syndesmosis (Fig. 66.22). On rare occasions the fibula will not fracture and the proximal tibiofibular articulation will dislocate. A high fracture at the fibular neck is known as a Maisonneuve fracture. A fibular fracture occurring entirely above the tibiofibular syndesmosis is a hallmark of this injury. However, blunt trauma to the lateral aspect of the leg may also create this type of fracture.

STAGE 4

Once the fibular shaft has failed and motion continues, the posterior inferior tibiofibular ligament is disrupted or avulsed from the posterior inferior tibia at Volkmann's triangle or the posterior inferior fibula (Fig. 66.23).

• • •

Other more simplified mechanisms have been formulated for classification of ankle fractures where ease of memorization and application is desired. The Danis-Weber classification is one of the more popular simplified descriptions and has been used by Scandinavian authors in describing internal fixation methods. This commonly used system may be directly correlated to the Lauge-Hansen classification system.

Danis-Weber Classification

Recognizing the importance of the fibular fracture in ankle injuries, the Danis-Weber classification is based on the relationship of the fibular fracture line to the ankle joint (15). Three groups of injuries are described on the basis of whether the fibular fracture line begins below the inferior

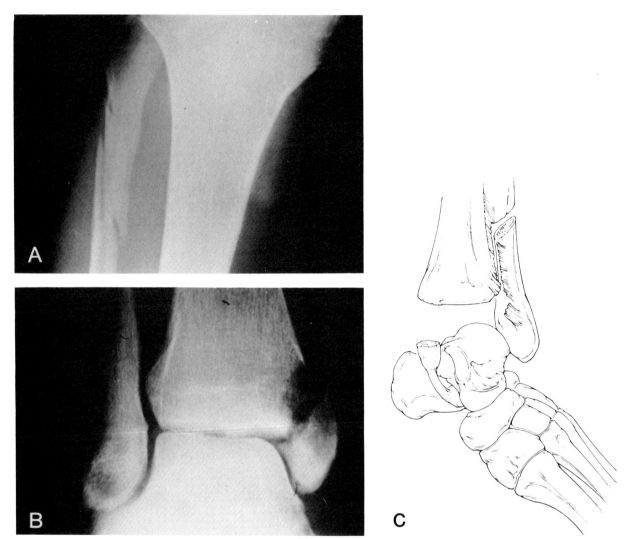

Figure 66.22. **A** to **C.** Pronation-eversion stage 3 injury with an avulsion fracture of the medial malleolus (stage 1), disruption of the anterior inferior tibiofibular syndesmosis (type A), at the level of the syn-desmosis (type B), or above the syndesmosis (type C). Generally the higher the fibular fracture, the more extensive the damage to the tibiofibular ligaments and the greater the degree of instability at the ankle mortise. Therefore the severity of injury to the ligamentous complex and the severity of the malleolar fracture increases progressively from fracture type A to fracture type C (8).

tibiofibular ligament and tibiofibular interosseous membrane (stage 2), and a classic high fibular fracture (stage 3).

The medial malleolus may be intact or fractured, with the fracture line somewhere between the horizontal and the vertical. The posterior edge of the tibia is usually intact, although rarely is there a medial posterior fragment when there is a medial malleolar fracture.

The type A injury corresponds directly with the supination-adduction mechanism as described by Lauge-Hansen (11) (Figs. 66.1 to 66.4). When present, either transverse avulsion fractures of the fibula and/or relatively vertical fractures of the medial malleolus are hallmarks of these injuries. Fractures of this type are generally the easiest to treat.

TYPE A

The type A injury involves a transverse avulsion fracture of the fibula either at the level of the ankle joint or distally. It may also be represented by rupture of the lateral collateral ligaments with the fibula remaining intact.

The inferior tibiofibular ligamentous complex (anterior and posterior inferior tibiofibular ligaments) is always intact. Consequently, the tibiofibular interosseous membrane is also intact and there is never any tibiofibular diastasis with this injury.

TYPE B

The type B injury involves a spiral or oblique fracture of the fibula, beginning at the level of the inferior tibiofibular syndesmosis. The fracture may be smooth or comminuted, depending on the forces involved.

The inferior tibiofibular ligamentous complex is usually

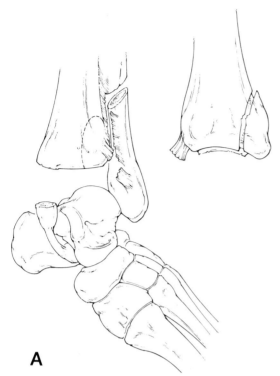

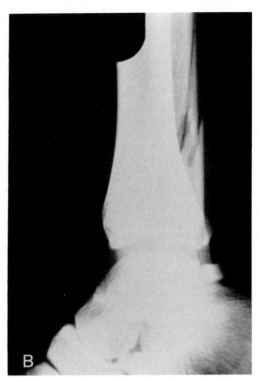

Figure 66.23. **A** and **B.** Pronation-eversion stage 4 injury with an avulsion fracture of medial malleolus (stage 1), disruption of the anterior inferior tibiofibular ligament and tibiofibular interosseous membrane (stage 2), classic high fibular fracture (stage 3), and an avulsion fracture of posterior inferior tibiofibular ligament from Volkmann's triangle.

partially disrupted. The anterior inferior tibiofibular ligament is either partially or completely torn or avulsed from its insertion to the anterior tibia (fracture of Tillaux-Chaput) or the anterior fibula (Wagstaffe fracture). The posterior inferior tibiofibular ligament is either intact or disrupted, depending on the force of the injury. The equivalent of a posterior inferior tibiofibular ligamentous disruption is an avulsion of the ligament from its attachment to the posterior tibia (Volkmann's fracture) or the posterior fibula. The tibiofibular interosseous membrane is intact.

The medial malleolus may be intact, or it may demonstrate an avulsion fracture of varying size. If the medial malleolus is intact, disruption of the deltoid ligament may be present.

Type B injuries correspond with both pronation-abduction (Figs. 66.5 to 66.9) and supination-eversion injuries (Figs. 66.10 to 66.15) in the Lauge-Hansen classification system. The Danis-Weber classification is, therefore, most variable in this type of injury. Furthermore, a shortcoming of the Danis-Weber system may be appreciated in that type B injuries encompass those created by two drastically different mechanisms (i.e., pronation-abduction and supination-eversion). This makes closed and open reduction of type B injuries haphazard unless the correlation to the Lauge-Hansen mechanism is appreciated.

TYPE C

The type C injury encompasses fibular fractures above the tibiofibular syndesmosis, anywhere between the fibular syn-

desmosis and the head of the fibula. Very rarely, it may appear as a dislocation of the proximal tibiofibular joint.

The inferior tibiofibular ligamentous complex is disrupted. The anterior and posterior inferior tibiofibular ligaments are either ruptured through their substance or avulsed from their bony attachments to the tibia or the fibula. The tibiofibular interosseous membrane is ruptured from the level of the ankle joint to the level of the fibular fracture. Thus tibiofibular diastasis is present. Medially, there is always associated injury—either a transverse avulsion fracture of the medial malleolus or disruption of the deltoid ligament.

The type C injury corresponds with the pronation-eversion mechanism of Lauge-Hansen (Figs. 66.15 to 66.23). The hallmark of the injury in both systems is the high fibular fracture with tibiofibular diastasis. These injuries are generally the most difficult to treat.

DIAGNOSIS

An understanding of the mechanisms of ankle fractures, combined with clinical and radiographic evaluation, enable the surgeon to accurately diagnose and classify ankle injuries. Standard radiographic evaluation includes a mortise view, or 20° medial oblique, as well as lateral and 45° medial oblique views. The ankle mortise view allows examination of the tibial and fibular malleoli, the fibular shaft, and the distal tibial epiphysis, as well as the talar dome and the tibial plafond. The lateral ankle view allows further assessment of the fibular fracture and the aforementioned structures, as well as the posterior malleolus (third malleolus) of the tibia. Further oblique views may be obtained to enhance evaluation of particular structures of concern, such as the tubercle of Tillaux-Chaput at the tibial attachment of the anterior inferior tibiofibular ligament. Radiographs of the superior aspect of the leg may also be indicated, as in the pronation-eversion fractures.

Stress radiography may be necessary to evaluate ligamentous stability. In abduction and eversion fracture mechanisms (types B and C), stress eversion radiography may be necessary to diagnose deltoid ligament rupture when the medial malleolus remains intact. Stress inversion radiography may aid the diagnosis of fibular collateral ligamentous disruption in supination-adduction (type A) injuries, when the lateral malleolus remains intact. Although the syndesmosis is always disrupted in pronation-eversion (type C) fractures, stress radiography may be helpful in confirming tibiofibular diastasis.

Finally, clinical examination will prove most helpful in diagnosing questionable ligamentous or osseous injuries. Localized edema, ecchymosis, and palpable tenderness will suggest probable injury to the astute clinician. Tomograms and magnetic resonance images may also be obtained to assess degrees of articular involvement or specific soft tissue structures. A combination of clinical and radiographic findings will establish the diagnosis.

TREATMENT

Once the patient has been examined, one must decide whether to treat the injury by open or closed methods. Many factors must be evaluated before a specific course of treatment can be established; these include the patient's age, health, occupation, and activity level. The patient's psychological makeup and intellectual capabilities should be evaluated. The surgeon's own experience and knowledge of ankle fractures are paramount if he or she chooses to undertake management of the injury.

Considering that ankle fractures are intra-articular injuries, every attempt should be made to accurately realign the joint in an effort to avoid painful and disabling posttraumatic arthrosis. Treatment must focus on restoration of the length of the fibula, realignment of the ankle mortise, evaluation of the talar dome and the tibial plafond, and reapproximation of supporting soft tissue structures. Of utmost concern is the exact restoration of the length of the fibula (16). Accurate reconstruction of the mortise and avoidance of arthrosis depend on an exact anatomical fit of the fibula into the fibular notch of the tibia. For this reason, the fibular fracture is termed the dominant fracture in those injuries that fit the Lauge-Hansen and Danis-Weber classifications. Repair and stabilization of the inferior tibiofibular syndesmosis take second priority after restoration of fibular length. Reduction and stabilization of the tibial components of the fracture, both posterior and medial malleoli, as well as repair of ruptured collateral ligaments, complete joint reconstruction. Although controversy exists as to whether certain ankle fractures should be treated open or closed, current literature, as well as the authors' own experience, tends to support open reduction with rigid internal fixation for unstable injuries that involve more than minimal displacement (17-22).

Nonoperative Treatment

Nonoperative treatment of ankle fractures consists primarily of closed reduction if necessary, followed by maintenance of the reduction. Although closed reduction and casting do not always result in anatomic reduction and some degree of arthrosis may ensue, the techniques should be fully understood and mastered by any surgeon who treats ankle fractures. Closed reduction serves a vital role in the emergency treatment of displaced ankle fractures involving distal neurovascular compromise (Fig. 66.24). Moreover, debilitated patients or those who are considered poor operative risks may also benefit from closed reduction. Furthermore, certain malleolar fractures with mild displacement, such as supination-eversion stage 2 injuries, have been shown to respond favorably to appropriate closed reduction (23-26).

Closed reduction can be a successful tool only in the hands of the surgeon who fully understands the mechanism of injury that created the specific fracture pattern. An understanding of the Lauge-Hansen classification system will, therefore, greatly facilitate closed reduction of malleolar fractures of the four basic types. Other factors that must be considered before closed reduction is attempted include the patient's level of comfort as well as skeletal muscle spasm and relaxation. Usually general anesthesia is best for controlling these factors. Frequently intravenous sedation and analgesia with diazepam or medazolam combined with meperidine may be used, especially in the emergency room. These agents require careful monitoring of the patient and are best administered with the assistance of other emergency room personnel or an anesthesiologist. Local tissue factors are also important when one is considering closed reduction because excessive soft tissue edema may make the procedure quite difficult.

Strong consideration should be given to the edema that will continue to develop after closed reduction. If an ankle fracture is treated within a short period of time after injury and the ankle is placed in plaster immobilization, the normal posttraumatic edema will soon fill the confines of the cast. Moreover, it is common practice to reduce the amount of padding lining the contoured cast when a fracture is treated with closed reduction and immobilization, thus allowing even less room for the accommodation of edema. For this reason, we recommend the use of a modified compression splint or plaster shell, contoured to maintain reduction, in the early phases of acute fracture care. Close observation of the extremity must follow, with attention paid to the patient's complaints in an effort to avoid pressure lesions and vascular compromise of the skin and other soft tissues. The surgeon must be prepared to bivalve or reapply the cast to accommodate increasing or decreasing edema. If the cast is applied to an edematous extremity, edema will eventually resolve, considerable motion may become available within

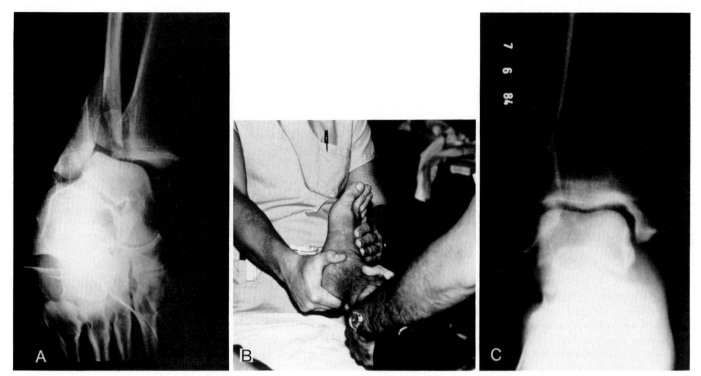

Figure 66.24. **A.** Radiograph of a displaced stage 4 supination-eversion fracture of a right ankle on presentation to the emergency room. The patient's complaints included numbness of the fourth and fifth toes and paresthesias involving the dorsolateral aspect of the tarsus. The dorsalis pedis pulse was markedly diminished compared with the contralateral limb. **B.** Emergency closed reduction with the patient sedated with intravenous diazepam and meperidine. **C.** Postreduction radiograph. The dorsalis pedis pulse improved and the paresthesias diminished. The patient was subsequently taken for emergency ORIF.

the cast, and reduction may be lost. Close monitoring of any fracture treated with closed reduction is mandatory.

The basic concept of closed reduction of any fracture is initially to recreate the injury, apply appropriate traction to the distal part, and then reverse the mechanism of injury to relocate the fracture fragments (27). The principles necessitate stabilization of the lower extremity with manual counterpressure and traction in the proximal calf region. The surgeon stands at the foot of the table and actually performs the reduction. Maintenance of the reduction and prevention of overcorrection depend on the intact soft tissue hinge (Fig. 66.25). Soft tissues (periosteum, capsule, ligaments, and tendons) on the concave side of the injury remain intact, whereas those on the convex side are considered ruptured. Appropriate traction places the intact soft tissues under tension and removes interposing soft tissues from between fracture fragments. On reversal of the fracture mechanism, the intact soft tissues effect a tension band or hinge that guides reduction and prevents subluxation in the direction of overcorrection. A fracture that displays no primary displacement does not require closed reduction.

After closed reduction, temporary stabilization is achieved manually or with a splint and radiographs are obtained to confirm adequate anatomical realignment. A cast with an appropriate amount of cotton padding is then applied. Only a curved cast will maintain the correction; therefore, a three-

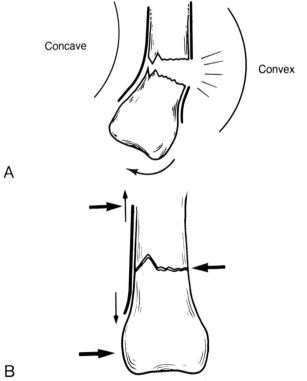

Figure 66.25. **A.** Soft tissue hinge. **B.** Its application during reduction.

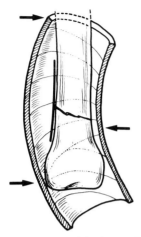

Figure 66.26. Curved plaster supplying three-point pressure to maintain reduction.

point pressure technique is used following manual reduction (Fig. 66.26). Closed reduction requires approximately 6 to 8 weeks of non-weight-bearing below-the-knee cast immobilization. For high fibular fractures and injuries involving extensive soft tissue disruption, the patient should be placed in an above-the-knee cast. Periodic radiographic evaluations should be made during the healing phase, and rehabilitative range of motion exercises are prohibited until the cast is removed.

SPECIFIC TECHNIQUES OF CLOSED REDUCTION OF ANKLE FRACTURES

Supination-Adduction Fracture (Type A)

In the supination-adduction injury, the surgeon should grasp the foot by the heel and midarch and rotate the heel and foot with an inverting motion. Distal traction is then applied, with the surgeon attempting to pull the foot away from the tibia and then reversing the direction of motion and everting the heel and forefoot to bring the foot and ankle back beneath the tibia. As the foot and ankle are everted, a tension band effect is created along the intact medial soft tissue structures, preventing lateral subluxation of the fracture fragments. This maneuver should relocate the medial and lateral malleolar components of this fracture.

Occasionally, in more severe injuries or in certain variations of the supination-adduction mechanism, there may be entrapment of soft tissue structures, such as the peroneal or the tibialis posterior tendons within the fracture gap. This condition could make closed reduction impossible.

After closed reduction and radiographic evaluation, the reduction is maintained by application of the cast by a three-point reduction (pressure) technique. Medial pressure is applied to the heel, forcing the foot into eversion, while a lateral counterpressure is applied just above the lateral malleolus. The surgeon manually applies pressure at these two areas. The third point of pressure is the proximal extent of the cast itself, the proximal tibia being forced against the

medial aspect of the cast. This three-point pressure, or curved cast, is critical to maintenance of the reduction.

Pronation-Abduction Fracture (Type B)

The technique for reduction of the pronation-abduction fracture is the opposite of that used for closed reduction of the supination-adduction injury. The surgeon recreates the injury by everting the heel and foot. Distal traction is applied to the foot, after which the heel and foot are rotated into inversion, thereby reducing both fibular and tibial malleolar fractures. The intact lateral soft tissues create a tension band effect that maintains the reduction. The same principles and three-point reduction concept pertain to the application of the immobilizing cast.

Supination-Eversion Fracture (Type B)

Reduction of the supination-eversion ankle fracture requires a complex maneuver to obtain accurate anatomical reduction. While the proximal tibia is stabilized, the surgeon grasps the foot and heel with the internal hand (the surgeon's left hand when reducing a fracture of the left ankle) at the posterior aspect of the heel, and the external hand (the surgeon's right hand when reducing a fracture of the left ankle) at the lateral aspect of the forefoot.

The injury is recreated by external rotation of the foot with slight eversion. A strong distal traction is applied, after which the calcaneus is pulled forward while the foot is strongly rotated in the direction of internal rotation and slight plantarflexion. This maneuver will initially open the fibular fracture and allow distraction. The forward pull on the calcaneus will allow closed reduction to occur around the posterior surface of the fibular fracture. Plantarflexion is necessary to maintain distal traction on the fibular malleolus as the internal rotation closes the gap. This can be a difficult fracture to treat by closed reduction because of the shortening that occurs with the fibular fracture and valgus shift of the ankle, especially in stage 3 and 4 lesions. After reduction, the foot and leg are incorporated into a curved plaster cast for immobilization. Good long-term follow-up results have been reported after closed reduction of stage 2 supination-eversion fractures (23, 24).

Pronation-Eversion Fracture (Type C)

The surgeon will generally find the pronation-eversion fracture quite easy to reduce because usually there is considerable soft tissue instability. The injury is recreated by external rotation of the foot with slight pronation or eversion. The reduction technique is essentially identical to that used for the supination-eversion fracture, with distal traction and slight anterior pull on the calcaneus. The foot is then forced through internal rotation with supination and slight plantarflexion. Because of the torque-induced rotary nature of this fracture, the soft tissue restraints that would be used as tension banding structures are often destroyed. Overcorrection of this fracture with less than anatomical reduction is quite possible. Furthermore, the high degree of instability associated with the pronation-eversion fracture makes it quite easy to lose the reduction in the process of cast application or at any time after the reduction.

Once an acceptable reduction has been accomplished, it is imperative that the correction be monitored during the healing phase. If any unacceptable shift is identified, the surgeon must consider an additional closed reduction or an open surgical reduction.

Operative Treatment

For many years the Swiss AO and others have espoused open reduction with rigid internal fixation as the treatment of choice for most ankle fractures (17, 20-24). The principles and techniques described here for the operative treatment of ankle fractures are those originally developed by the AO. The primary advantages of these techniques are direct visualization of the injury and the ability to obtain accurate anatomical reduction. The internal fixation devices provide rigid maintenance of the reduction and allow active rehabilitation of the fractured ankle during the healing phase. This avoids the condition of cast disease by preventing excessive loss of soft tissue mass and strength and by preventing the development of immobilization-induced arthrosis.

The ideal time for open reduction and internal fixation in the healthy individual is immediately after the injury, before the traumatized ankle becomes excessively edematous. Early surgical intervention allows evacuation of hematoma and prevents further edema and internal hemorrhage. Optimally, if the patient is seen within 6 hours after injury, surgery is quite feasible. Often if treatment is postponed beyond 6 to 12 hours, the ankle will respond with reactive edema, internal hemorrhage, and compromise of circulation to the skin. This may make wound closure very difficult, predisposing the patient to infection. However, the prompt application of a Jones compression cast and the institution of ice, elevation, and bed rest will typically prevent excessive edema from developing while the patient awaits surgical reduction.

If the patient has considerable edema and hematoma, it is often recommended that conservative therapy be initiated and continued for several days. Progressive hematoma, on the other hand, suggests vascular injury requiring surgical exploration and institution of hemostasis. Otherwise, therapy should involve closed reduction as necessary, application of a modified Jones compression dressing, and maintenance of elevation, ice, and rest. Certain injuries may benefit from skeletal traction or application of an external fixation frame. Once the reactive edema and commonly associated skin conditions such as fracture blisters (Fig. 66.27) have resolved, surgical intervention may be considered. The delay may be from 5 days to 2 weeks, depending on the nature of the injury and the success in controlling post-traumatic edema and hematoma.

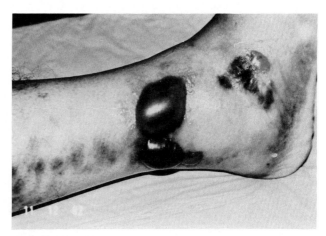

Figure 66.27. Severe fracture blisters associated with pronation-eversion ankle fracture.

SURGICAL APPROACHES

The primary goal of operative treatment is to restore the length of the fibula, followed by repair of the inferior tibiofibular syndesmosis and anatomical reconstruction of the ankle mortise. Surgical treatment begins laterally by open reduction and stabilization of the fractured fibula. The patient is positioned on the table in the contralateral decubitus position on the vacuum pack with the fractured fibula upward. One must be careful to pad the contralateral common peroneal nerve at the proximal aspect of the fibula. Alternatively, the limb may be placed in the supine position with knee flexion and the proximal portion of the leg supported with a bump or sling device. Typically, a long curvilinear skin incision, starting approximately 3 to 5 cm superior to the lateral malleolus and just posterior to the shaft of the fibula, is used (Fig. 66.28A). The incision is continued distally, gently curving anteriorly over the tip of the lateral malleolus and terminating approximately 3 cm distal and inferior to the malleolus. The tissues are dissected in anatomical layers, with care to avoid injury to both the sural and intermediate dorsal cutaneous nerves. This exposure allows visualization of the fibula, the anteroinferior tibiofibular ligament, and the fibular collateral ligaments, as well as the lateral aspect of the talar dome and the tibial plafond. A posterior malleolar fracture (Volkmann's fracture) of the tibia may also be directly reduced and fixated through this incision, although elongation may be necessary.

After reduction and fixation of the fibula and repair of the anterior syndesmosis, the vacuum pack is deflated and the patient is turned to the supine position. The fractured limb is allowed to rotate externally, thus presenting the medial aspect of the ankle. Typically, a curvilinear skin incision, starting just posterior and superior to the medial malleolus and gently curving anteriorly as it approaches the tip of the medial malleolus, is used (Fig. 66.28B). This incision terminates approximately 2 to 3 cm distal to the tip of the malleolus. The tissues are dissected in anatomical layers, with care taken to avoid damage to the saphenous vein and

Figure 66.28. **A.** Lateral exposure for access to the distal fibula, anterior-inferior tibiofibular ligament and fibular collateral ligaments, talar and tibial articular surfaces, and direct reduction of a posterior triangle fracture. **B.** Medial exposure for access to the medial malleolus, deltoid ligament, and articular surfaces.

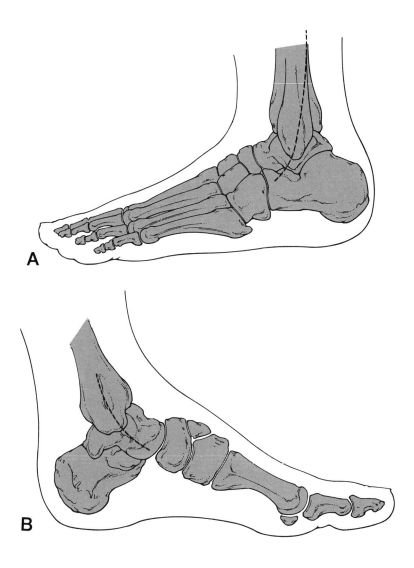

nerve as the deep fascia over the malleolus is exposed. This exposure allows visualization of the medial malleolus and the deltoid ligament, as well as the medial aspect of the talar dome and the tibial plafond. Furthermore, direct reduction and indirect fixation of a large posterior malleolar fragment (Volkmann's fracture) of the tibia may be performed through this incision after proximal elongation. The medial approach may also be designed so that the skin incision starts at the anterosuperior margin of the medial malleolus, gently curving posteriorly as it traverses the tip of the malleolus to end approximately 2 to 3 cm distal to the malleolus. This anteromedial exposure allows indirect fixation of a large posterior triangle fragment of the tibia after direct reduction of the posterior fragment via the posterolateral exposure.

SPECIFIC TECHNIQUES OF OPEN REDUCTION INTERNAL FIXATION OF BASIC ANKLE FRACTURES

The discussion that follows focuses on reduction and fixation of the four basic malleolar fracture patterns of the Lauge-Hansen classification system. The discussion is also organized to portray the practical benefits of the Danis-Weber classification system. Open reductions with internal fixation (ORIF) begin at the lateral aspect of the ankle with realignment and fixation of the fibula and repair of the syndesmosis, followed by inspection and repair of the medial and posterior aspects of the joint as necessary. In all cases the articular surfaces of the tibial plafond and the talar dome should be examined during surgery, and ankle range of motion and ligamentous stress resistance should be periodically assessed. Intraoperative radiographs should be obtained to confirm proper reduction of the fragments, once temporary reduction has been achieved. Another set of radiographs should be taken before wound closure to confirm final osseous alignment and placement of fixation devices.

Supination-Adduction Fracture (Type A)

FIBULAR REPAIR. Stage I of the supination-adduction injury involves a transverse avulsion fracture of the fibula at or distal to the joint line (inferior to the syndesmosis) or disruption of the lateral collateral ligaments of the ankle. The

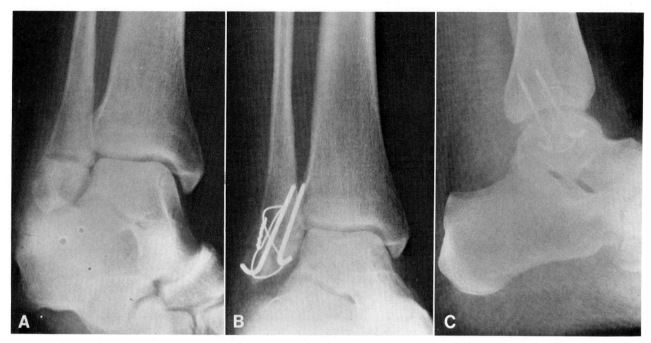

Figure 66.29. **A.** Stage 1 supination-adduction right ankle fracture. **B** and **C.** Postoperative mortise and lateral radiographs. Note the parallel relationship of the axial Kirschner wires.

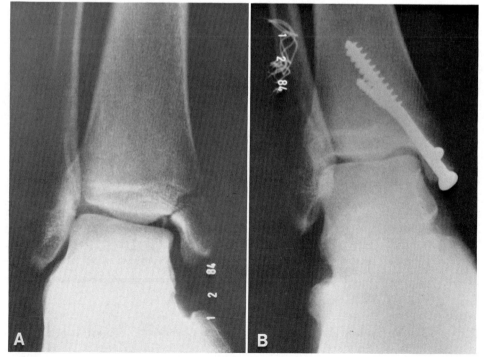

Figure 66.30. **A.** Stage 2 supination-adduction fracture with impaction of the medial aspect of tibial plafond. **B.** Fixation with two interfragmental lag screws following local shift of cancellous bone to restore subchondral support of the tibial plafond.

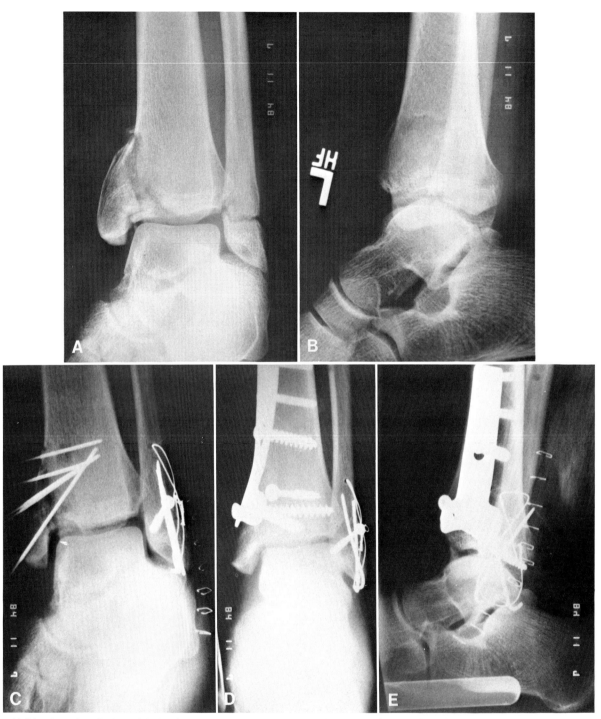

Figure 66.31. Stage 2 supination-adduction fracture with extensive medial marginal comminution and impaction of the tibial pilon. **A** and **B.** Mortise and lateral views. **C.** Intraoperative view of fibular stabilization and temporary fixation of the tibia. **D** and **E.** Postoperative mortise and lateral views showing restoration of the tibial articular surface and buttress plating.

syndesmosis remains intact, and diastasis does not occur. After open reduction, fixation of the fibula is usually obtained with two 0.062-inch axial Kirschner wires (K-wires) and a 20- or 22-gauge figure-of-eight or box stainless steel tension band wire loop (Fig. 66.29). Intraoperative radiographs should confirm that the K-wires have not entered the synovial cavity of the ankle. In the absence of a fibular fracture, the lateral collateral ligaments should be evaluated preoperatively by means of stress manipulation and radiography. If necessary, primary repair of the collateral ligaments can be performed with a combination of 0 and 2-0 absorbable and nonabsorbable sutures.

MEDIAL REPAIR. Stage 2 of the supination-adduction injury produces a vertical push-off fracture of the medial malleolus, in conjunction with distal tibial articular impaction that may propagate extensively into the metaphysis. The orientation of the articular disruption of the tibia varies greatly with the sagittal plane position of the ankle and the intensity of axial impaction at the time of injury. When the ankle is in a position of dorsiflexion at the time of injury, the anterior margin of the distal tibial plafond typically sustains impaction and comminution. Similarly, if the ankle is plantarflexed, the posterior margin of the distal tibia becomes impacted and is shorn off. Before reduction of the fracture, the medial, anteromedial, or posteromedial margins of the distal tibial bearing surface must be examined for subchondral impaction. Adequate reconstruction requires realignment of the subchondral cortical bone plate and local transfer of metaphyseal cancellous bone to fill the underlying subcortical defect, thereby providing a supportive mold for articular cartilage regeneration. Furthermore, the talar dome should be evaluated for transchondral fractures. The push-off fracture fragment of the tibia is then reduced and is ideally fixed with two interfragmental lag screws directed perpendicular to the fracture line and parallel to one another (Fig. 66.30). If there is extensive marginal pilon comminution, buttress plating or other forms of osteosynthesis may be required (Fig. 66.31).

Pronation-Abduction and Supination-Eversion Fractures (Type B)

FIBULAR REPAIR. Type B fractures, also known as transsyndesmotic fractures, vary primarily with respect to the orientation and length of the fibular fracture. The fixation of the fibula varies with the fracture configuration. Generally speaking, the short oblique transsyndesmotic fracture is not amenable to interfragmental lag screw fixation and requires stabilization with a one-third tubular plate. As the length of the transsyndesmotic fracture increases, it becomes advantageous to employ the antiglide effect achieved by positioning the plate on the posterior aspect of the fibula. If the fibula displays a very long spiral transsyndesmotic fracture, fixation is best achieved with three or more interfragmental lag screws, each oriented perpendicular to the plane of the fracture at equally spaced intervals along the fibula.

Stage 3 of the pronation-abduction injury is exemplified by the transsyndesmotic short oblique fracture of the fibula originating at the level of the inferior tibiofibular articulation. After open reduction of the fibula, fixation may be achieved with an axial compression plate because the fracture is usually too short to allow placement of an interfragmental lag screw. On rare occasions it may be possible to orient an interfragmental screw by placing it through one of the plate holes. However, this technique is generally not applicable to short oblique fibular fractures, and attempts at this form of fixation for this particular fracture may compromise stability. The configuration of this fracture is amenable to stabilization with a well-contoured one-third tubular plate applied to the lateral or posterior aspect of the fibula (Fig. 66.32). Fine-thread 3.5 mm cortical screws are used to purchase both fibular cortices, thereby lagging the plate to the fibula. Once again, as the length of the oblique transsyndesmotic fracture increases, it is beneficial to position the plate on the posterior aspect of the fibula so as to take advantage of the antiglide effect. Indeed, many surgeons prefer to routinely apply the posterior antiglide plate to any type B fracture (28).

The short oblique fracture configuration is well suited to stabilization by the load-screw method of axial compression

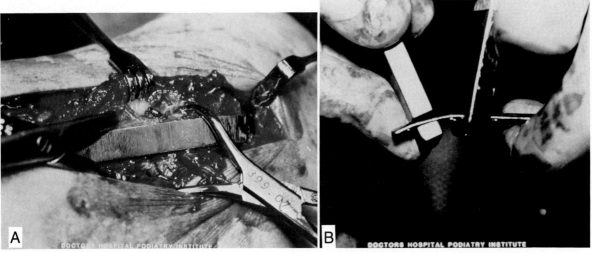

Figure 66.32. **A.** Aluminum template used to ascertain the contour of the fibula for subsequent plate bending. **B.** Twisting a one-third tubular plate to accurately fit the contour of the distal fibula.

(Fig. 66.33). After the plate is fixed to the proximal fragment of the fibula, the most proximal drill hole in the distal fragment is placed through the plate hole and offset away from the fracture line. The offset orientation of this screw allows the countersink portion of the screw head to engage the plate eccentrically as the screw seats into the concentric plate hole, thereby placing on the plate an extrinsic load that tends to push the plate away from the fracture line. However, the rigid plate, being anchored to the proximal portion of the fibula, does not elongate or move relative to the proximal portion of the fibula. Tightening of this offset screw will effect tension in the plate, which is converted to

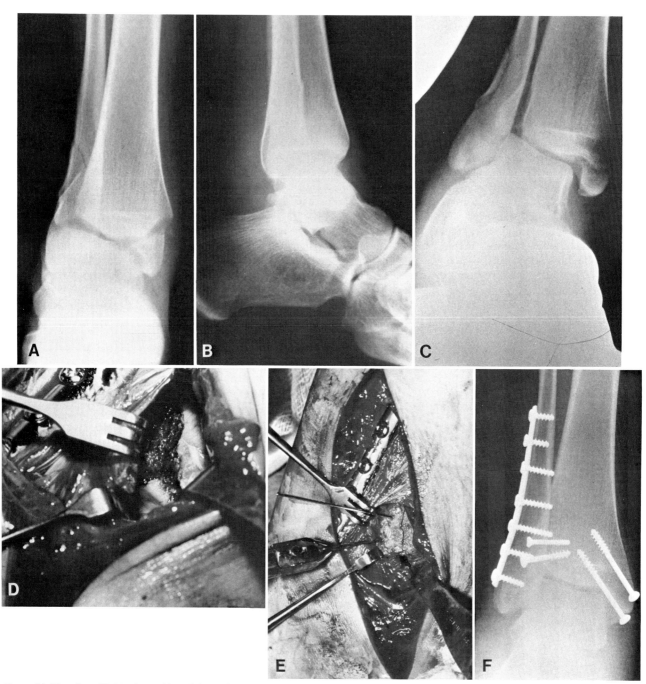

Figure 66.33. **A** and **B.** Mortise and lateral views of short oblique type B fibular fracture. **C.** Valgus stress radiograph reveals significant subluxation of ankle mortise with talar dome impaction of distal tibia but no tibiofibular diastasis. **D** and **E.** Lateral marginal impaction of the distal tibial articular surface requiring cancellous bone grafting to effect subcortical support, followed by direct internal fixation. The fibula has already been stabilized with an axial load-screw plate. **F.** Postoperative mortise view.

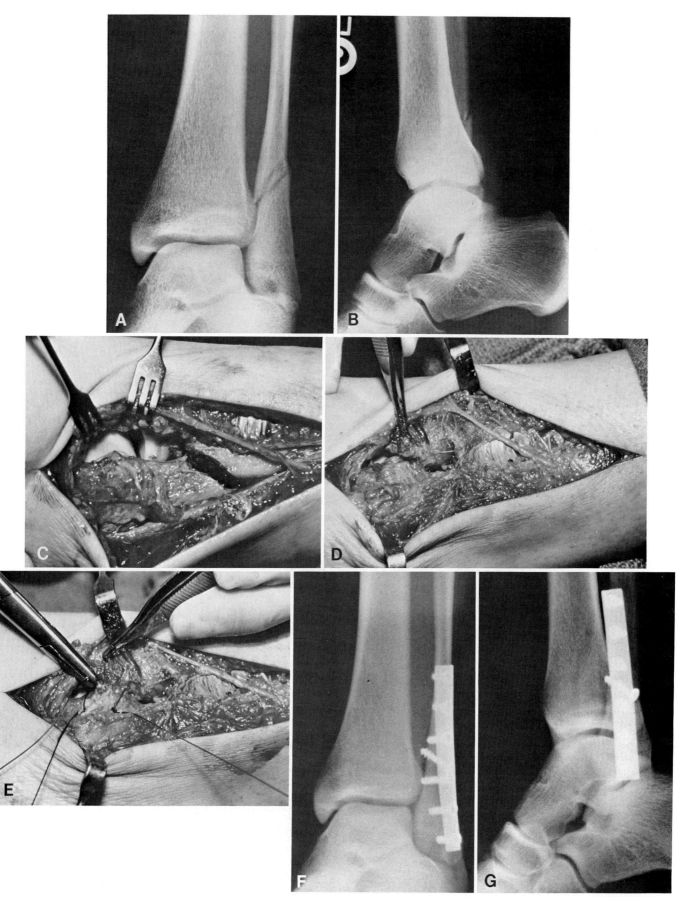

Figure 66.34. **A** and **B.** Mortise and lateral radiographs of stage 2 supination-eversion left ankle fracture. **C.** Intraoperative view of oblique fracture of the fibula with proximal and posterior spike and visualization of tibial and talar articular surfaces. **D.** Midsubstance tear of anterior-inferior tibiofibular syndesmotic ligament noted after the repair of the fibular fracture. **E.** Repair with intraosseous nonabsorbable suture. **F** and **G.** Postoperative mortise and lateral views. Note the perpendicular relationship of the interfragmental screw and the neutralization plate.

axial compression between the fracture fragments (load screw method), thereby increasing friction between the fragments and enhancing rigidity.

A small amount of additional axial compression may be achieved by application of the load screw method to the second most proximal screw stabilizing the distal fragment. Application of this second offset screw requires loosening of the first load screw a small amount, just prior to purchasing the second load screw. After achieving full purchase with the second load screw, the first screw in the distal fragment is retightened to full purchase.

The remaining drill holes in the distal fragment of the fibula are drilled concentrically. At the level of the lateral malleolus, it becomes necessary to prevent screw penetration into the distal tibiofibular articulation and the ankle joint cavity. Therefore, when a laterally positioned plate is used, only the lateral cortex of the fibula should be purchased distally with 3.5 mm cortical (fine-thread) screws.

Stage 2 of the supination-eversion injury involves the classic spiral fracture of the fibula originating at the level of the inferior tibiofibular articulation. The spiral fracture is actually an elongated variation of an oblique fracture that propagates through the fibula from anterior to posterior as it ascends the distal portion of the shaft, thereby creating a posterior-proximal spike of bone (Fig. 66.34). After anatomical reduction of the fibular fracture, fixation can be achieved with interfragmental 4.0 mm cancellous lag screws or 3.5 mm fine-thread cortical screws used in a lag fashion,

augmented with the application of a well-contoured one-third tubular neutralization plate (Figs. 66.34 and 66.35). The neutralization plate should be positioned oblique to, or as close as practical to, 90° from the plane of the interfragmental screws. The more posterior the plate application, the more it will resist proximal gliding of the distal fragment on the proximal fragment. The neutralization plate is anchored to the fibula with concentrically drilled 3.5 mm fine thread cortical screws. Occasionally the orientation of the spiral fracture allows application of an interfragmental compression screw through a central hole in the plate. Care must be taken to avoid entrance of the screws into the tibiofibular articulation or the ankle joint proper.

Very long spiral fractures of the fibula are best stabilized with multiple (three or more) interfragmental lag screws independently oriented perpendicular to the fracture interface at the level of screw insertion (Fig. 66.36).

The posterior antiglide plate, with or without interfragmental screw placement, may also be used to rigidly stabilize the long oblique fibular fracture (Fig. 66.37) and is considered the ideal form of stabilization in cases involving advanced osteoporosis (28, 29). Pure application of the posterior plate avoids the need to purchase soft fibular malleolar cortex with screw threads. The contour of the posterior plate is modified distally to effect a small amount of anterior bending that either cups the distal contour of the malleolus or actually penetrates the soft cortex, thereby providing purchase of the distal fragment. The plate is then lagged to the

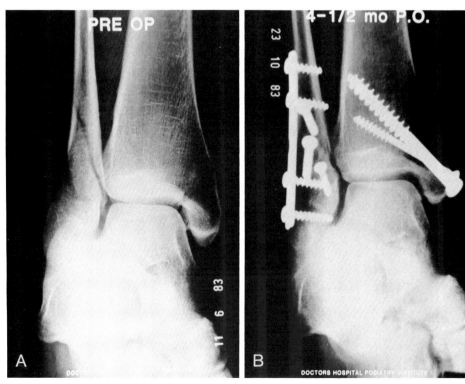

Figure 66.35. Stage 4 supination-eversion fracture, right ankle. **A.** Preoperative radiograph. **B.** Postoperative radiograph revealing interfragmental compression screws oriented 90° to the neutralization plate used to stabilize the fibula.

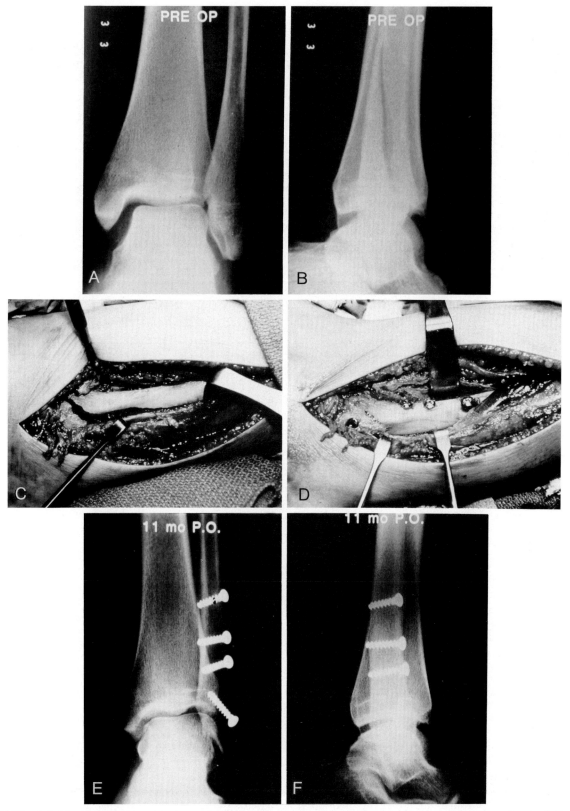

Figure 66.36. Spiral fracture of fibula originating at the level of the anterior inferior tibiofibular ligament. **A** and **B.** Preoperative radiographs. Note that the fracture propagates from anterior to posterior as it ascends the fibular shaft. **C** and **D.** Lateral exposure used for open reduction with internal fixation using four 3.5 mm cortical screws in a lag fashion. **E** and **F.** Postoperative radiographs. Note the orientation of each screw so that each traverses fracture line in a perpendicular fashion as the fracture spirals up the fibular shaft.

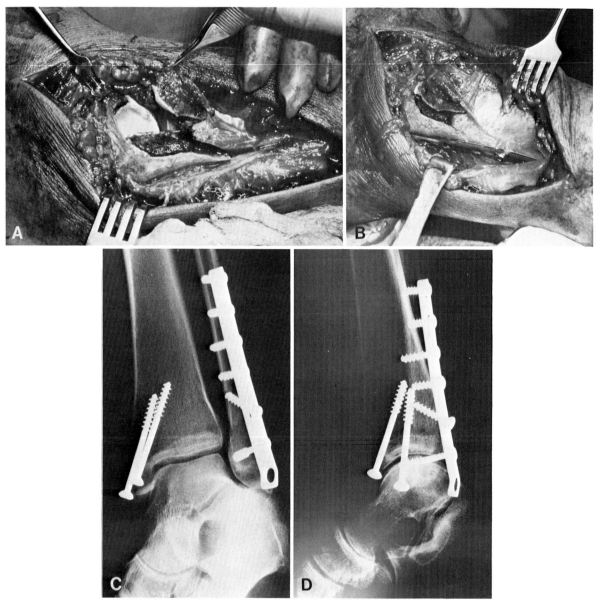

Figure 66.37. **A** and **B.** Intraoperative identification of a type B oblique fibular fracture with a large Wagstaffe fragment (in forceps) and reduction and stabilization with a posterior antiglide plate. Prior to tightening the screws anchoring the plate to the fibula, the Wagstaffe fragment is anatomically reduced and then fixated with an interfragmental lag screw directed through the plate. **C** and **D.** Postoperative mortise and lateral views. Note the bend in the distal tip of the posterior plate and the orientation of the interfragmental lag screw stabilizing the Wagstaffe fragment (second most distal screw in the plate).

posterior aspect of the proximal portion of the fibula. The most distal screw in the proximal portion of the fibula is termed the "trick screw" (28), and its purchase effects anatomic reduction and rigid stabilization of the distal fragment. If possible, the remaining plate holes in the distal fragment are further secured with lag screws.

In very soft bone with comminution, it may be beneficial to augment stability with the addition of Kirschner wire or Steinmann pin splintage (Figs. 66.38 and 66.39). Depending on the surgeon's preference, this form of fibular fixation may be applied for many type B fractures in patients with good bone stock.

The severely osteoporotic fibular fracture may also be stabilized with multiple 0.062-inch K-wires with or without a tension band wire loop. Oblique transfixation of the fibula to the tibia with these wires does not effect compression but does add to the stability of the mortise (21). Transsyndesmotic wires must be removed before weight bearing is resumed.

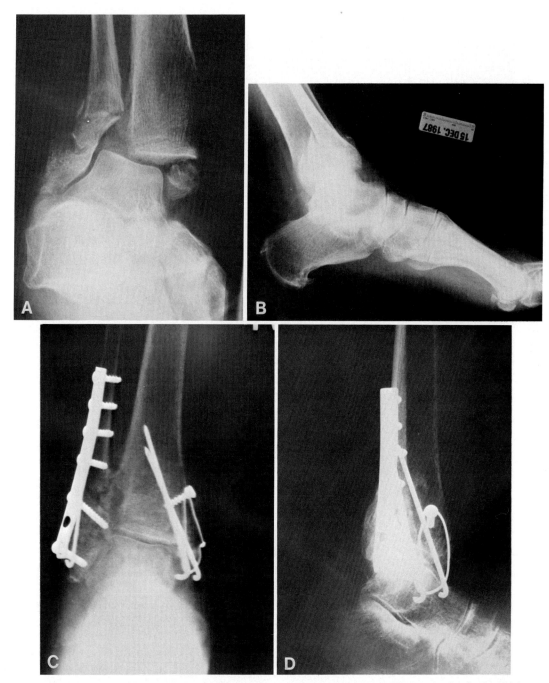

Figure 66.38. **A** and **B.** Mortise and lateral radiographs of a stage 4 supination-eversion trimalleolar fracture in a 77-year-old woman with osteoporosis. Note the severe displacement and comminution of the fibula and the lateral aspect of the tibia. **C** and **D.** Postoperative mortise and lateral views reveal modified tension band wire with hanging screw stabilizing the medial malleolus, and a posterior antiglide plate with an axial Kirschner wire fixating the fibula. The anterior syndesmotic ligament was primarily sutured.

Syndesmosis Repair. After open reduction and fixation of the type B oblique fibular fracture, the syndesmosis must be evaluated. Stage 2 of the pronation-abduction injury involves partial or complete rupture of the anterior and posterior inferior tibiofibular ligaments or avulsion fractures of the ligamentous attachments from the tibia or the fibula.

Similarly, stage 1 of the supination-eversion mechanism involves disruption of the anteroinferior tibiofibular ligament, and stage 3 of this injury causes posterior rupture or, more commonly, avulsion fracture of the posterior malleolus. Tibiofibular diastasis is not typically elicited with type B transsyndesmotic fractures because the interosseous membrane

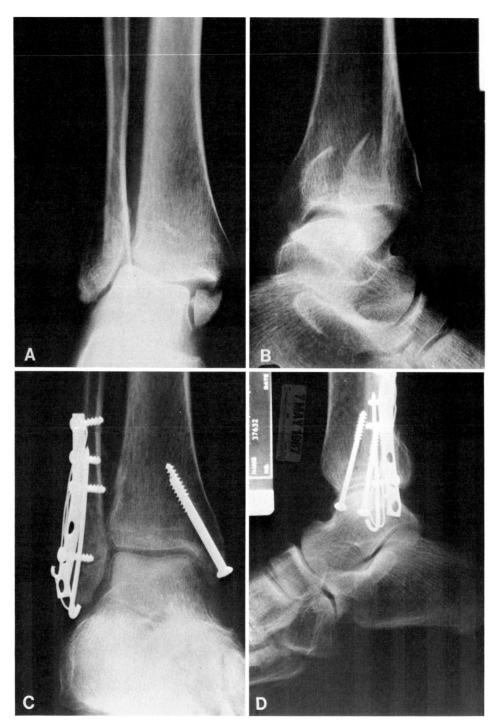

Figure 66.39.   Radiographic appearance of stage 4 supination-eversion trimalleolar fracture in an alcoholic patient with diminished bone stock. **A** and **B.** Initial mortise and lateral views. Note the high degree of lateral and posterior displacement of the foot on the leg. **C** and **D.** Postoperative views showing posterior anti-glide plate and modified tension band wire used to stabilize the fibula and two interfragmental lag screws fixating the medial malleolus. The posterior malleolar fragment is reduced and stabilized by virtue of its Vassal relationship to the fibula.

remains intact. However, anterior and posterior drawer signs indicative of anterior and/or posterior disruption of the syndesmosis may be elicited.

Anterior and posterior syndesmotic disruption may take various forms. Anteriorly, the tibiofibular ligament either tears through its midsubstance (Fig. 66.34) or tears from the tibia with a cortical avulsion fragment of the tubercle of Tillaux-Chaput (Fig. 66.40). Less commonly, the anterior ligament is avulsed from its fibular attachment with a resultant Wagstaffe fracture (Fig. 66.37). Posteriorly, the tibiofibular ligament usually pulls off the posterior tibial triangle (third malleolus), creating a Volkmann's avulsion fracture. Fracture of the posterior malleolus of the tibia is especially common in stage 3 of the supination-eversion and stage 4 of the pronation-eversion mechanisms, and the configuration of this fracture varies with respect to the sagittal plane position and axial loading of the ankle at the time of injury. Most often, the external rotary force created by the supination-eversion mechanism results in an avulsion fracture that occurs by virtue of the intact posterior-inferior tibiofibular ligament.

Techniques for repair of the syndesmosis vary with respect to the specific disruption pattern associated with the fibular fracture. Tears through the substance of the ligaments of the syndesmosis are primarily repaired with 0-gauge nonabsorbable suture material or stainless steel wire. This may be reinforced with 2-0 absorbable sutures or an intraosseous or transosseous wire suture anchored through drill holes in either the tibia, or the fibula, or both (Fig. 66.34), depending on the degree of isolated ligamen-

tous damage. Nonabsorbable sutures or wire used to repair the anterior inferior tibiofibular ligament may also be anchored around the implant used to stabilize the distal fibula. Avulsion fragments are best stabilized with interfragmental lag screws and may be positioned through an associated plate (Figs. 66.37 and 66.40). When ligamentous avulsion produces a very small cortical fragment, a polyacetal spiked washer with an interfragmental lag screw can be used to reattach the ligament to subcortical bone.

In most stage 3 supination-eversion injuries, the small posterior malleolar avulsion fracture will spontaneously reduce on reduction of the fibular fracture (Fig. 66.41). This occurs by virtue of the intact posterior tibiofibular ligament and classically exemplifies the Vassal principle. The small posterior triangle fragment rarely needs fixation because it is adequately stabilized by rigid internal fixation of the fibula in conjunction with surrounding soft tissue constraints. If excessive ankle mortise instability persists after fixation of the fibula and repair of the anterior aspect of the syndesmosis, or if the posterior avulsion fragment involves more than 25% of the distal tibial articular surface (14), then Volkmann's fracture can be directly reduced and fixated with interfragmental compression screws via the posterolateral exposure (Fig. 66.42). Indirect fixation of a large posterior malleolar fracture may also be performed through a modified anteromedial exposure after direct reduction of the fragment through the posterolateral exposure or through the posteromedial exposure after direct reduction via the same posteromedial access. Re-evaluation of the inferior syndesmosis should reveal adequate stability after re-

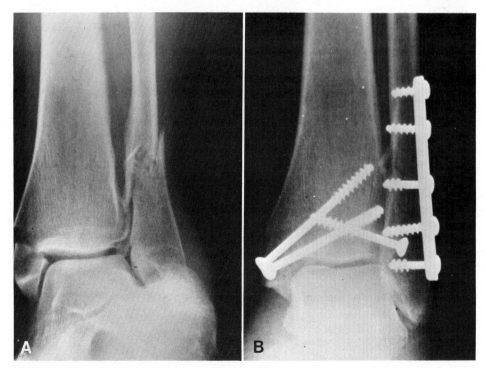

Figure 66.40. **A** and **B.** Preoperative and postoperative views of comminuted stage 4 supination-eversion fracture with a large Tillaux-Chaput avulsion fragment repaired with an interfragmental lag screw.

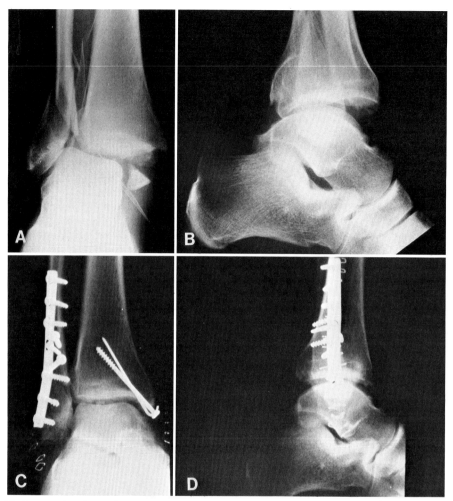

Figure 66.41. **A** and **B.** Preoperative views of displaced stage 4 supination-eversion trimalleolar fracture. **C** and **D.** Postoperative view reveals reduction of the posterior fragment reduction (lateral view) via the Vassal principle and secondary stabilization of the medial malleolus with an interfragmental lag screw and an anti-rotation Kirschner wire.

pair of the anterior, lateral, and posterior aspects of the joint.

After repair of the syndesmosis, stability of the mortise should be reassessed by means of anterior and posterior drawer and valgus stress manipulation of the ankle.

MEDIAL REPAIR. Stage 1 of the pronation-abduction injury and stage 4 of the supination-eversion injury involve a transverse avulsion fracture of the medial malleolus at or inferior to the tibiotalar articulation or rupture of the deltoid ligament. The fracture is reduced and temporarily stabilized with two K-wires. After intraoperative radiographic evalu-

ation, the fracture is ideally fixated with two parallel interfragmental 4.0 mm cancellous bone screws lagged perpendicular to the fracture interface (Figs. 66.33, 66.37, 66.39, 66.40, and 66.42). The K-wires are used as a guide for screw direction and placement. A secondary form of fixation may be used should the avulsion fragment be very small or the bone soft. A single interfragmental screw may be combined with an antirotational K-wire for small fragments (Fig. 66.41). Alternatively, two 0.062 inch axial K-wires and a 20- or 22-gauge stainless steel tension band wire loop may be used to effect rigidity. Because of the glabrous contour of

Figure 66.42. **A** and **B.** Mortise and lateral views of a stage 4 supination-eversion fracture with a large posterior malleolar fragment. **C** and **D.** Intraoperative view of the type B fibular fracture and radiographic appearance of the fixation with interfragmental screws and neutralization plate. **E.** Intraoperative appearance of an avulsion fracture of the medial malleolus and a large posterior marginal fragment. **F** and **G.** Intraoperative radiographic views of temporary fixation of the reduced tibial fractures. **H.** Intraoperative appearance of direct interfragmental screw fixation of tibial malleolar fractures. **I** and **J.** Postoperative mortise and lateral views.

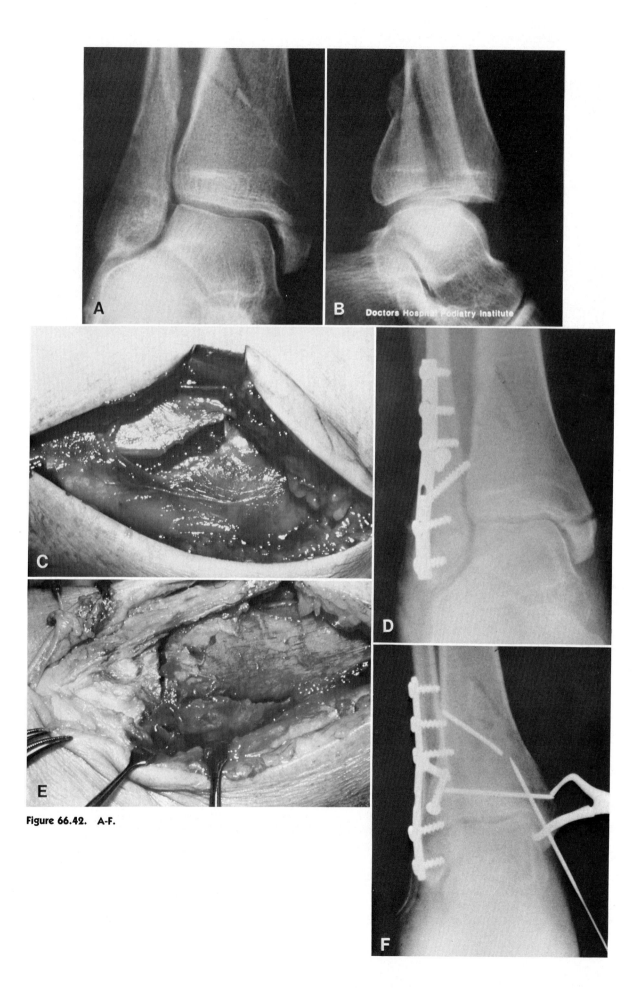

Figure 66.42. A-F.

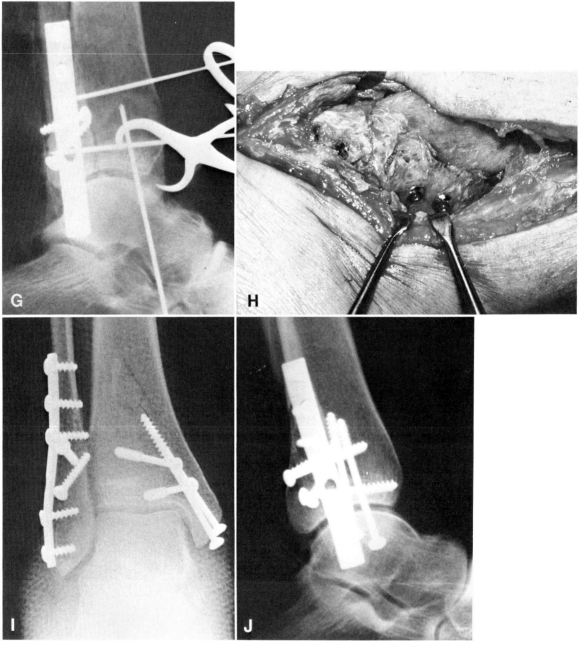

Figure 66.42. G-J.

the tibia at the junction of the metaphysis and medial malleolus, it is often easier to secure the tension band wire loop around an isolated proximal screw than through intraosseous channels (Fig. 66.38). The proximal screw in this application is referred to as the hanging screw, and tension wire stability may be enhanced with the use of a small washer.

Should the medial malleolus not be fractured, consideration should be given to repair of the deltoid ligament. Primary repair should be performed if ligament interposition prevents anatomic relocation of the mortise or if there

is radiographic evidence of tibial or talar osteochondral fracture or avulsion fragments between the medial malleolus and the talus (16, 30). The deltoid ligament is repaired with a combination of 0 and 2-0 absorbable and nonabsorbable sutures.

Pronation-Eversion Fractures (Type C)

Stage 3 of the pronation-eversion injury involves the classic high fibular fracture. The fracture is typically oblique or spiral in nature and, depending on the degree of rotary forces involved, may become comminuted, with the production of one or more butterfly fragments. Open reduction and fixation of the fractured fibula varies with the exact position of the fracture above the anteriorinferior tibiofibular ligament and the degree of comminution. The high fibular fracture may occur at basically three levels: *(a)* distal diaphysis, *(b)* approximately mid-diaphysis, and *(c)* very high, near the neck of the fibula, where the defect is called a Maisonneuve fracture. Direct reduction may be achieved for those fractures at or below the mid-diaphyseal level. After anatomic reduction the fibula is fixated with interfragmental 4.0 mm cancellous screws or with 3.5 mm fine-thread cortical screws used in a lag fashion. This fixation is augmented with the application of a well-contoured one-third tubular neutralization plate oriented approximately 90° from the plane of the lag screws. The more posterior the plate application, the more the plate will resist proximal gliding of the distal fragment on the proximal fragment. In the event of marked comminution, length and alignment of the fibula are maintained by means of a six- to eight-hole one-third tubular buttress plate or application of an external skeletal frame.

Direct open reduction is generally not recommended for the Maisonneuve fracture because of the potential for post-incisional common peroneal entrapment neuropathy. In the rare event that this fracture remains seriously displaced or unstable, ORIF may be indicated. Indirect reduction and fixation of the high fibular fracture will usually provide adequate reduction and stabilization. This entails restoration of the length of the fibula, with direct visualization of the fit of the fibula into the fibular notch of the tibia as a guide to the reduction. Once reduced, the fibula is temporarily transfixed to the tibia with two 5/64-inch Steinmann pins or large K-wires. The reduction may be reassessed by comparing postreduction intraoperative radiographs of the fractured ankle with preoperative radiographs of the contralateral ankle. The syndesmosis and interosseous membrane are then repaired, followed by final transfixation of the fibula to the tibia with two fully threaded 3.5 mm positional screws.

SYNDESMOSIS REPAIR. Stabilization of the ankle mortise in the pronation-eversion injury also varies with the level of fibular fracture. In stage 2 of this fracture, the anterior inferior tibiofibular ligament ruptures through its substance, avulses the tubercle of Tillaux-Chaput, or creates a Wagstaffe fracture. This is followed by tearing of the interosseous membrane up to the level of the fibular fracture with resultant tibiofibular diastasis. Evaluation of the ankle mortise after open reduction and internal fixation of the fractured fibula or temporary transfixation of the Maisonneuve fracture will reveal diastasis as well as anterior and posterior drawer signs. The anterior ligament should be repaired as previously described. The interosseous membrane should then be visualized and any defects primarily repaired. Usually the membrane tears away from the tibial shaft. Nonabsorbable 0-gauge suture material is used to reapproximate tibial periosteum to the intact portion of the interosseous membrane in an over-and-over or mattress

fashion. This may be reinforced with 2-0 absorbable sutures. Frequently small defects in the interosseous membrane may not be repaired when transfixation screws are planned.

After primary repair of the fibular fracture and the anterior aspect of the inferior syndesmosis and the interosseous membrane, mortise stability is again evaluated. Tibiofibular diastasis should not occur; however, disruption of the posterior aspect of the inferior syndesmosis will enable the surgeon to elicit a posterior drawer sign and, to a lesser degree, an anterior drawer sign. Stage 4 of the pronation-eversion fracture pattern involves rupture of the posterior inferior tibiofibular ligament or, more commonly, fracture of the posterior tibial malleolus (Volkmann's fracture). A small posterior triangle fragment results from avulsion fracture of the posterior syndesmotic ligament. This usually can be adequately reduced and stabilized by virtue of the Vassal principle after fixation of the fibula.

As the degree of ankle plantarflexion and axial loading increases at the moment of injury, the posterior malleolar fracture becomes more of a push-off injury and tends to involve more of the articular surface of the distal tibia. Repair of the posterior malleolus varies primarily with the degree of articular involvement, and it is recommended that fracture fragments representing 25% to 30% of the distal tibial bearing surface be rigidly stabilized to allow early post-surgical rehabilitation (14). If the posterior fragment is large and unstable, it should be directly reduced and fixated through the posterolateral exposure. Impacted areas of subchondral bone should be elevated and packed with autogenous cancellous bone from an adjacent area of the tibial epiphysis before reduction.

Direct fixation of the large posterior fragment is performed with two interfragmental 4.0 mm cancellous bone screws directed perpendicular to the fracture line and parallel to one another. Indirect fixation of a very large posterior triangle fragment may be performed through the modified anteromedial exposure after direct reduction through the posterolateral exposure or through the posteromedial exposure after direct reduction through the same posteromedial exposure.

TIBIOFIBULAR TRANSFIXATION (TRANSFIXION). Ideally, there should be no tibiofibular diastasis nor anterior or posterior drawer signs after repair of the fibula and the anterior and posterior aspects of the inferior syndesmosis. Intraoperatively, tibiofibular diastasis is assessed by means of a bone hook to purchase the medial fibular cortex above the syndesmosis and a lateral pull to separate the fibula from the tibia. If ankle mortise instability persists, then tibiofibular transfixation is required. Although transfixation of the fibula to the tibia is best avoided if it is not necessary, the added stabilization is beneficial when the hook test reveals persistent diastasis.

The goal of tibiofibular transfixation is to stabilize the mortise without compression. Two fully threaded 3.5 mm cortical screws are used to rigidly position the fibula in relation to the tibia. A single 4.5 mm fully threaded screw may also be used successfully. The screw direction should be from posterolateral to anteromedial at an angle of 25°

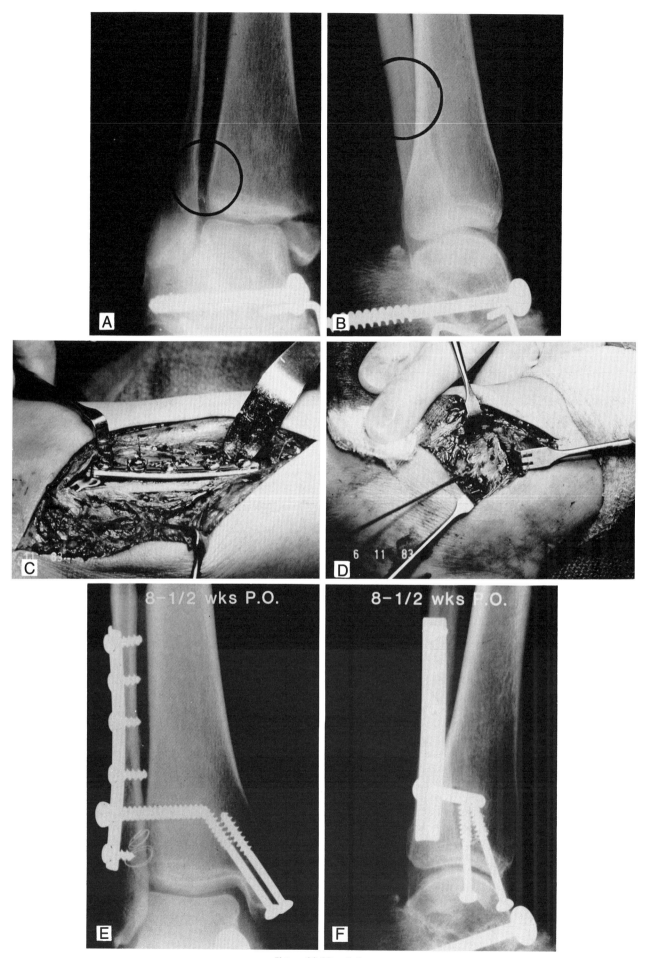

Figure 66.43.   A-F.

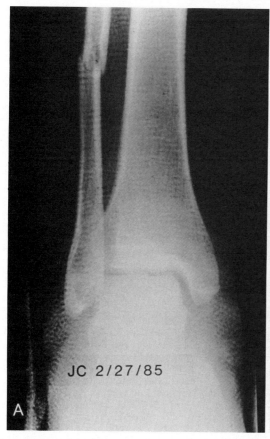 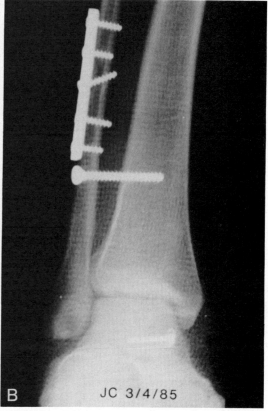

Figure 66.44. Pronation-eversion fracture, right ankle. **A.** Preoperative radiograph after closed reduction. **B.** Postoperative radiograph. Note the transfixation screw placement distal to the plate. Note the small cortical screw and polyacetal washer used to reattach the deltoid ligament to the talus.

to 30° from the sagittal plane of the leg. Moreover, the transfixation screw must purchase both cortices of the fibula and the lateral cortex of the tibia. The medial cortex of the tibia may be purchased for added stability, although this is not mandatory. It is important to assure accurate distal articulation of the fibula with the tibia in an effort to prevent maintenance of diastasis by the transfixation screw.

Placement of tibiofibular transfixation screws varies with the level of the fibular fracture. When the distal diaphysis of the fibula is fractured and fixated with a one-third tubular plate, the transfixation screw is incorporated through a hole in the plate located 3 to 5 cm proximal to the anterior inferior tibiofibular ligament (Fig. 66.43). When the fibula is fractured at a mid-diaphyseal level and fixated with a one-third tubular plate, the transfixion screw or screws may be placed distal to the plate and yet 3 to 5 cm proximal to the

syndesmosis (Figs. 66.44 and 66.45). In the case of a Maisonneuve fracture, two 3.5 mm cortical screws are placed 3 and 5 cm proximal to the syndesmosis. Two positional screws, in conjunction with repair of the syndesmotic ligaments, are necessary to achieve adequate transfixion and indirectly fixate the high fibular fracture.

MEDIAL REPAIR. Following open reduction and internal fixation of the fibula and stabilization of the ankle mortise, either the medial malleolus or the deltoid ligament must be repaired as previously described above.

POSTOPERATIVE CARE OF ANKLE FRACTURES

Closed suction drainage is used throughout the first 24 to 48 hours postoperatively. The extremity is extrinsically stabilized in a modified Jones compression dressing and is kept

Figure 66.43. Pronation-eversion fracture, right ankle, 6 months after triple arthrodesis. **A.** Preoperative anteroposterior radiograph. Note the transverse medial malleolar fracture (stage 1) and avulsion of tubercle of Tillaux-Chaput (stage 2) (circled). **B.** Preoperative lateral radiograph. Note the high fibular fracture (circled). **C.** Lateral exposure for ORIF high fibular fracture. **D.** Medial exposure for ORIF of the medial malleolus. **E** and **F.** Eight and one half weeks' follow-up radiographs. Note 4.5 mm cortical screw used for transfixation, and wire suture repair of anterior inferior tibiofibular ligament.

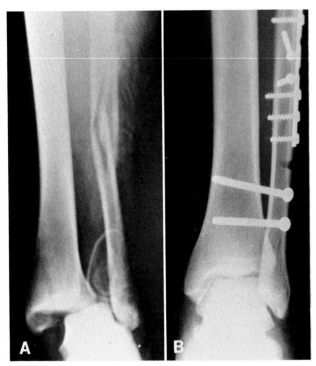

Figure 66.45. **A.** Preoperative mortise view of stage 4 pronation-eversion fracture with midshaft comminution of the fibula. **B.** ORIF with two fully threaded 3.5 mm transsyndesmotic positional screws stabilizing the mortise.

iced and elevated. The dressing is usually changed on the third postoperative day, and a below-the-knee synthetic cast is applied. In cases with marked soft tissue disruption or a very high fibular fracture, an above-the-knee cast may be used. The patient bears absolutely no weight on that leg for 6 to 8 weeks. Active range-of-motion exercises are initiated as early as the first postoperative day. Transfixation screws are generally removed before full weight bearing begins at 6 to 8 weeks. Ankle hardware may be removed 4 to 6 months postoperatively, or any time thereafter, as desired.

References

1. Bohler L: Diagnosis, pathology and treatment of fractures of the os calcis. *J Bone Joint Surg* 13:75, 1931.
2. Warwick R, Williams PL (eds): *Gray's Anatomy*, ed 35 (British). Philadelphia, WB Saunders, 1973, pp 460-461.
3. Wagstaffe WW: An unusual form of fracture of the fibula. *St Thomas Hosp Report* 6:43, 1875.
4. Pankovich AM: Fractures of the fibula at the distal tibiofibular syndesmosis. *Clin Orthop* 143:138-147, 1979.
5. Tillaux: Recherches cliniques et experimentales sur les fractures malleolaires (Rap de Gosselia). *Bull Acad Med* 1:817, 1872.
6. Chaput V: *Les Fractures Malleolaires due Cou-de-pieds et Les Accidents du Travail*. Paris, Masson & Cie, 1907.
7. Earle J: Forward dislocation of the tibia with a small portion of its edge fractured. *Lancet* 2:348, 1828.
8. Muller ME, Allgower M, Schneider R, Willenegger H (eds): *Manual of Internal Fixation*, ed 2. New York, Springer-Verlag, 1979, pp 284-285.
9. Dias LS, Tachdjian MO: Physeal injuries of the ankle in children: classification. *Clin Orthop* 136:230-233, 1978.
10. Ashurst APC, Bromer RS: Classification and mechanism of fractures of the leg bones involving the ankle. *Arch Surg* 4:51-129, 1922.
11. Lauge-Hansen N: Fractures of the ankle. II. Combined experimental-surgical and experimental-roentgenologic investigations. *Arch Surg* 60:957-985, 1950.
12. Lauge-Hansen N: Fractures of the ankle. IV. Clinical use of genetic roentgen diagnosis and genetic reduction. *Arch Surg* 64:488-500, 1952.
13. Lauge-Hansen N: Fractures of the ankle. III. Genetic roentgenologic diagnosis of fractures of the ankle. *Am J Roentgenol* 71:456-471, 1954.
14. Yde J: The Lauge-Hansen classification of malleolar fractures. *Acta Orthop Scand* 51:181, 1980.
15. Weber BG: *Die Verletzungen des Oberen Sprungelenkes*. Bern, Verlag Hans Huber, 1972.
16. Yablon IG, Heller FG, Shouse L: The key role of the lateral malleolus in displaced fractures of the ankle. *J Bone Joint Surg* 59A:169-173, 1977.
17. Burwell HN, Charnley AD: The treatment of displaced fractures at the ankle by rigid internal fixation and early joint movement. *J Bone Joint Surg* 47B:634-659, 1965.
18. Cedell CA: Is closed treatment of ankle fractures advisable? *Acta Orthop Scand* 56:101-102, 1985.
19. Wheelhouse WW, Rosenthal RE: Unstable ankle fractures: comparison of closed versus open treatment. *South Med J* 73:45-50, 1980.
20. Meyer TL, Kumler KW: ASIF technique and ankle fractures. *Clin Orthop* 150:211-216, 1980.
21. Heim U, Pfeiffer KM: *Small Fragment Set Manual*, ed 2. New York, Springer-Verlag, 1982.
22. Hughes JL, Weber H, Willenegger H, Kuner EH: Evaluation of ankle fractures: nonoperative and operative treatment. *Clin Orthop* 138:111-119, 1979.
23. Cedell CA: Ankle lesions. *Acta Orthop Scand* 46: 425-445, 1975.
24. Ramsey PL, Hamilton W: Changes in the tibio-talar area of contact caused by lateral talar shift. *J Bone Joint Surg* 58A: 356-357, 1976.
25. Bauer M, Jonsson K, Nilsson B: Thirty-year follow-up of ankle fractures. *Acta Orthop Scand* 56:103-106, 1985.
26. Kristensen KD, Hansen T: Closed treatment of ankle fractures: stage II supination-eversion fractures followed for 20 years. *Acta Orthop Scand* 56:107-109, 1985.
27. Charnley J: *The Closed Treatment of Common Fractures*, ed 3. New York, Churchill-Livingstone, 1974.
28. Vogler HW: Type B Danis-Weber ankle fracture: the anti-glide plate. In Scurran BL (ed): *Foot and Ankle Trauma*. New York, Churchill-Livingstone, 1989, pp 627-638.
29. Schaffer JJ, Manoli A: The antiglide plate for distal fibular fixation. *J Bone Joint Surg* 69A:596-604, 1987.
30. Baird RA, Jackson ST: Fracture of the distal part of the fibula with associated disruption of the deltoid ligament. *J Bone Joint Surg* 69A: 1346-1349, 1987.

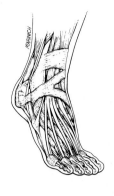

CHAPTER **67**

Pilon Fractures

George Gumann, D.P.M.

Pilon fractures are very complex injuries, and successful treatment of them requires great expertise. By definition, a pilon fracture involves the distal tibial metaphysis with extension into the ankle joint. There is usually, but not always, an associated fibular fracture. This injury, also called an explosion fracture of the distal tibia, is by nature a high-velocity injury in which the talus forcibly impacts the distal portion of the tibia. Common mechanisms of injury include motor vehicle accidents, falls from heights, and skiing accidents.

Ruedi and Allgower (1) have established the most commonly used classification system for pilon fractures. The system is divided into three fracture types (Fig. 67.1). Type I is a fracture of the distal tibia without significant displacement (Fig. 67.2). Type II is a fracture of the distal tibia with significant displacement (Fig. 67.3). Type III is a fracture of the distal tibia with severe comminution, significant displacement, and loss of the cancellous weight-bearing portion of the distal tibial plafond (Fig. 67.4). Lauge-Hansen (2) also attempted to describe this fracture pattern with his classification of pronation-dorsiflexion injuries, which has four stages (Fig. 67.5). Stage I is a fracture of the medial malleolus. Stage II is a fracture of the anterior aspect of the tibia. Stage III is a supramalleolar fracture of the fibula. Stage IV is a transverse fracture of the posterior aspect of the tibia. Kellam and Waddell (3) suggested two distinct fracture patterns that were correlated to the mechanism of injury. Type A was a rotational fracture with two or more large tibial articular fragments, minimal or no anterior tibial comminution, and usually a transverse or short oblique fracture of the fibula above the tibial plafond. This fracture pattern is produced by a primary rotation force with minimal axial compression. Type B was a compressive fracture demonstrating multiple tibial fragments, a narrowed ankle joint, significant anterior tibial comminution, and superior migration of the talus. It is caused by a severe axial compression force but is not always associated with a fibular fracture. Tile (4) agrees with the above description but identifies an axial compression fracture, a shear (tension) fracture, and a combined pattern. Tile (4) agrees with Kellam and Waddell (3) that the rotational or shear type of fracture has the better prognosis.

Because of the complex nature of the pilon fracture, one must be able to employ a variety of different treatment modalities. Some pilon fractures are best treated nonsurgically because they are either nondisplaced or are so comminuted that surgical repair is not possible. Others can be anatomically reduced and rigidly internally fixated. Finally, some may benefit from a limited surgical intervention to improve the position somewhat. Sometimes several different treatment options may be combined to produce the desired end result. The key to managing these difficult injuries is to carefully evaluate the fracture configuration and then select the best treatment modality for that specific patient.

With any trauma, a good history and physical examination are necessary. Since a percentage of these patients have polytrauma, life-threatening injuries must be identified and take precedence. The diagnosis of a pilon fracture is not difficult to make. There may or may not be gross deformity of the ankle region. It is essential to ascertain whether the fracture is closed or open. Careful observation is necessary for even pinpoint defects in the skin indicating an open

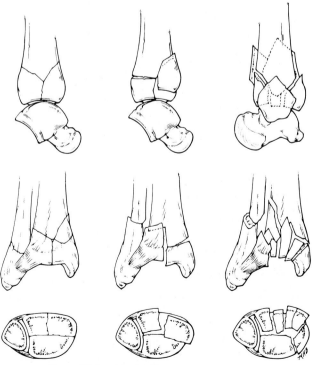

Figure 67.1. AO classification of pilon fractures.

The private views/opinions of the author are not to be construed as reflecting official policy of the Department of Defense or the Army Medical Department.

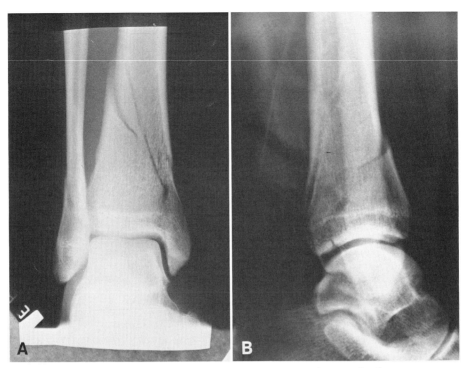

Figure 67.2. **A** and **B.** Anteroposterior and lateral views of type I pilon fracture.

fracture (Fig. 67.6). The entire distal tibia, ankle, and rear-foot region will be tender to palpation. There will be tenderness on attempted gentle range of motion of the ankle. The neurovascular status distal to the injury must be evaluated, but it usually remains intact. Initially edema and ecchymosis may be slight, but in time both will increase significantly. This can result in formation of fracture blisters and skin necrosis, which will delay or in some cases prevent operative intervention. Even without skin complications, severe edema will delay surgery, as wound closure may not be possible. Obviously, open fractures are surgical emergencies, and the patients need to be taken to the operating room immediately.

Radiographs readily demonstrate the fracture and should include anteroposterior, mortise, and lateral views of the ankle (Fig. 67.7). Other radiographs of the leg and foot should be obtained if indicated. In polytrauma patients, the first radiographs obtained should include, at a minimum, an anteroposterior view of the chest, a lateral cervical-spine view, and an anteroposterior view of the pelvis. An understanding of the pilon fracture configuration can be enhanced by tomograms and/or a computed tomography (CT) scan. The author recommends both. The frontal and transverse fracture planes are very well delineated with a CT scan, but the indirect sagittal plane reconstructions done by CT are poor (Fig. 67.8). However, lateral tomograms have been helpful in demonstrating the sagittal plane fracture deformities, especially the anterior and posterior tibial plafond fragments. The goal of the radiographic examination

is to help decide which fractures are surgically reducible by observing the degree of comminution present and any articular step-offs within the joint surface. One must identify the key fragments that would aid in restoration of the distal tibial articular surface.

The initial treatment after resuscitation of the patient, history and physical examination, and radiographic evaluation is stabilization of the fracture. Assuming that the fracture is closed, any gross deformity should be reduced. This can usually be performed with the patient under intravenous sedation in the emergency room. A modified Jones compression dressing of alternating layers of cast padding and elastic bandages is applied, followed by a below-knee cast. A plaster AO or posterior splint is also acceptable, but the compression dressing will provide greater comfort and more uniform compression. Occasionally the injury may have to be reduced with the patient under general anesthesia in the operating room. An open fracture requires only temporary stabilization with a splint, as the patient will be taken quickly to the operating room. Obtaining tomograms and a CT scan is often a time-consuming process, so many patients who require operative reduction are treated on a delayed basis. Once the results of the radiographs, tomograms, and CT scan are evaluated, a definitive treatment plan can be devised.

How does one decide the best treatment alternative? Many factors need to be analyzed, including the patient's age, physical health, activity level, postinjury expectations, ability to handle complications, osseous involvement, and soft tis-

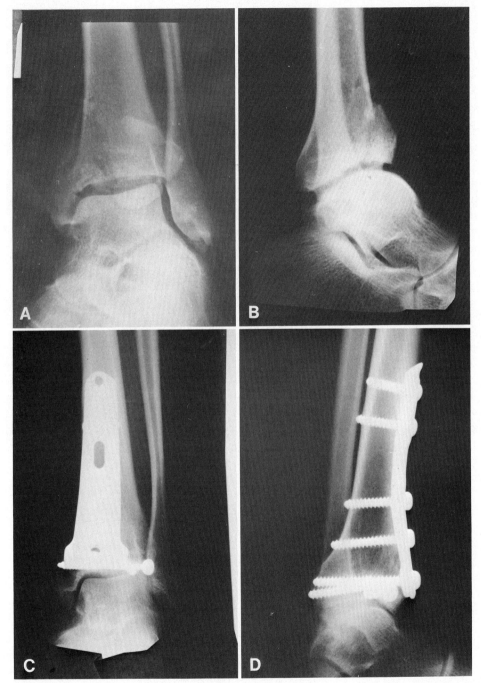

Figure 67.3.   A and **B.** Mortise and lateral views of type II pilon fracture. **C** and **D.** Anteroposterior and lateral views of fixation.

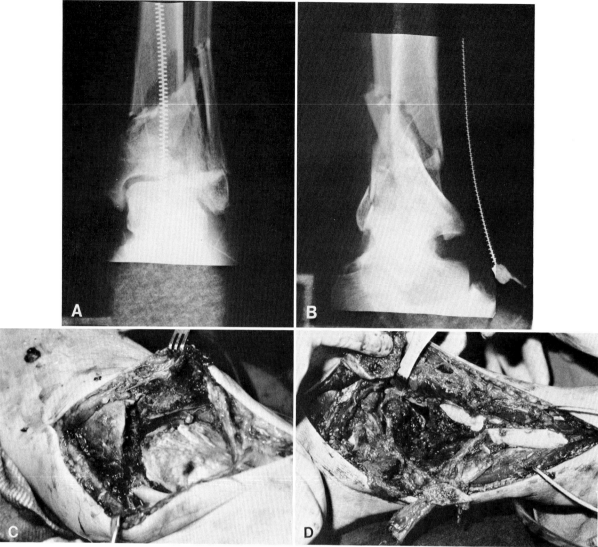

Figure 67.4. **A** and **B.** Anteroposterior and lateral views of type III pilon fracture. **C** and **D.** Medial and lateral incisions demonstrating the severe comminution associated with these fractures.

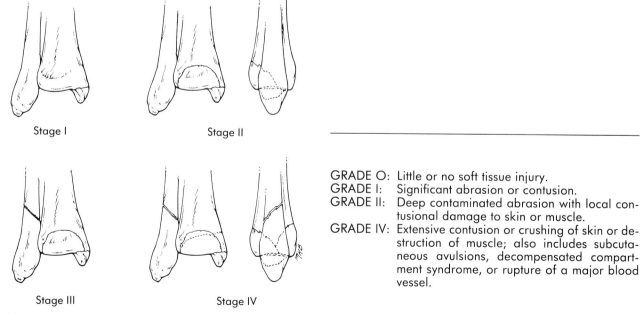

Stage I

Stage II

Stage III

Stage IV

Figure 67.5. Lauge-Hansen classification of pronation-dorsiflexion fractures.

GRADE O: Little or no soft tissue injury.
GRADE I: Significant abrasion or contusion.
GRADE II: Deep contaminated abrasion with local contusional damage to skin or muscle.
GRADE IV: Extensive contusion or crushing of skin or destruction of muscle; also includes subcutaneous avulsions, decompensated compartment syndrome, or rupture of a major blood vessel.

Figure 67.6. Grading of soft tissue injury by Tscherne and Gotzen.

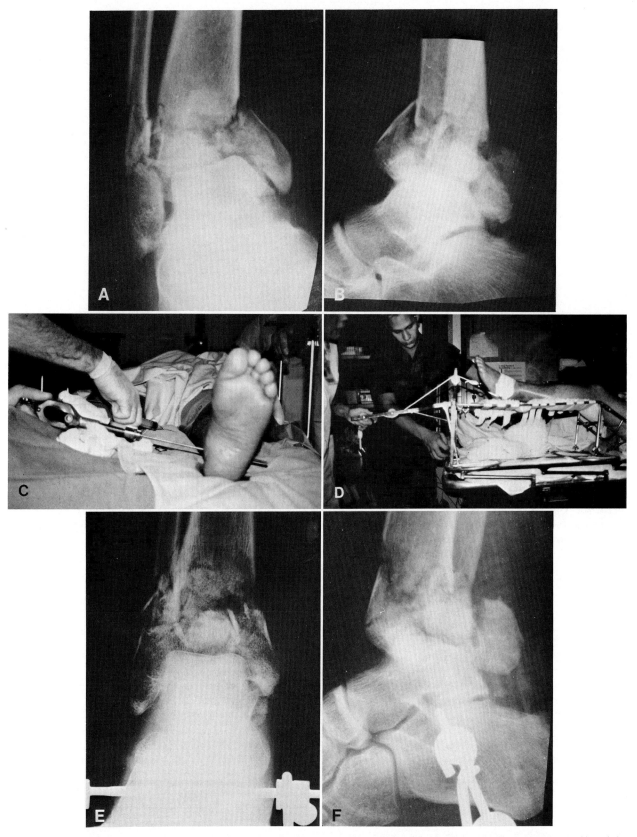

Figure 67.7. **A** and **B.** Mortise and lateral views of a closed type III pilon fracture with severe comminution of the tibial plafond and destruction of the articular surface. Injury was sustained in a parachute jump, which resulted in bilateral pilon fractures. **C.** Placement of Steinmann pin into calcaneus for traction. **D.** Placement of patient with calcaneal pin traction in a Bohler-Braun frame. **E** and **F.** Anteroposterior and lateral views in calcaneal pin traction. Note that the varus deformity has been corrected but that traction has not anatomically restored the tibial plafond. **G** and **H.** Mortise and lateral views one year after injury. There is mild tenderness diffusely about the ankle and good position for an ankle arthrodesis.

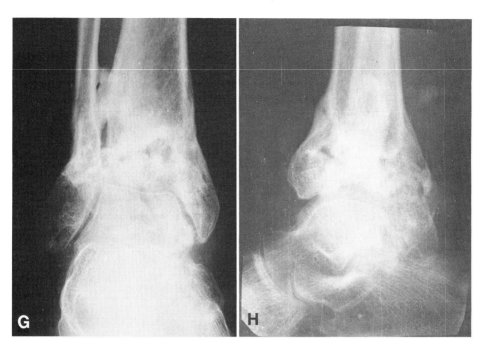

Figure 67.7.   G-H.

sue damage. Tile (4) has discussed the individual features of pilon fractures, which need to be carefully assessed. What is the quality of the bone? Is it solid in a younger patient and able to support internal fixation, or is the person elderly with osteoporotic bone that would not allow screw purchase? What is the state of the soft tissue? Tscherne and Gotzen (5) have developed a grading system for soft tissue damage (Fig. 67.6). Remember, the soft tissue envelope about a fracture is crucial to its osseous consolidation. One should not operate in the presence of severe edema, fracture blisters, skin necrosis, or severely contused skin. The distal ends of the tibia and fibula are very subcutaneous and healing can be precarious. Consequently, the timing of surgery and use of an atraumatic technique are important to the healing of the fracture. What technical difficulties will be encountered? Here the expertise of the surgeon comes into play. How comminuted are the articular surface and the distal tibia? Are they reconstructible? How good is the surgeon's knowledge of atraumatic technique and AO fixation principles? Is there an appropriate selection of implants?

On review of the literature, Ruoff and Snider (6) recommended traction as the best treatment option. Fourquet (7) reported a 50% functional outcome, while Bonnier (8) reported 43% in a large series with both conservative and

surgical treatment. However, in l969 Ruedi and Allgower (1) reported a series of 84 consecutive pilon fractures treated by the principles of the Swiss study group. These principles include the following:

1. Reconstruction of the fibular fracture
2. Reconstruction of the tibial articular surface
3. Cancellous bone graft to fill the distal tibial metaphyseal defect
4. Buttress plate application to the medial or anterior aspect of the tibia.

They reported 74% good and excellent functional results an average of 4 years after surgery. In a second study of the same group of patients 9 years postoperatively, Ruedi (9) indicated that a number of patients showed even better results than they did 4 years after surgery. Heim and Naser (10), in 1977, reviewed a series of 128 cases with good functional results in 90%. Heim was the principal surgeon in most cases, and 90% of the injuries were caused by skiing accidents. In the study by Ruedi (9) 75% of the fractures were caused by skiing accidents. In 1979 Ruedi and Allgower (11) reported on 75 patients seen at the University of Basle with a 69.4% good or excellent functional result. Also in

Figure 67.8.   A and **B.** Mortise and lateral views of a closed type III pilon fracture sustained in a fall. There is gross valgus deformity with significant displacement of the tibial articular surface. The patient was determined not to be a candidate for surgery, although the fracture is reconstructible. **C** and **D.** Frontal and transverse plane views of CT scan.

E and **F.** Mortise and lateral views after closed reduction performed in cast room and treatment with a calcaneal pin incorporated into a plaster cast. The valgus deformity has been corrected, but the tibial plafond is not anatomically reduced.

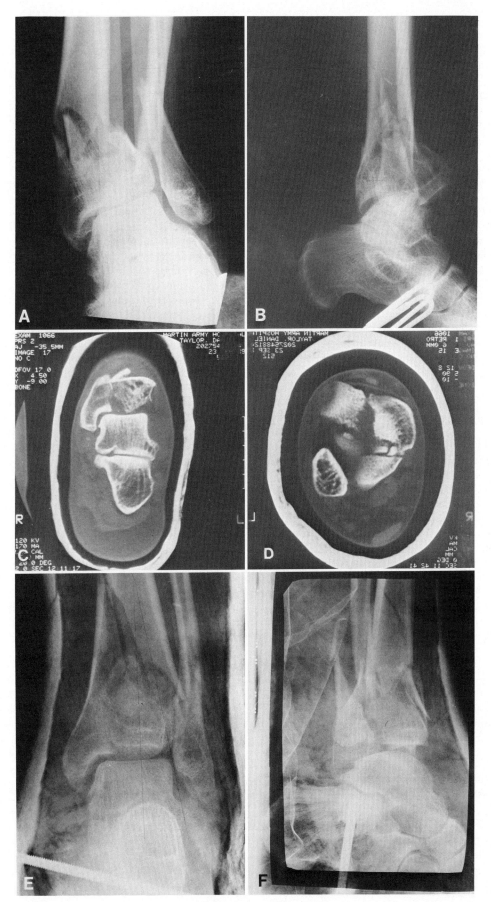

Figure 67.8.   A–F.

1979, Kellam and Waddell (3) reported their results in 26 cases of pilon fractures. Surgical treatment of a shearing, rotational type of pilon fracture without major articular impaction yielded good results in 84%. However, among fractures of the axial compression type with impaction and comminution, good results were achieved in only 53%. From these statistics, it was concluded that the type of fracture had a significant impact on the final result.

Kellam and Waddell (3) also confirmed what Ruedi and Allgower (1) had reported: traumatic arthritis will occur within 1 year after injury in all patients in whom it is going to occur. This is directly related to the degree of articular damage sustained at the time of injury and the congruity of the tibial articular surface. Kellam and Waddell (3) speculated that avascular necrosis of the smaller, comminuted fragments of subchondral bone readily led to progressive deformity, thus accelerating the arthritic process.

There are several methods that can be used to treat pilon fractures. As discussed previously, many factors should be considered before advancing to a specific form of treatment. The different treatment modalities are cast/splint/fracture brace, calcaneal pin traction, pins in plaster, limited internal fixation with or without external fixation, and open reduction with internal fixation.

CAST/SPLINT/FRACTURE BRACE

This treatment is best indicated for type I pilon fractures. Since the fracture is without significant displacement, the alignment cannot be substantially improved. This type of fracture is usually stable and can be maintained in a cast. The patient must refrain from weight bearing for 10 to 12 weeks, depending on the consolidation of the fracture. If the patient is noncompliant, a long leg cast with the ankle neutral and the knee flexed 90 degrees should be applied. This position will make it difficult to bear weight. If the patient is trustworthy, a below-knee cast will suffice. If the fracture is consolidating, early cast removal and the use of a splint/fracture brace or bivalved cast will allow the patient to mobilize the injured extremity. An example would be to use a below-knee cast for 4 to 6 weeks until the fracture is healing and then convert to a bivalved cast/splint/fracture brace for the final 6 to 8 weeks. If the fracture is very stable and nondisplaced and the patient is trustworthy, one could use the splint/fracture brace for the entire 10 to 12 weeks. Obviously, since pilon fractures tend to be high-velocity injuries, it is uncommon to find type I fractures. As with any fracture that is treated conservatively, radiographs should be taken on a weekly basis for up to 4 weeks to check for loss of position. Closed reduction and cast treatment can also be used for type III fractures with severe comminution, which would defy operative reduction and internal fixation. The fracture may be aligned by closed manipulation into as satisfactory a position as possible with the understanding that the reduction is not anatomic but will provide a better relationship for later fusion.

Finally, this might be an acceptable treatment option in a patient with a type II or III fracture that is surgically repairable but for other reasons the patient is not a candidate for surgery.

CALCANEAL PIN TRACTION

Calcaneal pin traction is best used for those severe type III fractures that are not surgically reconstructible (Fig. 67.7 A and B). A Steinmann pin is placed in the calcaneus with the patient under local anesthesia with sedation in the emergency room or under regional/general anesthesia in the operating room. Placement of the Steinmann pin is easily performed with the aid of local anesthesia. After a sterile preparation, the skin is anesthetized on the medial aspect of the heel and then the periosteum on the medial aspect of the calcaneus. A stab incision is made in the anesthetized area, starting on the medial side where it is easier to avoid the neurovascular structures. Next the soft tissue is spread with a hemostat to create a tunnel down to the medial wall of the calcaneus. A large-diameter Steinmann pin is advanced with a drill through the calcaneus to exit the lateral cortical wall and tent the skin on the lateral side of the heel. The skin is then anesthetized laterally, a stab incision is made, and the Steinmann pin is advanced until an equal amount is exposed on both sides of the heel (Fig. 67.7C). The Steinmann pin is placed posterior to the vertical axis of the tibia, as this will help prevent any tendency of the talus to sublux anteriorly. If the talus has subluxed posteriorly, however, the pin should be positioned more anteriorly. After insertion of the calcaneal pin, traction is applied in a Bohler-Braun frame or suspended overhead (Fig. 67.7D). Initially, 7 to 10 pounds of traction is applied. Radiographs are then obtained to evaluate the position so that any necessary adjustments can be made (Fig. 67.7 E and F). Calcaneal pin traction should be used for 4 to 8 weeks until the fracture shows some evidence of consolidation. At that time, the Steinmann pin can be removed and the fracture placed into a cast, or the pin can remain in place and be incorporated into the cast. Incorporation of the Steinmann pin in the cast is a good idea if the traction must be discontinued before osseous consolidation.

The advantage of calcaneal pin traction is that it allows range of motion of the ankle (Fig. 67.7 G and H). This technique can be valuable as a temporary means of stabilization of a fracture for which the surgeon plans surgical reconstruction but needs time for the soft tissues to become favorable. Calcaneal pin traction may also be employed in a case in which the fracture was reduced by surgical intervention but the fixation is not completely stable. Pin traction can be used to take forces off the repair and allow range of motion. Radiographs should be obtained weekly to check position. It should be noted that occasionally this treatment option can make the position of the fracture worse. One of the potential problems with calcaneal pin traction is the tendency of the fracture to drift into valgus position if the fibula is fractured. One way to help this situation is to fixate the fibula and then treat the tibial component with pin traction.

PINS IN PLASTER

Pins in plaster is a very old orthopedic technique that in some ways could be considered a "poor man's external fixator." This technique could be considered in the severely comminuted type III fractures that would defy operative reconstruction. A Steinmann pin is placed in the calcaneus as described previously, the fracture is reduced as much as possible, and a plaster cast is applied (Fig. 67.8). A second Steinmann pin may occasionally be placed in the proximal tibia for additional control or even distraction. Again, alignment of the foot and leg would be achieved. Although not necessarily an anatomic reduction, an improved position would be achieved for a delayed fusion.

The problems with this technique include potential pin tract infection, loosening of the Steinmann pins, inability to obtain an anatomic reduction, and inability to mobilize the ankle. This technique may be combined with a limited operation that would fixate the fibula to prevent valgus drift while attempting to control the tibia with the pins in plaster.

PRIMARY ARTHRODESIS

It is the author's opinion that primary arthrodesis is rarely indicated. If the pilon fracture is so comminuted that it is not possible to perform an anatomic reduction, the author would still prefer to use one of the other described treatment options. This is because some patients will do reasonably well for a period of time, even without an anatomic reduction and early arthritic findings. Older, more sedentary patients will tolerate arthritic changes better than younger, active ones. Consequently, the author employs ankle arthrodesis on a delayed basis when warranted by symptoms. Another reason not to consider primary arthrodesis is that, for successful fusion, compression is important. This is not possible with a severely comminuted pilon fracture. This view is supported by Kellam and Waddell (3) as well as by Tile (4).

LIMITED OPEN REDUCTION

Limited open reduction is a treatment option that is reserved for type III fractures that are not amenable to anatomic reduction and can combine several different techniques. In these cases, it is usually impossible to reduce the tibial component anatomically, whereas the fibula is reconstructible. The fibula is usually fixated with a combination of cortical screws inserted in lag fashion for compression and a one-third tubular plate. As previously discussed, after fibular fixation, calcaneal pin traction can be employed and will allow range of motion. Another technique would be to use a calcaneal pin incorporated into a cast or to drive a Steinmann pin from the inferior aspect of the calcaneus superiorly through the talus into the tibia. A third option would be to place the patient into an external fixator. The EBI (Orthofix) external fixator has an attachment that can allow range of motion of the ankle. In select cases, besides fixation of the fibula, it may be possible to piece together some of the major tibial articular components, securing them with

K-wires or lag screws, and then to use one of the options described above (Fig. 67.9).

OPEN REDUCTION WITH INTERNAL FIXATION

Open reduction with internal fixation is best used for type II injuries and those type III fractures that can be anatomically reduced (Fig. 67.10). The most important decision is to determine which fractures are amenable to successful surgical reconstruction and which ones should have some other kind of treatment. Failure to achieve an anatomic reduction and stable fixation in a restorable fracture results in a traumatized extremity with an increased risk of complications and perhaps precludes other treatment options. As previously indicated, it is necessary to evaluate the quality of the bone, the degree of comminution of the tibial articular surface, the possibility of reconstructing the tibial metaphysis, the state of the soft tissues, and the general health of the patient.

If the patient is deemed a candidate for surgery, then the next question is when to perform the surgery. Should it be done immediately, or on a delayed basis? Immediate surgery is best if possible. This may not be possible, as it takes time to obtain tomograms and a CT scan for some patients, whereas other patients are seen late, after soft tissue complications have occurred. Also, this is not the type of surgery that should be started in the middle of the night by an exhausted surgical team. If surgery is delayed, then one must wait 7 to 10 days for the local skin conditions to stabilize. If fracture blisters develop, the delay may be further prolonged.

As already indicated, any gross deformity is treated by closed reduction followed by the application of a compression dressing and a below-knee cast, posterior splint, or AO splint. The reduction is performed with the patient under intravenous sedation in the emergency room, although occasionally a general anesthetic is required. The patient is admitted, and the extremity is treated with ice and elevation in either a Bohler-Braun frame or overhead traction. Preoperative blood work as well as both tomograms and a CT scan are obtained, if desired. If surgery is to be delayed, the patient is monitored for possible compartment syndrome. If fracture blisters develop, they are debrided and treated with a combination of wet-to-dry saline dressings with periodic air drying. This can be done through windows cut in the cast or with alternative treatment methods, such as calcaneal pin traction, to allow access for wound care. Tile (4) has recommended that if the lateral skin is in good condition but the anterior and medial skin is not, then one might initially fixate the fibula alone. The skin on the tibial side should be determined to have improved prior to tibial fixation. Fixation of the fibula will help gain length, prevent valgus drift, and afford partial stability, and it can be incorporated into other forms of treatment if the soft tissue condition does not improve.

Obviously, open pilon fractures require immediate surgical intervention for debridement and irrigation. Appropriate cultures have to be obtained, and the patient must

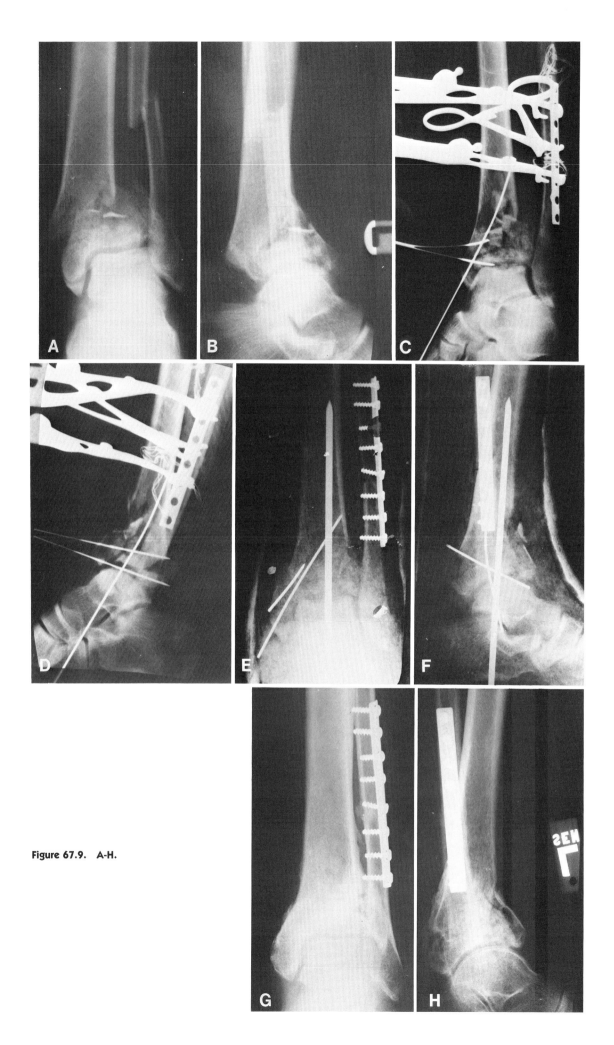

Figure 67.9. A-H.

Figure 67.9. **A** and **B.** Anteroposterior and lateral views of a severely comminuted, closed type III pilon fracture sustained in a parachute jump. **C** and **D.** Mortise and lateral views of intraoperative position after reduction and provisional stabilization of the fibula along with provisional K-wire stabilization of the larger tibial fragments. The articular surface of the tibia was destroyed, and there was a large defect in the metaphysis, which required a bone graft. **E** and **F.** Mortise and lateral views of final reduction with vertical Steinmann pin transfixation. **G** and **H.** Anteroposterior and lateral views of fracture 1 year after injury. The fracture has consolidated, and there is mild tenderness with reduced range of motion. The position is good for a future ankle arthrodesis.

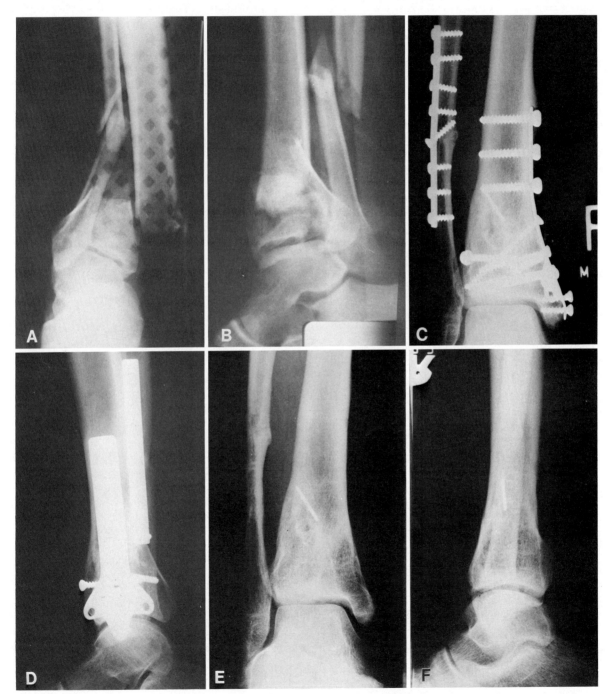

Figure 67.10. **A** and **B.** Anteroposterior and lateral views of an open type III pilon fracture sustained in a fall off a ladder. (Gumann G : Ankle Fractures in Scurran BL (ed): *Foot and Ankle Trauma*, Churchill Livingstone, New York, 1989, p. 608, reproduced with permission). **C** and **D.** Mortise and lateral views 19 months postoperatively demonstrating osseous consolidation. Postoperative course was complicated by a soft tissue infection which required incision and drainage 2 months after initial surgery. Both the tibia and the fibula were bone grafted at a third operation about 1 month after debridement. **E** and **F.** Mortise and lateral views 38 months postoperatively. The internal fixation has been removed, and there is no evidence of traumatic arthritis.

be placed on a regimen of therapeutic antibiotics. The tetanus status of the patient should be addressed. A detailed discussion of open fracture management is beyond the scope of this chapter, but the typical antibiotic is usually a first-generation cephalosporin. This will be supplemented with an aminoglycoside or even triple antibiotic coverage if indicated. The antibiotics are usually prescribed for 3 days and then discontinued. A controversy exists with regard to the placement of internal fixation devices on either a primary or a delayed basis. The author favors primary internal fixation at the time of the initial debridement, if feasible. Reasons for not employing primary internal fixation might be severe contamination or the likelihood that additional dissection would be required, which may devitalize osseous fragments. Patients with significant open fractures (grades II and III) should be returned to the operating room in 48 hours for a second debridement, followed by additional debridement as indicated. If fixation is not performed primarily, it can be accomplished on a delayed basis in 5 to 7 days along with delayed primary closure of the wounds.

At surgery, incision placement is important. If only the tibia is fractured, a single incision may be required. It can be placed anteriorly, anteromedially, or posteromedially, depending on which area of the tibia needs to be approached. Sometimes two incisions are necessary. If both the tibia and the fibula are fractured, then two incisions are required (Fig. 67.11). The important thing to remember is to maintain a 5 to 10 cm bridge between the two incisions to prevent skin necrosis. The fibula is approached through a posterolateral incision. The standard tibial approach is by a long incision, which starts about 1 cm lateral to the tibial crest proximally and extends distally, curving over the anteromedial aspect of the medial malleolus. However, incisional placement may have to be modified according to the fracture configuration. To help prevent necrosis, full-thickness flaps are raised, including both skin and adipose tissue. In open fractures, the incisions may have to be modified to either avoid the wound or be incorporated into it. Once through the skin, the fracture fragments are approached along the disrupted periosteum. The bony fragments should be reflected on a periosteal hinge, much like opening a book. The periosteum should not be completely stripped, as this will devitalize the bony fragments.

The principles for surgical reconstruction of a pilon fracture have been established by Ruedi and Allgower (1) (Fig. 67.12A). These include *(a)* reconstruction of the fibula (Fig. 67.12B), *(b)* reconstruction of the articular surface of the tibia (Fig. 67.12C), *(c)* placement of a cancellous autograft

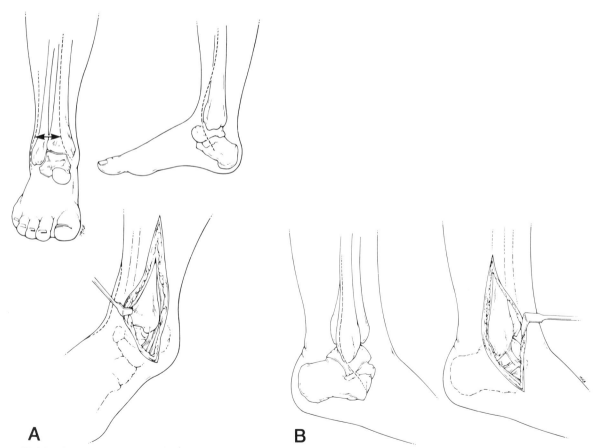

Figure 67.11.   A. Two-incision approach with elaboration of the anteromedial incision. The surgeon should remember to maintain a 5 to 7 cm skin bridge between the two incisions to prevent skin necrosis. **B.** Placement of posterolateral incision.

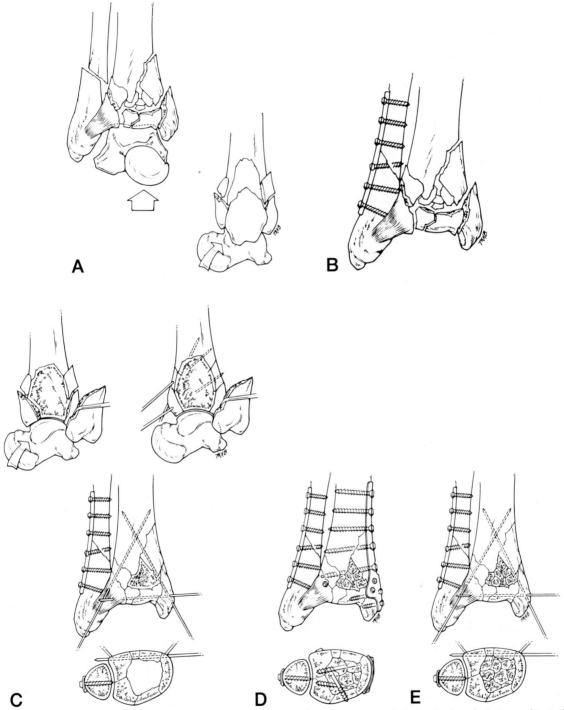

Figure 67.12. **A.** Type III pilon fracture. **B.** Fibular reconstruction. **C.** Reconstruction of the tibial plafond using the talus as a template with provisional stabilization. **D.** Tibial metaphyseal defect packed with can-cellous iliac bone graft. **E.** Application of a buttress plate to the tibia to prevent late varus deformity.

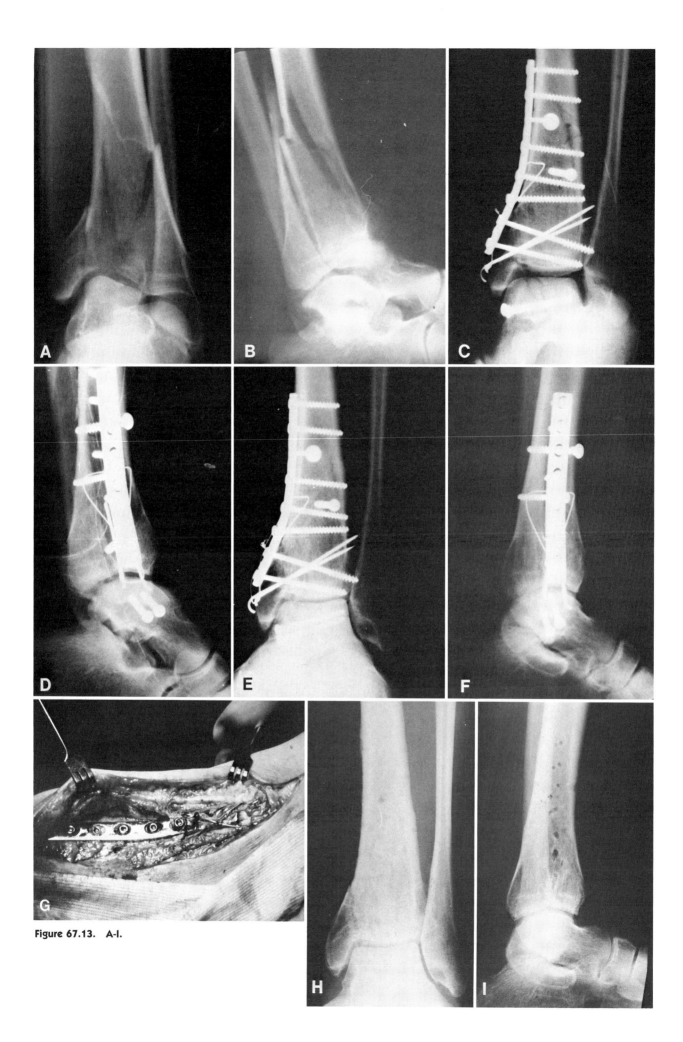

Figure 67.13. A-I.

into the tibial metaphyseal defect (Fig. 67.12D), and *(d)* application of a buttress plate to the tibia (Fig. 67.12E). These principles are critical for successful reconstruction of the pilon fracture. All are applicable for type III injuries; however, some type II pilon fractures do not require bone grafting.

Fibular Reconstruction

In 20% of pilon fractures, the fibula remains intact, so one can proceed with reconstruction of the tibia (Figs. 67.13 and 67.14). In the other 80% of the cases, fibular reconstruction takes priority. Successful reconstruction of the fibula restores the proper length and rotation to the ankle. This is also important because the key tibial fragment is usually attached to the fibula and aids in tibial reconstruction. The fracture configuration of the fibula can be transverse, oblique, or spiral. The transverse and oblique fractures tend to be more commonly associated with the axial compression mechanism of injury. The spiral fracture is usually associated with the rotational injury. The fibula is usually fixated with a combination of interfragmentary compression screws, cortical screws, and a one-third tubular plate for neutralization. However, Tile (4) indicates that noncomminuted transverse or short oblique fractures can be fixated with an intramedullary Rush rod or Steinmann pin since rotational stability is less important with pilon fractures than with ankle fractures. The advantage is quickness, a short incision, and little soft tissue dissection. Surgical intervention should begin with the tibia if the fibula is severely comminuted and cannot be anatomically restored. After tibial reconstruction, an attempt is made to impart the proper length to the fibula by stabilization with a one-third tubular plate.

Tibial Articular Reconstruction

If available, it is important to use the tomograms and the CT scan to identify the key fragments of the tibia. If the anterior syndesmosis is intact (usually with compression fractures), then the key anterolateral fragment will be attached to the fibula and in a more anatomic position after fibular reconstruction. Provisionally, the tibial fragments should be stabilized with K-wires using the talus as a template if necessary. If the fragments are large, they can be fixated with several lag screws or a bone-reduction forceps (Fig. 67.15). If the metaphysis is too comminuted to reconstruct, one should concentrate on restoring the congruity of the articular surface. Once provisional stabilization is ac-

complished, radiographs should be obtained to confirm the adequacy of the reduction. In cases of significant comminution with several large fragments that are positioned anteriorly and posteriorly, there are two techniques that can be of benefit. First, one may place two 6.5 mm cancellous screws from anterior to posterior, one lagging fragments on the medial side and the other on the lateral side. The screws are allowed to protrude posteriorly and a cerclage wire is placed around the tips of the screws. Alternatively, the threads of the 6.5 mm cancellous screws can engage the holes of a one-third tubular plate that has been placed along the posterior aspect of the tibia (Fig. 67.16).

Cancellous Bone Graft

In type III pilon fractures the large defect in the tibial metaphysis must be treated with a bone graft. The best source of bone is the iliac crest. This graft will support the tibial articular surface and prevent collapse during the consolidation phase. This is not the ideal situation for an allogeneic bone graft, but it may be used if autogenous bone is unavailable.

Buttress Plate Application to the Tibia

To prevent late varus deformity, a buttress plate should be applied to the tibia (Fig. 67.17). It may be applied to the medial or anterior aspect, depending on the fracture configuration. Several different styles of implant are available. On the medial side, one can employ the cloverleaf plate (Fig. 67.10 C and D), the T-plate (Fig. 67.15 G and H), or a dynamic compression plate (Figs. 67.13 C and D and 67.14 J and K). If the implant must be applied anteriorly, then either the spoon plate (Fig. 67.3 C and D) or the T-plate (Fig. 67.15 G and H) may be used. After the plate has been applied to the tibia, final intraoperative radiographs are obtained with the hope that they will demonstrate an anatomic reduction with good position of the fixation devices.

The author has seen parachute injuries caused by axial loading in addition to rotational forces that produce complex ankle fractures with major tibial fragments, especially posteriorly and medially. These fractures are called mini-pilons but are essentially type II pilon fractures. No large cancellous defects are created. These fractures have been successfully treated without bone grafting and with multiple lag screw fixation without buttress plating (Fig. 67.18). No late varus drift has been noted.

Incisions must be closed without tension. Since these in-

Text continued on p. 1671.

Figure 67.13. **A** and **B.** Anteroposterior and lateral views of a closed type II pilon fracture without associated fibular fracture. There is also a sagittal plane shearing fracture of the talus. This injury was sustained in a helicopter crash. **C** and **D.** Mortise and lateral views of intraoperative reduction. The reductions of both the tibia and the talus are anatomic. A dynamic compression plate has been applied to buttress the medial aspect of the tibia. **E** and **F.** Mortise and lateral views 10 months after surgery demonstrating fracture consolidation with no avascular necrosis of the talus. **G.** Intraoperative photograph at time of hardware removal demonstrating the dynamic compression plate and tension band wire. **H** and **I.** Mortise and lateral views 21 months after initial surgery; the patient is free of symptoms.

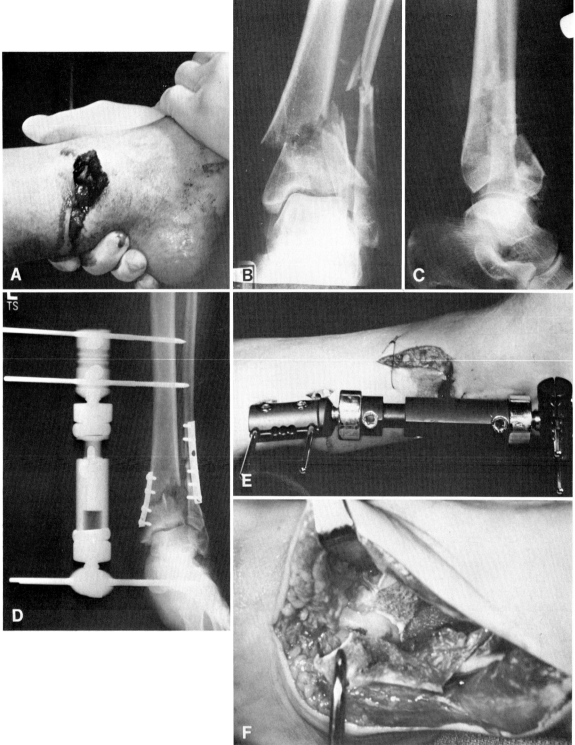

Figure 67.14. **A.** Grade III open pilon fracture sustained by a 45-year-old white woman who fell while climbing into a deer stand. Leaves, dirt, and the patient's sock were embedded in the wound. **B** and **C.** Mortise and lateral radiographs of open type III pilon fracture. **D.** Initial surgery on the day of admission involved debridement with reduction and internal fixation of the fibula with a one third tubular plate and provisional stabilization of the tibia with a one third tubular plate and an external fixator. **E.** Photograph of external fixator applied medially for provisional stabilization. Note early necrosis of the proximal skin flap. **F.** Intraoperative photograph through lateral incision demonstrating comminuted tibial metaphysis. **G** and **H.** Mortise and lateral views of reduction with provisional K-wire fixation during operation for definitive fixation 10 days after initial injury. The patient had several debridements prior to this surgery. **I.** Intraoperative photograph through medial incision showing final tibial fixation after bone graft with 3.5 mm dynamic compression plate. **J** and **K.** Anteroposterior and lateral radiographs of final reduction and fixation. **L.** Medial incision 14 days after injury following debridement of necrotic skin flaps. The wound is granulating, but part of the plate is exposed. The patient was referred to a plastic surgeon for wound coverage but was discovered to have osteomyelitis. She subsequently had radical debridement and application of an Ilizarov frame at the referral institution, and soft tissue coverage has been delayed.

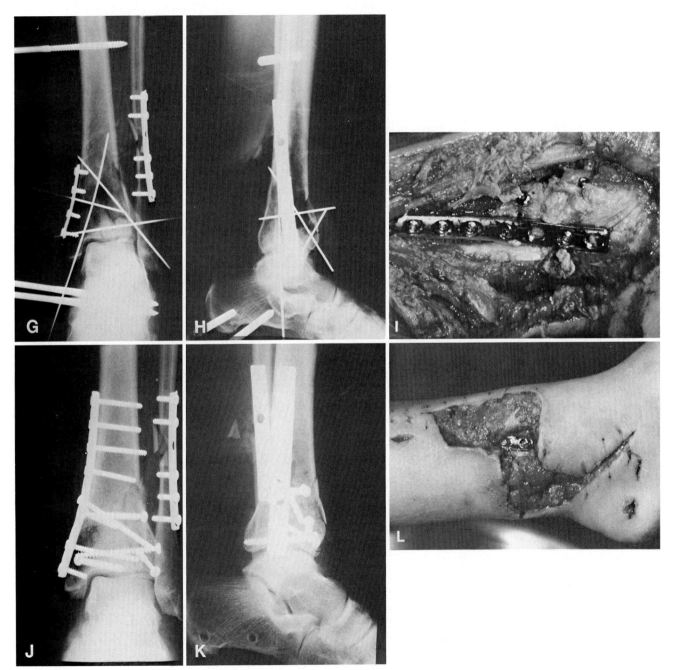

Figure 67.14.   G-L.

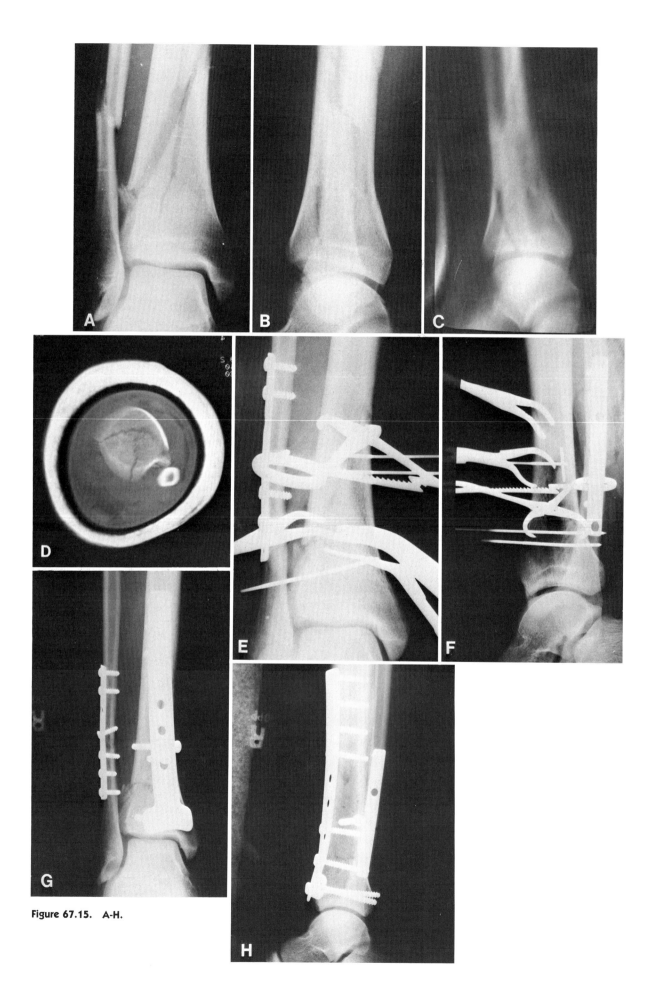

Figure 67.15. A-H.

Figure 67.15.   **A** and **B.** Mortise and lateral views of a closed type II rotational pilon fracture. **C.** Lateral tomogram demonstrating gaping of the tibial articular surface and superior displacement of the anterior fragment. **D.** CT scan revealing tibial fragments. **E** and **F.** Mortise and lateral intraoperative views with reduction of the fibula followed by reduction of the tibial plafond and provisional stabilization with K-wires and bone reduction forceps. **G** and **H.** Mortise and lateral views of final reduction, which is anatomic with application of an anterior buttress plate. No bone graft was required.

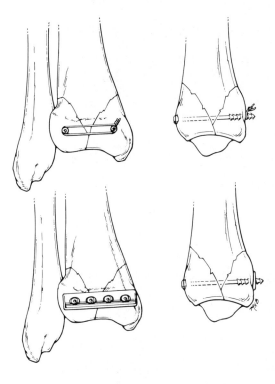

Figure 67.16.   Techniques of stabilizing a comminuted tibial plafond, which has major fragments anteriorly and posteriorly.

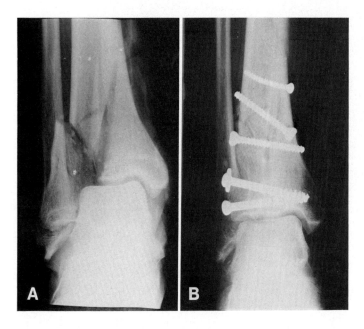

Figure 67.17.   **A.** Closed type II pilon fracture. **B.** Fracture was fixated without a buttress plate. Despite fracture consolidation, there is late varus deformity and the superior screw is bent. The patient contributed to the problem with premature weight bearing.

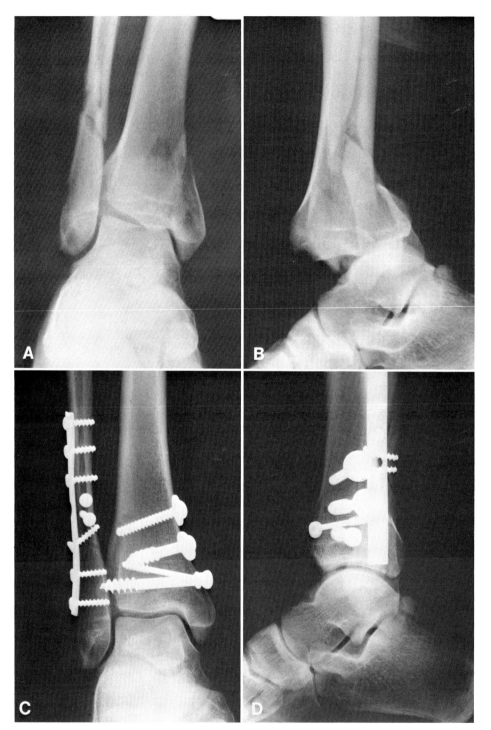

Figure 67.18.   A and **B.** Mortise and lateral views of a closed complex fracture dislocation of the ankle, which we describe as a minipilon fracture. The injury was sustained in a parachute jump. **C** and **D.** Mortise and lateral views of open reduction with internal fixation. No varus deformity ensued, despite the fact that no buttress plate was used. Also, no bone graft was required.

juries are complex and often necessitate prolonged operative time, significant edema may occur, especially if the tourniquet has been released. This can make closure difficult to obtain. The medial incision must be closed, as it will lie over the major implant. The lateral incision can always be addressed as a delayed primary closure. Ideally, both incisions can be closed primarily in most cases. A suction drain should be used in each incision.

Postoperatively, the patient is placed in a compression dressing and a cast or splint. Prophylactic antibiotics, which were begun intravenously before surgery for closed fractures, are continued for 24 hours. The usual choice is a first-generation cephalosporin. The extremity is elevated, and ice is applied. Postoperative analgesics are prescribed. The dressing is removed and the operative site is examined in 48 hours. The suction drains are removed at this time. Range-of-motion exercises are begun, both actively and passively, under the guidance of a physical therapist. It is important to begin motion exercises only if fixation is truly stable. If stable fixation is not present, then the patient can be treated in a cast or calcaneal pin traction can be employed. If the reduction is stable, the compliant patient can be treated in a removable fracture brace/splint in order to continue motion exercises or be placed in a below-knee cast. It is important to splint the ankle at 90 degrees to prevent an equinus contracture. Either way, the patient must refrain from weight bearing for a minimum of 3 months to allow fracture consolidation. This should be determined by clinical examination and with serial radiographs. It is also important to use elastic support hose to help control edema.

The most common late complication of pilon fractures is traumatic arthritis. As mentioned previously, it will usually develop within 1 year in those patients in whom it will develop. The obvious surgical treatment for this problem is ankle fusion when symptoms warrant. Other complications include loss of motion, prolonged edema, incisional scarring, skin necrosis, soft tissue and/or osseous infection, delayed union/nonunion, implant failure, nerve entrapment, phlebitis, and malunion. Axial malalignment can be addressed by supramalleolar osteotomy.

The potential risk of infection cannot be understated. The soft tissue trauma, extensive bony comminution, devascularized bony fragments, extensive dissection, long incisions, and prolonged operating time combine to facilitate the development of infection. These factors can be further complicated by an open injury. The worst possible scenario would be an infected nonunion. In the case of soft tissue infection, the incisions are opened, appropriate cultures are taken (gram stain, aerobic and anaerobic cultures), appropriate intravenous antibiotic therapy is instituted, debridement and irrigation of the wounds are completed, and stable fixation is left in place. If the fixation is unstable, an attempt is made to obtain stable fixation. Alternatively, fixation is changed to a different form of stabilization, such as an external fixator or a cast. If the fracture has consolidated, then the fixation can be removed. The wounds are left open for delayed primary closure. If the tibial incision is directly over the implant, however, wound closure might be considered over a suction irrigation drain. This is because it is very difficult to encourage granulation tissue or skin to grow over a large metallic implant. In the case of osteomyelitis or an infected pseudarthrosis, a below-knee amputation may be the best reconstructive procedure. If an attempt is made to salvage this situation, it can require such complex procedures as radical debridement and application of an external fixator, a Papineau bone graft, a free fibular graft, or a free composite graft. A surgeon trained in microvascular procedures can be helpful in attempting to resolve this complex problem.

References

1. Ruedi TP, Allgower M: Fractures of the lower end of the tibia into the ankle joint. *Injury* 1:92, 1969.
2. Lauge-Hansen N: Fractures of the ankle. *Arch Surg* 56:250, 1948.
3. Kellam JF, Waddell JP: Fractures of the distal tibial metaphysis with intra-articular extension: the distal tibial explosion fractures. *J Trauma* l9:250, 1979.
4. Tile M: Fractures of the distal tibial metaphysis involving the ankle joint: the pilon fractures. In Schatzker J, Tile M: *Rationale of Operative Fracture Care.* New York, Springer-Verlag, 1987, pp 343-369.
5. Tscherne H, Gotzen L: *Fractures With Soft Tissue Injuries.* New York, Springer-Verlag, 1984.
6. Ruoff AG, Snider RK: Explosion fractures of the distal tibia with major articular involvement. *J Trauma* 11:86, 1971.
7. Fourquet D: Contribution a l'etude des fractures recentes du pilon tibial. *Thesis.* Paris, 1959.
8. Bonnier P: Les fractures du pilon fracture. *Thesis.* Lyons, 1961.
9. Ruedi T: Fractures of the lower end of the tibia into the ankle joint: results 9 years after open reduction and internal fixation. *Injury* 5:130, 1973.
10. Heim U, Naser K: Fractures du pilon tibial: resultats de 128 osteosynthesis. *Rev Chir Orthop* 63:512, 1977.
11. Ruedi T, Allgower M: The operative treatment of intra-articular fractures of the lower end of the tibia. *Clin Orthop* 138:105-110, 1979.

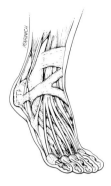

CHAPTER **68**

Physeal Injuries

Alan S. Banks, D.P.M.

"Fractures in children are different." This simple statement by Blount (1) explains why the practitioner must be cognizant of the basic principles involved when facing a physeal injury. The biology and management of these injuries is different and requires that one look at the child as something other than an adult counterpart. With this in mind, discussion will begin with the anatomical considerations involved in injuries to the physis and then proceed to the diagnosis and treatment of these conditions.

ANATOMY

Each long bone may be divided into three separate sections. The *diaphysis*, or primary growth center, is the lengthy central aspect of the developing bone. The diaphysis expands at each end to form regions known as the *metaphyses*, which are more involved in active bone growth. *Epiphyses*, or secondary ossification centers, lie adjacent to the metaphysis and are separated from it by the growth plate or *physis*. The opposite side of the epiphysis articulates with the adjacent joint. When considered together, the epiphysis and physis will hereafter be known as the epiphyseal complex (Fig. 68.1).

Epiphyseal Complex

Within the lower extremity there are two types of epiphyseal complexes: pressure and traction. Pressure complexes are located at the end of long bones as just described. The primary purpose of these particular structures is to provide for rapid longitudinal growth to the developing body. Other functions include provision of the proper configuration necessary for joint function and correct axial relationship

and distribution of weight-bearing or compressive forces through the limb or part. Traction epiphyseal complexes serve as sites for muscular attachment and, therefore, are subject to tremendous tensile forces. They may also be known as apophyses. Examples are the posterior tubercle of the calcaneus at the insertion of the Achilles tendon and the tibial tuberosity at the insertion of the quadriceps. These complexes are not articular and do not contribute to longitudinal growth, although they may provide additional shape or contour to the bone.

Metaphysis

The metaphysis is a wider portion of the osseous shaft interposed between the epiphyseal complex and the diaphysis. Newly ossified material is refined in this region as bone migrates away from the physis. The cortical bone is thinner than that of the diaphysis and exhibits greater porosity. Fenestrations within the cortex allow for the passage of the additional vascular elements needed to supply the metabolic demands of the region. Naturally, this means that the developing metaphysis will be susceptible to certain types of injury. However, these fenestrations do allow the periosteum to firmly adhere to the cortex, thereby offering some degree of stability.

Physis

The physis is a radiolucent cartilaginous plate located between the metaphysis and the epiphysis, and it is a primary structure of concern in pediatric and adolescent skeletal trauma. Trauma to the physis is commonly labeled as epiphyseal injury. This is actually a misnomer, however, as it is not the epiphysis but the physis that, when damaged, may cause growth arrest. The physis has a characteristic arrangement of cells that progresses in an orderly manner from resting chondrocytes to ossified medullary bone (Fig. 68.2).

The area of the physis adjacent to the epiphysis makes up the *zone of growth*. This area of cartilage consists of resting chondrocytes and a layer of actively dividing cells directed towards the metaphysis. The resting chondrocytes were at one time thought to actively supply the cells necessary for growth. Newer evidence shows that the resting cells rarely replicate. However, each has a large endoplasmic reticulum, suggesting a high level of protein synthesis in this area. Currently it is believed that these cells are responsible for providing the nutrients and materials required for the areas

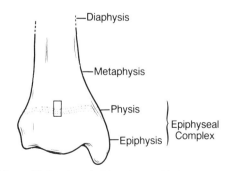

Figure 68.1. A typical long bone with three regions.

- Diaphysis

- Metaphysis

- Physis

- Epiphysis

} Epiphyseal Complex

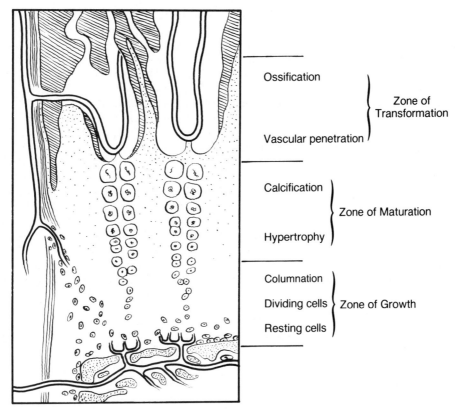

Figure 68.2. Microscopic anatomy of the physis.

involved with active growth (2). Within this zone there is also an abundant intercellular matrix containing chondroitin sulfuric acid, hyaline, and collagen, all of which add considerable strength and nutritive support to the area (3, 4).

Increased mitosis occurs in the adjacent layer of actively dividing cells. Here the chondrocytes will begin to organize into pallisades or longitudinal rows parallel to the long axis of the bone.

The next region encountered is the *zone of cartilage maturation*. The chondrocytes, which are now well organized into columns, will hypertrophy and the previously rich intercellular matrix will become sparse. Concomitantly, the random order of the collagen fibrils within the intercellular matrix will assume an orderly arrangement between the cell columns (4, 5). Previously it was assumed that the chondrocytes degenerated before absorbing hydroxyapatite crystals and undergoing calcification. However, it now appears that these hypertrophic cells assume an active role in the calcification process (2). The relative loss of intercellular matrix in this region, as well as the loss of intracellular substance, makes this the weakest area of the physis. It is especially susceptible to shearing, bending, and tension stresses but more resistant to compression (6).

Once calcification has occurred, the cells will enter the *zone of cartilage transformation*. When sufficient calcification is reached, vascular mesenchyme will invade the tissues and

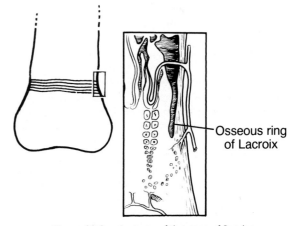

Figure 68.3. Anatomy of the zone of Ranvier.

the process of ossification and remodeling will begin. Although this area is also relatively weak, the initiation of calcification increases its strength as compared to the zone of cartilage maturation.

Zone of Ranvier

Ranvier was the first to describe the circumferential groove surrounding the periphery of the physis (7) (Fig. 68.3).

Composed of fibroblasts, fibrocytes, undifferentiated mesenchymal tissue, and the osseous ring of Lacroix (an extension of the metaphyseal cortex), this groove is most noticeable in the younger patient and gradually disappears as the child matures. Its functions are to render support to the physis and to provide for appositional expansion at its periphery (4, 7) so that latitudinal and longitudinal growth of the physis may proceed in harmony. At the same time, this zone acts as a peripheral restraint to physeal growth (8). The periosteum of the metaphysis adheres firmly to these tissues and thus acts to bind the epiphyseal complex and the metaphysis together.

Periosteum

The periosteum of the child is more highly vascularized, more osteogenic, thicker, and stronger than that of the adult. The periosteum is loosely attached at the diaphyseal level, being separated from the cortex by a layer of soft osteogenic tissue. The development of Sharpey's fibers does not occur until the child approaches maturation. It is at this time that the periosteum establishes its intimate contact with the diaphyseal cortex. There are two reasons for this delay. One is that the periosteum is much more active in osteogenesis in the diaphysis of the child. Second, the musculature derives most of its origin from the periosteum rather than from the cortex. This arrangement allows for coordinated growth of osseous and muscular tissues that otherwise would not be possible.

At the metaphysis the periosteum becomes much more firmly attached to the cortical bone, as was discussed earlier. This intimate relationship between the bone and the periosteum continues along the periphery of the physis and into the zone of Ranvier, as well as the epiphyseal perichondrium. Even at this level, muscular attachment is still primarily served by the periosteum rather than by the cortex.

The ligaments surrounding the joint insert into the perichondrium of the epiphysis, as well as into the zone of Ranvier. This allows for coordinated growth of osseous and soft tissues and also reduces the tensile forces on the epiphyseal complex.

The periosteum adds considerable strength to the epiphyseal complex and the adjacent metaphysis, especially against shearing forces. Several investigators have shown that, once the periosteum is removed from this area, the physis may be separated relatively easily (8-10). However, Ogden (6) pointed out that this layer has a secondary role in load distribution because the periosteal membrane has a lower elastic modulus.Thus it acts primarily as a checkrein once a fracture has occurred.

Vasculature

The metaphysis derives its blood supply from several sources. The first is via the nutrient arteries of the diaphysis. These branch and form a circulatory plexus at each end of the long bone, which supplies the central aspect of the metaphysis, whereas the more peripheral regions will be nourished by vessels from the periosteum and the perichondrium. This metaphyseal circulation will form capillary loops that may extend as far as the margin of the hypertrophic cells of the physis.

The epiphysis derives its blood supply from separate nutrient arteries that enter the epiphysis proper. These vessels will form a rich vascular plexus to supply the epiphysis and, after penetrating the subchondral bone plate, will extend so that they also supply the reproductive cells of the cartilaginous physis.

The physis derives its blood supply in part from the two previously mentioned sources, as well as from the perichondrial vessels of the zone of Ranvier. Although these three systems are independent, anastomoses may infrequently occur within the cartilaginous region of the physis.

Traditionally, the metaphyseal vessels were not thought to supply the replicative cartilage cells of the physis. Thus interruption of the blood supply to this system would only temporarily interrupt the process of cartilage maturation and would have little influence on overall growth. The cartilage cells would continue to reproduce but would fail to become ossified. Therefore, once disturbed by injury, it will be about 3 to 4 weeks before the metaphyseal circulation can be restored, at which time ossification will resume. When the epiphyseal vessels are disturbed, the germinal cells of the physis lose their blood supply and degenerate. Obviously, the cell division necessary for growth cannot continue. This will result in premature fusion of the physis, either totally or partially. However, more recently one study has demonstrated that both metaphyseal and epiphyseal circulations may be necessary for predictable growth at the physeal level (11).

Disruption of the perichondrial vessels surrounding the growth plate may also cause growth arrest. These vessels are necessary for continued *appositional* growth at the periphery of the physis. Certain types of injury (fractures, burns, radiation, degloving injury) may disrupt this supply and subsequently lead to premature fusion of all or, more frequently, parts of the physis.

Classification of Injury

Several different classifications have been proposed for evaluating physeal injuries (4, 12-15), but the most universally accepted is that of Salter and Harris (4). Since the inception of this system, however, additions have been made to more accurately explain the events of physeal injury and the associated prognosis. The classification used henceforth will be that of Salter and Harris with the modifications supplied by Ogden (6, 16).

TYPE I

The type I injury is a complete separation of the epiphysis from the metaphysis, with the line of fracture traversing through the physis between the layers of cellular hypertrophy and degeneration (Fig. 68.4). This fracture line need not be smooth, and it may involve small regions from other

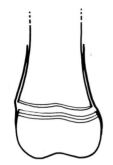

Figure 68.4.   Type IA fracture.

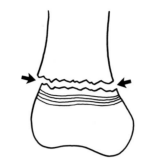

Figure 68.5.   Type IB fracture.

zones of the physis from tiny pieces of the primary spongiosa of the metaphysis. Usually the resting cells are left undisturbed and are avulsed with the epiphysis. Displacement of the epiphysis is usually minimal because the thick periosteum is strongly adherent to the zone of Ranvier. Often the only radiographic evidence of fracture will be an apparent increase in thickness at one end of the physis without other signs of displacement. At other times the injury will not be evident radiographically, and the diagnosis must be based on clinical symptoms and examination alone.

The injury just described has been designated a type IA fracture. This is most common in infants with limited development of the epiphysis. Type IB fractures occur in children who have systemic disorders that impair endochondral ossification. Disease entities most commonly associated with type IB fractures are myeloproliferative disorders such as leukemia and thalassemia, as well as various neuromuscular disorders manifesting with sensory deficits (6, 16, 17). At times this fracture may be the first indication of the disease process. The plane of cleavage with this injury is primarily through the layer of degenerative cartilage cells or through primary spongiosa (Fig. 68.5). In both types IA and IB the primary germinal elements are undisturbed; once healing has occurred, normal growth resumes.

A further subclassification, type IC, describes a fracture in which there is an associated injury to some of the germinal cells of the physis. This is a crush injury to all cell layers in the affected portion of the growth plate and occurs when the force propagating through the limb abruptly shifts (Fig. 68.6). Osseous bridging will result once the epiphysis expands and reaches the damaged region. Type I injuries usually occur in children under the age of 2 years. After that age a type II injury is more likely to result as the forces shift while propagating through the physis. Fractures of this type may also be associated with rickets, scurvy, osteomyelitis, and endocrine imbalances (4, 6, 16, 18).

TYPE II

The type II injury is the most common acute physeal injury and, like type I, is caused by a shearing or avulsion force. As the child matures, two things happen that favor the occurrence of a type II injury as opposed to type I. First, the relatively planar subchondral bone plate between the epiphysis and the physis will begin to contour in response to the

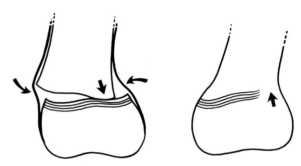

Figure 68.6.   Type IC fracture.

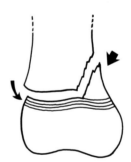

Figure 68.7.   Type IIA fracture.

various biomechanical stresses surrounding the joint. Second, cartilaginous extensions from the physis, known as mamillary processes, will begin to develop and reach into the metaphysis. These two events supplement the overall stability of the physis against shearing forces and tend to redirect disruptive stress propagating through the physis into metaphyseal bone. Thus, in a type II fracture, the plane of cleavage enters the physis at the same level as the type I injury (between the hypertrophic and degenerative cell layers) and propagates through the growth plate until such time as the force is redirected into metaphyseal bone. This results in a portion of the metaphysis being avulsed with the epiphysis. This flag or fragment is known as the Thurston-Holland sign. The periosteum will be torn on the convex side of the fracture where the deforming force entered, and the periosteum will remain intact on the concave side of the fracture that holds the metaphyseal fragment. As with type I injuries the germinal cells of the physis are attached to the epiphysis and are not damaged. Ogden has classified this as the type IIA fracture (Fig. 68.7).

In type IIB fractures the metaphyseal fragment that accompanies the epiphysis is a free fragment (Fig. 68.8). In type IIC injuries a thin layer of metaphysis is present across the entire epiphyseal fragment (Fig. 68.9). This is more common in the phalanges because the trabeculae within these small bones are oriented in a transverse direction instead of longitudinally. The plane of cleavage in type IIC fractures is through the primary spongiosa of the metaphysis. Type IID fractures involve an element of compression against the physis, usually at the point where the fracture force turns to exit through the metaphysis. This will damage all layers of the growth plate and may lead to premature closure (Fig. 68.10).

TYPE III

The fracture line in the type III injury begins at the joint surface of the epiphysis and progresses through the secondary ossification center until it reaches the physis. There it will turn approximately 90° and run through the layer of hypertrophic cells to the periphery. This fracture pattern is also caused by a shearing force and is seen more frequently in older children where the physis is nearing fusion (Fig. 68.11). Type IIIB differs from this in that when the fracture turns toward the periphery a small layer of primary spongiosa is avulsed with the epiphysis (Fig. 68.12). Other than the few growth cells that are cleaved by the fracture line, the germinal elements are intact; however, one must be concerned with possible interruption of the blood supply to the free fragment, as well as the congruity of the joint surface.

TYPE IV

A type IVA injury occurs when the fracture line begins at the articular surface of the epiphysis, extends directly through it, and continues through all layers of the physis into the metaphysis (Fig. 68.13). This injury may not be apparent radiographically unless the epiphysis has reached a fair degree of ossification. Accurate reduction is necessary

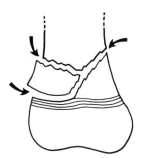

Figure 68.8. Type IIB fracture.

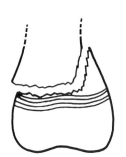

Figure 68.9. Type IIC fracture.

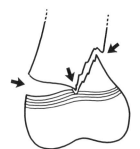

Figure 68.10. Type IID fracture.

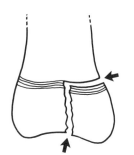

Figure 68.11. Type IIIA fracture.

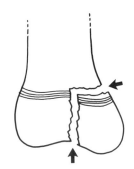

Figure 68.12. Type IIIB fracture.

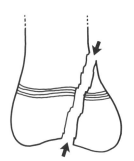

Figure 68.13. Type IVA fracture.

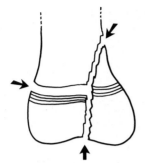

Figure 68.14. Type IVB fracture.

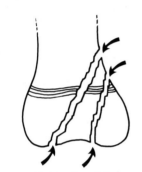

Figure 68.15. Type IVD fracture.

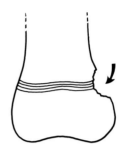

Figure 68.16. Type VI fracture.

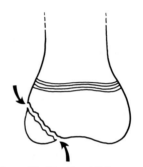

Figure 68.17. Type VII fracture.

to restore proper joint congruity, as well as architectural integrity, to the physis. The subtypes of the type IV injury mainly involve multiple fragments of the avulsed bone (Figs. 68.14 and 68.15).

TYPE V

Salter and Harris (4) were the first to describe the type V injury in their classification system. This fracture is said to occur after a severe crushing force and thus destroys the structural integrity to all cell layers of the physis. Subsequently, premature fusion will occur. On initial examination, there is no radiographic evidence of the injury and diagnosis must be based on history followed by watchful waiting to determine whether premature fusion develops. Patients must be re-evaluated frequently since growth disturbance may occur up to several years after the injury. Type V fractures are rare and are said to be most often associated with the ankle and knee because these joints have primarily one plane of motion in addition to being weight-bearing joints.

However, Peterson and Burkhart (19) have questioned whether the type V injury as described by Salter and Harris exists. Their theory was based on several points: *(a)* the finding of only two possible cases of type V injury in the Mayo Clinic files and the fact that these were not without question; *(b)* the relative absence of reports of such injuries in the literature; *(c)* the speculative assumption that premature closure is caused by compression when initial ra-

diographs show no abnormality; and *(d)* the fact that all cases of type V injury reported in the literature concerned the knee. Of the many documented cases of premature closure of the proximal tibial epiphysis, the common factor underlying each was prolonged immobilization. Thus their conclusion was that the type V classification as described by Salter and Harris was not valid and that a more appropriate mechanism must be found to explain this injury. Symmetrical premature closure of a physis is therefore more likely caused by a localized ischemia secondary to immobilization as opposed to damage to the germinal cells at the time of trauma.

Other forms of injury may cause symmetrical growth arrest of the physis. These other injuries include electrical burns (20), radiation (21), and frostbite (22, 23).

TYPE VI

Originally described by Rang (24), the type VI injury involves the zone of Ranvier and the associated periphery of the physis rather than the unit as a whole (Fig. 68.16). Certain types of trauma, such as burns or degloving processes, may disturb the peripheral areas of the physis and, accordingly, lead to partial growth arrest. Localized contusion may similarly disrupt normal anatomy. Radiographically, initial examination may show no osseous damage, but an osseous bar or bridge will develop peripherally where the perichondrial ring was disrupted, with the potential for resultant angular deformity.

TYPE VII

The type VII injury is an avulsion fracture of a piece of the epiphysis without involvement of the physis. At times this injury will have to be distinguished from a possible secondary ossification center, especially at the fibular or tibial malleolus. These are relatively rare fractures, and growth deformity is not a concern. This injury is mentioned only for the sake of completeness (Fig. 68.17).

GENERAL PRINCIPLES OF DIAGNOSIS AND TREATMENT

Diagnosis

Any child who is seen with an acutely painful extremity should be suspected of having a physeal injury until proven otherwise. The symptoms and complaints at the time of presentation are variable, with pain and swelling usually most noticeable overlying the physeal area. However, the degree of visible clinical findings may be relatively subdued. An important step in evaluating the painful extremity is adequate visualization of the part with radiographs. At least three different views of the affected area are usually in order, because many times the fracture may not be apparent with standard anteroposterior and lateral views. Contralateral films for comparison may be helpful in certain instances.

At times the only radiographic evidence of a type I injury will be either an apparent increase in the width of the physis at one end or a slight interruption in the continuity of the bone as the cortex is followed from the metaphysis to the epiphysis. Epiphyses may rotate after a type I or type II fracture, and it is essential that this rotation be recognized if joint integrity is to be restored. It is common to have a type I fracture in which the epiphysis is avulsed and then spontaneously reduced once the deforming force is relieved. This may be erroneously diagnosed as a sprain and is seen frequently in the distal fibula. In addition, one must remember that a type I injury may be the first sign of a more serious systemic disorder. Patients with previous type I fractures or presenting with a suspicious history may require further medical evaluation to rule out a pathological process or perhaps child abuse.

In type II fractures the metaphyseal fragment may be of variable size. Often it is so small that it is not noticed. If the epiphysis has spontaneously reduced into its anatomical position as in a type I fracture, then the only radiographic evidence present may be a fine lamellar piece of metaphyseal bone that was avulsed with the epiphysis. Visualization of this fragment may require close scrutiny; when demonstrated, it is known as the Werenskiold sign (25) (Fig. 68.18). At other times a larger piece of metaphyseal bone is readily apparent, and this is termed a Thurston-Holland or flag sign. These two findings are diagnostic of a type II fracture.

Type III and type IV fractures should be recognized, provided adequate radiographs have been taken. The incidence of the traditional type V injury as described by Salter and Harris is in question. However, severe crush injuries have been known to occur on rare occasions in which the metaphysis is actually driven through the physis and into

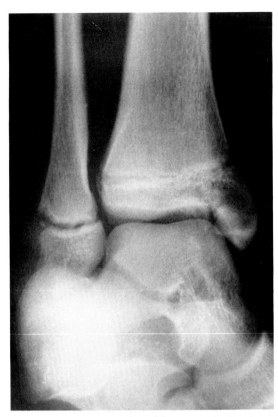

Figure 68.18. The small metaphyseal fragment at the lateral aspect of the fibula is called the Werenskiold sign and indicates a type IIA fracture.

the epiphysis or beyond. Such an injury will be obvious, and radiographs may show comminution of the epiphysis or displacement of the metaphysis into or through the physis.

SOFT TISSUE INJURY

Traditionally, most clinicians have believed that soft tissue injury in the child is rare, as the ligaments have been thought to be the stronger elements of joint anatomy. Therefore, after pediatric trauma, physeal injury would be the ensuing event. Although one would not argue about the integrity of the ligamentous structures, the number of associated ligamentous disruptions witnessed by those at many institutions cannot be casually dismissed. In particular, total disruption of the lateral ankle ligaments in children has been seen fairly often. Partial or total disruption of the anterior talofibular and calcaneofibular ligaments may occur without disruption of the distal fibular physis in an inversion injury. Damage to these structures has also been seen in association with Salter-Harris type III injuries to the medial aspect of the tibial physis without associated fracture of the fibula. Total disruption of the lateral ankle ligaments is a significant injury, and proper therapy depends on an accurate diagnosis. Generally, a good clinical examination is all that is required, as these two injuries are associated with distinctly different anatomic areas.

Salter (26) has recommended stress radiography when there is marked local tenderness over the physis without evidence of fracture in standard views. However, others have questioned its necessity (18, 27).

Treatment

Type I and II injuries generally respond well to closed reduction. When closed reduction is attempted, care should be taken so that undue trauma is not exerted on the fracture fragments. Although the germinal cells may have been preserved at the time of fracture, excessive or aggressive manipulation in reduction may disrupt their continuity. This is especially true when one is evaluating an older fracture. After 7 to 10 days callus formation has become well established, and manipulation at this time may prove more detrimental than beneficial. At this point, it is probably better to accept any ensuing deformity and treat it appropriately than to incur a growth arrest through forceful manipulation. In some instances soft tissue interposition between the metaphysis and the associated epiphyseal fragment may prevent closed reduction and open reduction will be necessary.

Reduction of type I and type II injuries does not have to be exact because remodeling of any residual minor displacement will occur, provided the child has 2 or more years of growth remaining and the resulting deformity is in the same plane as the movement of the affected joint. Rotational deformities should not be expected to remodel (28). Obviously, common sense will also dictate what is to be done. Residual deformity is much more acceptable in the lesser digits because the sequelae of poor alignment may or may not cause symptoms and if a problem arises treatment usually consists of simple arthroplasty. The ankle joint will require more precise reduction, however, with surgical intervention being required in instances in which adequate closed reduction cannot be obtained.

Type III and IV fractures should be accurately reduced; open, anatomical reduction is preferred for type IV injuries of major joints.

An additional consideration in type III and IV injuries, other than anatomical restoration of the physis is preservation of the congruity of the affected joint surface. When open reduction is attempted, then the following principles should be followed. The soft tissues, especially the periosteum, should be handled with care. This will maintain circulation to an area in which it has already been partially disrupted. Excessive stripping of periosteal tissue may disrupt the cells that provide appositional growth at the zone of Ranvier. If possible, threaded screws or wires are not to be placed across the physis. If needs dictate that fixation devices cross the growth plate, then only the smallest possible smooth Kirschner wires should be used. Early removal after healing is required. Preferably, all of the fixation devices should be maintained in the metaphysis rather than in the epiphysis.

When reduction is accomplished, casting should be used for at least 3 to 4 weeks, and up to 6 weeks in the older child. Symptoms may dictate that a longer period of immobilizaton is needed in some cases.

Although the existence of the traditional Salter-Harris type V fracture is in question, the patient who has a history suggestive of this type of injury should be placed in a non-weight-bearing cast for 3 to 4 weeks. It would seem plausible to initiate aggressive range-of-motion exercises after casting to counteract the possible development of premature fusion secondary to immobilization as was noted earlier.

Specific Injuries

FOOT

The flexibility of the child's foot tends to either resist injury or transmit the traumatic forces to a more proximal area. As a result most of the physeal injuries in the foot will involve a crushing mechanism, although this varies as the patient ages and becomes more active. Of particular importance are the various anatomical anomalies that may be present within the foot. Such variants may at times present a dilemma when one is examining a patient. Enumeration of these anomalies is beyond the scope of this chapter, and other sources have addressed the subject well (29).

Fractures of the phalanges are fairly common physeal injuries seen in the foot. The mechanism of injury is no different from that which causes digital fractures in the adult (e.g., jamming of the digit against some type of furniture or a crush from a heavy object). Fractures of the physis of the proximal phalanx of the hallux may also be seen on occasion and require more attention as open reduction may be necessary if a large part of the joint surface is involved. No matter which technique is used, immobilization and abstinence from weight bearing are in order. If the physis has been crushed, then prophylactic antibiotics are recommended, since a higher incidence of osteomyelitis has been associated with such injuries (6). This is because small cutaneous fissures are purportedly created by the trauma and serve as a portal of entry for the bacteria.

Several normal variants of this epiphysis have been documented, including fissures or fragmentation and sclerosis. Idiopathic fissures are most common and usually fuse without incident, whereas fracture of this epiphyseal complex is associated with a high incidence of hallux rigidus (30).

Avulsion of the nail from the proximal nail fold should alert the clinician of the potential for an associated physeal injury. This type of injury is usually seen after a stubbing of the digit in a barefooted child. If the magnitude of force was sufficient to disrupt the nail, a radiograph should be obtained to determine whether a fracture of the distal phalangeal physis has occurred (Fig. 68.19). Generally a nail bed laceration is present, thus constituting an open fracture. Appropriate treatment consists of avulsion of part or all of the nail, thorough irrigation, and repair of the nail bed laceration. A drain of some type is placed beneath the nail fold, and a course of oral antibiotics is prescribed (31). Experiences with the hand have shown that failure to recognize

Figure 68.19.   Lateral radiograph of a 9-year-old girl after a stubbing injury of the hallux with avulsion of the proximal nail. A type IIA fracture is demonstrated. (From Banks AS, Cain TD, Ruch JA: *Physeal fractures of the distal phalanx of the hallux. J Am Podiatr Med Assoc* 78:310-313, 1988, by permission).

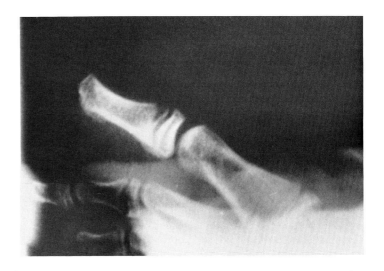

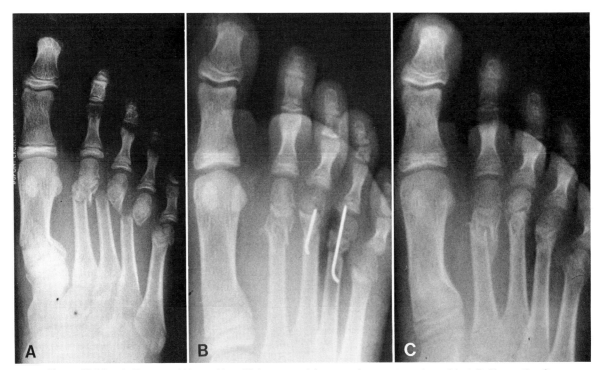

Figure 68.20.   **A.** Ten-year-old boy with multiple metatarsal fractures after a motorcycle accident. **B.** Six months after ORIF for relocation of the third and fourth metatarsal heads. **C.** After the removal of Kirschner wires.

the osseous injury or to provide adequate local care may lead to infection (32).

Patients with physeal fractures of the lesser metatarsals seen at Northlake Regional Medical Center have most often been associated with motorcycle or bicycle accidents and falls. As often as not, the fracture involves the metaphysis proximal to the growth plate. Most of these fractures will be transverse in nature, conferring a certain inherent stability. Indirect soft tissue attachment of the deep transverse intermetatarsal ligament to the metatarsal head also tends

to stabilize the fragment. For individual fractures, closed reduction is generally acceptable. Once multiple metatarsal fractures have occurred, however, the stabilization rendered by the deep transverse ligament is negated. Therefore displaced fractures may require internal fixation with smooth Kirschner wires. One question that has yet to be answered concerns the degree of displacement that is acceptable in these weight-bearing bones without risking the later development of plantar lesions or metatarsalgia (Fig. 68.20).

Fractures of the first metatarsal have most commonly been

greenstick injuries of the diaphysis and the metaphysis. These will generally do well with immobilization. Variations have been seen, however, and the specific consideration is the subsequent function of the first ray. Therefore, a more aggressive approach may be indicated.

ANKLE

Following the example of Lauge-Hansen (33), Dias and Tachdjian (34) have developed a classification system for physeal fractures involving the ankle. As in the Lauge-Hansen classification, the specific fractures are diagnostic of cer-

tain injury mechanisms, and when these mechanisms are understood, closed reduction may be greatly facilitated. The first part of each hyphenated term in the nomenclature designates the fixed position of the foot at the time of injury, while the latter term denotes the direction of force being transmitted through the ankle (Fig. 68.21).

A supination-inversion fracture involves a simple inversion force applied to the supinated foot. Grade I is a type I or type II separation of the distal fibular epiphysis or rupture of the lateral ankle ligaments. Grade II is a continued progression of the inversion force, resulting in a type III or type IV fracture of the distal tibial epiphysis (Fig.

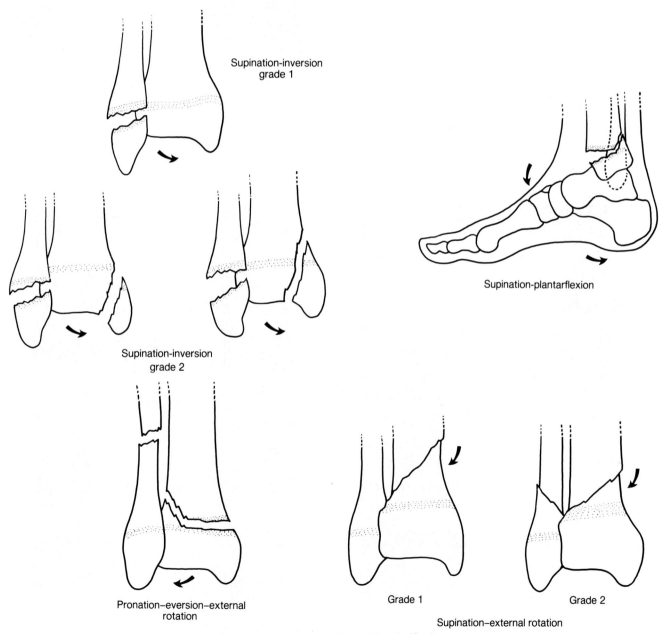

Figure 68.21.   The Dias and Tachdjian classification.

68.22). Type IV patterns may be particularly difficult to diagnose in some instances because of the small metaphyseal fragment (35).

Special attention should be directed towards the type III or IV injury of the medial malleolus because a high percentage of partial growth arrest or subsequent deformity has been reported, even when closed reduction is anatomical (35, 36). Chadwick and Bentley (37) attribute this to the force involved with most of these injuries. Generally this is associated with a supination-inversion mechanism. The medial malleolar fracture is evoked by a compressive force of the talus against the malleolus and growth plate. Therefore, this element of compression is more likely responsible for growth arrest than is the specific alignment. Anatomic reduction with screw fixation was advocated to minimize risk of subsequent problems. It has been postulated that, even if the physis was irreparably damaged, anatomic reduction would act to prevent adhesions between the epiphysis and the metaphysis. The cartilage that remains serves as a physiologic interposition to prevent growth arrest. Other authors have similarly recommended open reduction and internal fixation of these injuries (35, 36). Conversely, Landin and associates (38) noted that only two of twenty patients had minor problems after type III or IV medial malleolar fractures.

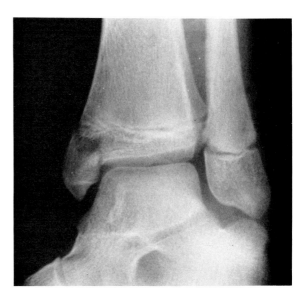

Figure 68.22. Supination-inversion grade II injury—type IA fracture, distal fibular physis. Type IIIA fracture, distal tibial physis.

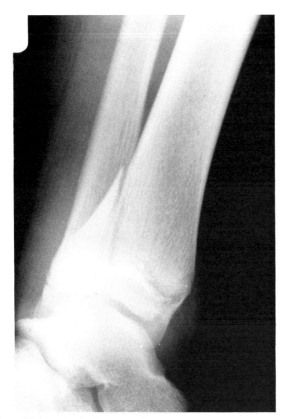

Figure 68.23. Supination-plantarflexion injury—type IIA fracture, distal tibial physis. The large metaphyseal fragment attached to epiphysis is the Thurston-Holland or flag sign.

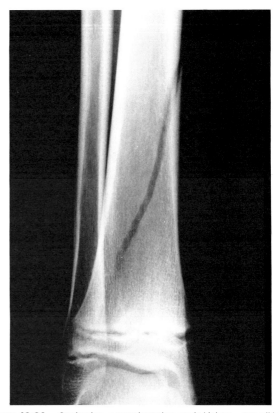

Figure 68.24. Supination-external rotation grade I injury—type IIA fracture, distal tibial physis. Notice how the fracture line starts laterally and runs superomedially.

A supination-plantarflexion fracture occurs with the foot supinated and the ankle receiving a plantargrade force. Grade I is a type II or occasionally a type I fracture of the distal tibial epiphysis (Fig. 68.23).

A supination-external rotation fracture occurs when the foot is supinated and an external rotatory force is applied. Grade I is a type II fracture of the distal tibial epiphysis with a long spiral fracture of the distal tibia. This may be differentiated from the supination-plantarflexion injury by the anteroposterior view. In this fracture the line will start at the lateral aspect of the distal tibia and run both proximally and medially (Figs. 68.24 and 68.25).

Grade II demonstrates a spiral fracture of the fibula without injury to the fibular epiphysis. The fibular fracture starts medially and runs posterosuperiorly (Figs. 68.26 and 68.27).

A pronation-eversion-external rotation fracture is a combination of eversion and external rotation forces applied to a pronated foot. Grade I is a type II fracture of the distal tibial epiphysis in which the metaphyseal fragment is often located laterally or posterolaterally. There may also be a fibular fracture without involvement of the physis (Fig. 68.28).

Two particular fracture patterns are not included within the Dias and Tachdjian classification system. The first is a type III fracture of the lateral aspect of the distal tibial physis. This is the equivalent of the Tillaux fracture in the

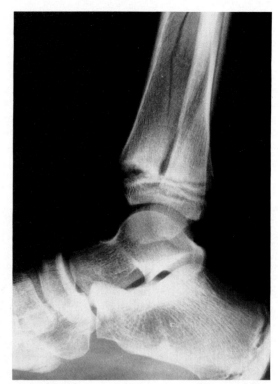

Figure 68.25. Supination-external rotation grade I, lateral view.

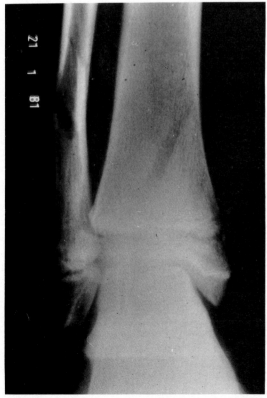

Figure 68.26. Supination-external rotation grade II, type IIA fracture of distal tibial physis, spiral fracture of fibular shaft.

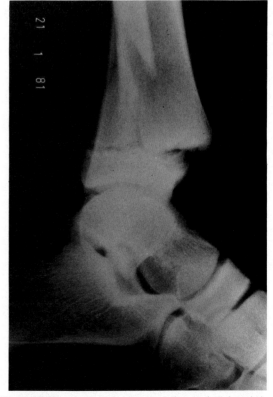

Figure 68.27. Supination-external rotation grade II, lateral view.

adult (Fig. 68.29). The other fracture pattern without classification is the triplane fracture. This may be seen as an apparent type III injury in an anteroposterior radiograph and as a type II fracture in the lateral radiograph. It is actually a type IV fracture that involves all three coronal body planes; hence the name *triplane fracture* (39). Marmor (40) originally described the three fragments associated with the injury: *(a)* the tibial shaft with the attached medial aspect of the distal tibial epiphysis, *(b)* an anterolateral tibial fragment, and *(c)* the remaining portion of the epiphysis with a posterior metaphyseal fragment (Figs. 68.30 and 68.31).

However, later authors have described several triplane fractures consisting of two fragments (41).

Kleiger and Mankin (42) were the first to note that an important anatomical factor involved with this fracture is the process of physiological epiphysiodesis of the distal tibial physis. Rather than fusing uniformly, the physis fuses over a period of about 18 months, starting in the middle, then progressing medially, and continuing until the anterolateral aspect of the physis fuses last (Fig. 68.32). The pattern of injury exhibited by these two fracture types is directly related to the sequence of physiological epiphysiodesis at the distal end of the tibia. A relatively weak area exists temporarily at the anterolateral aspect of the distal tibial physis and serves as the site for fracture propagation. However, triplane fractures have also been seen in patients with completely open growth plates (43). Most of these individuals had a hump or elevation in the medial aspect of the distal tibial physis, which appeared to be the site of the epiphyseal fracture. It was proposed that this anatomic feature stabilized the medial aspect of the physis in a manner similar to medial fusion of the growth plate in older children.

These injuries were originally described as a consequence of lateral rotation (42). Confirmation was provided by later authors. As the talus rotates laterally within the ankle mortise, the anterior inferior tibiofibular ligament applies tension to the distal tibial epiphysis and initiates the fracture.

Fortunately, most of these fractures heal uneventfully whether open or closed reduction is employed; even when premature fusion is encountered, the residual deformity is usually small because the physis has almost physiologically fused. The chief concern is with preservation of the integrity of the ankle joint mortise. Either tomograms or CT scans may be considered in questionable cases. The multiplanar

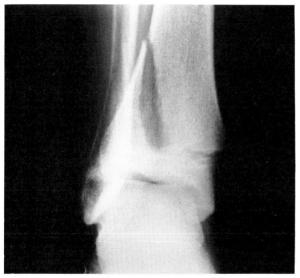

Figure 68.28. Pronation-eversion-external rotation fracture. Metaphyseal fragment is posterolateral in this type of injury.

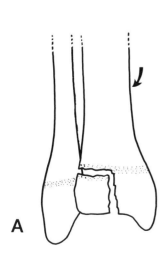

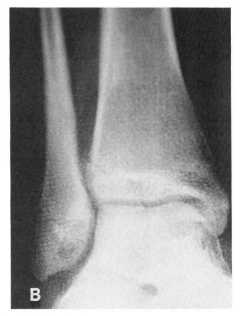

Figure 68.29. A and **B.** Tillaux fracture.

configuration of the fracture tends to afford inherent stability and resistance to displacement.

Yao and Huurman (44) have noted that tomography demonstrated significant fracture displacement in a juvenile Tillaux fracture, which was not appreciated on routine radiographs. Other authors have also found more sophisticated radiographic study to be of value in determining the most appropriate management of these injuries (45, 46). Generally, displacement of 2 mm or less has been regarded as acceptable for conservative management, with open reduction recommended for greater degrees of separation (43, 47-49).

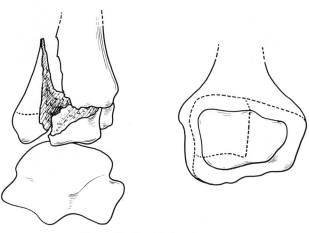

Figure 68.30.   Triplane fracture.

TORUS FRACTURES

Although torus fractures do not involve the growth plate, they are unique to children and, therefore, merit consideration within this context. Torus fractures, also referred to as greenstick fractures, are radiographically characterized by buckling of the metaphyseal cortex (Figs. 68.33 and 68.34). However, microscopic study of this injury has revealed that what actually occurs is a plastic deformation of bone on one side with a concomitant complete fracture of the opposite cortex (50). The fracture typically occurs at the transitional area from the more porous metaphyseal cortex to the dense diaphyseal bone. Anatomically, this appears to be the most susceptible area of the pediatric skeleton to compressive or impaction stress.

Torus fractures generally heal well with cast immobilization and abstinence from weight bearing. Angular deviation may remodel, and later surgical intervention may be considered for residual deformity.

FOLLOW-UP

After a physeal fracture the patient should generally be monitored with sequential radiographs to ensure that residual deformity does not develop. If closed reduction has been employed, it is important to perform radiographic studies after several days to ensure that good apposition has been maintained. Once the initial swelling has subsided, the cast may loosen and, in doing so, disrupt the fragments. A useful tool for evaluating the progress of posttraumatic healing in the child is the Harris growth-arrest line (51). This line will become evident in the metaphysis as growth is resumed after

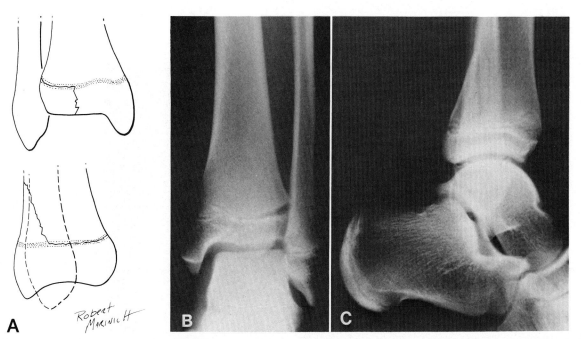

Figure 68.31.   **A.** Anteroposterior view of a triplane fracture appears as a type III injury. In the lateral view the fracture may appear as a type II injury. In actuality, it is a type IV injury. **B** and **C.** Radiographs of a typical triplane fracture.

Figure 68.32. Normal fusion of distal tibial physis. Notice how the central aspect of the physis has attained a greater degree of fusion, followed by the medial, and then the lateral aspects of the physis.

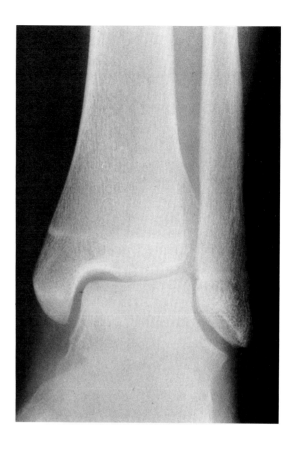

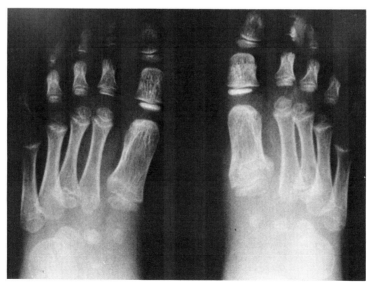

Figure 68.33. Torus fracture of the first metatarsal base.

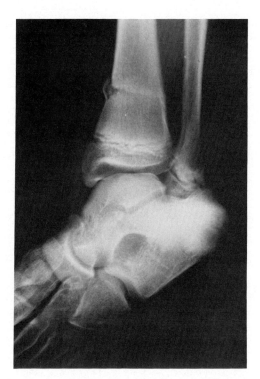

Figure 68.34. Torus fracture of the tibia following a fall from playground equipment.

injury. When the physis is damaged, growth is temporarily arrested; however, the minerals needed for ossification will continue to be deposited at the metaphyseal side of the fracture. When growth resumes, a region of denser bone is present as a thin white line traversing the bone. In some instances the line will become evident as early as 6 weeks after injury (52). This Harris line should remain parallel to the physis as it continues to migrate farther and farther away until it gradually becomes reabsorbed (Fig. 68.35). Should an angular deformity develop, then the Harris line will become oriented in an oblique fashion in relation to the physis. Should partial arrest occur, the Harris line will be seen to converge into the physis at the point of premature fusion. It has been suggested that accurate predictions of the nature of future growth may be made as early as 3 months after a fracture (50).

SUMMARY

Communication between the physician and the parents is essential, and the possibility of partial or complete growth arrest should be discussed. Although most children do well after physeal fractures, alerting the parents to the risks of such injuries may serve two purposes: *(a)* it may ensure that the child is more careful in observing postinjury precautions, and *(b)* it may diffuse hostility toward the physician in the event of growth arrest. Although the potential complications of physeal injuries are fearsome, fortunately they

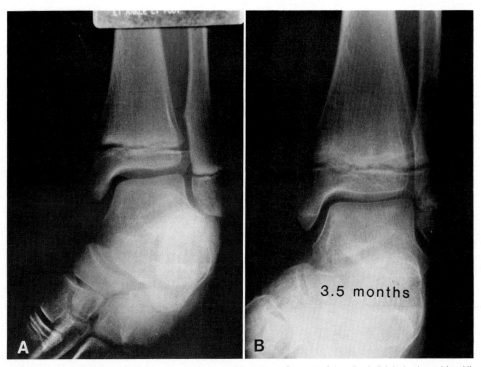

Figure 68.35. **A.** Pronation type injury in this patient with a type I fracture of the distal tibial physis and buckling of the fibular shaft. **B.** Three and one half months after the injury, with the growth arrest line already visible.

are not commonly seen in cases in which proper initial care has been instituted.

References

1. Blount WP: *Fractures in Children*, Huntington, NY, Robert E. Krieger, 1977.
2. Robertson WW: Newest knowledge of the growth plate. *Clin Orthop* 253:270-278, 1990.
3. Siffert RS: The growth plate and its affectations. *J Bone Joint Surg* 48A:546-563, 1966.
4. Salter RB, Harris WB: Injuries involving the epiphyseal plate. *J Bone Joint Surg* 45A:587-622, 1963.
5. Von der Mark K, Von der Mark H: The role of three genetically distinct collagen types in endochondral ossification and calcification of cartilage. *J Bone Joint Surg* 59B:458-463, 1977.
6. Ogden JA: *Children's Fractures*, ed 2. Philadelphia, Lea & Febiger, 1983.
7. Shapiro F, Holtrop ME, Glimcher MJ: Organization and cellular biology of the perichondrial ossification groove of Ranvier. *J Bone Joint Surg* 59A:703-723, 1977.
8. Haas SL: Further observations on the transplantation of the epiphyseal cartilage plate. *Surg Gynecol Obstet* 52:958, 1931.
9. Morscher E, Desaulles PA, Schenk R: Experimental studies on tensile strength and morphology of the epiphyseal cartilage at puberty. *Ann Pediatr* 205:112, 1965.
10. Morscher E: Strength and morphology of growth cartilage under hormonal influence of puberty. Animal experiments and clinical study on the etiology of local growth disorders during puberty. *Reconstr Surg Traumatol* 10:3, 1968.
11. Tomita Y, Tsu-Min T, Steyers C, Ogden L, Jupiter JB, Kutz JE: The role of the epiphyseal and metaphyseal circulations on longitudinal growth in the dog: an experimental study. *J Hand Surg* 11A:375-382, 1986.
12. Poland J: *Traumatic Separation of the Epiphysis*. London, Smith, Elder, and Co, 1898.
13. Aitken AP: The end result of the fractured distal tibial epiphysis. *J Bone Joint Surg* 18A:685-691, 1936.
14. Aitken AP: Fractures of the epiphysis. *Clin Orthop* 41:19-23, 1965.
15. Carothers CO, Crenshaw MA: Clinical significance of a classification of epiphyseal injuries at the ankle. *Am J Surg* 89:879-889, 1958.
16. Ogden JA: Injury to the growth mechanisms of the immature skeleton. *Skeletal Radiol* 6:237-253, 1981.
17. Exarchou E, Politou C, Vretou E, Pasparakis D, Madessis G, Caramerou A: Fractures and epiphyseal deformities in beta-thalassemia. *Clin Orthop* 189:229-233, 1984.
18. Rang M: *Children's Fractures*, ed 2. Philadelphia, JB Lippincott, 1983, p 16.
19. Peterson HA, Burkhart SS: Compression injury of the epiphyseal growth plate: fact or fiction? *J Pediatr Orthop* 1:377-384, 1981.
20. Brinn LB, Moseley JE. Bone changes following electrical injury. *AJR* 97:682, 1966.
21. Argvelles F, Gomar F, Garcia A, Esquerdo J: Irradiation lesions of the growth plate in rabbits. *J Bone Joint Surg* 59B:85, 1977.
22. Dreyfus JR, Glimcher MJ. Epiphyseal injury following frostbite. *N Engl J Med* 253:1065, 1955.
23. Rang M: *The Growth Plate and Its Disorders*. ed 2. London, Churchill-Livingstone, 1983, p 231.
24. Rang M: *The Growth Plate and Its Disorders*. London, Churchill-Livingstone, 1969, p 206.
25. Werenskiold B: Contribution to the roentgen diagnosis of epiphyseal separations. *Acta Radiol* 8:419-426, 1927.
26. Salter RB: *Textbook of Disorders and Injuries of the Musculoskeletal System*, ed 2. Baltimore, Williams & Wilkins, 1983, p 461.
27. Jahss M: *Disorders of the Foot*. Philadelphia, WB Saunders, 1980, p 1671.
28. Rang M: *The Growth Plate and Its Disorders*, ed 2. London, Churchill-Livingstone, 1983, p 31.
29. Kohler A, Zimmer EA, Wilk SP: *Borderlands of the Normal and Early Pathologic in Skeletal Roentgenology*, ed 3. New York, Grune & Stratton, 1968.
30. Lyritis G: Developmental disorders of the proximal epiphysis of the hallux. *Skeletal Radiol* 10:250-254, 1983.
31. Banks AS, Cain TD, Ruch JA: Physeal fractures of the distal phalanx of the hallux. *J Am Podiatr Med Assn* 78:310-313, 1988.
32. Engber WD, Clancey WG: Traumatic avulsion of the fingernail associated with injury to the phalangeal epiphyseal plate. *J Bone Joint Surg* 60A:713-714, 1978.
33. Lauge-Hansen N: Fractures of the ankle. II. Combined experimental surgical and experimental roentgenologic investigations. *Arch Surg* 60:957, 1950.
34. Dias LS, Tachdjian MO: Physeal injuries of the ankle in children. *Clin Orthop* 136:230-233, 1978.
35. Cass JR, Peterson HA: Salter-Harris type IV injuries of the distal tibial epiphyseal growth plate, with emphasis on those involving the medial malleolus. *J Bone Joint Surg* 65A:1059-1070, 1983.
36. Kling TF, Bright RW, Hensinger RN: Distal physeal fractures in children that may require open reduction. *J Bone Joint Surg* 66A:647-657, 1984.
37. Chadwick CJ, Bentley G: The classification and prognosis of epiphyseal injuries. *Injury* 18:157-168, 1987.
38. Landin LA, Danielsson LG, Jonsson K, Pettersson H: Late results in 65 physeal ankle fractures. *Acta Orthop Scand* 57:530-534, 1986.
39. Lynn MD: The triplane distal tibial epiphyseal fracture. *Clin Orthop* 86:187-190, 1972.
40. Marmor L: An unusual fracture of the tibial epiphysis. *Clin Orthop* 73:132-135, 1970.
41. Piero A, Aracil J, Martos F, Mut T: Triplane distal tibial epiphyseal fracture. *Clin Orthop* 160:196-200, 1981.
42. Kleiger B, Mankin HJ: Fracture of the lateral portion of the distal tibial epiphysis. *J Bone Joint Surg* 46A:25-32, 1964.
43. Clement DA, Worlock PH: Triplane fracture of the distal tibia. *J Bone Joint Surg* 69B:412-415, 1987.
44. Yao J, Huurman WW: Tomography in a juvenile Tillaux fracture. *J Pediatr Orthop* 6:349-351, 1986.
45. Seitz WH, Andrews DL, Shelton ML, Feldman F: Triplane fractures of the adolescent ankle—a report of 3 cases. *Injury* 16: 547-553, 1985.
46. Dias LS, Giegerich CR: Fractures of the distal tibial epiphysis in adolescence. *J Bone Joint Surg* 65A:438-444, 1983.
47. Cooperman DR, Spiegel PG, Laros GS: Tibial fractures involving the ankle in children: the so-called triplane epiphyseal fracture. *J Bone Joint Surg* 60A:1040-1046, 1978.
48. von Laer L: Classification, diagnosis and treatment of transitional fractures of the distal part of the tibia. *J Bone Joint Surg* 67A:687-698, 1985.
49. Stefanich RJ, Lozman J: The juvenile fracture of Tillaux. *Clin Orthop* 210:219-227, 1986.
50. Light TR, Ogden DA, Ogden JA: The anatomy of metaphyseal torus fractures. *Clin Orthop* 188:103-111, 1984.
51. Harris HA: The growth of the long bones in childhood. *Arch Int Med* 38:784-806, 1926.
52. Hynes D, O'Brien T: Growth disturbance lines after injury of the distal tibial physis. *J Bone Joint Surg* 70B:231-233, 1988.

Postoperative Complications and Considerations

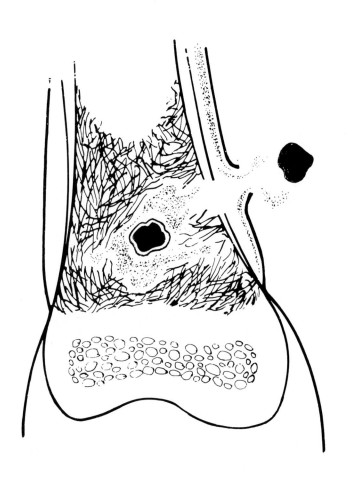

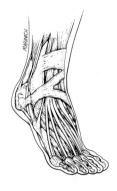

CHAPTER **69**

Edema, Hematoma, and Infection

Stephen J. Miller, D.P.M.

MANAGEMENT OF POSTOPERATIVE INFECTIONS

Whether surgery is performed in the hospital, in the office, or in an outpatient surgery center, there are basically three phases for the management of a surgical case: preoperative, intraoperative, and postoperative. Concern for wound sepsis involves all three phases. The prevention of surgical infections, as well as their management, begins with careful preoperative planning and includes several important considerations within the other two phases. The goal is to avoid infection by minimizing risk.

It is a well-established and proved concept that all wounds are contaminated, whether they are traumatically sustained or surgically induced in even the cleanest of situations. In fact, reactive culture specimens taken at the time of closure of clean surgical wounds have been reported in up to 85% of cases. However, not all wounds become infected (1, 2).

The triad necessary to produce a postsurgical infection includes a receptive host, contamination by microorganisms, and a wound culture medium. Each of these factors is associated with many exogenous agents (Tables 69.1 to 69.3). For example, the skin is a potent defense barrier to infection. Even when broken, it can withstand the assault of over 7.0 × 10⁶ bacteria. However, the presence of just one silk suture foreign body alters the resistance of the host so that only 10² bacteria will cause an infection (3). The difference is a factor of over 10,000 (Fig. 69.1). Similarly the degree of inflammation corresponds to the amount of drainage and the presence of foreign bodies (Fig. 69.2).

Thus each exogenous factor may in itself be of sufficient weight to tip the homostatic scale in favor of an infection.

If more than one factor is allowed to affect the surgical outcome, the risk of infection is greatly increased.

This section deals with means by which the surgeon may avoid infection and treat those that arise. It also involves a basic understanding of the defense mechanisms and host response involved in resisting sepsis. The goal for infection rate in clean, uncontaminated, elective operations should approach zero. Less than 1% is a current and probably achievable goal.

Today the important role of host resistance has been recognized in the prevention of infection. Methods of wound development and care are now designed to take advantage of these natural defenses. Thus total wound management must include operative techniques that minimize injury to the tissue and preserve local physiology and resistance.

HOST RESPONSE TO INFECTION

Defense Systems and Decisive Period

The basic host defense mechanisms against bacterial invasion are through specific or acquired (humoral) immunity and nonspecific or natural (cell-mediated) immunity (4, 5). Phagocytosis, the most important process in the control of infection, functions within each system (6).

Specific resistance, mediated through the lymphocyte and macrophage systems, is characterized by such elements as specific humoral antibody production, opsonins, delayed hypersensitivity reactions, and specific cellular immunities.

Table 69.1.
Factors Affecting the Host
(Compromising the Immune Response)

Extremes of age
Physical status—obesity
Dehydration
Shock
Malnutrition/vitamin deficiency
Anemia
Infection at remote site
Recent antibiotic therapy
Uncontrolled diabetes
Other systemic disease
Steroid therapy
Immunosuppression—drugs or disease
Anergy (to skin tests)

Table 69.2.
Factors That Influence Contamination

Preoperative hospitalization
Antiseptic agents
Hand preparation—time, agent, gloves
Preoperative skin preparation—shower, shave, technique
Perspiration
Surgical supplies and equipment
Lack of strict instrument sterilization
Drapes—gowns, materials, technique
Moisture—tissue fluids, irrigation
Breaks in sterile technique
Long hair/beard uncovered
Talking by scrub team members
Movement or talking by nonscrubbed personnel
Number of personnel in operating room
Duration of surgery
Dose of invading organisms
Virulence of invading organisms

Table 69.3.
Factors That Enhance the Wound As a Culture Medium

Ischemia
   Inadequate supply
   Vessel disruption
   Tourniquet of long duration
   Epinephrine—high concentration
   Tissue trauma
   Edema
Tissue necrosis
   Rough handling
   Dessication
   Electrocautery
Tissue type
   Skin
   Adipose
   Muscle
   Tendon, ligament, fascia
Foreign bodies
   Sutures
   Prostheses
   Fixation devices
Dead space—hematoma/seroma
Incubation period

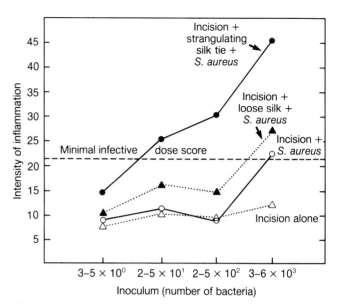

Figure 69.2. Degree of inflammation as related to compromising factors such as a silk suture (foreign body) and strangulating suture. (From Howe CW: Experimental studies on determinants of wound infection. *Surg Gynecol Obstet* 123:507, 1966.)

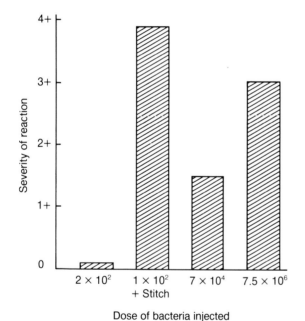

Figure 69.1. Ability of the skin to resist staphylococcal infection. Severity of the infection is adversely influenced by the presence of single silk suture (foreign body). (From Elek SD: Experimental staphylococcal infection in the skin of man. *Ann NY Acad Sci* 65:85, 1956.)

It is a learned activity that depends on the recognition of the invading organisms. Although its role in postoperative infection control is thought to be secondary, it is the mechanism most likely responsible for killing the bacteria immediately after contamination. It does so by way of a two-step procedure: a bacteriostatic first step or opsonization from substances already in the interstitial spaces and a bactericidal second step carried out by phagocytic cells (7). This whole process is aided by the immediate phase of increased vascular permeability that follows tissue injury and functions to deliver more humoral and cellular weapons.

This initial time during which the bacteria attempt to break through the local defenses of the host has been called "the decisive period in the defense against bacterial invasion" (5, 6, 8, 9) (Fig. 69.3). It occurs in an amazingly short time, usually about 3 to 4 hours. If the early host response is inadequate within this period, the number of bacteria that survive the initial killing within the tissue will determine the ultimate size of the mature lesion. At this point, more powerful secondary events take place for further defense.

The mechanisms of nonspecific immunity are those of the common process of inflammation. Its antimicrobial activity includes phagocytosis, intracellular killing by enzyme systems and myeloperoxidase, and extracellular killing by such substances as properdin, complement, and lysozyme (4, 5). It will overlap and complement the humoral system and is dominated by leukocytic phagocytosis.

Inflammatory Response

DEFINITION

Inflammation is a dynamic process, reflecting the attempt of injured tissues to regain homeostasis and restore themselves to a normal state. It involves four major events: *(a)* changes in vascular caliber and blood flow, *(b)* increased vascular permeability, *(c)* infiltration of the tissues by leukocytes, and *(d)* phagocytosis (10). Thus inflammation should not be regarded as a single process but rather as a collection of distinct mechanisms, each of which is designed

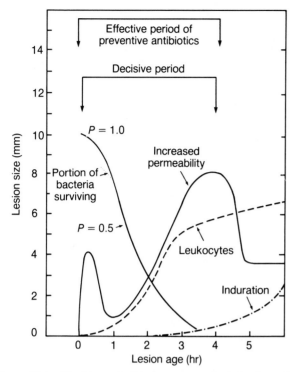

Figure 69.3. "Decisive period" is shown as a period of active antibacterial activity and is related to the arrival of leukocytes, beginning of induration, and increased permeability. (From Leak LV, Burke JF: Early events of tissue injury and the role of the lymphatic system in early inflammation. In Zweifach BW, Grant L, McCluskey RT (eds): *The Inflammatory Process*, ed 2, vol 3. New York, Academic Press, 1974, p 201.)

for the defense of the body against external injury but each of which has other uses as well (11).

FUNCTION

By its definition, inflammation is a universal response of tissue to injury, whether it be caused by trauma, thermal injury, surgery, or infection. More specifically, the early inflammatory lesion serves three purposes. First, it provides a massive humoral and phagocytic assault on a tissue area invaded by bacteria to accomplish bacterial killing. Second, it localizes and isolates the reactive area, thereby preventing or limiting the spread of bacteria to uninvolved tissues. Third, it functions as the initial clean-up mechanism, removing bacterial debris and dead tissue fragments; thus in this capacity it may be thought of as the first step in wound healing (7).

STIMULATION AND MEDIATION

The acute inflammatory response is initiated by tissue injury or by the presence in the tissue of materials recognized as foreign. Damaged endothelium, bacterial cell wall fragments, and urate crystals are examples of such. Once the response is triggered, vascular and cellular events take place, mediated by a variety of substances.

Inflammatory mediators are humoral, endogenous substances, whose levels increase at the site of the inflammatory trauma, in association with the appearance of at least one tissue response or structural change. These mediators are classified into three groups on the basis of their mode of action: *(a)* receptor mediators, which act via receptors, *(b)* lytic enzymes, which cause direct tissue damage, and *(c)* chemotactic factors, attracting cells to the site of inflammation (12). These pathways are depicted in Figure 69.4. As may be seen, the various mediators and chemotactic factors can be generated by *(a)* clotting of blood (kallikrein, plasminogen activator, fibrinopeptides), *(b)* injured tissues (collagen fragments), *(c)* complement (C5a being the most active and important), *(d)* bacteria (liberation of bacterial peptides), *(e)* lymphocytes (lymphokines derived from antigen-stimulated lymphocytes), and *(f)* prostaglandins (causing pain and further inflammation) (6). It is important to note that the various pathways are integrated with other cascades and processes.

LEUKOCYTIC INFILTRATION AND PHAGOCYTOSIS

Once the vascular phases are under way, the stage is set for leukocytic infiltration into the tissues. Initially the white blood cells become sticky and adhere to the endothelium of the blood vessels. Then, in response to various chemotactic factors, the leukocytes squeeze between the endothelial cells—a process known as *diapedesis*—and migrate into the tissues within a few hours. They move quite rapidly and are present in the tissues in large numbers in about 4 hours. Monocytes tend to migrate more slowly and become the prominent cell type within 12 to 24 hours.

When the leukocytes arrive at the site of the surgical wound or bacterial invasion, they must recognize the invaders. Such recognition is facilitated by coating the bacteria with opsonins, primarily the C3 component from the complement system and IgG component from the humoral system. Following opsonization the leukocytes can then attach themselves to the bacteria, invaginate their outer cell wall, and engulf the organism, forming an intracellular phagocytic vacuole or phagosome (Fig. 69.5).

Once inside the cell the bacterium is attacked by two types of enzyme-containing granules. Destruction occurs when the granules fuse to the phagosome and release their powerful contents, an anaerobic process known as degranulation. The primary or azurophilic granules release lysosomal enzymes, peroxidase (myeloperoxidase), lysozyme, and cationic protein. They are oxygen-dependent microbicidal agents. The secondary or specific granules contain lysozyme, lactoferrin, and alkaline phosphates (6, 10, 11, 13). Thus intracellular killing occurs by both oxygen-dependent and oxygen-independent mechanisms.

Prophylactic Antibiotics

After many studies and literature reviews, there is no doubt that prophylactic antibiotics reduce the infection rates for selected indications (14-22). However, ideal timing for their

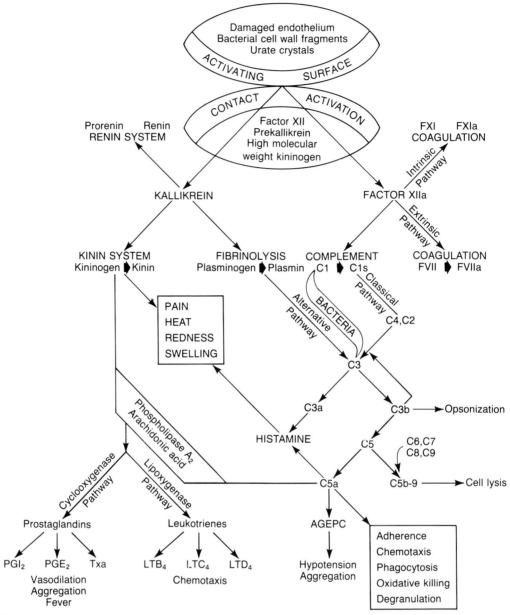

Figure 69.4. Diagrammatic overview of the principal pathways of inflammation, illustrating the interrelationship between important mediation systems and their specific inflammatory effects. (Redrawn and modified from Kalter ES: Inflammatory mediators and acute infection. *Resuscitation* 11:133-140, 1984.)

administration to enhance host defenses should coincide with the decisive period, when the success of antibacterial activity is so critical. This is termed the "effective period of preventative antibiotics" during which antibiotics function to augment the natural mechanisms of bacterial resistance in tissue (Fig. 69.3). They affect bacteria directly without interfering with host defenses. Thus both forces, natural host resistance and antibiotics, are additive or even synergistic in preventing or reducing the final size of bacterial lesions (4, 5, 23). The important concept is that the anti-biotics must be in the tissue *before* the wound is opened and exposed to contamination.

In general, the indications for clean foot and ankle surgery are procedures in which foreign materials are implanted in the tissues; procedures of long duration, greater than 3 hours; procedures involving extensive dissection, potential dead space, and sequestered hematoma formation; and in high-risk patients such as those with diabetes mellitus, obesity, vascular insufficiency, or immunosuppression or those receiving steroid therapy.

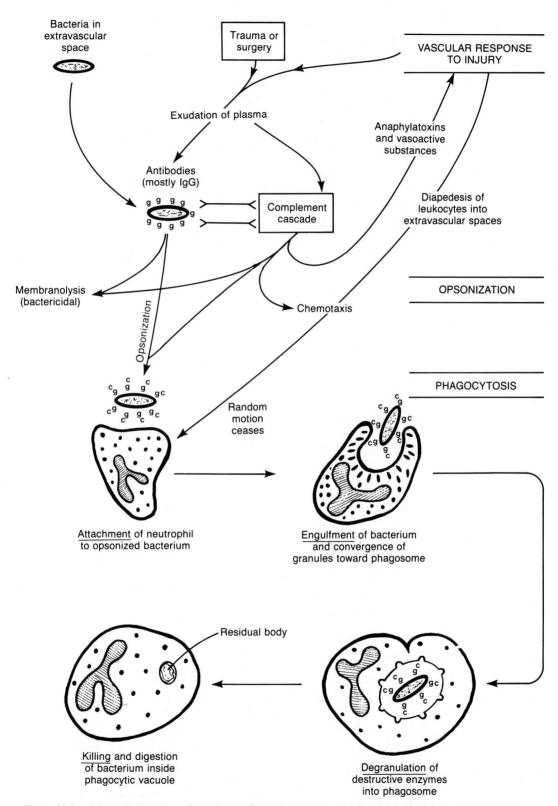

Bacteria in extravascular space

Trauma or surgery

VASCULAR RESPONSE TO INJURY

Exudation of plasma

Anaphylatoxins and vasoactive substances

Antibodies (mostly IgG)

Diapedesis of leukocytes into extravascular spaces

Complement cascade

Membranolysis (bactericidal)

Opsonization

OPSONIZATION

Chemotaxis

PHAGOCYTOSIS

Random motion ceases

Attachment of neutrophil to opsonized bacterium

Engulfment of bacterium and convergence of granules toward phagosome

Residual body

Killing and digestion of bacterium inside phagocytic vacuole

Degranulation of destructive enzymes into phagosome

Figure 69.5. Schematic illustration of the phases of vascular response, opsonization, phagocytosis, and intracellular destruction of invading bacterium. *g,* gammaglobulin antibody; *c,* complement.

As of this writing the safest drug of choice is the broad-spectrum cephalosporin, cefazolin (14). Its relatively high serum levels, long duration, and bone penetration make it the most practical. However, because *Staphylococcus* is the most common offending organism, a more specific anti-staphylococcal agent may be selected from the penicillinase-resistant penicillins. If a violent penicillin allergy is present or suspected, vancomycin can be used.

The dose of cefazolin is 1 to 2 gm given intravenously before the first incision. If desired, two to three additional doses of 1 gm each every 8 hours administered postoperatively are sufficient to complete the prophylactic course. Any further administration has not been shown to yield any better results than the three to four doses. If oral antibiotics are necessary, 1 gm of an oral cephalosporin may be ingested 2 hours before surgery. The postoperative course remains the same.

FACTORS THAT INFLUENCE THE RISK OF INFECTION

Factors Affecting the Host

A number of host factors will adversely increase the risk of surgical wound infection (Table 69.4). Dehydration, shock, anemia, and malnutrition have been shown to lower host defenses enough to compromise the body's response to invading organisms. Malnutrition in this application is defined largely by inadequate protein, as well as vitamin deficiencies. Any recent weight loss of more than 10% of body weight or low levels of serum albumin and transferrin should lead to a suspicion of protein calorie malnutrition. Important vitamins and trace minerals that support the host response include vitamins A, B, and C and zinc (24, 25).

Uncontrolled diabetes mellitus compromises the host response because hyperglycemia impedes leukocytic phagocytosis. Ideally, blood glucose levels should be maintained at less than 180 mg/dl before any elective surgery is initi-

ated. There is also interference with white blood cell migration in diabetics.

Other systemic conditions that alter host resistance include malignancy and infections at remote sites. Immunosuppressive drugs or diseases or even radiation therapy are important factors (Table 69.5). A careful history will reveal clues to other possible infections or recent antibiotic therapy, both of which may increase the presence of pathogenic or opportunistic microorganisms.

Adrenal corticosteroids, whatever their source, retard the inflammatory reaction. In large doses, as in steroid therapy, they tend to weaken host resistance. Although rarely seen in the elective foot surgery patient, relative or complete anergy may be present, significantly altering the immunocompetence of the host. Anergy refers to a lack of normal response of the humoral system to five or more common antigens found in the dermis of the patient. Such high-risk patients may be identified by skin testing with a battery of delayed hypersensitivity antigens, although other more specific quantitative and functional tests are available (25).

Finally, the physical status of the patient may influence the host response to bacterial invasion. Obese patients have been shown to be at higher risk for infection after surgery. Age is another factor. In Cruse and Foord's study (26) patients over 66 years of age had a six times greater postop-

Table 69.4.
Factors Increasing the Risk of Surgical Wound Infection[a]

Host Factors		Surgical Factors	
Age > 60 years	3 × increase	Type of wound:	
Malnutrition	3 ×	contaminated	2 ×
Active infection	2-3 ×	dirty	4-6 ×
Obesity	2 ×	Preoperative hospitalization:	
Steroid therapy	2 ×	>2 weeks	4 ×
Diabetes	2 ×	1-2 weeks	2 ×
		Night-time or emergency operation	2-3 ×
		Duration of operation >3 hours	2-3 ×
		Shaving operative site	2 ×
		Electrosurgical knife	2 ×
		Penrose wound drain	2 ×

From Maki DG: The epidemiology of surgical wound infection—guidelines for prevention. *J Surg Pract* 6:10-23, 1977.
[a]Excerpted from two large multifactorial studies, each encompassing over 15,000 operated patients (*Ann Surg* 160 [Suppl]:1-192, 1964; *Arch Surg* 107:206-211, 1973).

Table 69.5.
Some Systemic Conditions That Reduce Both Natural and Acquired Immunity to Wound Infections

Congenital Defects

Agammaglobulinemia
Chronic granulomatous disease
White cell disorders

Acquired Defects

Diabetes mellitus, especially diabetic hyperosmolarity and acidosis
Cushing's syndrome (endogenous or exogenous)
Addison's disease
Leukemias and aplastic anemias
Severe hemolytic anemia
Hyposplenism syndromes
Obesity
Liver failure
Heart failure
Radiation sickness
Severe trauma
Active sepsis
Coagulation disorders
Malnutrition
    Long-standing bowel obstruction
    Malabsorption and short bowel disorders
Active tuberculosis, leprosy, fungal disease

Local Defects

Rheumatic heart valve defects
Congenital heart and great vessel disease
Chronic pulmonary disease
Radiation tissue damage
Poor local blood flow
Regional ischemia
Neuropathies

Table 69.6.
Classification of Wounds According to the Degree of Operative Contamination[a]

Class	Description
Clean	Surgical incisions made with no break in aseptic technique. No known contamination and no inflammation encountered
Clean-contaminated	Minor break in aseptic technique
Contaminated	Major break in aseptic technique. Fresh traumatic wound (<4 hours old)
Dirty or infected	Acute bacterial inflammation encountered with or without pus
	Traumatic wound with delayed treatment (>4 hours), retained foreign body, or from dirty source

[a]Adapted to lower extremity surgery from the National Research Council.

Table 69.7.
Microorganisms Harbored Within Skin

Location	Microorganisms
Cornified layers	Lipophilic and non-lipophilic yeasts, gram-positive cocci, aerobic and anaerobic diphtheroids, *S. aureus*, *S. epidermidis*, *Streptococcus*, gram-negative bacilli, pathogenic yeast, *Peptococcus* (anaerobic)
Cellular layers	Herpes virus, dermatophytes, pathogenic yeast, *Streptotoccus*, wart virus
Dermis layers	Pathogenic yeasts, streptococci
Hair follicles	*Corynebacterium*, dermatophytes, *S. aureus*, lipophilic yeasts, *Propionibacterium acnes* (anaerobic)
Eccrine sweat glands	Gram-positive cocci, *S. aureus*

From Abramson C: Normal "opportunistic" flora of the lower extremities related to postoperative surgical wound infections. *J Am Podiatry Assoc* 67:9, 1977.

erative infection rate than did patients between 1 and 14 years of age.

The factors just discussed are those that largely influence systemic resistance in the host (Table 69.1). The other two areas of concern in preventing or establishing wound infections are sources of contamination and factors affecting local resistance within the wound itself.

Factors That Influence Contamination

There are many sources of microorganisms that may contaminate surgical wounds (Table 69.2). This is a rather broad topic that begins with resident versus transient skin flora and proceeds through the control and dissemination of microorganisms during surgery. It is discussed more thoroughly in the section on preoperative considerations.

The initial consideration is the duration of stay in the hospital before surgery. Even with a 1-week stay, Cruse and Foord (26) found a twofold increase in the infection rate (Table 69.4).

Wounds may be classified according to the degree of contamination encountered at the time of surgery (Table 69.6). For clean or clean-contaminated wounds the source of the greatest contamination is usually the skin (Table 69.7). Normal resident or even transient microorganisms become opportunistic invaders when their equilibrium with the host is upset by extraneous factors. The skin itself is an excellent barrier to infection. Once broken or opened, a portal of entry for bacteria is established. Infection then is defined as the unfavorable result of the equation of the dose of bacterial contamination multiplied by virulence and divided by the resistance of the host (1, 26).

It is impossible to completely sterilize the skin, whether it be of the patient or the operator's hands. A 5-minute hand scrub has been shown to cause no greater infection rate than does a 10-minute scrub (27). Selection of an effective antiseptic agent is important, but regardless of the technique or the agent many bacteria will remain out of

reach, especially those in hair follicles and, to a lesser degree, within sweat glands (Fig. 69.6). For that reason presurgical scrubs the night before surgery are not recommended. First, the ecological balance will be upset and opportunistic pathogens may proliferate, and second, perspiration in the intervening period will carry bacteria to the skin surface. After surgery, wounds or dressings should not be covered with impermeable plastic bags that will allow the accumulation of perspiration. A preoperative shower with use of an antiseptic soap will lower the chances of infection. Shaving hair from the operative site should not be done until the time of surgery.

The scrub team itself represents a relatively minor source of infective organisms. Glove punctures are not a major source of contamination. In one study, it was found that 11.6% of gloves (141 of 1209) were punctured by the end of the surgery; yet not a single wound infection occurred in those 141 patients (16). More important in the cause of infection is any break in sterile technique. Any break at all in aseptic procedure should be reported at once, regardless of the status of the person reporting it and no matter who has to correct it.

Human activity, particularly by nonscrubbed personnel in the operating room, accounts for most of the microorganisms in the air. Technical control of the air-handling systems through multiple exchanges, filtration, and laminar flow has tended to deemphasize the need to control the behavior and number of nonscrubbed people in the operating room (Fig. 69.7). Excess movement, heavy in and out traffic, talking, and uncovered hair all lead either directly or indirectly to the dissemination of bacteria into the environment. The operating room door should be kept closed and movement through it limited.

Strict attention must be paid to instrument and equipment sterilization procedures (Table 69.8). Ideally, drapes should be impermeable; however, if there is good control of irrigation and tissue fluids, this is not mandatory. Adhesive plastic drapes that attach to the skin have not been shown

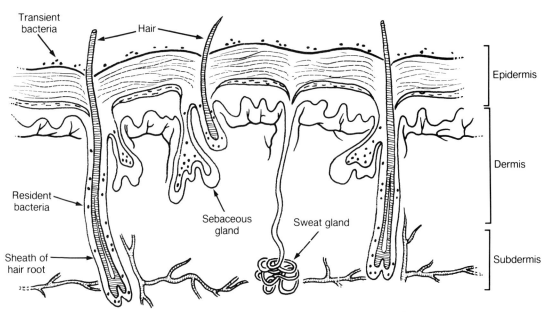

Figure 69.6. Schematic drawing showing transient bacteria on a surface that are easily removed by mechanical scrubbing, and deep resident bacteria that cannot be destroyed by skin antiseptics. (Redrawn from Sabiston DC [ed]: *Davis-Christopher Textbook of Surgery. The Biological Basis of Surgical Practice.* Philadelphia, WB Saunders, 1977, p 328.)

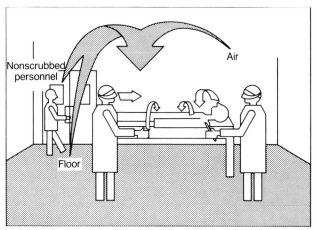

Figure 69.7. Schematic drawing showing in relative proportions sources of potential contamination in the operating room. Greatest contributions come from nonscrubbed personnel. (From Burke JF: Infection. In Hunt TK, Dumphy JE [eds]: *Fundamentals of Wound Management.* New York, Appleton-Century-Crofts, 1979.)

to decrease wound infection rates and are therefore not recommended (26). However, they may be used to isolate toenails, which harbor many microorganisms (28). Draping technique is very important. Surgical supplies and equipment may be vectors for contamination. They should be handled with strict aseptic technique.

Finally, there has been shown to be a direct relation between the length of time of a surgery and the infection rate. With every hour of operating time the rate of infection roughly doubles (26). It becomes obvious that control of no one factor alone will greatly influence the risk of postoperative infection. More important, it is the attention paid to the whole combination of risk factors—the attention to detail—that significantly contributes to the goal of a zero infection rate.

More critical than contamination of the wound by bacteria is the physiological state of the local tissues before and after the surgical intervention.

Factors That Enhance the Wound As a Culture Medium

First and foremost of importance relative to wound physiology is circulation. Without adequate local perfusion the tissues lack sufficient oxygen and nutrients to cope with the infliction of a surgical wound. Factors that may contribute adversely to local ischemia include tourniquets of long duration, high concentrations of epinephrine, vessel disruption, unnecessary trauma, and excess edema (Table 69.3).

Necrosis of local tissues through rough handling, desiccation, or overzealous electrocautery will provide a bacterial medium. Frequent irrigation with physiological solutions is essential. The implantation of a foreign body, whether it be a suture, a prosthesis, or a bone fixation device, may greatly diminish host resistance in the local wound. The dose of bacteria necessary to establish an infection is reduced by a factor of 10,000.

The type of tissue injured is very important. Skin itself has the greatest resistance to infection. Adipose subcutaneous tissue dies quickly when its circulation is cut off; necrotizing fasciitis can develop within this layer. Because the

Table 69.8.
Some Acceptable Methods of Sterilization and Disinfection Commonly Used for the Operating Room

Basic Principle: Initial cleanliness, adequate contact, sufficient time, and the use of an efficacious agent are the controlling factors in effective sterilization and disinfection.

Method	Typical Uses
Autoclave (pressurized wet heat) Normal sterilization cycle 121°C 30 min 15 lb/sq in Flash sterilization cycle 134°C 3 min 29.4 lb/sq in	Sterilization of drapes, gowns, sheets, towels, surgical instruments, lap pads, surgical needles and other items not damaged by intense heat. For unwrapped, open instruments only, with no linen in tray.
Ethylene oxide gas Chemical sterilization under carefully controlled time, temperature and humidity conditions. Items incorporating rubber, plastic and other nonmetallic materials must be aerated for up to 24 hours after sterilization to dissipate toxic residual gas ("gas aerator" can reduce aeration time).	Sterilization of lensed instruments, ampules, catheters, anesthesia face masks and tubing, pacemakers and other heat-labile items. (For implantable items up to 72 hours of aeration may be required depending on composition of plastic materials.)
Activated gluteraldehyde Cold chemical solution effective against vegetative organisms (5 min), TB bacilli (10 min) and spores (10 hr). Items must be rinsed in sterile water before contact with human tissue.	Disinfection of lensed instruments, anesthesia face masks and tubing, and other heat-labile nonporous items.
Povidone-iodine Kills vegetative organisms (10 min) and TB bacilli (20 min) but is not sporicidal.	Patient skin preparation and hand scrubbing.
70% Ethyl alcohol Kills vegetative organisms and TB bacilli in 5 min. Not sporicidal. Dissolves cement in lensed instruments.	Disinfection of polyethylene tubing, other plastic items and electrical cords.
Phenolics Kill vegetative organisms and TB bacilli when properly applied in effective concentrations for sufficient time.	Cleaning and disinfection of environmental surfaces such as floors, walls and furniture.

From Burke JF: Infection. In Hunt TD, Dumphy JE (eds): *Fundamentals of Wound Management.* New York, Appleton-Century-Crofts, 1979.

dense collagenous structure of tendon, fascia, and ligament is difficult to perfuse, the demise of these tissues leads to a culture medium. Finally, muscle that is crushed and devitalized provides a wound that is ideal for anaerobic infection because of its reduced oxidation-reduction potential. The resulting infection, such as clostridial myonecrosis or gas gangrene, may be catastrophic because it can then easily extend into normal uninjured muscle.

Dead space or potential cavities are dangerous because they may easily fill with blood or serum, which becomes a pabulum for microorganisms. In addition, hematoma has

been shown to reduce host resistance by interfering with opsonization, a process essential to efficient phagocytosis. Excess iron as a blood breakdown product has also been shown to interfere with the host response. Incomplete hemostasis, retained blood clots, and necrotic or traumatized tissue may convert a wound that would ordinarily resist millions of contaminating bacteria into one susceptible to hundreds.

Finally, an important factor to consider regarding the establishment of a postoperative wound infection is the incubation period. This refers to the time necessary for the invading organisms to multiply sufficiently to overcome the local host resistance and establish a wound infection. For most aerobic organisms the incubation period is roughly 72 hours; for clostridial myonecrosis it is 12 hours to 3 days; for necrotizing fasciitis it is 12 to 72 hours; and for tetanus it is 1 to 2 weeks.

DIAGNOSIS OF INFECTION

Cardinal Signs

The most obvious clinical sign of infection is inflammation. However, inflammation is a fundamental response to surgical incisions, traumatic wounds, crystal arthropathies, and a variety of other disorders. Because a surgical wound is already present, the inflammatory reaction is in progress. The real challenge to the surgeon is to understand and recognize the subtle clues as to when an infection is establishing itself in the postoperative inflammatory setting.

The four cardinal signs of inflammation, as described by Celsus (30 BC to 38 AD), are *tumor* (swelling), *rubor* (redness), *calor* (heat), and *dolor* (pain). Virchos (1858) subsequently added a fifth sign termed *functio laesa* or loss of function (11). Although these are well known in the healing arts, it is their *intensity* that will indicate the presence of a current or incipient infection. Especially notable is an unusual amount of pain at the surgical site by the second or third postoperative day, pain that is unresponsive to even the strongest of analgesics and often described as throbbing. Other possible causes of such intense pain are hematoma, excessively tight dressings, swelling within the restriction of a cast, and an acute gouty attack that may be instigated by the trauma of the surgery itself. These causes must be considered and measures taken to quickly rule them out. Obviously intense peri-incisional edema, erythema, and radiating heat should also heighten suspicion of an infection (Fig. 69.8).

FEVER

Body temperature is elevated when the "setpoint" or "thermostat" in the hypothalamic thermoregulatory center is raised. It does so in response to a variety of stimuli, but accumulated research suggests that these different activators cause fever by stimulating the release of endogenous pyrogen from leukocytes and Kupffer's cells (29). Specific stimuli include bacterial endotoxin (lipopolysaccharide component of gram-negative bacteria), phagocytosis (central feature of the inflammatory reaction), and certain immune reactions. The endogenous pyrogen then stimulates the hypothalamic center to raise the setpoint and body temperature increases through physiological mechanisms (Fig. 69.9). Chills and shivering are two signs that the setpoint has been raised.

Gram-negative bacteria tend to cause more of an intense fever because of the strong stimulus of their endotoxin, resulting in a direct release of endogenous pyrogen from leukocytes. Gram-positive bacteria, on the other hand, tend

to evoke a profound inflammatory response within the extravascular tissue and thereby cause the release of endogenous pyrogen by way of leukocytic phagocytosis.

It has been suggested that perhaps a threshold concentration of endogenous pyrogen is necessary to cause fever, whether the stimulus is bacteria or the inflammatory process itself (30). For this reason fever is often not seen in conjunction with postsurgical foot infections, particularly in their early stages. Other possible causes of temperature elevations must be considered (Fig. 69.10). The chronological sequence of postoperative temperature changes as they are most likely to occur is depicted in Table 69.9.

Blood Tests

An elevated erythrocyte sedimentation rate (ESR) is rather nonspecific in that it simply confirms the presence of an active inflammatory process. More informative is a complete blood count (CBC) with attention directed especially to the white blood cell (WBC) portion.

Although not always present during postoperative wound infections, a progressive neutrophilic leukocytosis with a WBC count of over 10,000 indicates active infection. When there is a "shift to the left" in the white cell differential, it means that so many leukocytes have been activated by the infection that younger developing forms from the blood pool are showing up prematurely in the general circulation. The more severe the infection the greater the left shift as immature leukocytes arrive in greater numbers. The more localized the infection the less pronounced is the neutrophilia and vice versa.

Anemia may occur in both acute and chronic infections, because of the effect of bacterial toxins on the bone marrow. This is rarely seen in postoperative wound infections.

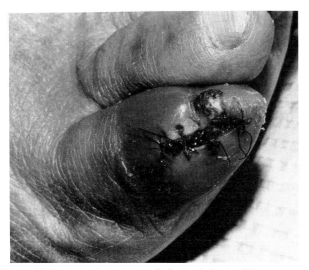

Figure 69.8. Early physical signs of infection following fifth toe surgery. Swelling, redness, drainage, and dehiscence should instigate prompt management.

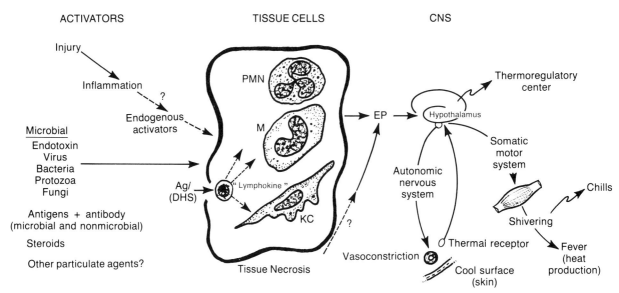

Figure 69.9. Schematic illustration of postulated pathway of chills and fever pathogenesis. *PMN*, granulocyte; *M*, monocyte; *KC*, Kupffer cell; *DHS*, delayed hypersensitivity; *EP*, endogenous pyrogen. (Redrawn from Atkins E, Bodel P: Fever. In Zweifach BW, Grant L, McCluskey RT (eds): *The Inflammatory Process*, ed 2, vol 3. New York, Academic Press, 1974, p 507.)

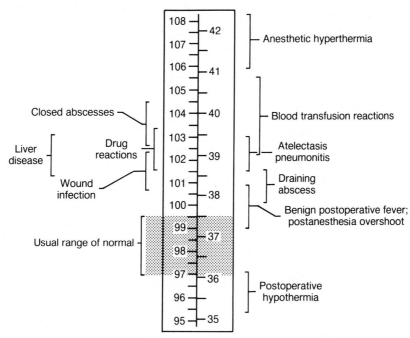

Figure 69.10.   General guide to some approximate postoperative temperature elevations. (From Miller SJ: Body temperature following podiatric surgery. *J Am Podiatry Assoc* 74:477-481, 1984. Reproduced with permission.)

Table 69.9.
Chronological Sequence of Postoperative Temperature Changes

Intraoperative	Heat pyrexia
	Malignant hyperthermia
	Hypothermia
First 12-24 hours	Postoperative hypothermia
Day 1	Postanesthesia overshoot
	Atelectasis/pneumonitis
Second 24 hours	Thrombophlebitis
Day 2	Pulmonary embolism
	Benign postoperative fever
Third 24 hours	Postsurgical infection
Day 3	Urinary tract infection
	Benign postoperative fever
	Constipation
Other causes appropriate to the	Drug fever
situation	Catheter fever
	Blood transfusion reaction
	Intravenous fever

From Miller SJ: Body temperature following podiatric surgery. *J Am Podiatry Assoc* 74:477-485, 1984.

Table 69.10.
Blood-Stream Infections

Term	Definition	Significance
Bacteremia	Simple presence in the blood stream of bacteria that have clinical manifestations	Method by which infections can be spread to distant foci
Septicemia	Clinical state in which in addition to bacteremia there are fever, chills, and other clinical symptoms	Represents the failure of the body to localize the infection
Toxemia	Clinical state produced by the effects of bacterial toxins	Not dependent on the presence of microorganisms in the blood

Modified from Witt CS: Clinical signs and symptoms of infection. In DiGiovanni JE, Smith SD (eds): *Decision Making in Foot Surgery.* New York, Stratton Intercontinental Medical Book Corp, 1976, pp 147-186.

Signs of recovery include a drop in the total leukocyte count, disappearance of the left shift, increase in the number of monocytes, and relative lymphocytosis.

Blood culture specimens should be taken only when the generalized spread of infection into the blood stream is suspected. High fever (over 103° F), chills, and hypotension in a generally prostrate and septic-appearing patient are indications for blood cultures. Because bacteremia normally precedes the development of fever and chills, multiple samples taken over a period of 24 hours may be necessary for specific diagnosis in intermittent bacteremia. The terminology used in blood stream infections is illustrated in Table 69.10. It is very important in obtaining blood samples that the skin be thoroughly cleansed with antiseptic agents before the venipuncture (31, 32).

Dehiscence and drainage together are prime signs that a postsurgical wound may be infected. When this is seen, even during dressing changes at 2 or 3 days after surgery, it is imperative that specimens be obtained for Gram's stain, as well as culture and sensitivity testing.

The Gram's stain is a valuable technique for the determination of the morphology of bacterial cells, as well as their taxonomic grouping, both of which may lead to a rapid presumptive diagnosis. The procedure is quite simple and may be readily performed in the office if a microscope is available. The specimen should be gently applied to a glass slide by rolling the swab or dispensing one or two drops of material so that a thin smear is created. It should be air dried first, then heat fixed by rapidly passing the slide over a clean flame two or three times. Once the Gram's stain technique (Table 69.11) has been applied—rigid timing is not necessary—the specimen is then viewed under a microscope. It should first be scanned with the low-power objective (10 ×) to locate the specimen material. Then an oil immersion lens (100 ×) is necessary with which to observe for bacteria.

Interpretation of a Gram's stain involves more than simply noting the presence or absence of bacteria in the specimen. If only a few bacteria are seen, then one should be suspicious of contaminating organisms. If polymorphonuclear leukocytes (PMNs) alone are seen, the only thing certain is the presence of an inflammatory reaction. However, if a large number of organisms are seen, especially if they are of one type, along with PMNs, then there is good evidence for infection. The Gram's stain will determine if the bacteria fall into the gram-positive or gram-negative categories, or if a mixed infection is present. Morphologically there are only four possibilities: gram-positive cocci, gram-negative cocci, gram-positive rods, and gram-negative rods. Gram-positive cocci in clusters are characteristic of *Staphylococcus* species; chains are characteristic of *Streptococcus* species.

With this limited but valuable information, along with clinical impressions, empirical selection may be made of one or more antibiotics so that prompt treatment may be initiated. It also allows time for the incubation of specimen cultures and the determination of microorganism sensitivities.

Culture and Sensitivity Studies

No culture report is better than the specimen submitted. A culture will yield useless or misleading information if it is improperly collected or transported to the laboratory. First, the specimen must be collected before the initiation of antimicrobial therapy. The area peripheral to the wound should be cleansed with an antiseptic before a culture specimen is obtained. This will limit contamination by resident flora.

Whether a swab or needle aspiration technique is used, the instrument should be accurately plunged into the involved tissues to obtain an adequate amount of the invading organism. If necessary for patient comfort, a proximal ankle block with local anesthetic should be performed. When non-draining cellulitis is present, it may be necessary to inject a small amount of sterile physiological saline solution into the tissues and then aspirate them to obtain a specimen. Finally, the specimen should be placed in an appropriate support medium, identified, and transported promptly to the laboratory where it should be cultured immediately. Forty-eight hours are usually necessary to identify a culture.

If the wound is foul-smelling, contains gas, or has other characteristics of a possible anaerobic infection, such as a suspicious Gram's stain finding, diabetic foot, or compromised circulation, then an anaerobic culture should be taken. Ideally it should be swabbed from deep within the wound after the surface is cleansed with an antiseptic, or it should be aspirated with a needle from the edge of the advancing lesion. The needle must be sealed immediately with a sterile cork or rubber stopper. If a swab is used, it must be placed deep within an anaerobic culture medium. In either case the specimen must be transported to the laboratory immediately and cultured at once. Contact with free oxygen will destroy anaerobic bacteria. Several bacteriological clues will help identify the presence of an anaerobic infection (Table 69.12).

Once the organism is isolated and identified it may be necessary to perform antibiotic sensitivity testing to determine the most efficacious chemotherapeutic agent. This test is not necessary if the organism's susceptibility is known. For example, group A streptococci remains highly sensitive to penicillin; thus further testing is not indicated if it is the infecting organism. Also, if known normal flora are grown in the culture, they are not tested for susceptibility to antibiotics.

The most common method of antibiotic susceptibility test-

Table 69.11.
Gram's Stain Technique

Solution	Procedure	Effect
Bucker's ammonium oxalate crystal violate	Flood slide with primary Violet stain. Rinse immediately with tap water.	Stains all bacteria violet.
Acetone or ethanol (alcohol) or mixture	Apply a few drops to slanted specimen. Acetone works more rapidly than ethanol. Rinse with tap water.	Decolorizes the gram-negative bacteria
Gram's iodine	Apply iodine solution to slide. Rinse with tap water.	Iodine complexes with the crystal violet
Safranin	Apply counterdye and rinse quickly with tap water. Allow to air dry or blot with clean absorbent towel.	Stains gram-negative organisms red

Table 69.12.
Clinical Clues to Anaerobic Infection

1. Intense pain without discharge
2. Foul-smelling putrid discharge
3. Necrotic tissue or gangrene
4. Gas in tissue, crepitus, or on x-ray film
5. Infection involving muscle or tissue destruction
6. Infection related to the use of aminoglycosides
7. Bacteremic picture with jaundice
8. Black discoloration of blood-containing exudates

ing is that of impregnated disk diffusion. The area of no growth around the disk is known as the zone of inhibition. After 18 to 24 hours of incubation the exact size or diameter is measured and translated into *susceptible, intermediate,* and *resistant* categories based on prior studies using dilution tests. "Susceptible" or "sensitive" implies that the organism may be treated with that particular antibiotic agent with the minimal inhibitory concentration (MIC) dosages recommended for that type of infection and infecting species. "Resistant" means that the strain is not completely inhibited within the usual therapeutical dose range (33). Some laboratories report all intermediate strains as resistant.

Disk diffusion testing does not quantitatively determine the degree of sensitivity. Sometimes antimicrobial therapy must be carefully titrated. In these instances it is necessary to know the MIC—the minimal concentration of the agent that inhibits the growth—or the minimal bactericidal concentration (MBC)—the concentration necessary for killing 99.9% of the microorganisms in the initial inoculum during 24 hours of incubation. Laboratory requests may be made for tube dilution sensitivity studies that are used to measure the MIC and MBC values and also to determine the antibiotic sensitivity of slowly growing or fastidious microorganisms that cannot be measured by the disk diffusion method (33).

Sometimes it is necessary to determine the concentration of the antimicrobial agent in the patient's serum. These assays are performed when the difference between the therapeutical and toxic concentrations of antibiotics is very narrow. In addition, they are used in patients with renal failure who may accumulate unusually high levels of antibiotics in their blood. Performing these tests may then determine if the therapeutic level of the antibiotic has been reached without reaching or exceeding the toxic level. This primarily applies to aminoglycosides to avoid ototoxicity and occasionally to treatment with very high doses of penicillins to avoid neurotoxicity (33). Serum is taken at the time of anticipated peak blood level following the administration of the antibiotic, and then its concentration is assayed.

Determination of Bacterial Beta-Lactamase Activity

Certain strains of *Staphylococcus aureus* and *Haemophilus influenzae* have become resistant to penicillins and cephalosporins by producing enzymes called beta-lactamases (penicillinases), which destroy the beta-lactam nucleus of these antibiotics (34, 35). Rapid laboratory methods for detection of beta-lactamase production by bacterial cultures are available. Testing may be done as soon as cultures are isolated, often 12 to 24 hours before susceptibility tests are available (36).

Clavulanic acid is an inhibitor of beta-lactamases, which-works by irreversibly binding with the said enzymes. It has been introduced in combination with some penicillins (e.g., amoxicillin-clavulanic acid or ticarcillin-clavulanic acid) for the treatment of infections caused by certain beta-lactamase-producing organisms (37, 38).

Determining the Organism

Although a Gram's stain may provide specific but limited information, preliminary attempts at identifying the infecting organism require a knowledge of the more common bacteria that cause wound sepsis. Further information can be gleaned by careful examination of the wound and the dressing, as well as from the clinical experience of the surgeon. The odor and character of exudates, amount of swelling, color of the skin and exposed tissues, and time since surgery may be valuable clues.

AEROBIC ORGANISMS

Coagulase-positive *Staphylococcus aureus* has consistently been the most common infecting organism in postoperative infections (28, 39-41). This also applies to foot and ankle surgery (42) and corresponds in general to the causative agents found in infections of the foot (43-45). Closely following this is the less but increasingly virulent organism, coagulase-negative *Staphylococcus epidermidis*. Postsurgical tissue infected with colonized *Staphylococcus* becomes intensely erythematous, swollen, tender, and localized. Abscesses may form consisting of thick, creamy yellow pus from *S. aureus* and white pus from *S. epidermidis*. Considerable tension is placed on the suture line, which usually leads to dehiscence and suppurative discharge.

Without pus, the wound infection usually appears quite similar to that caused by beta-hemolytic group A streptococci. This aerobic organism is an enzymatically active bacterium that can spread rapidly through the tissues, resulting in an intense cellulitis. Infection may develop as rapidly as within 12 to 24 hours of contamination but may occur as long as 1 or 2 weeks later. It can easily dissolve fibrin clots, even in lymphatic vessels, leading to proximally progressing lymphangiitis seen on the skin as red streaks. Tender lymphadenopathy in the popliteal fossa or groin is a diagnostic sign. Wound discharge may be present, but it is usually more serious. Untreated, it may lead to generalized septicemia.

Gram-negative bacilli as a cause of wound infections increased by a factor of 14 from 1965 to 1970 (43). A survey of data on postsurgical wounds reported between 1972 and 1975 showed that *Escherichia coli, Klebsiella, Proteus, Pseudomonas, Enterobacter,* and *Serratia* were the most frequently isolated gram-negative bacteria (28). This is consistent with other surveys of pathogens causing foot infections (43-45). The particular anatomical location of the lower extremities makes them constantly susceptible to showers of alimentary tract organisms. These bacteria tend to reside and colonize in the toe webs, the nail folds, the periungual areas, and the dorsal and plantar skin surfaces of the foot (46).

Gram-negative rods are rarely transmitted as airborne contaminants. They usually require contact or manipulation of the wound or dressing and are highly probable causes of infection when a dressing has become wet, such as in a bath or shower, during the early stages of wound healing. Exposure to soil or areas fertilized with animal feces, such as gardens, also make these organisms likely culprits. The skin and tissue response to gram-negative rod infection is usually a nonspecific suppurative reaction that may be indistinguishable from that caused by staphylococci. They frequently cause a more serious drainage that is mildly malodorous. *Pseudomonas* will yield more of a greenish exudate with a characteristic odor.

These three groups, staphylococci, streptococci, and gram-negative bacilli, cause the majority of postoperative wound infections. Other organisms that may be responsible include *Corynebacteria* or diphtheroids, *Acinetobacter, Candida*, and anaerobic bacteria. It should be remembered that many wounds have a mixture of infecting agents because some organisms such as *Candida* and *Enterobacter* gain secondary entry after an infection is already underway.

ANAEROBIC ORGANISMS

When anaerobic or even facultative bacteria are involved in postoperative wound sepsis, their rapidly destructive abilities make a swift clinical diagnosis critical to successful treatment. The presence of one or more clues (Table 69.12) should heighten suspicion; intense tissue destruction is not always evident. Radiographs should be taken to look for gas within the tissues. Remember that facultative and aerobic organisms may act in concert to provide a more favorable environment for anaerobic growth by using up the oxygen or by contributing substances that lower the oxidation-reduction (redox) potential of the local tissues. Healthy tissues maintain an oxidation-reduction potential (E_h) of $+120$ MV and, because this will not support anaerobes, it is one of the body's major defenses against such microbes (47). Organisms involved in this synergistic polymicrobic process include *S. aureus, S. epidermidis, Peptococcus, Peptostreptococcus, Corynebacterium, Bacteroides* (especially *B. fragilis*), and a variety of species of *Clostridium* and gram-negative rods.

ANAEROBIC INFECTIONS

The clinical features of various anaerobic infections are listed in Table 69.13.

Clostridial Myonecrosis (Gas Gangrene)

This is probably the most severe infection caused by anaerobes. It results from gram-positive spore-forming bacilli that may be found in the soil and that are part of the normal human bowel flora, making the extremities most susceptible. These saprophytic clostridial bacteria include *Clostridium perfringens (welchii), C. histolyticum, C. novyi*, and *C. bifermentans*. Frequently anaerobic infections contain a mixture of these organisms. As with all histotoxic *clostridia*, their virulence is a product of the toxins they produce. For example, the alpha-toxin produced by *C. perfringens* is a potent lecithinase that is both hemolytic and necrotizing. The incubation time is 12 hours to 3 days (47, 48).

Table 69.13.
Differentiating Characteristics of Certain Anaerobic Infections of Skin and Soft Tissue[a]

	Clostridial Myonecrosis (Gas Gangrene)	Synergistic Nonclostridial Anaerobic Myonecrosis	Anaerobic Streptococcal Myositis	Infected Vascular Gangrene	Necrotizing Fasciitis	Anaerobic Cellulitis
Incubation	Usually less than 3 days	Variable, 3-14 days	3-4 days	More than 5 days, usually longer	1-4 days	Almost always more than 3 days
Onset	Acute	Acute	Subacute or insidious	Gradual	Acute	Gradual
Toxemia	Very severe	Marked	Severe only after some time	Nil or minimal	Moderate to marked	Nil or slight
Pain	Severe	Severe	Variable, as a rule fairly severe	Variable	Moderate to severe	Absent
Swelling	Marked	Moderate	Marked	Often marked	Marked	Nil or slight
Skin	Tense, often very pale	Minimal change	Tense, often with a coppery tinge	Discolored, often black and desiccated	Pale-red cellulitis	Little change
Exudate	Variable, may be profuse, serous and blood stained	"Dishwater" pus	Very profuse, seropurulent	Nil	Serosanguineous	Nil or slight
Gas	Rarely pronounced except terminally	Not pronounced, present in 25% of cases	Very slight	Abundant	Usually not present	Abundant
Smell	Variable, may be slight, often sweetish	Foul	Very slight, often sour	Foul	Foul	Foul
Muscle	Marked change	Marked change	At first little change except edema	Dead	Viable	No change

[a] Facultative bacteria may also produce some of these infections.
From Finegold SM, Sutter VL: *Anaerobic Infections.* Kalamazoo, MI, Upjohn Co, 1983, p 52.

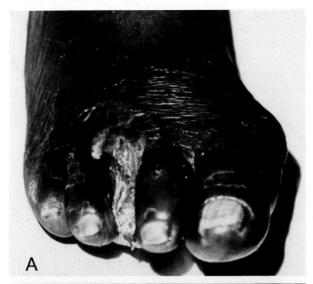

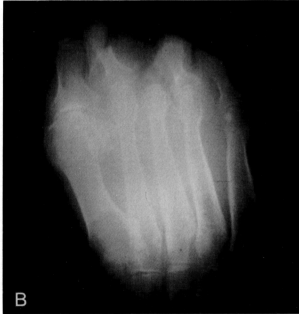

Figure 69.11. **A.** Anaerobic infection at amputation site. **B.** Presence of radiolucent areas near the head of the second metatarsal indicates gas in the tissues.

Clostridial myonecrosis is distinguished by involvement of normal uninjured muscle. It is usually associated with delayed or inadequate surgical intervention, poor blood supply, or damage and contamination of muscle tissue. The surrounding skin shows signs of ecchymosis, necrosis, and edema, and early intense pain is common. Characteristically, gas is produced within the infected soft tissues (Fig. 69.11), and brown, watery, foul-smelling exudate may be evident. Untreated, a rapidly fatal toxemia may develop.

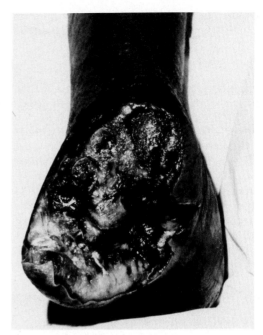

Figure 69.12. Foot with infected vascular gangrene partially amputated at Lisfranc's joint. Notice the characteristic black and desiccated gangrenous tissue. (Courtesy of Stanley R. Kalish).

Synergistic Nonclostridial Anaerobic Myonecrosis

Also called synergistic necrotizing cellulitis (49), this is a virulent polymicrobial soft tissue infection involving skin, subcutaneous tissue, fascia, and muscle. It is caused by *Bacteroides* species or anaerobic *streptococci*, or both, in collaboration with aerobic or facultative gram-negative bacilli. Characteristics are similar to those of gas gangrene. Overall mortality is 76%. Prognosis is poorer in patients treated by simple incision and drainage than in those treated by wide excision, which may necessitate hip disarticulation (48).

Anaerobic Streptococcal Myositis

This infection has much more of an insidious onset, developing slowly over 3 to 4 days. It is caused primarily by the gram-positive microaerophilic *Peptostreptococcus*, the anaerobic counterpart of *Streptococcus* (50). The same organism is responsible for a nonclostridial crepitant cellulitis, which is a connective tissue infection that does not involve muscle and is associated with abundant gas formation and minimal systemic toxicity (51).

Infected Vascular Gangrene

Infected vascular gangrene occurs primarily with loss of blood supply; and infection occurs in conjunction with or as a result of ischemic (dry) gangrene. There is usually little or no discharge, but the tissue is crepitant, foul-smelling, and often black and desiccated (Fig. 69.12). The infection may be caused by a number of anaerobes, including *C. perfringens* and *B. fragilis*, as well as facultative organisms.

Necrotizing Fasciitis

Necrotizing fasciitis is a life-threatening infection that may arise spontaneously, especially in patients with diabetes, peripheral vascular disease, or some other deficiency in host response (52). The most frequent anaerobic pathogen isolated is *Peptostreptococcus*. However, *S. aureus* or *S. pyogenes* may be involved, as well as the anaerobes, *Clostridium* and *Bacteroides*. The infection begins rapidly, within 24 to 72 hours after surgery or injury, with widespread dissection through deep fascial planes and necrosis of subcutaneous tissue. Probing beneath the surface will demonstrate wide undermining of the skin with separation from the fascia overlying the muscle. The subcutaneous fascia will appear gray and necrotic, but muscle will not be involved.

Anaerobic Cellulitis

Anaerobic cellulitis is defined as a localized infection of soft tissue that does not involve muscle (53). Foul odor and abundant gas in the tissues characterize the sepsis that can spread rapidly. Causative agents include *Clostridium*, gas-producing non-spore-forming anaerobes, and facultative organisms.

Meleney's Ulcer (Chronic Undermining Ulcer)

The chronic undermining or burrowing ulcer of Meleney is a deep indolent subcutaneous infection that spreads diffusely, producing multiple sinuses and necrotic ulcers as it undermines the skin (54). It may begin in surgical wounds, and healing is very slow even with antibiotic therapy. Muscle necrosis is not a feature. Causative organisms are microaerophilic hemolytic streptococci, although anaerobic organisms can be found as well.

Tetanus

Infections caused by *Clostridium tetani* have been reported following surgical procedures on the foot (55). The spores for this organism may grow in a sealed anaerobic environment especially when necrotic tissues and clotted blood are present as culture media. An average incubation period of 4 to 21 days is followed by a prodromal phase characterized by restlessness, yawning, headache, stiffness of the neck and jaw muscles, twitching in muscle around the wound, and increased reflexes in the wounded extremity, as well as diaphoresis, anxiety, and tachycardia. Tonic spasm of the skeletal muscles usually follows within 12 to 24 hours, causing the classical lockjaw (trismus), facial distortion (risus sardonicus), opisthotonus, and rigidity—the result of the powerful neurotoxin, tetanospasmin, released by the organism.

Immunization against tetanus requires two 0.5-ml subcutaneous injections of adsorbed tetanus toxoid 4 to 6 weeks apart. A third toxoid injection is given 6 to 12 months later. The patient is then considered actively immunized, and an adequate immune response may be expected for up to 10 years. "Booster" toxoid injections may then be given to stimulate the immune system to raise the serum antitoxin levels.

Table 69.14.
Initial Selection of Antibiotic Based on Gram's Stain and Likely Pathogen

Gram's Stain	Most Likely Bacteria	Initial Choice of Antibiotic	Comments
Gram-positive cocci in clumps	*Staphylococcus aureus*	Penicillinase-resistant penicillin: Oral: dicloxacillin, cloxacillin Parenteral: nafcillin or oxacillin (methicillin may cause interstitial nephritis)	Penicillin allergy: hives, urticaria: cephalosporin Possible anaphylaxis: vancomycin
Gram-positive cocci in chains	*Streptococcus pyogenes* (group A) *Streptococcus faecalis* (enterococcus) *Peptostreptococcus* *Staphylococcus epidermidis*	Oral: penicillin V Parenteral: penicillin G	Penicillin allergy: erythromycin
Gram-negative rods	*Escherichia coli, Klebsiella, Proteus, Pseudomonas, Enterobacter, Serratia*	Ampicillin or amoxicillin	Penicillin allergy: hives, urticaria: cephalosporin Possible anaphylaxis: trimethoprim-sulfamethoxazole *Klebsiella* is not sensitive to penicillin; cephalosporin is DOC If *Pseudomonas* is suspected, add amikacin or gentamicin
Gram-positive rods— large	*Clostridia* species	Oral: ampicillin, amoxicillin or bacampicillin Parenteral: penicillin G	Penicillin allergy: metronidazole, clindamycin, or chloramphenicol
Gram-positive rods— pleomorphic	*Bacteriodes fragilis*	Metronidazole	Secondary choices include clindamycin, chloramphenicol, cefoxitin; metronidazole does not cover aerobes or facultative anaerobes

TREATMENT OF POSTOPERATIVE INFECTION

Initial Considerations

In the face of as little as one sign of postoperative wound infection, procrastination may lead to disastrous complications. Prompt decisions are essential. Empirical antibiotics must be initiated promptly on the basis of clinical impressions, Gram's stain results, and the surgeon's own experience in determining the most likely pathogen (Table 69.14). Attention should also be paid to the bacteria and antibiotic sensitivity reports derived from statistics at local hospitals, especially with regard to resistant strains. If *Staphylococcus* is suspected, it should be considered penicillinase-resistant until the results of the culture and sensitivity studies are available.

Radiographs should be taken if sufficient time has elapsed for bony changes or if anaerobic gas production is suspected. Technetium 99 bone scans may be ordered if there is still some question as to osseous involvement. However, results will be equivocal if bone surgery was performed.

Whether hospitalization is required depends on the seriousness of the infection, the likely organism involved, and the medical status of the patient. For severe infections or infections requiring prolonged parenteral antibiotics, consultation should be sought with an internist, preferably an infectious disease specialist. This is important not only for selection, dosage, and management but also for monitoring allergic and toxic reactions, as well as changes in bacterial equilibrium.

Local Treatment

The simplest approach to the local treatment of postoperative infections is to apply the three Ds: decompression, drainage, and debridement. Decompression may involve the removal of one or more sutures or the release of pus from the wound. Opening the tissues is necessary to allow drainage, a procedure vital to successful treatment. If the wound or cavity is large, it should be packed with sterile gauze that may be impregnated with iodophor or some other antiseptic that is not irritating to the tissues. Further encouragement of fluid removal may be performed with the use of various types of drains. Gauze strips, Penrose drains, or silicone rubber catheters are ideal. They should not be used longer than 24 to 48 hours.

Finally, debridement is essential when necrotic debris is present. Incision and drainage alone will be ineffectual against many types of anaerobic infecting agents. If pain is a deterrent to this surgical therapy, then proximal nerve blocks may be performed. If necessary the patient may be returned to the surgery suite for spinal or general anesthesia so that a thorough debridement can be performed. Liberal irrigation is a helpful but often neglected part of the procedure. Various solutions may be used, such as Ringer's, normal saline (NS), NS and hydrogen peroxide, or NS and povidone-iodine solution. When *Pseudomonas* is involved, weak acetic acid (vinegar) solution will inhibit growth of the organism. All of these measures are directed at increasing circulation and improving local host defenses. Other forms of treatment may also be considered.

Limiting the patient's activities by prescribing rest and elevation will help prevent dissemination of the infection. Bulky compression dressings and splints may be used for protection. Elevation encourages venous and lymphatic drainage to reduce edema and improve local blood flow.

Wet-to-dry dressings with the use of the various irrigation solutions already described serve several purposes. They encourage and absorb fluid exudates, protect the wound against further contamination, provide a physiological environment, and debride necrotic tissue when they are removed. Povidone-iodine mixed with NS is especially effective because the elemental iodine released is bactericidal and will kill spores. Organic mercurial antiseptics (Mercurochrome, Merthiolate) are not good for local treatment of infections because they are primarily bacteriostatic, relatively ineffective at killing spores, and penetrate tissues poorly (1). When povidone-iodine-soaked gauze dries, it also provides a good splint for the wound, which is especially effective for the forefoot and toes.

Soaks with or without the aid of a whirlpool may be used when all other measures have been instituted and there is no danger that water will further contaminate the wound. Such treatment is soothing to the tissues, provides some measure of debridement, and kills superficial bacteria when an antiseptic is added to the water.

Definitive Systemic Antibiosis

TREATMENT LOCATION

When oral antibiotics are indicated for infection therapy, office care should be sufficient. In more serious infections for which parenteral antibiotics are required, the hospital is the ideal setting for establishing and maintaining intravenous administrations.

The hospital is an especially important location for treatment when the patient has sepsis or suffers from other medical disorders concurrently. However, with the focus on containing the rising costs of medical care, outpatient parenteral antibiotics therapy is becoming more widely accepted (56).

Whether the administration is by a home nurse or by the trained patient, central venous access may be maintained even for long periods, with use of a variety of modern devices and techniques (Fig. 69.13). For example, three types of "tunneled" catheters for long-term intravenous access are the Hickman, the Broviac, and the Groshong catheters. Each requires a surgical procedure for installation (57).

SELECTION AND ADMINISTRATION OF ANTIBIOTICS

Once the organism and its antimicrobial sensitivities are identified, an appropriate antibiotic may be selected for systemic therapy. This may require a change from the empirically selected agent already in use. The ideal drug should have the following characteristics:

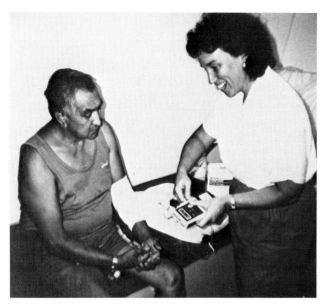

Figure 69.13. Nurse instructing a patient in the use of a CADD-PLUS (continuous ambulatory drug delivery) intravenous pump for self-administration of antibiotics. (Courtesy of O.P.T.I.O.N. Care, Bellingham, WA. CADD-PLUS, registered trade mark, Pharmacia, Inc, Piscataway, NJ 08855.)

1. Exhibit selective and effective activity against the organism involved
2. Be bactericidal as opposed to bacteriostatic
3. Have limited potential to induce bacterial resistance
4. Produce sufficient levels in the tissues involved
5. Not induce a hypersensitivity reaction
6. Have the least amount of potential for toxicity

Route of administration is an additional important consideration. Drugs given parenterally will reach generally higher tissue levels. However, some agents cannot be delivered except orally whereas certain organisms are susceptible only to parenteral antibiotics.

The ideal dosage of an antimicrobial agent has been defined as the least amount of drug to achieve the desired effect while producing no adverse reactions (58). However, one of the more common problems with antibiotic therapy is underdosing. Sensitivity studies determine only the inhibitory concentration of the infecting organism. Fortunately, this concentration is bactericidal for most antibiotics. However, for a few such as the aminoglycosides, the difference between the inhibitory and bactericidal concentrations can be quite large, leading to therapeutical failure. In addition, the course of treatment is frequently too short for adequate effect. This may lead to the development of resistant bacteria or even a relapse of the infection.

Adequate dosage requires several considerations: age and weight of the patient, time for peak blood levels, duration of effect of a single dose, rate and site of excretion of the drug, and ability of the antibiotic to reach the infected tissues. Except for severe foot and ankle infections or those involving bone, treatment should be for a minimum of 7 days and a maximum of 10 days. Prolonged therapy invites adverse effects of the drug. Such reactions include hypersensitivity, gastrointestinal toxicity, superinfection, and renal, hepatic, or hematopoietic dysfunction.

Although basic principles for managing infections have changed little in recent years, the development and availability of new antimicrobial agents have changed dramatically. As a result, it is difficult to make recommendations for specific antibiotics in a reference text such as this.

For selection and institution of specific anti-infection drugs, the reader is referred to current reviews and reference publications (36, 59-63). These publications should be consulted for appropriateness, characteristics, and recommended dosages of any antibiotic being considered for therapy. A sound understanding of antimicrobial agents is essential to their efficacious and safe use.

RESPONSE TO TREATMENT

The efficacy of antibiotic therapy should be evaluated frequently. If fever is present, it should fall within 12 hours of treatment initiation. The leukocytosis should reduce along with the neutrophilia although the monocytes may increase. Pain should subside within the same 12-hour period, and locally the wound should demonstrate a reduction in edema, erythema, and drainage.

If the patient is not responding to the antibiotic regimen, then several questions must be addressed: *(a)* is the isolated organism really the etiological agent? *(b)* are other organisms involved in the infection? *(c)* is the antibiotic being administered in adequate dosages? *(d)* is it reaching and penetrating the tissues? *(e)* have resistant bacteria emerged? and *(f)* has a superinfection developed? (1).

MANAGEMENT OF POSTOPERATIVE HEMATOMA

Definition

Hematoma refers to the collection or extravasation of blood, usually clotted, within a closed tissue space. It is caused by leakage from local vessels damaged by blunt trauma, local injury, or surgical dissection. Seroma, on the other hand, is a localized accumulation of serum, the clear portion of blood that remains after clotting has removed the fibrinogen and other elements. It is extravasated by locally damaged small vessels during the early stages of the inflammatory process.

In the postsurgical setting, a hematoma may be a very frustrating and often debilitating complication that can lead to infection or long-term swelling and disability. Understanding the etiology and pathophysiology of this problem will help in its prevention by alerting the surgeon to implement prophylactic measures. Management is not impossible but, in addition to prompt recognition and treatment, requires diligent adherence to the principles of healing and wound manipulation.

Etiology and Prevention

Blood supply lies between the surgeon's instruments and bone, and it is the operator's responsibility to provide the accurate anatomical dissection that will limit its disruption. Inadequate attention to hemostasis is the primary source of most postoperative hematoma. Dead space that has not been closed or drained will allow the accumulation of blood or serum (Fig. 69.14).

Arteries severed and not ligated during tourniquet hemostasis are ominous sources of bleeding. They may lead to a pulsating hematoma, also known as a false aneurysm. It is wise, then, to release the tourniquet and observe for complete hemostasis before wound closure. Reliance on pressure bandaging as a primary means of controlling internal bleeding is a weak substitute.

If complete control of bleeding is impossible at the time of surgery, then hemostatic agents should be implemented. Closed suction drains may be inserted if fluid accumulation is anticipated (Fig. 69.15).

A higher incidence of hematoma formation is seen in patients with myeloproliferative disorders, polycythemia vera, and coagulation defects, as well as in patients receiving anticoagulant therapy—even low-dose heparin prophylaxis or aspirin (64).

Diagnosis

Hematoma is a great mimicker of early wound infection. This occurs because the body response of intense local inflammation is almost identical in each case.

There is usually intense local pain caused first by the expansion of the hematoma itself and, second, by the extravasation of fluid and swelling of the tissues as the inflammation sets in. The pain and swelling occur much earlier than from infection, usually within the first 24 hours. They must be differentiated from the uncomplicated signs of inflammation seen during the early stages of normal healing.

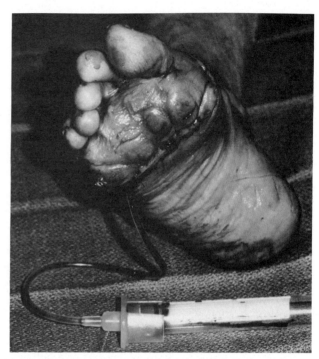

Figure 69.15. Closed suction drainage system following panmetatarsal head resections. (TLS Drain courtesy of Porox Medical, Fairburn, GA 30203.)

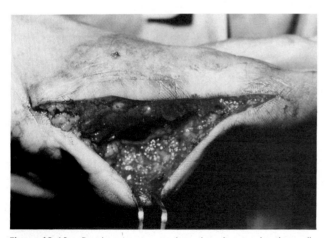

Figure 69.14. Dead space occurs where there is extensive tissue disruption or removal.

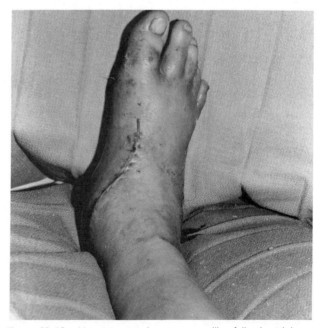

Figure 69.16. Hematoma causing excess swelling following triple arthrodesis procedure is common.

Pain, unresponsive to even the strongest of analgesics, including narcotics, points to hematoma, infection, or dressing pressure.

Swelling may be so intense as to cause a wound dehiscence, seen at redressing (Fig. 69.16). The inflammation may also radiate a large amount of heat from the wound site, with angry peripheral erythema. Ecchymosis may or may not be present.

Sequelae and Deleterious Effects

Aside from the intense and usually prolonged pain, hematoma may lead not only to wound dehiscence but also to frank skin slough if the local circulation is sufficiently compromised. Gross tissue edema results from the pressure obstruction of local capillaries, veins, and lymphatic vessels. This is usually difficult to eradicate (Fig. 69.17).

Over the long term, the additional tissue injury caused by hematoma simply leads to prolonged disability and rehabilitation. The overall result may jeopardize the success of the surgery, especially if the lesion is not promptly recognized and treated. The most deleterious effects of hematoma formation are infection and fibroplasia.

The fate of a formed hematoma depends on whether it is a localized and clotted pool of blood, compressing the local tissues into a sort of pseudocapsule, or disseminated diffusely through the tissue planes. The latter may be readily absorbed by the inflammatory process. The former, being largely devoid of blood supply, will undergo peripheral fibroplasia and then organize into dense scar tissue (65).

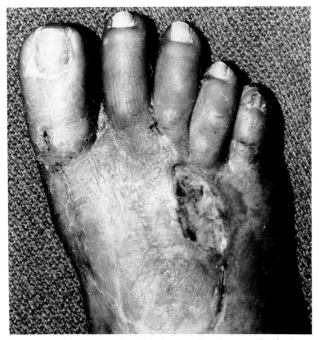

Figure 69.17. Skin slough and marked swelling about the forefoot were caused by hematoma. Patient fell during her convalescence, and swelling occurred within the cast as hematoma developed.

During the first 24 hours the reaction consists of pain, swelling, and possible dehiscence with little histological change observed. This is followed by the migration into the site of large numbers of polymorphonuclear leukocytes and mononuclear phagocytes to begin clean-up. The severity of this exudative stage may be reduced with the early use of steroids, which impede the laying down of fibrin. During the first 3 days after formation of a hematoma, mononuclear cells predominate. One of their most important jobs is to engulf the iron pigment or hemosiderin from the degraded blood and remove it from the tissues.

At about the third day, fibroblasts appear at the site. They are thought to arise from the hemosiderin-filled phagocytes or from adjacent connective tissue. They tend to increase rapidly in number as they begin the production of collagen. Absence of a fibrin lattice seems to inhibit fibroplasia. Thus to avoid excess fibrosis, steroids may be introduced because they interfere with the chain of events that leads to the production of a fibrin lattice.

The end result is organization and fibrosis that leads to adhesion formation or obliteration of the space with dense scar tissue. The scar may be penetrated with new capillaries, but it contains few cells and is relatively inert metabolically. Its induration is easily palpable. The insoluble calcium and iron salts are mute evidence of its origin from blood. Attraction of further calcium may lead to calcification. Ossifying hematoma within muscle must be differentiated from myositis ossificans.

Hematoma and Infection

There is no doubt that hematoma formation is associated with an increased incidence of postsurgical infection (66). A number of reasons for this have evolved through observation and research.

First, blood itself is an excellent culture medium for bacterial growth, especially when incubation is provided by the tissues. Indeed, blood is used in the laboratory to enhance certain bacterial culture media. Second, hematoma obstructs the migration of inflammatory cells. Virtually any condition that contributes to such a decreased delivery of phagocytic cells to an area of bacterial contamination will encourage development of an infection.

In addition, it is becoming clear that hematoma enhances bacterial virulence (67-72). It has been shown that certain strains of bacteria become much more effective or virulent in the presence of ferric ions that originate from the accumulated blood (64, 68, 71, 72). In fact this effect is even magnified, because hemoglobin is present (68, 73, 74). All bacteria need iron but normally find little free iron in the tissues for replication. They must secrete chelators to extract the iron from plasma transferrin and other iron-binding protein. Not only does the free iron from a hematoma eliminate this difficulty; it also inhibits some of the antibacterial activity within the granulocytes. Hence the enhancement of infection (75).

It also appears that by way of transport proteins, such as transferrin and lactoferrin, the body actually withholds iron from invading bacteria as a form of defense. This is termed *nutritional immunity* and it is indeed compromised by the presence of a local hematoma (71, 76).

Finally, it has been clearly shown that fluids collecting in surgical wounds are deficient in opsonic activity, therefore interfering with bacterial phagocytosis and killing by neutrophils (77). Such knowledge supports the necessity for avoidance of hematoma formation and encouragement of wound drainage.

Early Phase Management

EXTRAVASATION

Probably the simplest method of removing blood and clots from a wound is by applying gentle pressure to the wound edges and squeezing out the undesirable accumulations. This is most effective when local anesthesia is still in effect. The longer the time lapse since surgery the poorer the results of this treatment.

ASPIRATION

Use of a hypodermic syringe with a large-bore (20 gauge) needle may be used to withdraw fluid from within a hematoma (Fig. 69.18). It is more effective if applied early, before all the blood has clotted. Otherwise it removes only serosanguineous fluid. It will not remove clots. The more fluctuant the hematoma, the more amenable it is to aspiration. Aspiration is very useful for extracting seroma-type fluid from wounds in which there is considerable dead space. Because of the slightly increased chance of infection with the introduction of a needle into a fresh surgical wound, careful attention to asepsis is essential.

DRAINS

The ideal method of drainage is to insert the catheter of a closed suction system with the use of a sharp trocar under sterile technique. The trocar enters and exits the wound through separate punctures, drawing the catheter (preferably silicone) into place (78) (Fig. 69.19). Gravity or Penrose drains are not recommended because of the increased liability of retrograde contamination.

STEROID INFILTRATION

Short-acting corticosteroids infiltrated locally will help slow clotting, interfere with organization, and prevent much of the intense and painful inflammation associated with hematoma. Because of these drugs' inhibition of phagocytosis, there is the increased risk of infection, which dictates their judicious use.

ACCELERATED DEGRADATION

Hyaluronidase is a hydrolytic enzyme that cleaves hyaluronic acid, a viscous polysaccharide found in the interstices

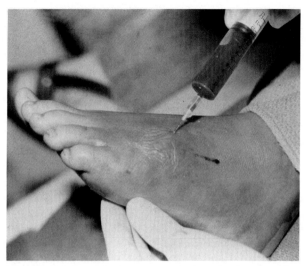

Figure 69.18. Evacuating hematoma with a hypodermic syringe. (Courtesy of John A. Ruch.)

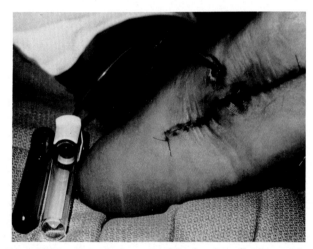

Figure 69.19. Evacuating hematoma following plantar fibroma resection with closed suction drainage system. (TLS Drain courtesy of Porox Medical, Fairburn, GA 30203.)

of tissues. There is no direct effect on the hematoma itself, but this enzyme will remove obstructions and thereby allow better diffusion of fluids within the tissues to enhance the inflammatory destruction. It should not be used when intense inflammation is already established.

Streptokinase is a nonenzymatic protein used for intravascular thrombolysis. It functions to dissolve existing thrombi through proteolytic action on the supporting fibrin network (79). It does so by activating the fibrinolytic systems, converting plasminogen to plasmin. Injected locally into a hematoma, it can function similarly to break up the fibrin network, although further research into this is needed. The enzyme urokinase is a similar thrombolytic agent.

WOUND REENTRY

When it is evident that the size or pressure of a hematoma will seriously impair healing, then it should be evacuated under sterile conditions (80). An aseptic surgical field should be established, with return to the operating room if necessary and the wound opened. Clots should be removed with liberal irrigation and all bleeders clamped and ligated or electrocoagulated. An optional closed suction drain may be inserted exiting from a separate puncture, and the wound closed in layers.

PROPHYLACTIC ANTIBIOTICS

When the diagnosis of postoperative hematoma is established, the increased risk of infection justifies the institution of prophylactic antibiotics. Because this is after the surgery and contamination is already present, a 5-to-7-day course is advised for oral antibiotics. Standard-dose regimens of parenteral antibiotics have been shown to penetrate hematoma in bactericidal concentrations (81-85). Some antibiotics, such as cefamandole, penetrate fibrin clots better than do others (86). One study showed that a hematoma can be penetrated by antibiotics given up to 4 days after its formation (87).

Management of Hematoma—Late Phase

COMPRESSION THERAPY

Firm but nonrestrictive compression dressings are an effective method of treating established hematoma. In addition to preventing further bleeding in the early stages, they also control swelling so that there is little interference with breakdown mechanisms (Fig. 69.20).

HEAT

Application of heat after the most intense inflammation has subsided and gentle warming of the tissues will accelerate the enzymatic degradation of the established hematoma, discouraging it from organizing.

PHYSICAL THERAPY

Range of motion exercises, massage, and ultrasound all serve to break up the fibrin network on which late organization depends. If the tissue is already firm or indurated, treatment is the same as for any dense scar tissue.

STEROID INFILTRATION

With or without hyaluronidase, longer-acting corticosteroid preparations may be used to soften the organized hematoma. Multiple needle penetration, or hypodermoclysis, will aid infiltration.

POSTOPERATIVE EDEMA

Edema or postoperative swelling is an alarming process to both the patient and the surgeon (Fig. 69.21). The cause is frequently associated with violations of surgical principles, although poor patient compliance in following postoperative instructions may certainly be instrumental. Understanding the pathophysiology greatly facilitates its prevention and management.

Definition

Postoperative swelling or edema is really the "tumor" portion of inflammation. It refers to the presence of excessive amounts of fluid within the intercellular tissue spaces, particularly the subcutaneous tissues. Because of the high protein content of fluid delivered from the vascular system into the inflamed tissues, it is considered an exudate. However, the actual protein content within the edematous interstitial

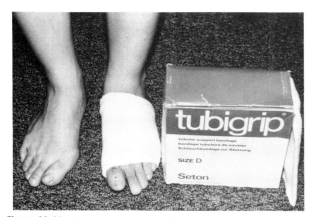

Figure 69.20. Late-phase treatment of hematoma with tubular compression bandage. A double layer is suggested.

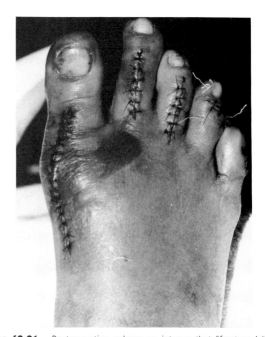

Figure 69.21. Postoperative edema so intense that "fracture blisters" containing serosanguineous fluid developed in skin.

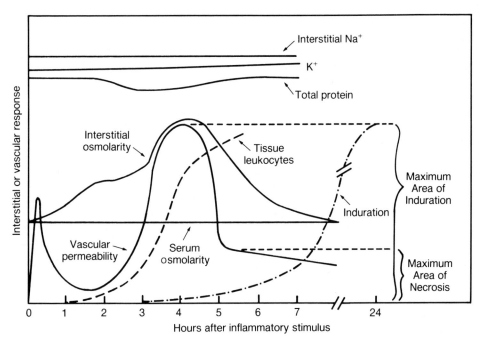

Figure 69.22. Times of occurrence of events in early inflammation showing the physiological development of edema. Changes in interstitial composition (osmolarity, electrolyte, and protein concentration) are compared with changes in vascular permeability and development of induration and leukocytosis. (From Leak LV, Burke JF: Early events of tissue injury and the role of the lymphatic system in early inflammation. In Zweifach BW, Grant L, McCluskey RT [eds]: *The Inflammatory Process,* ed 2, vol 3. New York, Academic Press, 1974, p 201.)

tissues remains somewhat constant for reasons that will be seen shortly (Fig. 69.22).

Pathophysiology

NORMAL PHYSIOLOGY

Under normal physiological conditions, body fluids move back and forth through the capillary endothelial wall, regulated by various tissue and fluid pressures. As can be seen in Figure 69.23, the pressure is consistently greater in moving the fluids out into the tissues although there is considerable capillary reabsorption.

Water and crystalloids are mainly absorbed at the venous limb of blood capillaries, whereas proteins, which continually pass across the capillary endothelial wall, are absorbed and removed by the lymphatic vessels. This helps maintain the colloid osmotic pressure gradient across the blood capillary wall (88). When surgical tissue damage and inflammation are imposed, there are some dramatic changes in interstitial fluid dynamics.

INCREASED VASCULAR PERMEABILITY

Surgical injury results in two basic types of increased vascular permeability. The first is rather short in duration, lasting only 15 to 30 minutes, and is caused by histamine and histamine-like permeability factors (serotonin, kinins, prostaglandins). It begins very early following injury, once the transient constriction of the damaged local vessels has

**PHYSICAL FORCES ACTING ACROSS
THE CAPILLARY WALL**
(approximate values in mm Hg)

Causing fluid to move out		Causing fluid to move in	
Intravascular hydrostatic pressure (average)	23	Osmotic pressure of plasma proteins	25
Osmotic pressure of tissue proteins and mucopolysaccharides	10	Hydrostatic tissue pressure	1–4
~33→		~26 to 29	

Figure 69.23. Physical forces acting across the capillary wall. (From Ryan GB, Majno G: *Inflammation.* Kalamazoo, MI, Upjohn Co, 1977, p 14.)

subsided (5 to 10 minutes). Although the arterioles dilate in response to the histamine vasoactive mediators, the increased permeability effected is not within the capillaries but through the walls of the venules. The endothelial cells in the walls tend to swell and "round up," creating separations between them. This allows large amounts of plasma with electrolytes and protein macromolecules to escape into the interstitial tissue spaces. All proteins in plasma will appear in inflammatory exudate (89-91). Immediately following this histamine-induced vascular response, the vessels return to their normal size.

The second type of vascular permeability is leakage caused by direct vascular injury. When there is considerable endothelial cell destruction, as by surgical dissection or sustained electrocautery, prolonged leakage from the vessels occurs. It may last for 1 or 2 days until the vessel is plugged by a thrombus or is repaired. Clearly the more damage sustained by the tissues during surgery, the greater and more protracted the edema from this type of prolonged vascular permeability.

ROLE OF THE LYMPHATIC VESSELS

The lymphatics have a key function in removing proteins and fluid from the extracellular tissue spaces. This role is greatly expanded during the early phases of inflammation. To compensate for the increased vascular permeability the lymphatic vessels rapidly dilate to a diameter several times their normal caliber (88).

Coincidentally, the volume of lymph draining from an injured area will increase five to twenty times or more with a considerable rise in the lymph protein concentration. Thus the inflammatory exudate is not simply a static pool but rather a pool of protein with a high turnover (91). The actual content of protein within the interstitial spaces remains somewhat constant (88).

As the tissues expand to accommodate more fluid during the development of the inflammation, a remarkable paradox occurs. The venules tend to be compressed while the lymphatics are greatly distended to remove excess local fluids, proteins, damaged cells, and bacteria and their toxins.

This amazing ability of lymphatics to dilate during early inflammation is the result mainly of structures known as lymphatic anchoring filaments, which maintain the capillary walls in close relationship to the surrounding interstitium, and to the presence of extensively overlapped adjacent endothelial cells that are free to slide past each other for relatively long distances. Thus, as the interstitial collagen bundles move relative to each other to accommodate increased fluid volume expansion, the anchoring filaments automatically dilate the lymphatic capillary lumen and the endothelial cells separate to accept the increased demand for fluid transport (88).

Prevention

ANATOMICAL DISSECTION

In reviewing the key role of the lymphatic vessels during inflammation, it is easy to understand why massive edema follows surgery in which unnecessary trauma and extensive dissection occur. The integrity of the lymphatic system must be preserved by gentle anatomical dissection and atraumatic technique if excess swelling is to be avoided. In addition, the more blood vessels that are damaged, the greater the prolonged permeability phase of inflammation.

INTRAOPERATIVE STEROIDS

Short-acting corticosteroids such as dexamethasone phosphate and betamethasone phosphate are often used to pre-

vent the postoperative pain associated with the inflammatory phase of healing. They should not become a crutch for wanton dissection, tearing of tissues, and unnecessary trauma. An additional benefit in limiting the intensity of early inflammation is the control of edema as well. It is the author's experience that edema is even further suppressed if the steroid is mixed with local anesthetic and infiltrated into the tissues before the first incision.

COMPRESSION DRESSINGS

Dressings designed to apply controlled compression as described in the chapter on postoperative management are very effective in preventing excess edema. They must be applied evenly, without wrinkles and without constriction. A certain amount of swelling must be tolerated to allow inflammation to take place (Fig. 69.24).

ELEVATION

The obvious benefit of elevation is to facilitate the massive lymphatic drainage. The foot is on the end of a dependent extremity that is, for the most part, immobilized after sur-

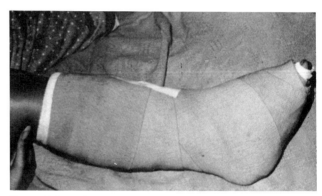

Figure 69.24. Controlled compression dressing to reduce edema utilizes alternating layers of cotton padding and elastic bandages.

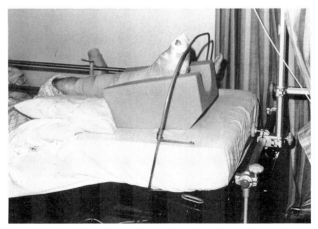

Figure 69.25. Elevation to relieve edema should place the feet at least above hips, preferably above heart.

gery. It must be elevated above the hip—or even above the heart—to give gravity the best advantage (Fig. 69.25).

ICE

The principal role of ice is to prevent swelling by local vascular constriction. This tends to limit the prolongation of vascular leakage. It is effective only during the very early phases of inflammation.

ANTIINFLAMMATORY DRUGS

The nonsteroidal antiinflammatory drugs (NSAIDs) effectively interfere with various aspects of the inflammatory process. However, it is difficult to measure their inhibition of edema in specific quantitative terms. One test for determining the relative potencies of the NSAIDs is the carrageenan-induced rat-paw edema assay. The relative ability of these drugs to reduce such edema does seem to reflect clinical experience (92) (Table 69.15). However, such ability must be weighed against any fluid retention potential the drug might have.

Management of Prolonged Postoperative Edema

One of the most difficult sequela to predict following lower extremity surgery is the duration of swelling. Even after scrupulous adherence to all operative principles, prolonged edema can frustrate both the surgeon and the patient. It is wise to make the patient aware of this before surgery. Treatment must be aggressive.

Elevation of the extremity as much as possible is essential. Range of motion exercises allow the muscles indirectly to pump lymphatic fluid through proximal channels and encourage vigorous circulation of the blood, enhancing transendothelial fluid exchange. The efficacy of oral enzymatic agents is equivocal. They do not appear to be withstanding the time test of clinical experience. Diuretics may be used if the patient is already known to retain fluids.

Compression therapy is central to the successful management of postoperative edema. Controlled compression dressings may be incorporated into the wound coverings initially. Once dressings are no longer necessary, the foot or even the foot and lower leg should be circumscribed with a double layer of tubular elastic bandage. This is a comfortable stockinette that provides even, relentless compression to the postsurgical tissue, continually milking the fluids from the interstitial spaces. Commercially available support hose of various strengths may be used for early return to work activity (Fig. 69.26).

Frequent massage of the local tissue helps reduce edema once postsurgical tenderness has subsided and healing is substantially advanced. Other physical therapy measures include therapeutical ultrasound and galvanic stimulation, both of which may be applied simultaneously with modern devices.

Ultrasound is defined as the cyclic pressure variation induced by mechanical vibration at frequencies above the limit

Table 69.15.
Effect of NSAIDs in the Carrageenin-Induced Rat-Paw Edema Assay

Drug	Dose (mg, kg, po)	% Inhibition	Potency[a] 95% Confidence Limits
Phenylbutazone	25.0	27	1
	50.0	39	
	100.0	57	
Acetylsalicylic acid	50.0	23	0.36 (0.13-0.85)
	100.0	32	
	200.0	40	
	400.0	43	
Tolmetin	6.25	38	2.17 (0.82-5.94)
	25.0	40	
	100.0	44	
Naproxen	0.78	16	15.5 (6.6-39.6)
	1.56	40	
	6.25	43	
	25.0	52	
	50.0	60	
Sudoxicam	0.37	7	24.1 (10.2-56.1)
	1.11	30	
	3.33	39	
	10.0	48	
Indomethacin	0.37	29	62.7 (26.1-148.5)
	1.11	38	
	3.33	46	
	10.0	47	

From Arrigoni-Martelli E: *Inflammatory and Antiinflammatories*. New York, Spectrum Publications, 1977, p 144.
[a]Weighted linear regression analysis.

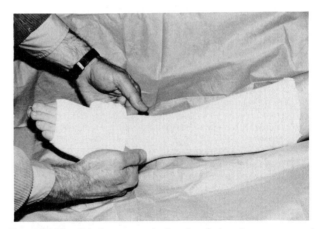

Figure 69.26. Tubular compression bandage for long-term management of prolonged postoperative edema.

of the human ear (93). Clinically, it is very effective in reducing postoperative edema provided it is applied frequently (e.g., every other day for 2 weeks). The exact physiological mechanism for its efficacy is unknown, but it has been shown to stimulate tissue repair and strengthen wounds following injury. Galvanic stimulation causes muscle contractions that function like a pump, as previously described.

References

1. Hugar DW: Management of infection. In Marcus SA, Block BH (eds): *American College of Foot Surgeons—Complications in Foot Surgery: Prevention and Management*, ed 2. Baltimore, Williams & Wilkins, 1984, pp 494-502.
2. Krizek TJ, Robson MC: Biology of surgical infection. *Surg Clin North Am* 55:1261-1267, 1975.
3. Elek SD, Cormen PE: The virulence of *Staphylococcus pyrogenes* for man: a study of the problems of wound infection. *Br J Exp Pathol* 38:573, 1957.
4. Burke JF: Infection. In Burke JF, Dunphy JE, Hunt TK (eds): *Fundamentals of Wound Management in Surgery*. South Plainfield, NJ, Chirurgecom, 1977.
5. Hunt TK, Dunphy JE (eds): *Fundamentals of Wound Management*. New York, Appleton-Century-Crofts, 1979.
6. MacLean LD: Systemic antibacterial mechanisms in trauma. *World J Surg* 7:119-124, 1983.
7. Leak LV, Burke JF: Early events of tissue injury and the role of the lymphatic system in early inflammation. In Zweifach BW, Grant L, McCluskey RT (eds): *The Inflammatory Process*, ed 2, vol 3. New York, Academic Press, 1974, pp 163-235.
8. Miles AA, Miles EM, Burker JF: The value and duration of defense reactions of the skin to the primary lodgement of bacteria. *Br J Exp Pathol* 38:79, 1957.
9. Miles AA: The inflammatory response in relation to local infections. *Surg Clin North Am* 60:93-105, 1980.
10. Ryan GB, Majno G: *Inflammation*. Kalamazoo, Mich, Upjohn Co, 1977.
11. Hurley JV: *Acute Inflammation*, ed 2. New York, Churchill-Livingstone, 1983.
12. Kalter ES: Inflammatory mediators and acute infection. *Resuscitation* 11:133-140, 1984.
13. Migliori V, Kanat IO: Surgical considerations in wound healing. *J Foot Surg* 23:377-381, 1984.
14. Conte JE, Jacob LS, Polk HC Jr: *Antibiotic Prophylaxis in Surgery. A Comprehensive Review*. Philadelphia, JB Lippincott, 1984, pp 1-25, 95-109.
15. Hunter WN, Borovoy M: Prophylactic antibiotics—control of implant contamination. *J Am Podiatry Assoc* 74:284-290, 1984.
16. Till K, Solomon MG, Kerman BL: Indications and uses of prophylactic antibiosis in podiatric surgery. *J Foot Surg* 23:166-172, 1984.
17. Okin S, Mehl S, DellaCorte M, Schechter D, Esposito F: The use of prophylactic antibiotics in clean podiatric surgery. *J Foot Surg* 23:402-406, 1984.
18. Norden CW: Critical review of antibiotic prophylaxis in orthopaedic surgery. *Rev Infect Dis* 5:928-932, 1983.
19. Nelson CL: Preventive antibiotics in orthopedic surgery. In Condon RE, Gorbach SL (eds): *Surgical Infections. Selective Antibiotic Therapy*. Baltimore, Williams & Wilkins, 1980, pp 125-130.
20. Green SA: Antibiotic update. *Adv Orthop Surg* 7:48-59, 1983.
21. Bowers WH: A rational plan for the use of preventative antibiotics in orthopaedic surgery In American Academy of Orthopaedic Surgeons: *Instructional Course Lectures* vol 16. St Louis, CV Mosby, 1977, p 30.
22. Pavel A, Smith RL, Ballard A, Larsen IJ: Prophylactic antibiotics in clean orthopaedic surgery. *J Bone Joint Surg* 56A:777, 1974.
23. Dineen P (ed): *The Surgical Wound*. Philadelphia, Lea & Febiger, 1981.
24. Neumann CG: Interaction of malnutrition and infection—a neglected clinical concept. *Arch Intern Med* 137:1364-1365, 1977.
25. Alexander JW: Infection, host resistance, and antimicrobial agents. In Dudrick SJ (ed): *American College of Surgeons, Committee on Pre and Postoperative Care: Manual of Preoperative and Postoperative Care*, ed 3. Philadelphia, WB Saunders, 1983, pp 106-136.
26. Cruse PJE, Foord R: The epidemiology of wound infection—a 10-year prospective study of 62,939 wounds. *Surg Clin North Am* 60:27-40, 1980.
27. Dineen P: An evaluation of the surgical scrub. *Surg Gynecol Obstet* 129:1181, 1969.
28. Abramson C: Normal "opportunistic" flora of the lower extremities related to postoperative surgical wound infections. *J Am Podiatry Assoc* 67:9-27, 1977.
29. Atkins E, Bodel P: Fever. In Zweifach BC, Grant L, McCluskey RT (eds): *The Inflammatory Process*, ed 2, vol 3. New York, Academic Press, 1974.
30. Miller SJ: Temperature regulation and postoperative fever: a preliminary study. *J Am Podiatry Assoc* 74:373-379, 1984.

31. Isenberg HD, Washington JA II, Balows A, Sonnenwirth AC: Collection, handling, and processing of specimens. In Lennette EH, Balows A, Hausler WJ Jr, Truant JP (eds): *Manual of Clinical Microbiology*. Washington, DC, American Society for Microbiology, 1980.
32. Clausen C: Diagnostic bacteriology. In Kelley VC (ed): *Practice of Pediatrics*, vol 2. Hagerstown, Md, Harper & Row, 1977.
33. Rosenblatt JE: Laboratory tests used to guide antimicrobial therapy. *Mayo Clin Proc* 58:14-20, 1983.
34. Richmond M, Sykes RB: The beta-lactamases of gram-negative bacteria and their possible physiologic role. In Rose AH, Tempest DW (eds): *Advances in Microbial Physiology*, vol 9. New York, Academic Press, 1973, p 31.
35. Sykes RB, Mathew M: The beta-lactamases of gram-negative bacteria and their role in resistance to beta-lactam antibiotics *J Antimicrob Chemother* 2:115, 1976.
36. Hermans, PE (ed): Symposium on antimicrobial agents. *Mayo Clin Proc* 62:788-1145, 1987.
37. Amoxicillin-clavulanic acid. *Med Lett* 26:98-100, 1984.
38. Clavulanic acid inhibits beta-lactamases. *FDA Drug Bull* 14:25, 1984.
39. Abramson C: The influence of hospital acquired infections on podiatric medical education. *J Podiatr Med Educ* 6:26, 1975.
40. Forgan-Smith WR: Antibiotics and surgery. *Br J Hosp Med* 14:529-540, 1975.
41. Shaw D: Infection associated with modern surgical procedures. *Postgrad Med J* 48:230, 1972.
42. Miller WA: Postoperative wound infection in foot and ankle surgery. *Foot Ankle* 4:102-104, 1983.
43. Curin G, Peters WJ, Tsoutsouris GV: A study of infections of the foot. *J Am Podiatry Assoc* 65:645-648, 1975.
44. Rubinlicht JR: Bacterial infections of the foot. A 30-month study. *J Am Podiatry Assoc* 66:393-407, 1976.
45. Curin G, Cowin RM, Riegelhaupt RW: The incidence and antimicrobial treatment of infections of the foot. *J Am Podiatry Assoc* 71:209-214, 1981.
46. Pollack M, Nieman RE, Reinhardt JA, Charache P, Jett MP, Hardy PH Jr: Factors influencing colonization and antibiotic resistance patterns of gram-negative rods. *Lancet* 2:668, 1972.
47. Finegold SM, Sutter VL: *Anaerobic Infections*. Kalamazoo, Mich, Upjohn Co, 1983.
48. Snelling CFT: Microorganisms and sepsis. In Kernahan DA, Vistnes LM (eds): *Biological Aspects of Reconstructive Surgery*. New York, Little Brown & Co, 1977, pp 107-118.
49. Stone HH, Martin JD: Synergistic necrotizing cellulitis. *Am Surg* 175:702, 1972.
50. Anderson CB, Marr J, Jaffe BM: Anaerobic streptococcal infections simulating gas gangrene. *Arch Surg* 104:186, 1972.
51. VanBeek A, Zook E, Yaw P, Gardner R, Smith R, Glover JL: Nonclostridial gas-forming infections. *Arch Surg* 108:552, 1974.
52. Rea WJ, Wyrick WJ Jr: Necrotizing fasciitis. *Am Surg* 172:957, 1970.
53. MacLennan JD: The histotoxic clostridial infections of man. *Bacteriol Rev* 26:177-276, 1962.
54. Meleney FL: *Clinical Aspects and Treatment of Surgical Infections*. Philadelphia, WB Saunders, 1949.
55. Brill LR, Harris GM, Kinberg P: Nosocomial postoperative tetanus infection. *J Foot Surg* 23:235-239, 1984.
56. Smego RA: Home intravenous antibiotic therapy [editorial]. *Arch Intern Med* 145:1001-1002, 1985.
57. Hadaway LC: Evaluation and use of advanced IV technology. I. Central venous access devices. *JIN* 12:72-82, 1989.
58. Albright J, Brand R (ed): *The Scientific Basis of Orthopaedics*, ed 2. Norwalk CT, Appleton & Lange, 1987.
59. The medical letter on drugs and therapeutics. *Handbook of Antimicrobial Therapy*, rev ed. New Rochelle, NY, The Medical Letter, Inc, 1984.
60. Kunin CM, Efron HY: Audits of antimicrobial usage—guidelines for peer review (Veterans Administration Ad Hoc Interdisciplinary Advisory Committee on Antimicrobial Drug Usage). *JAMA* 237:1001-1008, 1134-1137, 1241-1245, 1366-1367, 1481-1484, 1605-1608, 1723-1725, 1859-1860, 1967-1970, 1977.
61. Joseph WS: *Handbook of Lower Extremity Infections*. New York, Churchill Livingstone, 1990.

62. Abramson C, McCarthy DJ, Rupp MJ: *Infectious Diseases of the Lower Extremities*. Baltimore, Williams & Wilkins, 1991.

63. Gilman AG, Goodman LS, Gilman A: *Goodman and Gilman's The Pharmacological Basis of Therapeutics*, ed 6. New York, MacMillan, 1980, pp 1080-1248.

64. Hunter RL: Transferrin in disease II: defects in the regulation of transferrin saturation with iron contribute to susceptibility to infection. *Am J Clin Pathol* 81:748-753, 1984.

65. Roth D: Tissue injury due to extravasated blood. In Ulin AW, Gollub SS (eds): *Surgical Bleeding*. New York, McGraw-Hill, 1966, pp 71-79.

66. Schwartz S: Complications. In Schwartz S (ed): *Principles of Surgery*, ed 4. New York, McGraw-Hill, 1984, p 458.

67. Krizek TJ, Davis JH: The role of the red cell in subcutaneous infection. *J Trauma* 5:85, 1965.

68. Miles AA: The inflammatory response in relation to local infections. *Surg Clin North Am* 60:93-105, 1980.

69. Simmons RL, Howard RL (eds): *Surgical Infectious Diseases*. New York, Appleton-Century-Crofts, 1982, pp 467, 1024.

70. Miles AA, Pillow J, Khimji PL: The action of iron on local Klebsiella infection of the skin of the guinea-pig and its relation to the decisive period in primary infective lesions. *Br J Exp Pathol* 57:217-242, 1976.

71. Weinberg ED: Iron and susceptibility to infections. *Science* 184:952-956, 1974.

72. Polk HC Jr, Miles AA: Enhancement of bacterial infection by ferric iron: kinetics, mechanisms and surgical significance. *Surgery* 70:71, 1971.

73. Bornside GH, Cohn I Jr: Hemoglobin, a bacterial virulence-enhancing factor in fluids produced in strangulation intestinal obstruction. *Ann Surg* 34:63-67, 1968.

74. Bullen JJ, Rogers HJ: Effect of haemoglobin on experimental infections with *Pasteurella septia* and *Escherichia coli*. *Nature* 217:86, 1968.

75. Miles AA, Khimji PL, Maskell J: The variable response of bacteria to excess ferric iron in host tissues. *J Med Microbiol* 12:17-28, 1979.

76. Weinberg ED: Iron and infection. *Microbiol Rev* 42:45-66, 1978.

77. Alexander JW, Korelitz J, Alexander NS: Prevention of wound infections. A case for closed suction drainage to remove wound fluids deficient in opsonic proteins. *Am J Surg* 132:59-63, 1976.

78. Miller SJ: Surgical wound drainage system using silicone tubing. *J Am Podiatry Assoc* 71:287-296, 1981.

79. Thrombolytics. In *AMA Drug Evaluations*, ed 5. Chicago, American Medical Association, 1983, pp 829-835.

80. Hunt TK: Disorders of repair and their management. In Hunt TK, Dunphy JE (eds): *Fundamentals of Wound Management*. New York, Appleton-Century-Crofts, 1979, pp 133-134.

81. Barza M, Weinstein L: Penetration of antibiotics into fibrin loci in vivo. I. Comparison of ampicillin into fibrin clots, abscesses, and "interstitial fluid." *J Infect Dis* 129:59-65, 1974.

82. Barza M, Samuelson T, Weinstein L: Penetration of antibiotics into fibrin loci in vivo. II. Comparison of nine antibiotics: effect of dose and degree of protein binding. *J Infect Dis* 129:66-72, 1974.

83. Barza M, Brusch J, Bergeron MG, Weinstein L: Penetration of antibiotics into fibrin loci in vivo. III. Intermittent vs continuous infusions, and the effects of probenicid. *J Infect Dis* 129:73-78, 1974.

84. Nelson CL: Preventive antibiotics in orthopedic surgery. In Condon RE, Gorbach SL (eds): *Surgical Infections—Selective Antibiotic Therapy*. Baltimore, Williams & Wilkins, 1981, p 126.

85. Nelson CL, Bergfeld JA, Schwartz J, Kolczun M: Antibiotics in human hematoma and wound fluid. *Clin Orthop* 108:138-144, 1975.

86. Bergeron MG, Nguyen BM, Trottier S, Gauvreau L: Penetration of cefamandole, cephalothin, and desacetylcephalothin into fibrin clots. *Antimicrob Agents Chemother* 12:682-687, 1977.

87. Wilson FC, Worchester NN, Coleman PD, Byrd WE: Antibiotic penetration of experimental bone hematomas. *J Bone Joint Surg* 53A:1622, 1971.

88. Leak LV, Burke JF: Early events of tissue injury and the role of the lymphatic system in early inflammation. In Zweifach BW, Grant L, McClusky RT (eds): *The Inflammatory Process*, ed 2, vol 3. New York, Academic Press, 1974.

89. Bryant WM: Wound healing. *Clinical Symposia, CIBA Pharmaceutical Co* 29:1-36, 1977.

90. Ryan GB, Majno G: *Inflammation*. Kalamazoo, Mich, Upjohn Co, 1977, pp 12-23.

91. Hurley JV: *Acute Inflammation*, ed 2. New York, Churchill Livingstone, 1983, pp 29-57.

92. Arrigoni-Martelli E: *Inflammation and Antiinflammatories*. New York, Spectrum Publications, 1977, pp 111-115.

93. Dyson M: Stimulation of tissue repair by therapeutic ultrasound. In Dineen P (ed): *The Surgical Wound*. Philadelphia, Lea & Febiger, 1981, pp 206-214.

Additional References

Alexander JW: Infection, host resistance, and antimicrobial agents. In American College of Surgeons: *Manual of Preoperative and Postoperative Care*, ed 3. Philadelphia, WB Saunders, 1983, pp 106-136.

Alexander JW, Alexander NS: The influence of route of administration on wound fluid concentration of prophylactic antibiotics. *J Trauma* 16:488-494, 1976.

Alexander JW, Sykes NS, Mitchell MM, Fisher MW: Concentration of selected intravenously administered antibiotics in experimental surgical wounds. *J Trauma* 13:423-432, 1973.

Altemeier WA, Alexander JW: Surgical infections and choice of antibiotics. In Sabiston DC (ed): *Davis-Christopher Textbook of Surgery. The Biological Basis of Surgical Practice*. Philadelphia, WB Saunders Co, 1977, pp 340-362.

Artz C: Infections in surgery. In Artz CP, Hardy JD: *Management of Surgical Complications*, ed 3. Philadelphia, WB Saunders Co, 1975.

Axler DA, Dziarski R: Bacteria causing podiatric infections, and processing of clinical specimens. *J Am Podiatry Assoc* 75:1-12, 1985.

Baruch K, Beatie WH, Clarke WE, Cortese CJ, Dantcho AS, Duggar GE, Edgerton WC, Pappier MJ II, Pascalides JP, Ruch S, Stein N, Wattling WO: Infections. In American College of Foot Surgeons: *Complications in Foot Surgery*. Baltimore, Williams & Wilkins, 1976, pp 94-102.

Burke JF: Infection. In Hunt TK, Dunphy JE (eds): *Fundamentals of Wound Management*. New York, Appleton-Century-Crofts, 1979, pp 170-241.

Cohen A, Yourofsky R: Gangrene: a post-operative complication. *J Foot Surg* 19:202-206, 1980.

Cruse PJE: Incidence of wound infection on the surgical services. *Surg Clin North Am* 55:1269-1275, 1975.

Cruse PJE, Foord R: A five-year prospective study of 23,649 wounds. *Arch Surg* 107:206-210, 1973.

DiGiovanni JE, Smith SD: *Decision Making in Foot Surgery. Selected Papers from Fourth Annual Northlake Seminar*. New York, Stratton Intercontinental Medical Book Corp, 1976, pp 147-186.

Dudrick SJ (ed): *American College of Surgeons, Committee on Pre and Postoperative Care: Manual of Preoperative and Postoperative Care*, ed 3. Philadelphia, WB Saunders, 1983, pp 106-136, 169-181.

Edlich RF, Panek PH, Rodheaver GT, Turnbull VG, Kurtz LD, Edgerton MT: Physical and chemical configuration of sutures in the development of surgical infection. *Ann Surg* 177:679-688, 1973.

Elek SD: Experimental staphylococcal infections in the skin of man. *NY Acad Sci* 65:85, 1956.

Estersohn HS, Fuerstman R: The local use of antibiotics to prevent wound infection. *J Am Podiatry Assoc* 69:127-130, 1979.

Fitzgerald RH Jr: Current concepts in the prevention and management of the infected total joint arthroplasty. In Hughes SPF, Fitzgerald RH Jr (eds): *Musculoskeletal Infections: Recognition, Prevention and Management*, vol 3. New York, Advanced Therapeutics Communications, 1983.

Fitzgerald RH, Thompson RL: Current concepts review. Cephalosporin antibiotics in the prevention and treatment of musculoskeletal sepsis. *J Bone Joint Surg* 65A:1201-1205, 1983.

Gardner P: Reasons for "antibiotic failure." *Hosp Pract* 11:41-45, 1976.

Gerbert J, Spector EE, Clark JR, Sharpe DA: A case of deep wound infection in a postoperative site following a Silastic implant procedure of the first metatarsophalangeal joint. *J Am Podiatry Assoc* 64:804-817, 1974.

Green R: Pharmacology. In Marcus SA, Block BH (eds): *American College of Foot Surgeons—Complications in Foot Surgery: Prevention and Management*, ed 2. Baltimore, Williams & Wilkins, 1984, pp 78-87.

Hitchcock CR, Demello FJ, Haglin JJ: Gangrene infection. *Surg Clin North Am* 55:1403-1410, 1975.

Howe CW: Experimental studies on determinants of wound infection. *Surg Gynecol Obstet* 123:507-514, 1966.

Jawetz E: Four steps to correct antimicrobial drug choice. *Consultant* 17:42-48, 1977.

Krizek TJ, Robson MC: Evolution of quantitative bacteriology in wound management. *Am J Surg* 130:579-584, 1975.

Liu PV: Biology of *Pseudomonas aeruginosa. Hosp Pract* 11:139-147, 1976.

Lovell DL: Skin bacteria: their location with reference to skin sterilization. *Surg Gynecol Obstet* 80:174, 1945.

Maki DG: The epidemiology of surgical wound infection—guidelines for prevention. *J Surg Pract* 6:10-23, 1977.

Maki DG: The epidemiology of surgical wound infection—guidelines for prevention. In Condon RE, Gorbach SL (eds): *Surgical Infections. Selective Antibiotic Therapy.* Baltimore, Williams & Wilkins, 1980, pp 166-176.

Makris AT, Schwartz AR: The cephalosporins. *Am Fam Pract* 16:122, 1977.

Marks G, Mervine TB: Clinical experience with doxycycline in the treatment of surgical soft tissue infections. *Curr Ther Res* 16:424-430, 1974.

Mathieu A, Burke JF (eds): *Infection and the Perioperative Period.* New York, Grune & Stratton, 1982.

Meakins JL: Host defense mechanisms, wound healing, and infection. In Hunt TK, Dunphy JE (eds): *Fundamentals of Wound Management.* New York, Appleton-Century-Crofts, 1979, pp 242-285.

Miles AA, Miles EM, Burke J: The value and duration of defense reactions of the skin to the primary lodgement of bacteria. *Br J Exp Pathol* 38:79-86, 1957.

Miller JE (ed): Section I. Bone infections (symposium). *Clin Orthop* 96:1-287, 1973.

Miller SJ: Body temperature following podiatric surgery. *J Am Podiatry Assoc* 74:477-481, 1984.

Morris PJ, Barnes BA, Burke JF: The nature of the "irreducible minimum" rate of incisional sepsis. *Arch Surg* 92:367, 1966.

Mullens D: Bacterial infections in podiatry. I. *Arch Podiatr Med Foot Surg* 2:255-266, 1975.

Munster AM: Infections. In Hill GT (ed): *Outpatient Surgery,* ed 2. Philadelphia, WB Saunders, 1980, pp 134-159.

National Academy of Science–National Research Council: Postoperative wound infections: the influence of ultraviolet irradiation of the operating room and of various other factors. *Am Surg* 160:1, 1964.

Nelson JP: Musculoskeletal infection. *Surg Clin North Am* 60:213-222, 1980.

Nichols RL, Smith JW: Gas in the wound: what does it mean? *Surg Clin North Am* 55:1289-1296, 1975.

Pancoast SJ, Neu HC: Antibiotic levels in human bone and synovial fluid. Used in the evaluation of antimicrobial therapy of joint and skeletal infections. *Orthop Rev* 9:49-61, 1980.

Pankey GA, Cortez LM: Treatments of choice for bacterial infections of the skin. *Med Times* 105:92-98, 1977.

Pappas AM, Filler RM, Eraklis AJ, Bernhard WF: Clostridial infections (gas and gangrene). *Clin Orthop* 76:177-187, 1971.

Peacock EE: *Wound Repair,* ed 3. Philadelphia, WB Saunders, 1984, pp 1-7.

Polk HC Jr, Lopez-Mayor JF: Postoperative wound infection: a prospective study of determinant factors and prevention. *Surgery* 66:97, 1969.

Polk HC Jr, Miles AA: The decisive period in the primary infection of muscle by *Escherichia coli. Br J Exp Pathol* 54:99, 1973.

Ritter MA, Eitzen H, French MLV, Hart JB: The operating room environment as affected by people and the surgical face mask. *Clin Orthop* 111:147-150, 1975.

Ritter MA, French MLV, Eitzen HE: Bacterial contamination of the surgical knife. *Clin Orthop* 108:158-160, 1975.

Ryan GB: Inflammation and the localization of infection. *Surg Clin North Am* 56:831-846, 1976.

Schumacher GE: Pharmacokinetic and microbiologic evaluation of antibiotic dose regimens. *Clin Pharm* 1:66-75, 1982.

Schurman DJ, Burton DS, Kajiyama G, Moser K, Nagel DA: Sodium cephapirin disposition and distribution into human bone. *Curr Ther Res* 20:194-203, 1976.

Schurman DJ, Hirshman HP, Nagel DH: Antimicrobial penetration of synovial fluid in infected and normal knee joints. *Clin Orthop* 136:304-310, 1978.

Spector WG, Willoughby DA: *The Pharmacology of Inflammation.* New York, Grune & Stratton, 1968.

Tetzloff TR, McCracken GH Jr, Nelson JD: Oral antibiotic therapy for skeletal infections of children. *J Pediatr* 92:485, 1978.

Venge P, Lindbom A (eds): *The Inflammatory Process. An Introduction to the Study of Cellular and Humoral Mechanisms.* Stockholm, Almgvist and Wiksell International, 1981.

Wagner KF, Counts JW: The penicillins and cephalosporins—choosing among the newer agents. *Postgrad Med* 64:109-116, 1978.

Walter CW: Thirty-sixth Annual Charles V. Chapin Oration: The physician's role in cross infection. *RI Med J* 60:534-548, 1977.

Weinberg ED: Iron and susceptibility to infections. *Science* 184:954-956, 1974.

Zweifach BW, Grant L, McCluskey RT: *The Inflammatory Process,* ed 2, vols I-III. New York, Academic Press, 1974.

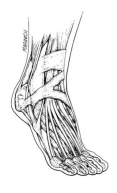

CHAPTER **70**

Osteomyelitis

David Edward Marcinko, D.P.M.

Allen Mark Jacobs, D.P.M., and Lawrence M. Oloff, D.P.M.*

The basic principles of management of contaminated bone have remained the same for more than 50 years, in spite of an explosion in medical technology. Early diagnosis remains vital to successful treatment and prevention of the acute process from becoming established as chronic osteomyelitis. The clinician must be able to identify and carefully monitor patients in whom a higher incidence of osteomyelitis is statistically known to occur. In addition, familiarity with such entities as delayed or late osteomyelitis after implant arthroplasty allows for a high index of suspicion and early diagnosis in a clinical situation that could easily be attributed to noninfectious disease.

Newer diagnostic modalities, such as computerized tomography (CT), magnetic resonance imaging (MRI), positron emission transmission (PET), and differential scintigraphy, are useful in the early diagnosis of osteomyelitis and may contribute valuable information in cases with nonspecific symptoms. Despite such advanced presumptive diagnostic modalities, the demonstration of organisms cultured from appropriately selected and retrieved bone remains the foundation of diagnosis. The treatment of osteomyelitis may be initiated in high-risk patients with minimal nonpathognomonic findings in whom antimicrobial prophylaxis is in reality the treatment of impending infection.

When osteomyelitis is established, incision, drainage, and the removal of all sequestered or sinister material is the sine qua non of surgical therapy. When osteosynthesis or polymeric or ceramic implanted materials are present, considerable judgment is required with regard to how best to resolve the infection without sacrificing the device.

Antibiotic selection remains subject to a variety of factors that must be seriously considered if one is to select the most appropriate agents. Selection of the best agent is far from exacting. The selected parenteral antibiotic weighs as heavily in the prognosis of many cases as does appropriate surgical therapy.

The long-term management of patients with osteomyelitis involves judgments that must be made in the face of sometimes conflicting clinical or empirical data. Clinical experience will ultimately determine the time of wound closure, placement and use of drains or irrigation systems, termination or continuation of antibiotic therapy, and other related decisions. Those who acquire such experience and

familiarize themselves with applicable medical literature are best able to make the appropriate decisions.

TERMINOLOGY AND DEFINITIONS

The term *osteomyelitis* appears to have been introduced by Nelaton (1) in 1844 to describe an infection of bone and marrow. Although osteomyelitis is primarily an infectious process of bacterial etiology, occasional cases occur as the result of fungal, viral, or parasitic infection (2-4). Suppuration of bone cortex without marrow extension is properly referred to as "suppurative" or "infectious" osteitis (5). Contamination of periosteum alone is "infectious" or "suppurative periostitis."

The differentiation of osteomyelitis, suppurative osteitis, and infectious periostitis is ordinarily difficult on a clinical and radiographic basis. In the presence of established infection, the clinical and radiographic signs and symptoms of osteomyelitis, infective osteitis, and periostitis may be strikingly similar. Bacterial and pustular accumulation below the periosteum, for example, may result not only in periosteal elevation or reaction that is confirmed by radiographic or radionuclide evaluation but also in an interruption of blood supply to the outer third of the bone cortex because of a loss of periosteal circulation. Confusion results because radiographic and radionuclide changes may occur in the absence of direct bone contamination. In addition, periosteal reaction or osteitis may occur in response to a variety of noninfectious disorders. In the presence of established soft tissue infection or ulceration, inflammatory radiographic or bone scanning changes may be indistinguishable from suppurative bone disease, despite the absence of direct bone or periosteal contamination.

A variety of terms have been used to classify the nature of bone infection and include acute, subacute, chronic, and residual osteomyelitis (6). The differentiation of osteomyelitis on the basis of temporal terminology may be difficult and does not imply cause or a specific treatment regimen. For example, acute symptoms in a previously symptom-free patient may be associated with radiographic or other signs consistent with chronic osteomyelitis, but recurrent episodes clinically consistent with acute disease may also occur (7, 8). As the result of such clinical and radiographic overlap in signs and symptoms, it has been suggested that the terms *initial* and *recurrent* be used to describe osteomyelitis (9). Acute osteomyelitic signs and symptoms may occur in a

**Appreciation is expressed to Allen Mark Jacobs, D.P.M., and Lawrence M. Oloff, D.P.M., who wrote this chapter in the first edition.*

previously symptom-free patient years after surgery with internal fixation or implantation of prosthetic devices. At the time of initial evaluation for acute symptoms, radiographic signs may be consistent with apparent chronicity of the infectious disease.

Recently an attempt has been made to classify and supersede the traditional classification concepts of osteomyelitis. For example, Cierny and associates (10), in 1980, developed a potential clinical staging system in adults using both an anatomic category (stage I, medullary; stage II, superficial; stage III, localized; and stage IV, diffuse) and a physiologic category (A-host, good systemic defense and local vascularity; B-host, systemic and local compromise; C-host, noncandidate for surgery with treatment more problematic than the disease process). With their method, 12 (4 × 3) different stages of osteomyelitis may be described in a pragmatic clinical scheme.

Finally, Buckholz (11), in 1987, developed his classification based on the definitions of osteomyelitis and osteitis. It included seven types of bone infection: (a) wound-induced, (b) mechanogenic infection, (c) physeal osteomyelitis, (d) ischemic limb disease, (e) a combination of types a to d, (f) septic arthritis with osteitis, and (g) chronic osteomyelitis with osteitis. Unfortunately, the classification jargon is not universally accepted and may result in confusion and misunderstanding (11). Thus there are still no precise classification models for the osteomyelitic process.

BACTERIAL RECOVERY AND ISOLATION

The conclusive bacteriological diagnosis of osteomyelitis rests on the obligatory isolation of the pathogen from bone or blood cultures (12). The specificity inherent in limited open biopsy of suspicious osseous tissue must be weighed against the risk of potential contamination of uninvolved tissues. In addition, the dissection required may result in nonhealing surgical wounds in the presence of compromised peripheral vascular perfusion or rheumatic inflammatory disorders.

Mackowiak and associates (13) have demonstrated that cultures obtained from draining sinus tracts and soft tissue specimens proximal to osteomyelitic bone frequently fail to demonstrate the organism responsible for contamination. In their study of 183 such cultures taken from 35 patients, 102 gave results that did not coincide with operative cultures, although results of repeated sinus cultures demonstrated a better correlation. Thus cultures obtained from neurotrophic ulcers or disrupted surgical wounds cannot be relied on to isolate and identify the cause of underlying infection. However, in retrospective studies on the causes of bone infections, operative cultures are often not available and a presumptive diagnosis of *Staphylococcus aureus*, for example, can be made if the organism is isolated from its associated sinus tract. Antibiotic therapy, initiated on the basis of such nonosseous cultures, may result in apparent resolution or diminution of soft tissue infection, although the osteomyelitic process of bone destruction continues.

Blood cultures represent a means of indirectly identifying the microorganisms responsible for osteomyelitis. Morrey and Peterson (14), Nade (15), and others demonstrated recovery of osteomyelitis-inducing bacteria in 50% of untreated acute cases of hematogenous osteomyelitis. This compared to microorganism recovery with limited bone biopsy or bone aspiration in 60% to 90% of cases (8). In the presence of spiking fever or other evidence of bacteremia, such as the sudden appearance of tachypnea and hypotension in a postoperative patient, blood culture may substantiate the hematogenous bacterial origin of the osteomyelitis. The cause of such contaminating organisms include colonized intravenous devices, urinary tract infections, and pulmonary infectious disease (16). A negative blood culture cannot prove that osteomyelitis is absent, and consideration should be given to limited open biopsy or aspiration when clinical and radiographic evaluation suggests a failure of therapy. Blood cultures may be useful in reflecting the potential source of bone pathogens from such origins as urinary tract or upper respiratory tract infections (17). Fitzgerald and associates (18) noted that when a sinus tract and drainage were present after implant arthroplasty, polymicrobic or pure gram-negative infections were often observed. This may be seen in cases of deep infection or osteomyelitis after surgery or in the presence of a healed surgical wound. In bone infection, with either a healed or a draining surgical wound, repeat cultures must be evaluated for changing bacterial flora as well as fluctuating antibiotic sensitivity patterns. Cultures should be obtained on removal of wound-packing materials, drains, or other apparatus, because superinfection from colonized bacteria may occur in as many as 30% of those cases in which such treatment material is used in the treatment of osteomyelitis (19).

In the presence of closed wounds or where open biopsy is not feasible, aspiration may be performed in an attempt to identify the organism(s) responsible for osteomyelitis or deep abscess (20). The risk of inadvertent bacterial seeding from infected soft tissue must be considered, and the surgical approach to questionable areas of bone should be through noninflamed and noninfected soft tissues. If performed percutaneously, a Jamshidi (Perfectum Corp., Hyde Park, NY) 11-gauge, 6-inch, self-contained bone needle biopsy kit is ideal for the task; it consists of an outer cannula and handle with an inner stylet for tissue penetration. The needle itself should be directed accurately toward the suspicious area under fluoroscopic guidance, as described by McLaughlin and Whitehill (21). In the absence of fluoroscopic equipment, needle position may be confirmed by standard radiographic techniques. Use of an imaging technique decreases the likelihood of aspiration or biopsy from uninvolved areas and aids in the prevention of damage to implanted polymers or fixation devices. If aspirated material cannot be obtained for Gram's stain or culture evaluation and radiographs confirm appropriate needle placement, the wound may be flushed with nonbacteriostatic saline solution and the wash aspirated for microbial analysis (8).

In summary, current literature argues in favor of bone biopsy, deep aspiration, or bone washing to establish the diagnosis of osteomyelitis. Successful management is ultimately the result of treatment directed at the invading pathogen(s) (20) (Table 70.1).

INFECTING ORGANISMS

Gram-positive cocci continue to represent the most common bacteria associated with postoperative and nonpostoperative osteomyelitis (6). *Staphylococcus aureus, Staphylococcus epidermidis,* and streptococci account for up to 73% of the osteomyelitis following musculoskeletal surgery (22). A higher incidence of mixed gram-positive and gram-negative or pure gram-negative infections is encountered in postoperative infections when prophylactic antibiotics have been used for the more commonly encountered gram-positive organisms (18, 23). When osteomyelitis or other infection occurs in a patient who received prophylactic antibiotics, it should be assumed that the infecting organism is not susceptible to the administered antibiotic (23).

S. epidermidis has been reported with increasing frequency as the causative organism of infection after implant arthroplasty. The onset of clinical *S. epidermidis* osteomyelitis may be delayed for months or even years. The organism can no longer be regarded as only a common skin contaminant (24, 25).

The organism most likely responsible for osteomyelitis is dependent on a variety of circumstances. Kalish and Mahan (26) demonstrated that *Pseudomonas aeruginosa* is a common cause of osteomyelitis after traumatic wounds, particularly in plantar puncture wounds (Fig. 70.1). Osteomyelitis as-

Table 70.1.
Flow Chart Protocol in Suspected Osteomyelitis

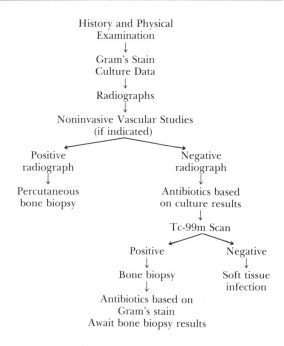

From Caprioli R, Testa J, Cournoyer RW, Esposito FJ: Prompt diagnosis of suspected osteomyelitis by utilizing percutaneous bone culture. *J Foot Surg* 25:263, 1986.

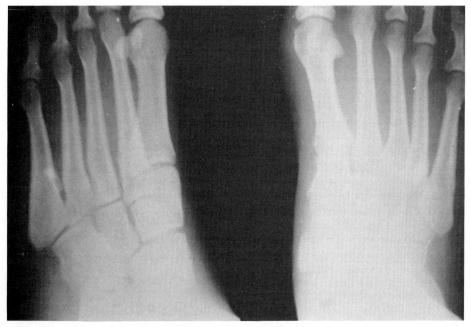

Figure 70.1. Radiographs of patient who had a puncture wound on plantar aspect of the left foot as a result of stepping on piece of glass. The left radiograph depicts a glass foreign body located between the proximal diaphyseal areas near the base of the fourth and fifth metatarsals. There should be a high index of suspicion for *Pseudomonas osteomyelitis* after puncture wounds of the foot, thus enabling earlier definitive treatment. Good results are reported with surgical debridement and drainage, curettage where indicated, tetanus prophylaxis, and proper antibiotic treatment.

sociated with diabetes mellitus and vascular compromise frequently involves gram-negative or mixed gram-positive and gram-negative infections (27). In addition, anaerobic bacteria occur with greater frequency in such patients (28, 29). The isolation of fastidious anaerobic bacteria such as *Bacteroides fragilis*, which may be found in up to 30% of all diabetic foot infections, is dependent on a careful culturing technique and efficient transport of specimens to the laboratory (30). Adeyokunna and Hendrickse (31) demonstrated a higher incidence of osteomyelitis caused by *Salmonella* species in patients with sickle cell anemia and related hemoglobinopathies. *Pseudomonas* and other gram-negative organisms, in either initial or recurrent osteomyelitis, are seen with greater frequency in drug addicts (9). Postoperative osteomyelitis has been reported with such unusual organisms as *Mycobacterium* (in renal transplant patients) (32), *Pasteurella multocida* (following trochanteric hip fracture with implant arthroplasty), *Salmonella typhi*, *Candida*, *Aspergillus*, *Fusarium*, and *Rhizopus* (33-35).

Hematogenous osteomyelitis remains a disease that is encountered primarily in children, although more cases of hematogenous osteomyelitis are being reported in older populations (6). A lack of phagocytic lining cells in the afferent metaphyseal loops of long bones, as well as the relatively inactive phagocytic lining cells in efferent metaphyseal loops, has been implicated in the development of hematogenous osteomyelitis (36-39). This peculiar osseous circulation in children is thought to play a major role in the development of hematogenous osteomyelitis and has been extensively described (10, 33, 36, 37). In any event, Jergeson (36) demonstrated that hematogenous osteomyelitis is usually caused by a single infecting organism that may be detected through the use of blood cultures. *S. aureus* remains the most commonly encountered cause in as many as 74% of all cases (15). In the presence of urinary tract infections, hematogenous osteomyelitis may be the result of streptococci or gram-negative organisms that frequently cause such urinary tract infections (9, 40). CT scanning and MRI studies may detect the earliest changes of hematogenous osteomyelitis before scintigraphy, which has a high false-negative rate (41).

In summary, *Staphylococcus* remains the most common cause of osteomyelitis. The colonization of soft tissues with more aggressive organisms, such as *Pseudomonas*, may belie the underlying organism responsible for bone infection. Although any microorganism may cause osteomyelitis, the more unusual organisms tend to be found in certain patient subsets (i.e., diabetic, immunocompromised, or vascularly deficient patients) or under special circumstances (i.e., puncture wounds, animal, fecal, or farmland contamination). These statistical patterns are by no means absolute, and every case must be evaluated for ultimate identification of the responsible organism.

PATIENT RISK FACTORS AND PATTERNS

It is well known that children and the elderly are at risk of hematogenous osteomyelitis (6, 16). Contiguous osteomy-

elitis, spreading from an adjacent soft tissue infection, is not unusual after surgery, ulceration, or puncture wounds of the foot (42, 43). In the presence of ischemic or neurotrophic ulceration, or after deep wounds, patients must be carefully monitored by serial, clinical, and radiographic examinations for the occurrence of osteomyelitis (44).

A variety of circumstances may place patients at higher risk of both hematogenous and contiguous osteomyelitis. Pinckney and associates (45) demonstrated that crush injuries to the toenail plate of children is frequently associated with osteomyelitis of the distal phalanx, so that careful bone monitoring appears judicious. In a retrospective study, Soave and Jacobs (personal communication) demonstrated a 20.8% infection rate in patients who underwent concurrent toenail and bone surgery, compared with an overall infection rate of 2.3% for all foot surgery at the same institution. Thus, when surgical procedures on both nail and bone are performed, the increased chance of infection mandates careful monitoring of such patients (Fig 70.2).

Ross and Ewald (46) demonstrated that patients with rheumatoid arthritis are at higher risk of postoperative osteomyelitis than other population subsets. Patients who are taking systemic corticosteroids or antimetabolites for dermatological, rheumatic, or neoplastic disease are likewise at similar risk (18, 47). Local depletion of immune factors such as complement, fibrosis, vasculitis, and the effects of immunosuppressive drugs (AZT) have also been implicated in higher infection rates.

The use of implanted materials has created another relative set of risk factors. Polymethylmethacrylate, for example, has been shown to decrease leukocyte migration to the site of infection as well as decrease the phagocytic and killing power of polymorphonuclear leukocytes (48). As a

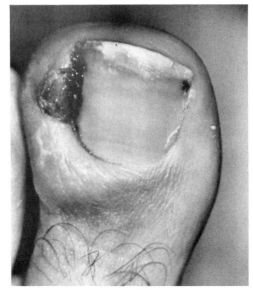

Figure 70.2. Acute osteomyelitis after toenail surgery is a rare occurrence. Partial nail avulsion with CO_2 laser matrixectomy of lateral hallucal border in which the phalanx became infected.

result, the failure to recognize osteomyelitis in the presence of luting agents or the inappropriate management of such cases may result in a protracted and therapeutically resistant bone infection.

It has been suggested that the presence of implanted materials at the site of osteomyelitis is markedly detrimental to the delivery of antibiotics, as well as interfering with normal immune defense mechanisms (49) (Fig. 70.3). In addition, the effects of bacteria and their toxins on the implanted metals or polymers must be considered. For example, infection and decreased tissue pH, along with the effects of released enzymes, are known to accelerate biocorrosion (50). Impairment of osseous vascular profusion, as well as the implants action as a nidus for the sequestration of bacteria, must also be considered (25). Reoperation through prior incisions is likewise associated with an increased risk of infection, especially when associated with questionable soft tissue changes (6).

The risk of infection in nonelective surgery is clearly higher than in elective surgery. A common example is that of bone resection under nonhealing ulcerations in patients with diminished vascular profusion. The operative management of fractures and open trauma is associated with a 13.9% infection rate, as compared with the 1% postoperative infection rate in elective musculoskeletal surgery (51). Fitzgerald and associates (18) were able to isolate bacteria from the operative site in 62% of the patients treated for open fractures. Osteomyelitis complicating open fracture management is not unusual and must be considered in the post-operative management of patients undergoing open fracture reduction.

Accordingly, the management of imminent osteomyelitis transcends the differentiation of prophylaxis and treatment. Effective early treatment requires recognition of patients at higher statistical risk, as well as an understanding of the most likely causative organisms. In elective foot surgery, prior surgery, lengthy or traumatic surgery, hematoma, inflammatory arthritis, nutritional or immune compromise, prosthetic devices, and the presence of peripheral vascular disease are all clearly predisposing factors to osteomyelitis.

In the presence of open injury or wound contamination, impending osteomyelitis is frequently established. Similarly, contiguous osteomyelitis may develop in the presence of soft tissue infections, wound ulcerations, or punctures or as a complication of infection after surgery.

Hematogenous osteomyelitis at the previously asymptomatic site of surgery, particularly when implanted materials have been used, has been reported with increasing frequency (40, 52). In such cases, consideration must be given to distant sites where hematogenous spread may predispose the implant site to infection months or even years after fixation or prosthetic device implantation (53).

CLINICAL SIGNS AND SYMPTOMS OF OSTEOMYELITIS

Hematogenous osteomyelitis not related to surgery is usually associated with the abrupt onset of increasing pain and tenderness as well as overt signs of inflammatory disease

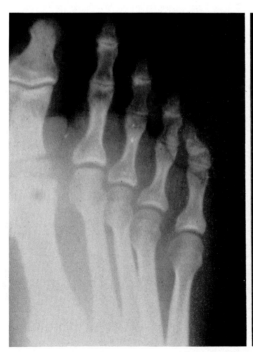
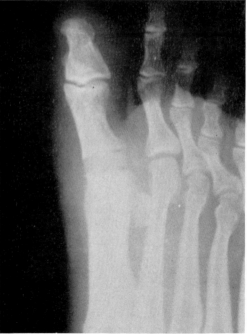

Figure 70.3. An important consideration with infected implant sites is whether the implant itself acts as a barrier to the healing process. Because a significant portion of the endosteal blood supply has been disrupted by intramedullary reaming for implant stems, this may leave the patient with somewhat impaired osseous vascular perfusion.

(54). Usually a disorder of children, the acute onset is associated with limping, guarding, fever, elevated acute phase reactants (ESR, C-reactive protein), and polymorphonuclear leukocytosis (10, 27). Evidence of coexisting infection at a site removed from the foot may be obtained through history, physical examination, and appropriate diagnostic studies. For example, the presence of urinary tract, dental, or pulmonary infection may indicate not only the source of the invading microorganism but also the likely pathogen. In the elderly, hematogenous osteomyelitis may be associated with the absence of local inflammatory signs or systemic manifestations, and the presentation may be surprisingly subtle (55). This is particularly true in patients with coexisting peripheral vascular disease. In the presence of peripheral neuropathy, pain and tenderness may be minimal or absent.

Hematogenous osteomyelitis may be responsible for a large percentage of bone infections at the site of implanted materials (56). For example, in one study hematogenous seeding occurred in 30% of postoperative infections after total joint arthroplasty of the hip and the knee. Infections that occur 24 months after surgery are believed to be of hematogenous origin (25). Hematogenous osteomyelitis may occur at the site of a previously asymptomatic prosthesis months or years after apparently successful surgery and uneventful recovery. In such cases increasing discomfort or local inflammatory findings may be difficult to differentiate from loosening of a prosthesis or fixation device (Fig. 70.4). Loading pain (poststatic dyskinesia) is frequently present with a loosened device. However, discomfort that is relieved after several minutes of weight bearing does not exclude a diagnosis of osteomyelitis (57).

An increasing volume of literature now suggests that areas in which fixation devices or prostheses have been used are particularly susceptible to delayed or late infection of hematogenous origin (16, 52, 53). This appears to be especially applicable when polymethylmethacrylate has been used as a fixation or luting device. Ultraclean surgical techniques, laminar airflow systems, and prophylactic antibiotics have been shown by Charnley (58) to reduce the incidence of not only acute postoperative osteomyelitis but also delayed and late infections. Despite the suggestion of original contamination inherent in such studies, many others indicate that hematogenous osteomyelitis is a distinct entity that results in delayed or late infection when polymethylmethacrylate has been used (59). For this reason, prophylactic antibiotics should be used when urinary tract, respiratory tract, or dental procedures are performed so as to reduce transient bacteremia and hematogenous contamination (60). Data that conflict with this concept have been reported recently, and no current guidelines exist (59).

Contiguous osteomyelitis of the foot is most often encountered in patients with previous lacerations, puncture wounds, or open trauma or after elective or nonelective surgical procedures (27, 61) (Fig. 70.5). Sinus tract formation and drainage are often present. In such cases, soft tissue infection is managed by careful evaluation of the underlying bone for the earliest indication of contamination. The expanded use of implant arthroplasty has also created an

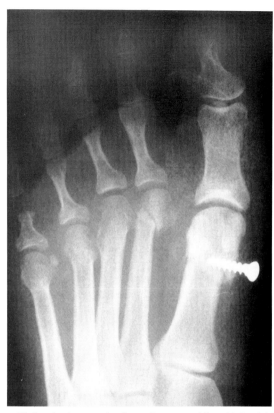

Figure 70.4. An increase in discomfort, especially with local inflammatory findings, may be difficult to differentiate from loosening of fixation device. Pain on initial weight bearing after a period of rest (poststatic dyskinesia) is often consistent with a loosened device; however, this does not exclude osteomyelitis. Sepsis alone may cause a fixation device or prosthesis to loosen.

equally expanded staging of postoperative osteomyelitis, which can be classified as acute, delayed, or late (10, 25). Acute postoperative osteomyelitis occurs within 1 month of implant arthroplasty and usually is accompanied by classic signs and symptoms of wound disruption, drainage, pain, inflammation, and systemic sequelae (62) (Fig. 70.6). Osteomyelitis under such circumstances may be the result of direct contamination at the time of surgery, hematogenous contamination from a remote site, or contiguous spread from an infected hematoma, a stitch abscess, or cellulitis (6). In such cases, the presence of soft tissue infection is usually recognized with ease and the patient is monitored appropriately for the earliest signs of osteomyelitis. Acute postoperative osteomyelitis, particularly in association with implant arthroplasty, occurs in only 40% of such infections, and in these cases the typical signs and symptoms are easily recognized (63).

In the majority of deep infections and osteomyelitis occurring after implant surgery, the infectious process is classified as delayed or late (52, 64). Delayed implant wound infection occurs between 1 month and 2 years after surgery, whereas late infection occurs 2 years or more after surgery

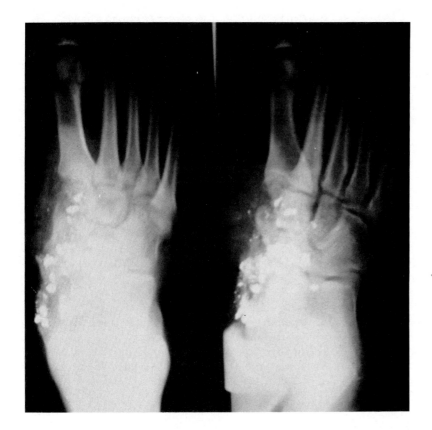

Figure 70.5. Contiguous osteomyelitis of foot may be seen with ulcerations, puncture or gunshot wounds, or open trauma and after both elective and nonelective surgical procedures. Radiographs demonstrate numerous scattered particles of lead shot as a result of a gunshot wound.

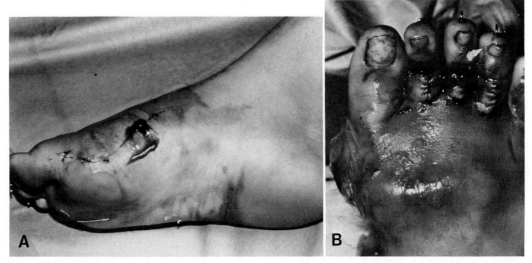

Figure 70.6. **A.** This infection occurred 1 week after forefoot reconstruction. A Scarf osteotomy was performed from a medial approach along with digital stabilization of all toes. **B.** The same foot 2 weeks after surgery. The classic signs and symptoms of wound disruption, pain, edema, drainage, heat, redness, and odor were present. Note extensive undermining of soft tissue planes about the first metatarsophalangeal joint. (Courtesy Dr. B. Holcomb, Atlanta, Ga.)

(53). As noted earlier, delayed or late osteomyelitis after surgery may be of hematogenous origin. Brause (62) demonstrated that 40% of the infections that arise at the bone-cement interface are of hematogenous origin. The seeding of bacteria at the site of previous surgery may be the result of persistent vascular response to surgical monomer or the mechanical effects of implants on bone. Some implanted materials create a chronic local subclinical inflammatory response that depletes local, humoral, and cellular defenses to otherwise controllable bacteria (48, 49). Radiolucency at the cement-bone interface may be caused by infection, loosening, reaction to monomer, or normal fibrous tissue response (65).

It has been suggested that a delayed or late infection may be caused by microorganisms that were introduced into the wound at the time of the original surgery (66). Why bacteria fail to initiate wound infection for 2 years or longer has been subject to speculation. Low organism virulence, or the decreased toxicity of their products, has been suggested (67). Some have suggested that, with time, local wound conditions may deteriorate so that optimal conditions eventually evolve for the growth of previously introduced but sessile bacteria (68). Examples include implant loosening, biocorrosion, or the deposition of polymer material in adjacent soft tissues. Regardless of the exact mechanism, the majority of infections that follow prosthetic implantation are delayed or late in presentation (69). The clinical similarities of osteomyelitis and corrosive metallic disease may include drainage and local inflammatory signs (50) (Fig. 70.7). Similarly, the loosening of an implant or a fixation device may be the result of osteomyelitis, but osteomyelitis may also be encouraged by loosening and local tissue damage. Delayed or late osteomyelitis may be difficult to differentiate from inflammatory arthritis, bursitis, rheumatoid nodules, tophaceous drainage or soft tissue inflammation secondary to the physical effects of the implanted material (detritic synovitis) (70, 71).

Acute osteomyelitis after surgery is usually associated with *Staphylococcus aureus* or other gram-positive cocci, although concurrent or pre-existing conditions alter the probability of discovering various pathogens (18). Late postoperative osteomyelitis, or osteomyelitis associated with a draining sinus tract, is more frequently associated with gram-negative or polymicrobic etiological agents (27).

DIAGNOSTIC RADIOGRAPHIC CONSIDERATIONS

The classic flat plate radiographic manifestations of osteomyelitis are well known and include soft tissue swelling, resorptive bone changes, periosteal reaction, bone destruction, and sequestra, involucrum, and cloaca formation (6). Normally the destructive process does not cross the epiphyseal line into the epiphysis, so that joint involvement is most often the result of soft tissue and capsular perforation. In some clinical settings, such as postoperative osteomyelitis associated with ulceration in the diabetic foot, both joint and diaphyseal and metaphyseal destruction may occur concomitantly (58). Unfortunately, radiographic manifestations of osteomyelitis follow the actual destruction of bone by days or weeks (11, 72). As a result, reliance on radiographs for the definitive evaluation of a patient in whom osteomyelitis is suspected may delay therapy while the infectious process continues to destroy osseous tissue. Similarly, a delay in the initiation of therapy until definitive radiographic findings are noted on sequentially comparative films may result in the establishment of major destruction before the initiation of appropriate medical and surgical therapy. Although the role of standard radiographic evaluation and sequential radiographic studies is significant, the diagnosis of osteomyelitis is established by a high index of suspicion and by indirect clinical evidence, bone biopsy, or aspiration (6).

Periosteal reaction may be seen in a variety of conditions, including soft tissue infection, in the absence of actual bone disease (73). Resorptive or frankly destructive changes may be noted in such disorders as rheumatoid arthritis or gout, whereas marked changes of the osteomyelitic type have been reported with increasing frequency in association with polymer implants, particularly those of the first metatarsophalangeal joint. Sclerosis, osteopenia, or fragmentation may

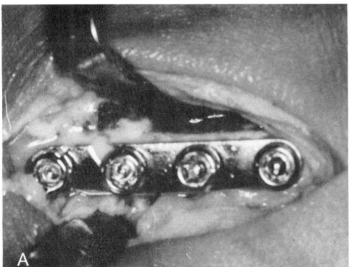

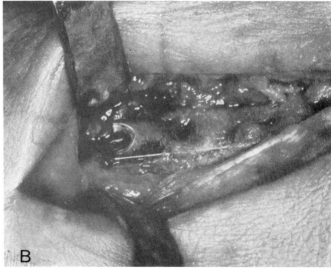

Figure 70.7. Clinical similarities of osteomyelitis and biocorrosion of metallic implants are remarkable and may include drainage along with local inflammatory signs. **A.** Representative of typical metallic implant. **B.** The same bone plate on removal several months later. Fracture of the device secondary to corrosion necessitated its removal. Note not only marked discoloration seen on the plate and bone, but the abnormal appearance of adjacent soft tissues as well. An attempt to culture microorganisms from this site was unsuccessful.

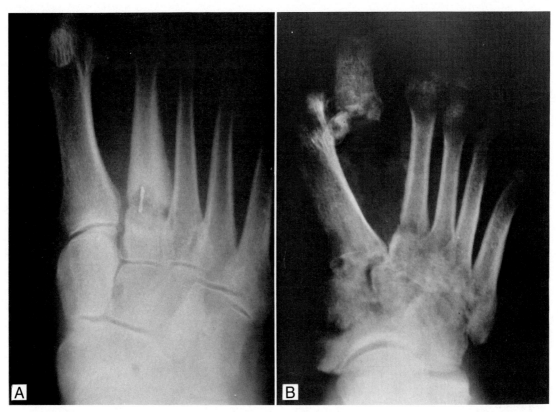

Figure 70.8. **A.** Radiograph reveals nonunion of osteotomy performed 7 months previously. A patient may progress to nonunion because of a smoldering low-grade infection that is not appreciated clinically. In this case, however, serial radiographs remained unchanged with regard to additional bone resorption, and gallium scans were negative. **B.** Typical radiographic presentation of a diabetic foot with severe neuropathy. The clinician must differentiate between osteoarthropathy, osteomyelitis, or a combination of both.

occur with implant failure, implant loosening, or metallic corrosion. Similarly, atrophic nonunion, hypertrophic nonunion, and osteomyelitis may be difficult to differentiate by radiographic evaluation early in the course of disease (74) (Fig. 70.8).

In the diabetic patient with an ulceration or deep infection, the changes visualized on radiographic evaluation may be associated with diabetic osteolysis, spontaneous fracture, reactive periostitis, or neurotrophic joint disease (72, 75). Thus, although seemingly logical to assume, it must be recalled that osseous change in the presence of soft tissue infection or ulceration represents presumptive evidence of osteomyelitis and is treated at a time when there is a paucity or absence of radiographic changes. Standard radiographs do not reveal the presence of the earliest disease since they lag behind the actual destructive process, and the full extent of bone involvement may be difficult to appreciate (Fig. 70.9). For this reason, a variety of other radiographic techniques may be applied to establish the presence and extent of early osteomyelitis although any evaluation is only as valuable as the clinical context in which it is placed. Even with the use of sophisticated diagnostic modalities, the final decision regarding treatment rests with a high index of suspicion.

Radionuclide Scintigraphy

Radionuclide bone imaging with sequential scintigraphy has had increasing success in the presumptive diagnosis of bone and soft tissue infections. Generally, a radiopharmaceutical agent is slowly injected intravenously and localizes in target tissues. A scintillation probe (detector) is then positioned over the target, and emitted gamma photons are converted into visible light and counted. A photomultiplier tube converts the light into an electronic pulse, and information is transferred to an electronic analyzer that differentiates among various gamma ray energies. A two-dimensional photodisplay unit records the image on retrievable film.

Historically, strontium-85 and strontium-87 were the first practical bone-imaging agents that localized in skeletal tissue through calcium exchange in bone matrix, although a low radionuclide count resulted in poor physical detail. The next agent, fluorine-18, was replaced by technetium-99m (Tc-99m), a derivative of molybdenum, which is the current agent of choice because of its low toxicity, lower cost, and greater availability. It is combined with an appropriate bone-imaging agent to form Tc-99m methylene diphosphate (MDP) and demonstrates osteoblastic absorption onto the surface of hydroxyapatite crystals. The agent's physical half-life is 6 hours, it is excreted by the kidneys, and it allows

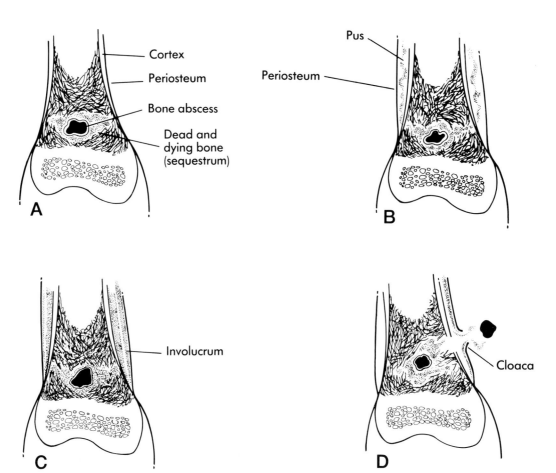

Figure 70.9. A. Sequestration (segmentation of dead bone from living bone) of devascularized bone due to Haversian and Volkmann canal destruction and osteocyte destruction. The process is highly suggestive of chronic osteomyelitis but may mimic osteoarthropathy in the diabetic foot. **B.** Infection eventually reaches subperiosteal tissues, causing elevation of periosteum due to purulent material. If close to a joint and intracapsular, septic arthritis may occur. **C.** Involucrum or new bone formation is suggestive of osteomyelitis. **D.** Cloaca formation, at bone-periosteal interface, for extrusion of sequestrum and necrotic products. (Reprinted from Downey MS: Osteomyelitis in the diabetic foot. *Reconstructive Surgery of the Foot and Leg—Update '89.* Tucker, GA, Podiatry Institute Publishing Co, 1989, p 204).

imaging 2 to 4 hours after intravenous injection. Normal uptake is seen at areas of tendon insertion, stress, osseous remodeling, and the epiphyseal plates of children. Regardless of the specific situation, the principles of differential scintigraphy remain the same. Its use in the diagnosis of osteomyelitis has been reviewed by Schlefman (76), while concepts of its use in the diabetic foot have been reviewed by Visser and associates (77).

Technetium methylene diphosphonate accumulates in areas of increased osseous vascularity and physiological activity (78). Intense uptake of this radiopharmaceutical may be consistent with osteomyelitis and is useful in localizing areas of suspected osseous disease and in determining the extent of involvement (79, 80). Scanning may be useful in establishing an early diagnosis of impending osteomyelitis at a time when standard radiographic evaluation reveals no abnormalities (81).

A positive technetium scan in a clinical setting of contamination suggests osteomyelitis provided there has been no recent bone trauma. However, technetium methylene diphosphonate uptake, particularly when not localized and intense, may be due to a variety of other causes. For example, increased technetium uptake may last for more than a year after loosening of a noninfected implant, bone reaction to polymethylmethacrylate, or the effects of an osteosynthesis device (82). Uptake from noninfectious periosteal reaction to adjacent soft tissue and bone infection, or extended patterns, may occur with radionuclide imaging. After osteotomies or arthrodeses, increased uptake of technetium may be seen until healing and remodeling have occurred (83, 84). When bilateral foot surgery has been performed, the marked uptake of technetium in the potentially infected foot, compared to an unimpressive or no accumulation in the contralateral limb, may be indicative of a pathologic condition (76). In cases of suspected osteomyelitis associated with trauma or ulceration, the accumulation of technetium may occur with osteolysis, reactive periostitis, neurotrophic joint disease, or normal bone healing (85).

Increased accumulation in soft tissues immediately after injection is indicative of hyperemia and inflammation but is not diagnostic of osteomyelitis (86).

The lack of specificity of technetium for osteomyelitis has resulted in a search for bone seeking radiopharmaceuticals specific for osteomyelitis. Gallium-67 citrate (Ga-67) has been shown to demonstrate a greater specificity for accumulation in areas of infection. It is not dependent on blood flow, as is Tc-99m MDP, and diagnostic imaging is performed 24 to 48 hours after injection. Its half-life is 78 hours, and it is excreted by the kidneys. Unfortunately, it has poor physical imaging characteristics, emitting many low-energy photons for each relatively large radiation dose. The mechanism of gallium-67 accumulation remains unclear, but it is thought to bind to white blood cells, plasma proteins, transferrin, ferritin, lactoferrin, and the siderophores that travel to areas of inflammation.

Although gallium uptake is more likely to be associated with infectious disease, it is not diagnostic of osteomyelitis and may accumulate in areas of inflammation or neoplasm. The original enthusiasm of gallium 67-citrate for the absolute early verification of osteomyelitis, as described by Deysine and associates (87), has been followed by increased reports of both false-positive and false-negative studies (88). Unlike technetium-99m, gallium-67 may accumulate in areas of soft tissue infection or inflammation (89, 90). Comparative studies of technetium and gallium uptake allow only inferences regarding the probability of osteomyelitis. An example of the sequential use of technetium and gallium may be found in the evaluation of a painful or tender implant arthroplasty, particularly in delayed or late infectious disease. A positive technetium-99m scan and a negative gallium-67 citrate scan are associated with an 85% probability that an infection is not present, whereas a positive technetium scan and a positive gallium scan represent a 70% certainty that osteomyelitis is established (91). A negative technetium scan and a positive gallium scan may represent cellulitis.

More recently, indium-111 (In-111) oxine (8-hydroxyquinoline) white blood cell and indium tropolene scanning has received endorsement for the early detection of both soft tissue and bone infection (92, 93). In-111 is an inflammatory imaging radiopharmaceutical that binds to cytoplasmic components of white blood cell membranes, although high radiation exposure is seen in the spleen and liver because of leukocyte destruction at these locations. Technically, autologous leukocytes are isolated from the patient's venous blood and labeled with indium-111 oxine. The prepared cells are then re-introduced to the patient and scanning is done 24 hours later. Indium studies appear to demonstrate greater specificity for infectious disease, and in the presence of abnormal indium accumulation infectious disease is usually present. However, false-positive accumulation of indium radiopharmaceuticals has been reported in noninfected bone grafts (88).

Radiopharmaceuticals offer the potential advantage of early detection of osteomyelitis and make determinations

possible before the onset of pathognomonic radiographic changes such as formation of sequestra or involucra (94). These studies therefore permit earlier and thus more effective therapy, particularly in cases of impending osteomyelitis. In the usual case, technetium is administered initially to evaluate the presence of bone disease (80, 95). The first phase of scanning is performed immediately after antecubital intravenous administration, and dynamic visualization of blood flow is achieved by rapid-sequence pictures, taken 1 to 3 seconds apart as the blood approaches the extremity. Information is obtained about the relative arterial supply of the area examined. During this immediate (radioangiogram) phase, the radiopharmaceutical is within the vascular system, and increased localization and intense uptake are consistent with hyperemia, inflammation, or infection. The second blood pool image phase (5 to 10 minutes after injection) quantifies the relative hyperemia or ischemia of the extremity through information about arterial blood present in the capillary and venous system and is a reflection of soft tissue inflammation. Interestingly, hematogenous (acute) osteomyelitis demonstrates a well-defined focus of increased radioactivity in the bone image with an identical area on the blood pool image. The third delayed image (2 to 4 hours) phase highlights the regional rate of bone metabolism and demonstrates osseous uptake only, because the radiopharmaceutical that has affinity for bone is removed from the soft tissues in 1 to 2 hours (86, 96). Finally, the fourth phase is a late delayed image taken 24 hours after injection. Theoretically, it will show greater bone activity and less soft tissue activity, especially in patients with marginal extremity vascularity.

Technetium methylene diphosphonate scanning may be useful as a solitary diagnostic tool. In the presence of osteotomy or implant discomfort, the failure to accumulate technetium is usually consistent with a problem of nonosseous origin (97). A high false-negative rate has been documented in hematogenous osteomyelitis, especially in pediatric patients (98, 99). When osseous surgery is contemplated contiguous to an ulcer, the failure of radionuclide accumulation may be assumed to be consistent with the absence of osteomyelitis or osteolysis (44). Radionuclide imaging is also useful for localizing the area of bone from which biopsy, culture, or aspiration material is to be obtained (78). When the early detection of osteomyelitis is considered, the sequential use of either gallium-67 citrate or indium-111, after a technetium scan is recommended (100). The second radioisotope is administered after completion of the technetium scan because it will clear from the body in 24 to 48 hours. Gallium or indium accumulation, particularly in the same area of bone in which technetium accumulated, is consistent with osteomyelitis (89). Sequential scanning is particularly useful in the evaluation of postoperative osteomyelitis, chronic or recurrent osteomyelitis, or osseous changes in the diabetic foot.

False-negative scans may occur because of vascular impairment to bone, preventing the delivery of radiopharmaceuticals to the infected area. The commonly used radiopharmaceuticals—technetium, gallium, and indium—all have associated false-positive and false-negative rates (88).

The sensitivity, specificity, positive predictive value, and negative predictive value of radionuclides in the evaluation of osteomyelitis are high when properly interpreted. Quadra-phasic technetium-99m scanning, with intense and focal uptake on all four phases (radioangiogram, blood pool image, delayed scan, and late delayed scan) is consistent with osteomyelitis. Although gallium is less sensitive than technetium, its specificity for osteomyelitis is higher (101). Indium 111 has a very high sensitivity for the presence of bone inflammation, demonstrating a high rate of false-positive studies and a decreased specificity (102).

The uptake of radiopharmaceuticals may reflect periosteal, endosteal, or osseous inflammatory disease distal or proximal to the actual level of an infectious process. Such extended or overflow patterns demonstrate less than intense and less well-localized accumulation of the agents (80, 81).

Decreased local osseous vascular perfusion, caused by compression from pus or frank microvascular infarction, may result in false-negative studies (103). This appears to be the problem most commonly encountered in acute pediatric hematogenous osteomyelitis. CT scanning and MR imaging may detect the early changes of hematogenous osteomyelitis in the face of negative bone scans (104).

Contrast studies and double-contrast studies have been described for the evaluation of osteomyelitis, particularly with reference to the evaluation of questionable clinical findings after implant arthroplasty (105). When polymethylmethacrylate has been used, infection typically occurs at the bone-cement interface (62). Loosening at the interface from bone resorption is common. The instillation of contrast media may demonstrate localization of the injected material between the implant and the cement or between the cement and the bone (106). The diagnostic specificity of arthroscopic and arthrographic techniques remains equivocal in many cases of osteomyelitis. When arthrography is performed for the evaluation of joint and bone infection, fluid should be obtained by aspiration for bacteriological examination before the introduction of contrast media. Synovial inflammation and the presence of capsular, tendinous, or soft tissue injury may be evaluated by arthrographic data (105, 107).

Sinograms and Fistulograms

Sinograms, bursagrams, and fistulography all may play roles in the evaluation of osteomyelitis (108). Injection of contrast media into a fistula may yield important information about the extent and origin of infection and therefore influence therapeutic considerations. A small flexible catheter may be securely placed within a cutaneous opening, or the contrast material may be injected through a standard syringe and a flexible needle of appropriate size, as long as the opening to the surface is occluded to prevent the spread of contrast media across the skin. The extent of fistulous involvement, as noted by the extent and distribution of contrast media,

must be carefully considered with regard to dissection across fascial planes. The possibility of spreading bacterial contamination to uninvolved tissues by the pressure of introduced contrast material must be considered while the patient is monitored for allergic phenomena and evidence of secondary contamination (52). Septicemia following fistulography has been reported, although it is considered unusual. When applicable, the use of contrast materials may be combined with CT scanning so that the combination of tests can yield detailed information that normally would not be available from the isolated use of either study individually (109).

Computerized Tomography Scans

CT scanning has been increasingly employed in the evaluation of osteomyelitis (72, 109). CT scanning can provide valuable anatomical detail that is not available with standard radiographic evaluation, particularly in the presence of complex fractures or fusions in the rearfoot. With an appropriate bone or soft tissue window, early subperiosteal medullary or endosteal changes may be visualized since the elevation of attenuated values in the marrow space is an early sign of acute osteomyelitis. In fact, trabecular bone mineralization changes may be detected with an accuracy of ±2% by high-resolution CT scanners. These changes, while indicative of cortical bone destruction and new bone formation, are not specific since aseptic necrosis, osteoporosis, arthrosis, and osteomalacia appear similar. Soft tissue techniques will allow for exceptional definition of the presence and extent of deep abscesses and periosteal reactivity, and they are particularly useful in the evaluation of deep plantar structures (Fig. 70.10).

Magnetic Resonance Imaging

MRI studies have the potential to reveal the definition, location, and extent of the anatomical bone destruction of osteomyelitis (104). This is based on the fact that water has a high proton content and MRI measures the water content of various body tissues (CT measures specific gravity). The more water (more protons), the higher the signal intensity. Therefore, such tissues as fat, muscle, tendon, ligament, nerves, and blood vessels have different imaging characteristics and are relatively ranked, according to the Spin-Echo Grayscale, from the brightest to the darkest. Medullary bone is white on a CT scan because of calcium (increased density) and white on an MRI scan because of high marrow content (increased intensity). Varying degrees of integrity or bone destruction are then compared and evaluated for diagnostic purposes.

Positron Emission Tomography

Positron emission tomography is an investigational modality for the administration of a positron-emitting radionuclide (biological tracer), such as carbon-11, oxygen-15, nitrogen-13, rubidium-81, rubidium-82, and gallium-68. These radionuclides penetrate and decay in precise depths when

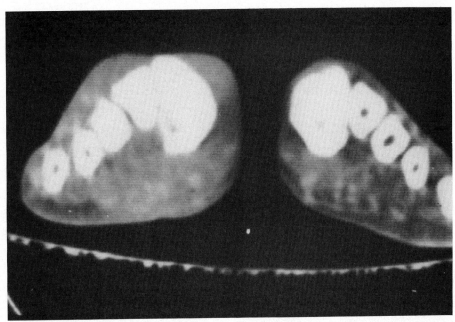

Figure 70.10. CT scanning has become an extremely valuable tool for anatomical detail not seen with standard radiographic technique. Early subperiosteal, medullary, or endosteal changes may be readily seen. Soft tissue techniques can provide adequate definition of the presence and extent of deep abscesses and are especially suited for evaluating deep plantar space infection or abscess. The patient whose foot is depicted on this CT scan had poorly controlled diabetes with suspected deep plantar space infection of his left foot. Note diffuse swelling of medial plantar aspect of the left foot. There is a lesser degree of edema along the dorsum of the left foot with air noted in soft tissues. Early obliteration of the medullary canal visualized by CT scan is an early finding in acute hematogenous osteomyelitis, which may precede positive bone scan changes.

passed through soft tissue and produce paired photons. The detection of these paired photons, referred to as annihilation coincidence detection, forms the basis of positron emission tomography. It is useful for the noninvasive study of regional tissue physiology and metabolic processes. Standards and definitions of soft tissue and bone infections are currently being formulated.

Miscellaneous Presumptive Tests

Magnified flat plate radiographs, xeroradiography, or diagnostic ultrasonography may be used selectively to provide additional information when needed in particular clinical circumstances (110, 111). Regardless of the radiographic modality employed, definitive diagnosis and management of infection rest in bone biopsy and the evaluation of clinical signs and symptoms. When time permits, or when invasive diagnostic procedures are avoided, radiographic and nuclear medicine studies may provide valuable adjunctive indirect information with regard to the presence and extent of osteomyelitis.

Radiographic magnification techniques may be particularly useful in the evaluation of early infectious disease in the small bones and joints of the forefoot (72). The early manifestations of such disorders as osteomyelitis, septic arthritis, or infectious osteitis may be evident on magnification views. Small areas of osteolytic foci or relatively minor and

previously unnoticed areas of subchondral bone disruption may be readily apparent on magnified views of the foot.

MANAGEMENT OF OSTEOMYELITIS

The management of osteomyelitis is dependent on a variety of factors peculiar to the clinical setting of each case. In general, treatment usually entails both medical and surgical therapy as well as local wound care. A variety of factors play roles in overall prognosis.

The key to the management of osteomyelitis is early recognition. In difficult circumstances any disruption of normal healing is regarded as suspicious, and treatment is frequently initiated in the presence of minimal signs and symptoms (Fig. 70.11). Terms such as *imminent, impending,* or *preosteomyelitis* have been applied when antimicrobial or surgical treatment is initiated for the management of osteomyelitis with an absolute minimum of specific signs and symptoms (112, 113). These signs may resolve before a firm diagnosis of osteomyelitis can be made. It is therefore difficult to substantiate successful treatment of impending or imminent osteomyelitis. However, the consideration of differential diagnoses in such cases and appropriate goal-oriented therapy will eliminate the unnecessary administration of parenteral antibiotics and unnecessary surgical experience for the patient. It would seem that the management of impending osteomyelitis is preferable to treatment that

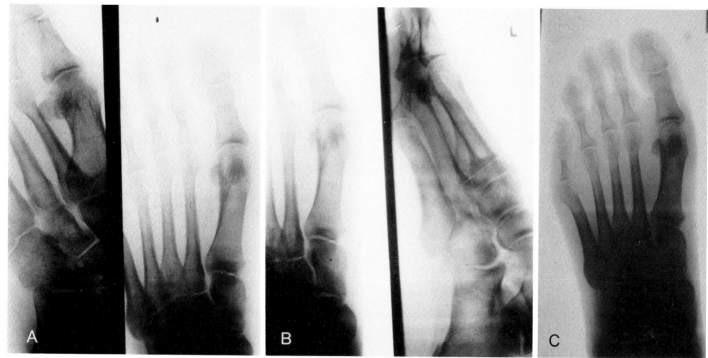

Figure 70.11. Early recognition is key to the management of osteo-myelitis. An astute clinician will regard any disruption of normal healing as suspicious and will frequently initiate treatment in the presence of minimal signs and symptoms. Such terms as *imminent, impending,* or *preosteomyelitis* have been assigned when antimicrobial therapy has been initiated in the presence of minimal signs and symptoms. These radio-graphs were taken after simple limited open bunionectomy on the left foot. Serial radiographs were taken approximately 4 weeks **(A)**, 6 weeks **(B)**, and 8 weeks **(C)** postoperatively. The patient was symptom-free with no overt clinical signs of gross infection. Minimal resorptive changes were noted at the distal medial aspect of the left first metatarsal head. The patient was given Duricef, 2 g orally daily for 3 months, at which time no continued osseous changes were noted. Use of oral antibiotics in this patient was made possible through early suspicion and recognition, which led to immediate incision and drainage.

is withheld until firm diagnostic signs and symptoms of es-tablished bone infection appear. The diagnosis of imminent or impending osteomyelitis is a clinical determination di-rected at preventing the conversion of acute osteomyelitis to chronic or recurrent osteomyelitis (6). Even with the ap-propriate management of osteomyelitis, an occasional pa-tient will proceed from rather abrupt onset to the demon-stration of a clinical condition consistent with chronic os-teomyelitis.

The Early Postoperative Period

Acute inflammatory signs and symptoms of superficial or deep infection, in the absence of osseous abnormalities that are radiographically demonstrable, are treated empirically. Incision and drainage is normally carried to the deep tissues without involving the periosteal, capsular tissues, or bone. Therapy is directed at organisms recovered from soft tissue cultures or blood cultures. Under such circumstances, it is generally believed prudent to monitor the patient carefully for any evidence of failure to respond to appropriate ther-apy. Under these circumstances, with the realization that soft tissue cultures may not reflect the underlying infecting

organism, bone biopsy and culture may have to be consid-ered. This is especially true in the face of expanding osseous radiographic change or the persistence of increased Ga-67 or In-111 uptake.

In the absence of frank culture material, therapy may be initially directed to *Staphylococcus aureus,* since it represents the most common pathogen (114, 115). Infecting *Staphylo-coccus* organisms should be considered to be coagulase-pos-itive and penicillinase-producing unless proven otherwise (116). It is often judicious to use either a first-generation cephalosporin or penicillinase-resistant semisynthetic pen-icillin until definitive cultures and sensitivities are obtained (117). In the presence of penicillin allergy, the parenteral use of cephalosporins must be considered. Cross-sensitivity between the cephalosporins and the penicillins is well known and can occur in 3% to 20% of patients (118). Clindamycin, lincomycin, erythromycin lactobionate, and vancomycin represent useful alternatives in the scenario of penicillin allergy and a reluctance to use a cephalosporin (119).

Surgical incision and drainage is performed to decom-press abscesses in either soft tissue or bone. In addition to frank decompression and removal of appropriate specimens for pathogen identification, all necrotic tissue is eradicated since debris within the wound is believed to present problems in treatment (9). Necrotic soft tissue serves to sequester bacteria, thus allowing progression as well as recurrence of the disease. Damage from vascular tissue pressure or abscess formation allows retention of persistent areas that are impenetrable to local body immune defenses and antibiotic agents (36, 120).

When appropriate, bone must be explored for medullary abscess or subperiosteal abscess by clinical evaluation and radiographic determination (6, 8). In the presence of an abscess, decompression should not be delayed for special studies such as scintigraphy (17). Periosteal tissue is incised, and the bone is inspected. Any area of devitalized or detached bone is removed. Decortication allows for inspection of the medullary canal. Any medullary abscess is drained, and all necrotic, devitalized, or questionable tissue is removed. Failure to remove areas of infection and necrosis will result in a delayed or poor clinical response. Necrectomy, when necessary, should be complete (121).

After debridement of infected and devascularized soft tissue and bone, difficult decisions must be made and there should be no vulnerable areas of access for resistant bacteria to invade (122). For example, the medullary canal of bone should not be left exposed. Rather, various techniques are employed to fill the defect. One example is the interpositioning of soft tissue, such as muscle, to prevent easy access to the areas of exposed bone (123, 124). In addition, such myofascial modifications are believed to play a role in successful revascularization of the bone and surrounding tissues (125).

Gentamicin-Impregnated PMMA Beads

For years, European authors advocated use of the antibiotic-impregnated polymethylmethacrylate (PMMA) bone cement to fill bone defects. However, the pressure of the cement allowed dissemination of bacteria during placement and prevented elution of the antibacterial agent into surrounding tissues, thus negating its effect. Because of this and other problems associated with gentamicin-impregnated cement, gentamicin PMMA beads have been developed. Self-generation in the operating room by the surgeon is questioned since quality is unknown. Gentamicin-impregnated polymethylmethacrylate has been used with or without concurrent parenteral antibiotics in the management of osteomyelitis and is generally an adjunct to treatment in this country.

The concept of using spherical PMMA beads to fill infected osseous defects was first described in 1972 by Klemm in cooperation with E. Merck Laboratories (Darmstadt) (126). According to Klemm, advantages of its use included a shorter downtime, reduced nursing staff work load, reduced incidence of secondary infections, and improved hospital hygiene. They combined the principles of high local antibiotic tissue levels with primary wound closure. Gentamicin is released in bactericidal concentrations at the site of infection, with only trace amounts detectable in the circulation, and there is a distinct difference between the local

application of gentamicin and the levels obtained by infusion. For example, gentamicin levels after injection are high in serum and urine samples and relatively low in tissues. Conversely, after implantation, extremely low serum and urine concentrations are seen but a high level in bone leads to therapeutic efficacy and fewer adverse effects. Bead implantation is contraindicated in cases of acute inflammation and as prophylaxis for open compound fractures or unstable fractures.

The indispensable first step in the treatment of any serious soft tissue or bone infection is the radical debridement of all necrotic tissue. Vital staining with disulfine blue, or other biologic dye, aids in the delineation of viable tissue since necrotic tissue will not incorporate the colored dye into its stroma because of a lack of vascular supply. A tourniquet is used to prevent blurring of vision by the stained blood. After removal of appropriate portions of bone cortex in the medullary canal, gentamicin-impregnated PMMA beads can be placed within the cavity to fill the osseous defect. The beads are placed within the osseous cavity in a precise fashion, rather than in random order, in accordance with the wound configuration to obtain a greater density and facilitate later removal. Usual arrangements include heaps, parallel chains, plates, or a meandering pattern (127).

The persistent local antibiotic levels of gentamicin after such a procedure are surprisingly high. Because of these levels, the usual classification of pathogens into sensitive or resistant strains may not be appropriate. This differentiation is based on the serum concentrations expected during systemic parenteral antibiotic administration. With levels 10 to 100 times higher, such levels may be bactericidal against pathogens that were previously assessed as resistant in the routine antibiogram. Examinations by Ritzerfield (128) proved that the antibiotic is effective against *S. aureus*, *Proteus*, *Pseudomonas*, and *E. coli*, but less so against *Enterobacter* and *Klebsiella*. The gentamicin itself may perfuse an area up to 2 cm surrounding the area of implantation, again reinforcing the concept of thorough preimplantation debridement.

Gentamicin-impregnated PMMA, available commercially since 1976, is produced in beads connected by several strands of stainless steel surgical wire. Gentamicin is the antibiotic of choice for combination with PMMA because it has good water solubility and intrinsic stability with respect to the high temperatures needed to produce the methacrylate beads (130° to 150° C). In addition, benefits of the aminoglycoside include a broad spectrum of antimicrobial activity, including both gram-positive and gram-negative organisms which are of increasing importance as problem pathogens resistant to other antibiotics. Gentamicin is bactericidal during both the proliferative and resting phases of growth. The PMMA serves as a vehicle for the antibiotic and allows protracted release of the agent into the surrounding local milieu at an initial rate of 400 to 600 μg/bead/day. Animal models have shown that on the tenth day after implantation 120 μg is detectable and that on the 20th day 50 μg remains. By the 80th day, only 10 μg of gentamicin base is released from one bead. The beads are available individually or strung in chains 10, 30, or 60 beads in length. The chains measure approximately 1 cm per bead. Marketed under the trade name Septopal (E. Merck Laboratories, Hawthorne, NY), the beads have a diameter of 7 mm, and each contains 7.5 mg of gentamicin sulfate along with 20 mg of zirconium dioxide as a contrast medium. A newer product is also available for use in smaller body parts. These smaller minibeads have been made by Ashe and are ideal for use in pedal structures (129). The minibeads are sterilized with ethylene oxide and packed in a double sachet envelope. The outer envelope is opened under sterile con-

ditions and, once contaminated, should not be reused or resterilized.

The beads may be placed in the area of bone or soft tissue infection and may be allowed to protrude from the skin (Fig. 70.12). After adequate debridement of bone and soft tissue, the beads may be allowed to remain in the wound for up to 14 days. The last bead of a chain should protrude above the skin level after primary wound closure to facilitate later removal. If the wound cannot be sutured closed, synthetic skin or multiple relaxation skin incisions should be used to accomplish coaptation. Before wound closure, an

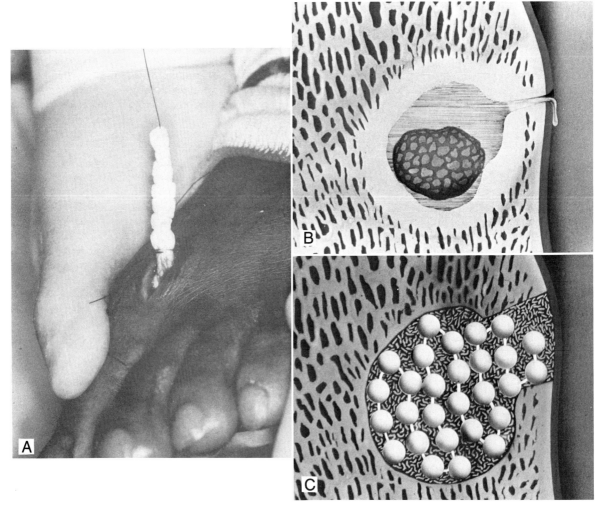

Figure 70.12. **A.** Photograph of a patient who had a total implant arthroplasty for severe degenerative joint disease. On his first postoperative visit, he had wound dehiscence and sinus tract draining with green-tinged exudate. On questioning, it was learned that the patient went out jogging in his old athletic footwear, starting on fourth postoperative day. Subsequent bone biopsy and culture revealed *Pseudomonas* osteomyelitis, and the implant was removed. The photograph shows gentamicin-impregnated polymethylmethacrylate beads on strand of 2-0 monofilament wire being placed in the space previously occupied by the implant and adjacent soft tissue, as well as bony structures. Beads are left in the wound for up to 14 days. Persistent local antibiotic levels may perfuse an area of up to 2 cm surrounding the area of implantation. Systemic antibiotics may be administered concurrently on the basis of the physician's experience and clinical judgment. **B.** Diagrammatic representation of sequestering osteomyelitis of the ankle joint with an open draining sinus tract and sclerosis of the cavity wall. **C.** After sequestrectomy and debridement, PMMA beads are implanted into the cavity. The last bead should lie outside the skin to facilitate removal 10 to 14 days later. (From Marcinko DE: Gentamicin-impregnated PMMA beads: an introduction and case review. *J Foot Surg* 24:116, 1985.)

overflow or gravity drain is placed into the cavity. As the gentamicin is released through diffusion, the hematoma should not be evacuated away since the primary purpose of the technique is to keep local tissue levels high. The purpose of drains is to guarantee a tension-free wound for closure, and drains are removed in a day or two. Although primary and tight closure of infected wounds seems to contradict conventional rules for the care of septic wounds, closure is very important. Because of the high local antibiotic concentrations, bacteria are killed almost immediately and general wound healing, as in aseptic conditions, may be expected.

Although the beads have been left in place for longer periods of time, it is generally recommended that they be removed no later than 14 days after implantation. Within this time frame the chains can be withdrawn easily, usually without anesthesia. If left in place for longer periods, their removal may be difficult since they become encapsulated in granulation tissue. If a bead or two breaks off the stainless steel chain, the decision to retrieve it is made with full knowledge of the risks of an additional surgical procedure; solitary beads have been left in place for years without apparent difficulty. After removal of the beads, small residual spaces fill in with connective tissue but larger voids must undergo cancellous bone grafting or endoprosthesis implantation.

Other antibiotics, such as vancomycin, may be used with polymethylmethacrylate beads. Antibiotics combined with polymethylmethacrylate must be heat stable and should not promote hypersensitive or allergic reactions.

In 1985, Marcinko (130) presented a case report of Septopal use in an infected diabetic patient and reviewed a report by Grieben of 1054 cases of osteomyelitis treated with gentamicin PMMA beads in 890 patients (personal communication, Darmstadt, Germany). Wound healing, freedom from sinus tract formation, and a normal erythrocyte sedimentation rate were parameters considered in the assessment of successful cases. With these criteria, a 6-year follow-up examination of 635 patients revealed that 535 remained free of infection. Failures were attributed to inadequate debridement and sequestration. Several patients required revisional debridement, although an overall therapeutic success rate of 97% was ultimately achieved. In addition, Wassner reported on another series of 161 patients treated with Septopal chains (131). One hundred thirty-three patients had postoperative wound infections, and 28 others had osteomyelitis. In the former group, wound healing was obtained in 124 patients and there were 9 failures. In the latter group treatment was successful in 25 patients, with only 3 failures. Most recently, Heard and Oloff (132) have successfully created an experimental model to establish the contiguous and remote antimicrobial effects of impregnated methacrylate. It will be useful in future studies comparing contact inhibition versus indirect antibiotic diffusion (133).

Closed Suction Irrigation

When there is a paucity of bone changes in an area of soft tissue debridement but a high index of suspicion of osteo-myelitis, several approaches may be taken. Fenestration or decortication of bone may be performed in association with the use of continuous closed suction irrigation. Continuous suction irrigation has attracted renewed interest after elucidation in the podiatric literature by Pressman (134) and the development of a dependable closed system with air venting shunt described by Schwartz and Marcinko (135) in 1985. Continuous closed suction irrigation was originally described in the management of pediatric hematogenous osteomyelitis, and in central Europe it is still used for periods of 3 to 5 weeks. It provides mechanical flushing of chronic and infected tissue from a wound, as well as direct antibiotic delivery to the infected area. The most efficient use of suction irrigation appears to be in treatment of chronic osteomyelitis. It is indicated when necrotic or infected tissue prevents diffusion of systemic antibiotics into the infected area. In some cases, continuous closed suction irrigation is applied as a prophylactic measure because recurrent symptoms may evolve despite the closure of a seemingly clean and appropriately debrided wound (136).

The widespread use of suction irrigation has been tempered with knowledge of potential side effects. One study demonstrated that bacterial colonization of the outflow (egress) tube occurred in 30% of the patients (137) and that the most common organism was *P. aeruginosa* or other gram-negative rods (134). Occasionally superinfection will occur because of the colonized tubing. For this reason, suction irrigation systems are generally removed as quickly as possible with continual monitoring for bacterial flora while the device is in use. A great deal of literature advocates the use of suction irrigation in association with infected implant surgery (138). When an attempt is made to salvage an implant device, debridement may be accompanied by primary closure over the drain when it is apparent that no residual necrotic or infected tissue exists (19).

The advantages of wound irrigation must also be weighed against a variety of commonly incurred technical problems (134). Seepage of the fluid into the incision or through the tubing portals is common and may cause wound maceration and a variety of local management problems. The successful use of such irrigation is dependent on an airtight system that is carefully monitored. Such problems as tube blockage must be recognized promptly. Multiegress tube systems are somewhat less problematical. In addition, reversal flow techniques as well as intermittent irrigation techniques have been used in an attempt to lessen the incidence of wound maceration and tube blockage (139). Finally, the use of a cold solution is not recommended since pain may result. A solution warmed to about 37° C is beneficial, and agents other than antimicrobials have been used to irrigate infected body parts.

The use of suction irrigation with bone decompression, decortication, or fenestration may be associated with other problems. After the decortication or fenestration, the possibility of fracture through the weakened bone must be considered and appropriate therapy rendered in terms of weight-bearing redistribution. Some authors advocate the use of PMMA beads or the introduction of myofascial tissues

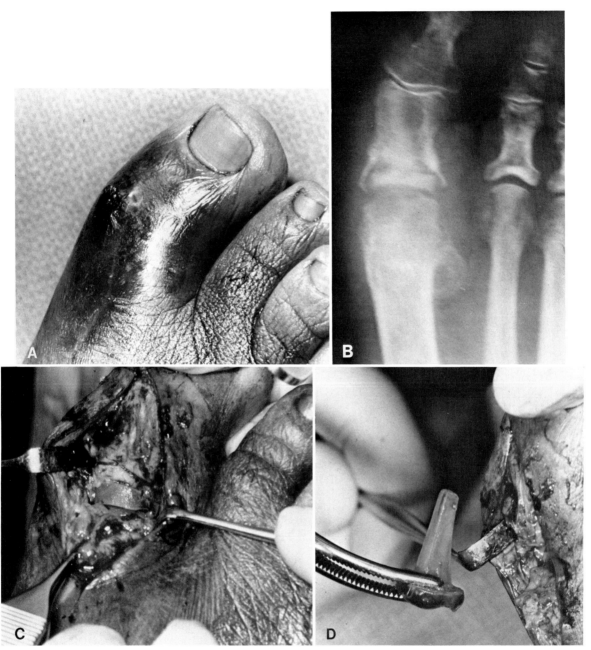

Figure 70.13.   A. Draining sinus tract located at the hallucal interphalangeal joint 2 weeks after surgery. Note edema, shiny skin appearance, and flexion deformity of the joint. **B.** Radiographic presentation with osseous engulfment of implant and erosive bone changes in the proximal phalanx. **C.** Salvage rates for joint implants involved in deep postoperative infection are variable and depend on the infecting organism. This patient had a deep infection at the site of hemi-implant arthroplasty of the first metatarsophalangeal joint. **D.** Implant removal is desirable if osteomyelitis has been established. In this case, implant removal was delayed until 4 weeks after discovery of the infection. Reimplantation can be performed as a single-stage exchange procedure from 6 months to 2 years after successful management of osteomyelitis. However, bone loss may preclude reimplantation.

into defects created by sequestrectomy (130, 140). Others advocate bone grafting, even in the presence of infection (141). It has been demonstrated that the main factor in graft take is the type of bone used and the local vascularity, rather than the presence of infecting bacteria (142). Regardless, fenestrated bone is prone to pathologic fracture, and grafting in such areas involves the use of a combination of periosteal cortical tissues and cancellous bone chips (143).

THE INFECTED PROSTHETIC DEVICE

As noted earlier, implant infections may be acute, delayed, or late. The presence of an implant at the site of infection is known frequently to prolong the course of treatment and resolution of the pathological process (53). This is because implant material creates areas through which antibiotics cannot readily diffuse. In effect, the implant serves to protect and cloister bacteria from exposure to antibiotics, but the effects of the invading organism on the implant itself must be considered. If removal of an implant is to be avoided, early diagnosis and parenteral antibiotic therapy must be accomplished together with early decompression. The use of suction irrigation under such circumstances is advocated in addition to early wound closure (144).

Salvage rates for deep postoperative implant infections are variable and are dependent on the infecting organism, the medical status of the patient, and early recognition of infection (52). Once osteomyelitis is established, however, it appears that the removal of commonly used implants is desirable (20) (Fig. 70.13). With the establishment of osteomyelitis, implants may be removed and, with appropriate debridement, replaced as a one-stage exchange procedure. If necrotic or infected tissue remains because of inaccessibility, reimplantation should not be considered (62).

The decision concerning wound closure and the use of drains or irrigation systems is totally dependent on the specific circumstances of each case and, therefore, is empirical. Sequential scintigraphy with technetium, gallium, or indium may be used to assess response (78). Reimplantation may be performed from 6 months to 2 years after successful management of the osteomyelitis (138). It is best to perform reimplantation after confirmation of sterility by culture. After treatment with parenteral antibiotics for 6 continuous weeks, reimplantation may be successful (62).

The possible recurrence of osteomyelitis after reimplantation must be weighed against the residual sequelae of simple resection arthroplasty or arthrodesis procedures after implant retrieval. Frequently, the extensive fibrosis that follows yields an arthrodesis-like effect that functions asymptomatically with appropriate mechanical control (Fig. 70.14).

Infection rates are known to be higher after surgery within areas known to have been previously infected (145). Consequently, a period of prophylactic antibiotic administration before reimplantation is warranted, as well as careful monitoring in the postoperative period.

In summary, the management of infection in the presence

of polymeric implants in the foot remains empirical. Soft tissue infection or imminent osteomyelitis does not require the removal of implants. In carefully selected cases, limited osteomyelitis may be treated with implant removal, debridement, and reimplantation as a one-stage exchange. When polymethylmethacrylate has been used, a sustained persistent response to unpolymerized monomer is known to occur at the site of the cement, increasing the incidence of delayed and late wound infection (48, 49). In a series of experiments, Petty (49) concluded that methacrylate decreased chemotactic and phagocytic properties of leukocytes (62) (Fig. 70.15). Under such circumstances, complete removal of methacrylate is necessary.

In biocorrosion of metallic implants, there may be radiographic and clinical findings similar to osteomyelitis, along with radiographically detectable bone changes (146). Similarly, recurrences of inflammatory arthritic disorders, such as gout, Reiter's syndrome, or rheumatoid arthritis, may be mistaken for delayed or late osteomyelitis associated with implant fixation (147, 148).

INFECTED SURGICAL OSTEOTOMIES OR FRACTURES

Osteotomies or fractures may heal in the presence of osteomyelitis by both external and internal callus formation (122). Traditionally, osteosynthesis devices were removed in the presence of bone or periosteal infection. In recent years, many authorities have advocated maintenance of internal fixation when possible (149). With the so-called active method of treatment, bone union is given priority over the infection (150). In the presence of stable internal fixation and evidence of response to local and systemic care, internal-fixation devices may be allowed to remain in place. When internal-fixation devices appear to be ineffective in maintaining anatomical alignment, compression, and fixation, they are generally removed (151).

In a recent study done by Lifeso and Al-Saati (149), 129 nonunited fractures were treated with rigid internal fixation and bone grafting. In 14 others, tibial nonunions were treated with posterior lateral bone grafting. In 37 actively infected cases, this was combined with sequestrectomy and appropriate antibiotics. The final success rate was 98.4%. Lifeso and Al-Saati concluded that active osteomyelitis is not a contraindication to internal fixation.

If the response to therapy appears to be impaired because of the presence of osteosynthesis devices, the latter may be removed before achievement of bony union or arthrodesis (152). Under such circumstances, a conversion to external fixation or other means of immobilization by external splintage may be used. It has been suggested that large internal-fixation devices may impair bone vascularity and therefore impede the delivery of parenterally administered antibiotics (153). Instability of a fracture or osteotomy site may itself contribute to decreased clinical response, and the maintenance of internal fixation is advocated when possible (150).

Increased corrosion of metallic devices, as well as the diminished physical properties of such devices, may occur as

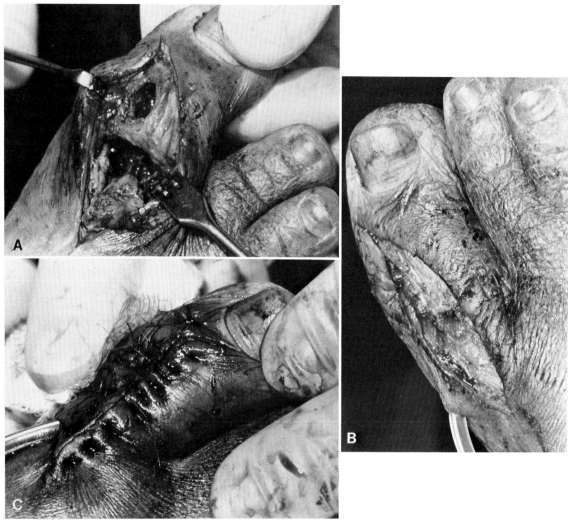

Figure 70.14. **A.** Bone after implant removal demonstrates extensive destruction of the proximal phalanx as a result of osteomyelitis. Extensive fibrosis resulted in a stiff interphalangeal joint. **B.** The wound is being closed, after debridement, with instillation of a suction drain system used in conjunction with appropriate parenteral antibiotics. **C.** Primary wound closure is important to maintain integrity of the closed system. The procedure is somewhat controversial because traditional concepts of wound sepsis are violated.

a result of exposure to the infectious processes (146). Therefore, in the presence of osteomyelitis, such devices are best removed when the purpose for which they were implanted has been achieved. Osteomyelitis at the site of metallic devices may be managed by debridement without disruption of the osteotomy or fracture site. When feasible, closure may be obtained with closed suction irrigation or gentamicin-impregnated PMMA beads, and failure to obtain soft tissue closure over the bone site does not necessitate removal of fixation devices (154). The fate of exposed bone has recently been reviewed, and it has been suggested that the time-honored tradition of sacrificing whatever soft tissues are necessary to obtain wound closure may be inappropriate (155). Union may be obtained by the placement of cancellous bone grafts on a good vascular bed, regardless of infection (141).

The conservative approach to infection in the presence of implants or fixation devices has generally yielded excellent results. A variety of studies indicate that in early, superficial, or deep infection, immediate excision of infected tissue, irrigation, and primary closure with appropriate antibiotics may often salvage the implant or fixation device (153). Indications for removal of foreign materials are difficult to establish. However, it appears clear that one indication is response failure, with increasing signs and symptoms of infection. After the seemingly successful management of infection, oral antibiotic coverage should be continued for a period of approximately 2 months after parenteral therapy and wound healing (153). Because recurrence of infection is high, careful monitoring through radiographic and radioisotopic studies appears essential (87, 88).

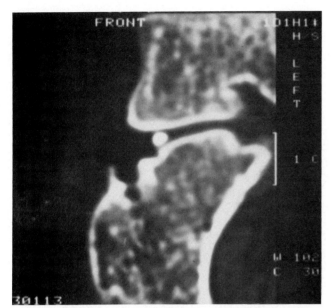

Figure 70.15. The presence of polymethylmethacrylate may play a role in infection at implant sites. Polymethylmethacrylate appears to decrease leukocyte phagocytic properties. Infection is most likely to occur at the bone-cement interface when polymethylmethacrylate is used as a luting agent. The CT scan depicted is from a patient who underwent a STA-PEG subtalar joint implant using polymethylmethacrylate for a flexible pes valgo planus deformity. In this particular case, the implant, as well as bone cement, may act as a barrier to delivery of antibiotics and to normal immune defense responses. The implant and bone cement can also serve as a nidus to harbor bacteria. Sepsis may result in loosening of the implant. The CT scan reveals a small, well-circumscribed sclerotic mass in the sinus tarsi, most probably a piece of polymethylmethacrylate that was not removed at time of surgery.

ANTIBIOTICS IN THE MANAGEMENT OF OSTEOMYELITIS

The use of parenteral antibiotics without surgery is generally reserved for the treatment of acute hematogenous osteomyelitis with no radiographic evidence of sequestration, involucra, or abscess formation. Traditionally, 4 to 6 weeks of parenteral antibiotic therapy is required, along with several months of oral antibiotic therapy (156, 157). The duration of oral antibiotic therapy is dependent on the degree of soft tissue and bone involvement at the time of the initial diagnosis, as well as on the success of surgical decompression and debridement. In the presence of avascular or fibrotic bone, antibiotics may be less effective because of failure of diffusion into sequestered bone. For that reason, medical and surgical therapy must be considered in each particular case. There is no evidence that established osteomyelitis can be managed with oral antibiotics alone. Hematogenous osteomyelitis has been successfully managed in large numbers of children with oral cephalosporin therapy (158).

Long-term intravenous or intramuscular antibiotic therapy may result in increased hospitalization costs, as well as a significant psychological burden on patients. Antimicrobial regimens of parenteral therapy for up to 2 weeks, followed by oral administration for 2 to 12 weeks, in children with acute disease have been described (159). Although the cure rate has approached 95%, this management cannot be used once evidence of chronicity is established or significant devitalization of tissue has occurred. Long-term antibiotic therapy includes monitoring for potential complications of intravenous coverage.

Initial medical therapy for osteomyelitis is dependent on a variety of factors. In the presence of urinary tract infection, for example, antibiotics directed at gram-negative organisms or streptococci may seem appropriate. Broad-spectrum agents or those directed at anaerobic or gram-negative infections may be appropriate for the initial treatment of patients with decreased peripheral vascular perfusion and diabetes mellitus. Specificity in the selection of antibiotics is dependent on the isolation of the organisms responsible for infection. In the absence of unusual circumstances, *Staphylococcus aureus* is the organism most often responsible for osteomyelitis (6). In the presence of methicillin-resistant *Staphylococcus*, vancomycin is the drug of choice (160). When penicillins appear to be the drugs of choice, semisynthetic penicillinase-resistant penicillins, such as oxacillin, methicillin, or dicloxacillin, are useful (8).

The selection of the appropriate antibiotic or the simultaneous use of multiple antibiotics is determined by the infecting organism(s) as well as by sensitivity patterns. Multiple drugs may be used simultaneously if cultures reveal the presence of more than one organism and these are not sensitive to the same antimicrobial agent. Similarly, severe infections of unknown etiology in neutropenic patients predisposed to polymicrobic infections (rheumatoid or diabetic patients) may be treated with more than one drug (9). In some situations, such as the management of *Pseudomonas aeruginosa*, combination drug therapy is associated with drug synergism, which increases treatment efficiency (10). The use of an aminoglycoside or third-generation cephalosporins with semisynthetic penicillins, such as piperacillin, ticarcillin, mezlocillin, or carbenicillin, is accepted in the management of *P. aeruginosa* (117).

Monitoring of bacterial flora, as well as serum peak and trough levels, is variably important, depending on the antibiotic and invading bacteria (114). *S. aureus* that eliminates penicillinase or β-lactamase will inactivate penicillin by destruction of its lactam ring. Only 20% of *S. aureus* infections are caused by bacteria sensitive to penicillins (161). Methicillin-resistant *S. aureus* will usually be resistant to aminoglycosides, cephalosporins, tetracyclines, and sulfonamides.

It is important to remember that the in vitro sensitivity of antibiotics may not be reflective of actual in vivo activity. In addition to serum testing and radiographic evaluation, the patient's clinical response is of great importance in the decision to continue antibiotic therapy. For example, the in vivo activity of aminoglycosides against staphylococcal organisms is less than one would expect from culture and sensitivity results (162). In the treatment of osteomyelitis, maintenance of therapeutic antibiotic levels at the mean bactericidal concentration is of great importance. The mean

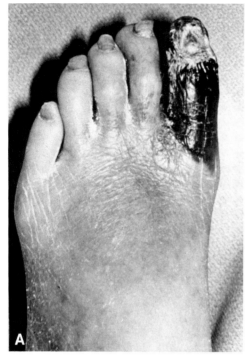
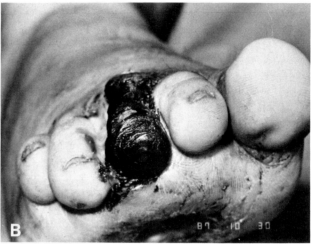

Figure 70.16. A and **B.** Amputation or radical resection of bone and necrotic tissue, to include at least the entire digit or ray, is indicated in these two cases of digital osteomyelitis with frank dry gangrene. Rarely does bone infection spread directly to neighboring joints. Vascular compromise with demarcation of infarcted tissue is dramatic.

bactericidal concentration is often many times the mean inhibitory concentration (15).

After the administration of parenteral antibiotics, oral antibiotic therapy is generally recommended, although the duration of therapy is empirical (8). When prosthetic or fixation devices remain, administration may continue for years. Norden (27) demonstrated that less than 3 to 4 weeks of parenteral antibiotic therapy is generally associated with failure to resolve infection. In the presence of chronic osteomyelitis, 6 weeks of parenteral antibiotic therapy appears to be necessary, with an oral follow-up of at least 2 months (163). Radiological changes will generally normalize after the stabilization of clinical signs and symptoms.

Patients who fail to respond on a clinical or radiological basis demonstrate an inadequate response to therapy (164). In such cases, the modification of antibiotic selection or further surgical intervention is required. Constant monitoring of bacterial flora is necessary because antibiotic substitution may be required to treat bacteria that have not been detected by initial culture and sensitivity techniques (165).

In certain situations modifications of traditional drug therapy may be required. Third-generation cephalosporins, for example, generally show increased activity against gram-negative organisms such as *P. aeruginosa* (166). Although combination therapy with aminoglycosides and such drugs as piperacillin or mezlocillin is generally first-line therapy against *Pseudomonas*, compromised renal status or hepatic function may necessitate the conversion to such drugs as third-generation cephalosporins. Strains of *Pseudomonas* that

are resistant to third-generation cephalosporins have been documented. The large sodium content of such drugs as carbenicillin or azlocillin may create problems in hypertensive patients (114, 167).

Drug costs also represent a major consideration in the management of osteomyelitis. Third-generation cephalosporins, as well as aminoglycosides, are expensive agents. Hospitalization length may be decreased and compliance increased through the use of outpatient antibiotic administration centers (168, 169).

AMPUTATIONS

In addition to the standard surgical and medical management regimens in the treatment of osteomyelitis, a variety of other therapies may be applied in particular cases. The use of electrogenerated silver ions and hyperbaric oxygen, both locally and systemically, in the management of osteomyelitis has been described (170, 171). Radical debridement or amputation is sometimes a necessary consideration. Ablative surgery, performed with an appropriate margin of safety between infected and noninfected tissue, results in a shorter antibiotic course and a shorter hospitalization (172). Benefits must be weighed against the effects of the loss of a particular part. Certainly, every practical attempt to preserve the pedal extremity should be made. However, in patients who are medically at risk of the side effects and sequelae of antibiotic therapy, or in whom the osteomyelitis might be quickly resolved by the elimination of a pedal appendage, amputation may represent a practical alternative. In patients with diminished peripheral vascular perfusion, well-localized osteomyelitis may be quickly resolved by amputation techniques (Fig. 70.16).

SUMMARY

The successful management of osteomyelitis depends on early recognition of imminent or impending infection. Prevention of acute bone infection from becoming chronic is also dependent on early and appropriate surgical and medical intervention. A variety of direct and indirect diagnostic and surgical techniques are available for the successful management of osteomyelitis. Parenteral antibiotic use is paramount.

References

1. Nelaton A: *Elements de Pathologie Chirurgicale*. Paris, Germer-Bailliere, 1844-1859.
2. Edwards EE: Severe candidal infections, clinical perspective, immune defense mechanisms, and current concepts of therapy. *Ann Intern Med* 8:91-106, 1978.
3. Chmel H, Grieco MH, Zickel R: Candida osteomyelitis; report of a case. *Am J Med Sci* 266:299-304, 1973.
4. Lefrock JL, Annangara DW: Treatment of infectious arthritis. *Clin Pharmacol Ther* 30:252-257, 1984.
5. Juttmann JW, Van der Slikke W: The treatment of osteitis complicating tibial fractures. *Br J Accident Surg* 13:210-215, 1980.
6. Waldvogel FA, Medoff G, Swartz MN: Osteomyelitis: a review of clinical features, therapeutic considerations and unusual aspects. *N Engl J Med* 282:198-206, 260-266, 316-322, 1970.
7. West WF, Kelly PJ, Martin WJ: Chronic osteomyelitis. I. Factors affecting the results of treatment in 186 patients. *JAMA* 213:1837-1842, 1970.
8. Armstrong EP, Rush DR: Treatment of osteomyelitis. *Clin Pharm* 2:213-222, 1983.
9. Waldvogel FA, Vasey H: Osteomyelitis: the past decade. *N Engl J Med* 303:360-370, 1980.
10. Cierny G, Mader JT, Penninck A: A clinical staging system for adult osteomyelitis. *Contemp Orthop* 10:17, 1985.
11. Buckholz JM: The surgical management of osteomyelitis: with special reference to a surgical classification. *J Foot Surg* 26 (Suppl): S17, 1985.
12. Jacobs JC: Acute osteomyelitis medical management in children. *NY State J Med* 78:910-912, 1978.
13. Mackowiak PA, Jones SR, Smith JW: Diagnostic valve of sinus tract cultures in chronic osteomyelitis. *JAMA* 239:26, 1978.
14. Morrey BF, Peterson HA: Hematogenous pyogenic osteomyelitis in children. *Orthop Clin North Am* 6:923-934, 1975.
15. Nade S: Choice of antibiotics in management of acute osteomyelitis and acute septic arthritis in children. *Arch Dis Child* 52:679-682, 1977.
16. Hall JE, Silverstein EA: Acute hematogenous osteomyelitis. *Pediatrics* 31:1033, 1963.
17. Pancoast SJ, Neu HC: Osteomyelitis—the initial treatment is crucial. *Med Times* 108:4, 1980.
18. Fitzgerald RH Jr, Nolan DR, Ilstrup DM, Van Scoy RE, Washington JA, Coventry MB: Deep wound sepsis following total hip arthroplasty. *J Bone Joint Surg* 59A:847-855, 1977.
19. Dombrowski ET, Dunn AW: Treatment of osteomyelitis by debridement and closed wound irrigation-suction. *Clin Orthop* 43:215-231, 1965.
20. Waldvogel FA: Treatment of osteomyelitis and septic arthritis. *Bull NY Acad Med* 58:733-746, 1982.
21. McLaughlin RE, Whitehill R: Evaluation of the painful hip by aspiration and arthrography. *Surg Gynecol Obstet* 144:381-387, 1977.
22. Ericson C, Lingren L, Lindberg L: Cloxacillin in the prophylaxis of post-operative infections of the hip. *J Bone Joint Surg* 55A:808-813, 1973.
23. Burnett JW, Gustile RB, Williams DN, Kind AC: Prophylactic antibiotics in hip fractures. *J Bone Joint Surg* 62A:457-461, 1980.
24. Nelson JP: Musculoskeletal infection. *Surg Clin North Am* 60:213-222, 1980.
25. Downes EM: Late infection after total hip replacement. *J Bone Joint Surg* 59B:42, 1977.
26. Kalish SR, Mahan KT: Complications following puncture wounds of the foot. *J Am Podiatry Assoc* 72:497-504, 1982.
27. Norden CW: Osteomyelitis. In Mandell GL, Douglas RG, Bennett JE (eds): *Principles and Practices of Infectious Diseases*. New York, John Wiley & Sons, 1979, pp 946-956.
28. Hall BB, Fitzgerald RH, Rosenblatt JE: Anaerobic osteomyelitis. *J Bone Joint Surg* 65A:30-35, 1983.
29. Raff MJ, Melo JC: Anaerobic osteomyelitis. *Medicine* 57:83-103, 1978.
30. Chow AW, Montgomerie JZ, Guze LB: Parental clindamycin therapy for severe anaerobic infections. *Arch Intern Med* 134:78-82, 1974.
31. Adeyokunna A, Hendrickse RG: Salmonella osteomyelitis in childhood: a report of 63 cases seen in Nigeria of whom 57 had sickle cell anemia. *Arch Dis Child* 55:175-184, 1984.
32. Lloveras J, Peterson PK, Simmons RL, NaJarian JS: Mycobacterial infections in renal transplant recipients. *Arch Intern Med* 142:888-892, 1982.
33. Bourguisnon RL, Walsh AF, Flynn JL, Baro C, Spinos E: Fusarium species osteomyelitis. *J Bone Joint Surg* 58A:722, 1976.
34. Porat S, Brezis M, Kopolovic J: Salmonella typhi osteomyelitis long after a fracture. *J Bone Joint Surg* 59A:687-689, 1977.
35. Tack KJ, Rhame FS, Brown B, Thompson RC: Aspergillus osteomyelitis. *Am J Med* 73:295-300, 1982.
36. Jergesen FH: Orthopedis. In Dunphy JE, Way LW (eds): *Current Surgical Diagnosis and Treatment*. Los Altos, CA, Lange Medical Publications, 1979, pp 907-978.
37. McHenry MC, Alfid RJ, Wilde AH, Levine MI, Medlar RC: Hematogenous osteomyelitis. *Cleve Clin Q* 42:125-153, 1975.
38. Hart UL: Acute hematogenous osteomyelitis in children. *JAMA* 41:671-680, 1937.
39. Trueta J: The three types of acute hematogenous osteomyelitis. *J Bone Joint Surg* 41B:671-680, 1959.
40. Winters JL, Cahen I: Acute hematogenous osteomyelitis: a review of sixty-six cases. *J Bone Joint Surg* 42A:691-704, 1960.
41. Fletcher BD, Scoles PV, Nelson AD: Osteomyelitis in children: detection by magnetic resonance. *Radiology* 150:57-60, 1984.
42. Fitzgerald RH Jr, Cowen JDE: Puncture wounds of the foot. *Orthop Clin North Am* 6:965-972, 1975.
43. Medoff G: Current concepts in the treatment of osteomyelitis. *Postgrad Med* 58:157-161, 1975.
44. Hetherington VJ: Technetium and combined gallium and technetium scans in the neurotrophic foot. *J Am Podiatry Assoc* 72:458-463, 1982.
45. Pinckney LE, Currarino G, Kennedy LA: The stubbed great toe: a cause of occult compound fracture and infection. *Radiology* 138:375-377, 1981.
46. Ross R, Ewald FD: Complications of total hip replacement arthroplasty in patients with rheumatoid arthritis. *J Bone Joint Surg* 58A:1130-1133, 1976.
47. Smith LW: Bone and joint infections. In Mandell GL, Douglas RG, Bennett JE (eds): *Principles and Practices of Infectious Diseases*. New York, John Wiley & Sons, 1979, pp 933-945.
48. Petty W: The effect of methylmethacrylate in chemotaxis of polymorphonuclear leukocytes. *J Bone Joint Surg* 60A:492-498, 1978.
49. Petty W: The effect of methylmethacrylate on bacterial phagocytosis and killing of human polymorphonuclear leukocytes. *J Bone Joint Surg* 60A:752-757, 1978.
50. Dunbleton JH, Black J: *An Introduction to Orthopedic Materials*. Springfield, IL, Charles C Thomas, 1975, pp 57-65.
51. Patzakis MJ, Ivler DL: Section III: Extra-abdominal surgery: antibiotic and bacteriologic considerations in open fractures. *South Med J* 70:46-48, 1977.
52. Ahlberg A, Carlsson AS, Lindberg L: Hematogenous infection in total joint replacement. *Clin Orthop* 137:69-75, 1978.

53. D'Ambrosia RD, Shoji H, Heater R: Secondarily infected total joint replacements by hematogenous spread. *J Bone Joint Surg* 58A:450, 1976.

54. Kahn DS, Pritzker KH: The pathophysiology of bone infection. *Clin Orthop* 96:12-19, 1973.

55. Harris NH: Some problems in the diagnosis and treatment of acute osteomyelitis. *J Bone Joint Surg* 42B:535, 1960.

56. Burton DS, Schurman DJ: Hematogenous infection in bilateral total hip arthroplasty. *J Bone Joint Surg* 57A:1004-1005, 1975.

57. Vanore J, O'Keefe R, Pikscher I: Silastic implant arthroplasty, complications and their classification. *J Am Podiatry Assoc* 74:423-433, 1984.

58. Charnley J: Post-operative infection after total hip replacement with special reference to air contamination in the operating room. *Clin Orthop* 87:167, 1972.

59. Ainscow DAP, Denham RA: The risk of hematogenous infection in total joint replacements. *J Bone Joint Surg* 66B:580-582, 1984.

60. Carlsson AS, Lidgren L, Lindberg L: Prophylactic antibiotics against early and late deep infections after total hip replacement. *Acta Orthop Scand* 48:405, 1977.

61. Riegler H, Routson G: Complications of deep puncture wounds of the foot. *J Trauma* 19:18, 1979.

62. Brause BD: Infected total knee replacement: diagnostic, therapeutic and prophylactic considerations. *Orthop Clin North Am* 13:245-249, 1982.

63. Fitzgerald RH (ed): *Musculoskeletal Infections, Recognition, Prevention and Management—Current Concepts in the Prevention and Management of the Infected Total Joint Arthroplasty.* New York, Adis Press, 1983, vol 3, p 6.

64. Inman RD, Gallegos KV, Brause BD, Redecha PB, Christian CL: Clinical and microbial features of prosthetic joint infection. *Am J Med* 77:47-52, 1984.

65. Reckling FW, Asler MA, Dillon WL: A longitudinal study of the radio-lucent line at the bone cement interface following total joint replacement procedures. *J Bone Joint Surg* 59A:355, 1977.

66. Gristina AG, Kolkin J: Current concepts review, total joint replacement and sepsis. *J Bone Joint Surg* 65A:128-134, 1983.

67. Eftekhar NS: Wound infection complications, total hip joint arthroplasty. Scope of the problem, and its diagnosis. *Orthop Rev* 8:49-64, 1979.

68. Hunter G, Dandy D: The natural history of the patient with an infected total hip replacement. *J Bone Joint Surg* 59A:847-855, 1977.

69. Hall AJ: Late infection about a total knee prosthesis. *J Bone Joint Surg* 56B:144, 1977.

70. Aptekar RG, Davie JM, Cattell HS: Foreign body reaction to silicone rubber: complication of a finger joint implant. *Clin Orthop* 98:231, 1974.

71. Coleman DL, King RN, Andrade JD: The foreign body reaction: a chronic inflammatory response. *J Biomed Mater Res* 8:199, 1974.

72. Schneider R, Freiberger RH, Chase G, Helman B, Ranawat CS: Radiologic evaluation of painful joint prosthesis. *Clin Orthop* 170:156-168, 1982.

73. Otto RC, Pouliadis GP, Kumpe DA: The evaluation of pathologic alterations of juxta osseous soft tissue by xeroradiology. *Radiology* 120:297-302, 1976.

74. Shereff MJ, Jahss MH: Complication for silastic implant arthroplasty in the hallux. *Foot Ankle* 1:95, 1980.

75. Kulowski J, Perlman R: Skeletal changes in malum perforans. *Pedis Arch Surgery* 32:1-21, 1936.

76. Schlefman BS: Radiology. In McGlamry ED (ed): *Fundamentals of Foot Surgery.* Baltimore, Williams & Wilkins, 1987, pp 136-163.

77. Visser HJ, Jacobs AM, Oloff L, Drago JJ: The use of differential scintigraphy in the clinical diagnosis of osseous and soft tissue changes affecting the diabetic foot. *J Foot Surg* 23:74-85, 1984.

78. Treves S: Skeletal scintigraphy in the diagnosis of acute osteomyelitis. *Hosp Pract* 55:66-73, 1979.

79. Gelfand MJ, Silberstein EB: Radionuclide imaging: use in diagnosis of osteomyelitis in children. *JAMA* 237:245, 1977.

80. Scoles PV, Hilty MD, Sfalcranakis GN: Bone scan patterns in acute osteomyelitis. *Clin Orthop* 153:210-217, 1980.

81. Howie DW, Savage JP, Wilson TG, Paterson D: The technetium phosphate bone scan in the diagnosis of osteomyelitis in childhood. *J Bone Joint Surg* 65A:431-437, 1983.

82. Williamson BR Jr, McLaughlin RE, Gwo-Jaw W, Miller CW, Teates DC, Bray ST: Radionuclide bone imaging as a means of differentiating loosening and infection in patients with painful total hip prosthesis. *Radiology* 133:723-725, 1979.

83. Fordham EW, Ramachandran PC: Radionuclide imaging of osseous trauma. *Semin Nucl Med* 4:411-429, 1974.

84. Rosenthal L, Lisbona R, Hernandez M, Hadjipavlou A: 99mtc-PP and 67/Ga imaging following insertion of orthopedic devices. *Radiology* 133:717-721, 1979.

85. Eymontt MJ, Alavi A, Dalinka MK, Kyle GC: Bone scintigraphy in diabetic osteoarthropathy. *Radiology* 140:475-477, 1981.

86. Gilday DL, Paul DJ, Paterson J: Diagnosis of osteomyelitis in children by combined blood pool and bone imaging. *Radiology* 117:331-335, 1975.

87. Deysine M, Rafkin H, Teicher I, Silver L, Robinson R, Manley J, Aufses AH: Diagnosis of chronic and postoperative osteomyelitis with gallium 67 citrate scans. *Am J Surg* 129:632-635, 1975.

88. Schauwecker DS, Park HM, Mock BH, Burt RW, Kerwick CB, Ruoff AC, Wellman HN: Evaluation of complicating osteomyelitis with tc99M MDP, IN-111 granulocytes, and Ga-67 citrate. *J Nucl Med* 25:849-853, 1975.

89. Staab EV, McCartney WH: Role of gallium 67 in inflammatory disease. *Semin Nucl Med* 7:219-234, 1978.

90. Tsan M, Chen W, Scheffel A, Gray HW: Studies of gallium accumulation in inflammatory lesions. 1. Gallium uptake by PMN leukocytes. *J Nucl Med Allied Sci* 19:34, 1977.

91. Duszynski DO, Kuhn JP, Afshani E, Riddlesberger MM: Early radionuclide diagnosis of acute osteomyelitis. *Radiology* 117: 337-340, 1975.

92. Propst-Proctor SL, Dillingham MF, McDougall IR, Goodwin D: The white blood cell scan in orthopedics. *Clin Orthop* 168:157-165, 1982.

93. McAfee JG, Thakus M: Survey of radioactive agents for in vitro labeling of phagocytic leukocytes II particles. *J Nucl Med* 17:488, 1976.

94. Sinn H, Silvester DJ: Simplified cell labelling with indium-111 acetylacetone. *Br J Radiol* 52:758-759, 1979.

95. Handmaker H, Leonards R: The bone scan in inflammatory osseous disease. *Semin Nucl Med* 6:95-105, 1976.

96. Shafer RB, Edeburn GF: Can the three-phase bone scan differentiate osteomyelitis from metabolic or metastatic bone disease. *Clin Nucl Med* 9:343-349, 1984.

97. Gilday DL: Problems in the scintigraphic detection of osteomyelitis. *Radiology* 135:791, 1980.

98. Conway JJ: Radionuclide bone imaging in pediatrics. *Pediatr Clin North Am* 24:701, 1977.

99. Gelfand MJ, Silberstein EB: Radionuclide imaging: use in diagnosis of osteomyelitis in children. *JAMA* 237:245, 1977.

100. Littenberg R, Tahita R, Alagraki N, Halpern SE: Gallium-67 for localization of lytic lesions. *Ann Intern Med* 79:403, 1973.

101. Ganel A, Horozowski H, Zaltzar S, Farie I: Sequential use of TC-99 MDP and Ga-67 imaging in bone infection. *Orthop Rev* 18:74, 1981.

102. Georgi P, Sinn H, Wellmann H, Strauss L, Sturm V: Clinical applications of In-111 acetylacetone labelled blood cells. In *Medical Radionuclide Imaging.* Vienna, Austria, International Atomic Energy Agency, 1981, vol 1, pp 477-480.

103. Jones DC, Cady RB: Cold bone scans in acute osteomyelitis. *J Bone Joint Surg* 63B:376-378, 1981.

104. Fletcher BD, Scoles PV, Nelson AD: Osteomyelitis in children: detection by magnetic resonance. *Radiology* 150:57-60, 1984.

105. Murray WR, Rodrigo JJ: Arthrography for assessment of pain after total hip replacement. *J Bone Joint Surg* 57A:1060, 1975.

106. McLaughlin RE, Whitehill R: Evaluation of the painful hip by aspiration and arthrography. *Surg Gynecol Obstet* 144:381-386, 1977.

107. Weiss MI, Coleman RE, McKee EK, Turner RJ: Radiology, radionuclide imaging and arthrography in evaluation of total hip and knee replacement. *Radiology* 128:677-682, 1978.

108. Goldman F, Manzi J, Carver A, Torre R, Richter R: Sinography in diagnosis of foot infections. *J Am Podiatry Assoc* 71:497-502, 1981.

109. Kuhn JP, Berger PE: Computed tomography diagnosis of osteomyelitis. *Radiology* 130:503-506, 1979.

110. Otto RC, Pouliadis GP, Kumpe DA: The evaluation of pathologic alterations of juxta osseous soft tissue by xeroradiography. *Radiology* 120:297-302, 1976.

111. Campbell CJ, Roach J, Grisolia A: A comparative study of xeroroentgenography and routine roentgenography in the recording of roentgen images of bone specimens. *J Bone Joint Surg* 39A:577-582, 1957.

112. Smith JK, Weiner SL: Osteomyelitis—drug therapy. *Hospitals* 6:63-66, 1981.
113. Bowers WH, Wilson FC, Greene WB: Antibiotic prophylaxis in experimental bone infections. *J Bone Joint Surg* 55A:795-807, 1973.
114. Eliopoulos GM, Moellering RC: Principles of antibiotic therapy. *Med Clin North Am* 66:3-15, 1982.
115. Hunt TK, Jawetz E: Inflammation, infection, and antibiotics: In Dunphy JE, Way LE (eds): *Current Surgical Diagnosis and Treatment*. Los Altos, CA, Lange Medical Publications, 1979, pp 122-146.
116. Meyer TL, Kieger AB, Smith WS: Antibiotic management of staphylococcal osteomyelitis, with particular reference to antibiotic-resistant infections. *J Bone Joint Surg* 47A:285, 1965.
117. Wilkowske CJ, Hermans PE: Actions and uses of antimicrobial agents in the treatment of musculoskeletal infections. *Orthop Clin North Am* 6:1129, 1975.
118. Barza M: Antimicrobial spectrum, pharmacology and therapeutic use of antibiotics. Part 2: Penicillins. In Miller RR, Greenblatt RB (eds): *Drug Therapy Reviews*. Philadelphia, Harper & Row, 1979, vol 2, pp 90-112.
119. Fekety R: Vancomycin. *Med Clin North Am* 66:175-181, 1982.
120. Nelson JP: Musculoskeletal infection. *Surg Clin North Am* 60:213-222, 1980.
121. Kelly PJ, Wilkowske CJ, Washington JA: Chronic osteomyelitis in the adult. *Curr Pract Orthop Surg* 6:120-130, 1975.
122. Hagen R: Osteomyelitis in a general surgical department. *Acta Orthop Scand* 40:673-674, 1969.
123. Neule HW, Stern PJ, Kreilein JG, Gregory RO, Webster KL: Complications of muscle-flap transposition for traumatic defects of the leg. *Plast Reconstr Surg* 4:512-517, 1983.
124. Ger R, Efron G: New operative approach in the treatment of chronic osteomyelitis of the tibial diaphysis: a preliminary report. *Clin Orthop* 70:165, 1970.
125. Serafin D, Sabatier RE, Morris RL, Georgiade NG: Reconstruction of the lower extremity with vascularized composite tissue: improved tissue survival and specific indications. *Plast Reconstr Surg* 66:230, 1980.
126. Klemm K: Treatment of chronic bone infections with gentamicin-PMMA chains and beads. *Accident Surg* 1:20, 1976.
127. Vecsei V, Barquet A: Treatment of chronic osteomyelitis by necrectomy and gentamicin-PMMA beads. *Clin Orthop* 159:201-207, 1981.
128. Ritzerfeld W: Discussions on infection treatment. In Contzen H (ed): *Munich Symposium on Accident Surgery*. Erlangen, VLE Verlag, 1977.
129. Ashe G: Suction drainage or gentamicin PMMA beads in the treatment of infected osteosynthesis. *Uhfallheikunde* 81:463, 1978.
130. Marcinko DE: Gentamicin impregnated PMMA beads: an introduction and review. *J Foot Surg* 24:116-121, 1985.
131. Wassner UJ: Principles and results of the treatment of soft tissue infections with Septopal. In *Local Antibiotic Treatment in Osteomyelitis and Soft Tissue Infections*. Amsterdam, Netherlands, Excerpta Medica, 1981.
132. Heard GR, Oloff LM: Antibiotic impregnated bone cement: an "in vitro" comparative analysis. *J Foot Surg* 28:54-59, 1989.
133. Jenny G, Taglang G: Local bone infection treatment with gentamicin PMMA-beads. *Beitr Orthop Traumatol* 27:3, 1980.
134. Pressman M: Continuous closed suction irrigation following post-operative infection of Silastic implant. *J Am Podiatry Assoc* 67:746-750, 1977.
135. Schwartz NH, Marcinko DE: Suction irrigation in podiatric surgery—construction and use of a dependable closed system. *J Am Podiatr Med Assoc* 74:216-221, 1984.
136. Dawyer RB, Eyring FJ: Intermittent closed suction-irrigation treatment of osteomyelitis. *Clin Orthop* 88:80, 1972.
137. Compere EL, Metzger WI, Mitra RN: The treatment of pyogenic bone and joint infections by closed irrigation with a non-toxic detergent and one or more antibiotics. *J Bone Joint Surg* 49A:614, 1967.
138. Sorto LA: The infected implant. *Clin Podiatry* 1:199-209, 1984.
139. Dilmaghani A, Close JR, Rhinelander FW: Method for closed irrigation and suction therapy in deep wound infections: preliminary report. *J Bone Joint Surg* 51A:323, 1969.
140. Shannon J, Woolhouse F, Eisinger P: The treatment of chronic osteomyelitis by saucerization and immediate skin grafting. *Clin Orthop* 96:98, 1973.
141. Juttman JW, Van der Slikke W: The treatment of osteitis complicating tibial fractures. *Br J Accident Surg* 13:210-215, 1982.
142. Meyer S, Weiland AJ, Willenegger II: The treatment of infected nonunion of fractures of long bones. *J Bone Joint Surg* 57A:836, 1975.
143. Coleman HM, Bateman JE, Dale GM, Starr DE: Cancellous bone grafts for infected bone defects: single stage procedure. *Surg Gynecol Obstet* 83:392, 1946.
144. McElvenny RT: The use of closed circulation and suction in the treatment of chronically infected, acutely infected, and potentially infected wounds. *Am J Orthop* 3:86-154, 1961.
145. Murray RA: Importance of soft tissue to treatment of chronic osteomyelitis. *JAMA* 180:198, 1962.
146. Dumbleton JH, Black J: *An Introduction to Orthopedic Materials*. Springfield, IL, Charles C Thomas, 1975, pp 162-185.
147. Buckholz HW, Elson RA, Engelbrecht E, Lodenkamper H, Rottger J, Siegel A: Management of deep infection of total hip replacement. *J Bone Joint Surg* 63B:342-353, 1981.
148. Willert HG, Judwig J, Semlitsch M: Reactions of bone to methylmethacrylate after hip arthroplasty. *J Bone Joint Surg* 56A:1363-1382, 1974.
149. Lifeso RM, Al-Saati F: The treatment of infected and uninfected nonunion. *J Bone Joint Surg* 66B:573-579, 1984.
150. Weber BG, Cech O: *Pseudoarthrosis, Pathology. Biomechanical Therapy, Results*. Berne, Switzerland, Hans Huber, 1976, pp 243-273.
151. McNeur JC: The management of open skeletal trauma with particular reference to internal fixation. *J Bone Joint Surg* 52B:54-60, 1970.
152. Alho A, Koskinen EVS, Malmberg H: Osteomyelitis in non-operative and operative fracture treatment: a survey of 49 adult patients. *Clin Orthop* 82:123-133, 1972.
153. Macausland WR, Eaton RG: The management of sepsis following intramedullary fixation of fractures of the femur. *J Bone Joint Surg* 45A:1643-1653, 1963.
154. Vasconez LO, Bostwick J, McGraw JB: Coverage of exposed bone by muscle transposition and skin grafting. *Plast Reconstr Surg* 53:526, 1974.
155. Barfred T, Reumert T: Myoplast for covering exposed bone of joints on the lower leg. *Acta Orthop Scand* 44:532, 1973.
156. Gristina AG, Kolkin J: Current concepts review; total joint replacement and sepsis. *J Bone Joint Surg* 65A:128-133, 1983.
157. Boland AL Jr: Acute hematogenous osteomyelitis. *Orthop Clin North Am* 3:225, 1972.
158. Tetzlaff TR, McCraken GH, Nelson JD: Oral antibiotic therapy for skeletal infections of children. Part 2. Therapy of osteomyelitis and supportive arthritis. *J Pediatr* 92:485-490, 1978.
159. Bryson YJ, Connor JD, Laclerc M, Giammona ST, James DC: High dose oral dicloxacillin treatment of acute staphylococcal osteomyelitis in children. *J Pediatr* 94:673-675, 1979.
160. Watanakunakorn C: Treatment of infections due to methicillin-resistant *Staph aureus*. *Ann Intern Med* 97:376-378, 1982.
161. Sande MA, Mandell GL: Antimicrobial agents: general considerations. In Goodman LS, Gillman AZ (eds): *The Pharmacological Basis of Therapeutics*. New York, Macmillan, 1980, pp 1080-1105.
162. Sande MA, Mandell GL: Antimicrobial agents:the aminoglycosides. In Goodman LS, Gillman AZ (eds): *The Pharmacological Basis of Therapeutics*. New York, MacMillan, 1980, pp 1162-1180.
163. Hodgkin UG: Antibiotics in the treatment of chronic staphlococcal osteomyelitis. *South Med J* 68:817-823, 1975.
164. Grieco MH: Antibiotic resistance. *Med Clin North Am* 66:25-37, 1982.
165. Ellner PD: Laboratory procedures to determine infection in orthopedic surgery. *Orthop Rev* 8:37-45, 1975.
166. Quintillani R, French M, Nightingale CH: First and second generation cephalosporins. *Med Clin North Am* 66:183-197, 1983.
167. Barry AL, Thornberry C, Jones RN, Gerlaut EH: In vitro evaluation of LY127935 in comparison with 11 related beta-lactam compounds and two aminoglycosides. *Curr Chemother Infect Dis* 1:76-77, 1979.
168. Poretz DM, Eron LJ, Goldenberg RI, Fenton AG, Rising J, Sparks S: Intravenous antibiotic therapy in an outpatient setting. *JAMA* 248:336-339, 1982.
169. Kind AC, Williams DN, Persons G, Gibson JA: Intravenous antibiotic therapy at home. *Arch Intern Med* 139:413-415, 1939.
170. Davis JC, Hunt DK: *Hyperbaric Oxygen Therapy: Human Series*. Bethesda MD, Undersea Medical Society, 1977, pp 221-224.
171. Becker RO, Spadaro JA: Treatment of orthopedic infections with electrically generated silver ions. *J Bone Joint Surg* 60A:871-881, 1978.
172. Keys JA: Amputations for chronic osteomyelitis. *J Bone Joint Surg* 26:350, 1944.

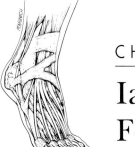

CHAPTER **71**

Iatrogenic Deformities in Foot Surgery

Dennis E. Martin, D.P.M.
E. Dalton McGlamry, D.P.M.

All surgeons, regardless of personal skill or the difficulty of a given procedure, must at some point deal with a deformity that was created by prior surgery. Unacceptable results are a consequence that all surgeons will occasionally face. Evaluation of the iatrogenic deformity requires honesty, imagination, and a thorough knowledge of the principal deforming influences. In fact, much can be learned about normal function and anatomy by evaluating surgical complications.

Iatrogenic structural complications after foot surgery can usually be classified into one or a combination of two broad categories. The original deformity may return or a secondary site of pathosis may develop as a result of the initial procedure. Complications may be attributable to inappropriate choice of the original procedure, poor technical execution of the procedure, a postoperative complication, or poor postoperative compliance by the patient. The genesis of the complication will greatly influence the approach to secondary surgical repair.

When planning secondary reconstruction, one must not only evaluate the current status of the foot but also attempt to trace the pathological history prior to the original procedure. In many instances an anatomically normal foot once existed but was subsequently altered by distorted mechanics. In other cases, the foot may have been structurally abnormal prior to surgical intervention (i.e., congenital or traumatic deformities). It will be important to make this distinction, as well as to develop an appreciation of the abnormal forces that have been acting on the foot to leave it in the state in which it is found. Although a return to normal structural alignment and function may be unrealistic, the goal of surgery should be to restore a functional symptom-free foot.

The cases that follow represent a cross-section of problems, each of which might have been prevented by careful preoperative planning and attention to technical detail. To add a sense of order, the discussion is divided into two parts: iatrogenic forefoot deformities and iatrogenic rearfoot sefomities.

IATROGENIC FOREFOOT DEFORMITIES

The forefoot presents a complex combination of anatomy and function. The myriad of osseous and soft tissue structures within the forefoot must act in concert with each other and with the intricate mechanics of the rearfoot to adapt to a variety of daily gait and activity requirements. When this balance is disrupted, whether it be from biomechanical, pathological, traumatic, or other mechanisms, a pathologic forefoot results. Depending on the feasibility of conservative therapy, surgical intervention may be necessary to repair the pathologic condition.

When one is planning surgical management of iatrogenic complications, it is important to determine whether the existing disorders are a result of continuing uncorrected pathological influences, a result of the original surgical procedure, or a combination of the two. Secondary procedures may need to address the original pathological processes that are still ongoing. In other instances, one will need to reverse the original procedure. In more severe cases, both the original pathosis and secondary complications will need to be rectified.

Three basic goals should be kept in mind as plans for secondary reconstruction are being made: *(a)* balanced metatarsal loading, *(b)* establishment of a functional metatarsophalangeal joint, and *(c)* creation of flexor power to a stable digit (1). These goals will be illustrated and more fully defined through a series of case studies.

The cases that follow demonstrate iatrogenic deformities occurring at various levels of the forefoot, including the digits, metatarsophalangeal joints, central (second, third, and fourth) metatarsals and the first and fifth metatarsals.

CASE 1

History and Objective Findings

A 28-year-old woman had recurrent bilateral digital deformities and lesser metatarsalgia. Approximately 19 months earlier she had undergone bilateral foot surgery for correction of multiple hammertoe deformities. The procedures performed included proximal phalangeal base resections of the second, third, and fourth digits on both feet. Since that time, the patient had continued to experience pain dorsally over the proximal interphalangeal joints of all the lesser digits as well as plantarly under the metatarsal heads. Although the recurrent deformities were bilateral, they were much more severe in the left foot.

Objectively, the patient demonstrated floating toe deformities with obvious extensor contracture at the second, third, and fourth digits on the left foot (Fig. 71.1). A moderate amount of hyperkeratosis was noted plantarly under metatarsal heads 2, 3, and 4, as well as dorsally over the proximal interphalangeal joints. Other abnormalities included mild hallux valgus deformity and an underlapping and varus de-

formity of the fifth digit. The patient's gait exhibited a significant antalgic limp on the left extremity. Radiographic examination revealed that the proximal phalangeal bases of the second, third, and fourth digits were absent (Fig. 71.2). Contractures were noted at both the interphalangeal and metatarsophalangeal joint level, making the floating toes quite obvious. Mild hallux abducto valgus was also evident.

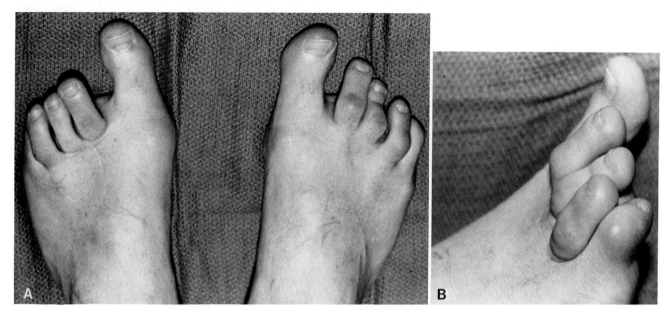

Figure 71.1. **A.** Dorsal view demonstrates floating toe deformities on the second, third, and fourth digits. **B.** Non-weight-bearing lateral view shows severe dorsal contracture of the intermediate toes.

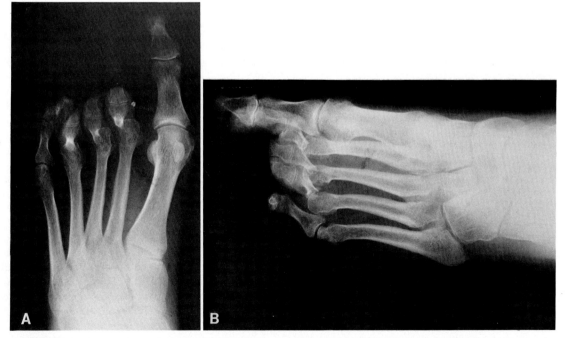

Figure 71.2. **A.** Preoperative dorsoplantar radiograph. Note the contracted lesser digits with absence of phalangeal bases. **B.** Preoperative oblique view shows degree of digital deformities.

Discussion and Treatment Options

In view of this patient's clinical and radiographic evaluation, aggressive salvage procedures, such as panmetatarsal head resections and digital stabilizations, would be feasible. This would allow the surgeon to create a balanced metatarsal load, reconstruct functional and symptom-free metatarsophalangeal joints, and re-establish flexor power to the digits by converting the long flexors to plantarflexors at the metatarsophalangeal joint. However, because of the patient's age, an alternative approach was presented with the understanding that if it were not successful then the salvage procedure would be required.

The alternative surgery included digital stabilizations by means of end-to-end arthrodesis of the proximal interphalangeal joints and transfer with reattachment of the long flexor tendons into the stumps of the proximal phalanges of the second, third, and fourth digits (Fig. 71.3). To help re-establish a functional metatarsophalangeal joint and re-create balanced metatarsal loading, metatarsophalangeal joint capsulotomies and plantar adhesiotomies were performed in conjunction with the digital arthrodeses (Fig. 71.4). After the flexor tendons were bluntly isolated, they were sutured into plantar drill holes in their respective phalangeal stumps under physiologic tension, with each digit held in a rectus position (Fig. 71.5). Kirschner wires were delivered through the metatarsophalangeal joints to help maintain the desired digital alignment. A derotation arthroplasty of the fifth proximal interphalangeal joint and an Austin bunionectomy of the first metatarsal were also performed. The first metatarsal osteotomy was oriented to allow for both lateral and plantar transposition of the capital fragment. This latter maneuver should aid in re-establishing balanced metatarsal loading by forcing the first ray to assume its share of weight bearing. Postoperative radiographs reveal excellent digital alignment with satisfactory wire position (Fig. 71.6).

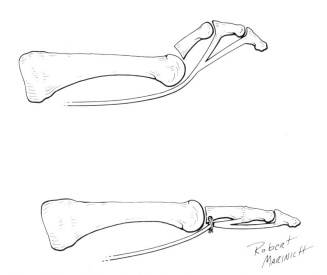

Figure 71.3. Attachment of the long flexor tendon into the proximal phalangeal stump will aid in stabilizing the digit and allow for toe purchase.

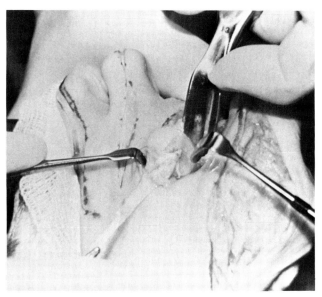

Figure 71.4. Use of the McGlamry metatarsal elevator to free any plantar adhesions.

Six months postoperatively, the patient related a dramatic relief of pain and was essentially free of symptoms. Clinical examination showed excellent maintenance of digital alignment and resolution of plantar keratoses (Fig. 71.7).

CASE 2

History and Objective Findings

A 63-year-old woman complained of recurrent digital pain and deformity of all the lesser digits on the right foot. Approximately 6 months previously, she had undergone surgical reconstruction for multiple digital contractures, including a medially dislocated second metatarsophalangeal joint (Fig. 71.8). The initial procedures included digital stabilization with peg-in-hole arthrodesis and metatarsophalangeal joint capsulorrhaphy of the second, third, and fourth digits. To aid in relocating the medially dislocated flexor plate apparatus of the second ray, an eversion capsulorrhaphy was performed through a combination of dorsal and plantar incisions (Fig. 71.9). A derotational arthroplasty was performed at the fifth proximal interphalangeal joint. Kirschner wire (K-wire) fixation was used across all the metatarsophalangeal joints to maintain the toes in slightly overcorrected alignment (Fig. 71.10).

The patient's initial postoperative course was essentially unremarkable with the exception of a moderate amount of persistent edema over the dorsal aspect of all the lesser digits. The K-wires were backed across the metatarsophalangeal joints into the toes at 3½ weeks and were completely removed from the digits at 6 weeks. At approximately 10 weeks, the dorsal edema persisted and severe tonic flexion contractures were noted involving toes 2 through 5. At the metatarsophalangeal joint level, motion was extremely lim-

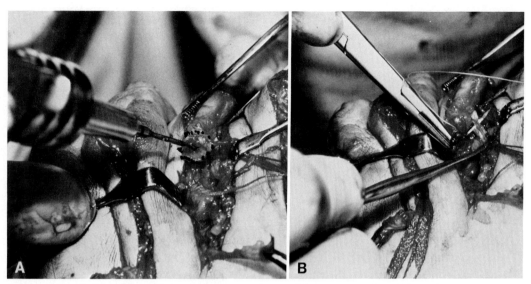

Figure 71.5. **A** and **B.** Intraoperative reattachment of flexor apparatus into phalangeal stump.

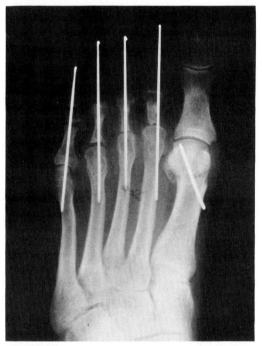

Figure 71.6. Immediate postoperative radiographs show rectus alignment to all digits with Kirschner wires across the metatarsophalangeal joints.

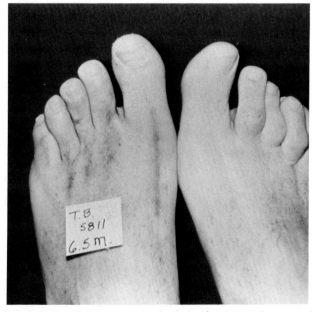

Figure 71.7. Clinical appearance 6 months after surgery shows good maintenance of digital alignment.

ited and a progressive abductus was evident. A trial of conservative therapy was attempted, including digital strappings, manipulation and stretching, and diathermy. Three months postoperatively, the lesser metatarsophalangeal joint limitus and abductus deformities were severe and nonreducible. The flexor plate apparatus of each ray had obviously dislocated laterally under the respective metatarsal heads. The cause of this dislocation was never definitively

identified. The patient also exhibited a significant hallux limitus deformity on the same foot (Fig. 71.11).

Discussion and Treatment Options

Because of the extensive soft tissue contractures and subsequent structural alterations throughout the entire forefoot, treatment options were limited. The patient had es-

Figure 71.8. Radiographic appearance before initial surgery demonstrates digital deformities with medially dislocated second metatarsophalangeal joint. The third metatarsophalangeal joint shows only mild adductus tendency.

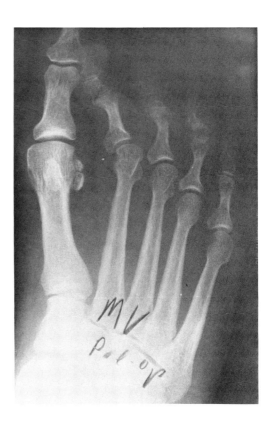

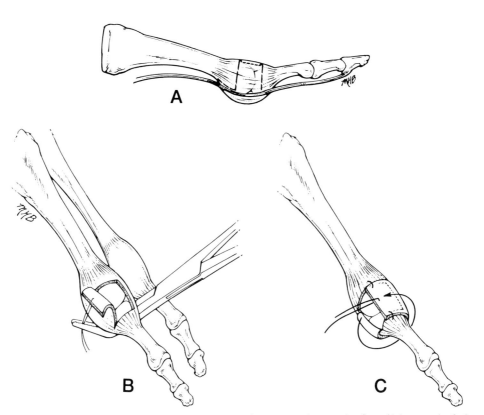

Figure 71.9. Illustration demonstrating eversion capsulorrhaphy technique. **A.** Flexor tendon displaced to side of joint. **B.** Capsulorrhaphy forceps grasping eversion flap of joint capsule. **C.** Capsular flap anchored laterally to retain the flexor apparatus under metatarsophalangeal joint.

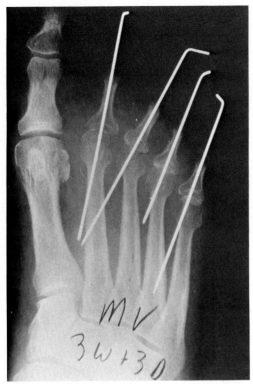

Figure 71.10. Postoperative radiograph 3 weeks 3 days after original digital reconstruction. Note the intentionally overcorrected position of the lesser digits.

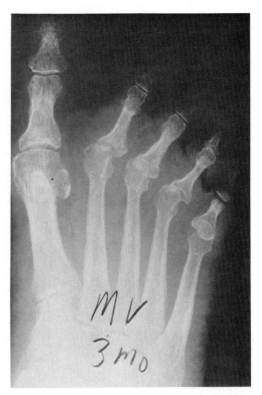

Figure 71.11. At 3 months a dorsoplantar radiograph demonstrates severe lateral angulation of the lesser metatarsophalangeal joints. Early degenerative changes are also noted at the first metatarsophalangeal joint.

sentially lost all motion at the metatarsophalangeal joint level. Secondary reconstruction in this circumstance requires aggressive arthroplasty techniques.

To restore an adequate pain-free range of motion to the lesser metatarsophalangeal joints, a panmetatarsal head resection was performed. Care was taken to develop a normal metatarsal parabola with an even distribution of weight plantarly. To restore a rectus digital alignment, the laterally dislocated flexor plates were reduced manually under their respective metatarsals and the toes were pinned in this position through the metatarsal stump. The hallux limitus deformity was addressed with a total implant arthroplasty of the first metatarsophalangeal joint (Fig. 71.12).

One year after the second surgery, motion at the lesser metatarsophalangeal joints had been maintained and the patient was free of symptoms. The digital alignment was satisfactory and showed no tendency toward recurrent deformity.

CASE 3

History and Objective Findings

A 44-year-old woman had undergone surgery at another medical center to alleviate a complaint of symptomatic, discrete lesions plantar to the second metatarsal heads of both feet. The surgeon at that time performed bilateral second

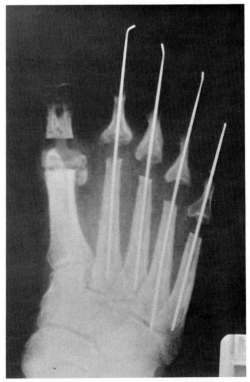

Figure 71.12. Postoperative radiograph after panmetatarsal head resections and total first metatarsophalangeal joint implant arthroplasty.

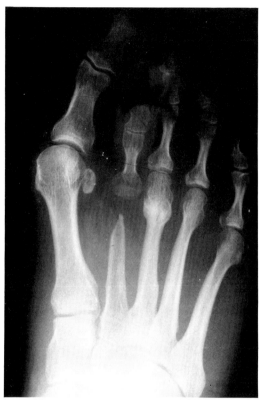

Figure 71.13. Radiograph demonstrating dramatically shortened second ray resulting from earlier metatarsal head resection.

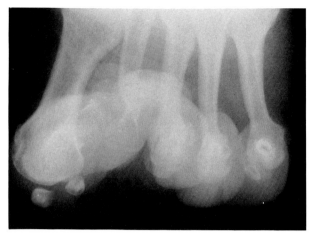

Figure 71.14. Metatarsal axial view showing disturbed transverse weight-bearing plane at metatarsal heads.

metatarsal head resections. Shortly after the initial surgery symptomatic transfer lesions developed plantar to the third metatarsal heads. A subsequent elevational osteotomy of the third metatarsal was performed. When the patient consulted us 13 years after her initial surgery, her chief complaint was of severe bilateral metatarsalgia. She was also concerned about a rapidly developing bunion deformity that had not been present before her initial surgery.

Examination demonstrated severe hyperkeratotic lesions plantar to the third and fourth metatarsal heads. A sulcus was present plantarly where the second metatarsal head had been removed. A moderate degree of hallux abducto valgus was present, along with a nonpurchasing second digit, and the patient's gait was markedly guarded. The patient had been unsuccessfully treated by conservative means and had been disabled for several years.

Radiographs demonstrate the degree of pathosis present in the patient's right foot. The dorsoplantar view (Fig. 71.13) shows a shortened second ray caused by resection of the metatarsal head and a large portion of the distal metatarsal. The shortening and associated contracture of the second digit may also be appreciated. Delayed union is evident at the osteotomy site of the third metatarsal, and the hallux has shifted into abducto valgus to occupy the space vacated by the unstable second toe. The metatarsal axial view (Fig. 71.14) demonstrates the disruption of the weight-bearing plane of the forefoot.

Discussion and Treatment Options

Several options were available for surgical reconstruction. Perhaps the easiest solution would be pan metatarsal head resections, with or without implant arthroplasty of the first metatarsophalangeal joint. However, to restore the metatarsal parabola, either the resection would have to be performed quite proximally or one of the resected metatarsal heads would have to be used as a graft to lengthen the severely shortened second metatarsal.

Another possible option might include implant arthroplasty of the first metatarsophalangeal joint after considerable shortening of the first ray combined with dorsiflexory osteotomies of the third, fourth, and possibly the fifth metatarsals. This latter approach would be difficult to control predictably.

Regardless of the metatarsal surgery chosen, fusion of the proximal interphalangeal joints of the third and fourth digits would be helpful in relieving the metatarsalgia by reducing the reverse buckling that was occurring at the metatarsophalangeal joints as a result of digital contractures.

Although the foregoing options might provide a pain-free foot, it is obvious that the ideal approach would return weight-bearing length to the shortened second metatarsal.

The approach chosen involved an autogenous bone graft to the second metatarsal, a Reverdin-McBride bunionectomy with adductor tendon transfer, and resection of the delayed union and realignment of the third metatarsal.

Autogenous bone was selected because it was thought that this would allow for more rapid incorporation of the graft. In addition, no joint capsule remained at the second metatarsophalangeal joint and consideration had to be given to the selection of a graft that would provide a suitable condylar end to the grafted metatarsal.

The graft also had to be suitable as a later recipient for implant arthroplasty, should this be necessary to restore joint motion. It was hoped that an asymptomatic pseudoarthrosis would develop, but provision had to be made for future implant arthroplasty in case it did not. To accept an implant stem, the distal aspect of the graft needed to have three strong cortical sides. The ideal donor site was judged to be the anterior aspect of the iliac crest. The dorsal cortex could be turned so that it provided a strong plantar support, and the anterior superior iliac spine could provide the strong cortical support at the distal aspect of the graft, should future implant arthroplasty be needed.

One may question the need for performing a bunion procedure in association with the bone graft. If normal function was to be restored to the second digit, then all deforming influences would have to be removed. Without correction of the hallux abducto valgus, there would always be a tendency for the second digit to be crowded into a dorsally displaced position.

Radiographs were taken on the third postoperative day after casting (Fig. 71.15). The patient's cast was bivalved so that ankle range-of-motion exercises could be initiated 10 days postoperatively. The patient bore no weight on the surgically treated foot throughout the entire recovery period.

Six months after surgery a vascular nonunion had developed at the graft site of the second metatarsal. The patient was then readmitted and surgery was performed to resect the fibrotic graft-host interface. At the same time a six-hole dynamic compression plate (DCP) was applied to

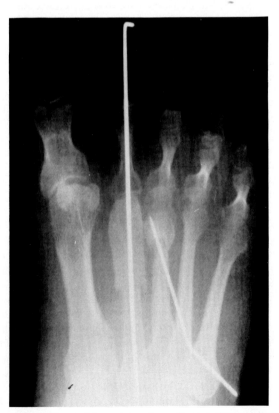

Figure 71.15. Immediate postoperative radiograph shows autogenous graft to second metatarsal and repair of third metatarsal delayed union with K-wire fixation to both.

the dorsum of the second metatarsal to provide rigid internal fixation (Fig. 71.16). It is interesting that the graft was found fully viable and quite vascular despite its fibrous union to the metatarsal stump. Two months after application of the compression plate, bony union was evident and weight bearing in a surgical shoe was initiated. Six months later the plate was removed and a lesser metatarsophalangeal joint hinge implant was inserted. The patient was able to return to comfortable walking and standing on the involved foot.

CASE 4

This case demonstrates a clinical and radiographic presentation very similar to that described in the foregoing example. However, the associated pathosis in the following example is considerably more severe.

History and Objective Findings

A 52-year-old female teacher was referred for evaluation of long-standing forefoot pain and deformity. Several years previously she had undergone surgical correction of a hallux valgus deformity as well as lesser metatarsalgia beneath the second metatarsal on the right foot. The procedures performed at that time included resection of the medial eminence of the first metatarsal, Akin osteotomy of the proximal phalanx of the hallux, and resection of the entire second digit as well as the second metatarsal head and a portion of the shaft. Since the original surgery, the patient had experienced constant forefoot pain and significant disability. Walking was limited and the patient was forced to teach from a sitting position.

On examination, the patient had a severe bunion deformity with a hallux elevatus component and with severe lesser metatarsalgia beneath the third and fourth metatarsals. Absence of the second digit with lateral deviation of the hallux was evident on clinical examination (Fig. 71.17). Compen-

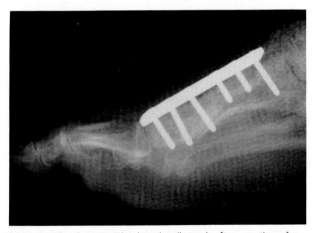

Figure 71.16. Postoperative lateral radiograph after resection of nonunion at graft interface and application of six-hole dynamic compression plate.

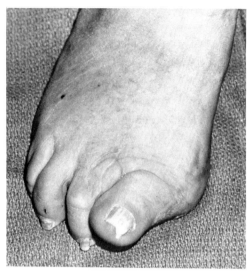

Figure 71.17. Clinical view of foot at initial presentation demonstrates absence of the second digit with extreme lateral deviation of the hallux.

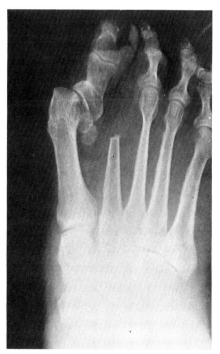

Figure 71.18. Preoperative radiograph demonstrating severe dislocation of the hallux and sesamoids into the first interspace. Also note the significant amount of second metatarsal shortening.

satory digital contractures were present at the proximal interphalangeal joints of the third, fourth, and fifth digits. The patient also exhibited a significant antalgic limp on the right extremity. Radiographic examination confirmed severe hallux valgus deformity with complete dislocation of the hallux and both sesamoids into the interspace (Fig. 71.18). The first metatarsal head had been staked, and all

of the second digit as well as the head and neck of the second metatarsal had been removed.

Discussion and Treatment Options

The list of possible treatment options for this patient was very similar to those in Case 3. The one obvious difference was the lack of a need to re-establish joint motion at the second metatarsophalangeal articulation in this case.

As in the previous case, the simplest solution would be panmetatarsal head resections with implant arthroplasty of the first metatarsophalangeal joint. However, the amount of shortening that would be required to restore a normal metatarsal parabola was once again the limiting factor to this approach, although there was the option of using a resected metatarsal head as a graft to lengthen the severely shortened second metatarsal.

Other less aggressive options might include hemi-implant arthroplasty of the first metatarsophalangeal joint and Reverdin osteotomy of the first metatarsal with excision of the fibular sesamoid. In an attempt to remove some of the retrograde buckling force occurring at the remaining lesser metatarsophalangeal joints, proximal interphalangeal joint arthrodeses could be performed on the third and fourth digits along with aggressive arthroplasty on the fifth digit.

Both of these options were rejected as failing to adequately address the pathological transfer of weight laterally under the third metatarsal. It is obvious that the ideal solution was to restore weight-bearing length and that this would involve grafting a second metatarsal. In view of the amount of shortening present, a substantial bone graft would be required.

The surgical approach chosen for this patient included a total implant arthroplasty of the first metatarsophalangeal joint with planned shortening of the hallux, peg-in-hole arthrodesis of the third and fourth digits with planned shortening, proximal interphalangeal joint arthroplasty of the fifth digit, and replacement of the second metatarsal with a frozen allogeneic osteochondral graft.

In contrast to the previous case, allogeneic bone was used in this patient. Because of the degree of shortening to the second metatarsal, it was decided to replace it with a compatible frozen osteochondral graft (Fig. 71.19). This type of graft permitted a significant degree of lengthening and provided an anatomic weight-bearing condyle at its distal end.

Because of the delay in union often associated with end-to-end grafting, such as used in the previous case, the graft-host link was varied in this patient. After adequate exposure of the entire second ray, bone was resected back to the level of the proximal shaft. The dorsal cortex and the dorsal half of the metatarsal stump was resected, leaving the plantar half of the bone intact. A matching L configuration cut was made in the metatarsal graft to allow for top-to-bottom grafting (Fig. 71.20). This type of relationship offered the advantage of greater bone-to-bone contact and allowed for the application of rigid internal compression fixation with three 2.0 mm cortical screws delivered in a dorsal-to-plantar direction and inserted in lag fashion.

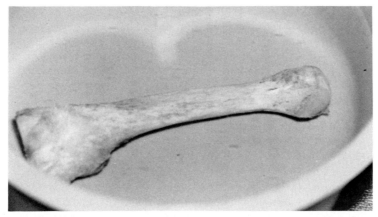

Figure 71.19. Fresh frozen allogeneic second metatarsal ready for grafting.

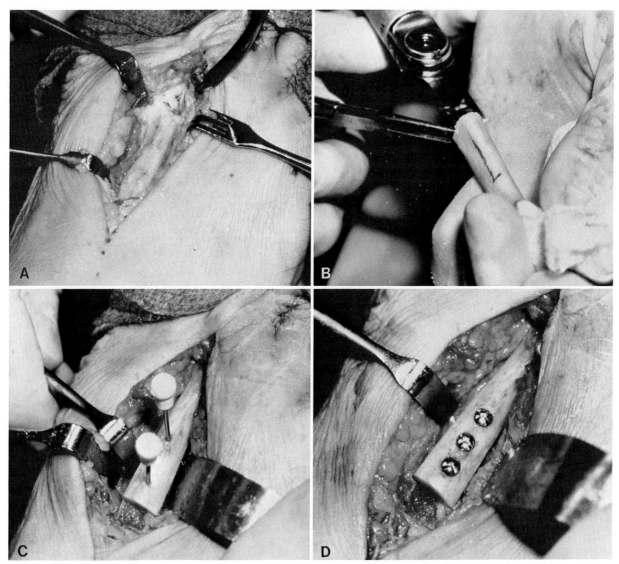

Figure 71.20. **A.** Exposure of second metatarsal stump. Note the degree of fibrosis distally at resection site. **B.** Remodeling of inverted graft into modified L configuration. **C.** Temporary fixation of graft with two K-wires. Note the top-to-bottom fit of the graft-host interface. **D.** Final fixation with three 2.0 mm cortical screws delivered from dorsal to plantar.

The combined restoration of a weight-bearing second metatarsal and stabilization of the third, fourth, and fifth digits allowed balanced metatarsal loading to be re-established. Digital alignment was restored and a functional, symptom-free first metatarsophalangeal joint was created with the total implant arthroplasty.

No weight bearing was allowed for a period of 3 months. Once radiographs demonstrated solid healing of the graft interface, the patient gradually returned to weight bearing. Initially she ambulated in a surgical shoe and eventually advanced to full weight bearing in a closed jogging-type shoe.

Follow-up radiographic examination revealed excellent incorporation of the second metatarsal graft and maintenance of digital corrections (Fig. 71.21). The first metatarsophalangeal joint remained in good position, with no signs of implant failure. Clinical evaluation at 3 months displayed little edema and good digital alignment (Fig. 71.22). It is now a little more than 3 years since the final reconstructive surgery, and the patient is functioning and free of symptoms. She continues to wear a silicone mold to fill the second toe space and add to the stability of great toe function.

CASE 5

This case also involves an iatrogenic deformity after lesser metatarsal surgery. Although the structural alterations in this patient were less severe than in the previous two examples, the resultant pain and disability were comparable.

History and Objective Findings

A 56-year-old woman had a chief complaint of pain involving her first metatarsophalangeal joint and the plantar aspect of her second metatarsal head. Additional concerns included cosmetically displeasing deformities at the first metatarsal and lesser digits, as well as an unstable gait (Fig. 71.23).

The patient's surgical history included elective bunionectomy 4 years earlier, followed by a revisional Keller-type bunionectomy 1 year later. Subsequent to the Keller procedure, the patient apparently developed a transfer lesion involving the second metatarsal, necessitating a dorsiflexory osteotomy. Further transfer occurred and involved a lesion under the third metatarsal. The surgeon then performed a third metatarsal dorsiflexory osteotomy, as well as a prophylactic fourth metatarsal osteotomy, in an effort to halt further progression of the transfer lesions. Postoperative management in each instance consisted of full and immediate weight bearing.

Clinical examination revealed a moderate hallux abductus deformity with dorsomedial bunion formation. Range of motion at the first metatarsophalangeal joint was decreased, painful, and crepitant. There was no purchase of the hallux in stance. Palpation of the lesser metatarsal weight-bearing parabola revealed severe elevatus deformity of the third and fourth metatarsal heads. The second metatarsal was most prominent plantarly with a resulting plantar adventitious bursitis. No plantar lesions were present because of the pa-

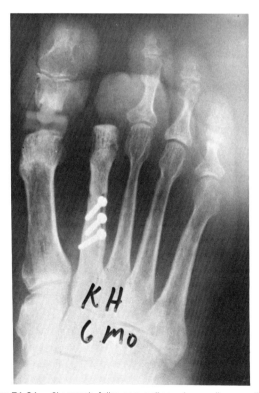

Figure 71.21. Six-month follow-up radiograph revealing excellent incorporation of graft and maintenance of digital alignment.

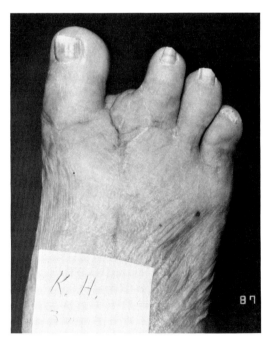

Figure 71.22. Clinical appearance of foot 3 months after reconstruction. Intentional shortening of the first, third, fourth, and fifth toes contributes to stability of the forefoot.

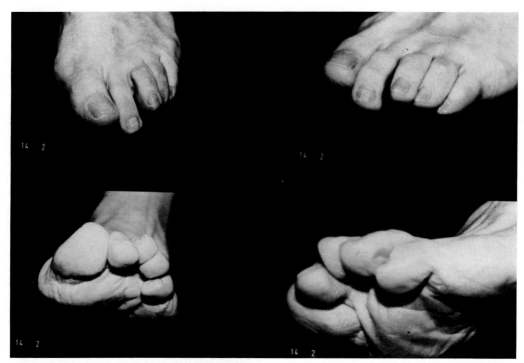

Figure 71.23. Clinical appearance of symptomatic foot after multiple earlier surgical procedures. All digits are hammered, and a large sulcus exists under the third and fourth metatarsal heads. Hallux abducto valgus deformity has recurred, and the third and fourth toes are floating.

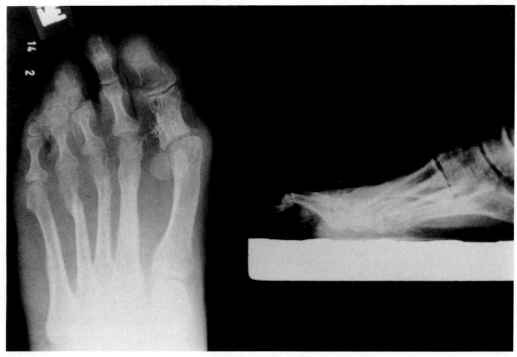

Figure 71.24. Dorsoplantar and lateral radiographs at initial examination of patient. Fibular sesamoid is well into the first interspace.

tient's unstable steppage gait, which had developed secondary to painful ambulation, and because of restricted weight bearing. All the lesser digits were contracted at the metatarsophalangeal joints and hammered. The third and fourth toes were floating without any ground purchase during ambulation (Fig. 71.23).

Radiographic examination of the left foot demonstrated hallux abducto valgus deformity with severe degenerative changes about the metatarsophalangeal articulation. Joint mice were evident (Fig. 71.24). The medial oblique radiograph best demonstrates results of surgical intervention about the distal metaphyseal areas of the second, third, and fourth metatarsals with resultant dorsiflexion (Fig. 71.25). An axial view is useful to correlate the relative degree of dorsiflexion of the metatarsal heads in relation to one another (Fig. 71.26).

Discussion and Treatment Options

Many complications and/or poor results after elective foot surgery are avoidable. One cannot say that the initial bunion procedures were incorrectly performed; however, experienced foot surgeons know that a nonpurchasing and dorsally contracted hallux with resulting second metatarsalgia is an often encountered sequela to a Keller-type hallux valgus repair. Many factors may be involved here, including failure to reattach the short flexor tendons, inadequate repair of the medial and dorsal capsule, severance of the long flexor tendons, and improper postoperative bandaging.

In the present clinical state, a revisional hallux valgus procedure is required, with attention to all the previously mentioned areas, as well as release of all lateral periarticular contractures. A hemi-implant can be inserted to re-establish hallux length and allow for a more functional propulsive hallux with pain-free range of motion. If the metatarsal head cartilage is found to be compromised, a total first metatarsophalangeal joint implant should be considered. Better purchase of the hallux in stance and push-off should also help alleviate the pain under the second metatarsal.

It is prudent to avoid metatarsal osteotomies when possible. Currently there does not appear to be an exact procedure or science governing lesser metatarsal surgery, and complications after such procedures are entirely too common. Such complications include pseudarthrosis, nonunion, malunion, transfer lesions, recurrence of lesions, exuberant bone callus formation, stress fracture, floating toes, and in-

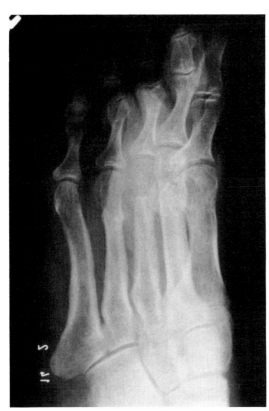

Figure 71.25. Medial oblique radiograph demonstrating evidence of old dorsiflexory osteotomies involving second, third, and fourth metatarsals distally.

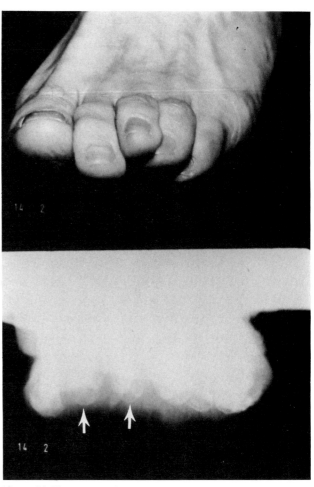

Figure 71.26. Metatarsal axial views are useful to gauge relative dorsiflexed position of one metatarsal versus another. Note dorsiflexed third and fourth metatarsals (arrows).

fection. This patient developed both transfer lesions and floating toes with secondary contractures of the digits at the metatarsophalangeal and proximal interphalangeal joints. Such contractures occur not only secondary to static deformity but also as a result of an unstable forefoot with grasping of the digits in an effort to purchase the supporting surface or to protect painful metatarsal heads. Weight bearing after a lesser metatarsal osteotomy (fixed or unfixed) is accompanied by an increased risk of complications as evidenced by excessive dorsiflexion of the distal part.

It was thought that the patient would benefit from plantarflexory osteotomies of the third and fourth metatarsals

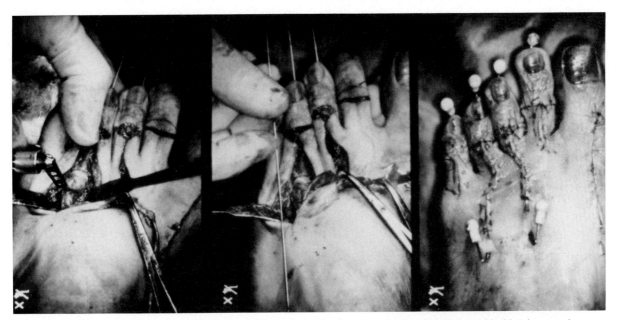

Figure 71.27.   Intraoperative photographs demonstrate extent of forefoot reconstructive procedures and incisional approaches.

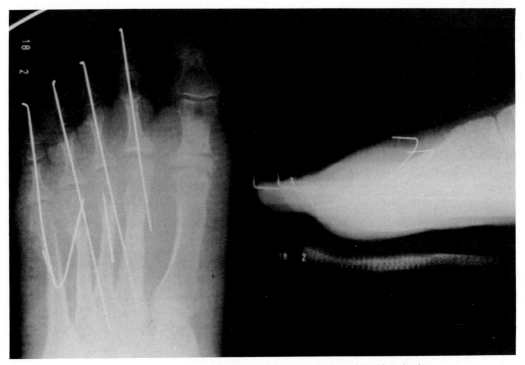

Figure 71.28.   Postoperative radiographs in dorsoplantar and lateral projections.

with stabilization and straightening of the second, third, and fourth digits by arthrodesis of the proximal interphalangeal joints and extensor soft tissue releases. Digital arthrodesis should serve to resist future metatarsophalangeal and interphalangeal joint contractures and will ultimately result in a more stable and propulsive forefoot.

The reconstructive procedures in this patient included a hemi-implant arthroplasty of the first metatarsophalangeal joint with fibular sesamoidectomy and reattachment of the flexor hallucis brevis and appropriate capsular repair, arthrodesis of the proximal interphalangeal joints of the second, third, and fourth digits with K-wire fixation, arthroplasty of the fifth digit, Reverdin osteotomy to correct a deviated proximal articular set angle, and plantarflexory distal metaphyseal osteotomies of the third and fourth metatarsals with K-wire fixation (Fig. 71.27). Any incisions crossing the metatarsophalangeal joint areas dorsally were curved so as to avoid a direct antitension line scar with a high probability of subsequent contracture. Transverse controlled-depth skin incisions were also made at the interphalangeal joints to remove redundant skin.

Postoperative radiographs show good alignment of all digits with adequate correction of the bunion and hallux abductus deformities (Fig. 71.28). Postoperative dressing change at 3 days revealed an excellent restoration of the transverse and sagittal weight-bearing metatarsal plane (Fig. 71.29). The patient was kept in a bivalved cast with no weight bearing until there was evidence of bony healing. However, she was instructed in early passive range-of-motion exercises of the first metatarsophalangeal joint to retain maximum range of motion.

The patient was followed closely throughout the postoperative period. Digital retainer devices were used to maintain correction during collagen remodeling (Fig. 71.30). Radiographs at 5 months revealed good transverse and sagittal alignment of the forefoot, with evidence of increased first metatarsophalangeal joint erosion and destruction (Fig. 71.31).

Because of continued degeneration, the patient returned 2 years after our initial surgery for total first metatarsophalangeal joint implant arthroplasty. All other symptoms had abated, and the patient was left with a stable forefoot and a good weight-bearing plane (Fig. 71.32). The total implant proved satisfactory in relieving the first metatarsophalangeal joint symptoms.

CASE 6

History and Objective Findings

A 53-year-old woman had a chief complaint of continued pain and swelling of 5 months' duration involving her right foot. The symptoms were located about the base of the first

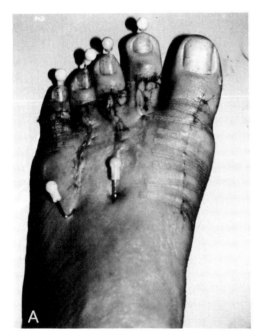
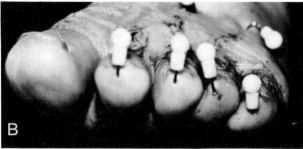

Figure 71.29. Postoperative clinical appearance of foot at 3 days. Overall transverse **(A)** and sagittal plane **(B)** forefoot relationships are much improved.

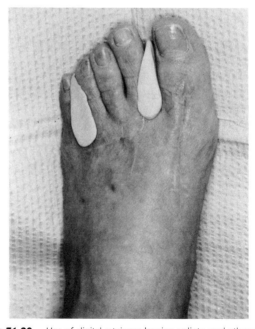

Figure 71.30. Use of digital retainers, bunion splints, and other devices is most important throughout postoperative period.

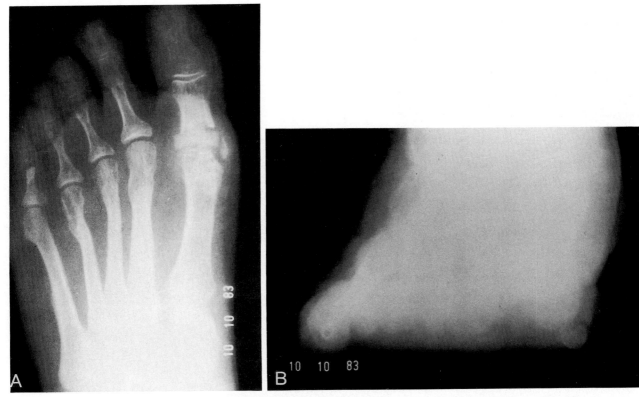

Figure 71.31. Dorsoplantar **(A)** and axial **(B)** radiographs at 5 months. Overall transverse and sagittal plane relationships are maintained. Some erosion and fragmentation about the medial first metatarsal head is evident.

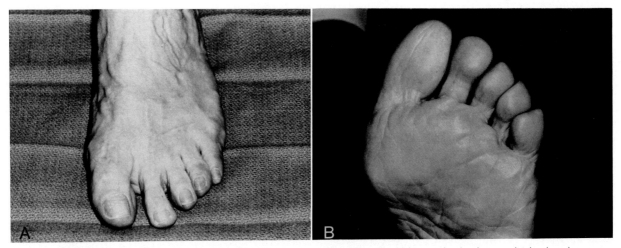

Figure 71.32. **A** and **B.** Clinical appearance of foot at 2-year follow-up. Surgical correction has been maintained, and the patient has a stable and functional forefoot.

metatarsal and were associated with increasing discomfort and tyloma developing beneath the heads of the second and third metatarsals.

Her past surgical history included correction of a moderate hallux abducto valgus deformity and severe metatarsus primus adductus and correction of a second-digit hammer-toe associated with metatarsophalangeal joint dislocation. The surgery had been performed 5 months earlier (Fig. 71.33). Procedures at that time included a modified Mc-Bride-Akin bunionectomy with a traditional transverse closing base wedge osteotomy of the first metatarsal. Fixation of the osteotomy was achieved with a dorsolateral loop of

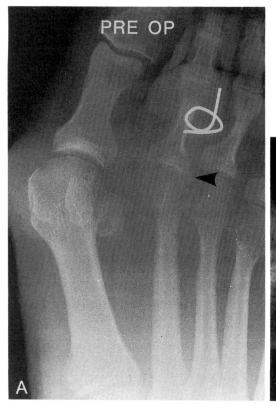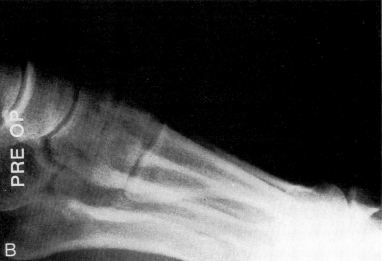

Figure 71.33.   Dorsoplantar **(A)** and lateral **(B)** radiographs of right foot prior to first surgery. Arrow depicts dorsal dislocation of second metatarsophalangeal joint.

28-gauge monofilament stainless steel wire and crossing 0.062-inch K-wires. An additional transverse 0.062-inch K-wire transfixed the first metatarsal to the second, third, and fourth metatarsals for additional stability. Arthrodesis of the second digit was performed along with metatarsophalangeal joint relocation (Fig. 71.34). Postoperatively, the patient was managed in a non-weight-bearing below-the-knee cast for a period of 4 to 6 weeks; however, the patient admitted to bearing weight on the cast periodically. After radiographic confirmation of healing, the patient was allowed to bear weight on the surgically treated foot.

On clinical examination, there was chronic edema of the right forefoot medially with increased warmth over the first metatarsal base. The first ray was noted to be extremely elevated with minimal hallux purchase. The second metatarsal head was very prominent plantarly. The transverse plane correction of the first metatarsal was excellent, and the first metatarsophalangeal joint range of motion was adequate. Motion was painful at the first metatarsal osteotomy site (Fig. 71.35).

Review of the radiographs (Fig. 71.36) revealed a hypertrophic nonunion at the base of the first metatarsal (arrows) with significant elevatus deformity of the first ray. Some relative shortening of the first ray was also evident. Transverse plane alignment of the first ray appeared good.

Discussion and Treatment Options

This case represents a common complication of hallux valgus surgery. Failure to understand the hinge-axis concept or improper surgical execution of the metatarsal osteotomy may result in an elevatus deformity (Fig. 71.37). In addition, a patient's failure to comply with instructions for total abstinence from weight bearing can lead to an elevated metatarsal and nonunion in spite of an excellent surgical repair and good cast immobilization.

Weak fixation techniques, such as dorsolateral stainless steel wire fixation, may allow easy fracture of a medial cortical hinge on reduction of the eccentrically loaded osteotomy. K-wire fixation was subsequently inadequate to provide stable internal fixation. This further enhanced the elevatus deformity and contributed to the nonunion. In fact, no form of fixation can be expected to tolerate weight bearing before bone healing has taken place.

With elevation of the first metatarsal, the first ray no longer bears its appropriate share of body weight during the stance and propulsion phases of gait. This fixed forefoot varus deformity subsequently leads to severe lesser metatarsalgia (Fig. 71.38). Additional complications may include stress fracture of the lesser metatarsals, hallux limitus and rigidus, hallux flexus, floating toes, and increased pronatory forces on the forefoot with a resulting increase in the hallux

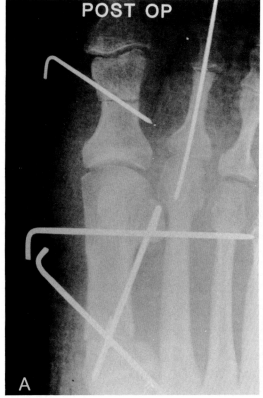

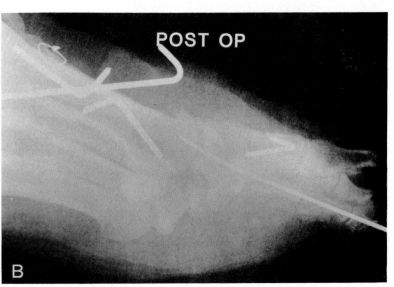

Figure 71.34. Postoperative dorsoplantar (**A**) and lateral (**B**) radiographs of right foot. Transverse plane alignment is acceptable. The medial cortical hinge is fractured, and the first metatarsal bone is elevated.

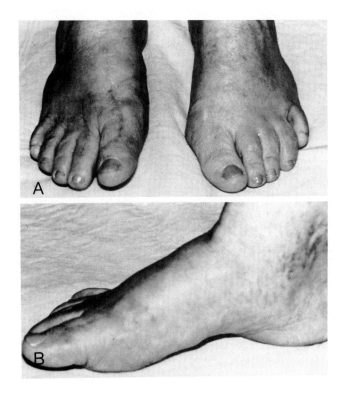

Figure 71.35. **A** and **B.** Clinical appearance of foot 5 months postoperatively reveals chronic brawny edema with mild erythema. Hallux is nonpurchasing in stance.

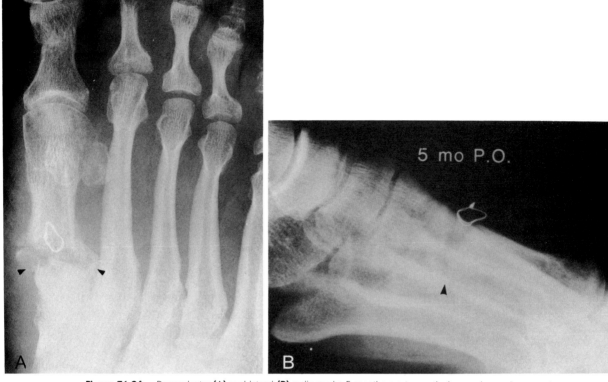

Figure 71.36.   Dorsoplantar **(A)** and lateral **(B)** radiographs 5 months postoperatively reveal vascular nonunion at previous osteotomy site with shortening and elevatus of first metatarsal.

Figure 71.37.   Intraoperative radiograph shows moderate elevatus deformity of first ray secondary to improper osteotomy axis and poor fixation technique. Osteotomy should be perpendicular to weight-bearing supporting surface in sagittal plane, and hinge should not be eccentrically loaded during fixation. Osteotomy is gaping plantarly.

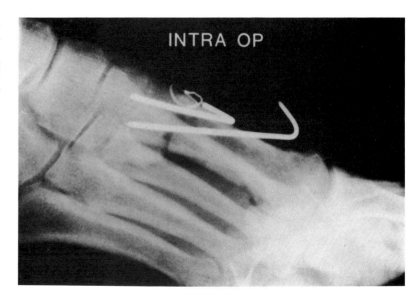

valgus deformity. Such symptoms may be more disabling than the original deformity.

When considering surgical reconstruction, one is faced with the mechanical problem coupled with a vascular or reactive nonunion. Theoretically, a vascular nonunion will heal if the patient bears no weight for an additional 4 to 8 weeks. At that time, however, one would have to deal with the elevatus and shortening of the first metatarsal, either by accommodative orthotic devices or by lesser metatarsal osteotomies. The latter approach may lead to further iatrogenic deformity. Attacking a new deformity without regard for the primary or causative problem would only end

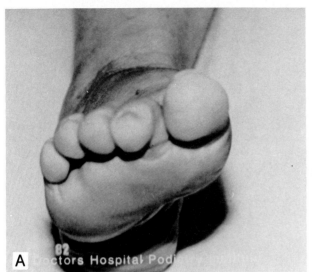
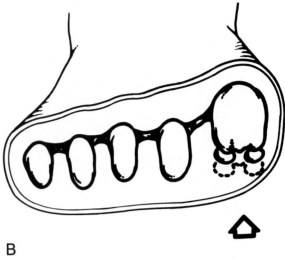

Figure 71.38. Axial clinical (**A**) and artistic representation (**B**) of first metatarsal elevatus deformity. Medial column of foot fails to bear its share of body weight. This results in increased pronatory influence and increased weight bearing under lesser metatarsals.

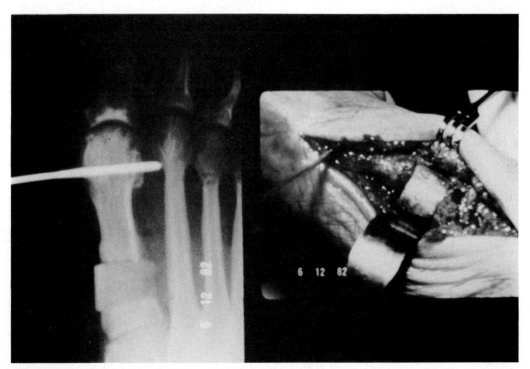

Figure 71.39. Intraoperative radiograph and clinical photograph showing allogeneic bone graft in place in area of previous nonunion. Metatarsal length and declination have been restored.

in further forefoot instability. One lesser metatarsal osteotomy would eventually lead to another, while all the digits, including the hallux, would contract in an effort to purchase the ground. This scenario was observed in the previous case. Hallux and lesser metatarsophalangeal joint limitus and/or rigidus would eventually develop, as well as a recurrence of the original hallux abducto valgus deformity.

The salvage procedures chosen for this patient included surgical resection of the nonunion site with insertion of a bone graft to correct the elevatus deformity of the first ray with restoration of its length (Fig. 71.39). This was accomplished with an allogeneic corticocancellous bone graft and a five-hole one-third tubular bone plate using axial compression in standard ASIF technique (Fig. 71.40). The patient

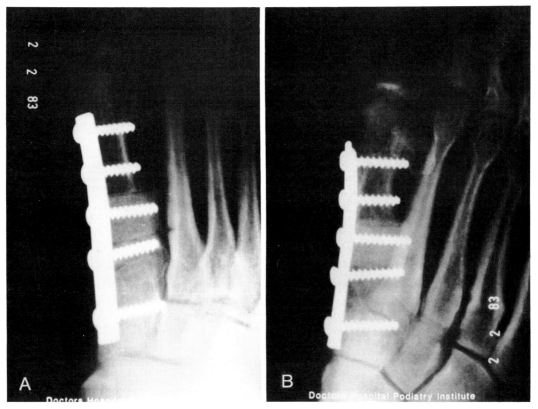

Figure 71.40.   Dorsoplantar **(A)** and medial oblique **(B)** radiographs at 11 weeks showing incorporation of bone graft.

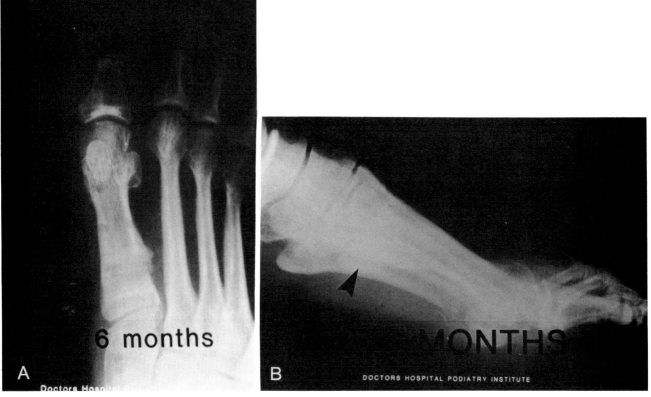

Figure 71.41.   A and **B.** Radiographic appearance of graft repair at 6 months.

abstained from weight bearing for approximately 11 weeks in a below-the-knee cast. She then began gradual weight bearing with removal of the plate and screws at 6 months postoperatively. The graft was fully incorporated, and the elevatus and shortening of the first ray were corrected (Fig. 71.41). The patient's forefoot is now much improved with an overall symptom-free propulsive gait (Fig. 71.42).

CASE 7

History and Objective Findings

A 49-year-old woman had a chief complaint of severe lesser metatarsalgia 2 years after Stone procedures were performed for bilateral hallux abducto valgus (radiographs suggested that more probably Mayo-type procedures had been performed). The patient had been disabled since the surgery and was unable to return to her occupation, which required standing on an assembly line. She also complained of low back pain secondary to her altered gait.

Physical examination revealed a markedly shortened first ray with a floating hallux. The second and third metatarsophalangeal joints were quite painful to palpation, and the patient's gait was markedly guarded (Fig. 71.43).

Discussion and Treatment Options

Before reconstruction, several surgical options were discussed. These included resection of the lesser metatarsal heads, implantation of the first metatarsophalangeal joint, and bone graft of the distal first metatarsal with restoration of its length, followed later by implantation.

Panmetatarsal head resection was a viable option but would result in a structurally weaker forefoot.

Implantation would restore part of the length of the first ray and possibly result in a hallux that was more plantar-

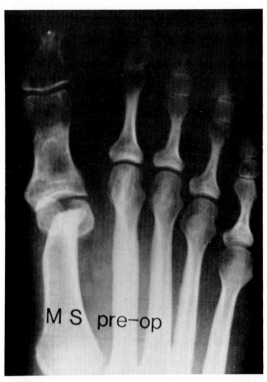

Figure 71.43. Preoperative dorsoplantar radiograph revealing aggressive first metatarsal head resection.

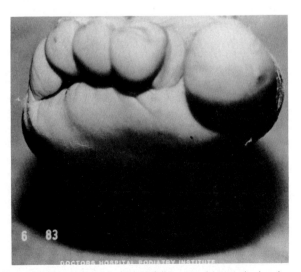

Figure 71.42. Long-term clinical follow-up photograph showing reduction of fixed forefoot varus deformity. Overall weight-bearing plane of forefoot is much improved. Hallux is plantargrade.

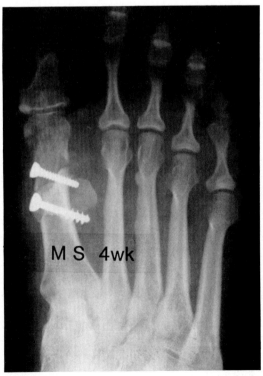

Figure 71.44. Autogenous grafting of proximal phalanx to remaining first metatarsal.

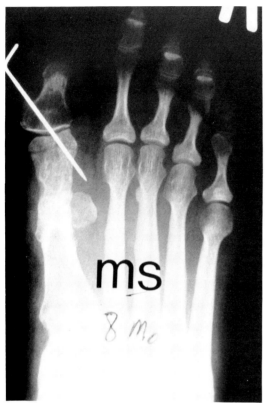

Figure 71.45. Postoperative dorsoplantar radiograph after dorsiflexory wedge osteotomy of new first metatarsal head with K-wire in place.

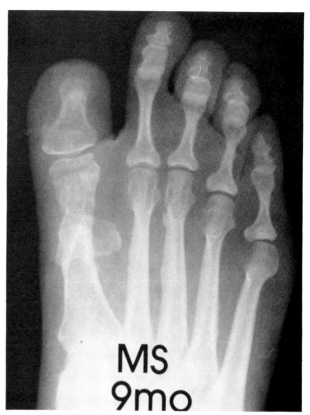

Figure 71.46. Dorsoplantar radiograph 9 months after final reconstruction.

grade. However, an implant is merely a spacer, not a weight-bearing device, and little or none of the lesser metatarsalgia would be relieved with this approach.

The final option was to graft bone to the first metatarsal to restore not only its length but its weight-bearing function as well. An autogenous graft is the preferred material, and it was judged likely to yield the quickest satisfactory result. Since the patient was more concerned with relief of pain than with cosmetic appearance, it was believed that the most easily available strong graft would be the proximal phalanx of the hallux. The end result would be a fusion of the proximal phalanx to the first metatarsal, with the interphalangeal joint of the hallux becoming the new metatarsophalangeal joint (Fig. 71.44).

The initial plan was that the new metatarsophalangeal joint would be implanted after successful healing of the arthrodesis. On examination 9 months later, implant arthroplasty was deemed unnecessary and a dorsally based wedge osteotomy was performed at the new metatarsal head to provide needed dorsiflexory range of motion. This resulted in satisfactory dorsiflexory range of motion (Figs. 71.45 and 71.46).

CASE 8

This case illustrates an iatrogenic deformity that followed improper surgical planning and technical execution.

History and Objective Findings

A 64-year-old man had a chief complaint of a painful "knot" involving the fifth metatarsal shaft of the right foot. He also described symptoms associated with a prominent third metatarsal head with pain on weight bearing. He stated that the entire right foot had a feeling of instability and rocking to the outside on weight bearing.

The surgical history included a fifth metatarsal osteotomy for correction of a tailor's bunion deformity. The surgery, which involved a minimal incision technique, had been performed 5 months earlier (Figs. 71.47 and 71.48). The patient related a history of immediate ambulation postoperatively in a surgical shoe, which he continued to wear for 4 months.

Clinical examination of the involved extremity revealed severe elevatus deformity of the fourth and fifth metatarsal heads with palpatory painless motion of the fifth metatarsal osteotomy. A tyloma was noted over the proximal lateral aspect of the fifth metatarsal, as well as over the third metatarsal head plantarly. Osseous spurring was palpable about the fifth metatarsal osteotomy area, and all toes were progressively clawing (Fig. 71.48). Biomechanical examination revealed a rather rigid forefoot valgus deformity with a supinatory rock in gait that resulted in compensation by dumping weight to the lateral border of the foot. The patient's ambulation was unsteady, with his lateral forefoot column giving way at midstance.

Radiographic study revealed a horse hoof type of nonu-

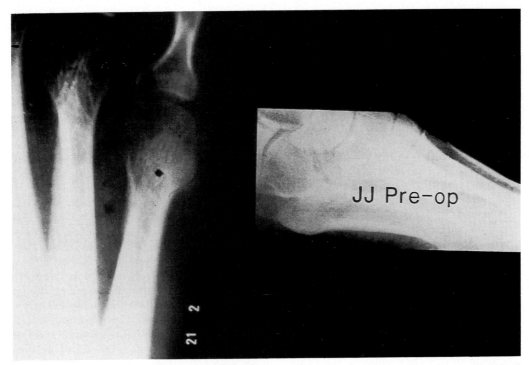

Figure 71.47. Preoperative dorsoplantar and lateral radiographs before minimal incision surgery to correct tailor's bunion.

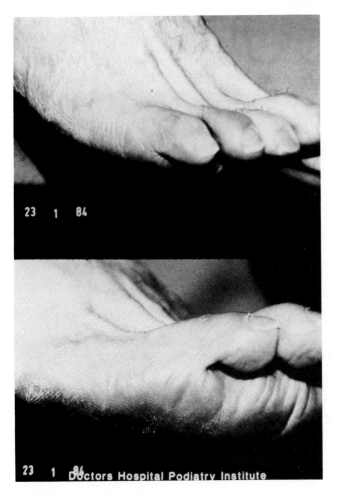

Figure 71.48. Clinical appearance 5 months after minimal incision surgery. Elevatus of fourth and fifth metatarsal heads is suspected, with callus developing under the fifth metatarsal nonunion as well as under the third metatarsal head.

nion involving the fifth metatarsal shaft with severe shortening and elevatus, some angulational deformity, and dorsolateral spurring. The fourth metatarsal, although not part of the planned original surgery, was obviously osteotomized unintentionally during the blind surgical procedure and had subsequently healed in an adducted and dorsiflexed position with some shortening (Fig. 71.49).

Discussion and Treatment Options

Unfortunately, this patient was subjected to lesser metatarsal osteotomies that did not serve to correct his initial problem of a rigid plantarflexed first ray. Continued ambulation postoperatively, along with subsequent compensation through subtalar joint supination, further enhanced dorsiflexion, adduction, and nonunion of the fifth metatarsal osteotomy.

Surgical considerations for salvage at this time included simple exostectomy, fifth metatarsal head and neck resection, metatarsal head resection with digital syndactyly, or revision of the nonunion and malunion with bone grafting and plate stabilization.

The patient opted for conservative care and was therefore treated with an accommodative orthotic device and ankle-high boots. His condition improved, but he continued to complain of instability during ambulation.

Three years later the patient returned for surgical intervention. Clinical examination again disclosed severe elevation of the fourth and fifth metatarsal heads with continued contracture of all the lesser digits. A large bursa was present

laterally over the shaft osteotomy site with an increased amount of palpable bone callus. Gait was unsteady, with the foot and ankle very unstable laterally (Fig. 71.50). Radiographs showed further enlargement of the fifth metatarsal nonunion with continued shortening and angulational deformity. Radiographic appearance of the fourth metatarsal malunion remained unchanged (Fig. 71.51).

The patient was taken to the operating room, and attempts were made to recreate a normal weight-bearing parabola of the forefoot. Initially, an autogenous corticocancellous iliac crest bone graft was harvested from the ipsilateral hip. The fifth metatarsal nonunion was then resected, and the bone graft was fashioned in such a manner as to lengthen and plantarflex the fifth metatarsal head. Rigid internal fixation was accomplished with a six-hole one-third tubular plate (Figs. 71.52 to 71.55).

The fourth metatarsal malunion was identified and a transverse osteotomy was performed at its apex. A triangulated bone graft was inserted in an effort to abduct and lengthen the metatarsal. Fixation and maintenance of plantarflexion of the ray were accomplished with a five-hole one-third tubular plate with appropriate contouring. Postoperative radiographs revealed adequate reconstruction of the forefoot parabola (Fig. 71.56). Clinically, the foot exhibited an acceptable transverse and sagittal plane relationship of the fourth and fifth metatarsals in relation to the others (Fig. 71.57).

The patient was managed in a non-weight-bearing bivalved short leg cast for approximately 3 months. Range-

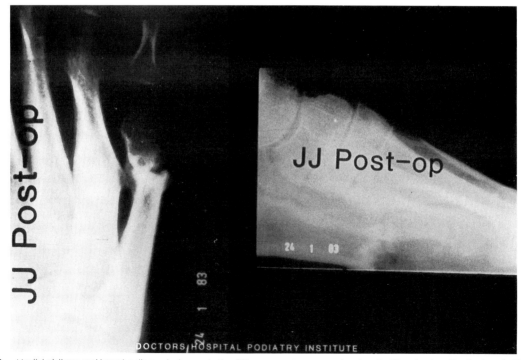

Figure 71.49. Medial oblique and lateral radiograph demonstrating fifth metatarsal nonunion as well as malunion of fourth metatarsal. Both seg- ments are noted to be significantly dorsally displaced. Fifth metatarsal is severely shortened.

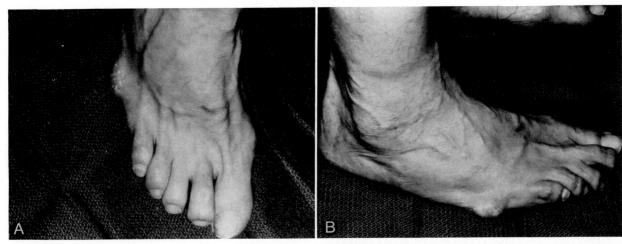

Figure 71.50. **A** and **B.** Clinical appearance of foot 3 years after initial consultation. Deformity is noted to be increasing rapidly because of overall instability of lateral column and continued compensation for rigidly plantarflexed first ray.

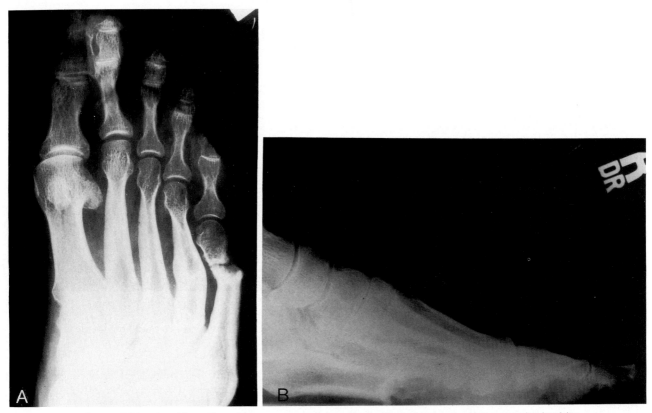

Figure 71.51. **A** and **B.** Radiographic appearance was consistent with persistent and enlarging nonunion involving fifth metatarsal. Elevatus of fourth and fifth metatarsal heads is clearly evident.

of-motion exercises were initiated at 2 weeks postoperatively to prevent cast disease. This was possible because the bivalved cast permitted removal for bathing once incisional healing occurred. After incorporation of the bone grafts, the patient required an appropriate orthotic device.

IATROGENIC REARFOOT DEFORMITIES

CASE 9

This case illustrates the importance of a thorough knowledge of the materials used during surgery.

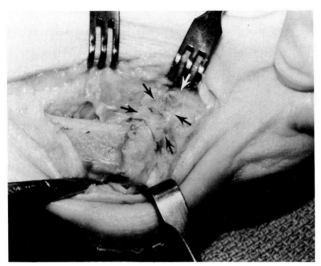

Figure 71.52. Fifth metatarsal nonunion site is exposed under tourniquet control. Note adducted and dorsiflexed distal capital fragment (arrows). Severe fibrocartilaginous spurring is noted about the proximal-lateral aspect of the nonunion site, which accounts for the bursa formation.

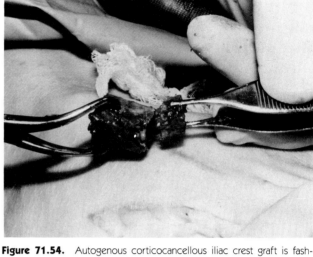

Figure 71.54. Autogenous corticocancellous iliac crest graft is fashioned for insertion.

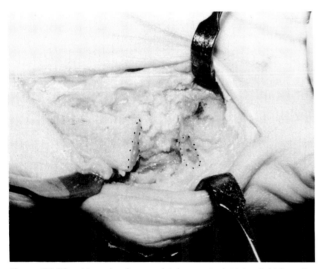

Figure 71.53. Nonunion is completely resected. Note slight beveling of the proximal segment as well as transverse resection in the frontal plane. These cuts will serve to plantarflex and straighten the distal metatarsal head after repair.

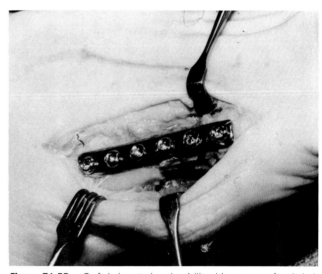

Figure 71.55. Graft is inserted and stabilized by means of a six-hole one-third tubular plate. Compression is achieved axially, and the plate is prestressed to prevent plantar gaping at the repair site.

History

The patient, a 32-year-old man with Charcot-Marie-Tooth disease, underwent a cavus foot reconstruction that involved triple arthrodesis, transfer of the tibialis posterior tendon through the interosseous membrane to the dorsum of the foot, and fusion of the interphalangeal joint of the hallux and the proximal joints of the three middle toes.

During surgery a small acetyl washer and a mated screw were used to anchor the tibialis posterior tendon into the navicular. The acetyl washer, which had not been previously sterilized, had to be flash autoclaved at the time of surgery. Otherwise, the surgery proceeded uneventfully.

Objective Findings and Subsequent Treatment

Routine postoperative radiographs demonstrated that the washer had dislocated from the screw head and was displaced dorsomedially (Fig. 71.58). The stability of the new tendinous insertion was also suspect, as the screw head alone was not adequate to maintain the tendon's insertional integrity during healing.

A second surgical procedure was required to retrieve and replace the dislocated washer for reinforcement of

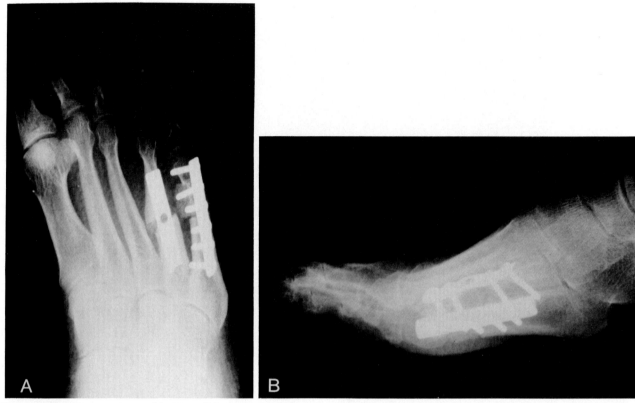

Figure 71.56. Postoperative medial oblique **(A)** and lateral **(B)** radiographs reveal adequate reconstruction of metatarsal length parabola, as well as correction of adduction deformities. The fourth and fifth metatarsal heads are returned to the plantar weight-bearing surface.

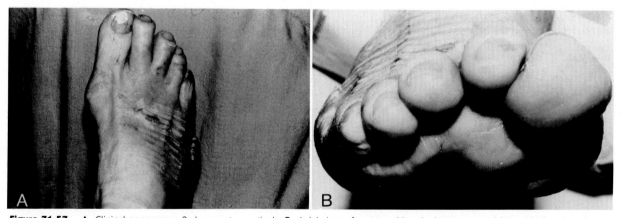

Figure 71.57. A. Clinical appearance 3 days postoperatively. **B.** Axial view of metatarsal heads shows acceptable weight-bearing plane.

the tendon attachment. Retrospective inquiry revealed that the manufacturer recommends that 24 hours should elapse between autoclaving and use of the washer in surgery. The acetyl washer temporarily loses its size memory and becomes somewhat elastic after heat sterilization and can be safely used only after a 24-hour recovery period.

Discussion

The foregoing illustrates a valuable point. Many times failure of implantable materials is caused not by an inherent property within the device but, rather, by improper application of the device or selection of the material. It is, therefore, most important that personnel working with implantable materials know the characteristics of those materials.

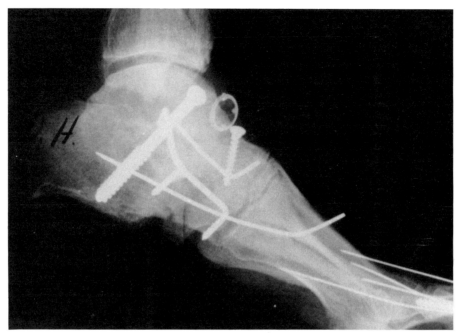

Figure 71.58. Postoperative view of foot after triple arthrodesis and tibialis posterior tendon transfer to dorsum of foot. A screw and an acetyl washer were used to anchor the tendon. The washer can be seen dislocated from the screw head.

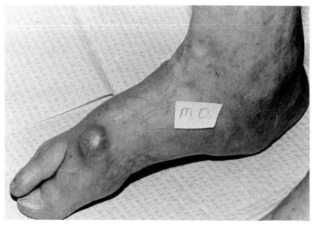

Figure 71.59. Dorsomedial clinical appearance of foot that was fused in a varus attitude 12 years earlier. Note the severe elevatus of the first metatarsal and the resultant dorsal bunion.

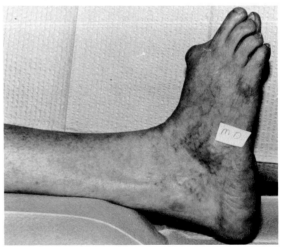

Figure 71.60. Lateral view of same foot as in Figure 71.59.

CASE 10

This case illustrates the importance of planning forefoot-to-rearfoot relationships when rearfoot and forefoot arthrodesis procedures are performed.

History

A 66-year-old woman had a chief complaint of severe pain along the entire lateral aspect of the right foot, as well as shoe irritation involving the dorsal aspect of the first metatarsal head. Symptoms were so severe that the patient had altered her entire life-style to avoid any unnecessary weight bearing. Twelve years earlier the patient had undergone triple arthrodesis for correction of a severe cavus foot deformity. Surgery had been performed on both feet at different times, but the right foot had never been satisfactory (Figs. 71.59 and 71.60).

Objective Findings

Clinical examination indicated tenderness to palpation along the lateral weight-bearing aspect of the calcaneus, under the base of the fifth metatarsal, and under the fourth and fifth metatarsal heads. The entire medial aspect of the foot failed to purchase the weight-bearing surface, and flexion contracture of the hallux had occurred as it attempted to stabilize the medial column. As the hallux plantarflexed, increased dorsal buckling occurred at the first metatarsophalangeal joint. Chronic irritation had resulted in a painful bursal sac over the dorsum of the first metatarsal head. The lateral radiograph demonstrates the deformities (Fig. 71.61).

Treatment and Discussion

The patient's chief complaints can be attributed to the fact that the foot healed in a varus position after the triple arthrodesis. It is axiomatic that when rearfoot joints are fused, both the rearfoot and the forefoot should be aligned in a slightly everted or valgus position. To do otherwise is to concentrate severe pressure on the lateral side of the foot. In this patient the residual elevatus of the first ray and the subsequent instability became a progressive deformity.

The authors have seen numerous such deformities resulting from triple arthrodesis. Once the problem develops, the alternatives for operative management of the problem may take one of two forms. The first is revision of the triple arthrodesis with derotation of both the rearfoot and the forefoot into mild valgus. With this approach a plantarflexory procedure of the first ray and hallux limitus repair may

also be necessary. A second approach is to perform plantarflexory osteotomies of the first through the fourth metatarsals in conjunction with a Dwyer calcaneal osteotomy. The authors have seen both approaches work, but revisional triple arthrodesis is a more direct approach to the problem.

In this instance the patient declined further surgery and has been helped somewhat by molded shoes and the use of a cane on the affected side.

CASE 11

This case illustrates the importance of always having a secondary form of internal fixation available. No one system or technique is going to be adequate for all situations.

History

The patient, a 51-year-old woman, was admitted to the hospital with a disabling pes valgus deformity that had culminated in rupture of the tibialis posterior. She subsequently underwent triple arthrodesis. Fixation was provided by three cancellous bone screws, one across each fusion site. The authors had used the three-screw fixation technique effectively for a number of years. It had been found to provide good, rigid internal fixation. In this case, however, as the screw was inserted across the calcaneocuboid joint, it contacted the talocalcaneal screw, making good compression impossible (Fig. 71.62). A ⅛-inch deficit remained laterally and plantarly at the calcaneocuboid joint after the screw had achieved maximum compression, but the fixation appeared to be quite secure. The small remaining void was packed

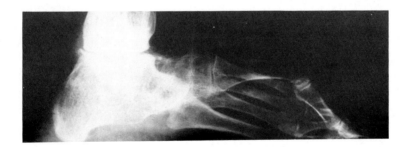

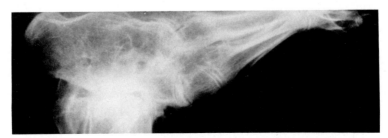

Figure 71.61. Lateral radiograph showing severe varus deformity.

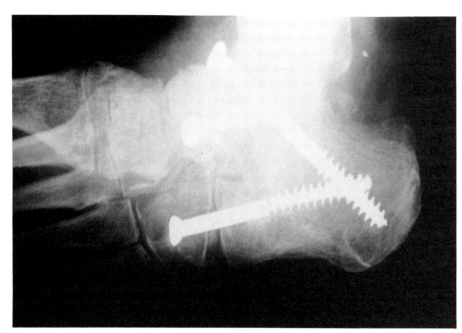

Figure 71.62. Oblique radiograph shows gaping of calcaneocuboid joint and broken screw.

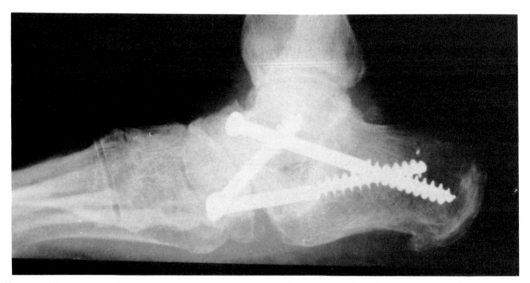

Figure 71.63. Lateral radiograph of foot showing mild rocker-bottom configuration after calcaneocuboid joint distraction.

tightly with cancellous bone chips with the expectation of uneventful healing. Bridging of the calcaneocuboid joint failed to occur, and the joint gap increased during healing.

Treatment and Discussion

At surgery, an attempt could have been made to forcibly advance the screw at the risk of fracturing the cortex of the cuboid, stripping the threads in the calcaneus, or perhaps breaking one of the two screws. An available alternative was redrilling the hole in a slightly different direction. The latter idea seemed unwise in the presence of rather soft bone. In

retrospect, removal of the calcaneocuboid screw and the use of two staples would have provided a more dependable alternative form of fixation.

After the void was packed with autogenous bone chips, the patient was placed in an above-the-knee cast and gait trained with strict instructions to bear no weight on the surgically treated extremity. She was seen 1 month after surgery, at which time she entered the office walking on the cast. Her family indicated that she had been walking on the cast for more than 2 weeks. X-ray examination showed that the calcaneocuboid screw had broken and further widening of the calcaneocuboid joint interface had occurred (Figs.

71.62 and 71.63). The patient went on to develop a symptomatic delayed union but declined further surgery. She did consent to a cast brace and cane-assisted weight bearing for 6 additional months, during which time solid union occurred. The fixation failure allowed opening of the calcaneocuboid joint along with lowering of the calcaneal inclination to a negative angle. Because of the negative calcaneal position, the patient requires a depth oxford with a full-length accommodative mold to avoid pressure beneath the midtarsal joint.

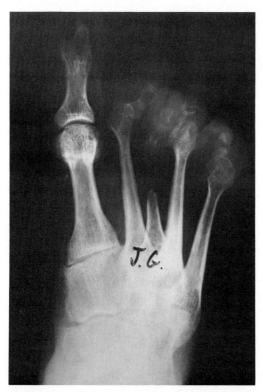

Figure 71.64. Dorsoplantar radiograph of patient with severe plantar symptoms beneath second and fourth metatarsals. The third metatarsal was previously resected to relieve plantar keratosis, thus transferring pressure to the second and fourth metatarsals. Proximal phalangectomies have also been performed.

It is important in all cases to have an alternate plan of fixation available. However, there is no fixation that is designed to withstand the forces of weight bearing.

CASE 12

This case illustrates the importance of understanding the cause of forefoot deformities before attempting to treat them.

History

A 33-year-old man was referred to the authors with severe pain under the second and fourth metatarsal heads and along the lateral border of the foot and with all the lesser toes dislocated. The patient had been born with claw feet and had been treated from earliest childhood.

The surgical history revealed that the patient had undergone multiple procedures on both feet, which included triple arthrodesis twice on each foot. More recent surgery had consisted of a resection of the third metatarsal head and neck, ostectomies of the proximal phalanges, and two Jones suspensions, all performed bilaterally (Figs. 71.64 and 71.65). The forefoot surgery had attempted to relieve intractable plantar keratoses beneath the third metatarsals and to correct clawtoe deformities.

Objective Findings

Clinical examination demonstrated osseous equinus of the ankle joint, along with marked limitation of motion and crepitus. Gait examination showed only partial heel contact with immediate heel lift and weight transfer along the entire lateral border of the foot to the ball area. A deep sulcus was present plantarly in the area normally occupied by the third metatarsal head. All the lesser toes were flail and unstable. Deep plantar keratoses were present beneath the second and fourth metatarsal heads.

Radiographic examination confirmed the osseous equinus along with absence of the third metatarsal head and neck and dislocation of all of the lesser toes (Figs. 71.64 and 71.65).

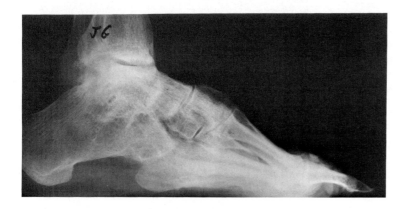

Figure 71.65. Lateral radiograph shows results of triple arthrodesis in which the rearfoot was fused in a varus position. The resulting osseous equinus appears largely responsible for the severe forefoot symptoms that subsequently developed.

Discussion and Treatment Options

An osseous ankle equinus developed after the patient's triple arthrodesis limiting ankle dorsiflexion and forcing weight to be thrust onto the forefoot in an abnormal manner. The equinus was a direct result of the position in which the rearfoot was fixed by arthrodesis. The patient's metatarsal surgery was ill advised. With limitation of ankle dorsiflexion, transfer of weight to the second and fourth metatarsal heads was bound to follow resection of the third metatarsal head. Furthermore, resection of the bases of the proximal phalanges of the lesser toes compounded pre-existing instability and led to complete loss of digital purchase. Subsequent buckling at the metatarsophalangeal joint increased pressure on the metatarsal heads and exacerbated the plantar lesions.

By the time we first saw the patient, our options for treatment were quite limited. We could perform panmetatarsal head resections of the first, second, fourth, and fifth metatarsals and graft lengthening of the excessively short third metatarsal bone. Syndactylization of the second and third toes and the fourth and fifth toes along with extensor tendon release might help to stabilize the toes. In addition, we could use a 1 inch heel raise to relieve some of the stress related to the ankle equinus. A metatarsal rocker sole could relieve much of the impact at the ball of the foot.

Because of the patient's poor medical status, it was elected to use a raised heel with a metatarsal level rocker sole combined with an accommodative orthotic device. The combination provided moderate, though far from adequate, relief.

CASE 13

This case illustrates the importance of overall alignment when an ankle arthrodesis is performed. Fusing the ankle in a plantarflexed position assures midfoot arthroses and forefoot deformities (Figs. 71.66 and 71.67).

History

A 35-year-old woman was referred for treatment of severe pain at Lisfranc's joint. She reported having had poliomyelitis at the age of 18 months with subsequent development of an unstable foot. She had undergone rearfoot arthrodeses at the age of 11 and arthrodesis of the ankle joint at the age of 16. Shortly after recovery from the ankle fusion she began to experience pain across Lisfranc's joint. The problem was diagnosed as degenerative arthritis of Lisfranc's joint and was treated by numerous conservative means. Prior treatment included orthotic devices and accommodative shoe corrections as well as anti-inflammatory medications.

Objective Findings

Clinical examination demonstrated a foot that was rigidly fixed in an equinus position with the heel unable to touch the ground. A rocker-bottom breech was present at Lisfranc's joint, and motion at that joint was greatly exagger-

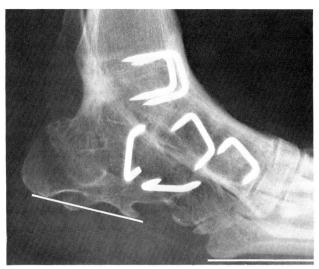

Figure 71.66. Lateral radiograph of foot that had undergone a pantalar arthrodesis many years earlier. Notice the negative calcaneal inclination, which is compensated by a breech at Lisfranc's joint.

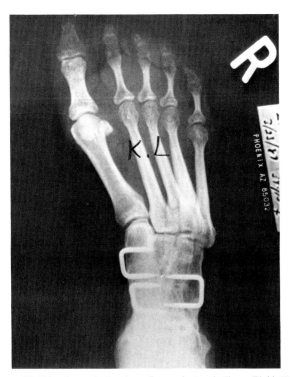

Figure 71.67. Dorsoplantar view of same foot as in Figure 71.66. Note increased joint space and adaptation at tarsometatarsal joints.

ated. The patient complained of pain across Lisfranc's joint on dorsiflexion and plantarflexion of the metatarsals.

Radiographic examination confirmed pantalar arthrodesis along with arthrodesis of the naviculocuneiform joints (Figs. 71.66 and 71.67). Marked joint adaptation and increased joint space were evident at all the tarsometatarsal

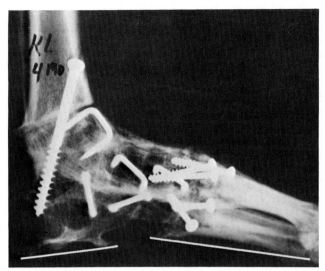

Figure 71.68. Postoperative radiograph. Dorsiflexory osteotomy at ankle joint has restored calcaneal inclination, permitting the heel to bear weight. Arthrodesis of the tarsometatarsal joints has restored forefoot stability and relieved painful arthroses at that level.

joints. Staples were present in the tarsal and ankle joint areas from the previous surgery. Of particular significance was the negative inclination of the calcaneus, which resulted in a rocker-bottom midfoot and severe bending force at the tarsometatarsal joints.

The patient had a toe-to-toe gait with no heel strike.

Treatment and Discussion

Ordinarily one would consider an accommodative heel lift along with prescription footwear and an accommodative orthotic device as appropriate. In this patient all such therapy had been given an adequate trial without subjective relief.

It was apparent that treatment should involve both appropriate surgical repair and long-term follow-up with accommodative orthoses and footwear. Surgical treatment included a dorsiflexory osteotomy at the distal tibia along with arthrodesis of the tarsometatarsal joints (Figs. 71.68 and 71.69). The distal tibial wedge was planned so as to both dorsiflex and evert the foot. Calcaneal inclination and forefoot declination were restored (Fig. 71.68). Arthrodesis of Lisfranc's joint was deemed necessary to relieve the painful arthrosis.

Postoperatively, the patient was placed in a shoe with a rocker sole designed to smooth the heel contact and to provide a roll-off at the metatarsophalangeal joint area.

Two years eight months after surgery the results were reported to be entirely satisfactory.

CASE 14

This case shows a rather rare complication of triple arthrodesis—avascular necrosis of the talus.

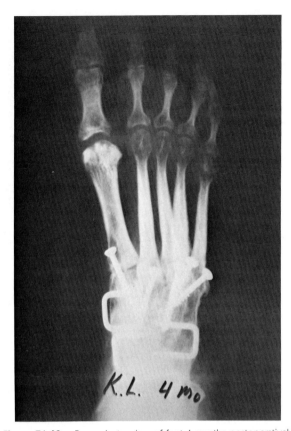

Figure 71.69. Dorsoplantar view of foot 4 months postoperatively.

History

The patient, a 32-year-old white woman with Charcot-Marie-Tooth disease, was referred for treatment of instability of the left foot and ankle. She had undergone tibialis anterior and tibialis posterior tendon transfers several years earlier. These had resulted in gross medial weakness and medial instability of the arch. The result was a foot that pronated in gait despite attempts at orthotic control. The patient was unwilling to wear an ankle-foot orthosis (AFO).

Objective Findings

Clinical examination confirmed the presence of anterior leg muscle function but the near absence of peroneus brevis function. Attempts at dorsiflexion of the foot resulted in dorsiflexion and eversion because of the lateral placement of the transferred muscles and loss of the original supinatory function of the tibialis posterior. Radiographs of the foot in relaxed stance appeared quite normal, although the patient controlled the position of the subtalar joint by external rotation of the leg (Fig. 71.70).

Treatment and Discussion

It was evident that any conservative treatment would require some type of upright brace, which the young woman re-

Figure 71.70. Preoperative lateral view of foot prior to triple arthrodesis. Neuromuscular instability of rearfoot provided indications for surgical stabilization of otherwise normal joints.

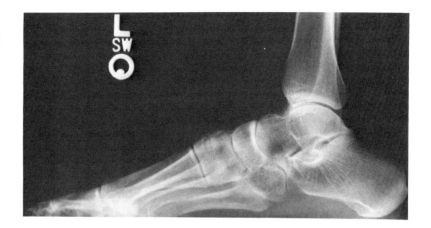

Figure 71.71. Immediate postoperative view.

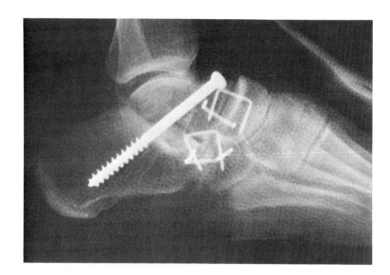

Figure 71.72. Lateral view 4 months later shows sclerotic changes in dome of talus.

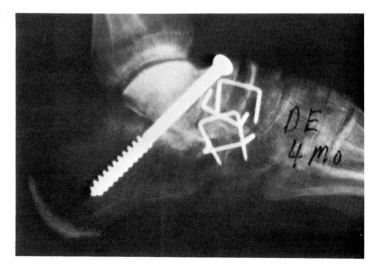

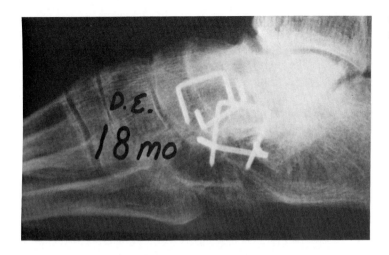

Figure 71.73. Avascular necrosis of talus 18 months after surgery. Note collapse of talus and flattening of trochlear surface.

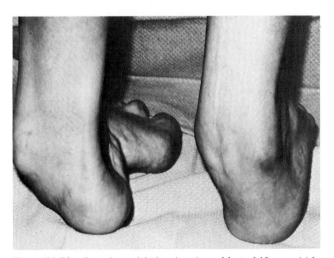

Figure 71.74. Posterior weight-bearing view of feet of 10-year-old female patient. Severe foot deformities are due to neuromuscular imbalance related to diastematomyelia.

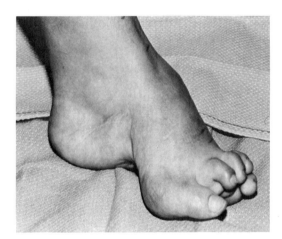

Figure 71.75. Medial view of left foot.

fused. Surgical treatment would have to provide stability of the rearfoot complex. It was thought that, with stabilization of the rearfoot, the muscles that had been previously transferred would be forced to function as true dorsiflexors rather than as dorsiflexors and evertors.

Surgery included triple arthrodesis (Fig. 71.71). At 4 months, postoperative radiographs showed marked sclerosis of the talus suggestive of avascular necrosis (Fig. 71.72). Despite attempts to limit weight bearing, the patient continued to walk and returned to work. Eighteen months after surgery the talus had collapsed to half its normal size and the trochlear surface had flattened (Fig. 71.73). By that time motion at the ankle was quite limited and the limb length was shortened.

When first identified, the avascular necrosis might have been treated by restriction of motion and elimination of weight bearing. Once the talus flattened with collapse of the

trochlear surface (Fig. 71.73), arthrodesis of the ankle became the only viable surgical alternative.

Case 15

This case illustrates the folly of relying on soft tissue releases alone to correct severe foot and ankle deformities in patients with neuromuscular diseases (Figs. 71.74 to 71.76).

History

The patient, a 10-year-old white girl, complained of poor balance and difficulty in weight bearing, even with bracing provided by two hightop molded shoes. In spite of excellent support, recurrent ulcerations were a problem. The patient's neurosurgeon had suggested that definitive correction of the feet could wait no longer because of the increasing severity of the deformities.

Medical history of note included diastematomyelia, which had resulted in progressive deformities of the feet. The deformities had increased rapidly along with growth.

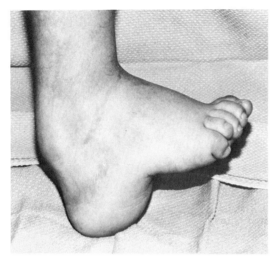

Figure 71.76. Lateral view of right foot. Note severe calcaneus deformity.

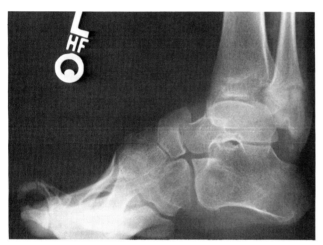

Figure 71.77. Preoperative lateral radiograph of left foot. A severe cavo adducto varus deformity is evident.

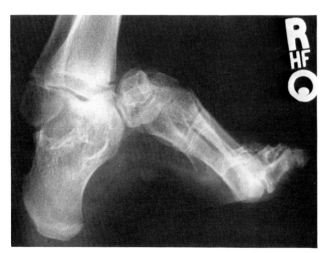

Figure 71.78. Preoperative lateral radiograph of right foot. Calcaneus deformity is evident, as is severe cavus deformity.

Surgical history included resection of the osseous protuberance from the spinal canal to relieve traction from the distal spinal cord. The patient had also undergone three Achilles tendon lengthenings on each lower extremity and three one-stage soft tissue and bone releases on each foot, including a talectomy on the right. Despite surgical correction, in each instance the deformity recurred rapidly.

Objective Findings

The patient appeared quite normal and well developed from the knees proximally. The left foot presented a cavo adducto varus deformity but with an associated severe first metatarsal equinus and hallux abducto valgus (Figs. 71.74 and 71.75). The right foot exhibited the unusual configuration of cavo calcaneo valgus deformity (Fig. 71.76). Hallux abducto valgus was also present on the right foot, as was first metatarsal equinus.

Radiographic evaluation confirmed clinical impressions concerning the left foot. On the right foot absence of the talus was revealed, along with nearly vertical orientation of the calcaneal inclination (Figs. 71.77 and 71.78).

Discussion and Treatment

Because of severe muscle imbalance related to diastematomyelia, it was believed that any effective treatment must involve arthrodesis of the appropriate joints. Any soft tissue release could be expected to provide only temporary relief because of the muscle imbalance associated with the underlying condition. Surgery in four stages was planned, with the rearfoot stabilization of one foot being followed by first ray realignment and metatarsophalangeal joint arthrodesis 3 months later (Figs. 71.79 and 71.80).

Postoperative treatment included accommodation of al-

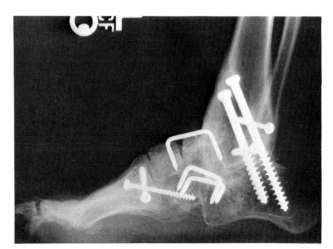

Figure 71.79. Postoperative radiograph of left foot 6 months after rearfoot and ankle stabilization and 3 months after arthrodesis of first ray and first metatarsophalangeal joint.

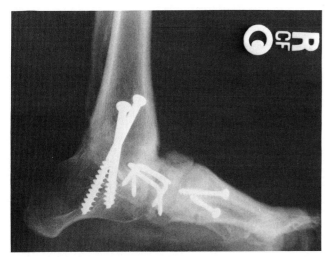

Figure 71.80. Postoperative radiograph of right foot 6 months after rearfoot stabilization and 3 months after arthrodesis of first ray and first metatarsophalangeal joint.

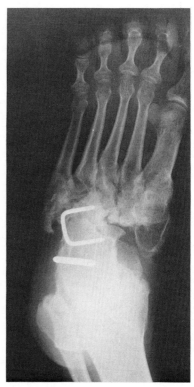

Figure 71.82. Dorsoplantar view helps one appreciate the instability of the midfoot that has resulted.

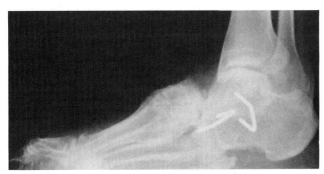

Figure 71.81. Lateral radiograph of patient with Charcot-Marie-Tooth disease who had undergone Lambrinudi-type triple arthrodesis several years earlier to control dropfoot deformity.

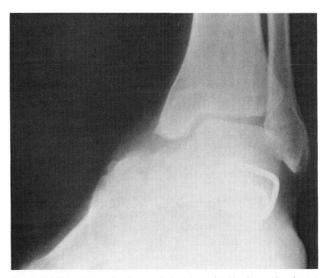

Figure 71.83. Relaxed anteroposterior view of ankle shows the degree of ankle instability that has developed.

tered length and configuration of the two feet. Appropriate footgear was provided with molded shoes and rocker soles, with the rocker placed at the metatarsal head level. The patient was also able to wear padded basketball shoes with rocker soles added. Creation of beveled rockers at the contact point of the heel and at the metatarsal level made possible a reasonably smooth gait.

A major consideration in the presence of neurological disorders that produce severe muscle imbalance is the unpredictability of the deformities. In this instance, the earlier surgery most likely failed because of the progressive nature of the deformities. Arthrodesis rather than muscle-tendon balancing is often chosen in cases in which neuromuscular imbalance makes soft tissue procedures unpredictable. In this case, the patient was a bit young to undergo the procedures that were performed. However, the severity of the deformities mandated the aggressive approach that was chosen.

CASE 16

This case illustrates the difficulty of stabilizing a rearfoot/ankle complex in the absence of muscle function about the ankle joint (Figs. 71.81 to 71.83).

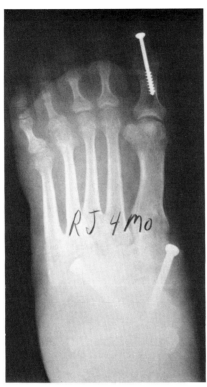

Figure 71.84. Dorsoplantar radiograph 4 months after surgery shows solid union of midtarsal joints and digital arthrodeses.

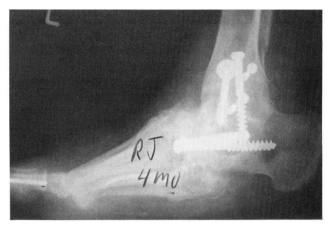

Figure 71.85. Lateral radiograph at 4 months shows solid union of pantalar arthrodesis with satisfactory alignment of foot to leg.

History

A 46-year-old man was admitted for arthrodesis of the left ankle and revisional arthrodesis of the midtarsal joint. Char-cot-Marie-Tooth disease had been diagnosed 11 years earlier. Four years earlier he had undergone a Lambrinudi-type triple arthrodesis in an attempt to stabilize the rearfoot and to provide a posterior stop at the ankle to prevent footdrop. After recovery from the arthrodesis, the patient found no improvement in the dropfoot disorder and noticed increasing instability in gait, with frequent ankle sprains.

Objective Findings

Clinical examination showed a severe steppage gait associated with an exaggerated knee lift and foot slap. Manual muscle testing revealed that all muscles of the anterior and lateral compartments were inadequate for the purposes of transfer. The posterior muscles were marginal. Examination of the ankle gave an impression of gross instability. The toes showed no extensor function, and barefoot walking was virtually impossible because of the toes folding under the forefoot.

Initial radiographs (Fig. 71.8l) showed a pseudoarthrosis at the talonavicular joint where a Lambrinudi-type arthrodesis had been attempted. The defect at the talonavicular joint can also be appreciated from the dorsoplantar view (Fig. 71.82). On a nonstressed anteroposterior view of the ankle, gross instability is evident (Fig. 71.83).

Treatment

The treatment plan as executed included ankle arthrodesis, revisional midtarsal arthrodesis, and arthrodesis of the interphalangeal joint of the hallux and the proximal joints of the second, third, and fourth toes (Figs. 71.84 and 71.85).

Discussion

Earlier treatment with triple arthrodesis appears to have failed to provide stability because the posterior process of the talus did not provide a stop against the posterior tibia at the ankle. At best, the Lambrinudi procedure is difficult to control accurately. In addition, the advanced state of muscle atrophy had precluded effective muscle tendon transfers. The loss of anterior compartment muscle strength resulted in a footdrop, and lateral compartment loss compounded the problem with added lateral ankle instability. In instances such as the foregoing, where no suitable muscles are available for transfer, pantalar arthrodesis offers a far more realistic approach to stabilizing the foot and aiding the patient's general sense of balance. The most frequent alternative is upright ankle-foot bracing.

REFERENCES

1. Smith TF: Surgical principles in the management of iatrogenic forefoot deformities. In McGlamry ED (ed): *Reconstructive Surgery of the Foot and Leg-Update '89*. Tucker, GA, Podiatry Institute Publishing Company, 1989, pp 279-286.

ADDITIONAL REFERENCES

Cavaliere RG, McGlamry ED: Iatrogenic deformities. In McGlamry ED (ed): *Comprehensive Textbook of Foot Surgery*. Baltimore, Williams & Wilkins, 1987, Vol I, pp 552-579.
McGlamry ED, Banks AS: Iatrogenic complications in foot surgery. In McGlamry ED (ed): *Comprehensive Textbook of Foot Surgery*. Baltimore, Williams & Wilkins, 1987, Vol I, pp 1066-1077.

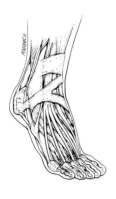

CHAPTER **72**

Augmentation of Bone Growth by Electromagnetic Field Stimulation

Allen M. Jacobs, D.P.M.
Ann M. Seifert, D.P.M.

The use of electrical energy in an effort to effect the healing of bone was initially described in 1812 when Hartshorne credited the healing of a tibial nonunion to "a shock of electric fluid" (1). In 1971 Friedenberg and associates (2) used direct current for the management of nonunion of the medial malleolus. In 1981, Brighton and co-workers (3) reported their results in a multicenter evaluation of the use of constant direct current for the management of osseous nonunion. The initial description of a totally implantable direct current bone stimulator appears to have been that of Duger and Wickham (4). Bassett and associates (5) in 1981 described the application of pulsed electromagnetic fields in the treatment of nonunion of bone using noninvasive methods.

A variety of therapeutic devices are currently available to provide electrical stimulation in the treatment of nonunions of bone. In addition, the same devices have been applied in the management of other clinical problems, including the treatment of osteonecrosis, congenital pseudarthrosis, failed arthrodesis, osteoporosis, chronic refractory tendonitis, and Charcot joints.

Electrical stimulation of nonunited fractures and osteotomies, particularly when applied in a noninvasive manner, is generally reported as being safe. A recent diagnostic and therapeutical technology assessment by the American Medical Association concluded "non-invasive electrical stimulation to be a safe treatment for fracture non-unions" (6).

Numerous retrospective studies appear to attest to the effectiveness of electrical stimulation in the management of osseous nonunion (7-9). However, the true value of electrical stimulation has been difficult to evaluate because of the paucity of controlled, randomized clinical studies. Barker and associates (10) reported the use of pulsed magnetic fields in a double-blind study of 16 patients. The remaining studies in which electrical stimulation has been used to achieve bone healing have reviewed cases in which immobilization, bone grafting, or other adjunctive methods were concurrently employed. Therefore the specific contribution of electrical stimulation to the healing of nonunion is difficult to ascertain.

BIOPHYSICS OF BONE HEALING

It is well known that changes in the environment or forces applied to bone and joints result in adaptation. Adaptation of bone in response to environmental factors is explained by Wolff's law, which states: "Modifications in the form and function of a bone are followed by changes in its internal architecture and secondary alterations in its external configuration in accordance with mathematical laws" (11). Numerous examples of osseous structural alteration in response to changes in stress are readily appreciated in clinical practice. Chronic abnormal function of the first metatarsophalangeal joint is associated with alteration in the structure of the first metatarsal head (12). Exercise programs have been shown to increase the bone mass of elderly nursing home residents (13), whereas an opposite alteration in osseous tissue occurs as the result of weightlessness (14).

Alterations in the radiographic appearance of bone in response to additional stress and the sequential changes of healing or remodeling of bone following fracture or osteotomy imply that from an engineering viewpoint, bone must possess a control system that is activated during various stages of physiological functions (15). In recent years, researchers studying the structural adaptations of bone to stress and other applied forces have focused on the electromechanical properties of osseous tissue as the means by which these alterations are mediated.

In 1957, Fuhada and Yasuda (16) demonstrated that when stress is applied to a bone in such a manner as to cause deformity, electrical potentials are generated within the bone. The appearance of electrical potentials within bone (or any material) to which an external force is applied is referred to as a piezoelectric property. The electrical signals generated within osseous structures in response to stress are known as endogenous stress-related potentials.

Endogenous Stress-Related Potentials

Two potential sources are known to exist that may explain the presence of endogenous stress-related potentials in bone. Stress applied to dry bone results in the generation of a measurable electrical potential, the result of the deformation of solid crystals within an asymmetrical lattice. These piezoelectric potentials arise from stress-induced orientation of electric dipoles within osseous material, primarily in the form of collagen (17). In addition, it has been demonstrated that endogenous stress-related potentials are electronegative in those areas of bone subjected to compression, and they are electropositive in those portions of osseous tissue subjected to tension (Fig. 72.1).

A second source of endogenous stress-related potential in bone is that of electrokinetic potentials. Electrokinetic potentials are generated at the interface of a solid and a fluid that contains ions (18). Within bone, an interface region exists between solids (e.g., hydoxyapatite) and the surrounding ionic fluids. Interactions at the interface result in the creation of a spatially varying electrical potential called the electric double layer (18). A slip plane or boundary exists between stationary fluids adsorbed to solid material and nonadsorbed moving ionic fluids. Therefore an electrical potential, the zeta potential, exists in the slip plane. When stress is applied to a bone, there is movement of nonabsorbed ionic fluids relative to the absorbed stationary fluid, resulting in stress-related bone potentials (Fig. 72.2).

To summarize, two sources of endogenous stress-related potentials appear to exist within bone, piezoelectric and electrokinetic. The potentials are biphasic, producing current flow in one direction with the application of stress and in the opposite direction when that stress is removed. These potentials are of a negative polarity in areas of compression and a positive polarity in areas of tension. Bone production occurs at electronegative areas whereas resorption occurs at electropositive areas.

Steady-State Potentials

In addition to stress-related potentials, a second type of endogenous bone electrical activity, steady-state or bioelectric potentials, are known to exist. Bioelectric or steady-state potentials may be recorded from the surface of a living bone when no stress has been applied. The electronegativity recorded from the surface of nonstressed living bone (steady-state or bioelectric potential) is dependent upon the presence of living cells (19). The presence of these steady-state potentials appears to be unaffected by denervation or arterial ligation.

Steady-state potentials are significantly electronegative at the site of growing bone, as exemplified by the physeal plates. In addition, strongly electronegative bioelectric potentials may be recorded throughout a fractured or osteot-

omized bone, with the peak electronegativity recorded at the site of bone healing (Fig. 72.3).

Cellular and Biochemical Response to Electrical Stimulation

Although stress-related and steady-state electrical potentials are very small, the discovery of these processes resulted in the hypothesis that Wolff's law was in effect mediated by electrical impulses. A theoretical strategy whereby the exogenous application of electronegative currents may stimulate osteogenesis is the basis upon which bone stimulation units are employed.

The effects of electromagnetic fields on osteogenesis at the site of nonunions have been reported. A variety of meth-

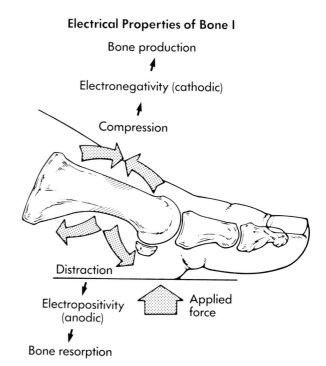

Figure 72.1. Stress-induced piezoelectric potentials. Stress applied to a bone generates a relatively electronegative (cathodic) area when bone is under compression and a relatively electropositive area (anodic) when bone is distracted (tension). Bone accretion occurs in areas of compression driven by the relative electronegativity. Bone resorption occurs in anodic areas of the tension side.

Figure 72.2. Stress-induced biokinetic potentials. When stress is applied to bone, motion of ionic fluids into pores occurs relative to adsorbed immobile fluids at the apatite/fluid interface. An electric potential, the zeta potential, occurs at the interface or slip layer between mobile and immobile fluids.

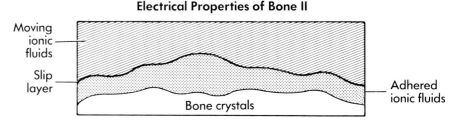

Electrical Properties of Bone III

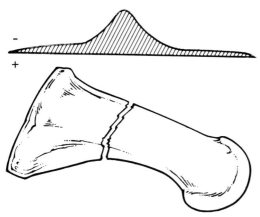

Figure 72.3. Steady-state potentials. Significant electronegative potential exists at the site of growing bone (physeal plate) or at the site of a healing fracture. When fracture healing occurs, the entire surface of the bone becomes electronegative, with maximal cathodic measurements at the level of the healing fracture.

ods to develop an exogenous electrical potential have been used, including constant direct current (20, 21), pulsed direct current (22, 23), electromagnetic stimulation (inductive coupling)(24, 25), and capacitively coupled electrical fields (26). Although all these devices administer exogenous electrical stimulation by different techniques, all have been associated with the healing of nonunions at a rate comparable with that of bone grafting (27).

A variety of mechanisms by which endogenous and exogenous electrical potentials stimulate bone healing have been proposed. The biochemical effects of pulsed electromagnetic fields, reviewed by Cheng (28), include significantly increased DNA synthesis by chondroblasts, increased collagen synthesis, an increased rate of amino acid transport functions across cellular membranes, enhanced H-noradrenaline release from nerve cell lines, and reduced cellular cAMP in mouse osteoblast cultures. These responses to pulsed electromagnetic fields indicate accelerated metabolic activity, implying the potential for rapid healing of connective tissue.

In addition, increased proteoglycan synthesis (29) in bone matrix, increased calcification of bone matrix, and increased proliferation of both osseous and cartilaginous cells have been noted in response to electrical stimulation (19).

At least 30 known or probable factors have been described to explain the cellular and mechanical responses of bone to electrical stimulation (30). Certain fundamental questions regarding the characteristics of administered exogenous electrical or electromagnetic energy and the concept of targeted biological response remain to be investigated. In normal bone growth or repair, endogenous electrical potentials serve to autoregulate osseous metabolic processes, with changes in the physical and electrochemical environment reflected by changes in potential within the bone. This is analogous to a rheostat light switch, which may be adjusted

to various levels between on and off. Whether a similar variability in exogenously administered electrical field is necessary remains unclear. It is possible, for example, that the electrical characteristics of recent nonunion, chronic nonunion, infected nonunion, nonunion with internal fixation, and the variety of qualitative and quantitative circumstances demand greater selectivity in the characteristics of the applied fields and their interactions with endogenous bone potentials.

INDICATIONS

Nonunion

The primary indication for electrically or electromagnetically induced osteogenesis is nonunion following fracture, osteotomy, arthrodesis, or infection. Electrical stimulation has been used as the primary modality for treatment in up to 40% of patients with nonunions (31). The use of electrical or electromagnetic stimulation of bone healing may be combined with other measures to enhance healing, including cast or brace immobilization, internal or external fixation, bone grafting, debridement and scarification, and the concurrent management of infection in bone or soft tissue.

No universal agreement exists as to the precise definition of a nonunion. A general understanding is a situation in which bone has failed to heal and all evidence of reparative processes has ceased. The precise differentiation of a delayed union from nonunion may be difficult to define clinically and radiographically. Asymptomatic cartilaginous or even fibrous union may occur within a bone that demonstrates the radiographic characteristics of nonunion. Under these circumstances, pain or other signs and symptoms that are extraosseous in nature may be used to determine the presence of a radiographically occult union.

A variety of temporal considerations have been proposed for the definition of a nonunion. The Food and Drug Administration defines a nonunion as an osseous discontinuity of 9 months' duration, in which there has been no evidence of osseous healing for 3 consecutive months. Others have advocated the use of electrical stimulation of bone "as soon as tardy union of bone is identified" (9). The argument is that early institution of electrical stimulation of a delayed union will reduce the disability time as well as the incidence of nonunion (32, 26).

Bassett and co-workers (33) have similarly suggested that an acute repair process following fracture may be augmented if the optimal pulse sequences can be identified. As was noted, the current forms of electrical stimulation appear to be suitable for the resolution of a chronic reparative process such as delayed union, yet may not be appropriate, and theoretically detrimental, for acute reparative processes.

Bone Grafting

Electrical stimulation may augment the normal incorporation of bone grafts (34), and a synergistic effect of bone grafting and electrical stimulation has been reported (35-

37). Bone grafting, in combination with electrical stimulation, should be employed if osseous defects exist inasmuch as electrical stimulation will not correct osseous malalignment or loss of bone substance (Fig. 72.4).

Fixation and Stabilization

The management of nonunions includes the stabilization of fracture, osteotomy, or arthrodesis sites in addition to the osteogenic stimulation provided by external electrical or electromagnetic fields. The use of fixation devices to achieve stability at the site of nonunion complements the use of electrical stimulation (37). Most cases described in the literature retrospectively evaluating the use of electrical bone stimulation have included the concurrent use of external immobilization and either internal or external fixation. It is for this reason that the actual role of electrical stimulation has been questioned (36) because only one controlled study appears to be available (10).

Infection

Electrical stimulation has been used with success for the management of infected nonunions (3, 38). Appropriate stabilization, as well as appropriate efforts to eradicate the microorganisms, must be concurrently employed as necessary. Therefore three problems exist that need be addressed: infection, osseous instability, and osteogenesis. In many cases, the existence of osseous infection necessitates the removal of fixation devices, so that control of infection takes priority to osteogenesis. The use of bone simulators allows for continued osteogenesis during active treatment of the infection.

Electrical stimulation has been noted to result in a reduction, a change in character, and resolution of drainage at the site of infected nonunions (9). Bone grafting, combined with electrical stimulation, has been demonstrated to successfully resolve signs and symptoms associated with infected nonunions (35, 39, 40).

In addition to the augmentation of osteogenesis, electrical

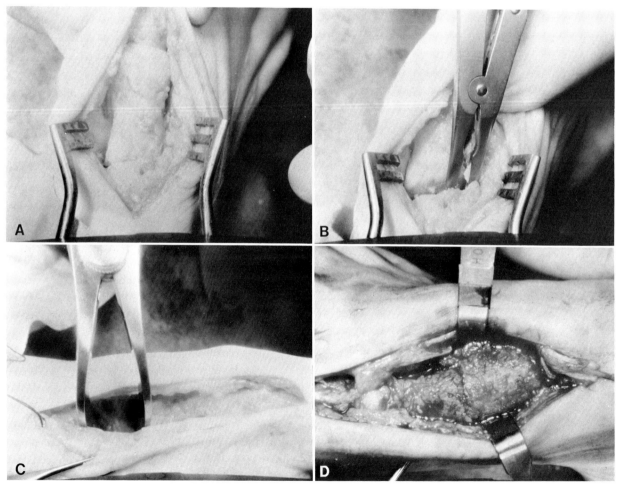

Figure 72.4. Technique for preparation of nonunion site. **A.** Atrophic nonunion of the first metatarsal secondary to osteotomy 2 years earlier. **B.** Following exposure of the osteotomy, complete debridement of dysvascular and necrotic tissue is performed. **C.** Site of the osseous defect following debridement. **D.** Autogenous bone graft is placed within the nonunion site. Appropriate fixation is then performed and treatment augmented with noninvasive bone stimulation.

stimulation may accelerate the resolution of infection by other, indirect means. A direct, bactericidal effect may be obtained with silver-tipped electrodes implanted directly into the site of the infected nonunion (41). The stimulation of a lymphocytic response occurs in vitro with exposures to pulsed magnetic frequencies (42). Increased vascularity has been reported (Yet-Patton G: The Effect of Electromagnetic Fields on the Rate of Healing of Injured Human Umbilical Vein Endothelial Cells. Master's thesis, University of Lowell, Lowell, MA, 1936)(43). The report details the use of electrical stimulation, an effort desirable for the delivery of antibiotics as well as cellular and humoral immune mechanisms.

Failed Arthrodesis

Electrical stimulation may be used to resolve symptoms associated with failed arthrodesing procedures, with a success rate of 85% (44, 45). Fixation devices that were used for the original arthrodesis should be examined as a potential source of distraction. If this is apparent, then these devices should be removed. The most important aspect in the use of electrical stimulation for failed arthrodesis is in the management of patient care after what appears to be a healed arthrodesis. Following the determination that osseous union has occurred at a fusion site, unrestricted weight bearing should not be allowed. Most fusions performed in the foot do not place joints in a position whereby loading produces axial compressive forces of a repeated nature. The mechanically immature tissue may eventually fail by progressive crack propagation with repetitive cyclical loading. Similarly, ankle arthrodesis may fail after seemingly successful clinical or radiographic union when early resumption of heel-toe gait is encouraged.

When consolidation has been obtained following the use of electrical stimulation at a failed arthrodesis site, care must be taken to protect the fusion from distraction forces with appropriate axial compression exercises, intermittent periods of non-weight bearing, and particularly following ankle arthrodesis, a peg-leg or heel-weight bearing gait (30). The use of weight-bearing casts or braces may also be of assistance.

Neuropathic (Charcot) Joint Disease

Electrical stimulation has been reported as effective in the management of neuropathic (Charcot) joint associated with diabetes mellitus or alcoholic neuropathy (30, 46). The use on non-weight-bearing immobilization in combination with pulsed electromagnetic frequency may result in a termination of joint inflammation, reduction of edema, and foot stability.

Charcot joint disease is characterized by progressive bone resorption and osteoclastic activity, with both processes reduced by electrical stimulation of bone because of a decrease in the cellular response to parathyroid hormone (47). In addition, improvement in ulcer healing rates and sensation related to electrical field-triggered alterations in neural re-

generation and axon transport rates have been reported (48, 49).

Avascular Necrosis

A variety of osteonecroses may affect the foot, including posttraumatic avascular necrosis of the talus, second metatarsal (Frieberg's disease), navicular (Köhler's disease), or dysvascular change after metatarsal osteotomy. As noted, electrical stimulation of bone increases angiogenesis while promoting osteogenesis. In addition, electrical stimulation diminishes osteoclastic resorption of bone associated with osteonecrosis, which is responsible for the bone collapse and fragmentation.

Electrical stimulation has been shown to be an effective alternative to arthroplasty for the management of avascular necrosis of the hip (50-52), and its use is crucial after distal first metatarsal surgery, thus avoiding the development of overt collapse and deformity, at which point resection arthroplasty may be necessary.

FUTURE APPLICATIONS

Several investigators have advanced the concept of stimulating osteogenesis by the implantation of electrically charged materials in direct apposition to bone (53-56). A variety of piezoelectric materials have been demonstrated to produce osseous growth when in contact with bone, including Teflon film, polyvinyllidene fluoride, and polymethyl L-glutamate.

An additional concept for the augmentation of bone repair through direct stimulation of bone healing is the incorporation of a piezogenic material within fixation devices such as bone plates (57). The use of an excitable material within fixation devices, which may be externally stimulated by methods such as ultrasound, has also been proposed (58).

Evidence exists that electrical stimulation may be of benefit in the management of chronic refractory tendinitis such as Achilles tendinitis. Electrical stimulation has been demonstrated to be effective in the treatment of similar problems of the rotator cuff (59). Chronic, refractory Achilles tendinitis may be commonly encountered, particularly in athletes. Marked similarities between this condition and refractory tendinitis of the rotatory cuff exist, including a tenuous vascular supply, chronic degenerative changes (tendinosis), calcium deposition, disabling pain, and possible rupture. Therefore, electrical stimulation may theoretically ameliorate the symptoms associated with chronic refractory Achilles tendinitis.

DEVICES AND METHOD OF APPLICATION

Devices for the electrical stimulation of bone healing all consist of a power source, electrodes or other means of delivering the energy to bone, and a means to record the time and dosage (current) employed.

Three broad categories of devices are available: invasive (implanted), semiinvasive (percutaneous), and noninvasive.

Noninvasive bone growth stimulators may be subdivided into two groups: those that produce current within bone by inductive coupling and those that produce current by capacitative coupling (Tables 72.1 and 72.2). Noninvasive techniques are primarily used for patient convenience in the management of foot and ankle conditions. Proper fracture management concurrent with the use of bone growth stimulation is essential. In most cases, immobilization of the fracture or arthrodesis site is essential. The control of infection with debridement, antibiotic therapy, antibiotic-loaded bone cement, and the stabilization of the morbid site with internal or external fixation must be considered as appropriate to each case.

Implantable (Invasive) Devices

Friedenberg and co-workers (2) first reported the successful healing of a nonunion (medial malleolus) with use of an implanted cathode. The use of implanted cathodes grew directly from laboratory experimentation with direct current. The use of implantable bone growth stimulators is generally not practical for the management of foot disorders because of the size of the cathode, the required surgical exposure of the nonunion site, and the compliance and care required by the patient. Therefore this modality has generally been discarded in favor of noninvasive techniques. In addition, the use of implanted biomaterials in the presence of active infectious processes has generally been discouraged. The technique has been reported as successful in at least one large series in which infected nonunion with chronic discharge was present (60).

When implantable cathodes are employed for persistent infection at the site of a nonunion, the prevailing observa-

Table 72.1.
Indications for Bone Growth Stimulators

Indication	Reference No.
Nonunion, aseptic	9, 23, 33, 35, 36
Nonunion, septic	3, 9, 39, 62, 36, 40, 41
Failed arthrodesis	32, 46, 47
Charcot joint disease	31, 48, 49
Osteonecrosis	52, 53, 54
Chronic refractory tendinitis	31, 61
Osteoporosis	31

Table 72.2.
Types of Bone Stimulators

Classification	Current	Example
Invasive	Direct	Orthogen/Osteogen (EBI)
Semiinvasive	Direct	DCBGS Osteogenesis System (Zimmer)
Noninvasive		
Inductive	Indirect	Physiostim (AME), EBI Bone Healing System (EBI)
Capacitative	Indirect	Orthopak (Bioelectron)

tions have been that drainage will cease and be followed by evidence of osteogenesis. Several months may be required before drainage stops, and replacement of the cathode may be necessary.

Bone grafting may be performed concurrently with the use of implantable cathodes (61). The overall success rate of implanted bone growth stimulation in the treatment of nonunions with and without drainage has been reported to be as high as 89%, with bone union obtained at an average of 16 weeks for noninfected sites and at 35 weeks for infected nonunions (60).

In general, the nonunion is approached directly by longitudinal incision of soft tissue and periosteum. The integrity of the soft tissues at the operative site may complicate the surgical approach. Approximately 1.5 to 2 cm of cortical bone is symmetrically removed from the nonunion site. Multiple bone culture and bone biopsy speciments should be obtained. All suspicious-appearing bone and soft tissue, including fibrous tissue and sclerotic bone, must be removed so that a clean medullary tunnel crosses the osteotomy site. The cathode is wound into a helical shape and placed into the surgical bone defect so as to cross the entire nonunion site. In addition, the ends of the cathode should be placed in such a manner as to discourage early displacement. Appropriate fixation techniques or bone grafting may be performed. The cathode should not touch the fixation devices.

A second incision is required at an appropriate location, usually the lower portion of the leg, in which the generator may be implanted below the fascia. Following connections of the generator to the cathode by subcutaneous tunneling the cathode is attached to the generator with a microconnector. Intraoperative radiographs should confirm the location of the cathode and generator before wound closure is performed. The leg should be placed in a cast and managed with non–weight bearing or weight bearing as deemed appropriate. Clinical and radiographic monitoring is necessary for confirmation of osseous healing and resolution of infection.

Semi-Invasive (Percutaneous) Techniques

The technique employs an insulated cathode whose exposed end is placed at the site of nonunion. Depending on the size of the bone and nonunion to be treated, up to four electrodes may be implanted within the area. In general, the electrodes can be inserted under fluoroscopic guidance, with minimal surgical dissection required. The cathode's insulated wire is then connected to a power pack that is generally incorporated within an applied cast (60). The technique is not appropriate for acute or chronically infected nonunions. Appropriate weight bearing is permitted. The power pack must be regularly checked for the charge available, and the position of electrodes should be periodically confirmed. The technique uses direct current averaging 20 microamperes per cathode. When fixation devices are present, the electrode should not be in contact with metal, which may dissipate the energy and reduce the effectiveness of the device.

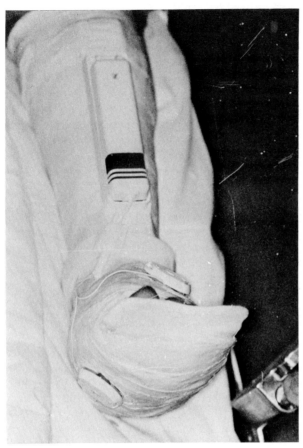

Figure 72.5. Capacitative-type noninvasive bone stimulator. The electrodes are placed on each side of the nonunion site. The unit is supplemented with a non-weight-bearing cast.

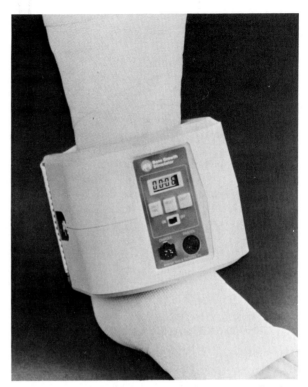

Figure 72.6. Induction bone stimulator used by placement directly over the nonunion site. The unit may be used with or without supplementary external immobilization as necessary. Such units are employed 3 to 10 hours per day for management of nonunion.

Non-Invasive Techniques

Success with noninvasive bone growth stimulators has resulted in an increased acceptance and use of this technique in the management of nonseptic and septic nonunions, failed arthrodeses, avascular necrosis, and neuropathic joint disease. With appropriate documentation, the cost of such devices are reimbursed by many insurance carriers. The technique is painless and can be used in the patient's home.

Two major types of noninvasive bone growth stimulators are presently available, inductive and capacitative coupling. A variety of such devices are available for clinical use. Capacitative bone growth stimulators consist of a power source, usually powered by a 9-volt alkaline battery, that contains visual or audio alarms for the patient, signifying poor skin contact of the electrodes or ineffective voltage. Most devices also include an elapsed time accumulator, which stores the number of days during which effective treatment was applied for reference by the clinician.

The unit delivers energy by means of two electrode disks that are directly attached to skin. Treatment with this technique requires a minimum of 3 months and a maximum of 6 months. Concurrent cast immobilization is necessary throughout the treatment period. Patients must be checked at the site of electrode attachment to the skin for evidence of skin irritation or sensitivity as a result of electrode gel or retained perspiration (Fig. 72.5).

Capacitative coupling allows the resumption of protected weight bearing on the casted extremity unless motion greater than 5° is present. Several studies have shown the technique to be successful in the healing of nonunions (62, 63).

The technique of application, which is rather simple, requires no surgery. The site of nonunion is confirmed, and an arbitrary axis that passes through the nonunion site is selected. The skin electrodes are placed on opposite sides of the nonunion site (180°). Errors in placement of up to 20° may be tolerated without loss of clinical effectiveness. A cast is applied and may be bivalved to allow access to the surface electrodes. The electrodes should be placed in such a manner as to avoid scars or areas of poor skin.

Cast guides may be used to provide an access hole within plaster or fiberglass and are incorporated within the cast. With hardening of the cast, the guides are removed. The bone stimulator (power source) may be mounted within the cast or on the cast or attached with a clip. Electrodes are then connected to the power source. The amplitude of the treatment current must be maintained between 5 and 10 milliamperes.

Inductive coupling uses external coils or electrodes that are placed at 180° and parallel to each other. The unit is placed over the nonunion site or cast. A time-varying programmed current is supplied to a treatment transducer, and the unit is simply plugged into a standard electrical outlet. The result is the creation of a pulsatile electromagnetic field (PEMF) that induces electrical currents at the nonunion site (Fig. 72.6).

Inductive coupling devices are easily used. The field generated has an average peak amplitude of 20 gauss. The system is used 3 to 10 hours daily until healing occurs, with an effective healing rate of 80%.

In general, the use of inductive coupling systems requires concurrent cast immobilization. However, if no motion is present at the site of nonunion, the transducer may be applied directly over the skin, with partial weight bearing allowed. The technique may be applied in the presence of fixation devices or infection.

CONTRAINDICATIONS AND CAVEATS

Malunion is not corrected by the use of electrical stimulation. Therefore, when rotational or angular deformity exists and is of clinical significance, consideration must be given to the eventual correction of this problem. Although rare, synovial pseudoarthrosis will not respond to electrical stimulation alone. The treatment of synovial pseudarthrosis requires surgical resection and grafting or compression in addition to electrical stimulation. As a general rule, electrical stimulation as an isolated treatment modality will not be successful if there is a deficit at the nonunion site greater than one half of the diameter of the bone.

Although the use of bone growth stimulators appears to be safe, their use during pregnancy or in children has not been established with certainty.

References

1. Peltier LF: A brief historical note on the use of electricity in the treatment of fractures. *Clin Orthop* 161:4-7, 1981.
2. Friedenberg ZB, Harlow MC, Brighton CT: Healing of a non-union of the medial malleolus by means of direct current: a case report. *J Trauma* 11:883-884, 1971.
3. Brighton CT, Block J, Friedenberg ZB: A multicenter study of the treatment of non-union with constant direct current. *J Bone Joint Surg* 63A:2-13, 1981.
4. Duger AF, Wickham CG: Direct current stimulation in spinal fusions. *Med J Aust* 1:73-75, 1974.
5. Bassett CAL, Mitchell SN, Gaston SR: Treatment of ununited tibial diaphyseal fractures with pulsing electromagnetic fields. *J Bone Joint Surg* 63A:511-523, 1981.
6. Cole HM: Questions and answers: noninvasive electrical stimulation for nonunited bone fracture. *JAMA* 261:917-919, 1989.
7. Bassett CA, Mitchell SN, Schink MM: Treatment of therapeutically resistant non-unions with bone grafts and pulsing electromagnetic fields. *J Bone Joint Surg* 64:1214-1220, 1982.
8. Pess GM, Waugh TR, Melone CP: Treatment of non-union with electrical stimulation. *Orthop Rev* 14:392-402, 1985.
9. Dunn AW, Rusk GA III: Electrical stimulation in the treatment of delayed union and non-union of fractures and osteotomies. *South Med J* 1530-1534, 1984.
10. Barker AT, Dixon RA, Sharrud WJ: Pulsed magnetic field for tibial non-union: interim results of a double blind trial. *Lancet* 1:994-996, 1984.
11. Evans FD, Rydel N: Studies on the anatomy and function of bone and joints. In *Intravital Measurements of Forces Acting on the Hip Joint*. New York, Springer-Verlag, 1966, pp 52-58.
12. Root ML, Weed J, Orion B: *Normal and Abnormal Function of the Foot*. Los Angles, Clinical Biomechanics Corp, 1977.
13. Smith EL, Reddon W: Physical therapy—a modality for bone acretion in the aged. *AJR* 126:1297, 1976.
14. Basset C: The effects of force on skeletal tissues in physiological basis of rehabilitation medicine. Philadelphia, WB Saunders, 1971, pp 283-288.
15. Hastings GW, Mahmud FA: Electrical effects in bone. *J Biomed Eng* 10:515-521, 1988.
16. Fuhada E, Yasuda I: On the piezoelectric effect of bone. *J Physiol Soc Jpn* 12:1158-1162, 1957.
17. Kennedy A: Changes in the mechanical and electrical environment and the effect on bone. *Orthopedics* 10:3-14, 1984.
18. Pollack SR: Bioelectrical properties of bone endogenous electrical signals. *Orthop Clin North Am* 15:13-14, 1984.
19. Brighton DT, McClusky WP: Cellular response and mechanisms of action of electrically induced osteogenesis. *Bone Mineral Res* 4:213-254, 1986.
20. Bassett C, Pawluck RJ, Becker RO: Effects of electric currents on bone in vivo. *Nature* 204:652-654, 1964.
21. Becker RO, Spadaro J: Experience with low current/silver electrode treatment for non-union. In Brighton C (ed): *Electrical Properties of Bone and Cartilage*. New York, Grune & Stratton, 1979, pp 631-638.
22. Jorgenson TE: The effect of electrical current on the healing time of crural fractures. *Acta Orthop Scand* 43:421-437, 1972.
23. Von-Satzger, Garbor H.: Surgical and electrical methods in the treatment of congenital and post-traumatic pseudoarthrosis of the tibia. *Clin Orth* 161:82-104, 1981.
24. Basset C: Pulsing electromagnetic field treatment in ununited fractures and failed arthrodeses. *JAMA* 247:623-628, 1982.
25. Bassett C: Pulsing and electromagnetic fields: a nonoperative method to produce bony union. In Academy of Orthopaedic Surgeons: *Instructional Course Lectures*, vol 31. St Louis, CV Mosby, 1982, pp 88-94.
26. Brighton C, Pollack S: Treatment of recalcitrant nonunion with a capacitively coupled electrical field *J Bone Joint Surg* 67A:577-589, 1985.
27. Becker R: Electrical osteogenesis. In Galasko C (ed): *Principles of Fracture Management*. New York, Churchill Livingstone, 1984, pp 162-174.
28. Cheng N: Biochemical effects of pulsed electromagnetic fields. *Bioelectrochem Bioenergetics* 14:121-129, 1985.
29. Okihina H, Shimomura Y: Effect of direct current on cultured growth cartilage cells in vitro. *J Orthop Res* 6:690-694, 1988.
30. Bassett CA: Fundamental and practical aspects of therapeutic uses of pulsed electromagnetic fields. *Crit Rev Biomed Eng* 17:451-529, 1989.
31. Brighton CT: Symposium: Electrical stimulation of nonunion. *Contemp Orthop* 11:3, 1985.
32. Compore CL: Electromagnetic fields and bones [editorial]. *JAMA* 247:699, 1982.
33. Bassett C, Valdos MG, Hernandez E: Modification of fracture repair with selected pulsing electromagnetic fields. *J Bone Joint Surg* 64A:889-895, 1982.
34. Bassett C, Hess K: Synergistic effects of pulsed electromagnetic fields and fresh canine cancellous bone grafts. *Orthop Trans* 8:341, 1984.
35. Stein GA, Anzel SH: A review of delayed unions of open tibial fractures treated with internal fixation and pulsing electromagnetic fields. *Orthopedics* 7:428-436, 1984.
36. Barker AT: Electromagnetic stimulation of bone healing: the need for multicenter collaboration. *J Med Eng Technol* 4:271, 1980.
37. Connolly JF: Selection, evaluation and indications for electrical stimulation of ununited fractures. *Clin Orthop* 161:39-53, 1981.
38. Paterson DC, Lewis GN, Cass CA: Treatment of delayed union and nonunion with an implanted direct current stimulation. *Clin Orthop* 148:117-128, 1982.

39. Kumpen JF, Silver RA: External electromagnetic fields in the treatment of non-union of bones. *Orthop Rev* 10:33, 1981.

40. Mulin J, Spaas F: Out-patient treatment of surgically resistant non-unions by induced pulsing currents—clinical results. *Arch Orthop Traumatol Surg* 97:293-301, 1980.

41. Becker RO, Spadara JA: Treatment of orthopedic infections with electrically generated silver ions: a preliminary report. *J Bone Joint Surg* 60A:871-881, 1977.

42. Cadossie R, Emilia G, Lorelli G, Ceccherelli S, Ferrari S, Ruggieci P: The effect of low frequency pulsing electromagnetic fields on the response of human normal lymphocytes to phytohaimoglobin. *J Electroanal Chem, Bioelectrochem Bioenerget* 14:115-119, 1985.

43. Yet-Patton G, Patten WF, Beer D, Jackobson B: Endothelial cell response to pulsed electromagnetic fields: stimulation of growth rate and angiogenesis in vitro. *J Cell Physiol* 134:37, 1988.

44. Bigliani L, Rosenwasser M, Caulo N, Schink M, Bassett C: The use of pulsing electromagnetic fields to achieve arthrodesis of the knee following failed total knee arthroplasty. *J Bone Joint Surg* 65A:480-491, 1983.

45. Bassett C, Mitchell S, Gaston S: Pulsing electromagnetic field treatment in ununited fractures and failed arthrodesis. *JAMA* 247:623-628, 1982.

46. Bier RR, Estersohn H: A new treatment for Charcot joint in the diabetic foot. *J Am Podiatr Med Assoc* 77:63-69, 1987.

47. Sieben R, Cain C, Chen M, Rosen D, Adey W: Effects of electromagnetic stimuli on bone and bone cells in vitro: inhibition of responses to parathyroid hormone by low energy, low frequency fields. *Proc Natl Acad Sci USA* 79:4180-4193, 1982.

48. Ito H, Bassett C: Effect of weak, pulsing electromagnetic fields on neural regeneration in the rat. *Clin Orthop* 181:283-291, 1983.

49. Orgel M, O'Bxan W, Murray H: Pulsing electromagnetic field therapy on nerve regeneration: an experimental study in the cat. *Plast Reconst Surg* 73:173-184, 1984.

50. Aaron R, Ciombor D: Treatment of osteonecrosis of the femoral head with pulsed external magnetic fields. *Ann NY Acad Sci* 435:367-372, 1985.

51. Aaron F, Lennox D, Bunce G, Ebert T: The conservative treatment of osteonecrosis of the femoral head. A comparison of pulsed electromagnetic fields and core decompression. *Trans Bioelectrical Growth Repair Soc* 8:24-41, 1988.

52. Sapkass J, Wang G: Experience with pulsed electromagnetic fields in the treatment of avascular necrosis of the femoral head. *Trans Bioelectrical Growth Repair Soc* 7:91-99, 1987.

53. Fukada E, Takamatsu T, Yasuda I: Callus formation by electret. *Jpn J Appl Phys* 14:2079-2080, 1975.

54. Yasuda I: Electrical callus and callus formation by electret. *Clin Orthop* 124:53-56, 1977.

55. Ficat J, Escourrow G, Fauran J, Durroux R, Ficat P, Sacabanne C: Osteogenesis induced by bimorph polyminyllidine fluoride films. *Ferroelectrics* 51:121-128, 1983.

56. Takamatsu T, Sadabe H, Okada K: Callus formation by piled polymer electret [Paper No. 38]: In Transactions of the Fourth Annual Brags. Kyoto, Japan, 1984. Biological Growth and Repair Society (Philadelphia).

57. Cochran G, Johnson M, Kadaba M, Palmieri B, Mahaffey G: Design consideration in development of a prototype, piezoelectric internal fixation plate: a preliminary report. *J Rehabil Res Dev* 24:39-50, 1987.

58. Cochran G, Kadaba M, Palmieri V: External ultrasound can generate microampere direct currents in vivo from implanted piezoelectric materials. *J Orthop Res* 6:145-147, 1983.

59. Binder A, Parr G, Hazelman B, Fitton-Jackson S: Pulsed electromagnetic field therapy of persistent rotator cuff tendonitis. A double blind controlled assessment. *Lancet* 635-697, 1984.

60. Brighton C: The semi-invasive method of treating nonunions with direct current. *Orthop Clin North Am* 15:33-34, 1984.

61. Paterson D, Simonis R: Electrical stimulation in the treatment of congenital pseudoarthrosis of the tibia. *J Bone Joint Surg* 67B: 454-462, 1985.

62. Paterson D: Treatment of non-union with a constant direct current: a totally implantable system. *Orthop Clin North Am* 15:47-59, 1984.

63. Brighton C, Pollack S: Treatment of non-union of the tibia with a capacitively coupled electrical field. *J Trauma* 24:153-155, 1984.

64. Brighton C, Pollack S: Fracture healing in the rabbit fibula when subjected to various capacitively coupled electric fields. *J Orthop Res* 3:331-340, 1985.

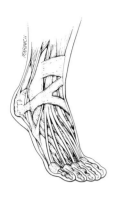

CHAPTER **73**

Prostheses After Lower Extremity Amputations

Richard P. Reinherz, D.P.M.

Limb amputations have been performed for centuries. Historically these resulted from rampant diseases (ergotism and leprosy), the effects of war, or gruesome judicial punishments (1). Original prostheses were crudely manufactured and served to replace useless parts, reduce invalidism, or save lives. As societies developed, peripheral vascular disease became recognized as a primary cause of extremity amputation. Improved techniques in determining the actual level of disease led to more distal amputations (2). Hence greater attention was directed toward cosmetic appearance and improved function as opposed to mere replacement.

The literature indicates that Aristophanes, as early as 500 BC, hired an actor with an artificial leg. Hegistratus, during the same era, escaped from prison by cutting off his chained foot and later designed a wooden replacement. Through the Middle Ages battle scars were considered indications of inferiority among warriors. Unless an appropriate alternative could be constructed, metal armor had to be altered to conceal the lost limb (1).

Ambrose Pare is credited for his foresight in identifying the fundamental principles in lower extremity prosthetic design. During the sixteenth century he described the essentials of fixed equinus, knee locks, adjustable sockets, and controls needed for lower limb function. This led to a variety of appliances being developed and improved through the nineteenth century. Prosthetic feet were then constructed from catgut cord and later solid rubber. Brigg in 1885 emphasized the importance of biomechanical alignment of artificial limbs with their body counterparts, especially in reference to the knee joint axis. By the end of that century a pneumatic rubber foot was developed that would allow the patient to overcome abrupt jerking movements (1).

During the twentieth century artificial limb architecture continued to improve. Surgeons recognized that certain operative techniques led to a better prosthetic fit. The appearance and integrity of a stump are critical. It should be conical, and in the past bone was covered solely with fascia and skin. Today some muscle tissue is sutured over the distal, rounded bones to provide total contact in the socket of the prosthesis. The incision should be placed transversely rather than vertically. The surgical scar should be freely mobile from underlying tissues and every attempt made to minimize adhesions.

Certain perioperative considerations are also important. Emotional factors can affect successful prosthetic use. Chil-

dren are especially vulnerable to curious gazes or thoughtless comments. Family and professional support is needed. An appliance is best dispensed early in life, or soon after an amputation, to maximize its therapeutic value.

MATERIALS

Various materials are used in constructing standard artificial limbs. Durability, ease of adjustment, moisture resistance, and weight are the factors that determine product usage. Willow, or balsa wood, is one of the oldest and best known materials. Steel was used for frames but has been replaced by aluminum. Thermoplastics offer lightweight materials that conform well to many anatomical surfaces and are moisture resistant.

Vulcanized rubber contributes to prosthetic design by its shock-absorbing qualities. Urethanes or synthetic rubbers possess a high tensile strength, are inert, resist abrasion, and adhere well to several surfaces. They absorb force by stretching, yet return to their original configuration (3).

Leather is common for straps, belts, and sometimes laced cuffs. It is easily managed and may be included as an internal lining. However, the material can become hot, heavy, and difficult to clean after staining by perspiration. Velcro is used as a fastener and replaces buckles in some applications.

PROSTHETIC DESIGN

The dramatic improvement in prosthetic design over the past decade has been noteworthy. Originating with the repair of oral and facial defects, multiple body organs including upper extremities, toes, feet, and entire legs have been artificially recreated without extrinsic, sometimes cumbersome, attachments. This can improve the patient's psychological adjustment and increase social and professional acceptance of the handicaps.

Silicone is the material of choice for replacement devices. The compound feels and appears as a human body part. It is durable, flexible, and resists stains (such as ink). Silicone is amenable to repair, and prosthetic longevity is between 2 and 8 years, based upon care and intended use (Buckner H, MDT, CDT, Life-Like Laboratory, Dallas, TX, personal communication).

The silicone prosthesis was briefly discussed in the literature by Engelmeier, who replaced the distal aspect of a

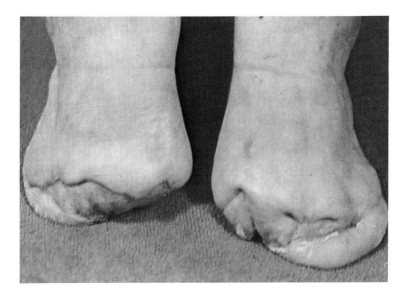

Figure 73.1. Bilateral forefoot amputation. Replacements are possible that are very lifelike. (Courtesy of H. Buckner, MDT, CDT, Life-like Laboratory, Dallas, TX.)

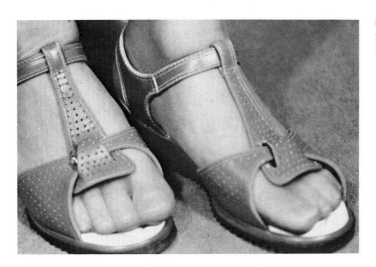

Figure 73.2. Same patient as shown in Figure 73.1, with prostheses in place, covered with shoes and stockings. (Courtesy of H. Buckner, MDT CDT, Life-Like Laboratory, Dallas, TX.)

third toe that was amputated after extensive mycotic disease (4). Engelmeier's intention was to allow the female patient to wear open-toed sandals and to avoid neighboring digital migration caused by the amputation. Biomechanical stability was maintained, and an ambulatory limp thereby was avoided.

A limited number of prosthetic laboratories in the United States actually fabricate custom-made silicone devices. One deterring aspect of this material is the necessity for a patient to be present from initial molding to final completion, compared with fabrication from a model taken by the referring physician or prosthetist. Various lower extremity amputation parts can be produced, including digits, a partial or complete forefoot, heel, and below- or above-the-knee leg (Figs. 73.1 and 73.2). Silicone or vinyl coverings are also available to place over prostheses produced from other materials.

One of the greatest feats in silicone prosthetic reconstruc-

tion is color matching to the remaining body parts. The device may be tinted or painted to simulate veins, nail details, or other inherent discolorations. Hair can be incorporated if the patient is referred directly to the laboratory (Buckner H, MDT, CDT, Life-Like Laboratory, Dallas, TX, personal communication)(Fig. 73.3). When a mold and color photograph are forwarded, the referring physician must be very careful. Limb position is important in deciding appropriate coloration. The amount of blood perceived in the skin varies with different positions, altering skin color. Thus it is imperative to determine the primary environment of the patient's limb to select appropriate coloration. Swatches of available color tones should be reviewed with the patient to determine the most accurate one. Darker paints are available from the designer for tone alteration (Reese CR, Realastic Professional Medical Products, Inc, Greenwood, SC, personal communication).

Prosthetic impressions are fabricated from a hydrocolloid

Figure 73.3. Amputated right forefoot with prosthetic replacement along side. Note realistic color and texture matchings. (Courtesy of H. Buckner, MDT, CDT, Life-Like Laboratory, Dallas, TX.)

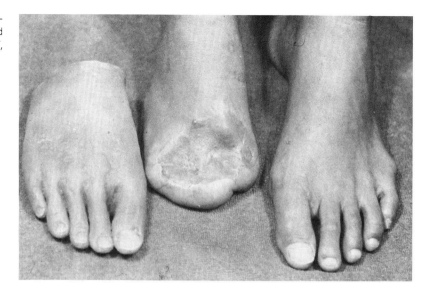

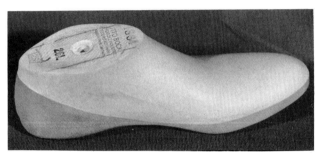

Figure 73.4. Solid ankle cushioned heel (SACH). Note the aperture in dorsal surface where a bolt is used to connect the ankle portion. Various densities of foam or rubber may be applied in the heel to gauge shock absorption.

such as flexinate, alginate, or other dental impression materials. The hydrocolloid is then filled with stone or gypsum and allowed to harden in order to provide a positive cast. A wax model may be sculpted prior to the silicone restoration by the experienced designer. Specific casting instructions are available from the laboratory when a model of the intended replacement is to be forwarded.

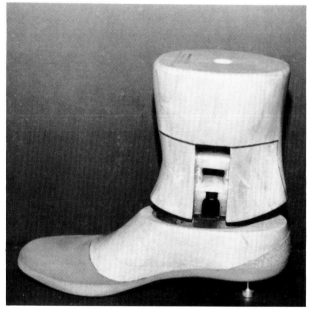

Figure 73.5. Greissinger Multi-Axis Foot, developed in Germany. (Courtesy of P. Leimkuehler, PEL Supply Co, Cleveland, OH.)

TRADITIONAL PROSTHESES

Artificial limbs have been termed static or dynamic. Those devices that passively replace a lost part are static. A dynamic device is one that is capable of actively expelling energy or determining sensations through electrodes attached to the body. Whether static or dynamic the connection between an amputee and the artificial part is important.

The socket of a prosthesis transfers the weight-bearing loads to the ground through the distal portion of the prosthesis, transmits power from the body to the artificial device for control, and provides a suspension to the prosthesis

when it is not in contact with the ground (5). These connections are known as sockets and appear as cuplike receptacles that enclose the amputated stump. They are often secured proximally by straps, bands, or suction.

The foundation of all lower limb prostheses is the foot. The most common pedal connection is the solid ankle cushioned heel (SACH) (Fig. 73.4). The bulk of the foot is constructed from wood or rubber. Varying densities of rubber or polyurethane are laminated into the SACH to provide different compressive capabilities. Prosthetic feet are constructed in an attempt to duplicate human biomechanics (6).

During the early stance phase of gait the leg internally rotates as the foot pronates. Later in the stance phase the leg externally rotates and the foot becomes fixed with respect to the ground. Extension of the toes creates tension on the plantar fascia, allowing the foot to convert into a semirigid lever (the windlass mechanism). This principle is also important for dynamic prosthetic design.

One study evaluated unilateral below-the-knee amputees using a SACH versus single axis foot (7). Interchanging the foot portion of the prosthesis did not significantly alter the gait patterns. However, the ankle demonstrated changes during the foot-flat phase of ambulation. A multiaxis foot and ankle joint has been described to provide a variety of rotational and sagittal plane movements (8)(Fig. 73.5).

Greater sophistication in prosthetic foot design has been mandated by an increasing popularity of aerobic sports. Burgess and associates (9) reported that 61% of 134 limb amputees participated in athletics, but only a few wore specifically designed recreational prostheses. The need for an efficient, dynamic appliance thus became evident. At least six brands of energy storing prosthetic feet are available in the United States (10). Most can be attached to a realigned conventional prosthesis such as the Seattle Foot. This appliance stores energy through compression as weight is applied. A series of fiberglass leaf-springs, with a rubber deflection bumper, initiate activity of the triceps surae, allowing for both energy storage and release. A cable limits the degree of limb extension. Those devices providing less energy storage than the Seattle Foot may be more suitable for less active persons or those with special needs, such as prolonged ambulation on uneven terrain (10).

Amputations through the foot have traditionally been frowned upon. This is based on a fear of potential equinus deformity from proximal muscle imbalances and the difficulty in achieving an adequate socket fit (11). However, more recently, authors have indicated that when a distal foot or ankle amputation can be performed, the increased energy required for ambulation after amputation can be minimized (12).

When a partial foot amputation is performed, one must ensure that dynamic function and intrinsic stability within shoe gear are both maintained. Rubin evaluated the partial

foot prosthesis (13) on the basis of length of stump, tissue viability, evidence of ulcerations, edema, sensory impairment, and deforming contractures. The location of amputation and the status of proximal tissue and contralateral limb are all considered. After resection of multiple digits, a

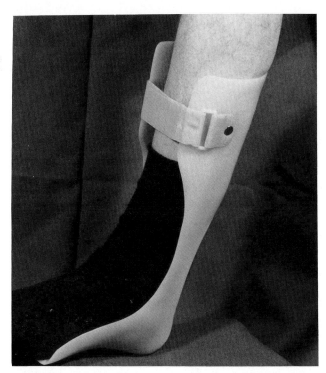

Figure 73.7. Molded plastic insert to protect against equinus deformities.

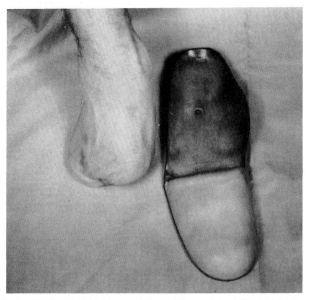

Figure 73.8. Partial foot amputation with accommodative insert prosthesis. The rivet indicates that a steel spring is incorporated within leather sole.

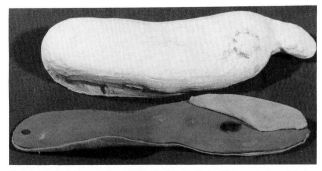

Figure 73.6. Insert with toe filler for lesser digits. Plantar accommodation for second metatarsal lesion is noted.

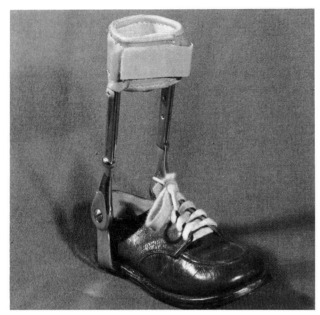

Figure 73.9. Double bar aluminum ankle-foot orthosis.

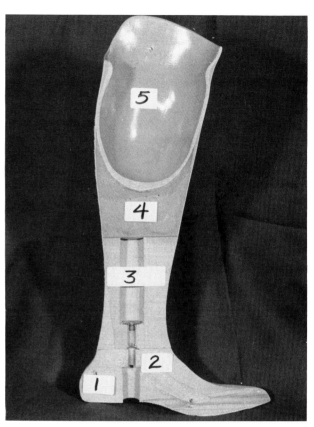

Figure 73.11. Hemisection of a patellar tendon-bearing prosthesis. *1.* SACH foot. *2.* Inflexible keel. *3.* Ankle block. *4.* Foam cushion. *5.* Connection with body part (socket). (Courtesy of S. Mersch, Post Rehabilitation, Kenosha, WI.)

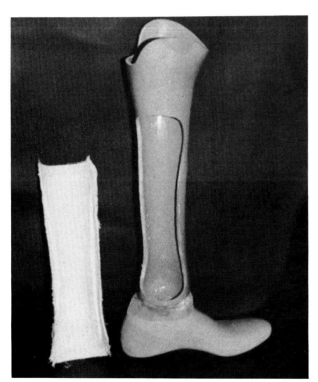

Figure 73.10. Symes prosthesis. **Left.** One can visualize how the medial opening permits insertion of a bulbous stump. (Courtesy of R. Selsberg, Orthopedic Braces and Appliances, Kenosha, WI.) **Right.** Prosthesis with intact window.

toe filler attached to a shoe insert was traditionally used. However, this may be inferior to forefoot prostheses. The silicone extension of these prostheses and pressure of the shoe cause a better unification between the prosthesis and the foot, avoiding irritations. When a toe filler is used, a shoe should be forwarded to the prosthetist for adequate fit. Any areas of plantar pressure must be identified for accommodation with the appliance (Fig. 73.6). The insole portion may consist of leather or plastazote. The toe filler must be soft enough to avoid irritation and may consist of cork with leather covering, rubber, or polyurethane foam. The degree of flexibility of the shoe to the sole must be compared with the length of the forefoot stump in order to improve gait and avoid irritation. Leg muscles above the injured foot must be exercised extensively, because they are visible beneath nylons in the female patient.

Amputations proximal to the metatarsal bases usually result in dorsiflexion and plantarflexion muscle imbalances, especially during ambulation (14). A molded plastic lower leg insert (Fig. 73.7), with a special shoe or with a toe filler and steel spring (Fig 73.8), will increase stability by avoiding equinus. A plastic laminated prosthesis for Chopart's amputations, known as the "clamshell," has been described

(14). For greater stability, a double bar aluminum ankle-foot orthosis (AFO) may be ordered (15) (Fig. 73.9). One argument against the use of the traditional AFO is that the immobilized ankle joint will become weak and stiff. The calf muscles will be thinner and may prevent a female from wearing a dress. Even if only the heel remains, a silicone foot prosthesis may be retained with an over-the-counter ankle support. If required, build-up to the heel and sole can reduce limp and lower back pain.

The Symes prosthesis may be used to accommodate total foot amputation. Disarticulation is performed immediately proximal to the cartilage of the distal tibia. The heel pad is fashioned, inclusive of the remainder of the posterior tibial nerve and vessels, as a weight-bearing stump. Appliances are constructed with a removable posterior or medial opening to permit insertion of the bulbous stump (Fig. 73.10). Some inherent strength is lost with a windowed prosthesis, and one may prefer an appliance with an expandable inner lining instead (16).

Amputations of the rearfoot, or amputation of the forefoot with an ulcerated plantar surface where no weight bearing is desired, are indications for a modification of the patellar tendon bearing (PTB) appliance (6, 14). Specific regions of the prosthesis transfer different loads. Vertical load, for example, is carried primarily by the socket near the patellar tendon (17). The PTB prosthesis is usually attached distally to a SACH foot (Fig. 73.11). Stresses can be transmitted between the socket and floor with maximal efficiency. A balsa wood variant is described for less active or lighter patients (18). This allows more efficient energy expenditure.

Successful management of a lower extremity amputation requires a team approach. This includes the surgeon, prosthetist, rehabilitative therapist, and often a biomedical engineer. Patients are no longer limited in their ability to participate in such activities as jogging or bicycling. Recent advancements in the fabrication of silicone replacements have resulted in increased cosmesis and greater acceptance of the deformity. Podiatric expertise dictates our active contribution to this important, continually progressive field of health care.

Acknowledgments

The author is indebted to Howard R. Reinherz, D.P.M., C.O. (Certified Orthotist), who provided extensive training on this subject and served as co-author during the initial writing. Blake Smith, D.P.M., podiatric resident at American International Hospital, Zion, IL, is recognized for aid in retrieval of information contained in this chapter. The author is indebted to Horst Buckner, M.D.T., C.D.T., who voluntarily critiqued this chapter and provided valuable insight.

References

1. Thomas A, Habban CC: *Amputation Prosthesis*. Philadelphia, JB Lippincott Co, 1945, pp 1-82.
2. Pritham CH: Suspension of the below-knee prosthesis: an overview. *Orthot Prosthet* 33:1-19, 1979.
3. Wilson MP: Clinical application of R.T.V. elastomers. *Orthot Prosthet* 33:22-29, 1979.
4. Engelmeier RL: Technique for prosthetic replacement of missing toes. *J Am Podiatry Assoc* 73:36-38, 1983.
5. Wilson AB: The connections. *Orthot Prosthet* 34:19-25, 1980.
6. Rubin G, Fischer E: Selection of components for lower limb amputation prostheses. *Bull Hosp J Dis* 1:39-67, 1982.
7. Doane NE, Holt LE: A comparison of the SACH and single axis foot in the gait of unilateral below-knee amputees. *Prosthet Orthot Int* 7:33-36, 1983.
8. American Academy of Orthopaedic Surgeons: *Atlas of Limb Prosthetics: Surgical and Prosthetic Principles*. St Louis, CV Mosby Co, 1981, p 9.
9. Burgess EM, Hittenberger DA, Forsgren SM, Lindh D: The Seattle prosthetic foot—a design for active sports: preliminary studies. *Orthot Prosthet* 37:25-31, 1983.
10. Wing DC, Hittenberger DA: Energy-storing prosthetic feet. *Arch Phys Med Rehabil* 70:330-335, 1989.
11. Pritham CH: Partial foot amputation—a case study. *Prosthet Orthot Clin* [Newsletter] 1:5-7, 1977.
12. Pinzio MJ, Kaminsky M, Sage R, Cronin R, Osterman H: Amputations at the middle level of the foot. *J Bone Joint Surg* 68A:1061-1064, 1986.
13. Rubin G: Indications for variants of the partial foot prosthesis. *Orthop Rev* 14:49-56, 1985.
14. Demopoulos JT: Orthotic and prosthetic management of foot disorders. In Jahss MH: *Disorders of the Foot*, vol 2. Philadelphia, WB Saunders Co, 1982, pp 848-854.
15. Reinherz RP, Reinherz HR: Orthopedic bracing for the lower extremities. *J Am Podiatry Assoc* 67:848-854, 1977.
16. Leimkuehler JP: Symes prosthesis—a brief review and a new fabrication technique. *Orthot Prosthet* 34:3-12, 1980.
17. Seliktar R, Bar A, Susak Z, Najenson T: A prosthesis for very short below-knee stumps. *Orthot Prosthet* 34:25-35, 1980.
18. Leimkuehler JP: A lightweight laminated below-the-knee prosthesis. *Orthot Prosthet* 36:46-49, 1982.

Index

Page numbers in *italics* denote figures; those by "t" denote tables

AAA bone graft, 1238–1239
Abduction, digital fracture in, 1492–1493, *1493*
Abduction deformity
  hallux, unrecognized, 588, *589*
  lesser metatarsophalangeal joint, 339–340, *340*
  pes valgo planus and, 777–778, *778*
  toe, 336, 366–367
Abductor digiti minimi muscle, flap from, 1286
Abductor hallucis muscle
  abnormal insertion, 841
  flap from, 1286
  hyperactivity, in metatarsus adductus, 830
  resection, in metatarsus adductus, 841, *842*
Abductor hallucis tendon
  abnormal insertion, in metatarsus adductus, 829–830
  release
    in clubfoot, 869
    in metatarsophalangeal joint arthrodesis, 561
  transfer, in hallux varus, 595, *596*, 597, 1317
Abrasion, definition, 1411, *1411*
Abrikossoff's tumor, 1167
Abscess
  biopsy, 1720
  in osteomyelitis, 1733
  in puncture wound, 1430, *1431*
  preoperative considerations, 196
Absorption
  bone, in neuropathic foot, 1359–1360, *1361–1362*
  by dressing, 206
  sutures (*see* Suture(s), absorbable)
Acanthoma, 1139
Acanthosis nigricans, 1140–1141
Accessory bones, navicular, vs. fracture, 1522–1523, *1523–1524*
Accessory ossicles (*see* Ossicles)
Acetaminophen, in postoperative pain, 215t, 217t
Acetyl washer, dislocation, complications, 1769–1771, *1772*
Acetylsalicylic acid, in edema prevention, 1715t
Achilles tendon
  advancement, 715–720, *715–719*
    in spasticity, 1316

anatomy, 448, 689, *690*, 1460
biomechanics, 690
blood supply, 1005–1006, 1450
bursa, superficial, 441–442, *442*
bursitis (*see* Haglund's deformity)
calcaneal fracture and, 1553–1554, *1557–1558*
calcification, 449, *450–452*, 453
corticosteroids effects on, 1460
examination, 1460, *1461*
exostosis at, 448–449, *450–452*, 453
incisional approaches, 1270, *1272*
laceration, 1417–1418, *1418*
lengthening, 720–726, *720–725*
  after transmetatarsal amputation, 1402
  in clubfoot, 865, *866*
  in congenital convex pes plano valgus, 886, 889
  in diabetes mellitus, 1378–1379, *1379*
  in midfoot amputation, 1402
  in muscular dystrophy, 968
  in pes valgo planus, 793, *794*, 795
magnetic resonance imaging, *36*, 39, *42*
necrosis, 1330
ossification, 1329–1330
repair, 449, *450–452*, 453, 1462
  polymer mesh in, 106, *106*
rupture, 1460–1462, *1461*
  after Haglund's deformity correction, 448
  in tendinitis, 1006
  weakness after, 1009, *1010–1011*, 1011
scarring, sural neuropathy in, 1110
skin coverage, 1290
splitting, surgical, 449, *450*
stress on, 448
tendinitis, electrical stimulation in, 1787
thickening, in arthritis, 453–454, *453–454*, 453t–454t
tight, causing hallux abducto valgus, 459
ultrasonography, 1451, 1454, *1454*, 1461
xanthoma, 1156, 1329
Acquired immunodeficiency syndrome (*see* Human immunodeficiency virus infection)
Acral lentiginous melanoma, 1148–1149, *1148*
Acrokeratoelastoidosis, 1156
Acrylic polymers, 106–107, *107*
  cement (*see* Polymethylmethacrylate)

Actinic keratosis, 1142
Adamantinoma, 1178
Adduction, digital fracture in, 1492–1493
Adduction deformity
  causing pes valgo planus, 777–778, *778*
  lesser metatarsophalangeal joint, 339–340, *340*
  toe, 336, 366–367
Adductor hallucis tendon
  detachment, 477–479, *477–481*
  release, in metatarsophalangeal joint arthrodesis, 561
  transfer, 488–490, *488–489*, 1317
    in Reverdin osteotomy, 501
Adductovarus deformity
  fifth toe, 330, *331*
  skin plasty in, 1290, *1290*
Adenoma, papillary eccrine, 1139
Adhesions
  in ankle equinus surgery, 728
  in hematoma, 1710
  in neuropathy, 1095
  in tendon healing, 1302–1303
  in tendon transfer, 1308–1309
Adhesive capsulitis, ankle, 991, *991*
Adipose tissue (*see* Fatty tissue)
Adiposis dolorosa, 1157–1158
Advancement skin flap, 1282–1283, *1283*
AFO (ankle-foot orthosis)
  in Charcot-Marie-Tooth disease, 978, *978*
  with prosthesis, *1796*, 1797
Age (*see also* Elderly persons; Pediatric patients)
  ankle equinus surgery, 708, *708*
  hallux abducto valgus appearance, 566
  nail changes and, 279
  surgical infection risk, 1696–1697, 1696t
  tendon transfer, 1306–1307, 1307t
AIDS (*see* Human immunodeficiency virus infection)
Akin osteotomy, 533–540
  bone resection, 534–535, *534–535*
  closure, 538
  complications, 539, *540*
  dissection, 533–534
  distal, 538–539, *538–539*
  failure, 533
  fixation in, 535–538, *536–538*
  in juvenile hallux abducto valgus, 576, *576*
  incision, 533–534